Essential Practice of Surgery

Springer
New York
Berlin
Heidelberg
Hong Kong
London
Milan
Paris
Tokyo

Essential Practice of Surgery
Basic Science and Clinical Evidence

With 259 Figures
With 61 Evidence-Based Tables

Edited by

Jeffrey A. Norton, MD
Professor of Surgery, University of California, San Francisco, San Francisco, California

R. Randal Bollinger, MD, PhD
Professor of Surgery, Professor of Immunology, Chief, Division of General Surgery, Duke University Medical Center, Durham, North Carolina

Alfred E. Chang, MD
Chief, Division of Surgical Oncology, Hugh Cabot Professor of Surgery, University of Michigan, Comprehensive Cancer Center, Ann Arbor, Michigan

Stephen F. Lowry, MD
Professor and Chairman, Department of Surgery, University of Medicine and Dentistry of New Jersey, Robert Wood Johnson Medical School, New Brunswick, New Jersey

Sean J. Mulvihill, MD
Professor and Chairman, Department of Surgery, School of Medicine, University of Utah Health Sciences Center, Salt Lake City, Utah

Harvey I. Pass, MD
Professor of Surgery and Oncology, Chief of Thoracic Oncology, Karmanos Cancer Institute, Wayne State University, Harper Hospital, Detroit, Michigan

Robert W. Thompson, MD
Professor of Surgery, Radiology, Cell Biology, and Physiology, Washington University School of Medicine, St. Louis, Missouri

Michelle Li, MD, Associate Editor

Illustrated by Mary K. Shirazi

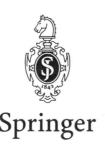

Springer

Jeffrey A. Norton, MD
Professor of Surgery, University of California, San Francisco, San Francisco, CA 94121-1598, USA

R. Randal Bollinger, MD, PhD
Professor of Surgery, Professor of Immunology, Chief, Division of General Surgery, Duke University
Medical Center, Durham, NC 27710, USA

Alfred E. Chang, MD
Chief, Division of Surgical Oncology, Hugh Cabot Professor of Surgery, University of Michigan,
Comprehensive Cancer Center, Ann Arbor, MI 48109-0932, USA

Stephen F. Lowry, MD
Professor and Chairman, Department of Surgery, University of Medicine and Dentistry of New Jersey,
Robert Wood Johnson Medical School, New Brunswick, NJ 08903-0019, USA

Sean J. Mulvihill, MD
Professor and Chairman, Department of Surgery, School of Medicine, University of Utah Health
Sciences Center, Salt Lake City, UT 84132, USA

Harvey I. Pass, MD
Professor of Surgery and Oncology, Chief of Thoracic Oncology, Karmanos Cancer Institute,
Wayne State University, Harper Hospital, Detroit, MI 48201, USA

Robert W. Thompson, MD
Professor of Surgery, Radiology, Cell Biology, and Physiology, Washington University School of
Medicine, St. Louis, MO 63110, USA

Library of Congress Cataloging-in-Publication Data

Essential practice of surgery : basic science and clinical evidence / editors, Jeffrey A.
Norton . . . [et al.].
   p.; cm.
  Includes bibliographical references and index.
  ISBN 0-387-95510-0 (alk. paper)
  1. Surgery. 2. Evidence-based medicine. I. Norton, Jeffrey A.
  [DNLM: 1. Surgical Procedures, Operative. 2. Evidence-Based Medicine. WO 500
E7781 2002]
RD31 .E72 2002
617—dc21   2002070547

ISBN 0-387-95510-0   Printed on acid-free paper.

9 8 7 6 5 4 3 2 1   SPIN 10880363

Springer-Verlag   New York Berlin Heidelberg
A member of BertelsmannSpringer Science+Business Media GmbH

To our families

Preface

We introduced the first edition of the textbook *Surgery: Basic Science and Clinical Evidence* two years ago. It is the first evidence-based surgical textbook and as such signaled a new focus in surgical education and practice. We want to thank the many residents, program directors, and surgeons who have used the text and recommended it to colleagues. We also wish to thank the authors for their comprehensive chapters; our collaborative efforts resulted in enthusiastic and supportive reviews in many journals, including the *New England Journal of Medicine*, the *Journal of the American Medical Association*, and *Archives of Surgery*. The publisher was also honored with the Best Clinical Medicine Book 2000 by the Association of American Publisher's Professional/Scholarly Publishing Division. An enormous amount of work from the authors, editors, and publisher resulted in *Surgery: Basic Science and Clinical Evidence*; we are proud of the fruits of our labor and grateful for your support of our endeavor.

We have heard from many of you, however, that a condensed, more portable version of our textbook would be of use to busy medical students, surgical residents, and practicing surgeons who need access to authoritative, evidence-based information during the course of their hectic workdays in the clinic and at the bedside. Thus, we have addressed these requests with the book you are holding in your hands, *Essential Practice of Surgery: Basic Science and Clinical Evidence*—an easy-to-use, companion spin-off

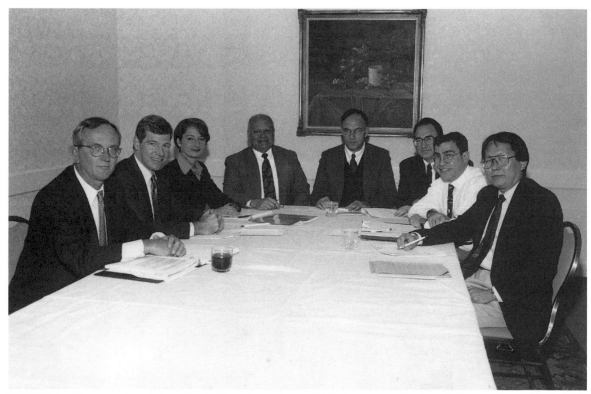

FIGURE 1. First meeting of the editorial board, October 1997 (Left to right: Stephen F. Lowry, Sean J. Mulvihill, Laura Gillan, R. Randal Bollinger, Jeffrey A. Norton, Robert W. Thompson, Harvey I. Pass, and Alfred E. Chang). (*Photo courtesy of Barbara Shapiro.*)

of our parent text. *Essential Practice* continues to emphasize the evidence-based practice of surgery. Working together with the contributors and my six coeditors, Dr. Randall Bollinger, Dr. Alfred Chang, Dr. Stephen Lowry, Dr. Sean Mulvihill, Dr. Harvey Pass, and Dr. Robert Thompson, along with UCSF department of surgery research resident Dr. Michelle Li, we have edited 57 of the most critical chapters from *Surgery: Basic Science and Clinical Evidence* into concise, abbreviated formats for quicker reference while retaining the most critical elements and best available evidence from the literature. Based on our discussions with residents and housestaff, we have focused on streamlining information from the larger volume with quick reading and referral in mind. The level of information covered in *Essentials* is intended to be ideal for board review or student courses in surgery as well as being useful for busy medical students, residents, and surgeons who want to read a more compact and portable but still very informative text. If the reader needs more information or has questions regarding certain issues, he or she may refer back to the parent textbook, *Surgery: Basic Science and Clinical Evidence.* We urge you to use the two books in cooperation with one another.

Again, we thank you for your enthusiastic support of *Surgery: Basic Science and Clinical Evidence.* Together with my six co-editors, we sincerely hope that all medical students, residents, and surgeons will embrace the evidence-based approach in *Essential Practice of Surgery: Basic Science and Clinical Evidence* and use it in the surgical care of their patients.

Jeffrey A. Norton, MD
San Francisco, CA
October 2002

Acknowledgments

The Editorial Board wishes to thank both the editorial and production staff at Springer-Verlag New York for their support and encouragement, Mary Shirazi, whose wonderful medical illustrations appear throughout the book, and Barbara Chernow and Kathy Cleghorn of Chernow Editorial Services for their outstanding work in coordinating the production of this text.

I personally would also like to thank my family members for their continued help and support, specifically Cathy, John, Meg, Pat, and Tim.

Jeffrey A. Norton, MD

The untiring support and encouragement of Monika Bollinger and the secretarial skills of Mary Ann Rohrer are gratefully acknowledged. I sincerely appreciate the superb work of each author who contributed to the Transplantation section and especially the participation of my former trainees, Drs. Stuart Knechtle, Allan Kirk, Bob Harland, and Betsy Tuttle.

R. Randal Bollinger, MD, PhD

To my wife, Lana, for her support in this effort.

Alfred E. Chang, MD

To Susette, Alex, Lorna, and Kate and to my mentors, Dick Kraft, Frank Moody, Murray Brennan, and Tom Shires who instilled a love of surgery.

Stephen F. Lowry, MD

To my assistant Eleanor Leveau for her tireless effort and calm efficiency, to my own mentor, Haile Debas, MD, for his teaching, advice and support, and to my wife, Kim, and sons, Michael, Jeffrey, and Timothy, for making my life complete.

Sean J. Mulvihill, MD

To my family, Helen, Eric, and Ally Pass, for their constant support.

Harvey I. Pass, MD

To my surgical mentors: Norm Thompson (dad), John Mannick, Ron Stoney, and Greg Sicard, for their inspiration and instruction. To my students, residents, and fellows, who keep me challenged, and to Della for keeping it all in order. To my wonderful wife, Michelle, and the joy of our lives, Taylor Alexandra, who makes it all worthwhile.

Robert W. Thompson, MD

Contents

Section Two   Gastrointestinal and Abdominal Disease

Section Three   Endocrine Surgery

Section Four   Vascular Surgery

Section Five   Cardiothoracic Surgery

Section Six   Transplantation

Section Seven   Cancer

Section Eight   Pediatric Surgery

Contributors

Craig T. Albanese, MD
Division of Pediatric Surgery, Department of Surgery, University of California, San Francisco, San Francisco, CA 94143-0570, USA

Andreas Amerhauser, MD
Department of Surgery, University of California, San Francisco, San Francisco, CA 94143-0144, USA

Carl L. Backer, MD
Division of Cardiovascular-Thoracic Surgery, Department of Surgery, Children's Memorial Hospital, Chicago, IL 60690-0022, USA

Paul E. Bankey, MD
Department of Surgery, University of Rochester Medical Center, Rochester, NY 14642, USA

Philip S. Barie, MD
Department of Surgery, Division of Critical Care and Trauma, Weill Medical College of Cornell University, New York Presbyterian Hospital, New York, NY 10021-4873, USA

B. Timothy Baxter, MD
Department of Surgery, University of Nebraska Medical Center, Methodist Hospital, Omaha, NE 68114, USA

Mark I. Block, MD
Department of Cardiothoracic Surgery, Medical University of South Carolina, Charleston, SC 29425, USA

William de Bois, MD
Department of Perioperative Services, New York Presbyterian Hospital, New York, NY 10021, USA

Carol R. Bradford, MD
Department of Otolaryngology, University of Michigan Medical Center, Ann Arbor, MI 48109-0312, USA

Edward G. Chekan. MD
Department of Surgery, University of Virginia Health System, Charlottesville, VA 22908, USA

Timothy A.M. Chuter, MD
Department of Surgery, University of California, San Francisco, San Francisco, CA 94143-0788, USA

Pierre-Alain Clavien, MD, PhD
Department of Visceral and Transplant Surgery, University Hospital Zurich, Zurich, Switzerland

J. Perren Cobb, MD
Department of Surgery, Burn, Trauma, Surgical Critical Care Section, Washington University School of Medicine, St. Louis, MO 63110-1093, USA

R. Duane Davis, Jr., MD
Department of Surgery, Division of Cardiothoracic Surgery, Duke University Medical Center, Durham, NC 27710, USA

James P. Dolan, MD
San Francisco VA Medical Center, San Francisco, CA 94121-1598, USA

David L. Dunn, MD
Department of Surgery, University of Minnesota Medical School, Minneapolis, MN 55455, USA

Rishad M. Faruqi, MD
Division of Vascular Surgery, SUNY Stony Brook Hospital and Medical Center, Stony Brook, NY 11794-8191, USA

Mitchell P. Fink, MD
Department of Critical Care Medicine, University of Pittsburgh Health System, Pittsburgh, PA 15261, USA

Matthew I. Foley, MD
Department of General Surgery, Oregon Health & Science University, Portland, OR 97201-3098, USA

Nicola A. Francalancia, MD
Department of Surgery, Division of Cardiothoracic Surgery, Brody School of Medicine, East Carolina University, Greenville, NC 27858-4354, USA

Joseph S. Friedberg, MD
Division of Thoracic Surgery, Department of Surgery, Thomas Jefferson University, Philadelphia, PA 19107, USA

Steven Gallinger, MD
Department of Surgery, University of Toronto, Toronto, Ontario M5G 1X5, Canada

Michael A. Golden, MD
Department of Surgery, Hospital of the University of Pennsylvania, Philadelphia, PA 19104-4227, USA

Jeffrey Hammond, MD
Department of Surgery, University of Medicine and Dentistry of New Jersey, Robert Wood Johnson Medical School, New Brunswick, NJ 08903, USA

Douglas W. Hanto, MD, PhD
Department of Surgery, Division of Transplantation, Harvard Medical School, Beth Israel Deaconess Medical Center, Boston, MA 02215, USA

Robert C. Harland, MD
Department of Transplant Surgery, University of Chicago Hospitals, Chicago, IL 60637, USA

David H. Harpole, Jr., MD
Department of Thoracic Surgery, Duke University Medical Center, Durham, NC 27710, USA

Hobart W. Harris, MD, MPH
Department of Surgery, University of California, San Francisco, San Francisco, CA 94110, USA

Alan Hemming, MD
Department of Surgery, University of Toronto, Toronto, Ontario M5G 1X5, Canada

Richard A. Hodin, MD
Department of Surgery, Massachusetts General Hospital, Boston, MA 02114, USA

Danny O. Jacobs, MD
Department of Surgery, Creighton University Medical Center, Omaha, NE 68131, USA

Daniel B. Jones, MD
Department of Surgery, University of Texas Southwestern Medical Center, Dallas, TX 75235, USA

K. Craig Kent, MD
Division of Vascular Surgery, Weill Medical College of Cornell University, New York Presbyterian Hospital, New York, NY 10021, USA

Allan D. Kirk, MD
Transplantation Section, National Institute of Diabetes, Digestive and Kidney Disease, National Institutes of Health, Bethesda, MD 20892, USA

Stuart J. Knechtle, MD
Department of Surgery, University of Wisconsin, Madison, WI 53792-7375, USA

Daniel Kreisel, MD
Department of Surgery, University of Pennsylvania, Philadelphia, PA 19104, USA

Kenneth A. Kudsk, MD
Department of Surgery, University of Wisconsin Hospital, Madison, WI 53792-7375, USA

Terry C. Lairmore, MD
Department of Surgery, Washington University School of Medicine, St. Louis, MO 63110, USA

Christine L. Lau, MD
Department of Surgery, Duke University Medical Center, Durham, NC 27710, USA

Hop N. Le, MD
Department of Surgery, University of California, San Francisco, San Francisco, CA 94143-0807, USA

Rayman W. Lee, MD
Department of Internal Medicine, Division of Pulmonary and Critical Care Medicine, University of Texas Medical Branch, Galveston, TX 77555-0561, USA

Alan T. Lefor, MD, MPH
Department of Surgery, Cedars-Sinai Medical Center, University of California, Los Angeles, School of Medicine, Los Angeles, CA 90048, USA

Marcel Levi, MD, PhD
Department of Internal Medicine, Academic Medical Center, University of Amsterdam, 1105 AZ Amsterdam, The Netherlands

Edward H. Livingston, MD
Division of General Surgery, University of California, Los Angeles, School of Medicine, Los Angeles, CA 90095-6904

Michael T. Longaker, MD
Department of Surgery, Stanford University School of Medicine, Stanford, CA 94305-5148, USA

H. Peter Lorenz, MD
Department of Surgery, Stanford University School of Medicine, Stanford, CA 94305-5148, USA

Robert C. Mackersie, MD
Department of Surgery, University of California, San Francisco, San Francisco, CA 94110, USA

Ronald V. Maier, MD
Department of Surgery, University of Washington, Harborview Medical Center, Seattle, WA 98104, USA

Kim A. Margolin, MD
Department of Medical Oncology, City of Hope Comprehensive Cancer Center, Duarte, CA 91010, USA

Jeffrey B. Matthews, MD
Department of Surgery, Harvard Medical School, Beth Israel Deaconess Medical Center, Boston, MA 02215, USA

Constantine Mavroudis, MD
Division of Cardiovascular-Thoracic Surgery, Department of Surgery, Children's Memorial Hospital, Northwestern University, Chicago, IL 60690-0022, USA

Robin S. McLeod, MD
Department of Surgery, University of Toronto, Mount Sinai Hospital, Toronto, Ontario M5G 1X5, Canada

Gregory L. Moneta, MD
Department of Surgery, Division of Vascular Surgery, Oregon Health & Science University, Portland, OR 97201, USA

Sean J. Mulvihill, MD
Department of Surgery, School of Medicine, University of Utah Health Sciences Center, Salt Lake City, UT 84132

Avery B. Nathens, MD, PhD, MPH
Department of Surgery, University of Washington, Harborview Medical Center, Seattle, WA 98104, USA

David G. Neschis, MD
Department of Vascular Surgery, Hospital of the University of Pennsylvania, Philadelphia, PA 19104, USA

Jeffrey A. Norton, MD
Department of Surgery, University of California, San Francisco, San Francisco, CA 92121-1598, USA

Theodore N. Pappas, MD
Division of General Surgery, Duke University Medical Center, Durham, NC 27710, USA

Helen A. Pass, MD
Breast Care Center, William Beaumont Hospital, Royal Oak, MI 48073, USA

Sheela T. Patel, MD
Department of Thoracic Surgery, Beth Israel Hospital, Boston, MA 02215, USA

Edward H. Phillips, MD
Department of Surgery, Division of Endoscopic Surgery, Cedars-Sinai Medical Center, University of California, Los Angeles, School of Medicine, Los Angeles, CA 90048, USA

Peter W.T. Pisters, MD
Department of Surgical Oncology, University of Texas, MD Anderson Cancer Center, Houston, TX 77030, USA

R. Lawrence Reed, MD
Department of Surgery, Loyola University Medical Center, Maywood, IL 60153, USA

Bruce R. Rosengard, MD
Department of Surgery, University of Pennsylvania Medical Center, University of Pennsylvania School of Medicine, Philadelphia, PA 19104-4227, USA

Todd K. Rosengart, MD
Department of Surgery, Division of Cardiothoracic Surgery, Evanston Northwestern Healthcare, Evanston, IL 60201, USA

William P. Schecter, MD
Department of Surgery, University of California, San Francisco, San Francisco General Hospital, San Francisco, CA 94110, USA

Daniel J. Scott, MD
Department of Surgery, Tulane University School of Medicine, New Orleans, LA 70112-2699, USA

C. Daniel Smith, MD
Department of Surgery, Emory University School of Medicine, Atlanta, GA 30322, USA

Vernon K. Sondak, MD
Division of Surgical Oncology, Department of Surgery, University of Michigan Medical School, Ann Arbor, MI 48109-0932, USA

David I. Soybel, MD
Department of Surgery, Harvard Medical School, Brigham and Women's Hospital, Boston, MA 02115, USA

Richard K. Spence, MD
Department of Surgical Education, Baptist Health System Program, Birmingham, AL 35211, USA

Thoralf M. Sundt, MD
Division of Cardiovascular Surgery, Mayo Clinic, Rochester, MN 55905, USA

Robert W. Thompson, MD
Department of Surgery, Radiology, Cell Biology, and Physiology, Washington University School of Medicine, St. Louis, MO 63110, USA

J.E. Tuttle-Newhall, MD
Division of Transplantation Surgery, Department of Surgery, Duke University Medical Center, Durham, NC 27710, USA

Robert Udelsman, MD, MBA
Department of Surgery, Yale University, Yale New Haven Hospital, New Haven, CT 06520-8062

John F. Valente, MD
Department of Surgery, Division of Transplantation, University of Cincinnati, College of Medicine, Cincinnati, OH 45267-0558, USA

Tom van der Poll, MD, PhD
Infectious Diseases, Tropical Medicine, and AIDS, Academic Medical Center, University of Amsterdam, 1105 AZ Amsterdam, The Netherlands

Madhulika G. Varma, MD
Department of Surgery, University of California, San Francisco, San Francisco, CA 94143-0144, USA

Ronald J. Weigel, MD
Department of Surgery, Stanford University Medical School, Stanford, CA 94305, USA

Mark L. Welton, MD
Department of Surgery, Stanford University Medical School, Stanford, CA 94305, USA

James F. Whiting, MD
Department of Surgery, Division of Transplantation, University of Cincinnati, College of Medicine, Cincinnati, OH 45267-0558

Brad A. Winterstein, MD
Department of Surgery, University of Nebraska Medical Center, Omaha, NE 68198, USA

Roger W. Yurt, MD
Department of Surgery, Weill Medical College at Cornell University, New York Presbyterian Hospital, New York, NY 10021-4873, USA

Joseph B. Zwischenberger, MD
Division of Cardiothoracic Surgery, University of Texas Medical Branch, Galveston, TX 77555-0528, USA

Evidence-Based Tables

All evidence-based tables are indicated in the text by an .

SECTION ONE

Care of the Surgical Patient

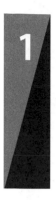

Evidence-Based Surgery

Robin S. McLeod

The term evidence-based medicine was coined by Sackett and colleagues[1] in the 1980s. They defined it as "the conscientious, explicit, and judicious use of current best evidence in making decisions about the care of individual patients." The practice of evidence-based medicine means integrating individual clinical expertise with the best available clinical evidence from systematic research. In short, evidence-based medicine means systematically searching for the best evidence rather than relying on expert opinion or anecdotal experience. In addition, Sackett and colleagues recognized the importance of the clinical expertise that most physicians possess and were explicit in stating that the evidence must be integrated with clinical acumen. Finally, the preferences and values of the patient must be considered in the decision making.

There are five linked ideas central to the practice of evidence-based medicine (EBM). First, clinical decisions should be based on the best available scientific evidence; second, the clinical problem, rather than the habits of protocols, should determine the type of evidence to be sought; third, identifying the best evidence means using epidemiological and biostatistical ways of thinking; fourth, conclusions derived from identifying and critically appraising evidence are useful only if put into action in managing patients or making health care decisions; and finally, performance should be constantly evaluated.[2]

Ultimately, there are many reasons to practice evidence-based medicine. First, most physicians want to do the best for their patients on an individual basis. To do so, one must be abreast of the current knowledge in the area. Second, patients are better educated and informed and are challenging physicians' views. Patients have access to the medical literature and can often cite it. Finally, if physicians wish to play a role in policy decision making and allocation of resources, they must have the evidence to justify the introduction and maintenance of these programs. Thus, physicians can no longer rely on their anecdotal experience.

Are We Practicing Evidence-Based Medicine?

It has been shown that even high-quality information published in the literature is often not applied by practicing physicians. Multiple studies have demonstrated varying rates of adoption of treatments that have proven to be effective in randomized controlled trials (RCT). "Convincing" evidence is often difficult to come by, but seems to be even more difficult to apply.

Requirements for Practicing Evidence-Based Surgery

Rosenberg and Donald have outlined some of the steps involved in the application of evidence-based practice.[3] First, the clinician must clearly identify and articulate a question that has arisen from clinical practice. External evidence is then sought, usually by performing a focused search of the literature. The information thus retrieved is subjected to critical appraisal, and finally the newly acquired knowledge is implemented in clinical practice. Thus, the necessary elements to practice evidence-based medicine are production and dissemination of high-quality evidence and retrieval and critical appraisal of the evidence. The remainder of this chapter discusses these two major issues.

Providing the Evidence

Various hierarchies have been proposed for classifying study design.[4,5] In simplest terms, studies can be classified as case series, case-control studies, cohort studies, and randomized controlled trials. The case series is the weakest and the randomized controlled trial the strongest for determining the effectiveness of treatment (Table 1.1).

TABLE 1.1. Hierarchy of Study Designs.

	Control group	Prospective follow-up	Random allocation of subjects
Case series	No	No	No
Case-control study	Yes	No	No
Cohort study	Yes	Yes	No
Randomized controlled trial	Yes	Yes	Yes

Case Series

Case reports (arbitrarily defined as 10 or fewer subjects) and case series are the typical surgical studies. There is no concurrent control group, although there may be a historical control group. Patients may be followed from the same inception point and followed prospectively, not necessarily for the purpose of the study but in the normal clinical course of their disease. Typically, data from patient charts or clinical databases are reviewed retrospectively. Thus, the outcome of interest is present when the study is initiated. Despite the limitations of this study design, the importance of results from case series should not be minimized. It is because of careful observation that innovations in surgical practice and techniques have been and continue to be made. However, results from case series should be likened to observations made in the laboratory. Just as those observations should lead to generation of a hypothesis and performance of an experiment to test it, a randomized controlled trial should be performed to confirm the observations reported in a case series. Case series are plagued with biases such as selection and referral biases, and because data are not collected specifically for the study they are often incomplete or even inaccurate. Therefore, incorrect conclusions about the efficacy of a treatment are common, and the mistake that surgeons make is relying solely on evidence from case series.

Case-Control Studies

The case-control study is the design used most frequently by epidemiologists to study risk factors or causation. There are two groups of patients: the case group is composed of subjects in whom the outcome of interest is present, whereas it is not present in subjects in the control group. Controls are selected by the investigator rather than by random allocation, so the likelihood of bias being introduced is real and thus there is a risk of making an erroneous conclusion. Generally the controls are matched to the cases with respect to important prognostic variables other than the factor that is being studied. It is important to match the subjects to avoid an incorrect conclusion about the significance of the factor being studied, but it is equally important not to overmatch the controls so a true difference is not observed. In case-control studies, as in case series, data are collected retrospectively. Thus, the outcome is present at the start of the study.

Cohort Studies

Cohort studies may be performed retrospectively or prospectively. There are two or more groups, but subjects are not ran-domly allocated to the groups. One group receives the treatment or exposure of interest, while the other group of subjects receives another or no treatment or exposure. The inception point may not be defined by the study, and the intervention and follow-up may be ad hoc. However, the outcome is not present at the time that the inception cohort is assembled. There is less possibility of bias than in a case-control study because cases are not selected and the outcome is not present at the initiation of the study. However, the likelihood of bias is still high because subjects are not randomly allocated to groups. Instead, there is some selection process, either by the subject or by the clinician, that allocates them to groups. For instance, subjects may be allocated to groups by where they live (when the effect of an environmental toxin is being studied), by choice (when a lifestyle factor such as dietary intake is being studied), or by the physician (when a nonrandomized study of a treatment intervention is being performed). Retrospective cohort studies differ from prospective cohort studies in that data analysis and possibly data collection are performed retrospectively but there is an identifiable time point that can be used to define the inception cohort. Such a date could be date of birth, date of first attendance at a hospital, etc. Cohort studies typically are performed by epidemiologists studying risk factors where randomization of patients is unethical. Although cohort studies are more powerful than case-control studies, subjects are not randomized, so the cohorts may potentially be biased. An example of a cohort study is the use of a database to follow patients who have had a mucosectomy versus no mucosectomy in restorative proctocolectomy to determine the long-term outcome.

Randomized Controlled Trials

The RCT is accepted as the best trial design for establishing treatment effectiveness. There are several essential components of the randomized controlled trial. First, subjects are randomly allocated to two groups: usually a treatment group (in which the new treatment is being tested) and a control group (in which the standard therapy or placebo is administered). Thus, the control group is concurrent and subjects are randomly allocated to the two groups. Second, the interventions and follow-up are standardized and performed prospectively. Thus, it is hoped that both groups are similar in all respects except for the interventions being studied. Not only does this guard against differences in factors known to be important, it also ensures that there are no differences caused by unknown or unidentified factors. This latter point is especially important. Statistical techniques such as multivariate analysis can be employed to adjust for known prognostic variables but obviously cannot adjust for unknown prognostic variables. There are multiple examples of studies showing differences between groups that cannot be accounted for by the known prognostic variables.[6]

Where differences in treatment effect are small, the RCT may minimize the chance of reaching an incorrect conclusion about the effectiveness of treatment. There are, however, some limitations to RCTs. First, RCTs tend to take a long time to complete because of the time required for planning, accruing, and following patients, and finally analyzing results. As a consequence, the results may not be available for many years. Second, clinical trials are expensive to perform, although their cost may be recuperated if ineffective treatments are abandoned and only effective treatments are implemented.[7] Third, the results may not be generalizable or applicable to all patients with the disease because of the strict inclusion and exclusion criteria and inherent differences in patients who volunteer for trials. As well, not all patients respond similarly to treatment. Fourth, in situations where the disease or outcome is rare or only occurs after a long period of follow-up, RCTs are generally not feasible. Finally, the ethics of performing RCTs is controversial, and some clinicians may feel uncomfortable with randomizing their patients when they believe one treatment to be superior even if that opinion is based only on anecdotal evidence.

There are elements common to all randomized controlled trials, as outlined in Table 1.2. The first and perhaps the most important issue in designing a RCT is to enunciate clearly the research question. Most RCTs are based on observations or experimental evidence from the laboratory. Always, RCTs should make biological sense, have clinical relevancy, and be feasible to perform. The research question determines who will be included, what the intervention will be, and what is to be measured. Frequently, a sequence of RCTs will be performed to evaluate a particular intervention. Initially, a rather small trial that is highly controlled using a physiological or surrogate endpoint may be performed. This trial would provide evidence that the intervention is effective in the optimal situation (efficacy trial). However, it might lack clinical relevance, especially if the endpoint were a physiological measure. However, if it were positive, it would then lead to another trial, with more patients and a more clinically relevant outcome measure. If this second trial were positive, a very large trial might be indicated to assess the effectiveness of the intervention in normal practice (effectiveness trial). Such an example would be studying the effect of a chemoprevention agent in colon cancer. Initially, the agent might be prescribed to a group of individuals at high risk for polyp formation (e.g., patients with familial polyposis coli) for a short time, with the outcome measure being a rectal biopsy for proliferative changes. A subsequent trial might observe polyp regression in this same cohort of patients, with subsequent trials aimed at the prevention of significant polyps in average-risk individuals who were followed for several years. As one can see, the

TABLE 1.2. Elements of a Randomized Controlled Trial.

1. Stating the Research Question
2. Selecting the Subjects
3. Allocating the Subjects
4. Describing the Maneuver
   a. The interventions
   b. Minimizing potential biases
   c. Baseline and follow-up maneuvers
5. Measuring Outcome
   a. Assessing treatment effectiveness
   b. Assessing side effects and toxicity
6. Analyzing the Data
7. Estimating the Sample Size
8. Ethical Considerations
9. Administrative Issues
   a. Feasibility of the trial
   b. Administration of the trial
   c. Data management
   d. Funding issues

selection of subjects, the intervention, the duration of the trial, and the choice of outcome measure may vary depending on the research question. Ultimately, however, investigators wish to generalize the results to clinical practice so the outcome measures should be clinically relevant. For this reason, quality of life measures are often included.

Although there are elements common to all randomized controlled trials, there are issues of special concern in surgical trials.[8] The issue of standardization of the procedure is of major importance in surgical trials. Standardization is difficult because surgeons may vary in their experience with and ability to perform a surgical technique; there may be individual preferences in performing the procedure, and technical modifications may occur as the procedure evolves. Moreover, differences in perioperative and postoperative care may also impact the outcome. There are two issues related to standardization of the procedure. First, there is the issue of who should perform the procedure: experts only or surgeons of varying ability. Second, there is the issue of standardization of the procedure so it is performed similarly by all surgical participants and it can be duplicated by others following publication of the trial results. The implications of these two issues differ, and strategies to address them also differ.

The first issue is analogous to assessing compliance in a medical trial. Thus, if the procedure is performed by experts only in a very controlled fashion, it is analogous to an "efficacy trial." The advantage of such a trial is that if the procedure is truly superior to the other intervention, then this design has the greatest likelihood of detecting a difference. The disadvantage, obviously, is that the results are less generalizable. As with most issues in clinical trials, there is no right or wrong answer. If the procedure is usually performed by experts, then it probably is desirable to have only experts involved in the trial. On the other hand, if a wide spectrum of surgeons usually perform the procedure, it would be appropriate not to limit surgical participation.

No matter how many surgeons are involved in the trial and that investigators want to mimic routine practice, there must be at least a certain amount of standardization so that readers of the trial results can understand what was done and duplicate the procedure in their own practice. There are several strategies to ensure a minimum standard. First, all surgeons should agree on the performance of the critical aspects of the procedure. It may not be necessary that there is agreement concerning all the technical aspects, but there should be consensus on those details deemed to be important. Furthermore, if there are aspects of the perioperative and postoperative care that impact on outcome (e.g., postoperative adjuvant therapy), these should be standardized. Teaching sessions may be held prior to starting the trial and feedback given to surgeons on their performance during the trial. As well, obtaining documentation that the procedure has been performed satisfactorily (for example, through postoperative angiograms to document vessel patency or pathology specimens to document resection margins and lymph node excision) may contribute to ensuring that the surgery is being performed adequately. Finally, patients are usually stratified according to surgeons or center to ensure balance in case there are differences in surgical technique between centers or surgeons.

Blinding is often a difficult issue in surgical trials. It may not be an issue if two surgical procedures are being compared but is a major issue if a surgical procedure is being compared with a medical therapy. There is often a placebo effect of surgery. The lack of blinding is especially worrisome if the primary outcome is a change in symptoms or quality of life rather than a "hard" outcome measure such as mortality or morbidity. In these situations, if a hard outcome measure is also measured and it correlates with the patient's assessment, there is less concern about the possibility of bias. Assessments may be performed by an independent assessor who is unaware of the patient's treatment group. Finally, if criteria used to define an outcome are explicitly specified a priori, it may minimize or eliminate bias (e.g., criteria to diagnose an intraabdominal abscess). Investigators may also choose in this situation to have a blinded panel review the results of tests to ensure that they meet the criteria.

The issue of timing of trials is difficult. Most surgeons would argue, that a learning curve exists in any procedure and that modifications to the technique are made frequently at its inception. By including these early patients, one would almost certainly bias the results against the new procedure. The introduction of laparoscopic cholecystectomy and the initially high rate of common bile duct injuries is a good example of this. On the other hand, it may be difficult to initiate a trial when the procedure is widely accepted by both the patient and the surgical community. The paucity of RCTs testing surgical therapies supports this latter contention. This dilemma arises because, unlike the release of medical therapies, there is no regulating body in surgery that restricts performance of a procedure or requires proof of its efficacy. Probably, RCTs should be performed early before they become accepted into practice, recognizing that future trials may be necessary as the procedure evolves and surgical experience increases. This plan is analogous to medical oncological trials in which trials are being planned as one is being completed. On the other hand, the procedure must be established adequately, because one certainly would not want to invest a large amount of money and time in a trial that produced results having no value at its completion.

Finally, patient issues may be of greater concern in surgical trials. In a medical trial, patients may be randomized to either treatment arm with the possibility that at the conclusion of the trial they can receive the more efficacious treatment if the disease is not progressive and the treatment is reversible. Surgical procedures, however, are almost always permanent. This point may be of particular concern if a medical therapy is being compared to a surgical procedure or the two surgical procedures differ in their magnitude or invasiveness. Patients may have a preference for one or the other treatment and therefore refuse to participate in the trial. There also tends to be more emotion involved with surgery, and patients may be less willing to leave the decision as to which procedure will be performed to chance. Surgeons themselves may feel uncomfortable in discussing the uncertainty of randomization with patients requiring surgery.[9] Thus, accruing patients for surgical trials may be more difficult than for medical trials.

Outcome Studies

Health services research, which includes outcomes research, has been defined by the Institute for Medical Studies as "a multidisciplinary field of inquiry, both basic and applied, that examines the use, costs, quality and accessibility, delivery, organization, financing and outcomes of health care services to increase knowledge and understanding of the structures, processes and effects of health services for individuals and populations."[10]

Health service research includes all types of evaluations including studies using the randomized controlled trial design. Outcomes research has been used to describe many different types of research. The term outcomes studies is usually used to describe those studies in which outcomes are assessed in large cohorts of patients, often using data from administrative databases. These cohorts may include patients registered in a HMO, those living in a specific geographic area, or some other defined group. Thus, outcomes studies, using the previously discussed hierarchy of study designs, are cohort studies. The strength and rationale for outcome studies is that they focus on populations or large groups of patients to minimize the selection and referral biases that are found in small institutional series. In addition, outcomes studies often use patient-based or patient-derived evaluations of care. The hope for the outcomes movement was that the information derived would improve decision making by clinicians, health care administrators, and patients and thereby lead to a cycle of improved care.

The number of outcomes studies evaluating surgical procedures in all disciplines has increased exponentially in recent years. While these have an important role, they should be viewed as being complementary to RCTs. Generally, a RCT is needed to establish the effectiveness of a treatment. The strength of the RCT is that conditions are tightly controlled to minimize bias and the risk of making an incorrect conclusion. However, because of this restriction, they also may lack generalizability. Variations in structure and process variables are minimized in RCTs, whereas outcomes studies try to determine what role these factors play in routine care because there is no control over the selection of patients and the practice of physicians.[11] Optimally, outcome studies can be used to determine whether services work as well in routine practice as they did in trials.

Although RCTs are the standard for determining treatment effectiveness, another potential role for outcome studies is in those situations where RCTs are not feasible (e.g., a rare condition) or are not ethical. The availability of large administrative databases and ready access to this information with modern computers and statistical software packages has allowed outcome studies to be performed. These databases have several important limitations. First, the data within a database may be inaccurate or incomplete. Second, the databases have usually been set up for administrative purposes and therefore clinically relevant data such as comorbid illness may be limited. Occasionally, it may be possible to link the administrative database to a clinical database that contains clinically relevant data. Alternately, additional information can be garnered by abstracting medical records or individual patient records. Finally, like clinical trials, outcome studies tend to be as good as the rigorousness of the methodology of the study. Thus, before embarking on the study, a hypothesis should be formulated, outcomes specified (e.g., length of stay, reoperative rate, readmission rate) plus comorbidities or risk factors (e.g., gender, age, hospital, surgeon) explicitly defined. Testing the database to ensure accuracy is also an important step. Finally, multivariate statistical tests and logistic regression analyses are performed to adjust for possible known confounders (i.e., control for the case mix).

There are several limitations of outcomes studies. Outcome studies are essentially observational studies, lacking the rigorous control of variables as in a randomized controlled trial. Thus, there is the risk of bias. If recognized, adjustments can be made in the analysis. However, unidentifiable factors may bias the results. Thus, inferences must be made cautiously because there may be unmeasured variations in the patients, practitioners, and processes that are the real explanation for differences in outcome. Second, often the available databases used have been set up for another purpose (such as health care delivery) and clinically relevant data may be limited. Optimally, patient-relevant outcomes such as quality of life should be measured. However, endpoints may be limited to length of hospital stay, operative mortality, reoperation rates, and readmission rates. In addition to the limited number of endpoints, comorbidity data may be inadequate or inaccurately recorded. Furthermore, it may be impossible to know whether a comorbidity was present preoperatively or occurred following surgery, which may limit the ability to adequately adjust the data for varying levels of risk or disease severity. Third, outcomes studies can only assess the impact of patient variables and practice patterns on the process of health care delivery. Because patient preferences are not recorded, their impact cannot be assessed but such certainly play a major role in both decision making and outcome. Finally, there may be large fluctuations in outcome from chance alone for low-frequency procedures, and rates may not be stable statistically.

The confusion surrounding outcome research includes not only these different design characteristics but also that the term has been applied to at least two other kinds of studies: assessing small area variation and assessing the relationship between volume and outcome.

Small Area Variation

Area variation describes the phenomenon of differences in the rates of medical and surgical services observed among geographic regions (so-called large areas). These variations have been recorded among countries, states, and provinces and among counties or health services areas (so-called small areas). These findings elicit concern because persons in areas of high volume may be receiving too much or inappropriate care (and thereby potentially be exposed to iatrogenic illness and postoperative death) while those in low-volume areas may be receiving too little care (and thereby not benefiting from modern medical care).[12]

The two main reasons cited for the variations have been differences in physician practice style and access to medical care. However, the variations may result from other causes including difficulties defining or diagnosing the disease, differences in the prevalence and severity of disease, and regional differences in patient preferences seeking and accepting medical care.[13] Variation in surgical rates is related to variation in physician opinion, and where differences in physician opinion do exist, there tend to be large geographic variations.

Recognizing these variations is only of value if the causes and consequences of variation can be ascertained so that strategies to minimize them can be implemented.[14] The conduct of RCTs to improve the quality of evidence available and development of evidence-based practice guidelines may be useful in this regard. An additional problem with the interpretation of area variation studies is knowing what the rate should be.[15] For some procedures, there may be no correct rate if patient preferences are considered.[16]

Volume–Outcome Differences

An increasing number of studies have shown that for complex operations, such as esophagectomy, Whipple procedure, low anterior resection and abdominoperineal resection, liver resection, and sarcoma surgery, surgical volume may have an impact on outcome.[17–20] However, outcomes of low-volume surgeons have been reported to be equivalent to those of high-volume surgeons if the low-volume surgeon worked at a high-volume hospital.[21] This finding suggests that the health care team and facilities may be as important or even more important than the individual expertise of the surgeon.

The implications of such studies are enormous and must be reviewed by policy and decision makers. Regionalization of more complex procedures has been suggested. Before doing so, however, one must be certain that the results of current studies are not biased and that observed differences are not caused by factors other than volume. Thus, rigorous volume–outcome studies with prospective collection of data and studies addressing patient preferences may be required for each procedure before such decisions can be made.

Levels of Evidence

There are several grading systems for assessing the level of evidence.[4,22] Most systems consider the a priori design of the study and the actual quality of the study. Studies in which there has been blinded random allocation of subjects are given highest weighting because the risk of bias is minimized. Thus, a randomized controlled trial will provide level I evidence provided it is well executed with respect to the issues discussed earlier in this chapter.

This system is of value because of its simplicity, but difficulties may arise when readers wish to pool results from several studies, either informally during their reading or when performing systematic reviews or developing guidelines. Decisions must be made on whether studies should be included or excluded depending on the quality of the study.[23] As well, the systems are not sensitive to the relevance of the findings of studies. For instance, neither the clinical relevance of the outcome measures, the baseline risk of the effect, nor the actual results of the studies (e.g., study results that are not consistent with results from other RCTs) are considered in any system.

In this volume, the quality of evidence is generally classified according to the system listed in Table 1.3.

What Is the Quality of Evidence Evaluating Surgical Practice?

As one would predict, repeated studies have shown that there is a predominance of case studies and a relative paucity of RCTs published in the literature. Concerns specific to the methodology of surgical trials, strong patient preferences, and inadequate funding have been cited as the primary reasons for this. Still, many important, well-designed surgical trials have been performed and continue to have a significant impact on treatment decisions.

TABLE 1.3. Levels of Evidence.

I	Evidence obtained from at least one properly randomized controlled trial
II-1	Evidence obtained from well-designed controlled trials without randomization
II-2	Evidence obtained from well-designed cohort or case-control analytic studies, preferable from more than one center or research group
II-3	Evidence obtained from comparisons between times or places with or without the intervention; dramatic results in uncontrolled experiments (such as the results of treatment with penicillin in the 1940s) could also be included in this category
III	Opinions of respected authorities, based on clinical experience, descriptive studies, or reports of expert committees

Assessing the Best Evidence

Systematic Reviews or Meta-Analyses

The terms systematic review and meta-analysis have been used interchangeably. However, systematic reviews or overviews are qualitative reviews, whereas statistical methods are used to combine and summarize the results of several studies in meta-analysis.[24] In both, there is a specific scientific approach to the identification, critical appraisal, and synthesis of all relevant studies on a specific topic. They differ from the usual clinical review in that there is an explicit, specific question that is addressed. In addition, the methodology is explicit and there is a conscientious effort to retrieve and review all studies on the topic without preconceived prejudice. The value of meta-analysis is that study results are combined so conclusions can be made about therapeutic effectiveness or, if there is no conclusive answer, to plan new studies.[25] They are especially useful when results from several studies disagree with regard to the magnitude or the direction of effect, when individual studies are too small to detect an effect and label it as statistically not significant, or when a large trial is too costly or time-consuming to perform. For the clinician, meta-analyses are useful because results of individual trials are combined so he or she does not have to retrieve, evaluate, and synthesize the results of all studies on the topic. Thus, it may increase the efficiency of the clinician in keeping abreast of recent advances.

Meta-analysis is a relatively new method for synthesizing information from multiple studies. Thus, the methodology is constantly evolving and like that of other studies, the quality of individual meta-analysis may be quite variable. There has been a call for standardization of the methodology used in meta-analysis.[26, 27] However, because the rigorousness of the methodology of many published meta-analyses may be quite variable, the clinician should have some knowledge of meta-analysis methodology and be able to critically appraise them. Published guidelines are available (Table 1.4).[28]

Some basic steps are followed in performing a meta-analysis. First, the meta-analysis should address a specific health care question. Second, various strategies should be used to ensure that all relevant studies (RCTs) on the topic are retrieved, including searching various databases such as MED-LINE and EMBASE. In addition, proceedings of meetings and reference lists should be checked and content experts and clinical researchers consulted to ensure all published and nonpublished trials are identified. Reliance on MEDLINE searches alone will result in incomplete retrieval of published studies.[29] Third, as in other studies, inclusion criteria should be set a priori. Fourth, data from the individual studies should be extracted by two blinded investigators to ensure that this is done accurately. As well, these investigators should assess the quality of the individual studies. Fifth, the data should be combined using various statistical techniques. Before doing so, statistical tests to determine the "sameness" or "homogeneity" of the individual studies should be performed.

Although some have embraced meta-analysis as a systematic approach to synthesizing published information from individual trials, others have cautioned about the results of meta-analysis and others have been skeptical of the technique completely.[30] In some cases meta-analyses on the same clinical question have led to different conclusions.[31] Some of these resulted from methodological problems. Failure to use sufficiently broad search strategies may result in exclusion of all relevant studies. Most commonly, unpublished studies are excluded, and these are more likely to be "negative trials" (so-called publication bias).[32] As well, there is evidence that omission of trials not published in English language journals may bias the results.[33] Finally, there is a strong association between statistically positive conclusions of meta-analyses and their quality (i.e., the lower the quality of the studies, the more likely that the meta-analysis reached a positive conclusion).[34] One of the values of meta-analysis is that the generalizability of the results is increased by combining the results of several trials. However, if there is great variation in studies, including patient inclusion criteria, dosage and mode of administration of medication, and length of follow-up (so-called heterogeneity), it may be inappropriate to combine results and doing so may produce invalid results. Other reasons for discrepancies may be the use of different statistical tests and failure to update the meta-analysis. Finally, meta-analysis has generally been restricted to combining the results of randomized controlled trials even though there is also a need for combining data from nonrandomized or observational studies.

The Cochrane Database of Systematic Reviews is a valuable source of high-level information for practicing clinicians. Unfortunately, this database is of somewhat more limited use

TABLE 1.4. Guidelines for Using a Review.

1. Did the overview address a focused clinical question?
2. Were the criteria used to select articles for inclusion appropriate?
3. Is it unlikely that important, relevant studies were missed?
4. Was the validity of the included studies appraised?
5. Were the assessments of the studies reproducible?
6. Were the results similar from study to study?
7. What are the overall results of the review?
8. How precise were the results?
9. Can the results be applied to my patient care?
10. Were all the clinically important outcomes considered?
11. Are the benefits worth the harms and costs?

Source: Adapted from Oxman et al.[28]

to surgeons because of the paucity of published surgical RCTs and meta-analyses.

Practice Guidelines

Practice guidelines have been defined by the Institute of Medicine (IOM) as "systematically developed statements to assist practitioner and patient decisions about appropriate health care for specific clinical circumstances."[35] Guidelines are not standards that set rigid rules of care for patients. Rather, guidelines should be flexible so that individual patient characteristics, preferences of surgeons and patients, and local circumstances can be accommodated.[36]

Guideline development has occurred for several reasons.[37] First, as discussed earlier there is growing evidence of substantial unexplained and inappropriate variation in clinical practice patterns, probably partly because of physician uncertainty. Second, there is evidence that the traditional methods for delivering continuing medical education are ineffective and that clinicians have difficulty in assimilating the rapidly evolving scientific evidence. Third, there is concern that as health care resources become more limited there will be inadequate funds to deliver high-quality care if current technology and treatments are used inappropriately or ineffectively.

Practice guidelines have been promoted as one strategy to assist clinical decision making to increase the effectiveness and decrease unnecessary costs of delivered health care services.[37] Many clinicians are wary of guidelines and believe that they are simply a means to limit resources and inhibit clinical decision making and individual preferences. Guidelines have also been criticized for being too idealistic and failing to take into account the realities of day-to-day practice. Critics argue that patients differ in their clinical manifestations, associated diseases, and preferences for treatments. Thus, guidelines may be too restrictive or irrelevant. Third, clinicians may be confused because of conflicting guidelines. Finally, guideline development may be inhibited because there is a lack of evidence upon which to base guidelines.

Many groups and organizations have begun to develop practice guidelines by using different methods.[38] Guidelines can be developed based on informal consensus. The criteria upon which decisions are based are often poorly described and there is no systematic approach to reviewing the evidence. More often, these guidelines are based on the opinion of experts. Readers are unable to judge the validity of the guidelines because even if a systematic approach was followed the process is not documented. In many instances, guidelines are self-serving and used to promote a certain specialty or expertise. The National Institutes of Health (NIH) and other bodies have produced guidelines based on a formal consensus approach. Although this approach tends to be more structured than the informal consensus, it suffers from the same potential flaws in that it is less structured and also susceptible to the biases of the experts.

Evidence-based guidelines are the most rigorously developed.[37,39,40] There should be a focused clinical question, and a systematic approach to the retrieval, assessment of quality, and synthesis of evidence should be followed. Guidelines development should also be a dynamic process with constant updating as more evidence is available. In addition to assess-

TABLE 1.5. Guidelines for Assessing Practice Guidelines.

1. Were all important options and outcomes clearly specified?
2. Was an explicit and sensible process used to identify select and combine evidence?
3. Was an explicit and sensible process used to consider the relative value of different outcomes?
4. Is the guideline likely to account for important recent developments?
5. Has the guideline been subject to peer review and testing?
6. Are practical, clinically important, recommendations made?
7. How strong are the recommendations?
8. What is the impact of uncertainty associated with the evidence and values used in guidelines?
9. Is the primary objective of the guideline consistent with your objective?
10. Are the recommendations applicable to your patients?

Source: Adapted from Hayward et al.[40]

ment of the literature, there is usually an interpretation of the evidence by experts, and the evidence may be modulated by current or local circumstances (e.g., cost/availability of technology).

Much attention has been paid to the preparation of guidelines, but there has been much less emphasis on the dissemination of and evaluation of the impact of guidelines. Unfortunately, there is some evidence that EB guidelines may not have as much impact on either changing physician behavior or improving outcome. Because there are many guidelines available, some with conflicting recommendations, clinicians require some skills to evaluate the guidelines and determine their validity and applicability (Table 1.5).[39,40]

Critically Appraising the Literature

Critical appraisal requires the clinician to have some knowledge of clinical epidemiology, biostatistics, epidemiology, decision analysis, and economics. While this knowledge is helpful, critical appraisal skills improve with practice and clinicians are encouraged simply to begin using the skills they already have in evaluating the literature and build on them.

To make decisions about a patient, clinicians generally need to know the cause of or risk factors for disease, the natural history or prognosis of disease, how to quantify aspects of disease (measurement issues), diagnostic tests and the diagnosis of disease, and the effectiveness of treatment. In addition, clinicians now need some knowledge of economic analysis, health services research, practice guidelines, systematic reviews, and decision analysis to fully appreciate the literature and all sources of information.

Generally, clinicians read articles so they can generalize the results of the study and apply them to their own patients. Two potential sources of error may lead to incorrect conclusions about the validity of the study results: systematic error (bias) and random error. Bias is defined as "any effect at any stage of investigation or inference tending to produce results that depart systematically from the true values."[41] For example, the term biased sample is often used to mean that the sample of patients is not typical or representative of patients with that condition. A number of biases might be present, not just those related to patient selection. It may be difficult for the reader to discern whether there is bias and if so its magnitude. The risk of an error from bias decreases as the rigorousness of the trial design increases. Because of the random allocation of patients as well as other attributes, the randomized controlled trial is considered the best design for minimizing the risk of bias. In observational studies, including outcomes research (where patients have not been randomized), various statistical tests (such as multivariate analysis) are frequently employed to adjust for differences in prognostic factors between the two groups of patients. However, it is important to realize that it is possible to adjust for only known or measurable factors. In addition, there may be other unknown and possibly important prognostic factors that cannot be adjusted. Again, only if patients are randomly allocated can one be certain that the two groups are similar with respect to all known and unknown prognostic variables.

The other type of error is random error. Random error occurs due to chance, when the result obtained in the sample of patients studied differs from the result that would be obtained if the entire population were studied.[41] Statistical testing can be performed to determine the likelihood of a random error. The type of statistical test used varies depending on the type of data. Some of the more common tests are shown in Table 1.6. There are two types of random error: type I and type II. The risk of stating there is a difference between two treatments when really there is none is known as a type I error. In the theory of testing hypotheses, rejecting a null hypothesis when it is actually true is called a type I error. By convention, if the risk of the result occurring due to chance is less than 5% (a p value less than 0.05), then the difference in the results of treatment is considered statistically significant and that there really is a difference in the effectiveness of the two treatments.

If a result is statistically significant, the clinician must determine whether it is clinically relevant or important.[42] Typically, treatment effects can be written as absolute or relative risk reductions. The absolute risk reduction (ARR) is simply the difference in rates between the control group and the experimental group, whereas the relative risk reduction (RRR) is a proportional risk reduction and is calculated by dividing the absolute risk reduction by the control risk. The advantage of the ARR is that the baseline event rate is considered. For instance, the RRR would be the same in two different studies where the rates between the control and experimental groups were 50% and 25% and 0.5% and 0.25%, respectively. In other words, while the ARR would be 25% in the first study and 0.25% in the second study, the RRR for both studies would be 50%. Although the RRR is the same in both studies, the treatment benefit in the second scenario may be trivial.

Recently, Sackett and colleagues have coined the term "number needed to treat" (NNT), which may make more intuitive sense to clinicians than thinking in terms of ARR and RRR.[43] It is calculated by dividing the ARR into 1. Thus, in the first example, 4 patients would have to be treated to prevent one bad outcome (the NNT is 2), whereas 400 would have to be treated to prevent one bad outcome (the NNT is 400) in the latter example. Determining whether the treatment benefit is clinically significant requires the judgment of the clinician. The statistician can only determine whether a treatment benefit is statistically significant. Whether the effect is clinically significant depends on the NNT, the frequency and severity of side effects (sometimes stated as the number needed to harm, NNH), and the cost of treatment and its feasibility and acceptability.

The other type of random error is the so-called type II error, which occurs when two treatments are, in reality, different but one concludes that they are equally effective. In the theory of testing hypotheses, accepting a null hypothesis when it is incorrect is called a type II error. It is not uncommon for clinicians to read a study in which the results are not statistically significant and to wonder whether the two treatments are equally effective or whether there is a type II error. When investigators plan a trial, they minimize the risk of a type II error by calculating a sample size to ensure that there is adequate power (1 − type II error) to show a difference if one really exists. To calculate a sample size, both the type I error and power are specified plus the mean and standard deviation or event rate in the control group and the size of the difference that one wishes to detect. Not surprisingly, the more variable the subjects, the less frequent the event rate, or the smaller the difference in the effects of the treatment, the more subjects that are necessary to be certain a treatment effect has not been missed. Conversely, fewer subjects are necessary if there is less subject variability, the outcome occurs more frequently, or one wishes to detect a large difference in treatment effect.

While a power calculation is performed a priori, a more useful measure for the reader interpreting the study results is the calculation of 95% confidence intervals (CI).[44] The 95% confidence interval means that one can be 95% certain that the true difference between the two treatments lies within this range of values.[41] Thus, suppose, in a study comparing stapled to hand-sutured anastomoses, the difference in leak rate was 2% with 95% confidence intervals of ±3%. In other words, one can be 95% certain that the true risk of an anastomotic leak is between 1% less than and 5% greater than with a stapled anastomosis. If so, one would be fairly confident that the two different anastomotic techniques are equally effective. On the other hand, if the confidence intervals were ±10%, so that the true difference in leak rates was somewhere between 8% less than and 12% greater than with a stapled anastomosis, one would be less likely to conclude that the anastomotic techniques were equal. Clinicians can interpret the negative result of a study much better when confidence intervals are calculated than when only a p value is given. The

TABLE 1.6. Types of Statistical Tests.

Data type	Statistical test (with no adjustment for prognostic factors)	Procedure test (with adjustment for prognostic factors)
Binary (dichotomous)	Fisher exact test or chi-square	Logistic regression (Mantel–Haenszel)
Ordered discrete	Mann-Whitney U-test	
Continuous (normal distribution)	Student's t-test	Analysis of covariance (ANCOVA) (multiple regression)
Time to event (censored data)	Log-rank Wilcoxon test	Log-rank (Cox's proportional hazards)

wider the confidence interval, the less certain one can be that the two treatments are really similar in effectiveness. Conversely, if the confidence intervals are narrow, one can be much more certain that the treatments are equally effective.

References

1. Evidence Based Medicine Working Group. Evidence-based medicine. JAMA 1992;268:2420–2425.
2. Davidoff F, Haynnes B, Sackett D, Smith R. Evidence based medicine. A new journal to help doctors identify the information they need. Br Med J 1998;310:1085–1086.
3. Rosenberg W, Donald A. Evidence based medicine: an approach to clinical problem-solving. Br Med J 1995;310:1126.
4. Canadian Task Force on Periodic Health Examination. The periodic health examination. Can Med Assoc J 1979;121:1193–1254.
5. Solomon MJ, McLeod RS. Clinical studies in surgical journals—have we improved? Dis Colon Rect 1993;36:43–48.
6. Shapiro S. Evidence of screening for breast cancer from a randomized trial. Cancer (Phila) (Suppl) 1977;39:2772.
7. Detsky AS. Are clinical trials a cost effective investment? JAMA 1983;262:1795–1800.
8. McLeod RS, Wright JG, Solomon MJ, Hu X, Walters BC, Lossing A. Randomized controlled trials in surgery; issues and problems. Surgery (St. Louis) 1996;119:483–486.
9. Taylor K, Margolese R, Soskolne CL. Physicians' reasons for not entering eligible patients in a randomized clinical trial of adjuvant surgery for breast cancer. N Engl J Med 1984;310:1363–1367.
10. Committee to Design a Strategy for Quality Review and Assurance in Medicare, Institute of Medicine. Medicare; a Strategy for Quality Assurance. Washington, DC: National Academy Press, 1990.
11. Greenfield S. The state of outcome research: are we on target? N Engl J Med 1989;320:1142–1143.
12. Health Services Group. Small-area variations: what are they and what do they mean? Can Med Assoc J 1992;146:467–470.
13. Eddy DM. Variations in physician practice: the role of uncertainty. In: Health Affairs, Vol. 3. XX: Project Hope, 1984:74–89.
14. Blais R. Variations in the use of health care services: Why are more studies needed? Can Med Assoc J 1994;151:1701–1719.
15. Wennberg JE. Which rate is right? (Editorial). N Engl J Med 1986;314:310–311.
16. Wright JG, Coyte P, Hawker G, Bombardier C, Cooke D, Heck D, Dittus R, Freund D. Variation in orthopedic surgeon's perceptions of the indications for and outcomes of knee replacement. Can Med Assoc J 1995;152(5):687–697.
17. Porter GA, Soskolne CL, Yakimets WW, Newman SC. Surgeon-related factors and outcome in rectal cancer. Ann Surg 1998;227:157–167.
18. Lieberman MD, Kilburn H, Lindsey M, Brennen MF. Relation of perioperative deaths to hospital volume among patients undergoing pancreatic resection for malignancy. Ann Surg 1995;222:638–645.
19. Simunovic M, To T, Theriault M, Langer B. Relation between hospital surgical volume and outcome for pancreatic resection for neoplasm in a publicly funded health care system. Can Med Assoc J 1999;160:643–648.
20. Gordon TA, Burleyson GP, Tielsch JM, Cameron JL. The effects of regionalization on cost and outcome for one general high-risk surgical procedure. Ann Surg 1995;221:43–49.
21. Birkmeyer JD, Finlayson SR, Tosteson AN, Sharp SM, Warshaw AL, Fisher ES. Effect of hospital volume on in-hospital mortality with pancreaticoduodenectomy. Surgery (St. Louis) 1999;125:250–256.
22. U.S. Preventive Services Task Force. Guide to Clinical Preventive Services. An Assessment of 169 Interventions. Baltimore: Williams & Wilkins, 1989.
23. Liberati A. Problems in defining hierarchies (levels) of evidence for studies to be included in systematic reviews of effectiveness of interventions. Presented at 2nd Symposium on Systematic Reviews: Beyond the Basics. Oxford, UK: January 1999.
24. Cook DJ, Sackett DL, Spitzer WO. Methodologic guidelines for systematic reviews of randomized controlled trials in health care from the Potsdam consultation on meta-analysis. J Clin Epidemiol 1995;48:167–171.
25. L'Abbee KA, Detsky AS, O'Rourke K. Meta-analysis in clinical research. Ann Intern Med 1987;107:224–233.
26. Spitzer WO, ed. The Potsdam International Consultation on Meta-analysis. J Clin Epidemiol 1995;48:1–171.
27. Chalmers TC, Altman DG, eds. Systematic Reviews. London: British Medical Journal Publishing Group, 1995.
28. Oxman AD, Cook DJ, Guyatt GH. Users' guides to the medical literature. VI. How to use an overview. Evidence-Based Medicine Working Group. JAMA 1994;272:1367–1371.
29. Solomon JS, McLeod RS. Should we be performing more randomized controlled trials evaluating surgical operations? Surgery (St. Louis) 1995;118:459–467.
30. Feinstein AR. Meta-analysis: statistical alchemy for the 21st century. J Clin Epidemiol 1995;48:71–79.
31. Moher D, Olkin I. Meta-analysis of randomized controlled trials: a concern for standards. JAMA 1995;274:1962–1964.
32. Dickerson K, Scherer R, Lefebvre C. Identifying relevant studies for systematic reviews. Br Med J 1994;309:1286–1291.
33. Moher D, Fortin P, Jadad AR, Juni P, Klassen T, Le Lorier J, Liberati A, Linde K, Penna A. Completeness of reporting of trials published in languages other than English: implications for conduct and reporting of systematic reviews. Lancet 1996;347:363–366.
34. Jadad AR, McQuay HJ. Meta-analyses to evaluate analgesic interventions: a systematic qualitative review of their methodology. J Clin Epidemiol 1996;49:235–243.
35. Committee to Advise Public Health Service on Clinical Practice Guidelines (Institute of Medicine). Clinical Practice Guidelines: Directions for a New Program. Washington, DC: National Academy Press, 1990:58.
36. Wright JG, McLeod RS, Mahoney J, Lossing A, Hu X. The Surgical Clinical Epidemiology Group. Surgery (St. Louis) 1996;119:706–709.
37. Browman GP, Levine MN, Mohide A, Hayward RSA, Pritchard KI, Gafni A, Laupacis A. The practice guidelines development cycle: a conceptual tool for practice guidelines development and implementation. J Clin Oncol 1995;13:502–512.
38. Wolff SH. Practice guidelines, a new reality in medicine. II. Methods of developing guidelines. Arch Intern Med 1992;152:946–952.
39. Guyatt GH, Sackett DL, Sinclair JC, Hayward R, Cook DJ, Cook RJ, for the Evidence Based Medicine Working Group. Users' guides to the medical literature. IX. A method for grading health care recommendations. JAMA 1995;274:1800–1804.
40. Hayward RSA, Wilson MC, Tunis SR, Bass EB, Guyatt GH, for the Evidence Based Medicine Working Group. Users' guide to the medical literature. VIII. How to use clinical practice guidelines. Are recommendations valid? JAMA 1995;274:570–574.
41. Last JM. A Dictionary of Epidemiology. Oxford: Oxford Medical Publications, 1983.
42. Sackett DL, Richardson WS, Rosenberg W, Haynes RB. Evidence Based Medicine. How to Practice & Teach EBM. London: Churchill Livingstone, 1997.
43. Cook RJ, Sackett DL. The number needed to treat: a clinically useful measure of treatment effect. Br Med J 1995;310:452–454.
44. Guyatt GH, Jaeschke R, Heddle N, Cook D, Shannon H, Walter S. Basic statistics for clinicians: 2. Interpreting study results: confidence intervals. Can Med Assoc J 1995;152:169–173.

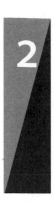

Nutrition

Kenneth A. Kudsk and Danny O. Jacobs

Implications of Nutrition Support for Clinical Outcome

To critically evaluate a specific therapeutic intervention, three criteria should be satisfied.[1–3] First, evidence should show that the treatment is better than no treatment in improving clinical outcome. Second, beneficial effects of the therapy should outweigh harmful effects. Third, compared with other alternatives, the treatment should represent wise use of resources. These issues are paramount in nutrition support because comprehensive studies of patients administered intravenous nutrition documented a 29% incidence of complications related to catheter placement (5.7%), sepsis (6.5%), metabolic (7.7%) and mechanical (9%) complications, and death (0.2%)[4] caused by fluid and electrolyte problems (e.g., refeeding syndrome with precipitous and sometimes lethal drops in potassium, phosphate, and magnesium levels), metabolic complications such as hyperglycemia, and other technical issues. Enteral complication rates have also been well documented and include aspiration, frequent tube dislodgement, and intraabdominal complications such as diarrhea, nausea, vomiting, and even intestinal necrosis.[5] The potential for serious and occasionally life-threatening complications dictates a close inspection of existing clinical data.

Determination of Nutritional Status

Significant limitations exist in clinicians' ability to quantify the degree of malnutrition, identify the degree of metabolic injury and stress, and measure the effectiveness of nutrition in reversing nutrition-related immunological and metabolic abnormalities. The benefits of therapy are very clear in some circumstances. Patients with short gut syndrome secondary to vascular disasters or recurrent resections as the result of chronic disease that leave no colon and less than 100 cm of jejunum or less than 50 cm of jejunum or ileum with an in-

tact colon cannot survive without parenteral nutrition.[6,7] In these circumstances, parenteral nutrition restores body composition, allowing a meaningful, productive existence,[8] but in other patients without such dramatic loss of the gastrointestinal tract or severely impaired nutritional status, improved clinical outcome with specialized nutrition support is less clear.

There is a strong inverse correlation between the body's protein status and postoperative complications in populations of patients undergoing elective major gastrointestinal surgery.[9,10] Measurement of protein status in an individual patient is inexact because of difficulties quantitating the degree of malnutrition and because disease processes themselves influence markers of malnutrition and clinical outcome.

Parameters including weight loss, albumin, prealbumin, and immune competence (measured by delayed cutaneous hypersensitivity or total lymphocyte count) have been used to classify patients into the states of mild, moderate, and severe malnutrition,[11–14] but by themselves individual markers may not accurately represent the nutritional status of the patient. Important information obtained during the history and physical examination is the amount of weight loss with the percentage of usual body weight calculated by these equations:

$$\% \text{ body weight loss} = \frac{\text{usual body weight minus current body weight}}{\text{usual body weight}} \times 100$$

or

$$\% \text{ usual body weight} = \frac{\text{current body weight}}{\text{usual body weight}} \times 100$$

In general, a weight loss of 5% to 10% over a month or of 10% to 20% over 6 months is associated with increased complications.[15] Although considered the single best serum marker of malnutrition in otherwise stable patients, serum albumin levels are influenced by synthesis rates, degradation rates, and vascular losses into the interstitium or through the gut and kidney. Delayed cutaneous hypersensitivity, a known marker of severe malnutrition, is influenced by injury, hepatic and renal failure, infections, edema, anesthesia, medications such as corticosteroids, coumarin, and cimetidine, and immunosuppressants.

As a predictive tool, combinations of these measurements have been used to quantify the risk for subsequent complications. The Prognostic Nutritional Index correlates with poor outcome in the following equation:

$$PNI\ (\%) = 158 - 16.6\ (ALB) - 0.78\ (TSF) - 0.20\ (TFN) - 5.8\ (DH)$$

where PNI is the risk of complication occurring in individual patient, ALB is serum albumin (g/dl), TSF is the triceps skinfold thickness (mm), TFN is serum transferrin (mg/dl), and DH is delayed hypersensitivity reaction to one of three recall antigens (0, nonreactive; 1, <5-mm induration; 2, >5-mm induration).[16] Because delayed hypersensitivity is uncommon in clinical practice, the equation has been simplified by substituting the lymphocyte score, using a scale of 0 to 2, where 0 is less than 1,000 total lymphocytes/mm^3, 1 is 1,000 to 2,000 total lymphocytes/mm^3, and a score of 2 is more than 2,000 total lymphocytes/mm.[17] The higher the score using either of these equations, the greater the risk of postoperative complications. The Prognostic Inflammatory Nutrition Index (PINI) appears to correlate with recovery from injury as the acute-phase protein response abates in the following equation: PINI = (CRP) (AAG)/(PA) (ALB), where C-reactive protein (CRP), α_1-acid-glycoprotein (AAG), and prealbumin (PA) are measured in mg/dl and albumin in g/dl.[18] The subjective global assessment clinically evaluates nutritional status by determining restriction of nutrient intake, changes in organ function and body composition, and the disease process.[19] There appears to be close interobserver agreement with good predictions of complications in general surgical patients, liver transplant patients,[20] and dialysis patients.[21]

In summary, there is no "gold standard" for determining nutritional status because of the influence of illness and injury on assessment parameters and the difficulty in isolating the individual influences of malnutrition and disease on clinical outcome. This conclusion was supported by nonrandomized prospective, retrospective, or case cohort-controlled studies.[22] Malnutrition appears to be a continuum that is influenced by the duration of altered nutritional intake and the degree of insult and metabolic stress during that time, as well as the ability of medical care to control or reverse the disease process and the metabolic perturbations induced by that disease process.

The Implications of Specialized Nutrition Support in Malnourished Versus Well-Nourished Patients

Although the effect of nutrition on outcome in patients with midrange degrees of malnutrition is unclear, there is significant class I data (class of evidence) describing the impact of nutrition support in nontrauma/noncritically ill general surgical patients at both ends of the nutritional scale. While perioperative nutrition in the well-nourished patient has resulted in either no significant impact or in increased infectious com-

plications, perioperative nutrition in the severely malnourished patient may result in improved postoperative morbidity (see Table 2.1).

Enteral Versus Parenteral Versus No Specialized Nutrition Support

Several class I randomized, prospective studies have investigated the route of nutrient administration in trauma and general surgical patients. Most of these studies were carried out in patients with blunt and penetrating trauma to the torso or head injuries. Most studies of blunt and penetrating trauma to the torso show improved outcome with early enteral feeding.[23–26] The benefits of reduced infectious complications with enteral feeding increase as the severty of injury increases.

The type of injury probably plays an important role. Only one[27] of five studies[28–31] of patients with severe head injury noted any benefit with early enteral feeding. Gastroparesis delayed advancement of successful enteral feedings in several of the studies. For the most part, closed-head-injury patients randomized to intragastric feeding received insignificant amounts of enteral diet for the first 10 days following injury, that is, they were severely underfed, but at this point, existing data would not suggest significant benefit of a neurological or infectious outcome with either very early enteral or parenteral feeding following severe closed-head injury. The gastroparesis often resolves within 4 to 5 days, allowing institution of early enteral feeding at that point. In patients in whom gastroparesis does not resolve within 6 to 7 days, parenteral nutrition or transpyloric placement of an enteral tube is clinically indicated (level III data) with transition to intragastric feeding as soon as the gastroparesis resolves.

Cognizant of the failure of enteral feeding with specialized diet to improve outcome in well-nourished patients following intestinal resection,[32] several authors have noted improved outcome in patients receiving enteral feeding following laparotomy compared with parenterally fed patients or patients receiving only intravenous fluids. Most of these included patients undergoing upper gastrointestinal surgery for carcinoma, and most showed benefit when nutrients were delivered via the gastrointestinal tract.

A study of ulcerative colitis patients, undergoing resection randomized to either polymeric enteral nutrition or an isonitrogenous, isocaloric parenteral nutrition solution, noted significant improvement in serum albumin rates with enteral feeding and more postoperative infectious complications with parenteral nutrition.[33] In a study of patients with Crohn's disease, polymeric enteral feeding achieved similar results with steroid treatment in inducing remission.[34]

Following liver transplantation, results have been inconsistent. Nutrition support has also been studied during acute pancreatitis. No differences were noted in the incidence of infectious complications or length of hospital stay between patients randomized to jejunal feeding or parenteral nutrition.[35] Duodenal feedings are contraindicated in patients with acute pancreatitis because of pancreatic stimulation caused by hormonal responses following intragastric and intraduodenal stimulation.[36] Intravenous feeding and jejunal feedings[37,38] do not appear to stimulate pancreatic secretions and can be given without fear of aggravating pancreatitis.

TABLE 2.1.

Perioperative and Early Feeding Studies with Substantial Number of Well-Nourished or Moderately Malnourished Patients.

Author	Year	Class of evidence	Conclusions
Veterans Affair Total Parenteral Nutrition Cooperative Study Group[120]	1991	1	Of 395 malnourished patients requiring laparotomy or noncardiac thoracotomy randomized to 7–15 days preoperative nutrition ($n = 192$) or no perioperative nutrition support ($n = 203$) and monitored for 90 days following surgery, the rates of major complications were similar in patients with mild or moderate degrees of malnutrition with more infectious complications in the TPN group ($p = .01$) but more noninfectious complications in the control group ($p = .02$); 90-day mortality rates were also similar. Only in severely malnourished patients did TPN significantly reduce noninfectious complications (5% vs. 43%, $p = .03$) with no increase in infectious complications.
Fan[121]	1994	I	A randomized prospective study of 124 patients undergoing resection of hepatocellular carcinoma randomized to perioperative intravenous nutrition with 35% branched-chain amino acids, dextrose, and lipid (50% medium-chain triglycerides) for 14 days in addition to oral diet or control group (oral diet alone). Postoperative morbidity rate reduced in perioperative fed group (34% vs. 55%) because of fewer septic complications (17% vs. 37%) and less deterioration of liver function as measured by indocyanine green. There were no significant differences in deaths although most of the benefit occurred in cirrhotic patients undergoing major hepatectomy.
Brennan[122]	1994	I	A prospective, randomized trial of 117 moderately malnourished patients randomized to postoperative parenteral nutrition ($n = 60$, albumin = 3.1, 5.8% preoperative body weight loss) or standard i.v. fluids ($n = 57$, albumin = 3.3, 6.8% preoperative body weight loss). Complications were significantly greater in TPN-fed patients with a significant increase in intraabdominal abscess and major complications.
Heslin[32]	1997	I	Of 195 well-nourished patients undergoing esophageal, gastric, pancreatic, or gastric resection randomized to jejunal feedings ($n = 97$; albumin 4.08 ± 0.04 g/dl) or i.v. feedings ($n = 98$; albumin = 4.1 ± 0.06 g/dl), no significant differences found in the number of major, minor, or infectious wound complications between groups and no difference in hospital mortality or length of stay. There was one small-bowel necrosis in the enterally fed group.
Doglietto[123]	1996	I	Their 678 patients with normal or mild malnutrition undergoing major elective abdominal surgery randomized to protein-sparing therapy or no specialized nutrition had similar operative mortality rates and postoperative complication rate.
Watters[124]	1997	I	Patients undergoing esophagectomy or pancreatoduodenectomy were randomized to postoperative early jejunal feedings ($n = 13$; albumin = 4.08 ± 5 g/dl) or no enteral feeding ($n = 15$; 4.1 ± 4 g/dl) during the first 6 postoperative days. Postoperative vital capacity and fractional expired volume were lower in the fed group and postoperative mobility was lower in the fed group in this well-nourished group of patients at low risk of nutrition-related complications. This study was confounded by increased epidural anesthesia in the enterally fed group.
Daly[55]	1992	I	Studied 85 patients randomized to standard ($n = 44$; albumin = 3.0 ± 1.2 g/dl) vs. supplemented ($n = 41$; albumin = 3.3 g/dl) enteral diets with 77 eligible patients. Infectious and wound complications ($p = .02$) and length of stay ($p = .01$) significantly shorter for supplemented group. Diets were not isonitrogenous.
Daly[125]	1995	I	Studied 60 patients with upper gastrointestinal lesions requiring resection randomized to standard enteral diet ($n = 30$) or diet supplemented with arginine, omega-3 fatty acids, and nucleotides ($n = 30$). Patients were moderately malnourished with albumins less than 3.4. Length of stay and infectious/wound complications significantly reduced ($p < .05$ for both) in supplemented group. Patients also randomized to jejunal feedings during radiation chemotherapy tolerated chemotherapy significantly better.

TPN, total parenteral nutrition.

Type of Nutrient Diet

Enteral Feeding

With the exception of burn patients in whom early intragastric feeding *prevents* gastroparesis,[39,40] patients undergoing laparotomy for major torso trauma or major intestinal surgery or patients sustaining severe closed-head injury developed a gastroparesis that preempts successful early intragastric feeding. When nutrition is delivered beyond the ligament of Treitz via nasojejunal, transgastric, or standard jejunostomy tubes, more complex formulas containing whole proteins, fiber, etc., are usually well tolerated with low rates

of distension, cramps, or diarrhea, although progression may be slower as the magnitude of insult increases, especially with trauma.[41]

During the hypermetabolism of stress and sepsis, experimental evidence suggests that specific substrates may be beneficial in supporting the metabolic and immunological responses following surgery, and thus specialty diets enhanced with various combinations of these nutrients have been developed and clinically tested. These "immune-enhancing" diets have been formulated containing various combinations of arginine, omega-3 fatty acids, nucleotides, glutamine, and branched-chain amino acids.

Glutamine production is increased during stress and sepsis while intracellular levels drop. As a substrate necessary for proliferating cells, it serves as a primary fuel for cells lining the gastrointestinal tract as well as immunological cells.[42]

Arginine promotes proliferating T cells after mitogen or cytokine stimulation in vitro and serves as a precursor for nitric oxide, nitrites, and nitrates, as well as putrescine, spermine, and spermidine.[43] Arginine also has beneficial effects on cellular immunity, increases fibroblast proliferation in wounds, and improves survival following injury and sepsis.[44,45] Arginine also is a secretagogue for growth hormone, insulin, prolactin, and glucagon.[46]

The polyunsaturated fatty acids induce immunological effects. Once released by phospholipases released in response to stress, the end products of omega-6 fatty acid metabolism result in increased levels of prostaglandin E_2, thromboxane A_2, and leukotriene B_4 of the 2- and 4-series prostaglandins and leukotrienes. These end products inhibit killer cell activity, antibody formation by immunological cells, and cell-mediated immunity.[47–49] Omega-3 polyunsaturated fatty acids displace polyunsaturated omega-6 fatty acids in the cell wall and, when released in response to the phospholipases, are metabolized to the 3- and 5-series prostanoids (prostaglandin PGI_3, thromboxane A_3, and leukotriene B_5) via the lipoxygenase pathway. In animal studies, these end products are neither proinflammatory nor immunosuppressive and, in animal models, both reduce bacterial translocation and mortality after burn injury and increase resistance to infection while promoting cell-mediated immunity.[50,51]

Nucleotides provide RNA necessary for cell proliferation and immune function, providing structural units for synthesis of DNA and RNA. Deprivation of nucleotides depress T-helper-cell function and IL-2 production and increases mortality following infection with *Candida albicans* or *Staphylococcus aureus*.[52,53]

Branched-chain amino acids are a primary energy source for muscle protein. Although clinical data do not substantiate the effectiveness of branched-chain amino acid supplementation alone in improving clinical outcome, they have been incorporated as another element in some of the immune-enhancing formulas.[54]

To date, several randomized, prospective studies comparing the various immune-enhancing diets versus standard enteral diets in trauma, burn, or general surgical patients have been published. Although there appears to be no benefit of these specialty formulas in well-nourished patients following elective surgery,[32] several well-controlled prospective studies suggest some benefit with these specialty formulas in high-risk trauma and, perhaps, some general surgical patients. Although not all studies compare isocaloric and isonitrogenous formulas,[55–58] there are enough current studies with matched, controlled diets to support their use in severely injured trauma patients.

Parenteral Feeding

Specialty parenteral formulas for hepatic failure, stress, and sepsis have been tested using branched-chain amino acids, different amino acid profiles, glutamine supplementation, and variations in the carbohydrate versus lipid mixture. Only glutamine-containing formulas appear to show potential for significant benefits from the published studies. Taking the few published, randomized studies into account, it appears that there may be some benefit of glutamine supplementation to the mucosal barrier to maintain normal permeability and immunological defenses. These studies are limited to small select populations and cannot be generalized to a broader range of general surgical patients.

Nonprotein energy sources have also been studied in parenteral formulas.[59–64] In patients receiving isocaloric, isonitrogenous parenteral solutions with varying concentrations of glucose and fat, either source of nonprotein calories appeared to produce similar effects on whole-body protein, kinetics, metabolic responses, and muscle protein degradation.[59] At higher doses, glucose appears to be more effective at suppressing gluconeogenesis than a high-fat diet.

Potential Mechanism for Reduced Infectious Complications with Enteral Feeding

The reduced incidence of sepsis and multiple organ dysfunction syndrome with enteral feeding of critically ill patients has become a focus of multiple investigations. Intravenous nutrition or lack of enteral feeding in association with stress is associated with bacterial translocation in animal models.[65] Clinically, bacterial translocation occurs in certain clinical setting such as bowel obstruction or hemorrhagic shock but does not appear to correlate with the development of extraintestinal infections.[66]

Significant changes in host defenses occur with parenteral feeding. Within the gastrointestinal tract, changes in mucosal architecture[67,68] and increases in permeability[69] have been documented. A critical component of the mucosal barrier defenses is the gut-associated lymphoid tissue, which lines all moist mucosal surfaces and composes approximately 50% of the body's total immunity. This system appears to be exquisitely sensitive to route and type of nutrition in the animal model.[70,71] Naïve T cells and B cells produced within the peritoneal cavity and bone marrow continually circulate through the Peyer's patches. If sensitized by antigens processed by antigen-producing cells within the Peyer's patches, these cells migrate to the mesenteric lymph nodes where they proliferate and are released into the thoracic duct. They subsequently enter the vascular tree[72] for delivery to the lamina propria and intraepithelial spaces of the small intestine as well as the upper and lower respiratory tract.[73] In these sites, the sensitized B cells become IgA-producing plasma cells while the sensitized T cells produce cytokines that upregulate or downregulate IgA production.[74] In addition to IgA, defensins, lactoferrin, and other innate defenses as well as mucin provide barriers to prevent attachment of bacteria to the mucosal surfaces. Intravenous parenteral nutrition significantly reduces the size and effectiveness of the gut-associated lymphoid tissue.[71]

Route of nutrient administration also affects peritoneal defenses. With intravenous feeding, blunting of the immunological response within the peritoneal cavity is manifested by reduced peritoneal immunological cell numbers, a blunted tumor necrosis factor (TNF) response, and impaired killing to a septic peritonitis with an increase in bacteremia and systemic TNF levels.[75]

Determining Dietary Requirements

There are certain issues common to both enteral or parenteral feeding in determining the nutrient prescription. Standard equations, such as the Harris–Benedict equation, multiplied by correction factors are used to determine nutrient goals. The use of indirect calorimetry, however, has shown that stress and activity correction factors frequently lead to overestimates of nutrient needs.[76,77] Increased oxygen consumption, increased CO_2 production, hepatic lipogenesis, immunosuppression, and other negative effects have been documented with overfeeding.[78,79] It is, thus, important to provide appropriate amounts of each nutrient.

Energy Calculations

Estimated energy requirements must consider organ function, body weight, and the clinical condition. Guidelines are noted in Table 2.2. To determine body weight for these calculations, actual body weight is appropriate for patients who are malnourished and for euvolemic or well-nourished patients expected to have delayed oral intake. Overfeeding can result when actual body weight is used to calculate injury requirements in obese patients, and an adjusted form should be used to avoid overfeeding.[80,81] [Adjusted body weight = ideal body weight + 0.25 (actual − ideal body weight).] In cases of significant fluid overload, an estimated dry body weight should be obtained by history from the patient or family.

Often the guideline calculations are compared with calculations using the Harris–Benedict equation based on gender, height, weight, and age to generate estimated body energy expenditure (BEE)[82] (Table 2.3A). Recent data from indirect calorimetry, however, have shown these correction factors often lead to overestimates of energy expenditure[76,77,83] with a more appropriate correction factor being approximately 15% greater than the BEE. Indirect calorimetry by portable metabolic carts uses expired gas analysis to determine overall resting energy expenditure (REE). By measuring carbon dioxide production (VCO_2) and oxygen consumption (VO_2), these values are applied to the Weir equation to determine REE. The metabolic rate in kilocalories as well as protein, carbohydrate, and fat oxidation can be calculated when the VO_2 and VCO_2 are combined with the urine urea nitrogen[84–86] (Table 2.3B).

The respiratory quotient (RQ) is the ratio of VCO_2 to VO_2, and a characteristic RQ exists for each fuel being metabolized: fat RQ = 0.7, glucose RQ = 1.0, and protein RQ = 0.8; lipogenesis has an RQ of approximately 8. If the RQ of a patient is greater than 1, it is a strong indicator of overfeeding.

There are limitations to indirect calorimetry. In critically injured patients who are mechanically ventilated, accuracy is

TABLE 2.3. Calculations Used to Determine Metabolic and Nutritional Parameters.

A. Male: BEE = 66 + (13.8 × W) + (5 × H) − (6.8 × A)
   Female: BEE = 655 + (9.6 × W) + (1.85 × H) − (4.7 × A)

   where W is the weight in kilograms, H is the height in centimeters, and A is the age in years.

B. Protein oxidation (g/d) = 6.25 × UUN
   Carbohydrate oxidation (g/d) = (4.12 × VCO_2) − (2.91 × VO_2) − (2.56 × UUN)

   Fat oxidation (g/d) = (1.69 × VO_2) − (1.69 × VCO_2) − (1.94 × UUN)

   If UUN is not available, MEE is calculated by
   MEE (kcal/d) = (3.9 × VO_2) + (1.1 × VCO_2)

   If UUN is available, the MEE is adjusted for protein metabolism in the equation:
   Adjusted MEE (kcal/d) = MEE − (2.17 × UNN)

C. Nitrogen balance = $\dfrac{\text{protein intake}}{6.25}$ − [(UUN × 0.8) + 1]

lost as the F_iO_2 increases because of potential measurement errors between inspired and expired oxygen levels. A 1% measurement error in the inspired or expired VO_2 in a patient receiving an F_iO_2 of 0.8 produces a 100% error in VO_2 calculation. Air leaks around tracheostomies, or through chest tubes, for example, are not uncommon in patients with high F_iO_2 levels and high positive end-expiratory pressures, which must be recognized in individual patient measurements. Indirect calorimetry is also labor intensive and requires dedicated personnel with defined protocols to provide reliable data.[87]

Because postsurgical patients usually have increases of 10% to 15% over the BEE calculated by the Harris–Benedict equation,[88,89] the current guidelines in Table 5.2 are adequate for most patients. If 30 kcal/kg is provided to most hypermetabolic patients, approximately 90% of them will attain their energy requirement, with minimal overfeeding in only 15% to 20%.[90]

Protein Requirements

The recommended daily allowance for protein intake in well-nourished, healthy individuals is approximately 0.8 g/kg/day[91] with each gram, providing 4.0 kcal/g. The recommended dose of amino acids (or protein with enteral feeding) for stressed or septic patients without renal dysfunction is 1.5 to 2 g/kg/day because of increased protein catabolism.[92,93] Although blood urea nitrogen (BUN) may increase to 40 mg/dl in some patients, this is without adverse metabolic consequences.

In nonhypermetabolic patients who have existing malnutrition or who are at risk of developing starvation-induced malnutrition, 1.0 to 1.5 g/kg/day of protein meets nutrient needs. In burn patients, excessive urinary and wound losses generally dictate administration of 2 to 2.5 g/kg/day. These administered doses, however, may need to be reduced in patients with chronic or acute renal failure. Under these conditions, it is prudent to provide 0.6 to 0.8 g of amino acids or protein/kg/day before dialysis and increase the dose to 1 to 1.2 g protein/kg/day once dialysis is instituted. The simultaneous administration with high caloric load (calorie/nitrogen ratio, 300–350:1) will often slow increases in serum

TABLE 2.2. Energy and Protein Needs for Surgical Patients.

Condition	Kcal/kg/day	Protein/kg/day	NPC:N
Normal to moderate malnutrition	(low stress) 25–30	1.0	150:1
Moderate stress	25–30	1.5	120:1
Hypermetabolic, stressed	30–35	1.5–2.0	90–120:1
Burns	35–40	2.0–2.5	90–120:1

loads of urea, phosphate, and potassium, allowing delayed dialysis.

Adequacy of protein administration may be assessed by a determination of nitrogen balance (Table 2.3C) in a 24-h urine collection. The UUN generally represents approximately 80% of excreted nitrogen, and additional nitrogen losses are estimated at 1 g/day.[94] Accurate urine collection and accurate records of protein intake determine the accuracy of this calculated value.

Glucose

The maximal rate of glucose oxidation is 4 to 5 mg/kg/min or approximately 7.2 g/kg/day. Total glucose administration in intravenous fluids, parenteral nutrition, or enteral nutrition should not exceed these levels.[95–97] In a 70-kg man, these needs are met by 2 l of 25% dextrose solution, providing 500 g of glucose. Blood sugar should ideally be maintained below 200 mg% whenever possible. It is suggested that infectious complications are increased with high blood sugars.[98,99] Administration of the glucose in these doses provides approximately 50% to 60% of total caloric requirements. Hydrated glucose in parenteral nutrition provides 3.4 kcal/g and oral carbohydrates provide 4.0 kcal/g.

Fat Requirement

The balance of nonprotein caloric requirements may be met by lipid infusion of approximately 1 g/kg/day. The maximum adult dose of intravenous lipid is 2.5 g/kg/day.[100] In an enteral form fat provides 9.1 kcal/g, whereas intravenous lipid provides 10 kcal/g because of the additional energy obtained from emulsifiers and glycerol. If overfeeding is suspected, total calories should be reduced. In patients with diabetes or receiving corticosteroids, high rates of fat administration may control glucose but induce hyperlipidemia, cholestasis, and perhaps immunosuppression.[101,102]

Intravenous lipid emulsion in the critically ill patient should be limited to 1 g/kg/day if triglyceride levels are less than 300 mg% and withheld in patients with hypertriglyceridemia, particularly if values are greater than 500 mg/dl.[98] There is no evidence that intravenous lipid emulsions aggravate acute pancreatitis so long as hyperlipidemia is not the cause of the pancreatitis and triglyceride levels are maintained in relatively normal ranges.

Organ System Complications of Overfeeding

PULMONARY FAILURE

Lipogenesis caused by overfeeding increases CO_2 production but rarely causes ventilator dependences in patients sustaining multiple trauma or sepsis. Under these conditions, failure to wean is usually the result of the increased metabolic rate, pneumonia, multiple rib fractures, pulmonary contusions, or sepsis.

HEPATIC FAILURE

Although the onset of hepatic failure generally carries a dismal prognosis, excessive protein restriction should be avoided. Intravenous amino acid solutions appear to be much better tolerated than enteral delivery of protein.

Enteral Nutrition

Both clinical and economic considerations suggest the use of the enteral route for feeding whenever possible.

Enteral Access

The majority of preoperative and postoperative patients tolerate intragastric feeding. Use of a polyurethane or silicone small-bore nasogastric (NG) tube is much better tolerated than large NG tubes. Small-bore tubes reduce the risk of complications such as esophageal stricture, reflux, or necrosis of the nasal alae. Styletted silicone tubes are particularly useful in placement, and their location can be confirmed with aspiration of gastric juice or confirmation via fluoroscopy or X-ray. Simple air insufflation is probably inadequate to confirm gastric placement because sounds transmitted from the left lung or distal esophagus may be auscultated in the left upper quadrant. In patients with an increased risk of aspiration due to reflux, advancement of the tube beyond the ligament of Treitz via endoscopic techniques or fluoroscopy may provide additional protection. Occasionally, use of a double-lumen tube allows gastric decompression as well as feeding beyond the pylorus and, ideally, beyond the ligament of Treitz. Unfortunately, nasojejunal or nasogastric tubes are frequently dislodged in uncooperative or confused patients, increasing the cost and complexity in providing enteral nutrition. In these situations, if laparotomy is not necessary, placement of an endoscopic gastrostomy with direct intragastric feeding may be preferable because it can be performed with minimal mortality and morbidity (Fig. 2.1A–E). This technique is especially useful in patients who require long-term intragastric feeding because of dysphagia or chronic neurological dysfunction after trauma or stroke but should be used with caution in patients with a history of previous esophageal reflux and aspiration. Direct gastric feeding is not suggested in neurologically impaired pediatric patients with recurrent pneumonia secondary to reflux. In these conditions, access distal in the gastrointestinal tract or surgical correction of the reflux is advisable.[103]

Laparotomy provides an opportunity to gain access beyond the ligament of Treitz for direct small-bowel feeding. Jejunostomies with direct small-bowel access using either a large-bore (14-, 16-, or 18-French) tube or needle catheter jejunostomies (5- and 7-French) allow direct administration of tube feedings in patients expected to have gastroparesis for a prolonged period of time. Needle catheter jejunostomies are predictably useful for 3 to 4 weeks following injury. Access points for all jejunostomies should be located at a site with a long mesentery so that abdominal distension does not tear the jejunostomy off the anterior abdominal wall as a result of the tethering effect at the ligament of Treitz. A loose Witzel tunnel should be constructed for a distance of about 4 cm and the jejunostomy sutured lateral to the rectus sheath with four to five sutures to minimize torsion or volvulus.

Standard enteral diets including those with fiber can be administered through both small- and large-bore needle catheter jejunostomies,[104] but protein supplement should not be added to formulas nor should immune-enhancing diets be used with a 5-French tube because of the risk of clogging. Tubes should be flushed at least four times a day, and no med-

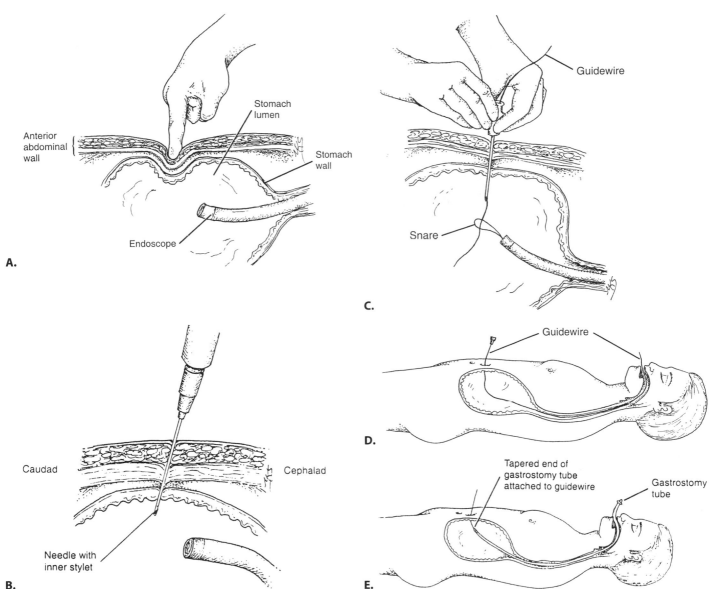

A.

B.

C.

D.

E.

FIGURE 2.1. **A.** The procedure for percutaneous endoscopic gastrostomy includes transillumination of the stomach and identification of the needle insertion site. **B.** A needle is inserted into the stomach across the abdominal wall under direct vision. **C.** A guidewire passed through the lumen of the needle is grasped with a snare. **D.** The ensnared guidewire is removed via the mouth. **E.** The tapered end of the gastrostomy tube is attached to the guidewire and pulled out through the stomach and abdominal wall to seal the button end. The external portion of the gastrostomy tube is then trimmed to fit the patient's body habitus as desired.

ications should be administered via the tube because elixirs containing these medications coagulate the enteral products and clog the tubes rapidly. Needle catheter jejunostomies usually cannot be replaced once they are lost. Larger-bore catheters can be replaced after 1 week and are more useful for long-term requirements.

Anastomosis above the site of enteral access or in the mid- or distal small bowel and colon provide no contraindication to direct small-bowel feeding, and there is no evidence of increased intraabdominal infection with small-bowel access in patients with no other hollow viscus violation.[105] Enteral feeding is not contraindicated in acute pancreatitis so long as nutrients are delivered beyond the ligament of Treitz.[35–38,105] Short-gut syndrome, uncontrollable diarrhea, distal bowel obstruction, or upper GI hemorrhage are relative contraindications, however, to direct enteral feeding.

Initiation of Tube Feeding

Direct intragastric feeding should be attempted in most patients without direct enteral access. In burn patients, intragastric feeding soon after admission prevents subsequent gastroparesis with a 95% success rate but must be started less than 18 h following admission. The highest success rate occurs when feedings are instituted within 6 to 8 h[39,40]; success decreases to less than 50% when intragastric feeding is instituted after 18 h.

Although gastric feedings can be administered as either bolus or continuous infusions, jejunostomy feedings should be continuously infused although long-term nursing home patients have been transitioned to bolus intrajejunal feeding over time. Intragastric and intrajejunal feedings are started at 25 to 30 ml/h and advanced over varying times to a goal meeting caloric and nutrient needs. With intragastric feeding, residuals are measured every 4 h and tube feeding advanced by 25 ml/h if residuals remain below 100 to 150 ml/h. With intrajejunal feedings, signs of intolerance include abdominal distension, diarrhea, and cramping. Most commonly, intrajejunal feedings are increased by 25 ml/h over 12- or 24-h increments to goal rate. Direct small-bowel feedings should be discontinued if feedings reflux back into the nasogastric tube, suggesting small-bowel intolerance.

Enteral Formulas

Choice of formula is determined by functional status of the gastrointestinal tract, patient nutrient requirements and limitations, or restrictions imposed by organ failure such as renal, hepatic, respiratory, or intestinal dysfunction. With an intact GI tract and mucosa, formulas with complex proteins, carbohydrates, and fats are well tolerated. Formulas that contain lactose should be avoided in patients who have undergone recent starvation or have not been fed via the gastrointestinal tract for a prolonged period of time.

Categories of Enteral Feeding Formulations

STANDARD, ISOTONIC FORMULAS

These formulas contain an appropriate balance of carbohydrate, protein, and fat (usually with a nonprotein calorie to nitrogen ratio of approximately 150:1). The macronutrients require digestion but provide adequate nutrition in a low volume with low osmolality (approximately 300 mOsm/l) with a caloric density of 1.0 kcal/ml. Approximately 1500 to 2000 ml are necessary daily to meet micronutrient requirements. These diets are considered low residue because they do not contain fiber. In general, these formulas are used in stable patients at risk of starvation-induced malnutrition or those with existing states of malnutrition who are neither stressed nor septic.

STANDARD FIBER-CONTAINING FORMULAS

These formulas are similar to the standard, isotonic products but contain a combination of both soluble and insoluble fiber, most often as soy polysaccharide. Fiber prolongs intestinal transit time, stimulates intestinal lipase activity, and provides the substrate for short-chain fatty acid metabolism by intraluminal bacteria.[106] These formulas are tolerated even in critically ill patients fed via needle catheter jejunostomies and appear to reduce the incidence of diarrhea compared with chemically defined diets. They do not occlude small-bore feeding catheters when catheters are properly flushed, and often have a high protein content appropriate for critically ill patients.

SPECIALTY, "IMMUNE-ENHANCING" FORMULAS

Several products enriched in nutrients such as branched-chain amino acids, glutamine, arginine, omega-3 fatty acids, nucleotides, or beta-carotene have been studied in clinical populations. These formulas are nitrogen rich, given the supplementation with arginine or glutamine. The proposed clinical functions of individual nutrients have been previously described.

HIGH-DENSITY FORMULAS

Patients requiring fluid restriction or very high calorie and protein requirements can benefit from formulas providing 1.5 to 2 kcal/ml. Smaller volumes are necessary to meet nutrient requirements, but osmolality is higher than that of isotonic formulas. Potential for diarrhea is greater, although in select patients nutrient needs can often be met with these formulas that cannot be met with standard isotonic formulas.

HIGH-PROTEIN FORMULAS

To meet the high protein needs of severely stressed and injured patients, formulas containing nonprotein calorie to nitrogen ratios of less than 125:1 are well suited for critically ill patients. Both isotonic and nonisotonic formulas are available.

ELEMENTAL/PEPTIDE-BASED FORMULAS

The products in these formulas have been predigested compared with formulas with intact micronutrients. Protein is provided in the form of mono-, di-, or tripeptides, fat is provided with MCTs and LCTs, and complex carbohydrates are limited. The fat content in some of these formulas is extremely low (less than 10% of total calories), which limits their long-term usefulness. However, these products are more readily absorbed in patients with maldigestion or malabsorption. In critically ill patients, these formulas should be started at a lower rate (15–20 ml/h) and advanced more slowly or initially diluted with water to produce a more isotonic formula; as rate increases, the concentration of these formulas can be increased.

RENAL FAILURE FORMULAS

These products contain only essential amino acids or a high ratio of essential to nonessential amino acids, and they are designed with a high calorie to nitrogen ratio to allow endogenous synthesis of nonessential amino acids from urea nitrogen. These formulas also contain moderate to low concentrations of the intracellular electrolytes potassium, phosphorus, and magnesium to control serum levels. These formulas are more expensive, and it is unclear whether there is significant clinical benefit over standard mixes of crystalline amino acids, but the restriction of electrolytes is often beneficial and cannot be achieved with other enteral formulas.

Applications of Enteral Feeding

The most common complications of tube feeding include diarrhea,[107,108] aspiration,[109] vomiting, distension, metabolic abnormalities, and tube dislodgment. Aspiration can be minimized by avoiding intragastric feeding in patients with severe reflux and prior evidence of aspiration. Elevation of the patient's bed by 30°, administration of prokinetic agents,[110–113] or institution of feedings beyond the ligament of Treitz may minimize these complications. Diarrhea occurs fairly frequently in tube-fed patients. The use of fiber-containing diets may reduce this incidence, providing substrates for the colonocytes. Not uncommonly, simultaneous administration of medications via the tube or use of antibiotics are the true cause of diarrhea in enterally fed patients.[114,115]

Metabolic complications can be aggravated with enteral nutrition. Hyperglycemia, hypophosphatemia, hyperkalemia or hypokalemia, and hypomagnesemia are not uncommon in postoperative patients who have preexisting nutritional deficiencies, renal failure, or diabetes mellitus requiring monitoring of fluid and electrolytes after institution of feeding.

Small-bowel necrosis and pneumatosis intestinalis have been associated with direct small-bowel feedings. Although the cause is unknown, speculation that inability to increase blood flow to the splanchnic bed when products are delivered into the small intestine may be one of the etiological factors. Although spontaneous necrosis has also been noted in similar patients not receiving tube feedings, it is prudent to delay jejunal feedings until hemodynamic stability is achieved and there is evidence of adequate splanchnic perfusion (adequate urine output). Intragastric feedings can be started in these conditions because high gastric residuals will reflect the small-bowel intolerance.

Parenteral Nutrition

Parenteral Access

Parenteral nutrient solutions with dextrose concentrations greater than 10% are hypertonic and must be administered into a large centrally located vein to avoid thrombophlebitis and venous sclerosis associated with administration of these hyperosmolar formulas. The superior vena cava is an ideal site in which to administer concentrated parenteral nutrition formulas. Infraclavicular transcutaneous puncture and cannulation of the subclavian vein usually accomplish access to the superior vena cava. Access to the superior vena cava can also be obtained by transcutaneous puncture of the external jugular or internal jugular veins, but catheters that exit in the neck are more difficult to care for, more uncomfortable for many patients, and probably more likely to become infected. Multiple lumen central venous catheters are usually inserted. Catheter infection rates are the lowest when catheters to be used for parenteral nutrition support are inserted under the strictest sterile conditions including use of a hat, mask, gown, and gloves.[116,117] Currently, safe practice dictates that a chest X-ray should be obtained to verify that the catheter tip is centrally located before concentrated dextrose solutions are administered. Once the line is inserted, at least one lumen should be reserved solely for the administration of the parenteral formulation because multiuse catheters appear to have higher infection rates.[118]

Access to the superior vena cava can also be obtained using catheters that are inserted peripherally in the upper extremity and threaded to the appropriate location. Such peripherally inserted central venous catheters, known by the acronym PICC lines, offer the ability to obtain central venous access without the risks associated with subclavian or jugular puncture. These lines can be used for several months and are often used for hydration or other parenteral therapy for home-bound patients.

Dedicated central venous access via the subclavian or jugular veins may rarely be impossible to obtain, for example, because of preexisting thrombosis or occlusion of the subclavian or innominate veins or superior vena cava or anatomical problems preventing safe puncture, or may be too risky, especially in patients with refractory coagulopathies and pulmonary insufficiency. In these circumstances, most institutions favor a policy whereby the dextrose concentration of parenteral nutrition solutions is limited to 15% or less.

Composition of Central and Peripheral Venous Solutions

The common macronutrients and their caloric densities and functions are presented in Table 2.4. Access to a large central vein is needed because these formulas usually have osmolarities greater than or equal to 1900 mOsm/kg and administration of the solutions into peripheral veins causes thrombophlebitis and venous sclerosis (Table 2.5). When infused into the central venous system, the nutrients are rapidly diluted to near isotonicity and then metabolized. These solutions usually contain about 1 kcal/ml. Typically, 2 to 3 l are administered over a 24-h period, thereby providing about 2000 to 3000 kcal/day. Occasionally, as for patients who will require home parenteral nutrition support, it may be advisable and feasible

TABLE 2.4. Caloric Densities, Sources, and Functions of the Major Macronutrients.

Macronutrient (caloric density)	Common sources	Functions
Carbohydrate (3.4 kcal/g)	Dextrose	Essential fuels used by glycolytic tissues; normally the major or sole energy source for the central nervous system, peripheral nerves, red blood cells, and some phagocytes. During prolonged starvation, the glucose requirement of the brain decreases as adaptation to ketone oxidation occurs. Are used by tissues that oxidize fat (e.g., muscle) when carbohydrates are administered as the major fuel source. Maintain hepatic glycogen stores, which may protect hepatocytes during hypoxia or exposure to toxins.
Lipids (10 kcal/g)	Polyunsaturated long-chain triglycerides from soybean oil or a safflower–soybean oil mixture	The most concentrated forms of energy. Stabilize, support, and protect vital structures. Complex with fat-soluble molecules like some vitamins; are used as structural components in biological membranes.
Protein (4 kcal/gm)	Crystalline amino acids	Major structural component of the body. Some are essential (histidine, isoleucine, leucine, valine, methionine, cysteine, phenylalanine, tyrosine, threonine, tryptophan, and lysine) because they cannot be synthesized by the body. Others are nonessential because they can be made from carbon and nitrogen precursors. Act as peptide hormones, enzymes, and antibodies. May join with carbohydrates to form glycoproteins, to serve as plasma proteins and immune globulins, and components of connective tissue cell membranes and mucous secretions.

TABLE 2.5. Central Parenteral Nutrition.

	Central	*Peripheral*
Daily calories	2000–3000	1000–1500
Protein	Variable	56–87 grams
Volume of fluid required	1000–3000 ml	2000–3500 mL
Duration of therapy	≥7 days	5–7 days
Route of administration	Dedicated central venous catheter	Peripheral vein or multi-use central catheter
Substrate profile	55%–60% carbohydrate 15%–20% protein 25% fat	30% carbohydrate 20% protein 50% fat
Osmolarity	~2000 mOsm/l	~600–900 mOsm/L

to administer the feeding solution over less than 24 h (a procedure known as cycling), if only to provide some time free from intravenous infusion.

Peripheral nutritional alimentation solutions typically have dextrose concentrations of 5%. Between 1000 and 1500 calories can be administered using this method, and the volume of fluid required to administer these calories is usually greater than 2 l/day. In contrast to the case central venous alimentation solutions, in which the substrate mixture is predominantly composed of carbohydrate, most of the calories from peripheral parenteral nutrition solutions are derived from fat. Peripheral nutritional prescriptions typically provide approximately 30% of calories as carbohydrate, 20% as protein, and at least 50% of calories as fat.

Peripheral parenteral nutrition is usually undesirable for several reasons. First, there is no evidence that this improves outcomes or significantly decreases nitrogen losses when it does not closely approximate a patient's energy needs. Second, the high-fat content typically administered as part of peripheral parenteral nutrition regimens may impair reticuloendothelial cell function and, therefore, immune responsiveness.[118]

Parenteral alimentation solutions are prepared by a pharmacist and typically combine 500 ml of 50% dextrose with 500 ml of a 10% to 15% amino acid mixture. Lipids should contribute no more than 30% of the total calories administered in nearly all circumstances. A typical prescription would administer 2 l of this standard solution each day. Administration of 500 ml of 20% fat emulsion for 1 day each week is sufficient to prevent essential fatty acid deficiency.

Once the basic solution is created, electrolytes are added as needed (Table 2.6). Sodium or potassium salts are given as chlo-

ride or acetate according to the requirements of the individual patient. Normally, equal amounts of chloride and acetate are provided. However, if chloride losses from the body are increased, such as may occur in patients who have nasogastric tubes, then most of the salts should be given as chloride. Similarly, more acetate should be given to patients when additional base is required because acetate generates bicarbonate when it is metabolized. Sodium bicarbonate is incompatible with parenteral nutrition solutions and so cannot be added to the mixture. Phosphate may be given as the sodium or potassium salt. Lipid emulsions contain an additional 15 mmol/l of phosphate.

Commercially available preparations of vitamins, minerals, and trace elements are added to the nutrient mix unless they are contraindicated. Both fat- and water-soluble vitamins should be given.

Trace element preparations that include zinc, copper, manganese, and chromium are added to the parenteral nutrition solution in amounts consistent with the AMA guidelines; 60 pg of selenium are also given daily. Because copper and manganese are excreted in the biliary tract, the dosages of these micronutrients should be modified or eliminated in patients with significant liver disease or biliary obstruction. Iron is not given to the critically ill because hyperferremia can increase bacterial virulence, after polymorphonuclear cell function, and increase host susceptibility to infection.[119]

Initiation and Maintenance of Infusion: Patient Monitoring

All patients should be metabolically and hemodynamically stable before parenteral nutrition support is begun. It is imperative that patients are provided adequate vitamins and trace elements while receiving parenteral nutrition.

Typically, one initiates parenteral nutrition with up to 2 l of the nutrient solution and 500 kcal as lipid. However, it may be advisable to start with 1 l of parenteral nutrition and then to increase the volume as indicated. Blood glucose concentrations should be less than 200 mg/dl, and abnormal electrolyte levels should be corrected, especially potassium, phosphate, and magnesium, before starting or advancing to the goal nutritional prescription. Obviously, patients with diabetes mellitus may need to be advanced more slowly to prevent severe glucose intolerance. Lipid can be infused as an alternative fuel source to fulfill energy requirements without increasing the glucose infusion rate. The solutions should be administered using a volumetric pump set at a constant rate up to the levels previously specified. It is important not to

TABLE 2.6. Electrolyte Concentrations in Parenteral Nutrition.

Electrolyte	Recommended central PN doses	Recommended peripheral PN doses	Usual range of doses
Potassium (mEq/l)	30	30	0–120 (CVL) 0–80 (PV)
Sodium (mEq/l)	30	30	0–150
Phosphate (mmol/l)	15	5	0–20
Magnesium (mEq/l)	5	5	0–16
Calcium (mEq/l) (as gluconate)	4.7	4.7	0–10
Chloride (mEq/l)	50	50	0–150
Acetate (mEq/l)	40	40	0–100

CVL, central venous line; PV, peripheral vein.

modify the infusion rate during any given day to try to compensate for excess or inadequate administration of the parenteral nutritional solution. A cyclic schedule (8–16 h/day) for patients requiring long-term parenteral nutrition can be initiated once the patient is metabolically stable. Cycling should be done gradually, and the last hour of infusion should be tapered to one-half the maintenance infusion rate to prevent rebound hypoglycemia.

Before central parenteral alimentation is discontinued, the volume of infusion should be decreased by at least half to avoid adverse effects that may occur secondary to relative hyperinsulinemia if the body is not allowed sufficient time to equilibrate. In emergency situations when the central parenteral nutrition solution must be suddenly discontinued, 10% dextrose should be given at the same infusion rate as was used for the parenteral nutrition unless there is severe hyperglycemia. When patients who are receiving parenteral nutrition require surgical operation, one can continue to administer the solution through the procedure but decreasing the infusion rate may make circulating glucose and electrolyte levels easier to control—especially in patients with glucose intolerance or other severe organ dysfunction.

During the initiation of central parenteral nutrition, serum chemistries must be monitored frequently. Once the patient has stabilized on his or her individual nutritional prescription, blood samples should be obtained at least twice weekly to measure chloride, CO_2, potassium, sodium, blood urea nitrogen (BUN), creatinine, calcium, and phosphate levels, and once weekly for liver function tests, albumin, total protein, uric acid, magnesium, and triglyceride levels. Patients should be weighed each day on the same scale. Urine or blood should be tested for sugar and acetone every 6 h initially and until blood glucose concentrations are stable. Electrolytes and other medications should only be added by the pharmacist when the parenteral nutrition solution is prepared.

Numerous common metabolic abnormalities may arise during the course of parenteral (or enteral) nutrition. Several of these are outlined in Table 2.7.

TABLE 2.7. Possible Etiologies and Treatment of Common Complications of Central Parenteral Nutrition.

Problem	Possible Etiology	Treatment
Glucose		
Hyperglycemia, glycosuria, hyperosmolar nonketotic dehydration or coma	Excessive dose or rate of infusion; inadequate insulin production; steroid administration; infection	Decrease the amount of glucose given; increase insulin; administer a portion of calories as fat
Diabetic ketoacidosis	Inadequate endogenous insulin production and/or inadequate insulin therapy	Give insulin; decrease glucose intake
Rebound hypoglycemia	Persistent endogenous insulin production by islet cells after long-term high carbohydrate infusion	Give 5%–10% glucose before total parenteral infusion is discontinued
Hypercarbia	Carbohydrate load exceeds the ability to increase minute ventilation and excrete excess CO_2	Limit glucose dose to 5 mg/kg/min. Give greater percentage of total caloric needs as fat (up to 30%–40%)
Fat		
Hypertriglyceridemia	Rapid infusion; decreased clearance	Decrease rate of infusion; allow clearance (~12 h) before testing blood
Essential fatty acid deficiency	Inadequate essential fatty acid administration	Administer essential fatty acids in doses of 4%–7% of total calories
Amino acids		
Hyperchloremia metabolic acidosis	Excessive chloride content of amino acid solutions	Administer Na^+ and K^+ as acetate salts
Prerenal azotemia	Excessive amino acids with inadequate caloric supplementation	Reduce amino acids; increase the amount of glucose calories
Miscellaneous		
Hypophosphatemia	Inadequate phosphorus administration with redistribution into tissues	Give 15 mm phosphate/1000 i.v. kcal; evaluate antacid and Ca^{2+} administration
Hypomagnesemia	Inadequate administration relative to increased losses (diarrhea, diuresis, medications)	Administer Mg^{2+} (15–20 mEq/1000 kcal)
Hypermagnesemia	Excessive administration; renal failure	Decrease Mg^{2+} supplementation
Hypokalemia	Inadequate intake relative to increased needs for anabolism; diuresis	Increase K^+ supplementation
Hyperkalemia	Excessive administration, especially in metabolic acidosis; renal decompensation	Reduce or stop exogenous K^+; if EKG changes are present, treat with Ca gluconate, insulin, diuretics
Hypocalcemia	Inadequate administration; reciprocal response to phosphorus repletion without simultaneous calcium infusion	Increase Ca^{2+} dose
Hypercalcemia	Excessive administration; excess vitamin D administration	Decrease Ca^{2+} and/or vitamin D administration
Elevated liver transaminases or serum alkaline phosphatase and bilirubin	Enzyme induction secondary to amino acid imbalances or overfeeding	Reevaluate nutritional prescription

Parenteral Nutrition for Patients with Abnormal Organ Function

DIABETES MELLITUS

In the insulin-dependent patient, the same amount of insulin that would normally be taken is added to the parenteral nutrition solution on the first day. Because as much as one-half of the insulin given binds to the container and intravenous tubing, the insulin given in this manner is almost always an underestimate of actual requirements. For example, if a patient's normal dose of regular insulin is 40 U/day for a 2000-kcal diet, then 20 U should be added to a parenteral nutrition solution of 1000 kcal. Thereafter, blood glucose concentrations obtained by finger-stick or blood sampling are determined every 6 h, and a sliding scale for subcutaneous regular insulin is used to provide supplementary insulin doses as needed. For the next day, one-half or all the insulin given on the previous day according to the sliding scale is added to the parenteral nutrition solution, depending on the level of control that is required.

For nondiabetic patients who develop hyperglycemia, a similar procedure is used whereby a sliding scale estimates the amount of insulin that is needed to maintain blood glucose levels below 200 mg/dl, and one-half this amount is then added to the next day's parenteral nutrition orders.

ACUTE RENAL FAILURE

In general, most patients with acute renal failure are catabolic with elevated energy requirements. Calories should be provided in sufficient quantities to minimize protein degradation. Traditionally, formulas designed for renal failure contained predominantly essential amino acids. However, the provision of nonessential amino acids may enhance protein synthesis and nitrogen retention. A balance of fat and carbohydrate should be provided. Lipid emulsions can be used as a source of concentrated energy in the patients who are fluid restricted. The contribution of fat to the total caloric intake should be no more than 30% while the remainder of the caloric requirements is provided by glucose.

Fluid and electrolyte balances are often impaired in patients with acute renal failure. Potassium, phosphate, and magnesium levels must be monitored carefully and should be added to parenteral nutrition if blood levels fall. Acetate salts of potassium or sodium can be administered to help correct a metabolic acidosis. Standard doses of the water-soluble vitamins and additional folic acid (1 mg/day total) should be added to the solution of patients who are undergoing dialysis because these substances are lost from the body in the dialysate bath. The supplementation of fat-soluble vitamins is usually not required, especially in patients who are also eating, because excretion is reduced in renal failure. In anuric patients, trace elements are not added to the nutrient solutions. However, for patients who require prolonged parenteral nutrition support and are dialyzed, trace elements and fat-soluble vitamins should be replaced. The various ultrafiltration techniques are also associated with highly variable but increased amino acid losses in the dialysate. In these instances, additional protein may be required to meet the patient's estimated needs. However, a portion of the patient's nonprotein calorie needs may be met by the dextrose contained in replacement solutions.

HEPATIC DYSFUNCTION AND LIVER FAILURE

Protein intake for patients with stable chronic liver disease depends on the patient's nutritional status and protein tolerance. Nutritionally depleted patients may require as much as 1.5 g of protein per kilogram estimated dry weight. However, protein intake may need to be decreased in patients with liver failure and encephalopathy. Protein-sensitive encephalopathic patients should be given 0.5 to 0.7 g protein per kilogram per day and increased gradually to 1.0 to 1.5 g/kg/day if possible.

Fluid restriction may be necessary in some patients with ascites and edema. In this instance the concentration of dextrose can be increased to maintain the amount of calories administered as carbohydrate. The amount of sodium given is reduced because these patients excrete nearly sodium-free urine. Administration of trace elements is often contraindicated because a major route of excretion for these substances, such as copper and manganese, is via the biliary system. Zinc deficiency is common in cirrhotic patients, and supplementation of this mineral may be necessary, especially if there are excessive gastrointestinal losses.

Common Complications and Their Management

CATHETER SEPSIS

Catheter sepsis is a very serious complication associated with central venous alimentation. Primary catheter sepsis occurs when there are signs and symptoms of infection and the indwelling catheter is the only anatomical focus of infection. Secondary catheter infections are associated with another focus or multiple infectious foci that cause bacteremia and seed the catheter.

Management of the patients with catheter infection depends on their clinical condition. If extremely ill patients with high fevers are hypotensive or have local signs of infection around the catheter site, the catheter should be removed, its tip cultured, and peripheral and central venous blood cultures obtained. In primary catheter sepsis, signs and symptoms should return to normal quickly. The organisms that grow from the catheter tip are the same as the ones that are identified in peripheral blood culture. Usually, more than 1×10^3 organisms are grown from cultures of the catheter tip.

Specific therapy should be initiated against the primary source in patients in whom a source of infection other than the catheter tip is present. If a secondary source is not identified and the symptoms persist, the catheter should be removed and its tip should be cultured. If the catheter tip culture returns positive or if the index of suspicion is high, appropriate antibiotic therapy is initiated. Central venous feeding can be resumed, maintaining blood glucose levels below 200 mg/dl.

OTHER COMPLICATIONS

Prolonged administration of parenteral nutrition may result in altered hepatic function tests and changes in liver pathological conditions that can lead to liver failure. Initially (1–2 weeks after initiation of parenteral nutrition), serum transaminases may be elevated. These abnormalities frequently resolve without any change in the composition or rate of parenteral nutrition administration. However, in patients receiving long-term parenteral nutrition (>20 days), serum transaminases levels may remain elevated, even after parenteral nutrition support is discontinued. Serum levels of alkaline phosphatase and bilirubin may also increase in some patients who receive long-term parenteral nutrition. Patients who do not receive some lipid as part of their parenteral nutrition may have more frequent and severe hepatic abnormalities. The provision of excess glucose increases insulin secretion, which stimulates hepatic lipogenesis and results in hepatic fat accumulation. Fatty infiltration is the initial histopathological change; it is readily reversible and may not be accompanied by altered liver function. Longer parenteral nutrition therapy may be associated with cholestasis and nonspecific triaditis and may progress to active chronic hepatitis, fibrosis, and eventual cirrhosis. The management of parenteral nutrition-related liver dysfunction is summarized in Table 2.7.

References

1. Wolfe BM, Mathiesen KA. Clinical practice guidelines in nutrition support: can they be based on randomized clinical trials? J Parenter Enteral Nutr 1997;27(1):1–6.
2. Eddy DM. Health system reform: will controlling costs require rationing services? JAMA 1994;272:324–328.
3. Eddy DM. Principles for making difficult decision in difficult times. JAMA 1994;271:1792–1798.
4. Wolfe BM, Ryder MA, Nishikawa RA, et al. Complications of parenteral nutrition. Am J Surg 1986;152:93–99.
5. Kudsk KA, Minard G. Enteral nutrition. In: Zaloga GP, ed. Nutrition in Critical Care. St. Louis: Mosby, 1994:331–360.
6. Nightingale JMD, Lennard-Jones JE, Walter ER, et al. Jejunal efflux in the short bowel syndrome. Lancet 1990;336:765–768.
7. Gouttebel MC, Saint-Aubert B, Astre C, et al. Total parenteral nutrition needs in different types of short bowel syndrome. Dig Dis Sci 1986;31:718–725.
8. Howard L, Anent M, Fleming CR, et al. Current use and clinical outcome of home parenteral and enteral nutrition therapy in the United States. Gastroenterology 1995;109:355–365.
9. Winsor JA, Hill GL. Risk factors for postoperative pneumonia: the importance of protein depletion. Ann Surg 1988;208:209–214.
10. King BK, Blackwell AP, Minard G, et al. Predicting patient outcome using preoperative nutritional markers. Surg Forum 1997;48:592–595.
11. Kudsk KA. Dear Miss Milk Toast (1998 Presidential Address—ASPEN). J Parenter Enteral Nutr 1998;22:191–198.
12. Pannen BHJ, Robotham JL. The acute-phase response. New Horizons 1995;3:183–197.
13. Rothchild MA, Oratz M, Schreiber SS. Albumin synthesis. N Engl J Med 1972;286:748–757.
14. Jeejeebhoy KN. Assessment of nutritional status. In: Rombeau JL, Caldwell MD, eds. Clinical nutrition: enteral and tube feeding. Philadelphia: Saunders, 1990:118–126.
15. Blackburn GL, Bistrian BR, Maini BS, et al. Nutritional and metabolic assessment of the hospitalized patient. J Parenter Enteral Nutr 1977;1:11–22.
16. Buzby GP, Mullen JL, Mathews DC, et al. Prognostic nutritional index in gastrointestinal surgery. Am J Surg 1980;139:160–167.
17. Niederman MS, Mantivonni R, Schoch P, et al. Patterns and routes of tracheobronchial colonization in mechanically ventilated patients. Chest 1989;95:155–161.
18. Ingenbleek Y, Carpentier YA. A prognostic inflammatory and nutritional index scoring critically ill patients. Int J Vitam Nutr Res 1984;55:91–101.
19. Detsky AS, McLaughlin JR, Baker JP, et al. What is subjective global assessment of nutritional status? J Parenter Enteral Nutr 1987;11:8–13.
20. Pikul J, Sharp MD, Lowndes R, et al. Degree of preoperative malnutrition is predictive of postoperative morbidity and mortality in liver transplant patients. Transplantation (Baltimore) 1994;57:469–471.
21. Enia G, Sicuso C, Alati G, et al. A subjective global assessment of nutrition in dialysis patient. Nephrol Dial Transplant 1993;8:1094–1098.
22. Klein S, Kinney J, Jeejeebhoy K, et al. Nutrition support in clinical practice: review of published data and recommendations for future research directions. J Parenter Enteral Nutr 1997;21(3):133–156.
23. Moore EE, Jones TN. Benefits of immediate jejunostomy feeding after major abdominal trauma—a prospective, randomized study. J Trauma 1986;26:874–879.
24. Moore FA, Moore EE, Jones TN, et al. TEN versus TPN following major abdominal trauma—reduced septic morbidity. J Trauma 1989;29:916–923.
25. Kudsk KA, Croce MA, Fabian TC, et al. Enteral versus parenteral feeding. Effects on septic morbidity after blunt and penetrating abdominal trauma. Ann Surg 1992;215:503–511.
26. Kudsk KA, Minard G, Croce MA, et al. A randomized trial of isonitrogenous enteral diets after severe trauma. An immune-enhancing diet reduces septic complications. Ann Surg 1996;224:531–540.
27. Grahm TW, Zadrozny DB, Harrington T. The benefits of early jejunal hyperalimentation in the head-injured patient. Neurosurgery (Baltim) 1989;25:729–735.
28. Rapp RP, Young B, Twym D, et al. The favorable effect of early parenteral feeding on survival in head injured patients. J Neurosurg 1983;58:906–911.
29. Hadley MN, Grahm TW, Harrington T, et al. Nutritional support in neurotrauma: a critical review of early nutrition in 45 acute head injury patients. Neurosurgery (Baltim) 1986;19:367–373.
30. Young B, Ott L, Twyman D, et al. The effect of nutritional support on outcome from severe head injury. Neurosurgery (Baltim) 1987;6:668–676.
31. Borzotta AP, Penning S, Papasadero B, et al. Enteral vs parenteral nutrition after severe closed head injury. J Trauma 1994;37:459–468.
32. Heslin MJ, Latkany L, Leung D, et al. A prospective, randomized trial of early enteral feeding after resection of upper gastrointestinal malignancy. Ann Surg 1997;226:567–577.
33. Gonzalez-Huix F, Fernandez-Banares F, Esteve-Comas M, et al. Enteral versus parenteral nutrition as adjunct therapy in acute ulcerative colitis. Am J Gastroenterol 1993;88:227–232.
34. Gonzalez-Huix F, de Leon R, Fernandez-Banares F, et al. Polymeric enteral diets as primary treatment of active Crohn's disease: a prospective steroid controlled trial. Gut 1993;34:778–782.
35. McClave SA, Greene LM, Snider HL, et al. Comparison of the safety of early enteral nutrition versus parenteral nutrition in mild acute pancreatitis. J Parenter Enteral Nutr 1997;21:14–20.
36. Ragins H, Levenson SM, Signer R, et al. Intrajejunal administration of an elemental diet at neutral pH avoids pancreatic stimulation. Am J Surg 1973;126:606–614.
37. Stabile BE, Borzatta M, Stubbs RS. Pancreatic secretory responses to intravenous hyperalimentation and intraduodenal elemental and full liquid diets. J Parenter Enteral Nutr 1984;8:377–380.
38. Bodoky G, Haranyi L, Pap A, et al. Effect of enteral nutrition in exocrine pancreatic function. Am J Surg 1991;161:144–148.
39. Raff T, Hartmann B, Germann G. Early intragastric feeding of seriously burned and long-term ventilated patients: a review of 55 patients. Burns 1997;23:19–25.
40. McDonald WS, Sharp CW Jr, Deitch EA. Immediate enteral feeding in burn patients is safe and effective. Ann Surg 1991;213:177–183.
41. Jones TN, Moore FA, Moore EE, et al. Gastrointestinal symp-

toms attributed to jejunostomy feeding after major abdominal trauma—a critical analysis. Crit Care Med 1989;17:1146–1150.

42. Souba WW, Smith RJ, Wilmore DW. Glutamine metabolism by the intestinal tract. J Parenter Enteral Nutr 1985;9:608–617.

43. Kirk SJ, Barbul A. Role of arginine in trauma, sepsis, and immunity. J Parenter Enter Nutr 1990;14:226S.

44. Saito H, Trocki O, Wang S-L, et al. Metabolic and immune effects of dietary arginine supplementation after burns. Arch Surg 1987;122:784–789.

45. Gianotti L, Alexander JW, Pyles T, et al. Arginine-supplemented diet improves survival in gut-derived sepsis and peritonitis by modulating bacterial clearance. Ann Surg 1993;217:644–654.

46. Barbul A. Arginine: biochemistry, physiology, and therapeutic implications. J Parenter Enteral Nutr 1986;10:227–238.

47. Kinsella JE, Lokesh B, Broughton S, Whelan J. Dietary polyunsaturated fatty acids and eicosanoids: potential effect on the modulation of inflammatory and immune cells: an overview. Nutrition 1990;6:24–44.

48. Peck MD. Omega-3 polyunsaturated fatty acids: benefit or harm during sepsis: New Horiz 1994;2:230–236.

49. Gurr MI. The role of lipids in the regulation of the immune system. Prog Lipid Res 1983;22:257–263.

50. Alexander JW, Saito H, Trocki O, et al. The importance of lipid type in the diet after burn injury. Ann Surg 1986;204:1–8.

51. Mascioli E, Leader L, Flores E, et al. Enhanced survival to endotoxin in guinea pigs fed IV fish oil emulsions. Lipids 1988;23:623–625.

52. Van Buren CT, Kim E, Kulkarni AD, et al. Nucleotide-free diet and suppression of immune response. Transplant Proc 1987;19:57–59.

53. Fanslow WC, Kulkarni AD, Van Buren CT, et al. Effect of nucleotide restriction and supplementation on resistance to supplemental murine candidiasis. J Parenter Enter Nutr 1988;12:49–52.

54. Naylor CD, O'Rourke K, Detsky AS, et al. Parenteral nutrition with branched-chain amino acids in hepatic encephalopathy. A meta-analysis. Gastroenterology 1989;97:1033–1042.

55. Daly JM, Lieberman MD, Goldfine J, et al. Enteral nutrition with supplemental arginine, RNA, and omega-3 fatty acids in patients after operation: immunologic, metabolic, and clinical outcome. Surgery (St. Louis) 1992;112:56–67.

56. Moore FA, Moore EE, Kudsk KA, et al. Clinical benefits of an immune-enhancing diet for early postinjury enteral feeding. J Trauma 1994;37:607–615.

57. Schilling J, Vranjes N, Fierz W, et al. Clinical outcome and immunology of postoperative arginine, omega-3 fatty acids, and nucleotide-enriched enteral feeding: a randomized prospective comparison with standard enteral and low calorie/low fat i.v. solutions. Nutrition 1996;12:423–429.

58. Saffle JR, Wiedke G, Jennings K, et al. A randomized trial of immune-enhancing enteral nutrition in burn patients. J Trauma 1997;42:793–802.

59. Smith RC, Mackie W, Kohlhardt SR, Kee AJ. The effect on protein and amino acid metabolism of an intravenous nutrition regimen providing seventy percent of nonprotein calories as lipid. Surgery (St. Louis) 1992;111:12–20.

60. de Chalain TM, Mitchell WL, O'Keefe SJ, et al. The effect of fuel source on amino acid metabolism in critically ill patients. J Surg Res 1992;52:167–176.

61. Chassard D, Guiraud M, Gauthier J, et al. Effects of intravenous medium-chain triglycerides on pulmonary gas exchanges in mechanically ventilated patients. Crit Care Med 1994;22:248–251.

62. Kohlhardt SR, Smith RC, Kee AJ. Metabolic response to a high-lipid, high-nitrogen peripheral intravenous nutrition solution after major upper-gastrointestinal surgery. Nutrition 1994;10:317–326.

63. Roulet M, Frascarolo P, Pilet M, et al. Effects of intravenously infused fish oil on platelet fatty acid phospholipid composition and on platelet function in postoperative trauma. J Parenter Enteral Nutr 1997;21:296–301.

64. Tappy L, Schwarz JM, Schneiter P, et al. Effects of isoenergetic glucose-based or lipid-based parenteral nutrition on glucose metabolism, de novo lipogenesis, and respiratory gas exchanges in critically ill patients. Crit Care Med 1998;26:813–814.

65. Deitch EA. Does the gut protect or injure patients in the ICU? Perspect Crit Care 1988;1:1–31.

66. Moore FA, Moore EE, Poggetti R, et al. Gut bacterial translocation via the portal vein: a clinical perspective with major torso trauma. Trauma 1991;31:629–638.

67. Johnson LR, Copeland EM, Dudrick SJ, et al. Structural and hormonal alterations in the gastrointestinal tract of parenteral fed rats. Gastroenterology 1975;68:1177–1183.

68. Levine GM, Derin JJ, Steiger E, et al. Role of oral intake in maintenance of gut mass and disaccharide activity. Gastroenterology 1974;67:975–982.

69. Purandare S, Offenbartl K, Westrom B, et al. Increased gut permeability to fluorescein isothiocyanate—dextran after total parenteral nutrition in rat. Scand J Gastroenterol 1989;24:678–682.

70. McGhee JR, Mestecky J, Dertzbaugh MT, et al. The mucosal immune system: from fundamental concepts to vaccine development. Vaccine 1992;10:75–88.

71. Li J, Kudsk KA, Gocinski B, et al. Effects of parenteral nutrition on gut-associated lymphoid tissue. J Trauma 1995;39:44.

72. Brandtgzaeg P, Halstensen TS, Kett K, et al. Immunobiology and immunopathology of human gut mucosa: humoral immunity and intraepithelial lymphocytes. Gastroenterology 1989;97:1562–1578.

73. Svanborg C. Bacterial adherence and mucosal immunity. In: Ogra PL, Lamm ME, McGhee JR, Mestecky J, Strober W, Bienenstock J, eds. Handbook of Mucosal Immunology. San Diego: Academic Press, 1974:71–78.

74. Tomasi TB Jr. Mechanisms of immune regulation at mucosal surfaces. Rev Infect Dis 1983;5:S784.

75. Lin M-T, Saito H, Fukushima R, et al. Route of nutritional supply influences local, systemic, and remote organ responses to intraperitoneal bacterial challenge. Ann Surg 1996;223:84–93.

76. Hunter DC, Jaksik T, Lewis D, et al. Resting energy expenditure in the critically ill: estimations versus measurement. Br J Surg 1988;75:875–878.

77. Hwang T-L, Hwang S-L, Chen M-F. The use of indirect colorimetry in critically ill patients—relationship with measured energy expenditure to injury severity score, a septic severity score, and Apache II score. J Trauma 1993;34:247–251.

78. Talpers SS, Romberger DJ, Bunce SB, et al. Nutritionally associated increased carbon dioxide production. Excess total calories vs high proportion of carbohydrate calories. Chest 1992;102:551–555.

79. Lowry SF, Brennan MF. Abnormal liver function during parenteral nutrition: relation to infusion excess. J Surg Res 1979;26:300–307.

80. Choban PS, Burge JC, Flancbaum L. Nutrition support of obese hospitalized patients. Nutr Clin Prac 1997;12:149–154.

81. Cicci A, Sunyecz LA, Mirtallo J, et al. A standardized system for assessment and delivery of nutrition support in a large teaching hospital. Nutr Clin Pract 1992;7:271–278.

82. Harris JA, Benedict FG. A biometric study of basal metabolism in man. Publication 279. Washington, DC: Carnegie Institution, 1919.

83. Garrel DR, Jobin N, deJonge LHM. Should we still use the Harris and Benedict equations. Nutr Clin Pract 1996;11:99–103.

84. Wilmore DW. The Metabolic Management of the Critically Ill. New York: Plenum Press, 1977.

85. Watters JM, Van Woert JH, Wilmore DW. Metabolism and nutrition. In: Greenfield LJ, Mulholland MW, Oldham KT, Zelenock GB, eds. Surgery: Scientific Principles and Practice. Philadelphia: Lippincott, 1993:38–85.

86. Weir JB de V. New methods for calculating metabolic rate with special reference to protein metabolism. J Physiol (Camb) 1949; 109:1–9.

87. Campbell SM, Kudsk KA. "High tech" metabolic measurements: useful in daily clinical practice? J Parenter Enteral Nutr 1988;12:610–612.

88. Elwyn DH. Nutritional requirements of adult surgical patients. Crit Care Med 1980;8:9–20.

89. Askanazi J, Carpentier YA, Elwyn DH. A controlled trial of the effect of parenteral nutrition support on patients with respiratory failure and sepsis. Clin Nutr 1983;2:97–103.

90. Fong Y, Marano MA, Barber E, et al. Total parenteral nutrition and bowel rest modify the metabolic response to endotoxin in humans. Ann Surg 1989;210:449–457.

91. Food and Nutrition Board, National Research Council. Recommended Dietary Allowances, 10th Ed. Washington, DC: National Academy of Sciences, 1989.

92. Kudsk KA, Teasley-Strausburg KM. Enteral and parenteral nutrition. In: Irwin RS, Cerra FB, Rippe JM, eds. Intensive Care Medicine, 4th Ed. New York: Lippincott-Raven, 1998.

93. Long CL, Lowry SR. Hormonal regulation of protein metabolism. J Parenter Enteral Nutr 1990;14:555–562.

94. Konstantinides FN. Nitrogen balance studies in clinical nutrition. Nutr Clin Pract 1992;7:231–238.

95. Nelson KM, Long CL. Physiological basis for nutrition in sepsis. Nutr Clin Pract 1989;4:6–15.

96. Wolfe R, Allsop J, Burke J. Glucose metabolism in man: responses to intravenous glucose infusion. Metabolism 1979;28:210–220.

97. Wolfe RR, Shaw JHF. Glucose and FFA in kinetics in sepsis: role of glucagon and sympathetic nervous system activity. Am J Physiol 1985;248:E236–E243.

98. Cerra FB. Metabolic and nutritional support. In: Mattox KL, Feliciano DV, Moore EE, eds. Trauma, 3rd Ed. Stamford: Appleton & Lange, 1996:1155–1176.

99. Pomposelli JJ, Baxter JK, Babineau TJ, et al. Early postoperative glucose control predicts nosocomial infection rate in diabetic patients. J Parenter Enteral Nutr 1998;22:77–81.

100. Pelham LD. Rational use of intravenous fat emulsions. Am J Hosp Pharm 1981;38:198–208.

101. Kinsella JE, Lokesh B, Broughton S. Dietary polyunsaturated fatty acids and eicosanoids: potential effect on the modulation of inflammatory and immune cells: an overview. Nutrition 1990;6:24–44.

102. Allardyce DB. Cholestasis caused by lipid emulsions. Surg Gynecol Obstet 1982;154:641–647.

103. Fonkalsrud E. Surgical treatment of gastroesophageal reflux (GER) syndrome in infants & children. Am J Surg 1987;154:11–18.

104. Collier P, Kudsk KA, Glezer J, et al. Fiber-containing formula and needle catheter jejunostomies: a clinical evaluation. Nutr Clin Pract 1994;9:101–103.

105. Dent D, Kudsk K, Minard G, et al. Risk of abdominal septic complications following feeding jejunostomy placement in patients undergoing splenectomy for trauma. Am J Surg 1993;166:686–689.

106. Palacio JC, Rombeau JL. Dietary fiber: a brief review and potential application to enteral feeding. Nutr Clin Pract 1990;5: 99–106.

107. Guenter PA, Settle RG, Perlmutter S, et al. Tube feeding-related diarrhea in acutely ill patients. J Parenter Enteral Nutr 1991;15: 277–280.

108. Eisenberg PG. Cause of diarrhea in tube-fed patients: a comprehensive approach to diagnosis and management. Nutr Clin Pract 1993;8:119–123.

109. Broe PJ, Toung TJK, Cameron JL. Aspirational pneumonia. Surg Clin North Am 1980;60(6):1551–1564.

110. Spapen HD, Duinslaeger L, Diltoer M, et al. Gastric emptying in critically ill patients is accelerated by adding cisapride to a standard enteral feeding protocol: results of a prospective, randomized controlled trial. Crit Care Med 1995;23:481–485.

111. Dive A, Miesse C, Galanti L, et al. Effect of erythromycin on gastric motility in mechanically ventilated critically ill patients: a double-blind, randomized, placebo-controlled study. Crit Care Med 1995;23:1356–1362.

112. Landry C, Vidon N, Sogni P, et al. Could oral erythromycin optimize high energy continuous enteral nutrition? Aliment Pharmacol Ther 1996;10:967–973.

113. Heyland D, Tougas G, Cook DJ, et al. Cisapride improves gastric emptying in mechanically ventilated, critically ill patients. A randomized, double-blind trial. Am J Respir Crit Care Med 1996;154:1678–1683.

114. Edes TE, Walk BE, Austin JL. Diarrhea in tube-fed patients: feeding formula not necessarily the cause. Am J Med 1990;88:91–93.

115. Lutomski DM, Gora ML, Wright SM, et al. Sorbitol content of selected oral liquids. Ann Pharmacother 1993;27:269–274.

116. Pemberton LB, Lyman B, Lander V, et al. Sepsis from triple- vs. single-lumen catheters during total parenteral nutrition in surgical or critically ill patients. Arch Surg 1986;121:591.

117. Miller JJ, Venus B, Mathru M. Comparison of the sterility of long-term central venous catheterization using single lumen, triple lumen, and pulmonary artery catheters. Crit Care Med 1984;12:634.

118. Pomposelli JJ, Bistrian BR. Is total parenteral nutrition immunosuppressive? New Horiz (US) 1994;2(2):224–229.

119. Kumpf VJ. Parenteral iron supplementation. Nutr Clin Pract 1996;11:139–146.

120. The Veteran Affairs Total Parenteral Nutrition Cooperative Study Group. Perioperative total parenteral nutrition in surgical patients. N Engl J Med 1991;325:525–532.

121. Fan St, Lo CM, Lai EC, et al. Perioperative nutritional support in patients undergoing hepatectomy for hepatocellular carcinoma. N Engl J Med 1994;331:1547–1552.

122. Brennan MF, Pisters PWT, Posner M, et al. A prospective, randomized trial of total parenteral nutrition after major pancreatic resection for malignancy. Ann Surg 1994;220:436–444.

123. Doglietto GB, Gallitelli L, Pacelli F, et al. Protein-sparing therapy after major abdominal surgery: lack of clinical effects. Ann Surg 1996;223:357–362.

124. Watters JM, Kirkpatrick SM, Norris SB, et al. Immediate postoperative enteral feeding results in impaired respiratory mechanics and decreased mobility. Ann Surg 1997;226:369–377.

125. Daly JM, Weintraub FN, Shou J, et al. Enteral nutrition during multimodality therapy in upper gastrointestinal cancer patients. Ann Surg 1995;221:327–338.

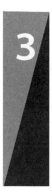

Perioperative Fluids and Electrolytes

Avery B. Nathens and Ronald V. Maier

Physiology

Body Fluid Compartments

Accurate replacement of fluid requires an understanding of the distribution of water, electrolytes, and colloid across the various body fluid compartments. Total body water (TBW) approximates 60% of total body weight, or 42 l in a 70-kg person. TBW is composed of the intracellular compartment and extracellular compartment. The intracellular compartment or intracellular volume (ICV) constitutes 40% of total body weight (28 l in a 70-kg patient) whereas the extracellular volume (ECV) makes up the remaining 20%. The ECV is composed of interstitial fluid (IF) and the intravascular or plasma volume (PV). Plasma volume constitutes 25% of ECV (5% of total body weight, or approximately 3.5 l), while the remainder is interstitial fluid. Red cell volume, approximately 2% to 3% of total body water, is part of the ICV. Thus, total blood volume is approximately 7% to 8% of total body weight, or approximately 5 l in a 70-kg patient (Fig. 3.1).

The solute and colloid compositions of the intracellular and extracellular fluid compartments differ markedly. The ECV contains most of the sodium in the body, with equal sodium concentrations in the PV and IF (140 mEq/l), while the intracellular [Na$^+$] is only 10 to 12 mEq/l. By contrast, the predominant intracellular cation is potassium, with the intracellular concentration [K$^+$] approximating 150 mEq/l in contrast to an ECV [K$^+$] of 4.0 mEq/l. Albumin represents the most important osmotically active constituent of the ECV and is virtually excluded from the ICV. Albumin is unequally distributed within the ECV; the serum concentration of albumin approximates 4.0 g/dl while the IF concentration averages 1.0 g/dl.

The distribution volume of various crystalloid or colloid solutions is that volume in which the administered solution will equilibrate over the short term. For example, TBW is the distribution volume for sodium-free water; ECV is the distribution volume for crystalloid solution in which [Na$^+$] approximates 140 mEq/l, whereas PV represents the distribution volume for most colloid solutions. To clarify this concept, assume a 70-kg patient has suffered an acute blood loss of 1000 ml, approximately 20% of the predicted 5-l blood volume. Any one of 5% dextrose in water (D5W), lactated Ringer's solution, or 5% albumin may be chosen to replace the lost blood volume. The formula describing the effects of fluid infusion on plasma volume expansion is as follows:

$$\text{Expected PV increment} = \frac{\text{volume infused} \times \text{normal PV}}{\text{distribution volume}}$$

Rearranging the equation would yield the following:

Volume infused
$$= \frac{\text{expected PV increment} \times \text{distribution volume}}{\text{normal plasma volume}}$$

In this example, the expected PV increment is 1 l (to replace shed blood) and the normal plasma volume is approximately 3.5 l. To restore blood volume using D5W, which distributes throughout TBW (42 l), it would be necessary to administer 12 l. By contrast, if lactated Ringer's solution (which distributes throughout ECV) were chosen, a 1-l PV increment would require approximately 4 l of crystalloid. Colloid solutions with similar oncotic pressures to plasma (e.g., 5% albumin) distribute within the intravascular space and thus have a distribution volume equal to the plasma volume. In this example, 1 l of 5% albumin would be required to replace the shed blood.

Maintenance Body Fluid and Electrolyte Requirements

Healthy adults require a minimal amount of fluid and electrolyte intake to maintain systemic homeostasis. Sufficient water is required to replace obligatory urinary losses of approximately 1000 ml/day and gastrointestinal losses of 100 to 200 ml/day. Additionally, insensible water losses must be

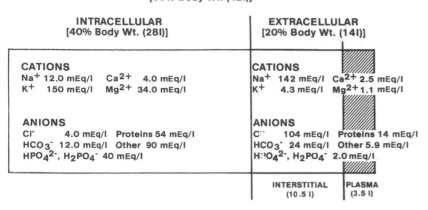

FIGURE 3.1. Distribution of body water and electrolytes in a healthy 70-kg male. (Adapted from Narins RG, Krishna GC. Disorders of water balance. In: Stein JH, ed. *Internal Medicine*, 2nd Ed. Philadelphia: Lippincott-Williams & Wilkins, 1987:794–805, with permission.)

taken into account. Insensible losses amount to 8 to 12 ml/kg/day and are equally divided into respiratory and cutaneous water loss. Cutaneous insensitive losses increase by approximately 10% for each degree of temperature greater than 37°C; thus these losses may become quite significant in the febrile patient. Respiratory insensitive water losses tend to be greater with inspiration of unhumidified air, as may occur with a tracheostomy. Overall maintenance fluid requirements are dependent on weight and are approximated using either of the approaches in Table 3.1. For example, a 60-kg patient would require approximately 100 ml/h of water (4 ml/kg × 10 kg plus 2 ml/kg × 10 kg plus 1 ml/kg × 40 kg) to keep up with obligatory water losses.

Daily sodium intake in normal individuals approaches 100 to 250 mEq/day. This intake is balanced by sodium losses in sweat, stool, and urine. However, renal conservation of sodium is extraordinary, and in cases of profound volume depletion urinary losses of sodium may be less than 1 mEq/day. In the perioperative period, adequate maintenance of sodium may be achieved with an intake of 1 to 2 mEq/kg/day. Normal potassium intake is approximately 40 to 120 mEq/day, approximately 10% to 15% of which is excreted as normal urinary losses. In individuals with normal renal function, body potassium stores can be maintained with an intake of approximately 0.5 to 1.0 mEq/kg/day.

Based on estimated maintenance requirements of Na^+ and K^+, there are several options for maintenance fluid replacement (Table 3.2). A 60-kg patient should receive approximately 60 to 120 mEq/day of sodium and 30 to 60 mEq/day of potassium. The most commonly used maintenance solutions are D5W 1/2 NS or 2/3 D5W 1/3 NS, which are relatively isotonic and provide the required amount of sodium over a 24-h period. Potassium is often added to these solutions at concentrations approximating 20 mEq/l to ensure that maintenance requirements are met. Although 0.9% saline is used quite frequently, the relatively high concentration of chloride results in a hyperchloremic metabolic aci-

dosis because of the inability of the renal tubule to excrete the excess Cl^-.

Perioperative Fluid Requirements

Appropriate management of fluids and electrolytes in the perioperative period requires a flexible yet systematic approach to ensure that fluid administration is appropriately tailored to the patient's changing requirements. The amount of fluids administered in the immediate postoperative period (within the first 12–24 h) must take into account the existing deficit, maintenance requirements, and any ongoing losses.

Estimation of the existing deficit must incorporate an approximation of intraoperative blood loss as well as fluid losses from evaporative and third-space, or extravascular, fluid sequestration. It is important to realize that the surgeon's estimated intraoperative blood loss is often 50% less than when calculated using more rigorous methods.[1,2] This discrepancy should be taken into account when estimating postoperative fluid requirements. Due to the shift of crystalloid from the intravascular space to the interstitium, crystalloid should replace blood loss in a 3:1 ratio.

Extravascular fluid sequestration represents another important source of intraoperative fluid loss. Extensive dissection at the operative site induces a localized capillary leak, the result of which is extravasation of intravascular fluid into the interstitium with edema formation. The loss of intravascular volume via this route depends on the extent of exposure and degree of dissection.

Ongoing fluid requirements usually represent gastrointestinal losses from stomas, tubes, drains, or fistulae. These losses may be accurately estimated by closely following recorded hourly outputs from any tube or drain. The electrolyte composition of the output depends on the source of effluent[3] (Table 3.3). The replacement fluid should be chosen to best approximate the composition of the ongoing losses. For example, nasogastric losses are typically replaced with normal saline supplemented with 10 mEq KCl/l, whereas losses from a duodenal fistula may best be replaced using lactated Ringer's solution.

Postoperative fluid orders should take into account the overall fluid balance in the operating room as an estimate of the existing deficit along with maintenance fluid requirements and any ongoing losses. The preferred approach is to reassess the patient frequently to determine intravascular volume sta-

TABLE 3.1. Maintenance Water Requirements.

Weight	ml/kg/h	ml/kg/day
First 10 kg	4	100
Second 10 kg	2	50
Each kilogram above 20 kg	1	20

TABLE 3.2. Options for Maintenance Fluid Replacement.

	Na^+ (mEq/l)	K^+ (mEq/l)	Cl^- (mEq/l)	Ca^{2+} (mEq/l)	Lactate[a] (mEq/l)	Glucose (g/l)
Normal (0.9%) saline (NS)	154	0	154	0	0	0
Dextrose 5% in water (D5W)	0	0	0	0	0	50
D5W 1/2 NS	77	0	77	0	0	50
2/3 D5W, 1/3 NS	50	0	50	0	0	33
Lactated Ringer's	130	4	109	3	28	0

[a]Lactate is used instead of Cl^- to maintain electroneutrality. It is converted to HCO_3^- by hepatic metabolism.

tus. In this regard, evaluation of heart rate, blood pressure, and most importantly hourly urine output provide an excellent measure of intravascular volume status. Orders for intravenous fluids should be rewritten frequently to maintain a normal heart rate, a urine output of approximately 1 ml/kg/h, and adequate blood pressure. It has become common practice to avoid potassium supplementation within the first 24 h. The rationale behind this approach is to prevent life-threatening hyperkalemia should oliguria become a significant problem in the early postoperative period. The preferred practice is to administer normal saline or lactated Ringer's in the first 24 h. The smaller volume of distribution of these solutions compared to dextrose-containing solutions ensures that adequate intravascular volume is maintained despite ongoing extravascular fluid sequestration. On the first postoperative morning, these solutions are switched to dextrose-containing solutions (2/3 D5W 1/3 NS or D5W 1/2 NS) supplemented with KCl, providing that urine output has been adequate.

Disorders of Sodium Homeostasis

Maintenance of a normal serum sodium concentration (135–145 mEq/l) is intimately associated with control of plasma osmolarity (P_{osm}). Plasma osmolarity is determined by the sum of the individual osmotically active substances as described in the following equation:

$$P_{osm} = 2 \times \text{plasma } [Na^+] + [\text{glucose}]/20 + [\text{BUN}]/3$$

Maintenance of the plasma osmolarity within normal limits depends on the ability of the kidneys to excrete water, thus preventing hypoosmolarity, and on a normal thirst mechanism with access to water to prevent hypernatremia. The ability to excrete maximally dilute urine (<100 mOsm/kg) allows the kidneys to excrete in excess of 18 l of water per day. In the presence of normal renal perfusion and intact renal function, antidiuretic hormone (ADH) is the principal regulator of serum osmolarity. A 1% to 2% reduction in P_{osm}

maximally inhibits ADH release, leading to a urine osmolarity that is maximally dilute. By contrast, a 1% to 2% increase in P_{osm} above normal or a 5% to 10% decrease in blood volume or blood pressure stimulates ADH release. Importantly, when both a low plasma osmolarity and low blood volume or pressure are present, the latter effect will dominate, resulting in an increase in ADH release. This is one of the principal mechanisms leading to the development of hyponatremia in patients with low intravascular volume. Additionally, changes in blood pressure or volume status will alter the osmolar set point and, to a lesser extent, the sensitivity of the osmotic response.[4]

Hyponatremia

The approach to hyponatremia begins with an assessment of the serum osmolarity[3] (Table 3.4). If serum osmolarity is high, it is important to consider the possibility of other effective plasma osmoles, the most common of which is glucose. In quantitative terms, for every 100 mg/dl rise in glucose the $[Na^+]$ falls by 1.3 mEq/l. Hyperglycemia shifts H_2O from cells, leading to dilutional hyponatremia. The treatment involves definitive management of the osmotically active agent, which, in the case of glucose, would be insulin. In rare cases the serum osmolarity may be normal. This phenomenon is referred to as pseudohyponatremia and is caused by hyperlipedemia or hyperproteinemia; it is an artifact of the laboratory assay. No treatment is required.

More frequently, a low $[Na^+]$ will be associated with reduced plasma osmolarity. The etiology and treatment of hypoosmolar hyponatremia may be classified into three groups depending on the extracellular volume status of the patient. A reduction in extracellular volume leads to an increase in ADH secretion, impairing the kidney's ability to excrete free water. Either administration of Na^+-free solutions or the ingestion of free water induced by thirst aggravates the resulting hyponatremia. The most common causes of hypovolemic hyponatremia are due to Na^+ loss. Typically, perioperative

TABLE 3.3. Volume and Composition of Gastrointestinal Fluid Losses.

Source	Volume (ml)	Na^+ (mEq/l)	Cl^- (mEq/l)	K^+ (mEq/l)	HCO_3^- (mEq/l)	H^+ (mEq/l)
Stomach	1000–4200	20–120	130	10–15	—	30–100
Duodenum	100–2000	110	115	15	10	—
Ileum	1000–3000	80–150	60–100	10	30–50	—
Colon (diarrhea)	500–1700	120	90	25	45	—
Bile	500–1000	140	100	5	25	—
Pancreas	500–1000	140	30	5	115	—

TABLE 3.4. Causes of Hyponatremia.

Pseudohyponatremia (normal plasma osmolality)
  Hyperlipidemia, hyperproteinemia

Dilutional hyponatremia (increased plasma osmolality)
  Hyperglycemia, mannitol

True hyponatremia (reduced plasma osmolality)
  Reduction in ECF volume

  Plasma, GI, skin, or renal losses (diuretics)

  Expanded ECF volume
    Congestive heart failure
    Hypoproteinemic states (cirrhosis, nephrotic syndrome,
      malnutrition)

  Normal ECF volume
    SIADH
    Pulmonary or CNS lesions
    Endocrine disorders (hypothyroidism, hypoadrenalism)
    Drugs (e.g., morphine, tricyclic antidepressants, clofibrate,
      antineoplastic agents, chlorpropamide, aminophylline, in-
      domethacin)
    Miscellaneous (pain, nausea)

SIADH, inappropriate antidiuretic hormone secretion.

isotonic losses (plasma, gastric losses) are replaced with hypotonic solutions in the face of mild hypovolemia. The treatment involves replenishing the extravascular volume with isotonic fluids in concert with restriction of free water.

Hyponatremia in the presence of an increased extravascular volume probably represents the next most common scenario in the perioperative period. Typically, these represent edematous states wherein there is a reduction in the effective circulating volume. Low cardiac output states, cirrhosis, and other hypoalbuminemic states are the more common etiologies. Both water restriction and Na^+ restriction are necessary. Depending on the severity of the hyponatremia, a loop diuretic may be required to increase both Na^+ and water loss; in most cases, this induces an excess of urinary water loss over Na^+ loss and should correct the hyponatremia.

Patients with a normal extracellular volume status and hypoosmolar hyponatremia may have the syndrome of inappropriate ADH secretion (SIADH). In the surgical patient SIADH is not often considered as a possible cause of hyponatremia, but nausea, pain, and narcotics, all of which are common in the postoperative period, may result in inappropriate ADH secretion and contribute to postoperative hyponatremia. Diagnosis is confirmed by demonstrating a low plasma hypoosmolarity, a less than maximally dilute urine ($U_{osm} > 100$ mOsm/l), and renal salt wasting ($U_{Na} > 20$ mEq/l).[3] Treatment includes management of the underlying cause and water restriction. Isotonic (0.9%) saline should not be administered to patients with the SIADH as it may cause the plasma $[Na^+]$ to fall.

The presence of symptoms in hyponatremia depends on the rate at which hyponatremia occurred. Symptoms of increased intracranial pressure from cerebral edema are the most prominent features and may be present at plasma $[Na^+]$ less than 125 mEq/l if the development of hyponatremia was rapid in onset. If the reduction in $[Na^+]$ occurs slowly, then symptoms may not be evident until plasma $[Na^+]$ drops as low as 110 mEq/l. Too rapid correction of plasma $[Na^+]$ may result in central pontine myelinosis, a process of demyelination caused by cell shrinkage that may result in irreversible brainstem injury. If the patient is asymptomatic or mildly symptomatic, the goal should be to raise the $[Na^+]$ by approximately 0.5 mEq/h; if symptomatic with coma or convulsions, then more rapid correction is necessary. The aim is to give sufficient Na^+ as 3% NaCl until either the symptoms have improved or the plasma $[Na^+]$ has increased by 5 mEq/l, whichever comes first. The following formula may be used to estimate the amount of Na^+ required to raise the $[Na^+]$ to a safe level (approximately 120 mEq/l):

$$Na^+ \text{ deficit} = 0.60 \times \text{lean body weight (kg)}$$
$$\times (120 - \text{measured plasma } Na^+)$$

Hypernatremia

Hypernatremia (plasma $[Na^+] > 150$ mEq/l) is far less common than is hyponatremia. Cellular shrinkage caused by fluid shifts from the intracellular space to the extracellular compartment may cause confusion, coma, and intracranial hemorrhage. Symptoms are usually not evident below a plasma $[Na^+]$ of 160 mEq/l.

Elevated plasma $[Na^+]$ occurs as a result of excessive free water loss and is thus frequently associated with hypovolemia and oliguria. Extrarenal losses represent the most common source of water loss. Excessive insensible losses caused by fever, hyperventilation, and burns or hypotonic fluid losses due to perspiration or severe diarrhea are the principal causes. If hypovolemia is sufficiently severe that tissue perfusion is compromised, then initial therapy should be isotonic saline until tissue perfusion is restored. If perfusion is adequate, then 0.5 normal saline or D5W is sufficient to return plasma $[Na^+]$ to normal.

Polyuria associated with excessive renal free water losses represents another frequent cause of hypernatremia. For example, osmotic diuresis induced by hyperglycemia or mannitol may cause profound hypernatremia if left unchecked. An inability to concentrate urine because of high output renal failure commonly associated with the recovery phase of acute tubular necrosis may also cause severe hypernatremia. In the context of the clinical scenario, the diagnosis is usually straightforward. Treatment simply involves measuring urinary electrolyte losses and providing adequate free water replacement. Central diabetes insipidus is not uncommon following neurosurgical operations or head injury and may cause profound hypernatremia. Administration of exogenous vasopressin in the form of dDAVP is both diagnostic and therapeutic.

Rapid correction of severe hypernatremia may cause irreversible neurological deficits. Plasma $[Na^+]$ should not be corrected at a rate faster than 0.5 to 1.0 mEq/l per hour. In the presence of convulsions, sufficient free water should be administered to either return the plasma $[Na^+]$ to the concentration documented before the convulsion or to reduce the $[Na^+]$ by about 6 mmol/l. The following formula may help to guide therapy:

$$\text{Water deficit} = \text{total body water}$$
$$\times \{(\text{plasma } [Na^+] \div \text{desired plasma } [Na^+]) - 1\}$$

Disorders of Potassium Homeostasis

Potassium is the major intracellular cation. Only about 2% of total body potassium is located in the extracellular fluid. Despite the small quantity of K^+ in the extracellular space, slight alterations in plasma $[K^+]$ may have dramatic effects on muscle contraction and nerve conduction, as the concentration gradient across the plasma membrane is the main determinant of membrane excitability. For this reason, abnormalities in plasma $[K^+]$ should be treated expeditiously.

Hypokalemia

Hypokalemia in the surgical patient is usually due to losses from the gastrointestinal tract, kidneys, or skin (Table 3.5). In the case of diarrhea, stool potassium losses represent the principal reason for hypokalemia. By contrast, the mechanism for hypokalemia in vomiting is more complex. The content of K^+ in gastric secretion is only about 10 mEq/l. As a result, massive vomiting would be necessary to cause hypokalemia. Typically, renal K^+ losses account for potassium depletion associated with vomiting. The extracellular volume contraction leads to elevated levels of aldosterone, which results in enhanced renal Na^+ reabsorption and increased K^+ secretion. Massive burns may also cause hypokalemia because of a combination of tissue breakdown and fluid loss.

The major danger associated with hypokalemia is cardiac arrhythmias. The potential for arrhythmias is exacerbated in the presence of a metabolic alkalosis, digoxin, or hypercalcemia. Electrocardiographic changes associated with hypokalemia correlate poorly with the plasma $[K^+]$ but typically are not manifest until the plasma $[K^+]$ drops below 3 mmol/l. Early changes include T-wave flattening or inversion and depressed ST segments, followed by the development of U waves and a prolonged Q-T interval. Hypokalemia may also manifest with weakness once plasma $[K^+]$ drops below 2.5 mmol/l.

Potassium replacement therapy should be geared toward rapid correction of plasma $[K^+]$, followed by slower repletion of the total body K^+ deficit. The potassium deficit may be quite large. For example, a fall in plasma $[K^+]$ from 4 to 3 reflects a total deficit of 100 to 400 mmol[3]. Too rapid correction may result in inadvertent hyperkalemia because it takes time for the administered K^+ to be transferred into cells. When possible, K^+ supplementation should be administered orally. However, if the plasma $[K^+]$ is less than 3.0 or enteral supplementation is not possible, then parenteral administration is indicated. Potassium can be administered intravenously into peripheral veins in concentrations as high as 40 mmol/l. Higher concentrations may cause phlebitis and thus should be administered into a central vein. The rate of administration in the absence of intractable arrhythmias should be no greater than 20 to 40 mEq/h. At this rate of administration, continuous ECG monitoring is indicated.

Hyperkalemia

Sudden increases in plasma $[K^+]$ are almost always caused by rapid administration or transcellular flux of K^+. By contrast, sustained hyperkalemia implies that there is impairment of renal K^+ excretion. It is important to be aware of pseudohyperkalemia, observed when the serum potassium (as measured by the laboratory) is spuriously elevated by potassium release from red blood cells or platelets after the blood specimen has been obtained. The diagnosis of pseudohyperkalemia can be made by demonstrating that the plasma $[K^+]$ is normal in a nonhemolyzed plasma sample in which clotting is prevented by drawing the blood into a heparinized tube.

Transcellular flux of K^+ from the cell into the extracellular fluid may occur in patients with severe metabolic acidosis, insulin deficiency (e.g., diabetes mellitus), or rhabdomyolysis as the intracellular potassium stores are released. Administration of succinylcholine may also cause a transient rise in plasma $[K^+]$ because of en masse muscle depolarization, particularly following paralysis or prolonged bed rest, such as is seen in severe burn injury.

The main risks associated with hyperkalemia are similar to those of hypokalemia: weakness and myocardial irritability. Electrocardiographic signs of hyperkalemia proceed from an increase in T-wave amplitude, leading to a narrow, peaked symmetrical T wave, followed by reduced P-wave amplitude and widening of the QRS complexes. If untreated, severe hyperkalemia may eventually cause a sinusoidal ECG complex and ultimately ventricular fibrillation. Signs or symptoms are rare at plasma $[K^+]$ below 6.0 mmol/l; beyond this, there is poor correlation with the serum potassium level and arrhythmias. The rate of rise of plasma $[K^+]$ appears to be extremely important; many patients with chronic renal failure tolerate plasma $[K^+]$ levels in excess of 6 or 6.5 without symptoms. Treatment is dependent on the presence or absence of electrocardiographic changes and the plasma $[K^+]$. Individuals with mild hyperkalemia (<6.0 mmol/l) can usually be treated conservatively by reducing daily intake. Active treatment to lower the plasma $[K^+]$ or to antagonize its effects on the cell membrane should be started if the $[K^+]$ has risen acutely to greater than 6.0 mmol/l or if any ECG manifestations of hyperkalemia are present. These therapeutic modalities should be used in conjunction with other methods to reduce total body potassium stores (Table 3.6).

Disorders of Mineral Homeostasis

In most surgical patients, abnormalities in the body fluid composition of calcium (Ca), magnesium (Mg), and phosphate (PO_4) are seldom extreme enough to cause concern. However, in the critically ill patient, these alterations may exacerbate potentially life-threatening situations.

TABLE 3.5. Causes of Hypokalemia.

Extrarenal losses
   Gastrointestinal (vomiting, nasogastric suction)
   Diarrhea
   Massive burns
   Profuse sweating
Renal losses
   Diuretic therapy
   Vomiting
   Tubular disorders (e.g., type I renal tubular acidosis)
   Drugs (cisplatin, amphotericin B)
Transcellular flux of K^+ into the cell
   Metabolic alkalosis
   Insulin administration
   β_2-adrenergic stimulation
Other
   Primary hyperaldosteronism
   Renal artery stenosis
   Cushing's syndrome

TABLE 3.6. Treatment of Hyperkalemia.

Treatment	Mechanism of action	Time frame
Intravenous calcium gluconate	Antagonizes effects of hyperkalemia on the cell membrane	Seconds to minutes
Glucose, insulin, sodium bicarbonate	Translocation of potassium into cells	30–60 min
Rectally or orally administered potassium-binding resins	Binds and hastens excretion of K^+ secreted into colon	1–4 h (rectal) >6 h (oral)
Dialysis	Movement across a concentration gradient and excreted	Immediate

Calcium Abnormalities

Total body calcium stores are approximately 1000 g, with almost 99% apportioned in bone. The remainder is located within the extracellular fluid and is either free (40%) or bound to albumin (50%) or other anions such as citrate, lactate, and sulfate. Only the free or ionized component is biologically active. Acid–base alterations affect the binding of calcium to albumin and account for the symptoms of hypocalcemia associated with hyperventilation. The resultant respiratory alkalosis increases the binding affinity of calcium for albumin, leading to a reduction in the serum ionized calcium levels. Similarly, changes in serum protein levels affect total serum calcium. The ionized calcium level (normal range, 4.5–5.5 mg/dl) can be estimated using the following formula:

$$\text{Ionized calcium (mg/dl)} = \text{total serum calcium (mg/dl)} - 0.8 \times \text{serum albumin (mg/dl)}$$

Routine supplementation or assessment in postoperative patients is usually not indicated. However, in patients with major fluid shifts, prolonged immobilization, alterations in GI absorption, or operative procedures on the thyroid or parathyroid, significant alterations in calcium homeostasis may arise.

Hypocalcemia

The most frequent cause of hypocalcemia is a low serum albumin. In this case, the ionized fraction remains normal and no treatment is indicated. Frequent alternate causes to consider include acute pancreatitis, massive soft tissue infection, small-bowel fistulae, and hypoparathyroidism. Massive blood transfusion induces hypocalcemia caused by chelation of calcium with citrate.

Manifestations of hypocalcemia may become evident at serum levels less than 8 mg/dl. The earliest symptoms include numbness or tingling in the circumoral region or at the tips of the fingers. Tetany or seizure may arise at more profound levels of hypocalcemia. A positive Trousseau's sign or Chvostek's sign may be suggestive of hypocalcemia. Hypocalcemia alters myocardial repolarization and results in a prolonged Q-T interval on the electrocardiogram. ECG monitoring may be useful to guide calcium supplementation in massive transfusion when rapid assays are unavailable.

The treatment of hypocalcemia depends on its severity. In symptomatic patients with an ionized calcium level less than 3 g/dl, intravenous replacement therapy should be administered: a 10-ml ampoule of either 10% calcium gluconate (93 mg elemental calcium) or calcium chloride (232 mg elemental calcium) should be administered in 50 to 100 ml D5W over 10 to 15 min. In less severe cases, oral supplementation may suffice and any oral preparation providing 1 to 3 g of elemental calcium per day will be adequate.

Hypercalcemia

There is an extensive differential diagnosis for hypercalcemia (see Chapter 38, The Parathyroid). Primary hyperparathyroidism and malignant disease account for 90% of cases, with the former more common in outpatients and the latter most common among hospitalized patients.[5] Hypercalcemia has protean manifestations including confusion, lethargy, coma, muscle weakness, anorexia, nausea, vomiting, pancreatitis, and constipation. Renal stones may develop in cases of prolonged hypercalcemia. Hypercalcemia may also induce nephrogenic diabetes insipidus and result in polyuria. Finally, electrocardiographic changes include a shortened Q-T interval. This alteration in cardiac repolarization predisposes the patient to fatal arrhythmias, particularly in the presence of digitalis.

A serum calcium concentration in excess of 15 mg/dl or in association with electrocardiographic changes requires urgent treatment. Most patients will respond to vigorous hydration with normal saline. Once the patient is rehydrated, furosemide may be administered to further increase calcium excretion. Rarely, adjunctive measures including administration of diphosphonates, calcitonin, or mithramycin may be necessary.

Magnesium Abnormalities

Magnesium is the principal intracellular divalent cation. Approximately 50% of total body magnesium is found in bone and is not readily exchangeable. Serum magnesium concentrations typically range between 1.5 and 2.5 mEq/l. Magnesium absorption occurs throughout the small intestine and is reabsorbed quite effectively in the renal tubules with renal excretion as low as 1 mEq/day. Hypomagnesemia may occur because of poor nutritional intake, malabsorption, or increased renal excretion due to diuretics. Hypomagnesemia is quite common in patients abusing alcohol. The signs and symptoms of hypomagnesemia are characterized by neuromuscular and CNS irritability, and in this respect are similar to those seen with hypocalcemia. Low serum magnesium levels appear to impair parathyroid hormone excretion and may induce hypocalcemia refractory to calcium supplementation unless the hypomagnesemia is corrected.[6]

Hypomagnesemia may be treated with either oral or parenteral magnesium preparations. If the serum magnesium level is less than 1 mEq/l or the patient is symptomatic, than parenteral treatment is indicated. In the presence of normal renal function, up to 2 mEq magnesium per kg of body weight may be administered daily.

Hypermagnesemia is extraordinarily rare in the absence of renal failure. Flaccid paralysis, hypotension, confusion, and coma may become evident at serum levels exceeding 6 mEq/l. Electrocardiographic features are similar to those seen in hyperkalemia. Emergency treatment of severe symptomatic hypermagnesemia involves administration of calcium as either calcium gluconate or calcium chloride. Calcium effectively antagonizes the effect of magnesium on neuromuscular function. Definitive treatment requires increasing renal magnesium excretion with a combination of hydration and diuresis. If renal function is impaired, then dialysis will be necessary.

Phosphate Abnormalities

Phosphate is the most abundant intracellular anion, and only 0.1% of total body phosphorus is in the extracellular fluid compartment. As a result, circulating plasma levels do not reflect total body stores. Hypophosphatemia may occur as the result of impaired intestinal absorption or increased renal excretion. Hyperparathyroidism may induce a drop in serum phosphate levels through an increase in renal excretion. Significant hypophosphatemia is very common following major liver resection, an effect caused by rapid phosphate utilization in the regenerating hepatocytes.[7] In this clinical setting serum phosphate should be measured frequently and treated appropriately. Careful monitoring of phosphate should also occur with the administration of parenteral nutrition after prolonged starvation because profound hypophosphatemia may result.[8] The potential adverse effects associated with severe hypophosphatemia include impaired tissue oxygen delivery due to decreased 2,3-diphosphoglycerate levels, muscle weakness, and rhabdomyolysis. Severe hypophosphatemia may be treated parenterally using potassium phosphate.

Hyperphosphatemia is most commonly seen in the setting of impaired renal phosphate excretion and in this scenario is frequently associated with hypocalcemia. Similarly, hypoparathyroidism reduces renal phosphate excretion, leading to an increase in serum phosphate levels. In these cases, treatment should be directed toward the underlying cause.

Acid–Base Abnormalities

The concentration of hydrogen ions in body fluids is maintained within an optimal pH range (7.35–7.45) to ensure adequate function of structural and enzymatic proteins. This narrow range is assured by the availability of several buffer systems including intracellular proteins and phosphates and the bicarbonate–carbonic acid system. The former functions primarily as an intracellular buffer and the latter as a buffer in the extracellular fluid. Further, alterations in excretion or retention of CO_2 or HCO_3^- through changes in minute ventilation or renal tubular handling of HCO_3^- provide an additional homeostatic mechanism for maintaining normal pH. By combining information on the various buffering systems, a nomogram can be constructed to describe the normal compensatory responses to acute and chronic acid–base disturbances (Fig. 3.2).

Metabolic Acidosis

Metabolic acidosis arises as a result of retention (or administration) of fixed acids or the loss of bicarbonate. In this way,

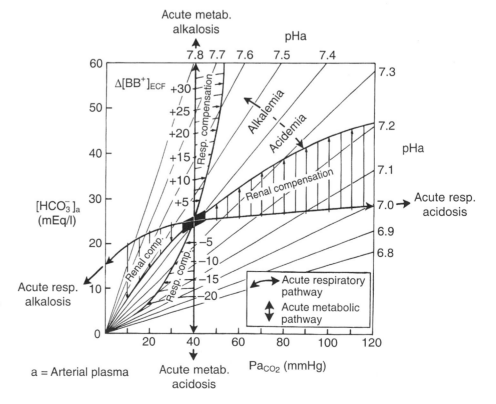

FIGURE 3.2. Compensatory responses to acute and chronic acid base alterations. $[BB^+]_{ECF}$ represents the base deficit. The *black diagonal box in the center* represents the normal range. As an example, if a metabolic acidosis develops such that a base deficit of −15 mEq/l occurs, the resulting acidosis would lower the pH to 7.1. However, normal respiratory compensation would reduce the Pa_{CO_2} to 27 mmHg and raise the pH to about 7.25. (From Johnson RL, Ramanathan M. Buffer equilibra in the lungs. In: The Kidney: Physiology and Pathophysiology. 2nd Edition. eds DW Seldin, G Giebisch. Philadelphia: Lippincott-Williams & Wilkins, 1992, with permission.)

TABLE 3.7. Metabolic Acidosis.

Anion gap	Non-anion gap

Renal failure	GI HCO_3^- loss
	  Diarrhea, ileus, fistula, and
	  ureterosigmoidostomy

Lactic acidosis	Renal HCO_3^- loss
	  Proximal renal tubular acidosis,
	  acetazolamide

Ketoacidosis
  Diabetic, alcoholic,
  starvation
	Failure of renal HCO_3^- production
	  Distal renal tubular acidosis

Toxic ingestions
  Salicylates, methanol,
  ethylene glycol,
  paraldehyde, toluene	

disorders associated with a metabolic acidosis are categorized by the presence or absence of an anion gap, in that addition of fixed acids results in an anion gap metabolic acidosis and bicarbonate loss results in an non-anion gap metabolic acidosis (Table 3.7). The anion gap (AG) refers to the difference between measured cations (Na^+) and measured anions (Cl^- and HCO_3^-):

$$AG = Na^+ - (Cl^- + HCO_3^-)$$

The normal anion gap ranges from 3 to 11 mM/l. These unmeasured anions consist of proteins (primarily albumin), sulfates, phosphates, and organic acids. A reduction in the plasma albumin concentration will reduce the baseline AG approximately 2.5 mEq for every fall of 1 g/dl in the serum albumin. Thus, a severely hypoalbuminemic patient may have an anion gap metabolic acidosis with an apparently "normal" anion gap if this is not considered.

Lactic acidosis represents the most frequent cause of acidosis in hospitalized patients. Most commonly, it arises as a result of impaired tissue oxygenation caused by a reduction in tissue perfusion or hypoxia. Hepatic dysfunction may also be associated with the presence of a lactic acidosis because of impaired lactate clearance. An anion gap acidosis is also a feature of renal failure. In uncomplicated renal failure, typically the anion gap does not exceed 23 and the serum bicarbonate does not drop below 12. If the acidosis extends beyond these parameters, another cause of acidosis should be considered.

The principal early manifestation of metabolic acidosis is an increase in minute ventilation primarily resulting from an increased tidal volume. The increase in minute ventilation serves to compensate for the metabolic acidosis by eliminating more CO_2. The appropriate ventilatory response should reduce $PaCO_2$ by 1 mmHg (from 40 mmHg) for every 1 mmol/l drop in HCO_3^-. If the reduction in CO_2 is less than expected, then ventilatory support should be strongly considered because any further aggravation of the acidosis may lead to rapid decompensation. As the pH drops below 7.2, loss of vasomotor tone and a reduction in myocardial contracility may lead to cardiovascular collapse.

Treatment of metabolic acidosis is dependent on the underlying etiology. In the case of lactic acidosis, efforts should be directed toward optimizing tissue perfusion through administration of crystalloid solutions or blood products. Administration of sodium bicarbonate is usually not indicated unless the acidosis is severe (pH < 7.15; $HCO_3^- < 12$ mmol/l). At this point the buffering capacity is markedly reduced and any further reduction in pH can lead to vasomotor collapse. Further, at a pH below 7.2, catecholamine resistance develops such that the myocardium and resistance vessels may not respond to either endogenous or exogenous catecholamines.

Metabolic Alkalosis

Primary metabolic alkalosis is characterized by an elevated plasma HCO_3^- concentration in the presence of an arterial pH greater than 7.4. Manifestations are rare, but when they do occur are chiefly those of excess neuromuscular excitability including paresthesias, carpopedal spasm, or light-headedness. Ventricular irritability may also be present at pH greater than 7.55. The expected respiratory response is a reduction in minute ventilation such that for every 1 mmol/l increase in plasma [HCO_3^-] there should be a 0.7 mmHg increase in $PaCO_2$.

An elevation in plasma [HCO_3^-] may occur as a result of one of three mechanisms: loss of acid from the gastrointestinal tract or urine; administration of HCO_3^- or a precursor, such as citrate (e.g., as occurs following massive blood transfusions); or loss of fluid with a high chloride/bicarbonate ratio. Treatment should be directed toward the underlying cause.

TABLE 3.8. Respiratory Acid–Base Disorders by Mechanism.

Respiratory acidosis	Respiratory alkalosis

Reduced respiratory drive
  Sedatives, hypnotics, narcotics
  CNS lesions
	Increased respiratory drive
	  Pain, fever, gram-negative sepsis, cirrhosis, CNS lesions,
	    pregnancy (progesterone effect) salicylates, theophylline

Increased work of breathing
  Restrictive lung disease: pulmonary
    fibrosis, pleural effusions,
    ankylosing spondylitis
  Obstructive lung disease: upper air
    obstruction, asthma
	Peripheral chemoreceptor stimulation
	  Hypoxia, hypotension

Myopathies
  Paralysis, Guillan–Barre syndrome
	Pulmonary receptor stimulation
	  Pneumonia, pulmonary edema, pulmonary embolus

Increased CO_2 production in concert with a fixed minute ventilation: e.g., fever, seizures, large pulmonary embolus	

Respiratory Acid–Base Disorders

Respiratory acid–base disorders are categorized as either acute or chronic. Chronic respiratory acid–base disorders differ from acute disorders because of the time available for renal alterations in either excretion of NH_4^+ or reabsorption of HCO_3^-. This renal compensatory response may occur after several hours or days. Chronic respiratory disorders have a renal response that leads to increased serum bicarbonate in respiratory acidosis and a decreased serum bicarbonate in respiratory alkalosis. By contrast, acute changes are characterized by significant changes in Pa_{CO_2} with minimal alterations in serum HCO_3^-.

In respiratory acidosis, a reduction in effective minute ventilation leads to an increase in Pa_{CO_2} and a reduction in pH. If the acidosis is acute, there should be no more than a 3 to 4 mEq/l rise in HCO_3^- as the result of cellular buffering. If chronic, there should be a 0.3 mEq/l increase in HCO_3^- for each 1 mmHg increment in Pa_{CO_2}. The most common cause of respiratory acidosis in postoperative patients is central respiratory depression due to excessive postoperative sedatives or narcotics (Table 3.8). In a patient with a fixed minute volume (e.g., on a mechanical ventilator), an increase in Pa_{CO_2} suggests either an increase in alveolar dead space (e.g., pulmonary embolus) or increased CO_2 production. The treatment of respiratory acidosis should be directed toward the underlying cause. If the cause is not easily correctable and the acidosis is severe, then assisted ventilation will be necessary. Administration of exogenous HCO_3^- may lead to a further increase in Pa_{CO_2} and is therefore not indicated.

Respiratory alkalosis is common in surgical patients. Typically, excessive pain, fever, or gram-negative sepsis lead to an increase in central respiratory drive, causing a reduction in Pa_{CO_2}, and, if chronic, a compensatory increase in serum HCO_3^- (Table 3.8). If the alkalosis is acute, then there should be no greater than a 3 to 4 mEq/l reduction in serum HCO_3^-. In chronic respiratory alkalosis, a reduction in HCO_3^- of 0.4 to 0.5 mEq/l for each 1 mmHg reduction in Pa_{CO_2} is expected. If treatment is indicated, it should be directed toward the underlying cause.

References

1. Brecher ME, Monk T, Goodnough LT. A standardized method for calculating blood loss. Transfusion 1997;37:1074.
2. Budny PG, Regan PJ, Roberts AH. The estimation of blood loss during burn surgery. Burns 1993;19:134–137.
3. Halperin ML, Goldstein MB. Fluids, Electrolytes and Acid-Base Physiology, 2nd Ed. Philadelphia: Saunders, 1998.
4. Robertson GL. Regulation of vasopressin secretion. In: Seldin DW, Giebisch G, eds. The Kidney: Physiology and Pathophysiology, 2nd Ed. New York: Raven Press, 1992.
5. Lafferty FW. Differential diagnosis of hypercalcemia. J Bone Miner Res 1991;6:S51–S59.
6. Fatemi S, Ryzen E, Flores J, Endres DB, Rude RK. Effect of experimental human magnesium depletion on parathyroid hormone secretion and 1,25-dihydroxyvitamin D metabolism. J Clin Endocrinol Metab 1991;73:1067–1072.
7. George R, Shiu MH. Hypophosphatemia after major hepatic resection. Surgery (St. Louis) 1992;111:281–286.
8. Solomon SM, Kirby DF. The refeeding syndrome: a review. J Parenter Enteral Nutr 1990;14:90–97.

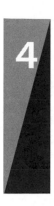

4

Hemostasis and Coagulation

Marcel Levi and Tom van der Poll

Basic Considerations

Current Insights into the Function of the Hemostatic System In Vivo

Blood coagulation can be divided into three parts: (1) primary hemostasis, consisting of the formation of a platelet plug and the occurrence of vasoconstriction, as a first line of defense of the body against bleeding; (2) fibrin formation, as a result of the activation of various coagulation proteins, which ultimately results in the generation of thrombin and subsequent fibrinogen to fibrin conversion; and (3) removal of fibrin, which is a function of the fibrinolytic system.[1,2]

PRIMARY HEMOSTASIS

After disruption of the integrity of the vessel wall, platelets adhere to the (sub)endothelium by means of their surface membrane glycoprotein receptor Ib. The ligand between this receptor and the vessel wall is the circulating protein named von Willebrand factor. As a consequence, the platelet becomes activated, which results in the expression of the platelet membrane surface receptor glycoprotein IIb/IIIa. Subsequently, platelets may aggregate with each other through this receptor, using circulating fibrinogen as a ligand. Red blood cells appear to play an important role in platelet adhesion and aggregation, potentially because of their physical capability to facilitate platelet transport to the surface (Fig. 4.1). Therefore, adequate function of primary hemostasis is dependent on a sufficiently high hematocrit.[3]

During the activation of the platelets and via a series of enzymatic reactions, arachidonic acid (from the platelet membrane) is converted into several eicosanoids, such as thromboxane A2 and various prostaglandins. These mediators may exert a vasoconstricting action and thus promote further activation of primary hemostasis. Another consequence of platelet activation is the release of various proteins from platelet storage granules, including (1) several platelet agonists (such as ADP and serotonin), (2) coagulation factors (such as von Willebrand factor and coagulation factor V), (3) heparin-binding proteins (such as platelet factor 4 and β-thromboglobulin), and (4) proteins with activity as a growth factor or chemokine (such as platelet-derived growth factor [PDGF], platelet transforming growth factor-β_1 [platelet TGF-β_1], epidermal growth factor, or thrombopoietin [TPO]). Last, the phospholipid membrane of the activated platelet provides an excellent surface on which the generation of thrombin and subsequent fibrin formation may take place.[4]

BLOOD COAGULATION

Although the coagulation system has traditionally been divided into an intrinsic and extrinsic pathway, such a division does not exist in vivo.[5] A schematic outline of the activation of coagulation in vivo is provided in Figure 4.2.

The principal route of activation of blood coagulation is via the tissue factor–factor VII pathway (the former "extrinsic system"). Tissue factor is a membrane-associated glycoprotein that is not in contact with the blood under physiological circumstances. Tissue factor is present at subendothelial sites and becomes exposed to the blood upon disruption of the normal architecture of the blood vessel. Alternatively, tissue factor can be expressed by endothelial cells or by mononuclear cells in response to certain stimuli, such as inflammatory mediators. After exposition of tissue factor to blood, a complex between tissue factor and factor VII occurs, upon which factor VII is converted into its active form (factor VIIa). The tissue factor–factor VII(a) complex subsequently binds and activates factor X, resulting in factor Xa. Once factor Xa is formed, it converts prothrombin (factor II) to thrombin (factor IIa). This enzymatic reaction requires the presence of factor V as a cofactor, and is most efficient in the presence of a suitable phospholipid surface, such as that provided by the activated platelet.

An alternative route for factor Xa activation by the tissue factor–factor VIIa complex is by the activation of factor IX. The importance of this "secondary" pathway for activation of coagulation is best illustrated by the striking hemorrhagic

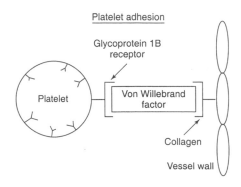

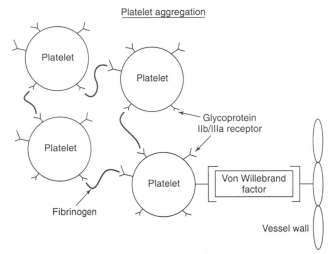

FIGURE 4.1. Platelet adherence to endothelium occurs via interaction of the platelet receptor and von Willebrand factor (*top*). This mechanism results in activation and expression of additional platelet receptors, which may aggregate via fibrinogen to other platelets (*bottom*).

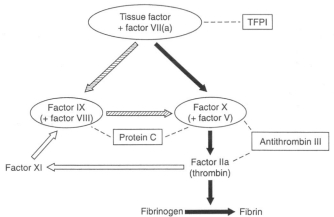

FIGURE 4.2. Schematic representation of the function of blood coagulation in vivo. The principal route of thrombin generation proceeds by the direct activation of factor X by the tissue factor–factor VIIa complex (*black arrows*). An alternative pathway is formed by the activation of factor IX by the tissue factor–factor VIIa complex and the activation of factor X by this activated factor IX (and cofactor VIII) (*shaded arrows*). A third amplifying pathway consists of the thrombin-mediated activation of factor XI, which can subsequently activate factor IX and X (*open arrows*). The point of impact of the three inhibitory systems (antithrombin III, the protein C and S system, and tissue factor pathway inhibitor [TFPI], respectively) are indicated with the *dotted lines*.

diathesis of patients with a deficiency of factor VIII or IX (hemophilia A and B, respectively; the incidence of hemophilia A and B is 1:10,000 and 1:70,000, respectively). A third amplifying pathway of the blood coagulation system consists of the activation of factor XI by thrombin. Factor XIa subsequently activates factor IX, resulting in further factor Xa and thrombin generation.

Thrombin is the key enzyme in the activation of coagulation. The presence of thrombin is not only essential for the conversion of fibrinogen into fibrin, but thrombin is also able to activate various coagulation factors and cofactors, thereby strongly facilitating its own formation. In addition, thrombin is a very strong activator of platelet aggregation. The formation of cross-linked fibrin is the ultimate step in the coagulation cascade. To further stabilize the clot, cross-linking of fibrin takes place by thrombin-activated factor XIII.

Synthesis of most of the coagulation factors takes place in the liver. Some coagulation factors (II, VII, IX, and X) require the presence of vitamin K for proper synthesis: in the absence of vitamin K, inactive precursor molecules are formed.

Natural Anticoagulant Mechanisms

Activation of the coagulation system is regulated at various points (see Fig. 4.2).[6] Inhibition of the tissue factor–factor VIIa complex may occur by the action of tissue factor pathway in-

hibitor (TFPI), a surface-associated protease inhibitor. Further regulation takes place by the protein C system. Activated protein C, assisted by its essential cofactor (protein S), proteolytically degrades the important cofactors V and VIII. Activated protein C is formed upon activation of circulating protein C by the endothelial cell-bound enzyme thrombomodulin in association with thrombin. Hence, thrombin not only plays a pivotal role in coagulation activation but is also involved in the inhibition of blood coagulation. Both protein C and protein S are vitamin K-dependent proteins. A third inhibitory system is formed by antithrombin III: This serine protease inhibitor forms complexes with thrombin and factor Xa, thereby losing their coagulant activity. The inhibitory action of antithrombin III on thrombin and factor Xa is strongly amplified in the presence of heparin.

A (usually hereditary) deficiency of antithrombin III, protein C, or protein S results in a procoagulant state, and patients with these deficiencies are prone to develop thrombosis. This development may occur in particular in situations with an enhanced thrombotic risk, such as the puerperium or postoperatively. A situation in which there is normal functional protein C but an impaired sensitivity of factor V to protein C is called activated protein C resistance (APC resistance) and is caused by a point mutation in factor V (factor V Leiden). The prevalence of this mutation is about 3% to 5% in the general population and may account for about 30% of all idiopathic venous thromboembolism.

Fibrinolysis

Fibrin plays only a temporary role and must be removed to restore normal tissue structure and function. The enzymatic degradation of fibrin is carried out by the fibrinolytic system, which is partly responsible for the unobstructed flow of blood. The function of the fibrinolytic system is schematically

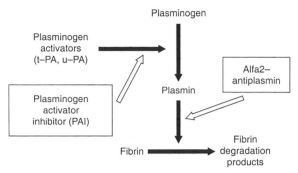

FIGURE 4.3. Schematic representation of the fibrinolytic system. Activation of fibrinolysis is indicated with *black arrows* and inhibition of the system by the *open arrows*.

represented in Figure 4.3. The pivotal event in the process of fibrinolysis is the conversion of the inactive zymogen plasminogen into the active protease plasmin, which cleaves cross-linked fibrin, resulting in the dissolution of a clot. Plasminogen activators, of which tissue-type plasminogen activator (tPA) and urokinase-type plasminogen activator (uPA) are most important, mediate the conversion of plasminogen into plasmin. Both activators are present in endothelial cells and may be released by various stimuli, including hypoxia and acidosis, as may occur during thrombotic occlusion. Inhibition of the fibrinolytic system may occur at the level of the plasminogen activators by plasminogen activator inhibitors (such as PAI-1) or at the level of plasmin by circulating protease inhibitors, of which α_2-antiplasmin is the most important one.

An imbalance between activators and inhibitors of the fibrinolytic system, resulting in a net antifibrinolytic state, may contribute to the development of thrombosis. The efficacy of postoperative pneumatic calf compression may be based not only on rheological advantages in the venous circulation but also result from the enhanced release of plasminogen activators from the vessel wall upon compression (and venous occlusion), thereby compensating for this fibrinolytic imbalance.

Anticoagulant Agents

ANTIPLATELET AGENTS

Platelets play a pivotal role in primary hemostasis and in the initiation of arterial and, to a lesser extent, venous thrombosis. Inhibition of platelet activity has been shown to be an effective strategy in the prevention and treatment of thromboembolic disease.

The antiplatelet effect of *aspirin* is based on the irreversible inhibition of the platelet membrane-associated enzyme cyclooxygenase. Cyclooxygenase is a crucial enzyme in the arachidonic acid metabolic pathway, and inhibition of this enzyme blocks the formation of thromboxane A_2, a potent platelet agonist and mediator of vasoconstriction. Low doses of aspirin preferentially inhibit the formation of platelet thromboxane A_2, whereas interference with the formation of other prostaglandins such as the platelet antagonist and vasodilator prostacyclin (PGI$_2$) by endothelial cells seems less prominent. The use of aspirin results in an irreversible (and relatively weak) inhibition of platelet aggregation; and may

be associated with significant impairment of primary hemostasis and a mild enhancement of bleeding as a consequence. In view of the life span of platelets (approximately 10 days), 5 to 7 days are usually required after termination of aspirin use to restore an adequate platelet function and effective hemostasis. The most important adverse effects of aspirin are bleeding and the occurrence of hemorrhagic gastritis or even gastric ulceration.

Dipyridamole exerts its antiplatelet effect by inhibition of phosphodiesterase, resulting in the intracellular accumulation of cyclic AMP, which has an antiaggregating effect. However, it has not shown any significant efficacy on the prevention of thromboembolic disease in large clinical trials. Another novel class of platelet inhibitors is represented by ADP-inhibitors, such as *Clopidogral (Plavix R)*.

Inhibitors of the glycoprotein receptor IIb/IIIa represent a new generation of antiplatelet agents that has been recently introduced. This group includes compounds such as tirofiban and the monoclonal antibody abciximax (Reopro®). These agents are potent inhibitors of platelet function. Their relative efficacy and safety are currently being evaluated in clinical trials.

VITAMIN K ANTAGONISTS (COUMARIN DERIVATIVES)

Oral anticoagulant agents are *coumarin* derivatives, such as warfarin, acenocoumarol, and phenprocoumon.[7] These compounds block the essential vitamin K-dependent carboxylation of coagulation factors II, VII, IX, and X, resulting in the formation of biologically inactive proteins and a decrease in the coagulant activity of these factors in plasma. The half-life of vitamin K-dependent coagulation factors ranges from 6 (factor VII) to 60 h (factor II); hence, the full effect of therapy is delayed for 2 or 3 days. Also, full restoration of normal coagulation after termination of coumarin therapy requires at least 3 to 5 days. The dose–effect relationship of oral anticoagulants may vary considerably both between patients (interindividual) and in any patient over time (intraindividual) as the result of changes in binding to plasma albumin, variable vitamin K intake, and variable clearance by the liver. Therefore, close monitoring of the intensity of anticoagulation is required. To do so, the prothrombin time (PT) determination is most often used. To correct for considerable differences in thromboplastin sensitivity, the International Normalized Ratio (INR) has been established. The INR corrects for the differences of the various thromboplastins used in the prothrombin time assays as compared to an international reference thromboplastin preparation. Increasing values of the INR represent higher intensities of anticoagulation, an INR of 1.0 indicating no anticoagulation. The most important side effect of coumarin treatment is bleeding.

HEPARIN AND LOW MOLECULAR WEIGHT HEPARIN

Heparin binds to antithrombin III, thereby potentiating the inhibitory effect of antithrombin III on coagulation factors IIa (thrombin) and Xa more than 1000-fold. The effect of heparin after intravenous administration is immediate, and heparin has a dose-dependent half-life: After the intravenous administration of a bolus dose of 5,000 units, the mean half-life is approximately 60 to 90 min. Also, the anticoagulant effect of heparin may be highly variable, and therefore frequent labo-

TABLE 4.1. Summary of Randomized Controlled Trials on the Efficacy and Safety of Low Molecular Weight Heparin in the Prevention of Postoperative Venous Thromboembolism in Patients Undergoing General Surgery, Major Orthopedic Surgery (Total Hip Replacement and Total Knee Replacement), and Trauma Surgery (level I evidence).

Type of surgery	No. of trials	No. of patients	Incidence of venous thromboembolism (95% CI)	Relative risk reduction of postoperative venous thromboembolism (compared with placebo)	Increase in total bleeding complications (compared with placebo) (95% CI)	Increase in major bleeding complications (compared with placebo) (95% CI)
General surgery	12	4386	5% (4–6)	80%	16%	3%
Major orthopedic surgery	30	4712	21% (20–22)	71%	7%	−1%
Trauma surgery	5	437	28%	44%	11%	0%

Source:
Koch A, Bouges S, Ziegler S, Dinkel H, Daures JP, Victor N. Low molecular weight heparin and unfractionated heparin in thrombosis prophylaxis after major surgical intervention. Update of previous meta-analyses. Br J Surg 1997;84:750–759.

Palmer AJ, Koppenhagen K, Kirchhof B, Weber U, Bergemann R. Efficacy and safety of low molecular weight heparin, unfractionated heparin and warfarin for thrombo-embolism prophylaxis in orthopaedic surgery: a meta-analysis of randomised clinical trials. Haemostasis 1997;27:75–84.

ratory monitoring is required. Usually the activated partial thromboplastin time (aPTT) is used to tailor heparin treatment. In special conditions, such as extracorporeal cardiopulmonary bypass, the whole blood activated clotting time (ACT) may be applied.

Low molecular weight heparins have recently been introduced that have an average molecular weight between 4 and 6 kDa.[8] In some situations these heparin fractions have shown a more favorable antithrombotic effect and induce less bleeding complications at therapeutic doses as compared to unfractionated heparin. In addition, low molecular weight heparins have a highly predictable inter- and intraindividual bioavailability and clearance, thereby precluding the need for frequent laboratory monitoring and frequent dose adjustments. The much longer half-life of low molecular weight heparins as compared to unfractionated heparin is advantageous in situations in which stable anticoagulation is required over a longer period of time. Large randomized controlled trials have demonstrated the efficacy and safety of low molecular weight heparin in the postoperative prevention of venous thromboembolism in various surgical patients (Table 4.1).

Bleeding is the most frequently encountered adverse effect of heparin treatment. In addition, heparin-induced thrombocytopenia (HIT) may occur. This entity is an immunological response to heparin characterized by the occurrence of thrombocytopenia and venous and arterial thromboembolism. HIT usually occurs at 5 to 7 days after initial exposure to heparin, but may be an immediate complication if the patient has received heparin previously. It is essential to immediately discontinue heparin in patients with HIT. Alternative anticoagulant therapy may consist of treatment with hirudin or heparinoids but not with coumarin derivatives, which may promote skin necrosis. Last, long-term use of heparin has been associated with the occurrence of osteopenia. These adverse effects appear to have a lower incidence if low molecular weight heparin is used.

THROMBOLYTIC AGENTS

Rapid dissolution of clots can be attained by the administration of thrombolytic agents. All thrombolytic agents are plasminogen activators, either recombinant endogenous plasminogen activators (such as recombinant tPA), administered at a dose that is 1000-fold higher than physiological concentration, or derived from exogenous sources, such as streptokinase. The most important side effect of thrombolytic treatment is bleeding.

Prohemostatic Agents

PLATELETS, PLASMA, AND COAGULATION FACTOR CONCENTRATES

Platelet transfusion may be considered in patients with severe thrombocytopenia and bleeding or a risk for bleeding. Platelet concentrates usually contain a mixture of the platelet preparation of the blood donation from six donors (6 units). After platelet transfusion, the platelet count should rise by at least 5×10^9/l per unit of platelets transfused. Guidelines for platelet transfusion are given in Table 4.2.

Fresh or frozen plasma contains all coagulation factors and may be used to replenish congenital or acquired deficiencies in these factors. For more specific therapy, or if the transfusion of large volumes of plasma is not desirable, fractionated plasma of purified coagulation factor concentrate is available.[9] Suggested guidelines for the use of fresh frozen plasma are given in Table 4.3.

Prothrombin complex concentrates (PCCs) contain the vitamin K-dependent coagulation factors II, VII, IX, and X. Hence, these concentrates may be used if immediate reversal of coumarin therapy is required.

Cryoprecipitate is fractionated plasma that contains mainly von Willebrand factor, factor VIII, and fibrinogen. However, because of problems in the production of cryopre-

TABLE 4.2. Suggested Transfusion Guidelines for Platelet Concentrates.

Platelet count $<10 \times 10^9$/l

Platelet count $<50 \times 10^9$/l with demonstrated bleeding or a planned surgical/invasive procedure

Documented platelet dysfunction (e.g., prolonged bleeding time) with (microvascular) bleeding or undergoing a surgical/invasive procedure and (assumed) insufficient efficacy of other interventions (e.g., desmopressin)

Bleeding patients or patients undergoing a surgical procedure who require more than 10 U of packed red cells

TABLE 4.3. Suggested Transfusion Guidelines for Fresh Frozen Plasma.

Correction of multiple or specific coagulation factor deficiencies in bleeding patients or if a surgical/invasive procedure is planned
> Congenital deficiencies of a specific factor (provided specific factor concentrates are not available, e.g., factor XI)
>
> Acquired deficiencies, e.g., related to liver disease, massive transfusion, or disseminated intravascular coagulation

Volume replacement in case of severe bleeding to avoid massive transfusion of gelatin or crystalloid solutions

Thrombocytopenic thrombotic purpura

cipitate, particularly with regard to standards to prevent the transmission of infectious agents, in most parts of the Western World cryoprecipitate is not readily available.

Purified concentrates containing only that specific factor are available for a selected number of clotting factors. These concentrates are particularly useful in cases of isolated (usually congenital) deficiency of a single clotting factor, such as factor VIII concentrate for the treatment of hemophilia A.

Clotting factor concentrates derived from plasma are of human origin. Potentially, these carry the risk of transmission of blood-borne diseases. Despite all current measures to prevent this complication, these risks are not fully eliminated. Hence, the use of these products should be limited as much as possible, especially if no strict indication is present or an alternative treatment is available.

DESMOPRESSIN

Deamino-D-arginine vasopressin (DDAVP, desmopressin) is a vasopressin analogue that induces release of the contents of the endothelial cell-associated Weibel–Palade bodies, including von Willebrand factor.[10] Hence, the administration of DDAVP results in a marked increase in the plasma concentration of von Willebrand factor (and associated coagulation factor VIII). DDAVP can be administered by different routes (intravenously, subcutaneously, and intranasally) but is usually administered by intravenous administration, resulting in an immediate prohemostatic effect. DDAVP is used for the prevention and treatment of bleeding in patients with von Willebrand disease or mild hemophilia A. It is also used in patients with an impaired function of primary hemostasis, such as those with uremia, liver cirrhosis, or aspirin-associated bleeding.

RECOMBINANT FACTOR VIIa

Given that activation of coagulation in vivo predominantly proceeds by the tissue factor–factor VII(a) pathway, recombinant factor VIIa has been developed as a prohemostatic agent and has recently become available for clinical use. Although no thrombotic complications of recombinant factor VIIa treatment have been reported thus far, the safety of this strategy in a general population remains to be established.

ANTIFIBRINOLYTIC AGENTS

Agents that exert antifibrinolytic activity are aprotinin and the group of lysine analogues.[11] The prohemostatic effect of these agents proceeds both by the inhibition of fibrinolysis (thereby shifting the procoagulant–anticoagulant balance to-

ward a more procoagulant state) and by a protective effect on platelets.

Aprotinin directly inhibits the activity of various serine proteases, including plasmin, coagulation factors or inhibitors, and constituents of the kallikrein-kinin and angiotensin system. The most important clinical side effect of aprotinin is a rarely occurring, but sometimes serious, allergic or anaphylactic reaction. The use of aprotinin is contraindicated in cases of ongoing systemic intravascular activation of coagulation, as in disseminated intravascular coagulation (DIC) and in patients with renal failure.

Lysine analogues (i.e., ε-aminocaproic acid and tranexamic acid) are potent inhibitors of fibrinolysis. The antifibrinolytic action of lysine analogues is based on the competitive binding of these agents to the lysine-binding sites of a fibrin clot, thereby competing with the binding of plasminogen. Impaired plasminogen binding to fibrin delays the conversion of plasminogen to plasmin and subsequent plasmin-mediated fibrinolysis. The use of lysine analogues is contraindicated in situations with ongoing systemic activation of coagulation (such as in DIC) and in cases of macroscopic hematuria because the inhibition of fibrinolysis may result in deposition of urinary tract-obstructing clots.

OTHER PROHEMOSTATIC AGENTS

Conjugated estrogen preparations may also improve primary hemostasis. Currently there is no sound evidence for the use of these agents to prevent or treat perioperative bleeding.

Fibrin sealant, usually consisting of a combination of human fibrinogen and bovine thrombin, may be used as a topical hemostatic agent. Although a number of controlled studies have shown the efficacy of this treatment in various surgical situations, there is no evidence that application of fibrin sealant results in a reduction of intraoperative or postoperative blood loss or other clinically significant outcome measures. In addition, fibrinogen is usually derived from human donor plasma and may carry the risk of transmission of blood-borne diseases. Further, the bovine origin of the thrombin may result in the formation of anticoagulation factor antibodies cross-reacting with human coagulation factors, resulting in a potentially severe bleeding tendency.

Monitoring of Blood Coagulation

For proper function of primary hemostasis, a platelet count of at least 30 to 50×10^9 is required. The function of the primary hemostatic system may be tested by performance of the bleeding time. However, clinical studies have shown that there is no correlation between the result of the bleeding time and the occurrence and intensity of perioperative bleeding.

Most frequently used screening tests for blood coagulation are the prothrombin time (PT) and the activated partial thromboplastin time (aPTT). Although both PT and aPTT are highly artificial and do not fully reflect coagulation in vivo, these tests are useful to screen for deficiencies of single or multiple coagulation factors. In case of an abnormal test result, assaying the coagulant activity of selected coagulation factors can be performed to more incisively analyze the function of blood coagulation. In addition, the PT is used to monitor coumarin treatment, whereas the aPTT is most frequently used to monitor the intensity of heparin anticoagulation.

Clinical Management of Coagulation Abnormalities and Bleeding

Conditions Associated with an Enhanced Risk of Perioperative Bleeding

CONGENITAL COAGULATION ABNORMALITIES

Congenital defects, either in primary hemostasis or in the blood coagulation system, may cause very serious intraoperative and postoperative bleeding. Albeit not an absolute rule, a defect in primary hemostasis will cause immediate hemostatic problems, whereas a defective blood coagulation system may cause postoperative bleeding up to 1 week after surgery.

The most frequently occurring congenital defect in primary hemostasis is a deficiency of von Willebrand factor, also called *von Willebrand disease.* (The incidence of severe von Willebrand disease is estimated at 1:25,000, but milder forms of this disorder may be present in 1 to 5 of 1,000 patients.) Low levels of von Willebrand factor are usually associated with low levels of factor VIII and a resulting impairment of blood coagulation. A typical patient with von Willebrand disease has a lifelong bleeding tendency, particularly of mucosal tissues (such as gingival or nose bleeding). Laboratory tests will reveal a prolonged bleeding time and low level of von Willebrand factor (and factor VIII) levels. Treatment of or prevention of bleeding in a patient undergoing an invasive procedure may consist of the administration of desmopressin, which will result in a two- to threefold increase in endogenous von Willebrand factor levels. If desmopressin has an insufficient effect when retested, von Willebrand factor concentrate may be administered. Also, adjunctive treatment with lysine analogues has proven to be effective.

Other congenital defects in primary hemostasis are *thrombocytopathies*, including the rarely occurring deficiencies of platelet membrane glycoproteins. The inability of platelets to release their contents upon activation (storage pool disease) is another cause of thrombocytopathy. No specific cause can be found in a considerable number of thrombocytopathies. All thrombocytopathies are detected by a prolonged bleeding time. Small uncontrolled trials indicate that a sufficient improvement of primary hemostasis may be achieved by the administration of desmopressin, potentially in combination with lysine analogues.[12] If this is not sufficient, a platelet transfusion should be considered. The best known congenital defects in blood coagulation are *hemophilia A* and *hemophilia B*, deficiencies of factor VIII and IX, respectively. Severe hemophilia (factor VIII or IX <1%) is characterized by a spontaneous bleeding tendency, particularly in muscles and joints. Moderate or mild hemophilia usually presents with bleeding after trauma or an invasive medical intervention. Spontaneous bleeding is rare. A deficiency in factor XI is a relatively frequent disorder and is associated with a bleeding tendency of a variable degree. Deficiencies in all other coagulation proteins do occur, but are relatively rare.

Coagulation factor deficiencies may be detected by prolonged clotting times (aPTT or PT), and subsequent analysis reveals a low level of the deficient factor. These screening tests do not detect a deficiency of factor XIII, which is characterized by rebleeding after initial adequate hemostasis. Treatment of coagulation factor deficiencies may be achieved by administration of coagulation factor concentrate. In case of a patient with hemophilia who must undergo a major sur-

gical intervention, coagulation factor administration should continue for at least 7 to 10 days.

LIVER FAILURE

Because the liver produces most coagulation factors, insufficient liver function is associated with low levels of coagulation factors.[13] A deficiency of vitamin K, as in cases of biliary tract obstruction or resulting from loss of storage sites in hepatocellular disease, may further lower levels of vitamin K-dependent factors. If liver failure is associated with portal hypertension and associated splenomegaly, a serious thrombocytopenia may also exist. In cirrhotic patients, impaired platelet function is often encountered. Because of these combined coagulation defects, patients with liver failure are at a considerable risk of perioperative bleeding.[14] Management of such patients includes perioperative assessment of the coagulation status by measuring platelet count, bleeding time, aPTT, and PT (and potentially one or two coagulation factors). A potential vitamin K deficiency should be treated with vitamin K_1. Correction of low levels of coagulation factors may be achieved by the administration of plasma or prothrombin complex concentrates. Large quantities of plasma, however, may precipitate hepatic encephalopathy or cause fluid overload. Patients with a severe thrombocytopenia (i.e., platelets <30–50×10^9/l) should receive a transfusion with platelet suspension. However, platelet concentrates may be effective only briefly because of the rapid removal of platelets by the enlarged spleen. In addition, small controlled studies have shown that the administration of desmopressin may result in an improvement of the bleeding time, although it is not clear whether this treatment reduces the risk of perioperative bleeding.[15]

RENAL FAILURE

Patients with renal failure often present with coagulation abnormalities and are at risk for enhanced bleeding. The hemorrhagic tendency in patients with uremia can be attributed to an impaired platelet adhesion, aggregation, and release. In addition, a low hematocrit in patients with renal failure may contribute to the impaired function of primary hemostasis.[16] The extent of the defect in primary hemostasis may be established by the bleeding time. The administration of desmopressin has been shown to result in a correction of the prolonged bleeding time in patients with uremia.[17] If an insufficient correction of the bleeding time is achieved, the administration of platelet concentrates could be added to the desmopressin treatment. Additional measures include the correction of anemia and execution of hemodialysis, which has been shown to (partially) restore the function of primary hemostasis.

VITAMIN K DEFICIENCY

Vitamin K is essential for the production of several coagulation factors (factor II, VII, IX, and X), and a deficiency in vitamin K results in low plasma levels of these factors. A vitamin K deficiency will result in a prolongation of global coagulation times, in particular the prothrombin time. Diagnosis of vitamin K deficiency can be made by administering vitamin K and observing the effect on the PT, which should be corrected within 24 h. Vitamin K_1 (usually 10 mg) can be administered orally and parenterally, but oral treatment is obviously not adequate in case of insufficient adsorption. Intravenous administration is preferred over intramuscular treatment (in view of the risk of muscle bleeds in patients with low levels of coagulation factors), but may be associated with a (small) risk of an adverse response. If immediate correction of deficiency of vitamin K-dependent coagulation factors is required, the administration of prothrombin complex concentrate will immediately restore the defect.

IMMUNE THROMBOCYTOPENIA AND OTHER IMMUNE COAGULATION DISORDERS

Immune thrombocytopenia (immune thrombocytopenic purpura, ITP) is caused by the presence of autoantibodies, usually directed against platelet glycoproteins. Increased platelet destruction and removal by the reticuloendothelial system may result in splenomegaly. In severe cases, the platelet count may be as low as 10×10^9 platelets/l, and autoantibodies to platelets are almost always detectable in serum. In general, patients with autoimmune thrombocytopenia have an enhanced bleeding risk, and retrospective data indicate that a platelet count of less than 50×10^9/l might predispose for an enhanced risk of perioperative bleeding.[18] Infusion with human immunoglobulin may provide a rapidly occurring but relatively short-lasting increase in the platelet count, and thus may be useful in case a nonelective major invasive procedure is necessary. Transfusion of platelets may cause the formation of other antiplatelet antibodies and should be reserved for emergency situations. The incidence of major bleeding complications in patients with autoimmune thrombocytopenia is very low following an appropriate preoperative preparation.

The development of (auto)antibodies to a coagulation factor (most frequently factor VIII) causes a rare but dangerous disorder.[19] This disorder is characterized by a severe bleeding tendency and is associated with high morbidity and mortality from bleeding. Laboratory tests will reveal a prolongation of the aPTT or PT that is not shortened after addition of normal plasma. A definitive diagnosis can be made by measuring the individual coagulation factors and by quantification of the inhibitor. Treatment may consist of (high doses) coagulation factor concentrate, activated prothrombin complex concentrates, or recombinant factor VIIa. The management of this disorder is complicated and should be carried out in a specialized center.

OTHER CONDITIONS ASSOCIATED WITH COAGULATION ABNORMALITIES

Other conditions associated with coagulation abnormalities include myeloproliferative or lymphoproliferative disorders, which may be associated with defective primary hemostasis caused by a combination of thrombocytopenia and impaired platelet function. Patients with malignancies may present with diverse coagulation abnormalities resulting from impaired primary hemostasis, low-grade disseminated intravascular coagulation (see following), or systemic hyperfibrinolysis.

How to Identify Patients at Risk for Bleeding

The cornerstone for recognition of a clinically significant coagulation disorder is the medical history, which should include an inquiry specifically about previous surgical procedures, bleeding complicating trauma, and bleeding after tooth extraction. A potential congenital coagulation disorder might be identified on the basis of a history of lifelong bleeding complications after minor trauma or interventions and a bleeding tendency in other members of the family. In addition, the history should particularly focus on the use of drugs that might affect hemostasis. During physical examination, abnormal bruising, petechiae, and splenomegaly are signs that might point to a defect in the coagulation system. Retrospective and prospective studies have shown that routine coagulation tests for most surgical procedures are not useful in patients with a negative medical history and normal physical examination. If the history is suspicious for bleeding disorders and if screening test results are abnormal, further analysis should be carried out. Table 4.4 summarizes the potential causes of abnormalities in the screening tests and suggests some followup tests to further analyze these abnormalities.

Consequences of the Preoperative Use of Anticoagulant Agents for Perioperative Bleeding Complications

Anticoagulant and antiplatelet agents are important in the primary treatment and secondary prevention of atherothrombotic cardiovascular disease and venous thromboembolism. A growing number of patients who must undergo a surgical procedure will be using aspirin, other antiplatelet agents, or oral anticoagulants.

A number of studies have addressed the question whether the preoperative use of aspirin results in an increased risk of perioperative bleeding. For major surgical procedures, most trials indicate that the preoperative use of aspirin resulted in enhanced perioperative bleeding, more transfusion of red blood cells and other blood products, longer operation times, and a higher incidence of reoperation because of excessive bleeding.[20,21]

However, more recent trials showed that the use of lower doses of aspirin that are currently in use (100 mg daily), albeit associated with increased perioperative blood loss, is without an increase in the transfusion need, incidence of reoperation due to bleeding, or duration of hospital stay.[22] A number of small clinical studies have shown that the administration of deamino-D-arginine vasopressin (DDAVP, Desmopressin) may effectively reduce the antihemostatic effect of aspirin.[23] Infusion of DDAVP (0.3 μg/kg) in patients who had used aspirin within 7 days before surgery resulted in a reduction of total blood loss and decreased red cell transfusion as compared to placebo. In cardiac surgery, a similar effect may be achieved by the administration of aprotinin.

Aspirin treatment should be interrupted at least 5 to 7 days preoperatively in case of elective surgery. For nonelective and emergency situations, minor procedures can be performed without any specific intervention. For major surgery or those procedures where even minor blood loss is not desirable, transfusion of platelets or administration of desmopressin should be considered.

Prospective studies have shown that the preoperative use of other nonsteroidal antiinflammatory agents is not associated with enhanced perioperative bleeding.[24] As far as the preoperative use of *oral anticoagulants* is concerned, earlier studies showed an unacceptable high incidence of perioperative bleeding, in particular in case of major surgery. Prospective clinical trials, however, show that surgery may be safely per-

TABLE 4.4. Common Causes for Abnormalities in Coagulation Screening Tests and Suggestions for Initial Further Analysis.

Finding	Potential cause	Further test
Thrombocytopenia	Immune thrombocytopenia (ITP)	Antiplatelet antibodies, thrombopoietin
	Impaired platelet production	Complete blood cell count and bone marrow analysis
	Disseminated intravascular coagulation	aPTT, PT, fibrin degradation products
	Heparin-induced thrombocytopenia	HIT test
Prolonged bleeding time	von Willebrand disease or thrombocytopathie	Platelet aggregation tests and von Willebrand factor
	Uremia, liver failure myeloproliferative disorder, etc.	—
aPTT prolonged, PT normal	Coagulation factor deficiency (factor VIII, IX, XI, or XII)	Measure coagulation factor
	Use of heparin	—
PT prolonged, aPTT normal	Coagulation factor deficiency (factor VII)	Measure coagulation factor
	Vitamin K deficiency	Measure factor VII (vitamin K-dependent) and factor V (vitamin K-independent) or administer vitamin K and repeat after 1–2 days
	(Mild) hepatic insufficiency	—
Both aPTT and PT prolonged	Coagulation factor deficiency (factor X, V, II or fibrinogen)	Measure coagulation factor
	Use of oral anticoagulants	—
	Severe hepatic insufficiency	Measure coagulation factors
	Disseminated intravascular coagulation	Platelets, fibrin degradation products
	Loss/dilution caused by excessive bleeding/massive transfusion	—

formed at low levels of anticoagulation (INR <1.5).[25] The dose of coumarin should be significantly reduced preoperatively to achieve these levels. In csaes where the interruption of anticoagulant treatment for recent venous thromboembolism may place the patient at high risk for recurrence in the postoperative period, it might not be desirable to interrupt anticoagulant treatment. In such cases, interruption of oral anticoagulation and simultaneous initiation of intravenous heparin should be contemplated. Shortly before the operation, heparin may be discontinued and may be restarted at 6 to 12 hours postoperatively.[26] In case of nonelective surgery, a rapid (12–24 h) reversal of coumarin therapy may be achieved by the administration of 10 mg of vitamin K. This treatment should be continued for 3 to 5 days, dependent on the half-life of the type of coumarin used. If necessary, immediate and complete correction of coagulation may be achieved by the administration of prothrombin complex concentrate.

The preoperative use of prophylactic (low molecular weight) *heparin* for the prevention of postoperative venous thromboembolism is not associated with an enhanced risk of intraoperative and postoperative bleeding in a large series of randomized controlled trials.[27] In patients treated with therapeutic doses of heparin, discontinuation of heparin will result in a near normalization of coagulation in approximately 3 to 4 hours. If rapid reversal of heparin treatment is needed (for example, in case of severe bleeding), this may be achieved by the administration of protamine.

Reduction of Perioperative Blood Loss by Interventions in the Coagulation System

CARDIAC SURGERY

Cardiac surgery may be associated with blood loss resulting from hemostatic imbalances. These mechanisms include (1)

the loss of platelets and impairment of platelet function caused by cardiopulmonary bypass, (2) hemodilution with associated decreased plasma concentrations of coagulation factors, (3) incomplete neutralization of heparin given during cardiopulmonary bypass, and (4) an inadequate function of the fibrinolytic system for which no clear explanation is presently available. A number of pharmacological agents have been used in an effort to diminish bleeding associated with cardiopulmonary bypass.

A number of studies have focused on the potential beneficial effect of *aprotinin* on the prevention of excessive bleeding in patients undergoing cardiac surgery. Randomized, controlled trials have invariably shown that administration of aprotinin resulted in a reduction of perioperative blood loss, postoperative chest tube drainage, the number of transfused units, and the number of patients receiving any transfusion. Most studies have demonstrated at least a 40% reduction in perioperative blood and a 50% reduction in transfusion requirements.

The potential to reduce blood loss by another antifibrinolytic therapy, *lysine analogues*, has also been investigated in a number of clinical trials. Generally, ϵ-aminocaproic acid showed insufficient efficacy relative to tranexamic acid, and most studies have focused on the latter agent. Tranexamic acid reduced bleeding after cardiac surgery, resulting in reduced transfusion requirements and a smaller number of patients who needed any transfusion.

A number of recent studies have directly compared aprotinin and tranexamic acid. A meta-analysis of these trials appear to indicate a higher efficacy of aprotinin as compared with lysine analogues, although the differences in the most important clinical endpoints, mortality and rethoracotomy, did not reach statistical significance. Several meta-analyses of controlled clinical trials with *desmopressin* in cardiac surgery showed a beneficial effect on blood loss and transfusion requirements, whereas the percentage of patients who need any transfusion, the incidence of reexploration, and mortality are not statistically affected by desmopressin.[28] Subgroup analysis of the various clinical trials suggests that desmopressin might be particularly effective in case of the preoperative use of aspirin, which is not uncommon in patients undergoing cardiac surgery. The effect of desmopressin, however, appears to be relatively small as compared with aprotinin and tranexamic acid.

At this time, a potential prothrombotic and graft-occluding effect of these interventions has not been clearly established.

LIVER TRANSPLANTATION

Major liver surgery, including orthotopic liver transplantation, may be associated with excessive blood loss. Factors that contribute to this complication are impaired synthesis of coagulation proteins by the diseased liver, a preexisting thrombocytopenia and thrombocytopathy, and impaired clearance of activated coagulation and fibrinolytic factors during the anhepatic phase. However, definitive place of prohemostatic agents in extensive liver surgery needs to be established.

Management of Postoperative Bleeding

A central issue for a patient who has excessive bleeding during or after surgery is the decision whether the bleeding is a result of a systemic hemostatic defect or a local problem in surgical hemostasis. In all cases of severe bleeding, a global coagulation screening (i.e., platelet count, aPTT, PT) should be carried out as soon as possible. If these tests show abnormal results, a brief trial of therapy with replacement of deficient hemostatic factors should be provided. However, unless there is prompt cessation of bleeding, this treatment should not delay the decision to reoperate if even the smallest suspicion of a local surgical problem exists.

Systemic coagulation defects in bleeding patients with a previously normal coagulation system generally arise by two different mechanisms: (1) loss of platelets and coagulation factors due to bleeding and dilution of these elements upon massive transfusion of red cells and plasma substitutes, and (2) consumption of platelets and coagulation factors in the framework of disseminated intravascular coagulation.

Patients with severe blood loss may require massive fluid replacement therapy with blood substitutes such as crystalloid, colloid, dextran, and starch solutions. The use of these synthetic plasma volume expanders in excess of 1 l/h may in some cases be associated with an impairment of primary hemostasis (most probably the result of interference with von Willebrand factor function) and the plasma coagulation system (due to dilution). Therefore, if there is need for massive expansion of circulating volume in bleeding patients or patients at risk for bleeding, use of these preparations should be accompanied by administration with fresh frozen plasma.

Transfusion with large amounts of packed red cells without concomitant replacement of platelets and coagulation factors may cause a generalized dilution coagulopathy,[29] which is readily established by a decrease in platelet count to usually 50 to $100 \times 10^9/l$ and a prolongation of global clotting times (aPTT and PT). Although there is no evidence from clinical studies to support this practice, it is generally recommended that patients who need massive transfusion of red cells receive 1 unit of plasma for every 2 to 3 units of red cells

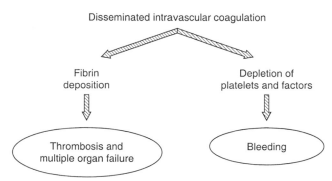

FIGURE 4.4. The clinical picture of disseminated intravascular coagulation (DIC), characterized by simultaneously occurring thrombosis and bleeding.

administered. Regarding low platelet count, retrospective analyses show that in bleeding patients with a platelet count lower than $50 \times 10^9/l$, transfusion of platelets is effective.[30] Hence, the threshold for platelet transfusion in patients with bleeding can be held at $50 \times 10^9/l$ unless defective platelet function is suspected.

Disseminated Intravascular Coagulation

Surgical patients may present with disseminated intravascular coagulation (DIC) because this is a frequent complication of a variety of disease states common in these patients, such as infection, severe trauma, or malignancies.[31] DIC is a syndrome and is always secondary to an underlying disorder. The syndrome is characterized by a systemic activation of the blood coagulation system, the generation and deposition of fibrin, microvascular thrombi in various organs, and in many cases the development of multiorgan failure (Fig. 4.4). Depletion of coagulation proteins and platelets resulting from the ongoing activation of the coagulation system may induce severe bleeding complications, although microclot formation may occur in the absence of severe clotting factor depletion and bleeding.[32] Severe bleeding from DIC poses a particular problem in trauma patients or during the early postoperative phase.

A spectrum of clinical entities have been associated with DIC, and the major conditions are listed in Table 4.5. Infection is the most common cause of DIC and, in patients with septic shock, DIC is a strong predictor of death.[33] Another cause of DIC is malignancy, although in that setting DIC usually is rel-

TABLE 4.5. Underlying Surgical Diseases Causing Acute or Chronic Disseminated Intravascular Coagulation (DIC)

Septicemia/infections

Polytrauma

Malignancies

Aortic aneurysm

Brain injury

Extended liver surgery

Extracorporeal circulation

Thermal injury/hypothermia

Fat embolism

Peritoneovenous shunt

Massive transfusion

atively mild. In contrast, the DIC that accompanies obstetrical catastrophes, such as abruptio placentae or amniotic fluid embolism, is very turbulent but usually self-limiting.

PATHOGENESIS OF DIC

DIC is characterized by widespread intravascular fibrin deposition resulting from enhanced fibrin formation and impaired fibrin degradation.[34] Enhanced fibrin formation is caused by tissue factor-mediated thrombin generation and simultaneously occurring depressing of inhibitory mechanisms (Fig. 4.5). That is, the normal counterbalance achieved by the anticoagulation systems (antithrombin III, protein C–protein S) is deranged, possibly due to increased factor consumption. Furthermore, impairment of endogenous fibrinolysis is mainly caused by high circulating levels of PAI-1, the principal inhibitor of plasminogen activation.

Thus, deposition of fibrin in the (micro)vasculature is caused by both the formation and its inadequate removal of intravascular fibrin. This inadequate removal is caused by an *impaired function of the fibrinolytic system.* Ultimately, the remarkable imbalance between coagulation and fibrinolysis results in a net procoagulant state.[35]

DIAGNOSIS OF DIC

No single laboratory test or combination of tests allows a definitive diagnosis of DIC. However, the clinical diagnosis can be made reliable by taking into consideration the underlying disease and a combination of laboratory findings. Hence, the diagnosis of DIC is usually based on markers of advanced consumption of coagulation proteins and platelets, that is, prolonged clotting times (aPTT and PT) and low platelets, in combination with tests that do not detect the generation but rather the degradation of fibrin (fibrin degradation products). Measurement of fibrinogen is commonly performed but has shown to be of no value for the diagnosis of DIC, especially because the acute-phase reactant properties of fibrinogen in many clinical situations may completely obscure ongoing fibrinogen consumption.

MANAGEMENT OF DIC

The cornerstone of DIC treatment is the specific and vigorous treatment of the underlying disorder. In some cases, DIC will completely resolve within hours after the resolution of the underlying condition, as, for example, in the case of DIC induced by abruptio placentae and amniotic fluid embolism. However, in other cases, such as in patients with sepsis and a systemic inflammatory response syndrome, DIC may be present for a number of days, even after proper treatment has been initiated. Under such circumstances, supportive measures to manage DIC may be necessary. Administration of coagulation factors or platelets may be useful, particularly in cases of persistent bleeding. In addition, therapeutic interventions aimed at the interruption of ongoing thrombin formation or at the inhibition of thrombin might have a beneficial effect. This effect might be further facilitated by administration of protease inhibitors, such as antithrombin III, levels of which may dramatically decrease in the course of DIC.

Treatment with *plasma or platelet concentrate* is guided by the clinical condition of the patient and should not be instituted on the basis of laboratory findings alone. Replacement may be indicated in patients with active bleeding and in those requiring an invasive procedure or otherwise at risk for bleeding complications. On the other hand, it has been suggested that transfusion of blood components may also be harmful by further stimulating the activated coagulation system. Despite the lack of evidence, most authors recommend treatment with fresh frozen plasma, at least when patients are bleeding or are at increased risk for bleeding.[36] To sufficiently correct the coagulation defect large volumes of plasma may be needed. The use of coagulation factor concentrates may overcome this need. However, these concentrates usually contain only a selected number of the various clotting factors, and they may be contaminated with traces of activated coagulation factors.

Although it has long been used, there is no sound evidence in favor of the use of heparin as routine therapy in patients with DIC. An exception may be made for patients with clinical signs of extensive fibrin deposition such as purpura fulminans, acral ischemia, or venous thrombosis. In such cases low-dose heparin (5–8 U/kg/h) is advocated, potentially in combination with plasma and, if appropriate, platelet replacement.[37] Future studies are needed to definitively indicate a potential role of LMWH in the supportive treatment of DIC patients. Use of antithrombin III has not proven conclusively to be clinically beneficial.

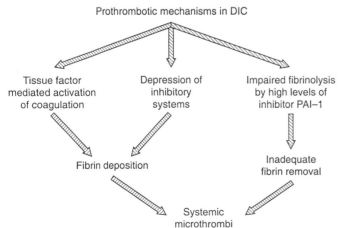

FIGURE 4.5. Schematic representation of the pathogenesis of DIC. Activation of coagulation depends on tissue factor-mediated thrombin generation and a simultaneously occurring depression of the physiological coagulation–inhibitory systems. Impaired function of the fibrinolytic system, caused by high levels of the fibrinolytic inhibitor PAI-1, further contributes to the procoagulant state.

References

1. Colman RW, Hirsh J, Marder VJ, et al. Hemostasis and Thrombosis. Basic Principles and Clinical Practice. Philadelphia: Lippincott, 1994.
2. Hathaway WE, Goodnight JR SH. Disorders of Hemostasis and Thrombosis. A Clinical Guide. New York: McGraw-Hill, 1993.
3. Colman RW, Cook JJ, Niewiarowski. Mechanisms of platelet aggregation. In: Colman RW, Hirsh J, Marder VJ, Salzman EW, eds. Hemostasis and Thrombosis: Basic Principles and Clinical Practice. Philadelphia: Lippincott, 1994.
4. Niewiarowski S, Holt JC, Cook JJ. Biochemistry and physiology of secreted platelet proteins. In: Colman RW, Hirsh J, Marder VJ, Salzman EW, eds. Hemostasis and Thrombosis: Basic Principles and Clinical Practice. Philadelphia: Lippincott, 1994.
5. Davie EW. Biochemical and molecular aspects of the coagulation cascade. Thromb Haemostasis 1995;74:1–7.

6. Davie EW, Fujikawa K, Kisiel W. The coagulation cascade: initiation, maintenance and regulation. Biochemistry 1991;30:10363–10370.
7. Hirsh J, Dalen JE, Deykin, et al. Oral anticoagulants. Chest 1995;108:231S–247S.
8. Weitz JI. Low molecular weight heparins. N Engl J Med 1997;337:688–698.
9. Edmunds LH, Salzman EW. Hemostatic problems, transfusion therapy, and cardiopulmonary bypass in surgical patients. In: Colman RW, Hirsh J, Marder VJ, Salzman EW, eds. Hemostasis and Thrombosis: Basic Principles and Clinical Practice. Philadelphia: Lippincott, 1994.
10. Mannucci PM. Desmopressin (DDAVP) in the treatment of bleeding disorders: the first 20 years. Blood 1997;90:2515.
11. Marder VJ, Butler FO, Barlow GH. Antifibrinolytic therapy. In: Colman RW, Hirsh J, Marder VJ, Salzman EW, eds. Hemostasis and Thrombosis: Basic Principles and Clinical Practice. Philadelphia: Lippincott, 1994.
12. Rao AK, Ghosh S, Sum L, et al. Mechanism of platelet dysfunction and response to DDAVP in patients with congenital platelet function defects. A double-blind placebo-controlled trial. Thromb Haemostasis 1995;74:1071–1078.
13. Levi M, Lensing A, ten Cate JW. Haemostasis, blood coagulation and fibrinolysis in liver disease. In: Tytgat GN, Lygidakis A, et al, eds. Hepatobiliary and Pancreatic Malignancies: Diagnosis, Medical and Surgical Therapy. Stuttgart: Thieme, 1988:173–178.
14. Marassi A, Manzullo V, Di Carlo V, et al. Thromboembolism following prothrombin complex concentrate and major surgery in severe liver disease. Thromb Haemostasis 1978;39:787.
15. Agnelli G, Parise P, Levi M, Cosmi B, Nenci GG. Effects of desmopressin on hemostasis in patients with liver cirrhosis. Haemostasis 1995;25:241–247.
16. Moia M, Mannucci PM, Vizzotto L, et al. Improvement in the hemostatic defect of uremia after treatment with recombinant human erythropoietin. Lancet 1987;2:1227.
17. Mannucci PM, Remuzzi G, Pusinri F, et al. De-amino-8-D-arginine vasopressin shortens the bleeding time in uremia. N Engl J Med 1983;308:8–12.
18 Kelton JG, Gibbons S. Autoimmune platelet destruction: idiopathic thrombocytopenic purpura. Semin Thromb Hemostasis 1982;8:83–104.
19. Cohen AJ, Kessler CM. Acquired inhibitors. Baillieres Clin Haematol 1996;9:331–354.
20. Watson CJ, Deane AM, Doyle PA, Bullock KN. Identifiable factors in post-prostatectomy haemorrhage: the role of aspirin. Br J Urol 1990;66:85.
21. Billingsley EM, Maloney ME. Intraoperative and postoperative bleeding problems in patients taking warfarin, aspirin, and nonsteroidal antiinflammatory agents. A prospective study. Dermatol Surg 1997;23:381.
22. Goldman S, Copeland J, Moritz T, et al. Improvement in early saphenous vein graft patency after coronary artery bypass surgery with antiplatelet therapy: results of a Veteran Administration cooperative study. Circulation 1988;77:1324.
23. Flordal PA. Use of desmopressin to prevent bleeding in surgery. Eur J Surg 1998;164:5.
24. Bartley GB, Warndahl RA. Surgical bleeding associated with aspirin and nonsteroidal anti-inflammatory agents. Mayo Clin Proc 1992;67:402.
25. Horskotte D, Schulte HD, Bircks W, et al. Lower intensity anticoagulation therapy results in lower complication rates with the St. Jude medical prosthesis. J Thorac Cardiovasc Surg 1994;107:1136–1145.
26. Kearon C, Hirsh J. Management of anticoagulation before and after elective surgery. N Engl J Med 1997;336:1506–1511.
27. Nurmohamed MT, Rosendaal FR, Büller HR, et al. Low molecular weight heparin versus standard heparin in general and orthopedic surgery: a meta-analysis. Lancet 1992;340:152–156.
28. Cattaneo M, Harris AS, Strömberg U, Mannucci PM. The effect of desmopressin on reducing blood loss in cardiac surgery. A meta-analysis of double-blind placebo-controlled trials. Thromb Haemostasis 1995;74:1064.
29. Lim RC, Olcott C, Robinson AJ, et al. Platelet response and coagulation changes following massive blood replacement. J Trauma 1973;18:577.
30. Roy AJ, Jaffe N, Djerassi I. Prophylactic platelet transfusions in children with acute leukemia: a dose-response study. Transfusion (Phila) 1973;13:283–290.
31. Levi M, Ten Cate H. Disseminated intravascular coagulation: Current concepts. N Engl J Med 1999;341:586–592.
32. Baglin T. Disseminated intravascular coagulation: diagnosis and treatment. Br Med J 1996;312:683–687.
33. Fourrier F, Chopin C, Goudemand J, et al. Septic shock, multiple organ failure, and disseminated intravascular coagulation. Compared patterns of antithrombin III, protein C, and protein S deficiencies. Chest 1992;101:816–823.
34. Levi M, ten Cate H, van der Poll T, et al. Pathogenesis of disseminated intravascular coagulation in sepsis. JAMA 1993;270:975–979.
35. Biemond BJ, Levi M, ten Cate H, et al. Endotoxin-induced activation and inhibition of the fibrinolytic system: effects of various interventions in the cytokine and coagulation cascades in experimental endotoxemia in chimpanzees. Clin Sci 1995;88:587–594.
36. Rubin RN, Colman RW. Disseminated intravascular coagulation. Approach to treatment. Drugs 1992;44:963–971.
37. Feinstein DI. Diagnosis and management of disseminated intravascular coagulation: the role of heparin therapy. Blood 1982;60:284–287.

Transfusion Therapy

Richard K. Spence

Risks of Blood Transfusion

Transfusion Reactions

The risks of allogeneic red blood cell transfusion include transfusion reactions, transfusion-transmission infectious disease, and immunomodulation. Transfusion reactions can be separated into three main groups: (a) acute intravascular immune hemolytic reactions from ABO incompatibility, (b) delayed immune hemolytic reactions, and (c) febrile reactions.[1] Reactions are estimated to occur in approximately 5% of transfusion recipients.

Symptoms of *ABO incompatibility reactions* can take many forms including hemoglobulinuria, fever, chills, coagulopathy, chest pain, and circulatory collapse. In the unconscious, anesthetized, euvolemic patient, acute reactions may present as either sudden hypotension or unexpected bleeding secondary to disseminated intravascular coagulation.[2] The majority of ABO transfusion reactions usually result from failure to correctly identify either the patient or the unit before transfusion.[3]

Delayed hemolytic reactions are caused by non-ABO antigen–antibody incompatibilities. Symptoms appear within 3 to 10 days after transfusion and include fever, malaise, hyperbilirubinemia, or a falling hematocrit. A falling hematocrit during the immediate postoperative period in a recently transfused patient is often attributed to recurrent or continued bleeding. A real danger exists in continuing to transfuse such patients with incompatible blood. An acute hemolytic reaction can be precipitated if blood has not been recross-matched since the original transfusion. A delayed hemolytic reaction should be ruled out by appropriate antibody testing in any patient with a falling, postoperative hematocrit and no overt evidence of continuing bleeding.[4,5]

Febrile reactions, the most common type, were once thought to be caused by circulating recipient antibodies to donor leukocyte or platelet contaminants. Recent evidence suggests that these reactions are cytokine mediated. The incidence of febrile reactions can be diminished greatly by the use of a leukodepletion filter.[6]

Graft-versus-host disease (GVHD) results from the engraftment of immunocompetent T lymphocytes, typically in a recipient who is immunosuppressed, although the syndrome has been seen following cardiac surgery, cholecystectomy, prostatectomy, and normal delivery.[7] GVHD is characterized by fever, skin rash, and gastrointestinal symptoms and is almost always fatal. GVHD is most common following directed donations from immediate family members who are either first-degree relatives or share an HLA haplotype. Fortunately, the offending lymphocytes are sensitive to gamma irradiation and can be eliminated by pretransfusion treatment with cesium-137 or cobalt-60 at doses that do not damage red cells.[7]

Transfusion-Transmitted Disease

Blood can carry and transmit a wide variety of viral, parasitic, rickettsial, and bacterial diseases. The estimated risk of contracting a specific disease from transfusion of blood products varies and depends upon many factors including the organism, patient risk factors, the screening processes used, the country of origin, and the overall vigilance of the blood provider[8–10] (Table 5.1).

Some viruses are common in blood donors but do not present a serious infectious risk. Cytomegalovirus (CMV), a member of the herpes family, is present in as many as one-half the units of allogeneic blood transfused.[11] This virus presents a small but troublesome risk, especially to specific groups of patients including premature infants, pregnant CMV-seronegative mothers, and seronegative adults who may need multiple transfusions, such as liver transplant recipients or blunt trauma victims. Clinical symptoms vary in severity and may include pulmonary, gastrointestinal, or systemic manifestations. Exposure to CMV can be reduced by eliminating unnecessary transfusions, screening for antibodies, and filtering leukocytes that carry the virus.[12,13]

Many other diseases can be transmitted by transfusion in-

TABLE 5.1. Risks of Allogeneic Transfusion

Type of risk	Units of blood transfused
Noninfectious	
Fatal ABO incompatibility reaction	1:1,000,000
Nonfatal hemolytic reaction	1:25,000
Febrile reaction	1:100
Immunosuppression	? (Potentially 1:1)
Graft-versus-host disease	Rare
Infectious	
HIV-1	1:493,000
HTLV	1:641,000
Viral hepatitis C	1:103,000
Viral hepatitis B	1:63,000
Bacterial infection	1:1,000,000
Chagas' disease	Unknown
Creutzfeld–Jacob syndrome	Unknown

Source: Data from references 11–21, 108–115.

cluding malaria, Chagas' disease, Q fever, Lyme disease, bovine spongiform encephalopathy, etc.[1,14] The risk of contracting these diseases is unknown, but is assumed to be low.

Immunomodulation

That immunomodulation occurs following allogeneic blood transfusion is not in question. What is in question is the clinical effect. Macrophage function is altered, resulting in decreased migratory capability and both eicosanoid and interleukin-2 production. Lymphocyte responses to both antigen and mitogen are suppressed; suppressor cell activity is increased with concomitant declines in helper to suppressor cell ratios. The immunomodulatory effect can occur following a single-unit transfusion, as noted in the renal transplantation experience, but also shows a dose–response relationship.[15]

A majority of investigators have found statistical support for either a causal relationship or an association between allogeneic blood transfusion and increased postoperative morbidity and mortality.[15–21] Still, the clinical impact of transfusion-related immunosuppression has not been established definitively, and the surgeon should be aware of the potential risks to patients. Whether the relationship is causal or merely an association, avoidance of allogeneic blood transfusion eliminates the risk, but this certainly is not possible in all patients. Mounting evidence implicates the leukocyte as the immunomodulatory agent, and reduction of leukocytes by filtration as an effective way to decrease the clinical impact.[22–25]

Storage Defects

Attention has been focused in recent years on the damage done to red blood cells and platelets during storage.[26] These so-called storage lesions may produce elevated levels of potassium or decreased levels of 2,3-diphosphoglycerate (2,3-DPG). Lack of 2,3-DPG results in a higher than desired red cell oxygen affinity, causing impaired release of oxygen to tissues.[27,28] Recovery of sufficient 2,3-DPG levels to correct this problem may take 24 to 48 h, depending on the length of pretransfusion storage. Platelets develop a progressive storage lesion during their 5-day residence in the blood bank, but this does not usually result in impaired effectiveness.[29] Red cells may be damaged by free radicals over time with loss of red blood

cell volume. Treatment of donors with antioxidants helps reduce this effect.[30]

Physiological Response to Anemia

The heart provides the primary response to acute, surgical anemia by increasing cardiac output, through either an increase in heart rate or an increase in stroke volume. Because the heart extracts approximately 80% of the oxygen delivered under normal conditions, its ability to increase output is determined by its ability to increase its own oxygen consumption. Cardiac oxygen extraction is improved by increasing coronary flow. To do this, the coronary arteries must dilate. In the presence of coronary artery disease, the heart may be unable to provide the work needed to increase total body oxygen delivery without risk to the myocardium. Continued demands on the stressed heart to provide oxygen in the face of anemia produce an anaerobic myocardium and infarction.[31]

Peripheral tissues may also compensate for anemia by increasing oxygen delivery, either by recruiting more capillaries or by increasing blood flow through existing beds. Some tissues, particularly those that are supply dependent, may compensate by increasing oxygen extraction.[32] Compensatory mechanisms are limited and dependent upon not only red cell mass but also circulating volume.[33] In the chronically anemic patient, increases in stroke volume and, therefore, in cardiac output are supplemented by increased levels of 2,3-DPG. These intracellular changes shift the oxyhemoglobin curve to the right, facilitating oxygen offload and increasing oxygen delivery.

In most clinical settings, oxygen consumption is relatively independent of hemoglobin level across a wide range of oxygen delivery (DO_2) values because of compensations made in oxygen extraction. As DO_2 decreases through a loss of Hgb, oxygen extraction should increase from a baseline of 15% to 25% to maintain a constant consumption. Any increase in circulating volume that improves cardiac output will also mathematically improve oxygen delivery regardless of hemoglobin level.

Transfusion Decisions in Surgery

The Hemoglobin Transfusion Trigger

Most transfusion decisions are made on the basis of isolated hemoglobin (Hgb) and hematocrit (Hct) values. The *National Institutes of Health Consensus Conference*, convened in 1988 to address the topic of perioperative red cell transfusion, focused primarily on the risks of transfusion and the need to modify our transfusion practices.[34] It also produced recommendations for a new transfusion trigger that represented an update of the traditional 10/30 rule that had existed for years.[35] The target, or trigger, hemoglobin was lowered to 8 g/dl, and guidelines for transfusion recommended use of clinical need and symptoms rather than numbers alone. Since then, much has appeared in the literature that has attempted to further define the transfusion trigger.[36–39] Investigators have focused on either defining an acceptable hemoglobin level, deriving a trigger from oxygen transport or metabolic variables, or describing the effect of transfusion in specific clinical settings. To date, no overriding consensus has been reached.

Symptoms as Transfusion Triggers

Symptoms of exertional dyspnea do not appear in the otherwise healthy individual until hemoglobin concentration reaches 7 g/dl. Even at this and lower levels, symptoms and signs are variable.

Metabolic Triggers

Other approaches to defining the transfusion trigger in metabolic terms have had limited success. Lactate levels have not proven useful in defining transfusion need following trauma,[40] acute myocardial infarction, or sepsis.[41]

Surgical Anemia: Approaches to Treatment

Although studies suggest that a Hgb value significantly lower than 10 g/dl is tolerated by many patients, this does not necessarily mean that a tolerable Hgb level should automatically be considered an acceptable level for use as a transfusion trigger in all patients. The decision to transfuse should be related to the specific patient's condition, assessing need on a case-by-case basis. This assessment should include a history and physical examination, a review of pertinent lab data, consideration of the operation planned and expectant blood loss, and analysis of risk factors that may contribute to increased morbidity and mortality. The history and physical examination should focus on preexisting diseases or conditions that may increase the risk of blood loss or the need for increased oxygen delivery. The presence of cardiac, pulmonary, and other atherosclerotic disease processes should be assessed and quantified when possible. Surgical patients with coronary artery disease and pulmonary hypoxia will most likely require higher perioperative Hgb levels than those without such problems.

If anemia is discovered during preoperative investigations, the surgeon must decide if the level of anemia and the risk of blood loss from the planned procedure are of enough merit to warrant action. If they are and if surgery can be postponed, the surgeon can use oral iron to correct the anemia. Oral iron therapy should also be used in patients undergoing autologous predonation of blood and those receiving erythropoietin.[42] If surgery cannot be delayed, the use of intravenous iron dextran may be considered.

Factors Affecting Blood Loss and Transfusion

Transfusion Practices

Several studies have demonstrated that the adoption of transfusion guidelines, practice policies, or transfusion algorithms can reduce the risk of exposure to allogeneic blood[43–45] (Table 5.2). The first step in this process is for the surgeon to review their transfusion practices to obtain an understanding of which patients are transfused and how much blood is used. Blood losses should be calculated, not estimated.[46] With this information, the surgeon can establish a blood ordering schedule

TABLE 5.2. Transfusion Practice Policies.

1. Assess transfusion need on a case-by-case basis.
   Develop a "transfusion prescription" or plan for each patient.
2. Limit patient exposure to allogeneic blood to appropriate need.
   Modify the hemoglobin level at which you transfuse, based on patient's history, clinical symptoms, and signs.
3. Prevent or control perioperative blood loss.
   Consider stopping anticoagulants and antiplatelet agents before surgery.
   Correct existing coagulopathy.
   Restrict perioperative phlebotomy.
   Consider use of regional and hypotensive anesthesia techniques.
   Maintain careful surgical hemostasis.
   Modify the surgical approach to minimize blood loss.
   Use local acting agents to stop bleeding.
   Consider the use of cautery, Argon beam, etc.
   Consider the use of antifibrinolytic drugs.
   Consider preoperative tumor embolization.
4. Use autologous blood as an alternative whenever possible.
   Schedule surgery to permit predonation of blood.
   Use acute normovolemic hemodilution.
   Use intraoperative and postoperative autotransfusion.
5. Maximize oxygen delivery to the patient.
   Treat underlying cardiopulmonary disease.
6. Increase or restore red cell mass by means other than transfusion.
   Consider iron, B_{12}, and folate replacement.
   Consider use of recombinant erythropoietin.
7. Involve the patient in the transfusion decision.
8. Record the reasons for and results of the transfusion in the patient's chart.
9. Develop hospital transfusion policies as a multidisciplinary effort.
10. Review individual and institutional policies on at least a yearly basis.

Source: Adapted from Reference 45.

that will serve as a personal guideline for both allogeneic blood use and institution of appropriate alternatives. The overall impact of such efforts awaits further, randomized trials using appropriate outcomes measures.[47]

Bleeding in the Surgery Patient

PREOPERATIVE ASPECTS

Preoperative measurement of hemoglobin and hematocrit will detect the presence of anemia, which can be analyzed further with red cell indices. Many surgeons measure prothrombin (PT) and partial thromboplastin times (PTT) in all patients who will receive heparin anticoagulation to screen for coagulopathy. A preferable approach is to question each patient about bleeding history, because most significant bleeding problems are congenital and have shown up in childhood, or are related to specific medications and disease processes.[48] All patients should be asked about the use of warfarin-based anticoagulants, aspirin, and nonsteroidal anti-inflammatory drugs because these all can lead to increased bleeding. When feasible, these agents should be stopped well in advance of any planned surgery.[49] Coagulation studies should be reserved for patients with clinical indications, such as a history of liver disease, malignancy, renal failure, or anticoagulant therapy.[50] Similarly, routine platelet measurements are of little value because deficiencies caused by abnormal production or increased destruction will be detected primarily by a good history and physical exam and qualitative defects will not be reflected in abnormally low counts.[51,52]

The presence of a major coagulation disorder such as hemophilia A or B or von Willebrand's disease is not an absolute contraindication to surgery. It has been reported that major surgical procedures can be performed with acceptable blood loss and outcomes in these patients so long as hemostasis can be corrected to normal or near-normal levels through the use of factor replacement therapy.[53]

ACUTE BLEEDING IN THE EMERGENCY PATIENT

Patients who present with active bleeding present a special challenge to the surgeon. Patients who fit into this category include those with bleeding varices, a ruptured aneurysm, or a variety of scenarios in the trauma patient.

Prompt diagnosis and timely surgical intervention directed at controlling hemorrhage are the mainstays of limiting allogeneic blood exposures in the patient with exsanguinating bleeding. Exsanguination remains the critical factor in determining outcome in isolated, major vascular injuries.[54,55] Autotransfusion equipment should be ready so that as much shed blood as possible can be salvaged and returned from the thoracic, abdominal, or thigh compartments. Even though the blood appears to have clotted, such losses can be successfully salvaged, washed, and returned as red cells to the patient. An estimate of blood lost should be made early so that appropriate replacements can be ordered from the blood bank.

In contrast to the trauma patient for whom early surgical intervention to stop bleeding is the norm, it is common practice in the patient with gastrointestinal bleeding to determine the need for surgery based on the number of units of blood lost or transfused within a 12- to 24-h period. By using such guidelines, not only do we magnify the risk of allogeneic blood exposure but we also increase mortality in direct proportion to the number of units transfused. Studies of such patients show a significant correlation between the amount of blood lost and/or transfused and death.[56]

INTRAOPERATIVE ASPECTS: TECHNIQUE

The choice of both anesthetic technique and operation can influence the amount of blood lost during surgery. Regional anesthetic techniques have been associated with decreased blood loss in orthopedic surgery. Oxygen consumption is reduced 15% to 20% under general anesthesia in most patients.[57] Narcotic anesthesia may add another 5% to 10% reduction, providing a greater margin of safety. If inhalational anesthetics are used, isoflurane is usually chosen because it has less inhibitory effect on the heart's conductivity. These anesthetic agents do not directly minimize blood loss, but they provide a somewhat safer environment for the stressed, anemic patient who may need increased cardiac reserves.

INTRAOPERATIVE ASPECTS: NONSURGICAL BLEEDING

Bleeding during surgery may also arise from hemostatic defects (Table 5.3). Coagulopathy in the patient with traumatic or massive bleeding and transfusion is partially dilutional in nature but is also related to both the degree and length of hypotension and hypoperfusion.[58,59] Tissue hypoxia following

TABLE 5.3. Hemostatic Causes of Intraoperative Bleeding.

Massive transfusion

Dilution from nonsanguineous fluids

Hemolytic transfusion reaction

Fibrinolysis/DIC

Undiagnosed bleeding disorder

Drugs

Hypothermia

injury or prolonged cross-clamping of visceral blood supply may also lead to release of plasminogen activators and thromboplastins.

Coagulation factor and platelet depletion is not so frequent a cause of intraoperative hemorrhage as is commonly perceived. Hypothermia may be a contributing factor.[60,61] It may be difficult to directly correlate the clinical observation of bleeding with prolongation of the PT and aPTT, which are reagent and temperature dependent.[62] Because coagulation testing is routinely performed at 37°C, rather than at the patient's actual in vivo temperature, normal coagulation tests can be obtained even in the presence of clinical evidence of a coagulopathy.[63] Normal test results in this setting suggest that sufficient clotting factors are available for coagulation if normothermia is restored.[64] Dilutional coagulopathy may be mistaken for or aggravated by the development of disseminated intravascular coagulation (DIC).[65–67] DIC in the setting of massive transfusion is reported to occur in 5% to 30% of trauma patients and is associated with high morbidity and mortality rates of nearly 70%.[68,69] Tissue injury and hemolysis with release of cytokines and tissue thromboplastin into the circulation may cause immediate activation of both the coagulation and the fibrinolytic systems, resulting in severe DIC.[62] At the present time no single laboratory test can be used to confirm or exclude the diagnosis of DIC. However, the combination of a low platelet count, a low fibrinogen, an elevated D-dimer, and the presence of soluble fibrin monomers in the context of the patient's underlying condition are the most helpful indicators of DIC.

Coagulation factors and platelets can be replaced as needed by infusing fresh frozen plasma or platelets. Stored, allogeneic blood maintains sufficient levels of all coagulation factors needed to prevent bleeding except V and VIII, which decrease over time.[70] If available, whole blood obtained via acute normovolemic hemodilution can be used to restore coagulation factors and platelets.

POSTOPERATIVE CARE

Unfortunately, blood loss frequently continues in the postoperative period in the form of phlebotomy for lab tests.[71] Standard order sheets that include standing orders for frequent and often unnecessary lab tests should be avoided.

Alternatives to Allogeneic Blood

Directed Donor Blood

Directed blood donations do not reduce the exposure to allogeneic transfusion. Directed donor blood carries significant risks including disease transmission and graft-versus-host disease. The use of directed donor blood may be an acceptable option in specific settings, such as neonatal or pediatric surgery. Surgeons should instruct patients about its potential dangers.

Autologous Predonation

Autologous predonation (PAD) is an alternative that has been proven to reduce dependence on allogeneic blood in multiple studies of a variety of surgical procedures.[72–74] It is considered the standard of care practice in orthopedic joint replacement surgery.[75]

Successful autologous predonation depends on (1) adequate time for donation, (2) hemoglobin level greater than 11.0 g/dl, (3) absence of significant patient disease, for example, severe aortic stenosis or active angina, (4) selection of appropriate patients based on anticipated blood loss and transfusion need, and (5) both patient and physician cooperation. The ideal patient for predonation is one who has an anticipated need for blood transfusion with a window of 2 or more weeks before surgery to donate. Relative contraindications to predonation include a history of congestive heart failure, valvular heart disease, recent myocardial infarction, angina, dysrhythmias, hypertension requiring multiple drug therapy, seizures, or cerebrovascular disease. An increased incidence of reactions is associated with donor age under 17 years, weight greater than 110 lb, female gender, and a history of previous reactions.[76]

Acute Normovolemic Hemodilution

Acute normovolemic hemodilution (ANH) is a strategy for obtaining fresh, whole, autologous blood without the difficult logistics and potential risks of PAD. The process involves the removal and temporary storage of blood in the operating room just before or immediately after the induction of anesthesia. Volume losses are replaced with either crystalloid or colloid solutions.

The removal of 1 to 4 units by ANH is possible in the patient with a normal hematocrit and results in a postdilutional hematocrit of 20% to 30%.[77] The amount of blood to be removed may be calculated from measured preoperative hematocrit and estimated blood volume (EBV).[78] The factor that limits nadir hemoglobin during hemodilution appears to be ventricular function. Patients with normal ventricular function can tolerate hematocrits of 15% to 22% without postoperative myocardial problems.[79,80] Those with left ventricular dysfunction may be at greater risk of ischemia during hemodilution.[81,82]

ANH appears to be cost-effective when compared to either allogeneic blood procurement and transfusion or PAD.[83,84] Hemodilution is most often used in combination with other techniques such as autotransfusion, preoperative use of erythropoietin, platelet sequestration, and modification of surgical technique.[85]

Autotransfusion

The value of autotransfusion, or collection and reinfusion of shed blood, in reducing the need for allogeneic blood transfusion has been documented in multiple retrospective analyses. Reports from surgeons who have used autotransfusion in more than 20,000 patients during a variety of elective surgical procedures show reduction in allogeneic blood use by as much as 75% of all transfusion needs.[86–88] Autotransfusion was the predominant intraoperative factor that correlated with decreased mortality in a series of 61 patients with ruptured abdominal aortic aneurysms.[89]

Intraoperative autotransfusion can be performed either with systems that collect blood directly, anticoagulate it, and reinfuse it through filters or with systems that collect the blood, wash it, and reinfuse a packed red cell product.[88] Systems without washing capability collect shed blood via a suction wand that simultaneously adds either heparin or citrate-phosphate-dextrose anticoagulant into a collection chamber. The collected blood is returned to the patient through a filter, relying on this as the only means of preparing the blood. Filters are capable of removing large debris, for example, bone chips and smaller particulate matter. Following filtration, the salvaged blood represents "red cells suspended in plasma," containing platelets, fibrinogen, and clotting factors.

Unwashed blood may contain vasoactive contaminants, activated clotting factors, fibrin degradation products, and free hemoglobin, all of which can be dangerous. Washing shed blood reduces but does not completely eliminate leukocytes from the infused product.[90] In spite of the problems associated with unwashed, shed blood, this product has been used successfully and safely in many patients to reduce allogeneic transfusion exposure.[91,92]

Systems that wash blood and concentrate the red cells have the advantage of providing a cleaner product, free of the contaminants found in unwashed blood. With these devices, blood is collected from the operative field, filtered, anticoagulated, and temporarily stored in a reservoir. The blood is transferred to a centrifuge bowl that spins at approximately 5000 revolutions per minute, separating the red cells from plasma. The cells are washed and resuspended in saline to attain a hematocrit of 40% to 60% before reinfusion.[93] Disadvantages of these systems include the loss of the plasma component, the need for expert help, setup time required, and expense.

Relative contraindications to the use of autotransfused blood, whether washed or not, include the presence of infection or bowel contamination, malignancy, and obstetrical procedures contaminated with amniotic fluid. When presented with such situations the surgeon must weigh the potential benefit obtainable from autotransfusion against the risks. Autotransfusion has been used successfully and without increased infectious risk with potentially contaminated blood.[94,95] Washing the blood appears to reduce the bacterial load; prophylactic antibiotics provide additional protection.[96] Autotransfusion has been used safely in cancer surgery in the Jehovah's Witness when the real risk of death from blood loss outweighed the theoretical risk of tumor cell dissemination.[97] The use of leukocyte reduction filters may eliminate viable cancer cells from shed blood.[98]

Although some controversy exists over when to use autotransfusion and which system to use, it is clear that this alternative does reduce allogeneic blood need in appropriately selected patients. Each surgeon would benefit from a systematic review of their own blood loss for specific procedures to provide a basis for a rational, cost-effective use of autotransfusion as well as other alternatives.

Pharmacological Agents Associated with Blood Loss and Transfusion

A variety of drugs that affect either blood loss or transfusion need are available to the surgeon. These drugs are grouped by their intended action into three broad categories: (1) those with the potential to increase bleeding, (2) those that help prevent or control perioperative bleeding, and (3) those which stimulate red blood cell production (Table 5.4).

Drugs with the Potential to Increase Bleeding

Aspirin, nonsteroidal antiinflammatory drugs (NSAIDs), warfarin, heparin, and similar anticoagulant drugs and thrombolytic are known to interfere with coagulation and to produce increased intraoperative bleeding. If the risk of increased blood loss caused by these drugs is greater than the risk of stopping them during the perioperative period, the drugs should be temporarily discontinued. Known coagulation disorders such as hemophilia and von Willebrand's disease should be identified preoperatively and an appropriate treatment regimen should be planned.

Drugs That Help Prevent or Control Perioperative Bleeding

Protamine is used intraoperatively to reverse the effects of heparin during major cardiovascular surgery. The dose administered is calculated initially from the amount of heparin given and is titrated against clotting times. Titration and administration of protamine based on specific, point-of-service measurement of coagulation factors may result in less postoperative bleeding and decreased transfusion need compared to a conventional regimen.[99,100]

Vasopressin can be used intraoperatively to reduce blood loss in patients with known varices who must undergo surgery. An infusion of 0.4 units/min of vasopressin started before making the skin incision produces subcutaneous vasoconstriction and limits bleeding.

A vasopressin analogue, desmopressin (1-desamino-8-D-arginine vasopressin, DDAVP), has minimal vasopressor activity. Its usefulness during surgery is based on its ability to elevate both factor VIII and factor VIII von Willebrand's factor two- to threefold over normal levels. The drug has a variety of side effects, which range from mild facial flushing to headache, tachycardia, hypertension, and tachyphylaxis. DDAVP can provide an advantage in the hemophiliac with low factor VIII levels.[53] However, its role in surgical patients is controversial. Desmopressin may have a limited usefulness in correcting identifiable platelet defects, such as those caused by aspirin.[101]

Aprotinin, a serine protease inhibitor, has been used successfully to reduce blood loss during cardiovascular surgery in a number of clinical trials. Aprotinin is thought to work by inhibiting kallikrein and plasmin or by preserving platelet adhesion membrane receptors during cardiopulmonary bypass.[102] Like desmopressin, aprotinin may have an important role in treating patients with aspirin-induced platelet abnormalities.

ϵ-Amino caproic acid and tranexamic acid have also been shown to be useful in reducing blood loss in cardiac surgery and liver transplantation in meta-analyses of the existing literature.[103,104] Bombesin, pentoxifylline, and prostacyclin are purported to work on the vascular system, bombesin by counteracting opioid-induced vasodilatation, and pentoxifylline and prostacyclin by improving microcirculatory flow and tissue oxygen delivery.[105] The clinical role of these drugs remains unproven, although the latter two may have some benefit in septic or critically ill patients who need to maximize peripheral oxygen consumption.

Fibrin glue is made by reacting fibrinogen, which can be obtained from a variety of sources including either human cryoprecipitate or autologous, platelet-rich plasma, with bovine thrombin to produce fibrin.[106] Fibrin sealants are generally commercially produced from processed human, animal, or synthetic sources. These materials adhere well to biological surfaces and have been shown to be effective in controlling bleeding in a variety of settings in randomized, controlled trials.[106] Insufficient information exists to determine if these products can reduce allogeneic blood transfusion when used alone. Unfortunately, fibrin glue derived from multiple, allogeneic donors may be a source of disease transmission. Whenever possible, autologous plasma should be used rather than allogeneic, if blood product exposure is to be avoided. Commercial produced, virus-free sealants may solve this problem. Combinations of fibrin sealant and a collagen matrix show promise.

Drugs That Stimulate Red Blood Cell Production

Recombinant human erythropoietin may provide a means of restoring red cells without either autologous or allogeneic transfusion. It is important when using erythropoietin to make sure that the patient's iron stores are replenished because existing iron is rapidly depleted. Iron dextran infusions to replace depleted iron stores can be used to treat acute, critical surgical anemia.[107]

Blood Substitutes

Blood substitutes, whether perfluorocarbon based or hemoglobin derived, are currently undergoing clinical trials and are not available for general use.

TABLE 5.4. **Pharmacological Agents Associated with Surgical Bleeding and Transfusion.**

1. Limit blood loss
   A. Vitamin K
   B. Protamine
   C. Desmopressin (DDAVP)
   D. Tranexemic acid
   E. ϵ-Amino caproic acid (EACA)
   F. Aprotinin
   G. Factor VIII/IX
   H. Vasopressin
   I. Topical agents
      1. Fibrin glue and sealant
      2. Surgical, Hemopad, etc.
2. Regenerate red blood cells
   A. Oral Fe
   B. Intravenous Fe
   C. Erythropoietin
   D. Steroids
   E. Intravenous nutrition
3. Blood substitutes
   A. Crystalloids
   B. Colloids
   C. Hemoglobin derivatives
   D. Perfluorocarbons

References

1. Klein HG. Allogeneic transfusion risks in the surgical patient. Am J Surg 1995;170(suppl 6A):21S–26S.
2. Sazama K. Reports of 355 transfusion-associated deaths: 1976 through 1985. Transfusion (Phila) 1990;30:583–588.
3. Linden JV, Kaplan HS. Transfusion errors: causes and effects. Transfus Med Rev 1994;8(3):169–183.
4. Seyfried H, Walewska I. Immune hemolytic transfusion reactions. World J Surg 1987;11:25–29.
5. Ramsey G. The pathophysiology and organ-specific consequences of severe transfusion reactions. New Horiz 1994;2(4):575–581.
6. Lane TA. Leukocyte reduction of cellular blood components. Effectiveness, benefits, quality control, and costs. Arch Pathol Lab Med 1994;118(4):392–404.
7. Davey RJ. Transfusion-associated graft-versus-host disease and the irradiation of blood components. Immunol Invest 1995;24(1–2):431–434.
8. Zeuzem S, Teuber G, Lee JH, Ruster B, Roth WK. Risk factors for the transmission of hepatitis C. J Hepatol 1996;24(suppl2):3–10.
9. Schmunis GA, Zicker F, Pinheiro F, Brandling-Bennett D. Risk for transfusion-transmitted infectious diseases in Central and South America. Emerg Infect Dis 1998;4(1):5–11.
10. Choudhury N, Ramesh V, Saraswat S, Naik S. Effectiveness of mandatory transmissible diseases screening in Indian blood donors. Indian J Med Res 1995;101:229–232.
11. Weber B, Doerr HW. Diagnosis and epidemiology of transfusion-associated human cytomegalovirus infection: recent developments. Infusionsther Transfusmed 1994;21(suppl 1):32–39.
12. Gunter KC. Transfusion-transmitted cytomegalovirus: the part-time pathogen. Pediatr Pathol Lab Med 1995;15(3):515–534.
13. Friedman LI, Stromberg RR, Wagner SJ. Reducing the infectivity of blood components—what we have learned. Immunol Invest 1995;24(1–2):49–71.
14. Leiby DA, Read EJ, Lenes BA, et al. Seroepidemiology of *Trypanosoma cruzi*, etiologic agent of Chagas' disease, in US blood donors. J Infect Dis 1997;176(4):1047–1052.
15. Houbiers JG, van de Velde CJ, van de Watering LM, et al. Transfusion of red cells is associated with increased incidence of bacterial infection after colorectal surgery: a prospective study [see comments]. Transfusion (Phila) 1997;37(2):126–134.
16. Tartter PI. Transfusion-induced immunosuppression and perioperative infections. Beitr Infusionsther 1993;31:52–63.
17. Triulzi D, Blumberg N, Heal J. Association of transfusion with postoperative bacterial infection. Crit Rev Clin Lab Sci 1990;28:95–107.
18. Quintiliani L, Pescini A, Di Girolamo M, et al. Relationship of blood transfusion, post-operative infections and immunoreactivity in patients undergoing surgery for gastrointestinal cancer. Haematologica 1997;82(3):318–323.
19. Heiss MM, Fasol-Merten K, Allgayer H, et al. Influence of autologous blood transfusion on natural killer and lymphokine-activated killer cell activities in cancer surgery: antibiotic and antithromboembolic prophylaxis in hip arthroplasty (a review of 700 primary implants). Vox Sang 1997;73(4):165–176.
20. Donohue JH, Williams S, Cha S, et al. Perioperative blood transfusions do not affect disease recurrence of patients undergoing curative resection of colorectal carcinoma: a Mayo/North Central Cancer Treatment Group study. J Clin Oncol 1995;13(7):1671–1678.
21. Gorog D, Toth A, Weltner J, Darvas K. [The effect of blood transfusion on the late results of the surgical treatment of rectal cancer.] Orv Hetil 1996;137(31):1693–1698.
22. Riggert J, Schwartz DW, Wieding JU, Mayr WR, Kohler M. Prestorage inline filtration of whole blood for obtaining white cell-reduced blood components. Transfusion (Phila) 1997;37(10):1039–1044.
23. Rapaille A, Moore G, Siquet J, Flament J, Sondag-Thull D. Prestorage leukocyte reduction with in-line filtration of whole blood: evaluation of red cells and plasma storage. Vox Sang 1997;73(1):28–35.
24. Blajchman MA, Bordin JO. The tumor growth-promoting effect of allogeneic blood transfusions. Immunol Invest 1995;24(1–2):311–317.
25. Manno CS. What's new in transfusion medicine? Pediatr Clin North Am 1996;43(3):793–808.
26. Karger R, Kretschmer V. [The importance of quality of whole blood and erythrocyte concentrates for autologous transfusion. A literature survey and meta-analysis of in vivo erythrocyte recovery]. Anaesthesist 1996;45(8):694–707.
27. Hebert P, Wells G, Teewdale M, et al. Does transfusion practice affect mortality in critically ill patients? Transfusion Requirements in Critical Care (TRICC) Investigators and the Canadian Critical Care Trials Group. Am J Respir Crit Care Med 1997;155(5):1618–1623.
28. Hsia CC. Respiratory function of hemoglobin. N Engl J Med 1998;338(4):239–247.
29. Muller-Steinhardt M, Janetzko K, Kandler R, Flament J, Kirchner H, Kluter H. Impact of various red cell concentrate preparation methods on the efficiency of prestorage white cell filtration and on red cells during storage for 42 days. Transfusion (Phila) 1997;37(11–12):1137–1142.
30. Greenwalt TJ. Recent developments in the long-term preservation of red blood cells. Curr Opin Hematol 1997;4(6):431–435.
31. Doak G, Hall R. Does hemoglobin concentration affect perioperative myocardial lactate flux in patients undergoing coronary artery bypass surgery? Anesth Analg 1995;80(5):910–916.
32. Guidelines for red blood cell and plasma transfusion for adults and children. Report of the Expert Working Group. Can Med Assoc J 1997;156(suppl 11):S5–56.
33. Erni D, Banic A, Wheatley AM, Sigurdsson GH. Haemorrhage during anaesthesia and surgery: continuous measurement of microcirculatory blood flow in the kidney, liver, skin and skeletal muscle. Eur J Anaesthesiol 1995;12(4):423–429.
34. Perioperative red cell transfusion. NIH Consensus Development Conference Statement. Bethesda: National Institutes of Health, 1988:1–17.
35. Adams R, Lundy JS. Anesthesia in cases of poor surgical risk. Some suggestions for decreasing the risk. Surg Gynecol Obstet 1942;74:1011–1019.
36. Wedgewood J, Thomas J. Peri-operative haemoglobin: an overview of current opinion regarding the acceptable level of haemoglobin in the peri-operative period. Eur J Anaesthesiol 1996;13(4):316–324.
37. Lundsgaard-Hansen P. Safe hemoglobin or hematocrit levels in surgical patients. World J Surg 1996;20(9):1182–1188.
38. Stehling L, Simon TL. The red blood cell transfusion trigger. Physiology and clinical studies. Arch Pathol Lab Med 1994;118(4):429–434.
39. Simon TL, Alverson DC, AuBuchon J, et al. Practice parameter for the use of red blood cell transfusions: developed by the Red Blood Cell Administration Practice Guideline Development Task Force of the College of American Pathologists. Arch Pathol Lab Med 1998;122(2):130–138.
40. Bannon M, O'Neill C, Martin M, et al. Central venous oxygen saturation, arterial base deficit, and lactate concentration in trauma patients. Am Surg 1995;61(8):738–745.
41. Astiz M, Rackow E, Falk J, et al. Oxygen delivery and consumption in patients with hyperdynamic septic shock. Crit Care Med 1987;15(1):26–28.
42. Van Wyck DB. Iron management during recombinant human erythropoietin therapy. Am J Kidney Dis 1989;14(2 suppl 1):9–13.
43. Eisenstaedt RS. Modifying physicians' transfusion practice. Transfus Med Rev 1997;11(1):27–37.
44. Morrison JC, Sumrall DD, Chevalier SP, Robinson SV, Morri-

son FS, Wiser WL. The effect of provider education on blood utilization practices. Am J Obstet Gynecol 1993;169(5):1240–1245.

45. Spence RK. Surgical red blood cell transfusion practice policies. Blood Management Practice Guidelines Conference. Am J Surg 1995;170(suppl 6A):3S–15S.

46. Brecher ME, Monk T, Goodnough LT. A standardized method for calculating blood loss. Transfusion (Phila) 1997;37(10):1070–1074.

47. Rutherford R. Vascular surgery—comparing outcomes. J Vasc Surg 1996;23(1):10–17.

48. Burk CD, Miller L, Handler SD, Cohen AR. Preoperative history and coagulation screening in children undergoing tonsillectomy [see comments]. Pediatrics 1992;89(4 pt 2):691–695.

49. Smith MS, Muir H, Hall R. Perioperative management of drug therapy, clinical considerations. Drugs 1996;51(2):238–259.

50. Erban S, Kinman J, Schwartz J. Routine use of the prothrombin and partial thromboplastin times. JAMA 1989;263(17):2428–2432.

51. Ratnatunga CP, Rees GM, Kovacs IB. Preoperative hemostatic activity and excessive bleeding after cardiopulmonary bypass. Ann Thorac Surg 1991;52(2):250–257.

52. McIntyre A. Blood transfusion and hemostatic management in the perioperative period. Can J Anaesth 1992;39(5):R108–R114.

53. Rudowski W, Scharf R, Ziemski J. Is major surgery in hemophiliac patients safe? World J Surg 1987;11:378–386.

54. Jackson M, Olson D, Beckett WJ. Abdominal vascular trauma: a review of 106 injuries. Am Surg 1992;58(10):622–626.

55. Lopez-Viego M, Snyder WD, Valentine R. Penetrating abdominal aortic trauma: a report of 129 cases. J Vasc Surg 1992;16(3):332–335.

56. Lee H, Hawker F, Selby W. Intensive care treatment of patients with bleeding esophageal varices: results, predictors of mortality, and predictors of the adult respiratory distress syndrome. Crit Care Med 1993;20(11):1555–1563.

57. Bjoraker D. Blood transfusion. What is a safe hematocrit? Probl Crit Care 1991;5(3):386–399.

58. Collins J. Recent developments in the area of massive transfusion. World J Surg 1987;11:75–81.

59. Hiippala ST. Myllyla GJ, Vahtera EM. Hemostatic factors and replacement of major blood loss with plasma-poor red cell concentrates. Anesth Analg 1995;81(2):360–365.

60. Ferrara A, MacArthur J, Wright H. Hypothermia and acidosis worsen coagulopathy in the patient requiring massive transfusion. Am J Surg 1990;160:515–518.

61. Bush H Jr, Hydo LJ, Fischer E, Fantini GA, Silane MF, Barie PS. Hypothermia during elective abdominal aortic aneurysm repair: the high price of avoidable morbidity. J Vasc Surg 1995;21(3):392–400.

62. Bick R. Disseminated intravascular coagulation and related syndromes: a clinical review. Semin Thromb Hemostasis 1988;14:299–305.

63. Rohrer MJNA. Effect of hypothermia on the coagulation cascade. Crit Care Med 1992;20:1402–1408.

64. Nicholls MD, Whyte G. Red cell, plasma and albumin transfusion decision triggers. Anesthol Intensive Care 1993;21(2):156–162.

65. Collins J. Problems associated with the massive transfusion of stored blood. Surgery (St. Louis) 1974;75:274–278.

66. Lucas C, Ledgerwood A. Clinical significance of altered/coagulation test after massive transfusions for trauma. Am Surg 1981;47:125–129.

67. Hewson J, Neame P, Kumar N, Ayrton A, Gregor P. Coagulopathy related to dilution and hypotension during massive transfusion. Crit Care Med 1985;13:387–392.

68. Humphries JE. Transfusion therapy in acquired coagulopathies. Hematol Oncol Clin North Am 1994;8(6):1181–1201.

69. Counts R, Haisch C, Simon T, Maxwell N, Heimbach D. Hemostasis in massively transfused trauma patients. Ann Surg 1979;190:91–96.

70. Spence R, Jeter E. Transfusion in surgery and trauma. In: Mintz R, ed. Transfusion Practice. Bethesda: AABB Press, 1998.

71. Smoller BR, Kurskall MS. Phlebotomy for diagnostic laboratory tests in adults. Pattern of use and effect on transfusion requirements. N Engl J Med 1986;314(19):1233–1235.

72. Britton L, Eastlund D, Dziuban S, et al. Predonated autologous blood use in elective cardiac surgery. Ann Thorac Surg 1989;47:529–532.

73. Spiess BD. Pro: autologous blood should be available for elective cardiac surgery. J Cardiothorac Vasc Anesth 1994;8(2):231–237.

74. D'Ambra M, Kaplan D. Alternatives to allogeneic blood use in surgery: acute normovolemic hemodilution and preoperative autologous donation. Am J Surg 1995;170(suppl 6A):49S–52S.

75. Nelson CL, Fontenot HJ. Ten strategies to reduce blood loss in orthopedic surgery. Am J Surg 1995;170(suppl 6A):64S–68S.

76. Spiess B, Sassetti R, McCarthy R, et al. Autologous blood donation: hemodynamics in a high-risk patient population. Transfusion (Phila) 1992;32:17–22.

77. Stehling L, Zauder HL. Acute normovolemic hemodilution. Transfusion (Phila) 1991;31(9):857–868.

78. Lisander B. Preoperative hemodilution. Acta Anaesthesiol Scand 1988;32(suppl 89):63–70.

79. Robertie P, Gravlee G. Safe limits of hemodilution and recommendations for erythrocyte transfusion. Int Anesthesiol Clin 1990;28(4):197–204.

80. Weiskopf RB, Viele MK, Feiner J, et al. Human cardiovascular and metabolic response to acute, severe isovolemic anemia (see comments). JAMA 1998;279(3):217–221.

81. Spahn DR, Schmid ER, Seifert B, Pasch T. Hemodilution tolerance in patients with coronary artery disease who are receiving chronic beta-adrenergic blocker therapy. Anesth Analg 1996;82(4):687–694.

82. Weisel R, Charlesworth D, Mickleborough L. Limitations of blood conservation. J Thorac Cardiovasc Surg 1984;88:26–38.

83. Roberts WA, Kirkley SA, Newby M. A cost comparison of allogeneic and preoperatively or intraoperatively donated autologous blood. Anesth Analg 1996;83(1):129–133.

84. Monk TG, Goodnough LT, Brecher ME, et al. Acute normovolemic hemodilution can replace preoperative autologous blood donation as a standard of care for autologous blood procurement in radical prostatectomy. Anesth Analg 1997;85(5):953–958.

85. Hallett JJ. Minimizing the use of homologous blood products during repair of abdominal aortic aneurysms. Surg Clin N Am 1989;69(4):817–826.

86. Keeling MM, Gray LA Jr, Brink MA, Hillerich VK, Bland KI. Intraoperative autotransfusion. Experience in 725 consecutive cases. Ann Surg 1983;197(5):536–541.

87. Williamson K, Taswell H. Intraoperative autologous transfusion (IAT): experience in over 8000 surgical procedures. Transfusion (Phila) 1988;28:11S.

88. Giordano GF, Giordano DM, Wallace BA, Giordano KM, Prust RS, Sandler SG. An analysis of 9,918 consecutive perioperative autotransfusions. Surg Gynecol Obstet 1993;176(2):103–110.

89. Marty-Ane CH, Alric P, Picot MC, Picard E, Colson P, Mary H. Ruptured abdominal aortic aneurysm: influence of intraoperative management on surgical outcome. J Vasc Surg 1995;22(6):780–786.

90. Perttila J, Leino L, Poyhonen M, et al. Leucocyte content in blood processed by autotransfusion devices during open-heart surgery. Postoperative inflammatory response after autologous and allogeneic blood transfusion. Acta Anaesthesiol Scand 1995;39(4):511–516.

91. de Varennes B, Nguyen D, Denis F, Ergina P, Latter D, Morin JE. Reinfusion of mediastinal blood in CABG patients: impact on homologous transfusions and rate of reexploration. J Cardiovasc Surg 1996;11(6):387–395.

92. Healy WL, Pfeifer BA, Kurtz SR, et al. Evaluation of autologous

shed blood for autotransfusion after orthopaedic surgery. Clin Orthop 1994;299:53–59.

93. Tawes R, Duvall T. Autotransfusion in cardiac and vascular surgery: overview of a 25-year experience with intraoperative autotransfusion. In: Tawes R, ed. Autotransfusion. Therapeutic Principles and Trends, Vol. 1. Detroit: Gregory Appleton, 1997;147–148.

94. Boudreaux J, Bornside G, Cohn IJ. Emergency autotransfusion: partial cleansing of bacteria-laden blood by cell washing. J Trauma 1983;23(1):31–35.

95. Ozmen V, McSwain NJ, Nichols R, et al. Autotransfusion of potentially culture-positive blood (CPB) in abdominal trauma: preliminary data from a prospective study. J Trauma 1992;32(1): 36–39.

96. Wollinsky KH, Oethinger M, Buchele M, Kluger P, Puhl W, Mehrkens HH. Autotransfusion—bacterial contamination during hip arthroplasty and efficacy of cefuroxime prophylaxis. A randomized controlled study of 40 patients. Acta Orthop Scand 1997;68(3):225–230.

97. Atabek U, Spence RK, Pello M, Alexander J, Camishion R. Pancreaticoduodenectomy without homologous blood transfusion in an anemic Jehovah's Witness. Arch Surg 1992;127(3):349–351.

98. Kongsgaard UE, Wang MY, Kvalheim G. Leucocyte depletion filter removes cancer cells in human blood. Acta Anaesthesiol Scand 1996;40(1):118–120.

99. Jobes DR, Aitken GL, Shaffer GW. Increased accuracy and precision of heparin and protamine dosing reduces blood loss and transfusion in patients undergoing primary cardiac operations. J Thorac Cardiovasc Surg 1995;110(1):36–45.

100. Despotis GJ, Joist JH, Goodnough LT. Monitoring of hemostasis in cardiac surgical patients: impact of point-of-care testing on blood loss and transfusion outcomes. Clin Chem 1997;43(9): 1684–1696.

101. Flordal PA. Pharmacological prophylaxis of bleeding in surgical patients treated with aspirin. Eur J Anaesthesiol Suppl 1997;14: 38–41.

102. D'Ambra MN, Risk SC. Aprotinin, erythropoietin, and blood substitutes. Int Anesth Clin 1990;28(4):237–240.

103. Laupacis A, Fergusson D, Brown RS, Thwaites BK, Mongan PD. Drugs to minimize perioperative blood loss in cardiac surgery: meta-analyses using perioperative blood transfusion as the out-come. The International Study of Peri-operative Transfusion (ISPOT) Investigators. Tranexamic acid is effective in decreasing postoperative bleeding and transfusions in primary coronary artery bypass operations: a double-blind, randomized, placebo-controlled trial. Anesth Analg 1997;85(6):963–970.

104. Fremes SE, Wong BI, Lee E, et al. Metaanalysis of prophylactic drug treatment in the prevention of postoperative bleeding. Ann Thorac Surg 1994;58(6):1580–1588.

105. Spence RK, Cernaianu AC. Pharmacological agents as adjuncts to bloodless vascular surgery. Semin Vasc Surg 1994;7(2):114–120.

106. Gibble J, Ness P. Current perspectives on the use of fibrin glue (sealant) in the United States in the 1990s. In: Tawes R, ed. Autotransfusion: Therapeutic Principles and Trends. Detroit: Gregory Appleton, 1997:250–260.

107. Goldberg MA. Erythropoiesis, erythropoietin, and iron metabolism in elective surgery: preoperative strategies for avoiding allogeneic blood exposure. Am J Surg 1995;170(suppl 6A):37S–43S.

108. Alter HJ. Transfusion transmitted hepatitis C and non-A, non-B, non-C. Vox Sang 1994;67(suppl 3):19–24.

109. Alter HJ, Nakatsuji Y, Melpolder J, et al. The incidence of transfusion-associated hepatitis G virus infection and its relation to liver disease (see comments). N Engl J Med 1997;336(11):747–754.

110. Wagner S. Transfusion-related bacterial sepsis. Curr Opin Hematol 1997;4(6):464–469.

111. Sanz C, Pereira A, Vila J, Faundez AI, Gomez J, Ordinas A. Growth of bacteria in platelet concentrates obtained from whole blood stored for 16 hours at 22 degrees C before component preparation. Transfusion (Phila) 1997;37(3):251–254.

112. Sarkodee-Adoo CB, Kendall JM, Sridhara R, Lee EJ, Schiffer CA. The relationship between the duration of platelet storage and the development of transfusion reactions. Transfusion (Phila) 1998;38(3):229–235.

113. Bradley J. The blood transfusion effect: experimental aspects. Immunol Lett 1991;29(1–2):127–132.

114. Klein HG. Immunologic aspects of blood transfusion. Semin Oncol 1994;21(2 suppl 3):16–20.

115. Blumberg N, Hea IJ. Transfusion-induced immunomodulation and its possible role in cancer recurrence and perioperative bacterial infection. Yale J Biol Med 1990;63:429–433.

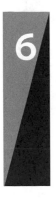

Diagnosis and Treatment of Infection

David L. Dunn

Microbes and Host Defenses

The complex process of host–microbe interactions can be conceptualized as an equation in which the risk of infection is directly proportional to a number of microbial factors and inversely proportional to the presence and vigor of various facets of host defenses. Microbial factors of importance include (1) number (inoculum size) and types of microbes, (2) rate of microbial proliferation, and (3) microbial virulence factors. These aspects are counterbalanced by host factors that include (1) strength of resident host defenses in the local environment at the site of microbial invasion, (2) magnitude and rate of recruitment of host defenses to the site of infection, and (3) potency of systemic host defenses should either local containment of microbes fail or should they be directly introduced into the bloodstream. This infection risk equation (see following) is useful to consider when determining whether or not intervention such as surgery, administration of antibiotics, or both should be undertaken.

$$\text{Infection} = \frac{\text{Microbial Invasion}}{\text{Host Defenses}} =$$

$$\frac{\text{Inoculum Size} \times \text{Species} \times \text{Division Rate} \times \text{Virulence Factors}}{\text{Potency (Resident/Recruited/Systemic)} \times \text{Recruitment Rate/Magnitude}}$$

Classification and Identification of Microbes

Microbes capable of causing infection may be encountered in the external environment or as part of the host microflora. The scope of potential pathogens that the surgeon may be called upon to diagnose and treat is enormous and includes many different bacteria, fungi, viruses, and parasites. These microbes are classified on the basis of a variety of characteristics that range from colonial morphology directly visualized without magnification to sophisticated genetic analysis. Microbiological diagnostic techniques of importance fall into several general categories: (1) differential staining, (2) isolation via colonial selection, (3) differential growth under various conditions, (4) observation of specific growth characteristics or traits, (5) direct identification of microbial antigens via immunological assays or demonstration of the presence of a host antibody response or, less commonly, a cellular immune response directed against them, and (6) identification of microbial genetic material.

Preliminary identification of bacteria and fungi within a sample of body fluid or tissue suspected of harboring infection is undertaken via microscopic observation using a number of different stains. Thereafter, in vitro growth in various types of media that facilitate isolation of the organism in pure culture takes place using standard techniques. Those microbes that do not readily replicate in vitro are identified either by antibody-based tests that serve to detect specific microbial antigens, or the host immune response to them, or both.

Particular species are identified according to their Gram stain and growth characteristics subsequent to isolation from a site of suspected or overt infection. The Gram stain is a simple but very important assay that can be performed rapidly by first fixing the specimen on a microscope slide using heat, staining it with crystal violet dye, fixing it with iodine-KI, then washing the specimen with either acetone or alcohol and counterstaining with a red dye such as safranin. Microscopic characteristics related to initial dye retention due to the structure of the bacterial cell wall serve to define bacteria according to color—gram-positive (blue) or gram-negative (red). Other parameters such as shape (round cocci, rodlike bacilli), patterns of division (single organisms, groups of organisms in pairs [diplococci], clusters [staphylococci] or chains [streptococci]), and presence and location of spores (e.g., terminal, central) facilitate initial identification (see Table 6.1).

Similar principles are applied for identification of fungi, although many of these microbes are dimorphic, replicating as single, separate cells (yeast) under certain nutrient and temperature conditions and as colonies in which the cells form long filaments (hyphae) under others. Occasionally, the presence of these pathogens can be deduced from the observation of characteristic large gram-positive microbes on Gram staining, but more commonly they are identified by use of special stains (e.g., KOH, India ink, Giemsa, methanamine silver).

Although growth in cell culture is possible for some pathogens, the presence of many viruses must be inferred by identification of the host immune (e.g., antibody) response. Use of a monoclonal antibody that is directed against a specific viral antigen and labeled with a marker (enzyme or immunofluorescent compound) can be useful for rapid microscopic identification of the presence of viral pathogens in body fluids or tissues. The presence of certain viral pathogens can be ascertained by use of routine light microscopy for identification of characteristic cytopathic abnormalities (e.g., CMV inclusion bodies) or via observation of characteristic viral particles via electron microscopy. Increasingly, viruses are being identified based upon the presence of viral genetic material using the polymerase chain reaction (PCR)–based test. As mentioned, the presence of parasites generally is confirmed by direct microscopic identification, by identification of a host antibody response to parasitic antigens, or the presence of these antigens by use of antibody-based tests, or by a combination of these assays.

Microbial Factors of Importance in the Development of Infection

One of the primary determinants of whether infection develops is the size of the initial microbial inoculum, which for bacteria is expressed in terms of colony-forming units (CFU). Two major reservoirs of microbes exist that can form the initial inoculum leading to infection in surgical patients: (1) host endogenous microflora, and (2) microbes within the external milieu, which often represents the nosocomial environment for hospitalized individuals.

The rate at which microbes proliferate in a specific environment represents a critical factor in the development of infection. Particularly in relation to bacteria and fungi, microbial division is dependent on ambient temperature and oxygen concentration, sources of nutrients, and inherent properties that determine the maximal division rate under optimal conditions. In addition, microbial growth is dependent on the capacity of one type of microbe to inhibit or promote the growth of another, the latter process being termed microbial synergy if associated with adverse effects greater than those caused by either organism alone during clinical infection. Finally, microbes may secrete toxins only under certain growth conditions, and some possess virulence mechanisms such as large polysaccharide capsules or leukocyte toxins that render them capable of evading or inhibiting host defenses.

The terms *pathogenicity* and *virulence* are relative designations and must be considered in relation to both host defenses and microbial virulence mechanisms (e.g., toxin secretion). Pathogenic microbes are those that are capable of causing disease; those that cause severe infection consistently are termed virulent. Low-virulence microbes are those that inconsistently cause infectious diseases in normal individuals. However, the host exists in a state of equilibrium with resident microflora and microbes within the environment that possess pathogenic potential but that are interdicted from causing disease by host defenses. Disruption or suppression of host defenses may allow invasion of microbes. Intriguingly,

TABLE 6.1. **Common Microbial Pathogens Capable of Causing Infection in Surgical Patients.**

Gram-positive bacterial aerobes
  Enterococcus faecium, faecalis
  Staphylococcus aureus, epidermidis
  Streptococcus pyogenes
  Streptococcus pneumoniae
  Streptococcus salivarius

Gram-negative bacterial aerobes
  Acinetobacter calcoaceticus
  Aeromonas hydrophila
  Citrobacter freundii
  Enterobacter cloacae, aerogenes
  Escherichia coli
  Hemophilus influenza
  Klebsiella pneumoniae
  Morganella morgagnii
  Proteus mirabilis
  Providencia stuartii
  Pseudomonas aeruginosa
  Pseudomonas cepacia, fluorescens
  Serratia marcescens
  Xanthomonas maltophilia

Fungi
  Absidia
  Aspergillus fumigatus
  Aspergillus niger, terreus, flavus
  Blastomyces dermatiditis
  Candida albicans
  Candida glabrata, krusei, parapsilopsis, torulopsis
  Coccidioides imitis
  Cryptococcus neoformans
  Fusarium
  Histoplasma capsulatum
  Mucor
  Pneumocystis carinii
  Rhizopus

Gram-positive bacterial anaerobes
  Clostridium perfringens, tetani, septicum
  Clostridium difficile
  Peptidostreptococcus
  Peptostreptococcus

Gram-negative bacterial anaerobes
  Bacteroides fragilis
  Bacteroides distasonis, thetaiotaomicron
  Fusobacterium

Acid-fast bacteria
  Mycobacterium avium-intracellulare
  Mycobacterium kansasii, chelonei
  Mycobacterium tuberculosis
  Nocardia asteroides and brasiliensis

Other bacteria
  Legionella pneumophila, micdadii
  Listeria monocytogenes

Viruses
  Cytomegalovirus
  Epstein–Barr virus
  Hepatitis B, C, and D viruses
  Herpes simplex virus
  Herpesvirus 6
  Human immunodeficiency virus
  Varicella zoster virus

only some species proliferate and cause infection, although even low-virulence organisms that rarely cause infection in an individual with intact host defense mechanisms can become pathogens in an immunosuppressed patient.

Host Defenses

Once a portal of entry for microbes is established (e.g., surgical wound, indwelling catheter, gut perforation), resident host defenses act to attempt to eliminate microbes that are present, and additional host defenses are recruited to the site of entry as microbes proliferate. These defenses consist of (1) physical barriers, (2) sequestration mechanisms, and (3) humoral and cellular host defenses in association with cytokines. All host defenses are tightly integrated such that the various components function as a complex, highly regulated system that is extremely effective in coping with microbial invaders. In addition, some elements of host defenses are redundant; however, despite this redundancy, perturbation of

one or more components may have a substantial negative impact upon resistance to infection.

PHYSICAL BARRIERS AND HOST MICROFLORA

The first line of host defense against both exogenous and endogenous microbes consists of physical, anatomical barriers. The hallmark of all barriers is that they possess either an epithelial (integument) or endothelial (respiratory, gut, urogenital) surface. These barriers serve to interdict the ingress of microbes into areas of the host that are sterile under normal circumstances. Microbes normally are associated with some but not all barriers, and in composite they are termed resident, endogenous, or autochthonous microflora. Common autochthonous microbes in various parts of the body are delineated in Table 6.2.

While barrier function remains intact, resident microflora are saprophytes, commensals, or symbionts; however, these same microbes often represent the initial inoculum of

TABLE 6.2. Common Autochthonous Microbes in Various Parts of the Body.

Region	Microbes[a]	Quantity[b]
Skin (all areas)	*Acinetobacter* *Brevibacterium* *Corynebacterium* *Micrococcus* *Pityrosporum* *Proprionibacterium* ***Staphylococcus aureus and epidermidis*** ***Streptococcus*** (nonenterococcal)	10^2-10^3
Skin (infraumbilical)	***Candida*** *Corynebacterium* ***Streptococcus faecalis, faecium*** ***Escherichia coli*** *Proprionibacterium* ***Staphylococcus aureus and epidermidis*** ***Streptococcus*** (nonenterococcal) ***Streptococcus faecalis and faecium***	10^2-10^5
Oropharynx	*Actinomyces* ***Bacteroides*** (non-*fragilis*) *Bifidobacterium* *Eubacterium* ***Fusobacterium*** ***Haemophilus*** *Moraxella* ***Peptostreptoccus*** *Porphyromonas* *Prevotella* ***Staphylococcus aureus and epidermidis*** ***Streptococcus*** (nonenterococcal) *Veillonella*	10^9-10^{11}
Stomach	***Candida*** ***Streptococcus*** (nonenterococcal)	10^2-10^3
Proximal small intestine	***Bacteroides fragilis*** and other spp. *Bifidobacterium* *Clostridium* ***Escherichia coli*** and other *Enterobacteriaceae* *Eubacterium* *Lactobacillus* ***Peptostreptococcus*** *Proprionibacterium*	10^3-10^7
Distal ileum	***Streptococcus faecalis, faecium***	10^5-10^8
Colorectum	*Veillonella*	$10^{11}-10^{12}$

[a]Potentially pathogenic organisms are designated in bold type.

[b]Colony-forming units (CFU)/ml or per gram feces.

pathogens when damage to or breach of a barrier occurs. This information is of considerable importance to surgeons, because prevention of infection is predicated on reducing the number of resident microbes before barrier disruption using topical microbicides or intraluminal antiseptics and/or antibiotics, plus systemic antibiotics to reduce the threat of microbial invasion and proliferation once wounding—either planned or traumatic—occurs.

First and foremost among the physical barriers is the integument. Besides acting to prevent ingress of pathogens, ancillary host defenses also exist as part of the integumentary barrier. For example, sebaceous glands secrete a variety of compounds that exhibit antimicrobial activity, which most likely both limits the number of resident microflora and prevents extensive colonization.

The respiratory tract possesses a number of host defense mechanisms, of which mucous secretion and ciliary action of specialized epithelial cells are the most critical. Mucus traps particles, including microbes, that are swept into the upper airways and oropharynx by ciliary action of specialized respiratory epithelial cells; coughing and expectoration follow. Any process that diminishes these host defenses can lead to microbial proliferation and invasion, usually eventuating in the presence of increasing numbers of microbes such that these organisms enter the distal branches of the respiratory tract, causing bronchitis or pneumonia.

The number of endogenous microbes varies throughout the gastrointestinal tract. Large numbers ($\sim 10^{11}$ CFU/ml) of aerobic and anaerobic bacteria are present at both ends of the gut, that is, oropharynx and colorectum, although the typical species differ somewhat among these two sites.[1] Few microbes ($\sim 10^2 - 10^3$ CFU/ml) are present within the normal stomach because of the low pH and initial slow transit that serve to promote microbial killing of ingested microbes in this highly acidic environment. Disease processes and drugs that inhibit gastric acidity may allow overgrowth of microbes in the stomach and thereby the small intestine, although in the absence of obstruction the relatively rapid transit time in the latter portion of the gut moves fluid, particles, and microbes aborally, counteracting overgrowth. Normally, the upper portion of the small-bowel lumen contains few microbes, but the number of resident microbes gradually increases aborally such that about 10^5 to 10^8 CFU/ml are present in the terminal ileum. The number of gut microbes present distal to the ileocecal valve increases exponentially such that within the sigmoid colon and rectum about 10^{11} to 10^{12} CFU/g feces are present. Anaerobes represent the predominant type of microbe, outnumbering aerobes by about 100 to 1. Large numbers of microbes exist within a dense layer of mucus that covers gut endothelial cells. Microbes adhere to gut endothelial cells, mucus, and to each other; and although these complex adherence interactions are not understood entirely, the autochthonous microflora create a highly anaerobic environment and act to prevent adherence, proliferation, overgrowth, and invasion of pathogens. This phenomenon is associated with the physical barrier and is termed colonization resistance.

SEQUESTRATION MECHANISMS

The mammalian host possesses a number of primitive host defenses that serve to sequester microbes at the site of in-

fection, thereby preventing dissemination. In any tissue, resident and recruited host defenses attempt to kill and eradicate all microbes, and the influx of inflammatory fluid contains fibrinogen, which during polymerization to fibrin traps bacteria in the extracellular milieu.[2,3] Also, within the abdomen, the omentum moves to a site of viscus perforation or inflammatory disease: this process, in conjunction with ileus and intestinal distension, serves to wall off infection. However, sequestration also partitions microbes from resident and recruited host defenses, the end result invariably being an abscess. The purulent material within the abscess represents the by-product of the death of both microbes and local and recruited humoral and cellular host defenses, and it is relatively impermeable to recruitment of additional host defenses or penetration of antibiotics. In addition, the presence of viable microbes within the abscess renders it a nidus for intermittent bacteremic episodes and complications related to its presence such as fever, pain, and bowel obstruction within the abdomen. Most likely, sequestration host defenses serve to convert serious, immediately life-threatening infections into more indolent, albeit chronic, types of infection. Invariably, an abscess requires some form of drainage although on occasion spontaneous discharge occurs. Rarely if ever can treatment be accomplished with antibiotics alone.

Finally, a number of proteins are present within the plasma and extracellular milieu that act to sequester nutrients that microbes require to divide. For example, transferrin and lactoferrin bind iron and thus limit the amount of this critical microbial growth factor. Low or high oxygen tension in certain parts of the body limits growth of aerobes or anaerobes, respectively.

HUMORAL AND CELLULAR IMMUNITY

Humoral immunity, so named because the components circulate within blood and body fluids as proteins, consists of two components: (1) antibodies (immunoglobulin, Ig), and (2) complement.[4] Antibodies are composed of a basic structure, two similar heavy (α, δ, ϵ, γ, or μ) and two similar light chains (κ or λ). Different antibodies may be capable of binding to different portions of an antigen, particularly if the antigen is a large, complex structure such as a microbe. The most limited antigenic region to which an antibody binds is termed an epitope, typically defined by competitive inhibition of binding of two or more distinct monoclonal antibodies. In humans, there are five different classes of antibodies—IgG, IgM, IgD, IgE, and IgA. There are four subclasses of IgG (IgG_{1-4}) and two of IgA ($IgA_{1,2}$). In addition, certain portions of the heavy chain of IgM and IgG possess the capacity to activate the complement cascade ($IgM \gg IgG$) once antigen binding occurs, and the terminal Fc portion of some subclasses of IgG is capable of binding to leukocyte receptors, markedly enhancing phagocytosis.

Antibodies are produced by B lymphocytes in response to the presence of substances including microbes that the mammalian host recognizes as a foreign antigen and not part of itself. In composite, B cells possess the ability to make a huge number of different Ig molecules ($>10^8$) via recombination and somatic mutation of genes that encode for the constant, variable, and hypervariable regions of each heavy and light chain. B-cell-bound IgD is capable of binding antigen directly, which triggers proliferation of a clone of B cells that secrete antibody; some of these cells circulate for long periods of time (memory cells). T-helper lymphocytes and macrophages interact with B cells, acting as accessory cells facilitating the antibody response. Some antigens are capable of directly stimulating B cells to produce antibody absent accessory cell interactions, although in general the response is less vigorous.

The humoral immune response serves to target multiantigenic pathogens for complement-mediated lysis and augmented phagocytosis. Most types of antigens engender production of antibody of the pentameric IgM class initially, but within about 2 to 3 weeks antibody of similar binding specificity but of the IgG class is secreted. Thereafter, if antigen persists or reexposure occurs after initial clearance, IgG of greater binding affinity is produced in ever larger amounts. Two subclasses of dimeric IgA (IgA_1, IgA_2) are secreted at mucosal surfaces by submucosal resident B lymphocytes, which act to prevent the ingress of antigens including pathogenic microbes, while IgE is present in small amounts in the circulation and is secreted into the respiratory tract. Although natural antibodies to many pathogens exist in low levels, initial contact followed by subsequent exposure to a particular pathogen triggers a more intense response because of the presence of memory cells. This phenomenon is the basis for vaccination against specific pathogens or toxins.

Complement consists of a large number of inactive proteins that circulate within the bloodstream. These proteins are activated and thereby modified in a specific sequence, several steps of which serve to trigger the production of large amounts of bioactive compounds. Activation of this cascade of proteins occurs by means of the binding of certain types of Ig to microbial antigens (IgM is extremely efficient), and via direct activation by specific components of the microbial cell wall such as gram-negative bacterial lipopolysaccharide (endotoxin, LPS) or yeast saccharides such as *Candida* mannan. Two different complement activation pathways (classical, alternate [Properdin]) lead to a single common pathway in which complement protein fragments play key roles in the host defense response. For example, C3b and C4b enhance Ig adherence, while C3bi and C1q serve as opsonins leading to enhanced phagocytosis of microbes by leukocytes. C5a...p, C3a, and C4a are anaphylatoxins (listed in order of potency) acting to increase vascular permeability and concurrent influx of additional proteins; C5a also is a chemoattractant causing phagocytic cell chemotaxis. Finally, C5b6–9 forms what is termed a membrane attack complex that creates a hole in microbes, leading to osmotic cell disruption and death.

Monocytes and polymorphonuclear leukocytes (PMNs) are capable of engulfing microbes, via the process of phagocytosis. Once internalized, that portion of the leukocyte membrane that has enveloped the pathogen (phagocytic vacuole) fuses with an intracellular structure termed the lysosome, which contains a variety of enzymes (e.g., lysozyme, cathepsin) and reactive oxygen metabolites (O^-_2, OH^-) that serve to kill and degrade the invading microorganism.

The body contains large numbers of resident macrophages within various tissues that serve as one of the first lines of host defense against microbial invasion. Microbial invasion also triggers the recruitment of PMNs to the site of infection via the aforementioned activity of the complement cascade and because of the presence of peptide sequences in which microbial derived *N*-formyl methionine is present. This leads to an influx of large numbers of these highly active phagocytic cells within 2 to 4 h of invasion, the magnitude and duration of this response being proportional to the size of the inoculum and ability of the microbes to proliferate and remain at the site of infection or spread. Both macrophages and PMNs secrete a number of highly bioactive substances into the internal milieu during cellular activation. Unfortunately, many of these compounds also exert deleterious effects upon the host. For example, the contents of lysosomes and reactive oxygen metabolites are extremely toxic to mammalian cells, and release of copious amounts of cytokines secreted by macrophages in response to bacterial cell wall products is thought to be responsible in large part for sepsis syndrome.

Cytokines function as regulatory molecules that play an important role during infection as follows: (1) coordination of cellular immunity with other aspects of host defense, and (2) regulation of host defense via augmentation and suppression of specific defense components, including their own activity. Bacteria and fungal cell wall compounds (e.g. endotoxins) trigger macrophages to synthesize and secrete large amounts of what are termed proinflammatory cytokines: tumor necrosis factor-α (TNF-α), interleukin-1β (IL-1β), interleukin-6 (IL-6), and interferon-γ (IFN-γ). Presumably because cytokines exert such potent effects within the local tissue environment and systematically, counterregulatory compounds are secreted in response to the release of proinflammatory cytokines.

Coordination of Host Defenses

Complex regulatory events occur in relation to the humoral, cellular, and cytokine components of host defense. As noted earlier, repeated antigenic stimulation leads to refinement of the antibody response such that high levels of increasingly high affinity IgG are produced. In addition, the host cellular response to infection is not confined to phagocytic cells. T lymphocytes have been thought to be an important defense mainly against intracellular pathogens such as *Mycobacteria tuberculosis*, but their role in defense against common bacterial infections has been elucidated as well. A paradigm in which a subset of T-helper lymphocytes (Th1) is associated with proinflammatory cytokines including IL-2, IFN-γ, and TNF-β has emerged, and this system is regulated by a separate subset of similar cells (Th2) that are associated with antiinflammatory cytokines such as IL-4 and IL-10.

Concurrent with the secretion of IL-1β and TNF-α during gram-negative bacterial infection and endotoxemia, a complex network of endogenous cytokine antagonists for these cytokines functions to dampen the host cytokine response. Interleukin-1 receptor antagonist (IL-1ra) is secreted, tumor necrosis factor-binding protein (TNF-BP) is shed from the cell surface (representing TNF RI), and other agents tightly regulate cytokine elaboration under normal circumstances, although during severe infection an exaggerated, dysregulated cytokine response can occur.[5–8]

Finally, certain parts of the body possess unique host defense mechanisms. For example, specialized areas on the peritoneal mesothelial surface of the diaphragm form stomata that lead into lymphatic channels, which in turn coalesce into large channels within the thoracic cavity that eventually drain into the thoracic duct.[9] Via this pathway, large volumes of fluid containing phagocytic cells, erythrocytes, or microbes can be pumped from the peritoneal cavity. However, if a large inoculum of microbes enters the bloodstream via this mechanism, sepsis syndrome can occur.

Antimicrobial Agents

The precepts of antimicrobial agent usage entail familiarity with the following: (1) microbes commonly encountered during the prevention or treatment of specific types of infections; (2) antibiotic class, mechanism of action, and spectrum of activity of index agents; (3) spectrum of activity of specific agents within a class; (4) prophylactic, empiric (preemptive), or therapeutic use coupled with duration of administration; (5) global, institutional, and unique care unit microbial antibiotic resistance patterns; (6) culture and antibiotic sensitivity patterns of organisms cultured from a specific site; and (7) clinical course of the patient.

β-Lactam Agents

Four subclasses of β-lactam drugs have been developed, all of which are bactericidal: penicillins, cephalosporins, monobactams, and carbapenems. These drugs act to inhibit bacterial cell wall synthesis by competitively inhibiting transpeptidation of the D-alanyl group of N-acteylmuramic acid residues. This step in microbial cell wall peptidoglycan synthesis and cross-linking is critical to microbial cell wall integrity.

Penicillin G is the index drug for this class; it possesses activity against many common gram-positive organisms, but resistant isolates have become increasingly common. Depot forms of the drug (procaine and benzathine penicillin) remain extremely useful agents, and penicillin V is available as an oral formulation. Ampicillin and amoxicillin exhibit activity against many enterococci and streptococci and a limited number of strains of gram-negative aerobes such as *Escherichia coli*. So-called semisynthetic penicillins such as methicillin exhibit substantial gram-positive activity, similar to penicillin G for streptococci plus enhanced activity against *Staphylococcus aureus*, although the prevalence of methicillin-resistant strains (MRSA) has increased substantially during the past decade. Carboxypenicillins (carbenicillin, ticarcillin) and ureidopenicillins (acylampicillins [piperacillin, azlocillin]) exhibit substantial activity against gram-negative aerobes including many strains *of Pseudomonas aeruginosa*, and the latter agents also are active against many strains of enterococci based upon their derivation from ampicillin.

Many microbes secrete enzymes that cleave the β-lactam ring of these agents, and several inhibitors of these virulence factors have been developed (clavulanate, sulbactam, tazobactam). These compounds have been combined with β-lactam antibiotics, and the combined drugs (ticarcillin-clavulanate, amoxicillin-clavulanate, ampicillin-sulbactam, piperacillin-tazobactam) possess an extended spectrum of activity that generally includes more strains of gram-positive and gram-negative aerobes than the parent antibiotic alone, plus potent anaerobic activity.

A large number of cephalosporins have been developed as well, and these agents are grouped into first-, second-, third-, and more recently fourth-generation drugs. A simple way to remember the spectrum of activity of the agents in each generation is that first-generation drugs exhibit considerable gram-positive aerobic activity including activity against methicillin-sensitive *Staphylococcus aureus* (MSSA), but little gram-negative aerobic activity. Gram-positive activity decreases progressively with second- and third-generation agents, whereas the gram-negative activity increases and selected second- and third-generation agents (ceftriaxone, cefoxitin, cefotetan) possess considerable activity against anaerobes. This activity occurs because bacterial enzymes located at the cell wall division plate to which different types of β-lactam antibiotics bind are distinct among gram-positive and gram-negative bacteria. Finally, cephalosporin agents do not possess any important degree of enterococcal activity.

A single monobactam agent has been developed (aztreonam), and this drug has activity against only gram-negative aerobes such as *E. coli* and many but not all strains of *Pseudomonas aeruginosa*. Carbapenem agents exhibit potent activity against many gram-negative aerobes including *P. aeruginosa* and most anaerobes. Imipenem-cilastatin is a combination drug in which cilastatin prevents degradation of the β-lactam component by renal tubular epithelial brush border dihydropeptidases. Meropenem is not degraded in this fashion while Ertapenem can be administered once daily.

Glycopeptides and Streptogramins

Vancomycin and teicoplanin are glycopeptides that act to kill bacteria by inhibiting bacterial cell wall synthesis in a fashion distinct from that of β-lactam drugs. These agents demonstrate potent activity against most strains of gram-positive pathogens including streptococci, many enterococci, MSSA, and MRSA. Bacteria resistant to one agent are generally resistant to the other. Vancomycin exhibits nephrotoxicity, and drug level and serum creatinine monitoring generally is required. Potential advantages of teicoplanin include reduced nephrotoxicity and less frequent dosing.

Streptogramins are a class of agents that act to prevent bacterial growth by inhibition of ribosomal synthesis. Streptogramins A and B act via two separate mechanisms, both of which are distinct from that of other protein synthesis inhibitors. Quinupristine-dalfopristine combines these two streptogramins and is active against many gram-positive pathogens.

Macrolides and Related Agents

Erythromycin is a macrolide antibiotic that acts to inhibit bacterial protein synthesis by binding to the 50S ribosomal subunit. It possesses activity against a number of gram-positive organisms and some degree of anaerobic activity. Azithromycin and clarithromycin also are macrolides and possess greater anaerobic activity. None of these drugs should be considered "first-line" agents for either staphylococci or streptococci, although they often are administered to patients who are allergic to β-lactam drugs. Clindamycin, chloramphenicol, and various tetracyclines are structurally unrelated but act to inhibit various steps in bacterial protein synthesis; they possess considerable activity against anaerobes as well as many gram-positive pathogens.

Aminoglycosides

The aminoglycosides are available only in parenteral formulation and are bactericidal, acting to inhibit microbial ribosomal protein synthesis plus a second poorly defined microbicidal mechanism, both of which lead to bacterial killing. Their spectrum of activity is primarily gram-negative aerobes including *Enterobacteriaceae* and pseudomonads, and they exhibit some degree of activity against some strains of gram-positive microbes. Their use is associated with nephrotoxicity, and for that reason many clinicians believe that drug levels and serum creatinine values should be monitored to avoid high peaks and troughs of drug levels if more than 3 days of therapy are needed or if the patient exhibits renal dysfunction before initial administration.

Quinolones

The quinolones act to inhibit bacterial replication by binding to one of several DNA synthase enzymes (DNA gyrase, DNA topoisomerase IV). Naladixic acid is the index agent, and this drug possesses activity primarily against gram-negative aerobic microbes. More recently, a number of fluoroquinolones have become available, all of which possess greater activity against gram-negative aerobes and some degree of gram-positive activity. Ciprofloxacin demonstrates excellent activity against gram-negative aerobes including *Pseudomonas aeruginosa*, while levofloxacin, ofloxacin, grepafloxacin, lomefloxacin, and sparfloxacin exhibit enhanced activity against gram-positive bacteria. Trovafloxacin and moxifloxacin demonstrate activity against gram-negative and gram-positive aerobes as well as anaerobes, but trovafloxacin is no longer available because of a low but significant incidence of severe hepatotoxicity associated with its administration.

Sulfonamides

Sulfonamide agents act by inhibition of microbial folic acid production, blocking the synthesis of tetrahydropteroid acid. A number of agents are available, and one of the most useful is sulfamethoxazole. When combined with trimethoprim, which inhibits the enzyme dihydrofolate reductase that catalyzes a later step in the same biosynthetic pathway, these drugs are extremely active against a wide spectrum of pathogens including gram-negative aerobes. This agent commonly is used to treat urinary tract infections and to prevent and treat infection caused by certain opportunistic pathogens in immunosuppressed patients.

Other Antibacterial Agents

Metronidazole is a drug that is available in oral and intravenous formulations and possesses potent activity against virtually all anaerobic bacteria, as well as gut parasites. It is often used to treat the anaerobic component of a polymicrobial infection; it is also effective against *Clostridium difficile*, and its oral formulation is used to treat colonic infection caused by this pathogen.

Antifungal Agents

A more limited number of agents are available to treat fungal pathogens; these consist of amphotericin B and several azole drugs. Amphotericin B acts to prevent fungal growth and kills fungi by binding to fungal cell wall sterols and causing cell death via lysis. However, this agent causes nephrotoxicity, the occurrence of which is related to the cumulative dose of drug administered. Several different liposomal preparations of this agent have been developed that allow administration of much higher (three- to fivefold) doses with less associated nephrotoxicity and equivalent or perhaps superior efficacy, albeit currently at higher cost. Azole agents inhibit fungal sterol synthesis that is critical to cell wall growth and therefore division. Agents such as ketaconazole are active against many routine fungi such as *Candida* as well as specific agents such as *Blastomyces dermatiditis*. Triazole drugs (fluconazole, itraconazole, voriconazole) and the echinocandin caspofungin are active against a wider array of fungi.

Antiviral Agents

Only a limited number of viral agents are available, although the number has increased in recent years. Acyclovir, ganciclovir, and their derivatives valacyclovir and valganciclovir exhibit activity primarily directed against herpesviruses. Amantadine is effective against influenza virus A (but not B), a pathogen that causes disease rarely even in immunosuppressed patients. Ribavarin is used to treat respiratory syncytial virus, and although it has been used to treat infection caused by adenovirus, its efficacy for this and other pathogens is limited.

The hepatitides are diseases caused by a diverse group of pathogens that are considered together because of their propensity to cause hepatocellular cytotoxicity, eventual cirrhosis and hepatic failure, and hepatocellular carcinoma. The most common pathogens among surgical patients are HBV and HCV, both of which can be transmitted via blood or body fluid exposure. Disease caused by HBV can be prevented by vaccination, and individuals at high risk for exposure (hemodialysis patients, and all surgeons and health care workers who participate in invasive procedures) should receive three doses of the recombinant vaccine.[10] Disease caused by HBV can range from asymptomatic infection identified solely by serological studies to fulminant hepatic failure. Postexposure prophylaxis of nonimmunized individuals consists of administration of hepatitis B immune globulin (0.06 ml/kg i.m. immediately and at 1 month), following which standard vaccination should take place. There is some evidence that progression of hepatitis can be ameliorated by use of lamivudine.

HCV is transmitted in a fashion similar to HBV, and also is identified via serological studies as well as RNA-based assays. IFN-α2b is used to treat chronic hepatitis caused by hepatitis C virus (3×10^6 U s.c. $3 \times$/week $\times$ 12 months), and a vaccine is being developed.[11] Various other hepatitis viruses (D and E) have been identified, most of which appear to be associated and to require HBV coinfection to cause disease. A series of agents have been developed against human immunodeficiency virus (HIV), including agents such as zidovudine, all of which act to prevent viral growth by inhibiting retroviral reverse transcriptase. Current recommendations for postexposure prophylaxis consist of administration of zidovudine for 1 month as a single agent for mucocutaneous exposure to HIV and in combination with other retroviral agents, lamivudine and indinavir, for serious or massive exposure including percutaneous injury.[12]

Appropriate Use of Antimicrobial Agents

Antibiotic usage in surgical patients can be categorized as prophylaxis, empiric (referred to as preemptive by some authors), and treatment. For surgical patients, antibiotics generally are used to prevent infection (prophylaxis) in situations in which the risk of wound infection is high. In this situation, one or more agents that possess activity against the most likely pathogens should be administered. So-called preemptive therapy entails the use of preoperative prophylaxis, following which postoperative doses are administered as well in a situation in which a large inoculum is likely to be present such as penetrating gastrointestinal tract trauma. Although antibiotics routinely are used to treat infection, it should be noted that for many disease processes the precise duration of therapy has not been established.

Basic tenets regarding antibiotic therapy in surgical patients are as follows: (1) define the disease process being treated, its severity, and set duration of antibiotic therapy from the outset; (2) reevaluate the patient's clinical course on an ongoing basis in relation to the need for antibiotic administration; (3) use antibiotics in conjunction with other treatment modalities such as drainage and debridement; (4) use stains, cultures, and sensitivity studies, and other laboratory tests to guide therapy but do not change agents or extend the antibiotic treatment course in a patient who is faring well solely on the basis of this information; (5) review the patient's drug allergy history carefully; (6) choose the least toxic drug appropriate for the infection; and (7) consider cost and, if equivalent agents are available, select the least expensive.[13]

Antibiotic Allergy

It is important to ascertain whether a patient has had any type of allergic reaction in association with administration of a particular antibiotic. Penicillin allergy is quite common, occurring in 7 to 40 of 1000 treatment courses. The incidence of cross-reactivity to other β-lactam drugs is difficult to ascertain because some initial cephalosporin preparations contained penicillin drugs as well. Although avoiding the use of any β-lactam drug is appropriate in patients who manifest significant allergic reactions to penicillins, the incidence of cross-reactivity appears highest for carbapenems, much lower for cephalosporins (~5–7%), and extremely small for monobactams.

Severe allergic manifestations to a specific class of agents, such as anaphylaxis, generally preclude the use of any agents in that class, except under circumstances in which use of an agent represents a life-saving measure.

Endocarditis Prophylaxis

Patients with valvular heart disease, prosthetic heart valves, or other cardiac defects should receive prophylactic antibiotics before undergoing dental, upper respiratory, and gastrointestinal or genitourinary procedures to prevent the occurrence of microbial endocarditis.

Antibiotic Resistance

The widespread use of antibiotics for the treatment of infectious diseases has led to significant improvements in morbidity and mortality rates, but has concomitantly heralded the appearance of microbes resistant to many different agents. Resistance patterns parallel the duration and extent of usage both of classes of agents and of a particular agent, particularly within an institution. It is imperative that the practitioner

become familiar with global, institutional, and care unit resistance patterns, which are of particular importance in surgical patients for whom prophylactic and preemptive therapy frequently is employed, the latter before culture and sensitivity results are available.

Surgical Infectious Diseases

Nosocomial Infections in Surgical Patients

Potential sites of such nosocomial infections in surgical patients include urinary tract infections (UTIs), pneumonia, surgical site (wound) infections (SSIs), and bloodstream infection bacteremia, the latter of which may occur with or without infection being identified at a specific site, including that of an intravascular device. Extensive survey data have been collected regarding the epidemiology of nosocomial infections that include (1) site-specific rates, (2) causative pathogens, and (3) associated morbidity and mortality (Table 6.3).[14] This information is useful in identifying and monitoring high-risk patients, implementing preventive strategies, and diagnosing and treating those infections that occur.

URINARY TRACT INFECTION AND PNEUMONIA

UTIs, the most common type of nosocomial infection, can occur in surgical patients as the result of underlying genitourinary disease or prolonged indwelling catheter drainage.[15] For that reason, every attempt should be made to remove this type of device after the initial operation. In general, this can be accomplished within 1 to 3 days even for major procedures. Significant infection can be diagnosed based upon the presence of more than 100,000 CFU/ml. Initial therapy should be directed against common gram-negative aerobic organisms such as E. coli, although UTIs caused by gram-positive bacteria such as Enterococcus faecalis and E. faecium are common as well. Meticulous aseptic technique during catheter insertion and tubing changes and daily meatal care serve to diminish the risk of such infections. If a UTI occurs during the postoperative period, it should be treated for 10 to 14 days with an antibiotic demonstrated to have efficacy based upon sensitivity testing, and a urine sample should be obtained for culture 3 to 5 days after completion of therapy. Identification

TABLE 6.3. Epidemiology of Nosocomial Infections in Patients in Surgical Intensive Care Units.

Nosocomial infection	Rate	Distribution[a] (%)
Urinary tract	5.3[b]	20.7
Surgical site	0.14–5.28[c]	13.2
Pneumonia	14.5[d]	31.4
Central line-associated bacteremia	4.9[e]	15.1
Other		19.6

[a]Percentage that each type of infection contributes to 100% of infections among surgical patients.
[b]Number of urinary catheter-days/number of patient days.
[c]Number of infections per 100 cases.
[d]Number of ventilator-days/number of patient days.
[e]Number of central line-days/number of patient days.
Source: Anonymous.[14]

of recurrent infection mandates a search for an underlying anatomical abnormality.

The occurrence of postoperative pneumonia in a surgical patient is a grave, potentially highly morbid event. In some patients the diagnosis is readily established based upon the presence of a discrete area of pulmonary consolidation on chest roetgenogram and a single organism being identified upon Gram stain and culture from a sample of sputum. In most hospitals, initial empiric therapy should be directed against gram-negative aerobic pathogens although gram-positive microbes such as *Staphylococcus aureus* also cause such infections. Patients who undergo prolonged tracheal intubation who develop fever and infiltrates on chest roetgenogram should undergo diagnostic bronchoscopy if routine sputum sampling does not reveal the presence of more than 25 PMNs per low-power field ($\times100$) via microscopic examination and a single causative organism using the former technique or routine culture. Postoperative pneumonia should be treated with a 14-21-day course of an appropriate parenteral antibiotic; it is associated with a mortality rate of more than 50% among patients requiring mechanical ventilation.[16,17]

SURGICAL SITE INFECTIONS

Surgical site infections are categorized according to whether they involve the superficial wound that constitutes the skin and subcutaneous tissue above the fascia, the deep wound that is the body cavity in which the procedure is performed, or both regions concurrently. Because of the importance of administering prophylactic antibiotics in reducing wound infection rates for certain types of procedures, surgical wounds are classified into three strata according to the potential risk of microbial contamination. Class I or clean wounds are those in which only skin microflora are likely to contaminate the operative field; because no hollow viscus that possesses endogenous microflora is entered, the risk of infection is low

($\sim$1–4%). A subset of class I wounds (I_D) are those in which prosthetic material such as mesh, a vascular graft, a cardiac valve, or a medical device is implanted; although the risk of infection is similar to other class I wounds, the consequences of wound infection can be dire, often defeating the purpose of the procedure. Class II clean contaminated wounds are those in which a hollow viscus likely to harbor microbes is entered (gut, biliary tract), such that both skin microflora plus resident microbes may be present in the wound, producing a slightly higher risk of infection ($\sim$3–6%). Class III wounds are those in which substantial microbial contamination (e.g., fecal soilage; traumatic heavily contaminated wound) may be present, and the overall wound infection risk is substantial ($\sim$4–20%), particularly if the skin edges of the superficial wound are apposed. Examples of operative procedures and ranges of wound infection rates are provided in Table 6.4. Wound classification systems are used by the surgeon to decide whether to administer prophylactic antibiotics, whether to select agents with activity against pathogens that are likely to contaminate the wound and cause infection, and whether to close the skin edges of the wound per primum.

A series of maneuvers appear, in composite, to reduce the rate of infection of either the superficial or deep portions of the wound or both sites. These include (1) preoperative patient skin preparation in the form of scrubbing the prospective wound area and showering using a topical microbicide; (2) clipping of hair, but avoidance of shaving the skin of the prospective wound site, particularly in advance of the procedure because microbial proliferation can occur in areas of epidermal damage; (3) surgeon handscrubbing and patient skin preparation using a topical microbicide immediately before the procedure; (4) instrument sterilization and avoidance of breaks in aseptic technique; (5) use of mechanical preparation, intraluminal antibiotics, or antiseptics for selected procedures to reduce the microbial inoculum within a hollow viscus that will be entered as part of the procedure; and

TABLE 6.4. Surgical Site Infection Risk Stratification and Rates of Infection.

Class	Definition	Examples	Rate (%)
I: Clean	Atraumatic wound No inflammation No break in aseptic technique No entry of biliary, respiratory, GI, or GU tracts	Herniorraphy Excision of skin lesion Thyroidectomy	1–4
I_D: Clean; prosthetic material implanted	Same as I, Clean	Vascular surgery with graft Cardiac valve replacement	1–4
II: Clean contaminated	Atraumatic wound No inflammation Minor break in aseptic technique Biliary, respiratory, GI, or GU tracts entered with either minimal spillage or prior preparation	Appendectomy without perforation Elective colectomy after bowel preparation Cholecystectomy	3–6
III: Contaminated	Traumatic wound with delay in therapy or exogenous contamination Inflammation or purulence Major break in aseptic technique Entry of biliary, respiratory, GI, or GU tract with gross spillage of contents	Colectomy for colonic perforation Open drainage of intraabdominal abscess	4–20

(6) administration of prophylactic antibiotics that possess activity against numerically common, albeit not all, potential pathogens that may contaminate the wound during the operation.

In current clinical practice, prophylactic usage of antibiotics consists of administration of an agent with activity against pathogens that could be present in substantial numbers, and in which the statistical likelihood of these microbes causing infection is low but measurable. For practical purposes this amounts to a risk of infection of more than 2% to 4%. Thus, standard practice entails administration of a prophylactic antibiotic 5 to 10 min before creating the skin incision for class I_D, II, and selected class III procedures.[18–21] In addition, the agent should be readministered during those procedures in which the duration of the operation exceeds the serum $t_{1/2}$ of the agent to ensure that microbial levels are continually present.

Whether systemic antibiotics should be administered to patients undergoing clean surgery continues to be debated. Several clinical trials have attempted to resolve this issue, but none have provided definitive evidence of the value of prophylactic antibiotics in reducing wound infection rates.[22,23] The subset of patients undergoing clean surgery in whom a prosthetic device is implanted into a tissue space (e.g., pacemaker, vascular graft) should receive an agent directed against skin microflora because in most cases wound infection is associated with considerable morbidity and occasional mortality.

The effect of prophylactic antibiotics has been most carefully examined in patients undergoing elective colonic resection. Initial studies provided evidence of the efficacy of mechanical preparation of the bowel using cathartics and enemas plus oral antibiotics administered on three occasions before the operation. Poorly absorbed agents directed against gram-negative aerobes (neomycin) and absorbable agents with activity against anaerobes (erythromycin, tetracycline, metronidazole) were examined, and clear benefit in reducing both superficial and deep wound infection rates were observed.[24] Current standard of care based upon survey results conducted during the past decade is the use of mechanical bowel preparation, two separate oral agents, plus a single dose of a parenteral agent with a spectrum of activity against aerobes and anaerobes.[25]

Superficial surgical wound infection must be treated by opening the wound, draining purulent material, debriding devitalized tissue, and instituting dressing changes that include packing the wound with gauze. Obtaining cultures and using of an antimicrobial agent should be reserved for patients who exhibit extensive cellulitis (>2 cm from incision margin) and immunosuppressed patients in whom unusual pathogens may be causative. Deep wound infections require percutaneous drainage if no ongoing source of infection such as a leaking anastomosis is present, although in some patients reexploration is required.

BLOODSTREAM INFECTIONS AND SEPSIS SYNDROME

Bloodstream infections occur frequently in the nosocomial environment; currently the incidence of nosocomial bloodstream infection is about 250,000 to 300,000 per annum in the United States.[14,26] Gram-positive microbes account for about 50 to 60% of events and gram-negative bacteria about 30%; fungemia, mainly caused by *Candida* sp., accounts for the remainder. Sepsis syndrome occurs in a subset of patients who manifest the systemic inflammatory response syndrome (SIRS) on the basis of infection. Currently, SIRS describes patients with two or more of the following: temperature above 38°C, heart rate greater than 90 beats/min, respiratory rate above 20 breaths/min, white blood cell count above 12,000 cells/mm^3, and the presence of more than 10% immature band forms of neutrophils on the peripheral blood smear.[27] It is highly likely, however, that most episodes of bacteremia and fungemia are both intermittent and transient, precluding isolation of the offending pathogens during every clinical event; less than 50% of patients who develop sepsis syndrome have a microbial pathogen cultured from their bloodstream. The term severe sepsis syndrome refers to the added presence of organ dysfunction. Septic shock is defined as the sepsis syndrome in association with hypotension that persists despite adequate fluid resuscitation.

Sepsis syndrome can progress to MSOF and is the thirteenth most common cause of death among patients in the United States, with as many as 400,000 cases occurring annually, and surgical patients account for about 30% of these cases.[28,29] Despite improvements in antimicrobial therapy and intensive care (e.g., aggressive fluid resuscitation, hemodynamic monitoring, and metabolic support), mortality associated with sepsis syndrome remains at about 40%, a statistic that has changed but little over the past several decades.

Because staphylococci are responsible for the majority of gram-positive bacteremic events, initial antibiotic therapy should target these organisms. Because of the appearance and rapid spread of VRE that has been associated with widespread vancomycin use, consideration should be given to the use of semisynthetic penicillins such as nafcillin or methicillin or a first-generation cephalosporin as initial empiric therapy. For the β-lactam-allergic patient or a patient who has developed a life-threatening infection, a short course (at most 3 days) of vancomycin should be administered, after which empiric therapy with this drug should be halted if no gram-positive organism is isolated either from blood or from a specific site of infection.

Bacteremia caused by gram-negative bacterial infections remains common, accounting for about 30 to 35% of cases. The mortality associated with gram-negative bacteremia in normal individuals is 10% and may exceed 50% in immunocompromised patients. Antibiotic therapy should be initiated if evidence of sepsis syndrome and a potential source of gram-negative bacterial infection are identified; therapy should not be delayed for culture documentation of bacteremia. The initial choice of antimicrobial agent should be based upon the institutional or care unit antibiotic resistance patterns.

Clinical trials in which febrile neutropenic patients were treated with either single agents or two agents in combination, usually a β-lactam drug plus an aminoglycoside, have provided evidence that the dual-agent therapy is more effective than single-agent therapy in this particular heavily immunosuppressed patient population. Currently, a single broad-spectrum β-lactam agent is used with or without vancomycin.[30,31] Although use of dual-agent therapy frequently is extended to other patient groups, no clinical trials have been performed to provide evidence of similar efficacy in the general patient population. When a microbe is identified that is typically highly resistant to many agents (e.g., *Pseudomonas* or *Xanthomonas* species), dual-agent therapy should be considered.[32]

C. albicans accounts for more than half the fungi cultured from clinical infections. Isolation of fungus from the bloodstream should prompt immediate initiation of antifungal treatment and a search for the source of infection. In nonneutropenic patients, either intravenous fluconazole or amphotericin B can be used initially, unless the isolate is known to be resistant to triazole drugs.[33] Fungemic patients who exhibit hemodynamic instability or neutropenia should receive amphotericin B as the initial therapeutic agent. Therapy for bacteremia or fungemia should be continued for 10 to 21 days, although the precise duration of therapy is unknown and has not been examined in clinical trials.

INTRAVASCULAR CATHETER INFECTIONS

Many patients undergo intravascular catheter placement at some time during their hospitalization, and epidemiological linear data indicate that among about 3 million central venous catheters inserted per annum in the United States, about 25% will become colonized and among about 5% (150,000) will be associated with bacteremia. Similar events are 10-fold less common when peripheral catheters are considered, probably because of their short duration of use.[34]

The risk of catheter infection is increased if inserted through infected or contaminated skin (e.g., burns), so these areas should be avoided if at all possible. Femoral vein catheters are more likely to become infected than subclavian or internal jugular vein catheters, probably related to both degree of skin contamination and catheter movement in and out of the exit site. Multilumen catheters may also have a higher rate of infection than single-lumen catheters, but this may not be clinically significant because multilumen catheters are typically used for short periods of time. Although tunneled or cuffed catheters initially were thought to decrease infection, several prospective studies have shown that these devices offer no advantage over noncuffed catheters.[35] In composite, the risk of infection increases significantly with the length of time a catheter is in place, although this is most probably a surrogate marker for catheter use and manipulation.

The use of routine catheter changes either via guidewire exchange or insertion at a separate site has been rigorously examined. The former increased infection rates, while the latter increased the incidence of mechanical complications.[36]

Superficial, limited intravascular catheter-related infections are diagnosed by the presence of redness, swelling, pain, and occasionally purulent exudate in proximity to the peripheral or central venous catheter exit or subcutaneous port site. Infection of a peripheral intravenous line site in general can be cured by removal of the catheter, and culture of the catheter tip or insertion site is unnecessary. Antibiotics directed against gram-positive microbes should be used to treat accompanying cellulitis or ascending lymphangitis, and the appearance of a doughy vein proximal to a peripheral catheter site is cause for concern because suppurative thrombophlebitis may be present. Under these circumstances, the catheter should be removed and the site examined; if more than 1 ml of purulent material is encountered, the patient should be taken to the operating room and this area explored.

The presence of purulent material and infected clot extending proximally in the vein mandates removal of the infected vein and treatment with a 14-21-day course of a parenteral antibiotic selected on the basis of initial Gram stain and subsequent culture and sensitivity data.

Purulent material at the catheter exit site should be cultured, and ultrasonography can be used to identify and percutaneously sample fluid within a subcutaneous port pocket. Demonstrably infected wounds should be locally explored and drained, and in most cases catheter removal is required. In the absence of obvious infection, however, blood cultures should be obtained peripherally and through the catheter, but the diagnosis is established unequivocally only by removing the device, demonstrating large numbers of microbes on the device itself, and observing resolution of the patient's signs and symptoms.

In the most commonly used semiquantitative method, the distal 2 cm of the catheter is rolled across an agar plate and growth of more than 15 colonies per plate is considered diagnostic of catheter infection. Because the most serious event with catheter infection is bacteremia, a positive blood culture is probably of the most practical importance. Blood cultures drawn through the catheter growing 5-10-fold more colonies than peripheral cultures obtained simultaneously verify the catheter as the source of bacteremia. In general, patients with signs of infection and a positive blood culture drawn through the catheter or a positive catheter tip culture (>15 colonies per plate) should be treated for catheter infection.

Patients should undergo catheter removal if catheter infection is suspected and the device can be readily removed without altering the patient's treatment course. However, if the catheter is required for ongoing treatment, the potentially infected line can be removed and the tip cultured, and a new catheter inserted over a guidewire. If the catheter tip culture shows that the original catheter was infected, a new catheter can be placed at a fresh site. Antibiotic therapy should be adjusted on the basis of culture data, including halting therapy among patients in whom neither bacteremia nor catheter colonization is identified, particularly in those individuals in whom systemic manifestations resolve rapidly.

Approximately 80% of catheter infections are caused by increasingly common gram-positive microbes, and about 75-85% can be successfully treated with a 14-21-day course of a parenteral antibiotic-absent catheter removal.[37,38] Initial empiric antibiotic therapy should not be extended more than 3 to 5 days without confirming the presence of a gram-positive microbe in blood or catheter exchange cultures. Antibiotic therapy should not be continued if the patient's clinical course fails to improve after 24 to 48 h. Under those conditions, the catheter should be removed.

VASCULAR AND CARDIOVASCULAR INFECTIONS

Infections involving the vascular system are rare and probably occur subsequent to hematogenous seeding of either a pathological abnormality or one created by operative intervention. *Salmonella* and staphylococcal infection can involve the great vessels on rare occasions, leading to "mycotic" aneurysm formation. This type of aneurysm can rapidly expand, and the risk of rupture is high. Acute and chronic infection of prosthetic vascular grafts is more common, occurring after about 2-6% of vascular procedures in which such material is implanted.[39] Complications associated with these infections include rupture, thrombosis, distal embolization, bacteremia, and sepsis syndrome. Standard care consists of removal of the infected portion of the graft and any surrounding infected tissue, concurrent vascular bypass to avoid recontamination (often extraanatomical), and administration of a 6-12-week course of an antimicrobial agent.

Native or prosthetic cardiac valvular infection initially is treated with a 6-12-week course of one or more antibiotics, but significant cardiac dysfunction, recurrent infection, particularly that associated with sepsis syndrome unresponsive to initial antimicrobial agent therapy, or fungal infection warrants valvular removal and replacement.[40] Every attempt should be made to reduce the inoculum size via administration of perioperative antibiotics, and the resected valve tissue should be examined microscopically for the presence of microbes and cultured. Generally, implantation of autogenous valves is preferred over prosthetic valves in this situation, and parenteral antibiotics should be continued for about 6 to 12 weeks after replacement of an infected cardiac valve in an attempt to reduce the likelihood of recurrent infection.

Skin and Soft Tissue Infections

Soft tissue infections are classified according to (1) tissue plane affected and extent of invasion, (2) anatomical site, and (3) causative pathogen(s) (Table 6.5).[41] Parameters such as rapidity of progression and clinical manifestations (e.g., septic shock) are important to consider as well. The most common of these diseases are superficial infections (cellulitis, erysipelas, lymphangitis, and furunculosis) caused by gram-positive aerobic skin microflora, although gram-negative bacteria and yeast also are capable of causing these infections, particularly in immunocompromised patients. Most commonly, erythema and mild cellulitis are associated with mild abrasive or penetrating trauma to the surrounding skin, the presence of dermatological disease, or a superficial surgical wound infection. These infections rarely progress to more serious infection and can be treated by a 3- to 5-day course of an oral first-generation cephalosporin or a semisynthetic penicillin. Superficial surgical wound infection must be treated by opening the wound, as previously mentioned.

More extensive cellulitis in which spread of erythema occurs is referred to as erysipelas. A life-threatening form of this disease occurs as the result of β-hemolytic streptococci in which rapid progression of disease from a single site occurs and systemic toxicity is severe because of bacterial exotoxin secretion.[42] Treatment consists of administration of 16 to 20 M_U/day of penicillin G i.v. and debridement of necrotic tissue. Spread of infection via lymphatic drainage channels manifests as "streaks" and is termed lymphangitis. Either of these types of infection should be treated with a parenteral antibiotic with gram-positive activity until resolution occurs. An

involved extremity should be elevated and mobility restricted until the infection is effectively treated. Furuncuolosis represents more extensive disease in which superficial subcutaneous abscesses form; treatment generally requires antimicrobial agent therapy and surgical incision and drainage if spontaneous drainage does not occur. In all patients with what appears to be superficial infection, a careful search for the presence of a more aggressive underlying soft tissue infection should be undertaken.

Aggressive infections involving the deep soft tissues can occur with or without the presence of a superficial infection, and the most difficult to diagnose and treat are those that involve only the deep tissue because few external manifestations occur. Deep soft tissue infections are classified as follows: (1) necrotizing fasciitis, (2) necrotizing myositis, (3) pyomyositis, and (4) parasitic muscle infections.[43,44] These infections are rare and difficult to diagnose, and it remains difficult to predict their occurrence.

The most common types of deep soft tissue infections are necrotizing fasciitis and necrotizing myositis. The former is a necrotizing infection of the fascia deep to the panniculus adiposus. Invariably there is rapid, extensive spread in the deep soft tissues that may secondarily involve the surrounding muscles. Necrotizing myositis primarily involves the muscles and will rapidly involve and impair the muscle bed and spread to adjacent soft tissues. Either of these types of infection can be caused by a single organism, most commonly *Streptococcus pyogenes* or *Clostridium perfringens*, and rarely gram-negative aerobes such as *Pseudomonas aeruginosa* or *Vibrio vulnificans*. More commonly, however, polymicrobial infections occur.

The clinical presentation of such infections often is indolent. Fever and confusion may be the first signs, and there may be pain out of proportion to any findings on physical examination, particularly if an extremity is involved. Drainage of watery, grayish fluid from the wound or an open sore, an odd coppery hue of the skin, brawny induration, and skin blebs and/or crepitus are pathognomonic of these infections, and rapid extension to adjacent sites can occur. Patients often exhibit high fever, tachycardia, hypotension, shock, and incipient MSOF with disseminated intravascular coagulation (most probably related to bacterial exotoxin secretion and bacterial synergistic interactions that occur during polymicrobial infections), and occasionally renal failure secondary to rhabdomyolysis.

Ascertaining the presence of a deep soft tissue infection can be difficult. Initially, the patient's history should be reviewed for the presence of any risk factors, and the patient should be thoroughly examined to determine whether possible entry sites, skin changes, or crepitus are present. Plain roentgenograms looking for gas in the soft tissue should be performed, and computerized tomography or magnetic resonance imaging can occasionally be helpful in establishing the diagnosis. However, radiological studies, particularly time-consuming scans, should not be performed if it seems highly likely that a deep soft tissue infection is present, particularly if the patient exhibits hemodynamic instability. Under those circumstances, rapid fluid resuscitation should take place and an incisional biopsy should be performed in the operating room, obtaining direct visualization of both the soft tissue and muscle. Fluid can be obtained for performance of Gram stain and cultures.

The presence of a deep soft tissue infection mandates radical debridement of all infected tissue, and the surgeon must

TABLE 6.5. Classification of Soft Tissue Infections.

Superficial soft tissue infections	Deep soft tissue infections
Cellulitis	Necrotizing fasciitis
Erysipelas	Necrotizing myositis
Furuncles	Parasitic muscle infections
Lymphangitis	Pyomyositis

be prepared to proceed with such intervention at the time of initial diagnostic exploration. For the most part, the surgeon must use his or her judgment to debride tissue to the point where all devitalized tissue has been removed. Some clinicians have advocated frozen section analysis, but it remains unclear whether this definitively provides information to assist with determining the extent of resection.[45] This type of surgery often is cosmetically disfiguring and may involve amputation of an extremity to save the patient's life. Planned reexploration and debridement must occur in almost all cases until the infection has been eradicated.

Antibiotic therapy initially should be directed against gram positive aerobes, gram-negative aerobes, anaerobes, and *Clostridium perfringens* until Gram stain and culture results are available. Antifungal therapy is often administered as well to immunosuppressed patients.

Deep soft tissue infections are associated with a mortality rate of about 50%, even with rapid diagnosis, radical debridement, and administration of appropriate antibiotics. Minimal debridement, incision and drainage plus antibiotics, or use of antibiotics alone is associated with approximately 80-100% mortality.[46] Higher rates of morbidity and mortality are associated with delay of diagnosis, less than radical debridement, initial selection of antibiotics that in retrospect prove to be ineffective against the pathogens encountered, and the occurrence of these infections in elderly, diabetic, or immunosuppressed patients.

Pyomyositis consists of abscesses deep within the muscle compartment. Patients develop fever and localized swelling. The surrounding muscle initially is not involved but may become infected subsequently. Causative organisms include *Staphylococcus aureus* and *Escherichia coli*.[47] Treatment consists of open drainage and debridement and antibiotics. Parasitic myositis is similar, but occurs as the result of *Trichinella* or *Toxocara* among patients in tropical environments or those infected with HIV. The presentation is more indolent, and treatment also consists of open-drainage administration of an antiparasitic agent.

Intraabdominal Infections

Infection within the abdominal cavity is termed microbial peritonitis and is classified according to etiology into primary, secondary, and tertiary forms. Effective treatment of this type of infection requires use of antimicrobial agents, operative intervention, or both.

Primary microbial peritonitis occurs without the presence of perforation of a hollow viscus and probably is caused by seeding of microorganisms, either directly or perhaps via bacterial translocation from the gut or via hematogenous dissemination, into the peritoneal cavity. This process is caused by a single type of organism (monomicrobial), and common causative pathogens include *E. coli* or other aerobic gram-negative bacilli, *Staphylococcus aureus*, *Enterococcus faecalis* and *E. faecium*, and, less frequently, *Candida albicans*. This disease process is associated with the presence of abnormal amounts of fluid within the peritoneal cavity, which normally contains only 50 ml or less. Thus, patients who develop hepatic cirrhosis and ascites and individuals undergoing peritoneal dialysis are prone to this type of infection. If suspected, abdominal paracentesis should be performed. Confirmatory evidence includes the presence of numerous PMNs and a single type of microbe on Gram stain. If polymicrobial flora are observed on Gram stain, the diagnosis of primary microbial peritonitis is incorrect and secondary microbial peritonitis most likely is present. Treatment of primary microbial peritonitis consists of administration of parenteral antimicrobial agents directed against the causative pathogen for 14-21 days. Removal of prosthetic material such as a peritoneal dialysis catheter generally is necessary, although it may be possible to treat some patients solely with antibiotics. Resolution of symptoms is the best indicator of successful therapy, although posttreatment paracentesis can be considered for severe or recurrent cases.

Secondary microbial peritonitis occurs subsequent to perforation of a hollow viscus in which endogenous microbes spill out into the peritoneal cavity, forming the initial inoculum. Not surprisingly, perforation of the colon is associated with higher infection rates compared to other types of perforation because of the large inoculum size, consisting of both aerobes and anaerobes. After such contamination, the clinical manifestations of infection include severe abdominal pain associated with distension, ileus, and fever, and evidence of free intraperitoneal air or leakage from the gut on routine radiographic studies or those using contrast mate-rial, respectively. At the time of abdominal exploration, fi-brinopurulent peritonitis is encountered that may be localized or diffuse. Subsequent to expeditious fluid resuscitation, patients who develop secondary microbial peritonitis should undergo surgery to alleviate the source of ongoing peritoneal soilage.

The optimal duration of therapy has proved difficult to ascertain among all patients who develop intraabdominal infection, although it has been determined for certain types of patients. In general, after appropriate surgical intervention patients with any type of localized peritoneal contamination can be treated with a 3-5-day course of an antimicrobial agent, whereas longer courses are indicated for immunosuppressed patients and patients with more extensive contamination. Currently, 10% or less of patients die if the initial therapy cures the disease; however, the mortality rate remains about 30-50% among those individuals in whom initial therapy is not successful.

Even after timely surgical intervention and preemptive antibiotic therapy, about 15-30% of patients demonstrate ongoing infection consisting of recurrent secondary microbial peritonitis, intraabdominal abscess, or tertiary microbial peritonitis. Parameters that should alert the surgeon to the presence of ongoing intraabdominal infection, particularly at the conclusion of antibiotic therapy, include fever (temperature >37.6°C), peripheral white blood cell (WBC) more than 10,000 cells/ml, and band forms on peripheral smear.[48,49] Note, however, that the presence of these indicators does not necessarily warrant continuance of antibiotics or alteration of agents to cure recrudescent infection; rather, it mandates an intensive search for a problem that may be rectified by further intervention (e.g., intraabdominal abscess, leaking anastomosis, UTI, catheter infection).

A subset of patients who develop secondary microbial peritonitis and who are unable to either eradicate or sequester intraabdominal infection develop what has been termed persistent or tertiary microbial peritonitis.[50] Many of these patients are immunosuppressed and require reexploration to ensure that a source of ongoing contamination is not present. Generally, cloudy infected peritoneal fluid is encountered and cultures reveal the presence of microbes that frequently are resistant to the antibiotics used to treat the initial episode of secondary microbial peritonitis. Treatment is directed against pathogens isolated at the time of reexploration, and frequent abdominal reexploration to perform lavage and debridement may be required. The mortality of this disease process remains above 50% despite use of potent antibacterial and antifungal agents and reexploration.

Patients who suffer gastroduodenal perforation and in whom *Candida* is isolated probably do not require antifungal therapy if surgical intervention is prompt. However, based upon retrospective analysis of patients in whom yeast was isolated from established intraabdominal infection, seriously ill immunocompromised patients probably benefit from such therapy with either amphotericin B (total dose, 300–500 mg) or a triazole drug.

Other Bacterial Infections

Mediastinal infection after cardiothoracic surgery requires exploration, drainage, and debridement. Gram-positive microbes cause most of these types of infection. Extensive infection may require open packing and eventual coverage using vascularized muscle flaps.

Large (>3–5 cm) hepatic, splenic, and pulmonary abscesses can be percutaneously drained. Concurrent antibiotic therapy against aerobes and anaerobes should be administered. Abscess drainage catheters should be left in place until such time as the output falls below about 30 to 50 ml/day, although some surgeons have noted that removal within 5 days is associated with recurrence, probably because collapse of the cavity has not occurred. However, the appropriate duration of catheter drainage treatment has not been rigorously examined.

Clostridium difficile colonization and infection can occur in hospitalized patients, and colonic and intestinal inflammatory disease caused by this pathogen is closely linked to antimicrobial agent usage, immunosuppression, and spread within the hospital environment. Treatment consists of oral metronidazole for 10-14 days. Recrudescence occurs in 10-15% of patients and should be treated with a 10- to 14-day course of oral vancomycin. Rarely, severe disease leads to severe colitis with sepsis syndrome, colonic necrosis, or perforation, any of which require subtotal or total colectomy.

Fungal Infections

Fungi are identified as a component of a polymicrobial infection or as sole pathogens. These types of infections can be classified according to (1) site of infection and (2) pathogenic and invasive potential of the causative microbe.

Common fungal infections encountered by surgeons include those caused by *Candida* and *Aspergillus*, and although other organisms bear mention they are less commonly cultured. UTIs, esophagitis, and fungemic events caused by *Candida albicans* can be treated with either a 14-21-day course of fluconazole or amphotericin B. Azole-resistant *Candida* should be treated with amphotericin B. *Cryptococcus neoformans* can cause cerebromeningitis in immunosuppressed patients and can be treated with either amphotericin B or fluconazole. More aggressive fungal infections caused by *Aspergillus* may manifest as pulmonary nodules or infiltrates in immunosuppressed individuals, although diffuse bronchoalveolar infection caused by this organism is common in this patient population. Although infections limited to a single site have been treated with itraconazole or voriconazole, most such infections require prolonged amphotericin B therapy (1.5–2.0 g total dose), concurrent with a reduction in immunosuppressive drug therapy in transplant patients. Lack of complete resolution within 3 to 4 weeks mandates consideration of surgical extirpative therapy.

Pulmonary infection caused by *Pneumocystis carinii* occurs in immunosuppressed patients and produces cough, tachypnea, and mild fever, and bilateral diffuse alveolar infiltrates or interstitial pneumonia on the chest roentgenogram. Bronchoscopy should be performed in patients who develop these manifestations; treatment consists of parenteral trimethoprim-sulfamethoxazole, trimethoprim-dapsone, or pentamidine even if the diagnosis is presumptive.

Viral Infections

Viral infections that come to the attention of surgeons include herpesviruses, HBV, HCV, HIV, and many other pathogens. Many of these types of infections occur in immunosuppressed solid organ and bone marrow transplant patients or in patients who have developed acquired immunodeficiency syndrome due to HIV. HSV and varicella zoster virus (VZV) generally cause mucocutaneous lesions that are self limited, while VZV can present as shingles. Either can be effectively treated with a 14-21-day course of acyclovir. Epstein–Barr virus (EBV) infrequently causes a primary mononucleosis syndrome that should be treated with high-dose acyclovir, but more commonly it is closely associated with posttransplant lymphoproliferative disorders (PTLD) in immunosuppressed patients. The incidence among solid organ transplant patients ranges from about 1-5% and appears to be correlated with the extent of exogenous immunosuppression. The optimal treatment of PTLD remains controversial.

Cytomegalovirus (CMV) remains a common problem in solid organ transplant patients, reported rates of infection being 50-75%, while clinical disease is somewhat less frequent (~15–25%).[51] CMV infection often presents as a very mild disease syndrome consisting of fever, myalgias, malaise, lethargy, leukopenia, and mild dyspnea. More serious illness may present initially as severe retinitis, interstitial pneumonia, gastrointestinal hemorrhage, hepatitis, or pancreatitis and may evolve into a lethal CMV syndrome consisting of severe hypoxia and respiratory failure caused by progressive pneumonitis, as well as hypotension, disseminated intravascular coagulation, massive gastrointestinal hemorrhage, multiple system organ failure, and death.

A series of randomized, prospective clinical trials have demonstrated that prophylactic administration of acyclovir, anti-CMV immunoglobulin, ganciclovir, and valacyclovir during the first 3 months after solid organ transplantation can reduce the incidence of CMV disease.[52–55] Patients who develop CMV disease should receive 14 to 21 days of parenteral ganciclovir, following which an additional 9 to 10 weeks of oral therapy is administered to prevent recurrent disease, which occurs in 10–25% of patients. Foscarnet is rarely used because of its nephrotoxicity.

Parasitic Infections

Entamoeba histolytica, *Echinococcus multilocularis*, and *E. granulosis* can cause hepatic abscesses.[56] Generally such abscesses are large and can become secondarily infected with bacterial pathogens. The diagnosis of infection caused by these pathogens should be established by examination of the stool, serological studies, and abdominal computerized tomography for amoebic disease, while only the latter two approaches are helpful in identifying echinococcal infection as humans are not definitive hosts. Treatment of amoebic abscesses consists of antiparasitic drugs such as metronidazole or tinidazole, although a number of alternative agents are available. Percutaneous drainage is not undertaken unless rupture seems imminent or there is no response to therapy within 72 h.

Echinococcal liver disease generally requires cyst excision via pericystecaomy and placement of omentum within the liver defect; hepatectomy is associated with higher rates of morbidity and mortality.[57] Initial sterilization of the cyst(s) can occur either preoperatively or intraoperatively using a scolicidal agent such as 3N saline or formalin, and antiparasitic agent therapy should be administered thereafter. Care must be taken to avoid cyst rupture and spillage, which can lead to widespread intraabdominal dissemination of daughter cysts containing viable scolices that are capable of peritoneal implantation and growth.

Occasionally, surgeons encounter biliary tract disease caused by the liver fluke *Chlonorchis senesis* or patients who develop acute abdominal pain from visceral larval migrans or bowel obstruction caused by helminths. Operative intervention invariably is required under these circumstances to treat the underlying disease in addition to therapy with antiparasitic agents. *Toxoplasma gondii* can cause necrotizing encephalitis, myocarditis, pneumonitis, and death in immunosuppressed patients, and a higher incidence of infection occurs among cardiac transplant patients. Treatment consists of administration of pyrimethamine and sulfadiazine.

References

1. Dunn DL. Autochthonous microflora of the gastrointestinal tract. Perspect Colon Rectal Surg 1990;2:105–119.
2. Dunn DL, Barke RA, Knight NB, Humphrey EW, Simmons RL. Role of resident macrophages, peripheral neutrophils, and translymphatic absorption in bacterial clearance from the peritoneal cavity. Infect Immun 1985;49:257–264.
3. Dunn DL, Simmons RL. Fibrin in peritonitis. III. The mechanism of bacterial trapping by polymerizing fibrin. Surgery (St. Louis) 1982;92:513–519.
4. Dunn DL, Meakins JL. Humoral immunity to infection and the complement system. In: Howard RJ, Simmons RL, eds. Surgical Infectious Diseases, 3rd Ed. Norwalk: Appleton & Lange, 1995: 295–312.
5. Giri JG, Wells J, Dower SK, et al. Elevated levels of shed type II IL-1 receptor in sepsis: potential role for type II receptor in regulation of IL-1 responses. J Immunol 1994;153:5802–5809.
6. Porteu F, Nathan CF. Shedding of tumor necrosis factor receptors by activated human neutrophils. J Exp Med 1990;172:599–607.
7. Pruitt J, Copeland E, Moldawer L. Interleukin-1 and interleukin-1 antagonism in sepsis systemic inflammatory response syndrome and septic shock. Shock 1995;3:235–251.
8. Aderka D. The potential biological and clinical significance of the soluble tumor necrosis factor receptors. Cytokine Growth Factor Rev 1996;7:231–240.
9. Dunn DL, Barke RA, Ewald DC, Simmons RL. Macrophages and translymphatic absorption represent the first line of host defense of the peritoneal cavity. Arch Surg 1987;122:105–110.
10. Barie PS, Dellinger EP, Dougherty SH, Fink MP. Assessment of hepatitis B virus immunization status among North American surgeons. Arch Surg 1994;129:27–31.
11. Anonymous. Recommendations for prevention and control of hepatitis C virus (HCV) infection and HCV-related chronic disease. Centers for Disease Control and Prevention. MMWR 1998; 47:1–39.
12. Anonymous. Update: provisional public health service recommendation for chemoprophylaxis after occupational exposure to HIV. MMWR 1996;45:468–472.
13. Sawyer MS, Dunn DL. Appropriate use of antimicrobial agents. Nine principles. Postgrad Med 1991;90:115–122.
14. Anonymous. National Nosocomial Infections Surveillance (NNIS) System report, data summary from October 1986–April 1998, issued June 1998. Am J Infect Control 1998;26:522–533.
15. Tambyah PA, Halvorson KT, Maki DG. A prospective study of pathogenesis of catheter-associated urinary tract infections. Mayo Clin Proc 1999;74:131–136.
16. Heyland D, Cook DJ, Griffith L, Keenan SP, Brun-Buisson C. The attributable morbidity and mortality of ventilator-associated pneumonia in the critically ill patient. The Canadian Critical Trials Group. Am J Respir Crit Care Med 1999;159:1249–1256.
17. Bowton DL. Nosocomial pneumonia in the ICU—year 2000 and beyond. Chest 1999;115:28S–33S.
18. Bold RJ, Mansfield PF, Berger DH, et al. Prospective, randomized, double-blind study of prophylactic antibiotics in axillary lymph node dissection. Am J Surg 1998;176:239–243.
19. Gonzalez RP, Holevar MR. Role of prophylactic antibiotics for tube thoracostomy in chest trauma. Am Surg 1998;64:617–621.
20. Midtvedt K, Hartmann A, Midtvedt T, Brekke IB. Routine perioperative antibiotic prophylaxis in renal transplantation. Nephrol Dial Transplant 1998;13:1637–1641.
21. Dobay KJ, Freier DT, Albear P. The absent role of prophylactic antibiotics in low-risk patients undergoing laparoscopic cholecystectomy. Am Surg 1999;65:226–228.
22. Platt R, Zaleznik DF, Hopkins CC, et al. Perioperative antibiotic prophylaxis for herniorrhaphy and breast surgery. N Engl J Med 1990;322:153–160.
23. Classen DC, Evans RS, Pestonik SL, Horn SD, Menlove RL, Burke JP. The timing of prophylactic administration of antibiotics and the risk of surgical-wound infection. N Engl J Med 1992;326:281–286.
24. Bartlett JG, Condon RE, Gorbach SL, Clarke JS, Nichols RL, Ochi S. Veterans Administration Cooperative Study on Bowel Preparation for Elective Colorectal Operations: impact of oral antibiotic regimen on colonic flora, wound irrigation cultures and bacteriology of septic complications. Ann Surg 1978;188:249–254.
25. Nichols RL, Smith JW, Garcia RY, Waterman RS. Holmes JW. Current practices of preoperative bowel preparation among North American colorectal surgeons. Clin Infect Dis 1997;24: 609–619.
26. Dunn DL. Gram-negative bacterial sepsis and sepsis syndrome. Surg Clin North Am 1994;74:621–635.
27. Bone RC, Balk RA, Cerra FB, et al. Definitions for sepsis and organ failure and guidelines for the use of innovative therapies in sepsis. The ACCP/SCCM Consensus Conference Committee. American College of Chest Physicians/Society of Critical Care Medicine. Chest 1992;101:1644–1655.
28. Burd RS, Cody CS, Dunn DL. Immunotherapy of Gram-Negative Bacterial Sepsis. Austin: Landes, 1992.
29. Dunn DL. Endotoxin antagonism. In: Baue AE, Faist E, Fry DE, eds. Multiple Organ Failure: Pathophysiology, Prevention, and Therapy. New York: Springer-Verlag, 2000.

30. Bodey G, Abi-Said D, Rolston K, Raad I, Whimbey E. Imipenem or cefoperazone-sulbactam combined with vancomycin for therapy of presumed or proven infection in neutropenic cancer patients. Eur J Clin Microbiol Infect Dis 1996;15:625–634.

31. Hathorn JW, Lyke K. Empirical treatment of febrile neutropenia: evolution of current therapeutic approaches. Clin Infect Dis 1997;24:S256–S265.

32. Gross PA, Barrett TL, Dellinger EP, et al. Quality standard for the treatment of bacteremia. The Infectious Diseases Society of America. Infect Control Hosp Epidemiol 1994;15:189–192.

33. Rex JH, Bennett JE, Sugar AM, et al. A randomized trial comparing fluconazole with amphotericin B for the treatment of candidemia in patients without neutropenia. Candidemia Study Group and the National Institute. N Engl J Med 1994;331:1325–1330.

34. Bullard KM, Dunn DL. Diagnosis and treatment of bacteremia and intravascular catheter infections. Am J Surg 1996;172:S13–S19.

35. Andrivet P, Bacquer A, Ngoc CV, et al. Lack of clinical benefit from subcutaneous tunnel insertion of central venous catheters in immunocompromised patients. Clin Infect Dis 1994;18:34–36.

36. Cobb D, High KP, Sawyer RG, et al. A controlled trial of scheduled replacement of central venous and pulmonary-artery catheters. New Engl J Med 1992;327:1062–1068.

37. Martinez E, Mensa J, Rovira M, Martinez JA, Marcos A, Almela M, Carreras E. Central venous catheter exchange by guidewire for treatment of catheter-related bacteraemia in patients undergoing BMT or intensive chemotherapy. Bone Marrow Transplant 1999;23:41–44.

38. Raad I, Bompart F, Hachem R. Prospective, randomized dose-ranging open phase II pilot study of quinupristin/dalfopristin versus vancomycin in the treatment of catheter-related staphylococcal bacteremia. Eur J Clin Microbiol Infect Dis 1999;18:199–202.

39. Henke PK, Bergamini TM, Rose SM, Richardson JD. Current options in prosthetic vascular graft infection. Am Surg 1998;64:39–45.

40. Reardon MJ, Vinnerkvist A, LeMaire SA. Mitral valve homograft for mitral valve replacement in acute bacterial endocarditis. J Heart Valve Dis 1999;8:71–73.

41. Dunn DL, Sawyer MD. Deep soft tissue infections. Curr Opin Infect Dis 1990;3:691–696.

42. Bilton BD, Zibari GB, McMillan RW, Aultman DF, Dunn G, McDonald JC. Aggressive surgical management of necrotizing fasciitis serves to decrease mortality: a retrospective study. Am Surg 1998;64:397–400.

43. Sawyer MD, Dunn DL. Deep soft tissue infections. Curr Opin Infect Dis 1991;4:649–654.

44. Sawyer MD, Dunn DL. Serious bacterial infections of the skin and soft tissues. Curr Opin Infect Dis 1995;8:293–297.

45. Stamenkovic I, Lew DP. Early recognition of potentially fatal necrotizing fasciitis. The use of frozen-section biopsy. N Engl J Med 1984;310:1689–1696.

46. Stone HH, Martin JD. Synergistic necrotizing cellulitis. Ann Surg 1972;175:702–711.

47. Hall RL, Callaghan JJ, Moloney E, Martinez S, Harrelson JM. Pyomyositis in a temperate climate. Presentation, diagnosis, and treatment. J Bone Joint Surg 1990;72:1240–1244.

48. Stone HH, Bourneuf AA, Stinson LD. Reliability of criteria for predicting persistent or recurrent sepsis. Arch Surg 1985;120:17.

49. Lennard ES, Dellinger EP, Wertz MJ, et al. Implications of leukocytosis and fever at conclusion of antibiotic therapy for intra-abdominal sepsis. Ann Surg 1982;195:19.

50. Rotstein OD, Pruett TL, Simmons RL. Microbiologic features and treatment of persistent peritonitis in patients in the intensive care unit. Can J Surg 1986;29:247.

51. Dunn DL, Mayoral JL, Gillingham KJ, et al. Treatment of invasive cytomegalovirus disease in solid organ transplant patients with ganciclovir. Transplantation 1991;51:98–106.

52. Dunn DL, Gillingham KJ, Kramer MA, et al. A prospective randomized study of acyclovir versus ganciclovir plus human immune globulin prophylaxis of cytomegalovirus infection after solid organ transplantation. Transplantation 1994;57:876–884.

53. Snydman DR, Werner BG, Heinze-Lacey B. Use of cytomegalovirus immune globulin to prevent cytomegalovirus disease in renal-transplant recipients. N Engl J Med 1987;317:1049–1054.

54. Balfour HH, Chace BA, Stapleton JT. A randomized, placebo-controlled trial of oral acyclovir for the prevention of cytomegalovirus disease in recipients of renal allografts. N Engl J Med 1989;320:1381–1385.

55. Lowance D, Neumayer HH, Legendre CM, et al. Valacyclovir for the prevention of cytomegalovirus disease after renal transplantation. International Valacyclovir Cytomegalovirus Prophylaxis Transplantation Study Group. N Engl J Med 1999;340:1462–1470.

56. Sharma MP, Dasarathy S. Amoebic liver abscess. Trop Gastroenterol 1993;14:3–9.

57. Di Matteo G, Bove A, Chiarini S, et al. Hepatic echinococcus disease: our experience over 22 years. Hepato-Gastroenterology 1996;43:1562–1565.

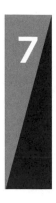

7

Wounds: Biology, Pathology, and Management

H. Peter Lorenz and Michael T. Longaker

Wound Biology

The overlapping segments of the repair process are conceptually defined as inflammation, proliferation, and remodeling. During the inflammatory phase, hemostasis occurs and an acute inflammatory infiltrate ensues. The proliferative phase is characterized by fibroplasia, granulation, contraction, and epithelialization. The final phase is remodeling, which is commonly described as scar maturation (Fig. 7.1).

Inflammation

Inflammation is the first stage of wound healing. After tissue injury, the lacerated vessels immediately constrict and thromboplastic tissue products, predominantly from the subendothelium, are exposed. Platelets aggregate and form the initial hemostatic plug. The coagulation and complement cascades are initiated. The intrinsic and extrinsic coagulation pathways lead to activation of prothrombin to thrombin, which converts fibrinogen to fibrin, which is subsequently polymerized into a stable clot.

As thrombus is formed, hemostasis in the wound is achieved (Fig. 7.2). The aggregated platelets degranulate, releasing potent chemoattractants for inflammatory cells, activation factors for local fibroblasts and endothelial cells, and vasoconstrictors (Table 7.1). Platelet adhesiveness is mediated by integrin receptors such as GPIIb/IIIa (αIIbβ3 integrin).[1–3]

Within minutes, the repair processes are initiated. After the transient vasoconstriction induced by platelet factors, local small vessels dilate secondary to the effects of the coagulation and complement cascades. Bradykinin is a potent vasodilator and vascular permeability factor that is generated by activation of Hageman factor in the coagulation cascade.[2] The complement cascade generates the C3a and C5a anaphylatoxins, which directly increase blood vessel permeability and attract neutrophils and monocytes to the wound. These complement components also stimulate the release of histamine and leukotrienes C4 and D4 from mast cells. The local endothelial cells then break cell-to-cell contact, which enhances the margination of inflammatory cells into the wound site.[2]

An efflux of white blood cells (first neutrophils, later monocytes) and plasma proteins enter the wound site (Fig. 7.3). The early neutrophil infiltrate scavenges cellular debris, foreign bodies, and bacteria. Activated complement fragments aid in bacterial killing through opsonization. The primary role of the neutrophil is to sterilize the wound. Accordingly, the initial neutrophil infiltrate is decreased in clean surgical wounds when compared to contaminated or infected wounds.

Within 2 to 3 days, the inflammatory cell population begins to shift to one of monocyte predominance (Fig. 7.4). Circulating monocytes are attracted and infiltrate the wound site.[3,4] These elicited monocytes differentiate into macrophages, and in conjunction with resident macrophages, orchestrate the repair process. Macrophages not only continue to phagocytose tissue and bacterial debris, but also secrete multiple growth factors. These peptide growth factors activate and attract local endothelial cells, fibroblasts, and keratinocytes to begin their respective repair functions. More than 20 different cytokines and growth factors are known to be secreted by macrophages, the primary cells responsible for regulating repair. (Table 7.2).[5,6] Depletion of monocytes and macrophages causes a severe alteration in wound healing with poor debridement, delayed fibroblast proliferation, and inadequate angiogenesis.[7]

Proliferation

FIBROPLASIA

The proliferative phase begins with the deposition of the fibrin and fibrinogen matrix and the activation and turnover of local fibroblasts (fibroplasia). The initial fibrin–fibrinogen matrix is populated with platelets and macrophages. These

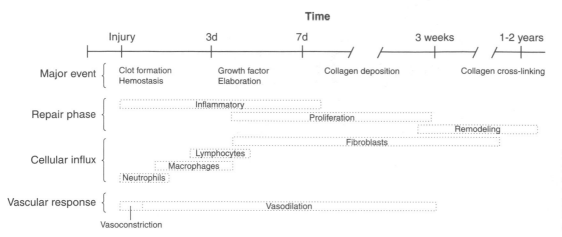

FIGURE 7.1. The temporal relationship of repair stages and cellular infiltrates into the wound. Overlap occurs between the stages, and the beginning and endpoints are approximate.

macrophages and the local extracellular matrix (ECM) release growth factors that initiate fibroblast activation. Fibroblasts migrate into the wound using the newly deposited fibrin and fibronectin matrix as a scaffold. Local fibroblasts become activated and increase protein synthesis in preparation for cell division. As fibroblasts proliferate, they become the prominent cell type by 3 to 5 days in clean, noninfected wounds (Fig. 7.5). After cell division and proliferation, fibroblasts begin synthesis and secretion of extracellular matrix products.

Integrins are transmembrane proteins with extracellular, membrane, and intracellular domains. They are heterodimeric and composed of alpha and beta subunits that interact to form the active protein receptor. Ligands include growth factors, ECM structural components such as collagen, elastin, and other cells. After ligands bind, a structural change occurs in the cytoplasmic domain of the integrin receptor and phosphorylation occurs. Signal transduction ultimately results in transcription factor synthesis and new gene expression resulting in new cellular function.

The initial wound matrix is provisional and is composed of fibrin and the glycosaminoglycan (GAG), hyaluronic acid.[4] Because of its large water of hydration, hyaluronic acid provides a matrix that enhances cell migration. As fibroblasts enter and populate the wound, they utilize hyaluronidase to digest the provisional hyaluronic acid–rich matrix, and larger, sulfated GAGs are subsequently deposited. Concomitantly, collagens are deposited by fibroblasts onto the fibronectin and GAG scaffold in a disorganized array.

Collagen types I and III are the major fibrillar collagens comprising the extracellular matrix and are the major structural proteins both in unwounded and wounded skin. There are now at least 19 different types of collagens described, each of which shares the right-handed triple helix as the basic structural unit.[8–12] Most collagen types are synthesized by fibroblasts; however, it is now known that some types are synthesized by epidermal cells.[13]

GRANULATION

Granulation tissue is present in wounds healing by secondary intention. This tissue is clinically characterized by its beefy-red appearance (i.e., "proud flesh"), which is a consequence of the rich bed of new capillary networks (neoangiogenesis) that have formed from endothelial cell division and migration. The directed growth of vascular endothelial cells is stimulated by platelet and activated macrophage and fibroblast products. One example is vascular endothelial growth factor, which is secreted by macrophages and acts to induce migra-

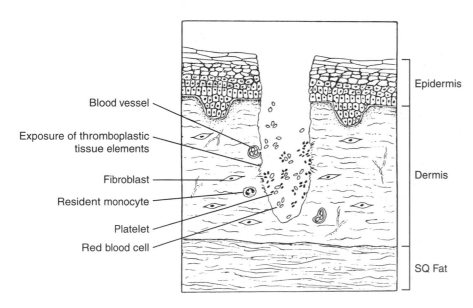

FIGURE 7.2. Immediately after tissue injury, hemostasis is stimulated by platelet degranulation and exposure of tissue thromboplastic agents.

TABLE 7.1. Platelets Contain Both Alpha and Dense Granules, Which Are Released at the Wound Site.

Substance	Biological effect
Alpha granules	
Platelet-derived growth factor	Matrix deposition
Transforming growth factor-β	Matrix deposition
Transforming growth factor-α	Epithelialization
Insulin-like growth factor-binding protein-3	Matrix deposition
Platelet factor-4	Activation of growth factors
β-Thromboglobulin	Activation of growth factors
Dense granules	
Adenosine diphosphate	Platelet aggregation
Calcium	Platelet aggregation
Serotonin	Vasoconstriction
Cytosol	
von Willebrand factor VIII	Mediator of platelet adhesion
Fibronectin	Ligand for platelet aggregation
Fibrinogen	Ligand for platelet aggregation
Thrombospondin	Ligand for platelet aggregation
Factor V	Hemostasis
Platelet-activating factor	Platelet activation
Thromboxane-A2	Vasoconstriction
12-Hydroxyeicosatetranoic acid (12-HETE)	Vasoconstriction

In addition, multiple activators and mediators of the hemostatic cascades are present on the platelet surface membrane (see Chapter 49). The substances released have myriad effects on the repair process. Vascular endothelial growth factor has recently been found to be present within platelets but its exact intracellular location is unknown.[26]

Source: Data were compiled from several sources (reviewed in References 1, 2, 3).

tion and proliferation of endothelial cells. Granulation tissue is a dense population of blood vessels, macrophages, and fibroblasts embedded within a loose provisional matrix of fibronectin, hyaluronic acid, and collagen.

The presence of granulation tissue is used as a clinical indicator that the wound is ready for skin graft treatment. Wounds that benefit from skin grafts are of sufficient size such that the healing time would be decreased. The high de-

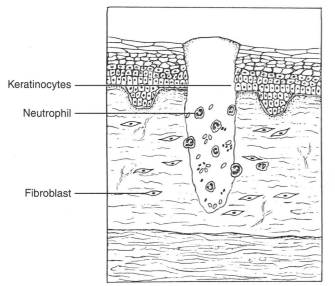

FIGURE 7.3. Within 24 hours, a neutrophil efflux into the wound occurs. The neutrophils scavenge debris, bacteria, and secrete cytokines for monocyte and lymphocyte attraction and activation. Keratinocytes begin migration when a provisional matrix is present.

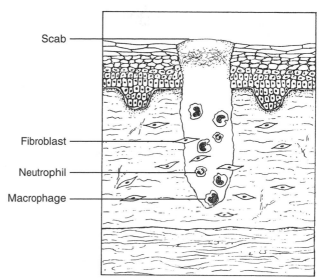

FIGURE 7.4. At 2 to 3 days after injury, the macrophage becomes the predominant inflammatory cell type in clean, noninfected wounds. These cells then regulate the repair process by secretion of a myriad of growth factors, including types that induce fibroblast and endothelial cell migration and proliferation.

gree of vascularity enables granulation tissue to readily accept and support skin grafts.

CONTRACTION

Open wounds are characterized by contraction, a phenomenon not present in closed surgical incisions. Open wounds occur after trauma, burns, and when previously closed wounds are secondarily opened because of infection. Contraction is the process in which the surrounding skin is pulled circumferentially toward the wound. Wound contraction decreases the size of the wound dramatically without new tissue formation. This repair component allows the wound to close, and thus heal much more rapidly than by epithelialization alone. In addition, the area of insensate scar is smaller.

The amount of contraction is related to the size of the wound and mobility of the skin. In humans, contraction is greatest in the trunk and perineum, least on the extremities, and intermediate on the head and neck. Up to 80% of wound closure can be caused by contraction in the trunk and perineum. These regional differences are thought to result from the relative differences in skin laxity in those areas.

Clinically, wound contraction can lead to contracture, which distorts tissue and leads to decreased function. For example, wound contraction across a joint can lead to a contracture in that joint. The range of motion, and thus function, of the joint is diminished. Contractures can develop in the extremities, eyelids, neck, spine, and fingers.

EPITHELIALIZATION

Within hours after injury, morphological changes in keratinocytes at the wound margin are evident. In skin wounds, the epidermis thickens, and marginal basal cells enlarge and migrate over the wound defect (see Fig. 7.5). Once these epithelial cells begin migrating, they do not divide until epidermal continuity is restored. New epithelial cells for

TABLE 7.2. A Partial List of Growth Factors Present at the Wound Site.

Growth factor	Cellular source	Target cells	Biological activity
TGF-β_1, TGF-β_2	Macrophages, platelets, fibroblasts, keratinocytes	Inflammatory cells, keratinocytes, fibroblasts	Chemotaxis, proliferation, matrix production (fibrosis)
TGF-β_3	Macrophages	Fibroblasts	Anti-scarring?
TGF-α	Macrophages, platelets, keratinocytes	Keratinocytes, fibroblasts, endothelial cells	Proliferation
TNF-α	Neutrophils	Macrophages, keratinocytes, fibroblasts	Activation of growth factor expression
PDGF	Macrophage, platelets, fibroblasts, endothelial cells, vascular smooth muscle cells	Neutrophils, macrophages, fibroblasts, endothelial cells, vascular smooth muscle cells	Chemotaxis, proliferation, matrix production
FGF-1, FGF-2, FGF-4	Macrophage, fibroblasts, endothelial cells	Keratinocytes, fibroblasts, endothelial cells, chondrocytes	Angiogenesis, proliferation, chemotaxis
FGF-7 (KGF)	Fibroblasts	Keratinocytes	Proliferation, chemotaxis
EGF	Platelets, macrophages, keratinocytes	Keratinocytes, fibroblasts, endothelial cells	Proliferation, chemotaxis
IGF-1/Sm-C	Fibroblasts, macrophages, serum	Fibroblasts, endothelial cells	Proliferation, collagen synthesis
IL-1α and IL-1β	Macrophages, neutrophils	Macrophages, fibroblasts, keratinocytes	Proliferation, collagenase synthesis, chemotaxis
CTGF	Fibroblasts, endothelial cells	Fibroblasts	Downstream of TGF-β_1
VEGF	Macrophages, keratinocytes	Endothelial cells	Angiogenesis

Redundant biological effects through both autocrine and paracrine mechanisms are apparent.

TGF-β, transforming growth factor-beta; TGF-α, transforming growth factor-alpha; TNF-α, tumor necrosis factor-alpha; PDGF, platelet-derived growth factor; FGF, fibroblast growth factor; KGF, keratinocyte growth factor; EGF, epidermal growth factor; IGF-1, insulin-like growth factor-1; Sm-C, somatostatin-C; IL-1, interleukin-1; CTGF, connective tissue growth factor; VEGF, vascular endothelial cell growth factor.

wound closure are provided by fixed basal cells in a zone near the edge of the wound.[14] Their daughter cells flatten and migrate over the wound matrix as a sheet (epiboly). Cell adhesion glycoproteins, such as tenascin and fibronectin, provide the "railroad tracks" to facilitate epithelial cell migration over the wound matrix. Following the reestablishment of the epithelial layer, keratinocytes and fibroblasts secrete laminin and type IV collagen to form the basement membrane.[13] The keratinocytes then become columnar and divide as the layering of the epidermis is established, thus reforming a barrier to further contamination and moisture loss.

Interestingly, keratinocytes can respond to foreign-body stimulation with migration as well. Sutures in skin wounds provide tracts along which these cells can migrate. Subsequent epithelial thickening and keratinization produce fibrotic reactions, cysts, or sterile abscesses centered on the suture. These are treated by removal of the inciting suture and epithelial cell sinus tract or cyst.

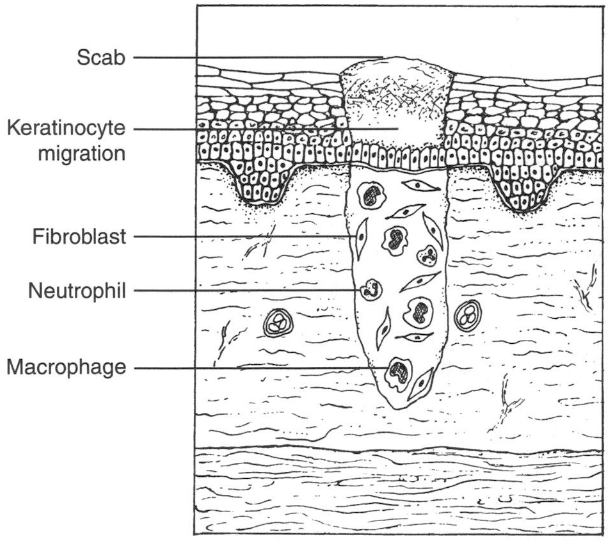

Remodeling Phase

The ECM is the scaffold that supports cells in both the unwounded and wounded states. The ECM is dynamic and during repair is constantly undergoing remodeling. The regulation of the remodeling is poorly understood, but simplistically can be conceptualized as the balance between synthesis, deposition, and degradation. Lysyl oxidase is the major intermolecular collagen cross-linking enzyme.[15] Collagen cross-linking improves wound tensile strength. Collagenases, gelatinases, and stromelysins are matrix metalloproteinases (MMPs) that degrade ECM components. The balance of collagen deposition and degradation is in part determined by the regulation of MMP activity. Proteins called tissue inhibitor of matrix metalloproteinases (TIMPs) specifically inactivate the MMPs.[16] Current investigation is examining the regulation of MMP–TIMP balance during wound ECM remodeling.[17,18]

Ultimately, the outcome of mammalian wound healing is scar formation (Fig. 7.6). Scar is defined morphologically as the lack of tissue organization compared to surrounding normal tissue architecture and is characterized by disorganized collagen deposition. New collagen fibers secreted by fibro-

FIGURE 7.5. Fibroblasts are activated and present at the wound by 3 to 5 days after injury. These cells secrete matrix components and growth factors that continue to stimulate healing. Keratinocyte migration (epiboly) begins over the new matrix. Migration starts from the wound edges as well as from epidermal cell nests at sweat glands and hair follicles in the center of the wound.

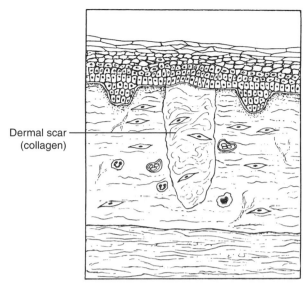

FIGURE 7.6. Scar formation is the outcome of healing in postnatal skin. Scar is composed of densely packed, disorganized collagen fiber bundles. Remodeling occurs up to 1 to 2 years after injury and consists of further collagen cross-linking and regression of capillaries, which account for the softening of scar and its color change from red to white.

blasts are present as early as 3 days after wounding. As the collagenous matrix forms, densely packed fibers fill the wound site. The ultimate pattern of collagen in scar is one of densely packed fibers and not the reticular pattern found in unwounded dermis.

During remodeling, wounds gradually become stronger with time. Wound tensile strength increases rapidly from 1 to 8 weeks post wounding. Thereafter, tensile strength increases at a slower pace and has been documented to increase up to 1 year after wounding in animal studies (Fig. 7.7). However, the tensile strength of wounded skin at best only reaches approximately 80% that of unwounded skin.[19] The final result of tissue repair is scar, which is brittle, less elastic than normal skin, and does not contain any skin appendages such as hair follicles or sweat glands. The major

benefit of repair by scar is the relatively rapid reformation of tissue integrity.

Regulation of Wound Repair

GROWTH FACTORS

Growth factors play a prominent role in the regulation of chemotaxis and wound healing. These polypeptides are released by a variety of activated cells at the wound site (see Table 7.2). They act in either paracrine or autocrine fashion to stimulate or inhibit protein synthesis by cells in the wound, and many have overlapping functions.

PLATELET-DERIVED GROWTH FACTOR

Platelet-derived growth factor (PDGF) is released from platelet alpha-granules immediately after injury. PDGF attracts neutrophils, macrophages, and fibroblasts to the wound and serves as a powerful mitogen. Macrophages, endothelial cells, and fibroblasts also synthesize and secrete PDGF. Platelet-derived growth factor stimulates fibroblasts to synthesize new extracellular matrix, predominantly noncollagenous components such as GAGs and adhesion proteins. PDGF also increases the amount of fibroblast-secreted collagenase, indicating a role for this cytokine in tissue remodeling.[20,21]

TRANSFORMING GROWTH FACTOR–BETA

Transforming growth factor–beta (TGF–β) directly stimulates collagen synthesis and decreases extracellular matrix degradation by fibroblasts.[22,23] It is released from platelets and macrophages at the wound. In addition, TGF-β is released from fibroblasts and keratinocytes. TGF-β acts in an autocrine fashion to further stimulate its own synthesis and secretion. TGF-β also chemoattracts fibroblasts and macrophages to the wound.

TGF-β is a profibrotic growth factor which accelerates wound repair at the expense of increased fibrosis. It has been implicated in pathological fibrosis in multiple different organ systems and is thought to be a factor in the formation of intestinal adhesions. TGF-β stimulates ECM synthesis and accumulation, increases integrin expression, and therefore enhances cell–matrix interactions.

FIGURE 7.7. Wound tensile strength as a function of time. Maximal wound tensile strength is 75%–80% of unwounded skin. (Modified from Levenson SM, Geever EF, Crowley LV, Oaks JF, Berard CW, Rosen H. The healing of rat skin wounds. Ann Surg 1965;161:293–308, with permission.)

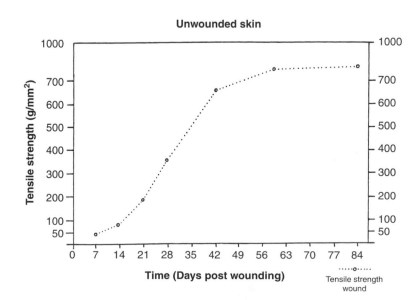

FIBROBLAST GROWTH FACTORS

Angiogenesis is stimulated by acidic and basic fibroblast growth factors (FGF-1 [or aFGF] and FGF-2 [or bFGF], respectively).[24] Endothelial cells, fibroblasts, and macrophages produce FGF-1 and FGF-2. The FGFs stimulate endothelial cells to divide and form new capillaries. They also chemoattract endothelial cells and fibroblasts.

VASCULAR ENDOTHELIAL GROWTH FACTOR

Vascular endothelial growth factor is also a potent angiogenic stimulus.[25,26] It acts in a paracrine manner to stimulate proliferation by endothelial cells after release from platelets, macrophages, fibroblasts, and keratinocytes.[27–29] Its expression is also increased in hypoxic conditions, such as those found at the wound site.[28]

OTHER GROWTH FACTORS

Epithelialization is directly stimulated by at least three growth factors: epidermal growth factor (EGF) and keratinocyte growth factors/–1 and –2 (KGF–1 and KGF–2).[24,30] EGF is released by keratinocytes to act in an autocrine fashion, whereas KGF is released by fibroblasts to act in a paracrine fashion to stimulate keratinocyte division and differentiation.

Multiple other growth factors affect wound repair. For example, insulin-like growth factor–I (IGF-I) stimulates collagen synthesis by fibroblasts, and IGF–I functions synergistically with PDGF and bFGF to facilitate fibroblast proliferation.[31] Interferon-gamma has been shown to downregulate collagen synthesis. The various interleukins mediate inflammatory cell functions at the wound site (see Chapter 4).[32]

THE EXTRACELLULAR MATRIX

The ECM is a depository of growth factors in latent forms under normal, unwounded conditions. With injury and matrix destruction, the previously bound and inactive growth factors are released in active form and thereby assist in initiating and regulating the repair process.

Scarless Repair: The Fetal Paradigm

Unlike the adult, the early-gestation fetus can heal skin wounds with regenerative-type repair and not with scar formation.[33,34] The epidermis and dermis are restored to a normal architecture in which the collagen matrix pattern is reticular and unchanged from unwounded dermis. The wound hair follicle and sweat gland patterns are normal.

Interestingly, inflammation plays a prominent role in postnatal repair, but it is not present in significant amounts in fetal skin wounds. An understanding of the biology of scarless fetal wound repair will help surgeons develop therapeutic strategies to minimize scar and fibrosis.

Wound Pathology

Nonhealing Wounds

Chronic or nonhealing wounds are open wounds that fail to epithelialize and close in a reasonable amount of time. These wounds are clinically stagnant and without evidence of further closure. There are likely many reasons why these wounds do not heal, but no broad, unifying theory exists. Simply put, chronic wounds may be thought of as lacking appropriate "start" signals. These wounds can be broadly categorized into three groups: pressure sores, lower extremity ulcers, and radiation skin injury.

PRESSURE SORES

Pressure sores develop over a bony prominence, usually in the immobile patient. These are frequently called "decubitus ulcers" or "bed sores." The sacrum, ischium, and greater trochanter are the most common locations affected.[35]

Pressure necrosis is a function of the amount of pressure on the tissue and duration of pressure. Microcirculation is compromised when the tissue pressure is greater than 25 to 30 mmHg, which blocks capillary perfusion pressure.[36] Necrosis can occur with as little as 2 h of sustained pressures at this level.[36] Skin is more resistant to pressure necrosis than the underlying fat and muscle, which explains the common finding of a small area of skin ulceration overlying a large area of subcutaneous fat and muscle necrosis.

To begin treatment of these patients, efforts should be made to control the factors leading to increased pressure. Paralyzed patients require periodic rotation and air mattress or other types of low-pressure beds. In addition, behavior and contractures may need to be addressed. Tight-fitting casts should be removed and replaced by those with no excess pressure. Other contributing factors should be identified and controlled, such as malnutrition, infection, and diabetes control. Necrotic tissue requires debridement.

With avoidance of pressure over the involved area, most pressure sores heal. However, they heal with scar formation, which is less resistant to trauma than intact skin. Thus, a higher incidence of recurrence exists after spontaneous closure of these wounds than if they are closed surgically with flaps of normal skin and muscle over the bony prominence.[37,38]

LOWER-EXTREMITY ULCERS

Leg ulcers generally arise from either one of two different vascular diseases: arterial or venous insufficiency. Most (80%–90%) result from venous valvular disease (venous insufficiency).[35,39,40] Increased venous pressure in the dependent lower extremity leads to localized edema and tissue necrosis. Tissue edema is thought to be a major inhibitor of repair at the ulcer site, but the exact mechanism is not known. Oxygen delivery and diffusion are likely impaired. Postcapillary obstruction leads to an increased perfusion pressure and hypoxia. Protein and red blood cell extravasation occurs, which further limits diffusion and oxygen delivery.

Arterial insufficiency to the lower extremity greatly impairs healing. Minor trauma, resulting from scratches and abrasions that would otherwise heal quickly in a normal patient, can progress into large wounds and ultimately necrotizing infection that is not only limb- but also life-threatening. A reliable clinical sign of adequate arterial inflow is the simple presence of an arterial pulse. If a single palpable pulse is present in the foot, then most wounds will heal. A nonhealing wound in an ischemic extremity is generally regarded as an indication for revascularization of that extremity.

RADIATION INJURY

External beam radiation through skin to treat deep pathology has both acute and chronic effects on skin. Acutely, a self-limiting erythema may develop that spontaneously resolves. Its late effect can be a more significant injury to fibroblasts, keratinocytes, and endothelial cells. DNA damage to these cells propagates over time and impairs the ability of these cells to divide successfully. Ultimately, a skin ulcer may occur spontaneously, but usually it occurs after repeated mild trauma such as abrasions.[41] If a surgical incision needs to be placed through an area of irradiated skin, then that incision is not likely to heal. Currently the only treatment modalities for these wounds are hyperbaric oxygen therapy or coverage with vascularized tissue flaps.

Clinical Factors Affecting Repair

INFECTION

Wound infection is an imbalance between host resistance and bacterial growth.[42] Bacterial infection impairs healing through several mechanisms.[43] At the wound site, acute and chronic inflammatory infiltrates slow fibroblast proliferation and thus slow ECM synthesis and deposition. Although the exact mechanisms are not known, sepsis causes systemic effects that can impede the repair processes.

Open wounds invariably become colonized by bacteria. The wound has no protective barrier to prevent bacterial adherence in the exposed dermis or subcutaneous fat and muscle. Colonization does not preclude healing. However, if bacterial infection occurs, then healing can be not only delayed but also stopped.

A threshold number of bacteria in the wound appears to be necessary to overcome host resistance and cause clinical wound infection. Bacterial contamination results in clinical infection and delays healing if more than 10^5 organisms per gram of tissue are present in the wound.[43,44] Skin grafts on open wounds are likely to fail if quantitative culture shows more than 10^5 organisms/g tissue, which provides further evidence that bacterial load impacts repair.[45] Similarly, well-vascularized muscle flaps heal open wounds successfully if bacterial loads are not greater than 10^5 organisms/g tissue.[46] These studies demonstrate that high levels of bacteria inhibit the normal healing processes.

Treatment of the closed, infected wound depends on whether fluid or necrotic tissue is present. If no fluid is draining or loculated, then cellulitis can be successfully treated with appropriate antibiotics. The wound should be opened, sutures removed, irrigated, and debrided if pus or necrotic tissue is present. Appropriate antibiotic administration following wound cultures treats surrounding cellulitis. Signs of wound infection include fever, tenderness, erythema, edema, and drainage.

NUTRITION

Wound healing is an anabolic event that requires additional caloric intake.[47] However, the precise calorie requirements for optimal wound healing have not been determined. Large injuries such as burns greatly increase metabolic rate and nutritional requirements.[48] Severely malnourished and catabolic patients clinically appear to have diminished healing; however, no studies have definitely proved this finding.[49]

Appropriate levels of vitamins C and A are necessary for proper fibroplasia, collagen synthesis, and cross-linking and epithelialization processes. Animal studies show that vitamin A also reverses the impaired healing that occurs with chronic steroid treatment.[50,51] While this is not proved conclusively in human studies, most surgeons administer vitamin A postoperatively to their patients on steroid therapy. Vitamin A is fat soluble and can be taken in toxic doses, so careful administration is essential. The oral dose is 25,000 U/day.[52]

Vitamin B_6 (pyridoxine) deficiency impairs collagen cross-linking.[53] Vitamin B_1 (thiamine) and vitamin B_2 (riboflavin) deficiencies cause syndromes associated with poor wound repair. Supplementation with these vitamins does not improve healing unless a preexisting deficiency condition is present.

Trace metal deficiencies such as zinc and copper have been implicated with poor wound repair because these divalent cations are cofactors in many important enzymatic reactions.[52] Zinc deficiency is associated with poor epithelialization and chronic, nonhealing wounds. Trace metal deficiency is now extremely rare in both enterally and parenterally fed patients.

Vitamin and mineral excess administration can be detrimental and cause toxicity, especially the fat-soluble vitamins. Adequate amounts are present in today's enteral feeding solutions and as supplemental additives to parenteral solutions. Supplemental administration is only necessary in deficiency states and certain unique clinical situations as described earlier.

OXYGEN AND PERFUSION

Wounds require adequate oxygen delivery to heal. Ischemic wounds heal poorly and have a much greater risk of infection.[54,55] Wound ischemia occurs secondary to a variety of factors: occlusive vascular disease, vasoconstriction, and hypovolemia. Excessive suture tension during wound closure will cause local wound ischemia and result in wound healing complications. Conversely, increased oxygen delivery at the wound improves wound healing.[54–57] Experimentally, collagen synthesis by fibroblasts is increased with supplemental oxygen.[58,59]

Anemia in the normovolemic patient is not detrimental to wound repair so long as the hematocrit is greater than 15%, because oxygen content in blood does not affect wound collagen synthesis.[58]

DIABETES MELLITUS AND OBESITY

Wound healing is impaired in diabetic patients by unknown mechanisms, although recent studies have implicated a lack of KGF and PDGF function in the wound.[60,61] Many of these patients have microvascular occlusive disease that may cause ischemia and impaired repair. Healing is enhanced if glucose levels are well controlled.[62] Obesity interferes with repair independently of diabetes.[63]

CORTICOSTEROIDS

Both topically applied and pharmacological steroid use impairs healing, especially when given in the first 3 days after wounding.[64,65] Steroids reduce wound inflammation, collagen synthesis, and contraction.[52] The exact mechanisms underlying how steroids impair healing are not fully understood. Because steroids decrease inflammation, they may decrease host bacterial resistance and thus increase wound infection complications. The entire repair process is slowed and risk of dehiscence and infection is increased. As stated previously, vitamin A administration can reverse this effect.[50,51]

RADIATION THERAPY

Both radiation and chemotherapeutic agents have their greatest effects on dividing cells. The division of endothelial cells, fibroblasts, and keratinocytes is impaired in irradiated tissue, which retards wound healing.

CHEMOTHERAPY

During the proliferative phase of repair, numerous cell types are active at the wound site. Antiproliferative chemotherapeutic agents act to slow this process and thus retard healing.[66] Following oncological surgical procedures, in most institutions chemotherapeutic agents are not administered until at least 5 to 7 days postoperatively to prevent impairment of the initial healing events.

Excessive Healing

Normal wounds have stop signals that halt the repair process when the dermal defect is closed and epithelialization is complete. When these signals are absent or ineffective, then the repair process may continue and result in a condition of excessive scar. The underlying regulatory mechanisms leading to excessive repair are not yet known.

To minimize visible scar on skin, elective incisions are least noticeable when placed parallel to the natural lines of skin tension (Langer's lines). This placement location has two advantages: the scar is parallel or within a natural skin crease, which camouflages the scar, and this location places the least amount of tension on the wound. Wound tension prevents thin scar formation. Sharply defined and aligned wound edges approximated without tension heal with the least amount of scar. Infection or separation of the wound edges with subsequent secondary intention repair also results in more scar formation.

HYPERTROPHIC SCAR

Hypertrophic scars and keloids are distinguished based on their clinical characteristics. Hypertrophic scars are defined as scars that have not overgrown the original wound boundaries, but are instead raised. They usually form secondary to excessive tensile forces across the wound and are most common in wounds across flexion surfaces, the extremities, breasts, sternum, and neck. Physical therapy with range-of-motion exercises is helpful in minimizing hypertrophic scar as well as joint contracture in the extremities.

Hypertrophic scar is a self-limited type of overhealing after tissue injury, and usually regresses with time. These scars generally fade in color as well as flatten to the surrounding skin level. There has never been a clear histological difference between hypertrophic scar and keloid. In general, both keloid and hypertrophic scar fibroblasts have an upregulation of collagen synthesis, deposition, and accumulation.[67]

Treatment options for hypertrophic scars include the application of pressure garments or topical silicone sheets, laser therapy, and reexcision with primary closure.[68–70] The latter option is most useful in cases of excess scar caused by infection or dehiscence. If the original wound was closed following the basic tenets described above, then reexcision with primary closure is not likely to result in an improved scar compared to the initial procedure. Recurrence of hypertrophic scar is quite high in these circumstances, and therefore most surgeons do not treat hypertrophic scar with excision and primary closure unless they plan adjuvant therapy.

KELOID

Scars that overgrow the original wound edges are called keloids. This clinical characteristic distinguishes keloid from hypertrophic scar. True keloid scar is not common and occurs mainly in darkly pigmented individuals with an incidence of 6% to 16% in African populations.[71] It has a genetic predisposition with autosomal dominant features. The keloid scar continues to enlarge past the original wound boundaries and behaves like a benign skin tumor with continued slow growth.

Keloids consist mainly of collagen. They are relatively acellular in their central portions with fibroblasts present along their enlarging borders. They do not contain a significant excess number of fibroblasts. Collagen scar deposition outpaces degradation, and the lesion continues to enlarge.

No uniformly successful treatment of keloid scar exists. Excision and primary closure invariably result in recurrence. Steroid injection directly into the keloid has the most benefit early in the course.[72]

Patients presenting with mature lesions of months to years duration that are slowly changing respond poorly to steroid injection. The only viable treatment options for mature keloids are to monitor and do nothing or to excise and administer adjuvant therapy.

Clinical Management of Wounds

Primary Intention

Primary intention healing occurs in closed wounds, which are wounds with the edges approximated. These wounds are usually closed in layers along tissue planes. Deep sutures are placed in collagen-rich layers such as fascia and dermis. These layers are strong and can hold sutures with a high degree of tension. Fatty tissue layers, such as subcutaneous fat, do not have significant collagen and cannot hold sutures under tension. For this reason, most surgeons do not close the subcutaneous fat layer, even in the morbidly obese patient.

To decrease scar formation and risk of infection, meticulous hemostasis should be performed. This step limits the amount of hematoma to be cleared, and thus decreases the inflammatory phase and likely decreases scar. Because hematoma is a culture media for bacteria, decreased bleeding also decreases the risk of infection. By limiting inflammation with sterile technique and tight hemostatic control, repair by activated fibroblasts can begin earlier and thus shorten the healing period.

Smaller surgical scars are achieved with no skin edge trauma and less resultant inflammation. Forceps crush-injury of the epidermis and dermis should be avoided by using fine forceps and skin hooks to retract and assist in dermal closure;

this decreases the amount of necrotic tissue at the wound edge and thereby reduces inflammation.

Uncomplicated wounds healing with primary intention epithelialize within 24 to 48 h. At this point, water barrier function has been restored and patients can be allowed to shower or wash. This stage has a psychological benefit during the postoperative recovery period. In addition, gentle cleansing removes old serum and blood, which reduces potential bacterial accumulation and infection risk.

Secondary Intention

Open wounds heal with the same basic processes of inflammation, proliferation, and remodeling as do closed wounds. The major difference is that each sequence is much longer, especially the proliferative phase. There is also much more granulation tissue formation and contraction. This type of healing process is referred to as secondary intention.

Open wound edges are not approximated but are instead separated, which necessitates epithelial cell migration across a longer distance. Before epiboly can occur, a provisional matrix must be present. Granulation tissue must form. There are variable amounts of bacteria, tissue debris, and inflammation present depending on wound location and etiology. Infection, with high protein exudative losses and acute and chronic inflammation, can disregulate repair and transform the healing wound into a clinically nonhealing wound.

During the proliferative phase of an uncomplicated course of secondary intention healing, a bed of granulation tissue is present. If no infection is present and the area is of sufficient size that healing will not be complete for at least 2 to 3 weeks, then placement of a partial or full-thickness skin graft should be considered. Grafts readily adhere to granulation tissue and will quickly speed the repair process. Partial thickness skin graft donor sites can heal in as little as 2 weeks, depending on graft thickness.

Topical Wound Treatment

LOCAL CARE

CLOSED WOUNDS
Closed wounds healing by primary intention require much less care than open wounds. Closed wounds should be kept

TABLE 7.3. Classes of Wound Dressings and Skin Replacements Currently Available.

Class	Composition	Characteristics/function	Commercial examples
Gauze	Woven cotton fibers	Permeable with desiccation; debridement; painful removal	Curity®
Calcium-alginates	Seaweed polymer that forms a gel when absorbs fluid	Absorbs exudate; nonadherent; nonirritating; requires a cover dressing (permeable)	Algisorb,® Sorbsan®
Impregnated gauzes	Fine mesh fabric (silicone, nylon) with dermal porcine collagens	Nonadherent; semipermeable	Biobrane II®
Films	Plastic (polyurethane); semipermeable	Allows water vapor permeation; adhesive	Opsite,® Tegaderm®
Foams	Hydrophilic (wound side) and hydrophobic (outer side); semipermeable	Necrotic/exudative wounds	Lyofoam,® Allevyn®
Hydrogels	Water (96%) and polymer (polyethyleneoxide)	Aqueous environment; requires secondary dressing; no adherence; not recommended if infection is present; semipermeable	Vigilon,® Aquasorb®
Hydrocolloids	Hydrophilic colloidal particles and adhesive	Absorbs fluid; necrotic tissue autolysis; little adherence; occlusive	Duoderm,® Intrasite®
Absorptive powders and pastes	Starch copolymers, hydrocolloidal particles	Absorbs exudate; used as a filler; good for deep wounds	Geliperm,® Duoderm granules®
Silicone	Silicone sheets	Sheet induces a localized electromagnetic field; decreases scar formation?	Sil-K®
Mechanical vacuum	Vacuum, sponge, plastic film	Sponge conforms to wound and vacuum removes edema fluid; stimulation of repair?	VAC® device
Dermal matrix replacements	Acellular matrix	Permeable; increased stimulation of repair?	Alloderm® (human, dermis), SIS® (porcine, small bowel submucosa), Integra® (bovine collagen, GAG, and silicone epidermal-type layer)
Dermal living replacements	Absorbable matrix populated with fibroblasts	Permeable; increased stimulation of repair?	Dermagraft®
Skin living replacement	Bovine collagen matrix populated with human fibroblasts with an outer layer of human keratinocytes	Impermeable; increased stimulation of repair?	Apligraf® (FDA approved 6/98)

A multitude of brands within each class are available, and only a few examples are listed. Recently, skin replacements have become available. Although expensive, they have great potential clinical usefulness. No particular brands are recommended in any class.

Source: Data partially taken from Feedar JA. Clinical management of chronic wounds. In: McCulloch JM, Kloth LC, Feedar JA, eds. Wound Healing Alternatives in Management. Philadelphia: Davis, 1995:137–185.

sterile for 24 to 48 h until epithelialization is complete. Tensile strength is only 20% of normal skin at 3 weeks when collagen cross-linking is becoming significant. At 6 weeks, wounds are at 70% of the tensile strength of normal skin, which is nearly the maximal tensile strength achieved by scar (75%–80% of normal; see Fig. 12.10).[19] Therefore, if absorbable suture is used to close deep structures that are under significant tension, such as abdominal fascia, the suture should retain significant tensile strength for at least 6 weeks before absorption severely weakens the suture. In addition, heavy activity should be limited for a minimum of 6 weeks while healing of deep fascial structures occurs.

OPEN WOUNDS

Necrotic material should be removed from open wounds on initial presentation and subsequently as it accumulates. Necrotic tissue serves only as a culture source for bacteria and does not aid healing. The only exception to immediate debridement is a dry, chronic, arterial insufficiency eschar without evidence of infection. These types of wounds may be best treated by revascularization before debridement.

Open wounds heal optimally in a moist, sterile environment. By keeping the wound covered and moist without infection, desiccation necrosis and healing delay are prevented.[73]

WOUND DRESSINGS

A plethora of wound dressings are available for all types of wounds. No type has conclusively been shown to accelerate healing more than the others. The optimal open wound dressing maintains a moist, clean environment that prevents pressure and mechanical trauma, reduces edema, stimulates repair, and is inexpensive. Less frequent dressing changes and prevention of skin irritation are also beneficial. At this time, no ideal dressing exists (see Table 7.3).

ENGINEERED SKIN REPLACEMENTS

With the biotechnology revolution, several dermal and skin replacements are now available through tissue engineering technology (Table 7.3). These products have the additional potential benefit of accelerating or augmenting repair by means of their biocomponents.

Pharmacological Treatment

ANTIBIOTIC OINTMENTS

Antibiotic ointments are commonly used in burn wound care as well as deep partial thickness injuries. They remain controversial in the nonburn patient because the risk of developing an invasive infection by resistant bacteria may be too high to justify their use. Open wounds are colonized by bacteria, and systemic antibiotics are only indicated if invasive infection is present. Nonburn wounds without infection will likely heal without topical antibiotic treatment so long as local care is adequate.

In burn patients, silver sulfadiazine is commonly used (see Chapter 20). It is inexpensive, has few side effects, and rarely induces bacterial resistance. It can be useful in chronic wound dressings as well. It is inexpensive and is well tolerated by pediatric and geriatric patients alike.

COLLAGENASES

The collagenases are useful to treat wounds that require fine debridement of necrotic tissue that is not amenable to surgical debridement, such as a thin layer of adherent exudate or small amounts of necrotic tissue remaining after a bedside wound debridement.

GROWTH FACTORS

Experimentally, exogenous application of several growth factors has been shown to accelerate normal healing as well as improve healing rates and efficacy in impaired models of healing.[24,74–83] The best-studied growth factors with the most promise to improve healing are PDGF, TFG-β, and members of the FGF family (see Table 12.2). Several obstacles must be overcome before widespread use, including efficacious application, vehicle development, and cost.

References

1. Ginsberg MH, Du X, Plow EF. Inside-out integrin signaling. Curr Opin Cell Biol 1992;4:766–771.
2. Roberts HR, Tabares AH. Overview of the coagulation reactions. In: High KA, Roberts HR, eds. Molecular Basis of Thrombosis and Hemostasis. New York: Dekker, 1995:35–50.
3. Wahl LM, Wahl SM. Inflammation. In: Cohen IK, Diegelmann RF, Lindblad WJ, eds. Wound Healing, Biochemical and Clinical Aspects. Philadelphia: Saunders, 1992:40–62.
4. Clark RAF. Wound repair. Overview and general considerations. In: Clark RAF, ed. The Molecular and Cellular Biology of Wound Repair. New York: Plenum Press, 1996:3–50.
5. DiPietro LA. Wound healing: the role of the macrophage and other immune cells. Shock 1995;4:233–240.
6. Riches DWH. Macrophage involvement in wound repair, remodeling, and fibrosis. In: Clark RAF, ed. The Molecular and Cellular Biology of Wound Repair. New York: Plenum Press, 1996:95–141.
7. Leibovich SJ, Ross R. The role of the macrophage in wound repair. A study with hydrocortisone and antimacrophage serum. Am J Pathol 1975;78:71–100.
8. Miller EJ, Gay S. Collagen structure and function. In: Cohen IK, Diegelmann RF, Lindblad WJ, eds. Wound Healing. Biochemical and Clinical Aspects. Philadelphia: Saunders, 1992:130–151.
9. Lodish H, Baltimore D, Berk A, Zipursky SL, Matsudaira P, Darnell J. Multicellularity: cell–cell and cell–matrix interactions. In: Molecular Cell Biology. New York: Scientific American, 1995:1123–1200.
10. Walchli C, Koch M, Chiquet M, Odermatt BF, Trueb B. Tissue-specific expression of the fibril-associated collagens XII and XIV. J Cell Sci 1994;107:669–681.
11. Hagg P, Rehn M, Huhtala P, Vaisanen T, Tamminen M, Pihlajaniemi T. Type XIII collagen is identified as a plasma membrane protein. J Biol Chem 1998;273:15590–15597.
12. Berthod F, Germain L, Guignard R, et al. Differential expression of collagens XII and XIV in human skin and in reconstructed skin. J Invest Dermatol 1997;108:737–742.
13. Marinkovich MP, Keene DR, Rimberg CS, Burgeson RE. Cellular origin of the dermal-epidermal basement membrane. Dev Dyn 1993;197:255–267.
14. Woodley DT. Reepithelialization. In: Clark RAF, ed. The Molecular and Cellular Biology of Wound Repair. New York: Plenum Press, 1996:339–350.
15. Kobayashi H, Ishii M, Chanoki M, et al. Immunohistochemical localization of lysyl oxidase in normal human skin. Br J Dermatol 1994;131:325–330.

16. Talhouk RS, Bissell MJ, Werb Z. Coordinated expression of extracellular matrix-degrading proteinases and their inhibitors regulates mammary epithelial function during involution. J Cell Biol 1992;118:1271–1282.

17. Moses MA, Marikovsky M, Harper JW, et al. Temporal study of the activity of matrix metalloproteinases and their endogenous inhibitors during wound healing. J Cell Biochem 1996;60:379–386.

18. Witte MB, Thornton FJ, Kiyama T, et al. Metalloproteinase inhibitors and wound healing: a novel enhancer of wound strength. Surgery (St. Louis) 1998;124:464–470.

19. Levenson SM, Geever EF, Crowley LV, Oates JF, Berard CW, Rosen H. The healing of rat skin wounds. Ann Surg 1965;161:293–308.

20. Pierce GF, Brown D, Mustoe TA. Quantitative analysis of inflammatory cell influx, procollagen type I synthesis, and collagen cross-linking in incisional wounds: influence of PDGF-BB and TGF-beta 1 therapy. J Lab Clin Med 1991;117:373–382.

21. Pierce GF, Mustoe TA, Altrock BW, Deuel TF, Thomason A. Role of platelet-derived growth factor in wound healing. J Cell Biochem 1991;45:319–326.

22. Pierce GF, Vande BJ, Rudolph R, Tarpley J, Mustoe TA. Platelet-derived growth factor-BB and transforming growth factor beta 1 selectively modulate glycosaminoglycans, collagen, and myofibroblasts in excisional wounds. Am J Pathol 1991;138:629–646.

23. Cromack DT, Pierce GF, Mustoe TA. TGF-beta and PDGF mediated tissue repair: identifying mechanisms of action using impaired and normal models of wound healing. Prog Clin Biol Res 1991;365:359–373.

24. Mustoe TA, Pierce GF, Morishima C, Deuel TF. Growth factor-induced acceleration of tissue repair through direct and inductive activities in a rabbit dermal ulcer model. J Clin Invest 1991;87:694–703.

25. Suh DY, Hunt TK, Spencer EM. Insulin-like growth factor-I reverses the impairment of wound healing induced by corticosteroids in rats. Endocrinology 1992;131:2399–2403.

26. Nissen NN, Polverini PJ, Koch AE, Volin MV, Gamelli RL, DiPietro LA. Vascular endothelial growth factor mediates angiogenic activity during the proliferative phase of wound healing. Am J Pathol 1998;152:1445–1452.

27. Banks RE, Forbes MA, Kinsey SE, et al. Release of the angiogenic cytokine vascular endothelial growth factor (VEGF) from platelets: significance for VEGF measurements and cancer biology. Br J Cancer 1998;77:956–964.

28. Frank S, Hubner G, Breier G, Longaker MT, Greenhalgh DG, Werner S. Regulation of vascular endothelial growth factor expression in cultured keratinocytes. Implications for normal and impaired wound healing. J Biol Chem 1995;270:12607–12613.

29. Fukumura D, Xavier R, Sugiura T, et al. Tumor induction of VEGF promoter activity in stromal cells. Cell 1998;94:715–725.

30. Werner S, Smola H, Liao X, et al. The function of KGF in morphogenesis of epithelium and reepithelialization of wounds. Science 1994;266:819–822.

31. Robertson JG, Pickering KJ, Belford DA. Insulin-like growth factor I (IGF-I) and IGF-binding proteins in rat wound fluid. Endocrinology 1996;137:2774–2781.

32. Heino J, Heinonen T. Interleukin-1 beta prevents the stimulatory effect of transforming growth factor-beta on collagen gene expression in human skin fibroblasts. Biochem J 1990;271:827–830.

33. Ferguson MW, Whitby DJ, Shah M, Armstrong J, Siebert JW, Longaker MT. Scar formation: the spectral nature of fetal and adult wound repair. Plast Reconstr Surg 1996;97:854–860.

34. Adzick NS, Lorenz HP. Cells, matrix, growth factors, and the surgeon. The biology of scarless fetal wound repair. Ann Surg 1994;220:10–18.

35. Young T. Pressure sores: incidence, risk assessment and prevention. Br J Nurs 1997;6:319–322.

36. Schubert V, Perbeck L, Schubert PA. Skin microcirculatory and thermal changes in elderly subjects with early stage of pressure sores. Clin Physiol 1994;14:1–13.

37. Relander M, Palmer B. Recurrence of surgically treated pressure sores. Scand J Plast Reconstr Surg Hand Surg 1988;22:89–92.

38. Kierney PC, Engrav LH, Isik FF, Esselman PC, Cardenas DD, Rand RP. Results of 268 pressure sores in 158 patients managed jointly by plastic surgery and rehabilitation medicine. Plast Reconstr Surg 1998;102:765–772.

39. Burton CS. Venous ulcers. Am J Surg 1994;167:37S–40S; discussion 40S–41S.

40. Margolis DJ, Cohen JH. Management of chronic venous leg ulcers: a literature-guided approach. Clin Dermatol 1994;12:19–26.

41. Bernstein EF, Harisiadis L, Salomon GD, et al. Healing impairment of open wounds by skin irradiation. J Dermatol Surg Oncol 1994;20:757–760.

42. Robson MC. Infection in the surgical patient: an imbalance in the normal equilibrium. Clin Plast Surv 1979;6:493–503.

43. Robson MC. Wound infection. A failure of wound healing caused by an imbalance of bacteria. Surg Clin North Am 1997;77:637–650.

44. Robson MC, Stenberg BD, Heggers JP. Wound healing alterations caused by infection. Clin Plast Surg 1990;17:485–492.

45. Robson MC, Krizek TJ. Predicting skin graft survival. J Trauma 1973;13:213–217.

46. Murphy RC, Robson MC, Heggers JP, Kadowaki M. The effect of microbial contamination on musculocutaneous and random flaps. J Surg Res 1986;41:75–80.

47. Barbul A, Purtill WA. Nutrition in wound healing. Clin Dermatol 1994;12:133–140.

48. Muller MJ, Herndon DN. The challenge of burns. Lancet 1994;343:216–220.

49. Albina JE. Nutrition and wound healing. J Parenter Enteral Nutrition 1994;18:367–376.

50. Ehrlich HP, Hunt TK. Effects of cortisone and vitamin A on wound healing. Ann Surg 1968;167:324–328.

51. Ehrlich HP, Tarver H, Hunt TK. Effects of vitamin A and glucocorticoids upon inflammation and collagen synthesis. Ann Surg 1973;177:222–227.

52. Levenson SM, Demetriou AA. Metabolic factors. In: Cohen IK, Diegelmann RF, Lindblad WJ, eds. Wound Healing, Biochemical and Clinical Aspects. Philadelphia: Saunders, 1992:248–273.

53. Masse PG, Pritzker KP, Mendes MG, Boskey AL, Weiser H. Vitamin B6 deficiency experimentally-induced bone and joint disorder: microscopic, radiographic and biochemical evidence. Br J Nutr 1994;71:919–932.

54. LaVan FB, Hunt TK. Oxygen and wound healing. Clin Plast Surg 1990;17:463–472.

55. Allen DB, Maguire JJ, Mahdavian M, et al. Wound hypoxia and acidosis limit neutrophil bacterial killing mechanisms. Arch Surg 1997;132:991–996.

56. Hopf HW, Hunt TK, West JM, et al. Wound tissue oxygen tension predicts the risk of wound infection in surgical patients. Arch Surg 1997;132:997–1004; discussion 1005.

57. Knighton DR, Hunt TK, Scheuenstuhl H, Halliday BJ, Werb Z, Banda MJ. Oxygen tension regulates the expression of angiogenesis factor by macrophages. Science 1983;221:1283–1285.

58. Jonsson K, Jensen JA, Goodson WH, et al. Tissue oxygenation, anemia, and perfusion in relation to wound healing in surgical patients. Ann Surg 1991;214:605–613.

59. Hunt TK, Pai MP. The effect of varying ambient oxygen tensions on wound metabolism and collagen synthesis. Surg Gynecol Obstet 1972;135:561–567.

60. Werner S, Breeden M, Hubner G, Greenhalgh DG, Longaker MT. Induction of keratinocyte growth factor expression is reduced and delayed during wound healing in the genetically diabetic mouse. J Invest Dermatol 1994;103:469–473.

61. Beer HD, Longaker MT, Werner S. Reduced expression of PDGF

and PDGF receptors during impaired wound healing. J Invest Dermatol 1997;109:132–138.

62. Goodson WH, Hunt TK. Wound healing in experimental diabetes mellitus: importance of early insulin therapy. Surg Forum 1978;29:95–98.

63. Goodson WH, Hunt TK. Deficient collagen formation by obese mice in a standard wound model. Am J Surg 1979;138:692–694.

64. Ehrlich HP, Hunt TK. The effects of cortisone and anabolic steroids on the tensile strength of healing wounds. Ann Surg 1969;170:203–206.

65. Marks JG Jr, Cano C, Leitzel K, Lipton A. Inhibition of wound healing by topical steroids. J Dermatol Surg Oncol 1983;9: 819–821.

66. Drake DB, Oishi SN. Wound healing considerations in chemotherapy and radiation therapy. Clin Plast Surg 1995;22:31–37.

67. Bettinger DA, Yager DR, Diegelmann RF, Cohen IK. The effect of TGF-beta on keloid fibroblast proliferation and collagen synthesis. Plast Reconstr Surg 1996;98:827–833.

68. Alster TS, West TB. Treatment of scars: a review. Ann Plast Surg 1997;39:418–432.

69. Ellitsgaard V, Ellitsgaard N. Hypertrophic scars and keloids: a recurrent problem revisited. Acta Chir Plast 1997;39:69–77.

70. Lee SM, Ngim CK, Chan YY, Ho MJ. A comparison of Sil-K and Epiderm in scar management. Burns 1996;22:483–487.

71. Murray JC, Pinnell SR. Keloids and excessive dermal scarring. In: Cohen IK, Diegelmann RF, Lindblad WJ, eds. Wound Healing, Biochemical and Clinical Aspects. Philadelphia: Saunders, 1992:500–509.

72. Maguire HC. Treatment of keloids with triamcinolone acetonide injected intralesionally. JAMA 1965;192:325–327.

73. Svensjo T, Pomahac B, Yao F, Eriksson E. Healing of full-thickness porcine wounds in dry, moist, and wet environments. Surg Forum 1998;48:150–153.

74. Greenhalgh DG, Sprugel KH, Murray MJ, Ross R. PDGF and FGF stimulate wound healing in the genetically diabetic mouse. Am J Pathol 1990;136:1235–1246.

75. Slavin J, Nash JR, Kingsnorth AN. Effect of transforming growth factor beta and basic fibroblast growth factor on steroid-impaired healing intestinal wounds. Br J Surg 1992;79:69–72.

76. Richard JL, Parer RC, Daures JP, et al. Effect of topical basic fibroblast growth factor on the healing of chronic diabetic neuropathic ulcer of the foot. A pilot, randomized, double-blind, placebo-controlled study. Diabetes Care 1995;18:64–69.

77. Steed DL. Clinical evaluation of recombinant human platelet-derived growth factor for the treatment of lower extremity diabetic ulcers. Diabetic Ulcer Study Group. J Vasc Surg 1995;21: 71–78; discussion 79–81.

78. Steed DL, Donohoe D, Webster MW, Lindsley L. Effect of extensive debridement and treatment on the healing of diabetic foot ulcers. Diabetic Ulcer Study Group. J Am Coll Surg 1996; 183:61–64.

79. Pierce GF, Tarpley JE, Allman RM, et al. Tissue repair processes in healing chronic pressure ulcers treated with recombinant platelet-derived growth factor BB. Am J Pathol 1994;145:1399–1410.

80. Lynch SE, de Castilla GR, Williams RC, et al. The effects of short-term application of a combination of platelet-derived and insulin-like growth factors on periodontal wound healing. J Periodontol 1991;62:458–467.

81. Antoniades HN, Galanopoulos T, Neville-Golden J, Kiritsy CP, Lynch SE. Injury induces in vivo expression of platelet-derived growth factor (PDGF) and PDGF receptor mRNAs in skin epithelial cells and PDGF mRNA in connective tissue fibroblasts. Proc Natl Acad Sci USA 1991;88:565–569.

82. Cromack DT, Porras-Reyes B, Purdy JA, Pierce GF, Mustoe TA. Acceleration of tissue repair by transforming growth factor beta 1: identification of in vivo mechanism of action with radiotherapy-induced specific healing deficits. Surgery (St. Louis) 1993;113:36–42.

83. Jones SC, Curtsinger LJ, Whalen JD, et al. Effect of topical recombinant TGF-beta on healing of partial thickness injuries. J Surg Res 1991;51:344–352.

Trauma: Priorities, Controversies, and Special Situations

Jeffrey Hammond

Trauma Management

Trauma remains the leading cause of death in all age categories from infancy to middle age (1–44 years) in the United States.[1] In 1984, trauma exceeded cancer and heart disease combined as a measure of years of potential life lost (YPLL) as determined by the Centers for Disease Control and Prevention.[2] By 1988, the estimated total annual cost of accidental trauma, including lost wages, medical expenses, and indirect losses, was estimated to be $180 *billion* in the United States alone.[3]

Advanced Trauma Life Support (ATLS) courses acknowledge the trimodal pattern of death after trauma. The first cohort, approximately 50% of trauma deaths, occurs in the immediate postinjury period, and represents death from overwhelming injury such as spinal cord transection, aortic disruption, or massive intraabdominal injuries.[4] Recognizing that there is little sophisticated treatment systems can do to salvage these patients, efforts should be directed at prevention.

In the second phase, deaths are usually caused by severe traumatic brain injury or uncontrolled hemorrhage, occur within hours of the injury, and represent perhaps one-third of all trauma deaths. Preventable death studies report reduction in preventable death rates from 20% to 30% to 2% to 9% upon institution of trauma system and/or trauma center development.[5] The third peak occurs 1 day to 1 month post injury and comprises approximately 10% to 20% of deaths. It is most often caused by refractory increased intracranial pressure subsequent to closed head injury or pulmonary complications. With aggressive critical care, nonpulmonary sources of sepsis, renal failure, and multiple organ failure as a cause of death are declining.

Thus, a cornerstone of trauma care is the timely identification and transport to a trauma center of those patients most likely to benefit, that is, the principle of triage. Trauma triage is founded upon the recognition that the nearest emergency room may not be the most appropriate destination.[6]

Current triage schema tend to assess the potential for life- or limb-threatening injury utilizing physiological, anatomical, and mechanism of injury criteria. In general, physiological criteria offer the greatest yield while anatomical criteria are intermediate and mechanism is low yield.[7] Highest yield criteria include prolonged prehospital time, a pedestrian struck at greater than 20 mph, the associated death of another vehicular occupant, and the physiological criteria of systolic blood pressure less than 90 mmHg, respiratory rate less than 10 or greater than 29 breaths per minute, or Glasgow Coma Score less than 13.

The basic tenets of trauma resuscitation focus on addressing the management decisions and algorithms that present in the second phase. To focus on this, the ATLS update retains the mnemonic **ABC**. Efforts during the initial, *primary*, survey are directed at establishing a secure **A**irway, using techniques of rapid sequence intubation (Table 8.1) if necessary, identifying that the patient has adequate **B**reathing by ruling out or treating immediately life-threatening chest injuries (Table 8.2), and ensuring adequate **C**irculation by control of obvious hemorrhage. Expeditious hemorrhage control, through operative and nonoperative means, has received increased emphasis over volume normalization through fluid administration and blood pressure maintenance in the new iteration. These treatment principles hold true in both the prehospital environment (EMS, emergency medical services) and the trauma center setting.

The *primary* survey is brief, requiring no more than 1 to 2 min. A cornerstone of the primary survey concept is the dictum to treat life-threatening injuries as they are identified.[8] Management during the primary survey relies heavily on knowledge of the expected patterns of injury based upon the mechanism of transfer of kinetic energy.[9] Laboratory tests and diagnostic radiology are not emphasized at this point.

Extending the alphabetical mnemonic, evaluation of **D**isability directs the resuscitation team to assess neurological function and assign a Glasgow Coma Score (GCS). The score derives from assessment of the patient's best motor, verbal, and eye-opening responses (Table 8.3). The patient is always

TABLE 8.1. Steps in Rapid Sequence Intubation.

1. Brief history and anatomical assessment
2. Prepare equipment and medications
3. Preoxygenate with 100% FiO_2
4. Premedicate with adjunctive agents (atropine, lidocaine)
5. Defasciculating muscle relaxant step
6. Sedation followed by induction of unconsciousness
7. Cricoid pressure
8. Muscle relaxation
9. Selleck maneuver
10. Intubation
11. Verification of endotracheal tube placement by CO_2 monitor
12. Secure ET tube; order chest x-ray; document

TABLE 8.3. Glasgow Coma Scale.

Component	Score
Best eye opening	
Spontaneously	4
To verbal command	3
To pain	2
No response	1
Best verbal response	
Oriented and converses	5
Disoriented	4
Inappropriate words	3
Incomprehensible sounds	2
No response or sounds	1
Best motor response	
Obeys commands	6
Localizes pain	5
Flexion-withdrawal	4
Decorticate flexion	3
Decerebrate extension	2
No motor response	1

assigned the most favorable score (e.g., if the patient is decorticate on one side and decerebrate on the other, the higher motor score is assigned) so that the score is reported as a finite number and not a range. Often, the trauma patient arrives in the emergency department intubated or therapeutically paralyzed. In these cases, the preintubation GCS should be elicited from the field personnel for use as the treatment baseline.

Implicit in this neurological assessment is the assumption that a spine injury is present until proven otherwise, dictating the need for vigilance in spine immobilization; this is especially true when concomitant head injury is present, and the head-and-neck axis should be considered as a single unit.[10] Evidence of a significant intracranial edema or space-occupying lesion, such as a GCS less than 8 or focal findings on cranial nerve exam, dictate early diagnostic imaging and neurosurgical consultation. Exposure directs the examiner to remove all clothing and log roll the patient to fully evaluate for injuries.

The *secondary* survey naturally follows the primary survey, and it is here that a more thorough head-to-toe examination is performed. Definitive hemorrhage control rather than normalization of volume status is again emphasized as the target of shock management. Blood loss may be estimated through assessment of blood pressure, heart rate, and skin color (Table 8.4). Invasive monitoring is not warranted. Hypovolemic hypotension requires >15% to 30% blood volume loss, but may be a late sign in younger patients with good compensatory mechanisms. Failure to correct hypotension or tachycardia after rapid infusion of 2 to 3 l of crystalloid solution suggests a volume deficit of greater than 15% or ongoing losses. Blood

TABLE 8.2. Life-Threatening Chest/Thoracic Injuries.

Immediately life threatening:
  Airway occlusion
  Tension pneumothorax
  Sucking chest wound (open pneumothorax)
  Massive hemothorax
  Flail chest
  Cardiac tamponade
Potential or late life threatening:
  Aortic injury
  Diaphragmatic tear
  Tracheobronchial injuries
  Pulmonary contusion
  Esophageal injury
  Blunt cardiac injury ("myocardial contusion")

Source: Adapted from ATLS (Advanced Trauma Life Support) class.

transfusion, using type O if type-specific blood is not available, should be considered when blood loss exceeds 1 l or if more than 3 l of crystalloid is needed to maintain blood pressure.

Prophylactic antibiotics should be started for penetrating trauma or open fractures.[11,12] The tetanus immunization status of the patient must be ascertained. If the immunization status is uncertain, or the patient has a tetanus-prone wound, tetanus immunoglobulin should be administered with the tetanus toxoid booster. Tetanus-prone wounds include those more than 6 h old, crush injuries, burns and electrical injuries, frostbite, high velocity missile injuries, devitalized tissue, denervated or ischemic tissue, or direct contamination with dirt or feces.[13]

Great care should be exercised during resuscitation efforts to protect against transmission of blood-borne diseases to the health care staff. Epidemiological studies have identified between 1% and 16% of trauma patients are infected with the human immunodeficiency virus (HIV) at time of presentation.[14,15] The incidence increases with the percentage of penetrating trauma within the case mix. The prevalence and risk of hepatitis B is even greater.

During the secondary survey, injuries are catalogued and potentially life-threatening or disabling injuries are identified. A treatment plan and priorities are set. A basic principle of trauma resuscitation is the need for continual reevaluation and reassessment. Some authors have published their experience with regard to a *tertiary* survey, which can identify a missed injury rate as high as 5% to 10%.[16] Finally, the leader of the resuscitation team must also be able to accurately assess his or her facility's ability to render definitive care and arrange for transfer to a tertiary facility or trauma center if warranted. Transfer to a higher level of care must be accomplished through physician-to-physician communication in a timely fashion and can be facilitated by preexisting transfer agreements.

Current Controversies

Not all trauma management decisions fit neatly into this paradigm, however. Within the Emergency Medical Services (EMS) community, the debate over "scoop and run" versus "stay and play" attempts at stabilization in the field continues.[17]

TABLE 8.4. Estimated Blood Loss Based on Physical Exam.

	Class I	Class II	Class III	Class IV
Blood loss (ml)	Up to 750	750–1500	1500–2000	>2000
Blood loss (% volume)	Up to 15%	15%–30%	30%–40%	>40%
Pulse rate	<100	>100	>120	>140
Blood pressure	Normal	Normal	Decreased	Decreased
Respiratory rate	14–20	20–30	30–40	>40
Urine output (ml/h)	>30	20–30	5–15	Negligible
Mental status	Slightly anxious	Mild anxiety	Anxious, confused	Lethargic

Regarding fluid resuscitation in the hypotensive patient, recent work by Mattox and colleagues in Houston supports the radical approach of limiting crystalloid infusion, even in the face of hypotension, in favor of a more rapid evacuation to a location for definitive care.[18] Conversely, Buchman and colleagues demonstrated a significant decrease in resuscitation times and increase in unexpected survival for the 5% of patients presenting in class III/IV shock utilizing a rapid infuser.[19] More to the point, Feero et al. identified that survival correlated with reduced scene time (defined as 10 min) for hypotensive patients with an Injury Severity Score (ISS) greater than 15, stressing the importance of triage and transport over interventions that may increase scene time.[20]

Similarly, the approach to diagnosis of blunt abdominal trauma is undergoing evolution. DPL is highly sensitive, approaching 97% in blunt trauma and 93% in penetrating trauma, with a 99% specificity.[21] Its high sensitivity was both an advantage as well as a disadvantage, however, as concern grew over the phenomenon of "nontherapeutic laparotomy."[22] Improvements in speed and resolution of computerized tomography (CT) led to this modality becoming the favored diagnostic approach for the *stable* trauma patient. Advantages of CT investigation of abdominal trauma include visualization of solid organ anatomy, including retroperitoneal structures, and the ability to grade and quantify injury.[23] This feature permits expectant nonoperative approach to solid organ injury. Disadvantages include the need to transport patients from the relative safety of the ED resuscitation area to the radiology suite, and the possible complications, such as allergic reaction or renal impairment, of administering a dye load. Moreover, the grading or staging of solid organ injury based on CT findings alone may poorly correlate with anatomical findings and should be considered in the context of vital signs indicative of hemodynamic status such as pulse and blood pressure.[24]

Ultrasound may replace DPL in the unstable patient.[25] Advantages of the Focused Abdominal Sonogram for Trauma (FAST) technique include its speed and immediacy; however, its true utility has not yet been established. Laparoscopy has not proved efficacious, with the exception of investigating penetrating trauma to the flank or back to rule out diaphragmatic injury, a condition for which neither DPL, CT, or FAST is accurate.[26]

The nonoperative management of traumatic brain injury is predicated on reducing brain edema in the absence of a space-occupying lesion that can be surgically attacked.

Steroids are contraindicated in these cases. Based on strong class II data, the use of intracerebral pressure monitoring for patients with GCS less than or equal to 8 mmHg is advocated. Ventriculostomies appear to be more efficacious than subarachnoid bolt monitors. This opinion is coupled with a recommendation against overaggressive hyperventilation to levels below a P_{CO_2} of 25 mmHg.

The role of CT scanning in so-called mild or minor head trauma (GCS 13–15) is unclear.[27] Use of the American Academy of Neurology (AAN) classification system for concussion (Table 8.5)[28] and neuropsychological follow-up are indicated.[29]

The use of steroids for acute spinal cord injury (SCI) remains a source of controversy.[30]

Special Situations

Trauma in the Elderly

For elderly Americans over age 65, trauma is the fifth most common cause of death.

Not only do the elderly tend to sustain different types of injuries, but their response to such injury and the ultimate outcome reflect the frequently occurring comorbidities and changes that occur in organ function over time.[31] The probability of a fatal outcome from trauma increases linearly with age, approximately 1% per year over age 65. Three types of events account for 75% of all injury-related deaths among the elderly: motor vehicle crashes, falls, and burns.

Obstacles to successful care of the elderly trauma patient include decreased physiological reserve, the likelihood of polypharmacy, and the probability of undisclosed or partially treated chronic diseases. The prevalence of preexisting medical conditions increases with age, up to 40% over age 65.

TABLE 8.5. Grades of Concussion: American Academy of Neurology (AAN) Guidelines.

Grade 1:
1. Transient confusion
2. No loss of consciousness
3. Concussive symptoms or mental status abnormalities resolve in *less* than 15 min

Grade 2
1. Transient confusion
2. No loss of consciousness
3. Concussive symptoms or mental status abnormalities (including amnesia) last *more* than 15 min

Grade 3
1. Any brief loss of consciousness
   a. Brief (seconds)
   b. Prolonged (minutes)

The presence of these preinjury comorbidities is tied to outcome, independent of age.[32]

Specific effects of aging contribute to the increased risk of poor outcomes after trauma.[33] Multifactorial cardiovascular changes include decreased coronary blood supply, slowed conduction, ventricular hypertrophy, decreased stroke volume, and increased systemic vascular resistance. The pulmonary system reflects decreased lung elasticity, decreased diffusion capacity, and increased destruction of alveolar septa. As a result, the aged lung has a decreased functional residual capacity despite little change in total lung capacity. Loss of protective airway reflexes and poor coughing effort contribute to a greater rate of aspiration. Over the five decades from age 30, the kidneys exhibit a progressive loss of renal mass, including both glomeruli and tubules. Renal blood flow and glomerular filtration rate decrease by nearly 50%. A concomitant decrease in concentrating ability translates into the need for greater urine volumes to ensure adequate excretion of acid and metabolite loads. Age-related dementia may be a confounding variable to the neurological exam. An age-related decrease in cerebral perfusion pressure accentuated the risk of hypotension. Loss of brain volume decreases the risk of cerebral contusion, but the increased space between brain and dura makes for an increased risk of subdural hemorrhage in which symptoms can be delayed or atypical. The tight adherence of the dura to the skull reduces the risk of epidural hematoma.

Aggressive approaches to surgery and critical care for the elderly trauma patient have lead to a good probability of return to independent function if survival is achieved.[34] These studies consistently report survival rates approaching 85% for patients older than 65 years, with 67% to 87% of these survivors returning to their prior level of independence at home, justifying aggressive intensive care management.

The Obese Trauma Patient

The National Center for Health Statistics and the National Health and Examination Nutrition Survey have identified 35% of Americans as overweight.[35] The physiological and anatomical effects of obesity within a critical care context are wide ranging.[36] Obesity is associated with increased work of breathing because of abnormal chest wall elasticity, increased chest wall resistance, abnormal diaphragm position, and need to eliminate a higher daily production of carbon dioxide. Ventilation-perfusion mismatching results in a widened aveolar-arterial oxygen gradient, derived in part from alveolar collapse and reduced functional residual volume. Tidal volumes (TV) based on actual body weight may result in high airway pressures and alveolar overdistension, however, so initial TV should be based on ideal body weight and adjusted according to airway pressures and oxygenation.[37]

Obese patients have a higher incidence of thromboembolic disease, in part the result of immobility, venous stasis, and increased thrombotic activity. This class of patients has been demonstrated to have impaired left ventricular contractility and ejection fraction. Drug dosing regimens are controversial, and there is disagreement and inconsistency in the literature. Although obese individuals have excess body fat, they are prone to develop protein energy malnutrition in response to stress, shifting to a preferential use of carbohydrates, which results in an increased respiratory quotient. Because energy expenditure equations are unreliable in the obese, in-

direct calorimetry should be utilized.[38] Nutritional support should not be withheld in the belief that weight reduction would be beneficial during critical illness or after injury. Obesity carries an increased risk of aspiration due to higher gastric volumes, prevalence of GE reflux, and increased intraabdominal pressure. Positioning the obese trauma patient to prevent this complication, or others such as skin breakdown, is made more difficult by the patient's body habitus.[39]

Obese patients have a higher likelihood of chest trauma, pelvic fracture or extremity fracture, and a decreased risk of head injury.[40] In addition, there is a statistically significant increase in pulmonary complications and mortality among the obese.

Trauma in the Jehovah's Witness

The Jehovah's Witnesses are a Christian sect whose current membership exceeds 3 million people worldwide. Most relevant to the medical community is their refusal to accept blood products on the basis of their religious beliefs.[41]

The Jehovah's Witness trauma patient represents unique management problems. Management decisions are based on several fundamental principles: (1) minimizing blood loss, (2) maximizing blood production, (3) maximizing oxygen delivery, and (4) decreasing metabolic requirements.[42] Minimizing blood loss starts by aggressively treating bleeding or potentially bleeding injuries. H_2 blockade to prevent gastrointestinal bleeding should be routine. Iatrogenic blood loss, most commonly from phlebotomy, should be kept to a minimum.

Procedures with a significant potential for blood loss should be delayed, if possible, until hemoglobin levels are adequate. If an operative procedure is to be performed, a red cell-salvaging device should be available and its potential use discussed with the patient or family. Efforts to maximize red blood cell production should begin immediately. The importance of nutritional status cannot be emphasized enough, and early enteral feeding is stressed. Supplemented iron should be administered to the anemic patient. The use of erythropoietin has gained wide popularity,[43] but its effect on hematopoiesis is not apparent for 1 to 2 weeks, limiting its benefit in the acute setting.

Maximizing oxygen delivery depends on circulating volume and oxygen content of blood. Crystalloid solutions are used for volume expansion but rapidly become distributed extravascularly. Synthetic colloids such as dextran and hespan may be added for volume expansion and are generally acceptable to the Jehovah's Witness.

An adjunctive strategy in the severely anemic patient is to decrease the metabolic rate, and thus the oxygen requirements.[44] Mild hypothermia of 30° to 32°C, neuromuscular blockage, barbiturates, and paralytics may be used to this end.

In all cases, medicolegal considerations dictate that there be clear documentation of the patient's religious preference and refusal to accept blood products, as well as the rationale for treatment decisions.

Trauma and Alcohol

Alcohol consumption is a major etiological factor in both intentional and unintentional trauma. Both acute and chronic alcohol use have a significant impact on mortality, and after motor vehicle trauma the link between alcohol use and death follows a dose–response curve.[45] It has been estimated that one alcohol-related fatality occurs every 22 min, and one-half of the $70 billion cost of motor vehicle crashes in the United States in 1988 was attributable to alcohol.[46]

Among the myths related to alcohol use is that alcohol protects against serious injury and that most people injured after consuming alcohol are social drinkers.[47] While intoxication is a legal issue, set in most states at a blood alcohol level (BAL) of 100 mg/ml, impairment can be demonstrated at levels of 0.05%.

Several quetionnaires have been developed to assess for at-risk behaviors and drinking patterns.

However, studies indicate little difference in the sensitivity and selectivity among these screening tests. The value of early identification cannot be overemphasized, however, and must be coupled with early intervention. After even one in-patient contact, professional treatment can obtain long-term (defined as 1 year) abstinence rates as high as 64% to 74%, compared to abstinence rates of 10% when treatment is delayed until referral after hospital discharge.

Trauma and the Prehospital Cardiac Arrest

The proper role of emergency department thoracotomy (EDT) in the management of severely injured and moribund trauma patients remains controversial. The physiological rationale and primary objectives are variously described as the ability to release pericardial tamponade, control intrathoracic hemorrhage, stop air emboli, open cardiac massage, and permit aortic cross-clamping for subdiaphragmatic hemorrhage. Since the 1980s, however, these indications have narrowed because the physiological assumptions underlying the procedure and the reported outcomes in various subgroups have not borne out the initial enthusiasm.[48]

In the normovolemic subject, open cardiac massage achieves 60% of baseline cardiac output compared to 25% for closed cardiac massage. In the face of hypovolemia, however, the state in which the trauma patient is most likely to be hypotensive, open massage does not afford significant advantage. An algorithm that reserves ED thoracotomy for patients with penetrating cardiac injury, other penetrating injury if signs of life are pres-ent, and selective application after blunt trauma can result in a significant reduction in performance of the procedure and its attendant costs without change in survival.

References

1. Eastman AB. Blood in our streets: status and evolution of trauma care systems. Arch Surg 1992;127:677–681.
2. Centers for Disease Control. MMWR 1989;38:27–29.
3. Rice DP, MacKenzie EJ. Cost of Injury in the United States: A Report to Congress. Atlanta: Centers for Disease Control, 1989.
4. Champion HR. Organization of trauma care. In: Kreis DJ, Gomez GA, eds. Trauma Management. Boston: Little, Brown, 1989:11–12.
5. Hammond JS, Gomez GA, Eckes J. Trauma systems: economic and political considerations. J Fla Med Assoc 1990;77:603–605.
6. Blaisdell FW. Trauma myth and magic: 1984 Fitts Lecture. J Trauma 1985;25:856–863.
7. Esposito TJ, Offner PJ, Jurkovich GJ, et al. Do prehospital trauma center triage criteria identify major trauma victims? Arch Surg 1995;130:171–176.
8. American College of Surgeons Committee on Trauma. Advanced Trauma Life Support. Chicago: American College of Surgeons, 1997.
9. National Association of Emergency Medical Technicians and American College of Surgeons Committee on Trauma. Prehospital Trauma Life Support, 4th ed. St. Louis: Mosby, 1999.
10. Kreipke DL, Gillespie KR, McCarthy MC, et al. Reliability of indications for cervical spine films in trauma patients. J Trauma 1989;29:1438–1439.
11. Eastern Association for the Surgery of Trauma. Practice management Guidelines for prophylactic antibiotics in penetrating abdominal injury. Website (www.east.org), 1998.
12. Eastern Association for the Surgery of Trauma. Practice management guidelines for prophylactic antibiotics in open fractures. Website (www.east.org), 1998.
13. Furste W. Tetanus prophylaxis in the United States. Bull Am Coll Surg 1992;77:22–26.
14. Kelen G, Fritz S, Qaquish B, et al. Substantial increase in HIV-1 infection in critically ill emergency patients. Ann Emerg Med 1989;18:378–382.
15. Hammond JS, Eckes JM, Gomez GA, et al. HIV, trauma and infection control: universal precautions are universally ignored. J Trauma 1990;30:555–561.
16. Enderson BL, Reath DB, Meadors J, et al. The tertiary trauma survey: a prospective study of missed injury. J Trauma 1990;30:666–669.
17. Smith JP, Bodai BI, Hill AS, et al. Prehospital stabilization of critically injured patients: a failed concept. J Trauma 1985;25:65–70.
18. Bickell WH, Wall MJ Jr, Pepe PE, et al. Immediate versus delayed fluid resuscitation for hypotensive patients with penetrating torso injuries. N Engl J Med 1994;331:1105–1109.
19. Buchman TG, Menker JB, Lipsett P. Strategies for trauma resuscitation. Surg Gynecol Obstet 1991;172:8–12.
20. Feero S, Hedges J, Simmons E, Irwin L. Does out-of-hospital EMS time affect trauma survival? Am J Emerg Med 1995;13:133–135.
21. Alyono D, Morrow CE, Perry JF. Reappraisal of diagnostic peritoneal lavage criteria for operation in penetrating and blunt trauma. Surgery (St. Louis) 1982;92:751–757.
22. Miller FB, Cryer HM, Chilikuri S, et al. Negative findings on laparotomy for trauma. South Med J 1989;82:1231–1234.
23. Pevec WC, Peitzman AB, Udekwu AO, et al. Computed tomography in the evaluation of blunt abdominal trauma. Surg Gynecol Obstet 1991;173:262–267.
24. Sutyak JP, Chiu WC, D'Amelio LF, et al. Computed tomography is inaccurate in estimating the severity of adult splenic injury. J Trauma 1995;39:514–518.
25. Rozycki G, Ochsner MG, Feliciano D, et al. Early detection of hemoperitoneum by ultrasound examination of the right upper quadrant: a multicenter study. J Trauma 1998;45:878–883.
26. Salvino C, Esposito TJ, Marshall WJ, et al. The role of diagnostic laparoscopy in the management of trauma patients: a preliminary assessment. J Trauma 1993;34:506–515.
27. Stein SC, Ross SE. Mild head injury: a plea for routine early CT scanning. J Trauma 1992;33:11–13.
28. Kelly JP, Rosenberg J. Practice parameter: the management of concussion in sport. Report of the Quality Standards Committee. Neurology 1997;48:581–585.
29. Brooks J, Fos LA, Greve K, Hammond JS. Assessment of executive function in patients with mild traumatic brain injury. J Trauma 199X;46:159–163.
30. Prendergast MR, Saxe J, Ledgerwood A, et al. Massive steroids do not reduce the zone of injury after penetrating spinal cord injury. J Trauma 1994;37:576–580.
31. Sacco WJ, Copes WS, Bain LW Jr, et al. Effect of preinjury illness on trauma patient survival outcome. J Trauma 1993;35:538–542.
32. Perdue PW, Watts DD, Kaufmann CR, et al. Differences in mor-

tality between elderly and younger adult trauma patients: geriatric status increases risk of delayed death. J Trauma 1998;45:805–810.

33. Schwab CW, Kauder DR. Trauma in the geriatric patient. Arch Surg 1992;127:701–706.

34. DeMaria EJ, Kenny PR, Merrian MA, et al. Aggressive trauma care benefits the elderly. J Trauma 1987;27:1200–1206.

35. Marik P, Varon J. The obese patient in the ICU. Chest 1998;113:492–498.

36. National Institutes of Health. Health implications of obesity. Ann Int Med 1985;103:147–151.

37. Almer L, Janzon L. Low vascular fibrinolytic activity in obesity. Thromb Res 1975;6:171–175.

38. Makk LJ, McClave DS, Creech PW. Clinical application of the metabolic cart to the delivery of total parenteral nutrition. Crit Care Med 1990;18:1320–1327.

39. Goodell TT. The obese trauma patient: treatment strategies. J Trauma Nursing 1996;3:36–44.

40. Boulanger BR, Milzman D, Mitchell K, et al. Body habitus as a predictor of injury pattern after blunt trauma. J Trauma 1992;33:228–232.

41. Fontanarosa PB, Giorgio GT. The role of the emergency physi-cian in the management of Jehovah's Witnesses. Ann Emerg Med 1989;18:1089–1095.

42. Mann MC, Votto J, Kambe J, et al. Management of the severely anemic patient who refuses transfusion: lessons learned during the care of a Jehovah's Witness. Ann Intern Med 1992;117:1042–1048.

43. Boshkov LK, Tredget EE, Janowska-Wieczorek A. Recombinant human erythropoietin for a Jehovah's Witness with anemia of thermal injury. Am J Hematol 1991;37:53–54.

44. Nearman HS, Eckhauser ML. Postoperative management of a severely anemic Jehovah's Witness. Crit Care Med 1983;11:142–143.

45. Anda RF, Williamson DF, Remington PL. Alcohol and fatal injuries among US adults: findings from the NHANES I epidemiologic follow-up study. JAMA 1988;260:2529–2532.

46. Wilson RF, Bender J, Gass J. Special problems of trauma in alcoholics. In Wilson RF and Walt A, eds. *Management of Trauma: Pitfalls and Practice.* Baltimore: Williams and Wilkins; 1996:167–172.

47. Waller JA. Management issues for trauma patients with alcohol. J Trauma 1990;30:1548–1553.

48. Cogbill TH, Moore EE, Millikan JS, et al. Rationale for selective application of emergency department thoracotomy in trauma. J Trauma 1983;23:453–460.

Shock and Resuscitation

Avery B. Nathens and Ronald V. Maier

Shock, at its most fundamental level, represents the clinical syndrome arising as a result of inadequate tissue perfusion. The discrepancy between substrate delivery and the cellular substrate requirement leads to cellular metabolic dysfunction. Inadequate oxygen delivery is implicated as the principal defect in shock states; the classification of which is listed in Table 9.1. The clinical manifestations of shock are caused by end-organ dysfunction secondary to impaired perfusion *and* the body's sympathetic and neuroendocrine response to an insufficient cellular supply/demand ratio for oxygen.

Timely restoration of perfusion and oxygen delivery usually reverses the shock state. However, the persistence or progression of shock may occur as a result of an ongoing occult perfusion defect, irreversible cellular injury, or a combination of the two phenomena. In addition, there is substantial clinical and laboratory evidence suggesting that cellular injury leads to the elaboration of proinflammatory mediators that may further compromise perfusion through functional and structural changes in the microvasculature. This form of secondary injury further impairs perfusion, creating a vicious cycle whereby cellular injury leads to impaired perfusion that further exacerbates cellular injury. Last, following recovery from the clinical shock state (i.e., total body hypoperfusion), there is diffuse activation of potent inflammatory cells that may lead to the systemic inflammatory response syndrome (SIRS). It is postulated that persistence of SIRS, through the secondary induction of global cellular dysfunction, may be causative in the development of the multiple organ dysfunction syndrome (MODS).[1-3]

Hypovolemic Shock

Hypovolemic shock is the most common cause of shock. It may arise as a result of one of two processes: either (1) hemorrhage, representing intravascular volume depletion through the loss of red blood cell mass; or (2) loss of plasma volume only through extravascular fluid sequestration *or* gastrointestinal, urinary, and insensible losses. Hemorrhage is the form of volume loss that can be most readily quantified and reproduced and thus represents the best understood form of shock, whereas extravascular fluid sequestration, also referred to as "third-space" fluid losses, is frequently underappreciated as a cause of shock. Third-space fluid losses are the principal cause of hypovolemia in the early postoperative period and in local inflammatory processes, such as pancreatitis, in which local changes in capillary permeability result in fluid extravasation from the intravascular space into the interstitium. Fluid sequestration is the principal cause of shock in patients with small-bowel obstruction. In this case, hypovolemia results from fluid loss into the interstitium, bowel lumen, and exudation of fluid into the peritoneal cavity. The clinical manifestations of nonhemorrhagic forms of hypovolemic shock are the same as with hemorrhage, although they can be more insidious in onset.

The physiological responses to hypovolemic shock are geared towards maintenance of cerebral and coronary perfusion and the restoration of effective circulating blood volume. The major compensatory mechanisms include an increase in sympathetic activity, release of stress hormones and expansion of intravascular volume through resorption of interstitial fluid, mobilization of intracellular fluid, and conservation of fluids and electrolytes by the kidney. The clinical manifestations are simply a reflection of the intense adrenosympathetic response and renal conservation of fluid. Microvascular hypoperfusion of selected vascular beds results from the combination of low intravascular blood volume, diminished cardiac output from a reduction in preload, and compensatory peripheral vasoconstriction.

A clinical staging system of hemorrhagic shock based on the percentage of acute blood volume loss has been described (Table 9.2).

Typically, classes I and II are referred to as compensated shock states in which the adrenergic response maintains a normal blood pressure. Passage from an initially compensated state of shock to class IV shock may occur rapidly, particu-

TABLE 9.1. Classification of Shock States.

Hypovolemic
Traumatic
Cardiogenic
Intrinsic
Compressive
Septic
Neurogenic
Hypoadrenal

larly in children and young adults. It is crucial to recognize compensated shock and intervene as early as possible. Decompensation of homeostatic mechanisms and inability to maintain systolic blood pressure above 90 mmHg after trauma-induced hypovolemia are associated with a mortality of more than 50%.[4] However, rapid and adequate restoration of circulating blood volume simultaneous with control of bleeding can reverse even severe hemorrhagic shock.

Hypovolemic shock is easily diagnosed when there is an obvious source of volume loss and when overt signs of hemodynamic instability and increased adrenergic output are present. The diagnosis is more challenging when there is an occult source or a slower rate of volume loss. In this particular situation, unreplaced gastrointestinal or urinary losses, excessive insensible loss, or intraabdominal fluid sequestration must be considered as alternate possibilities. Following trauma, blood loss in the chest, peritoneal cavity, retroperitoneum, pelvis, and thigh may be occult and should be considered in the evaluation of any hypotensive injured patient. Finally, plasma losses from tissue trauma or burns, free water deficit, or unreplaced insensible losses may lead to hypovolemia.

Laboratory evaluation may provide some diagnostic information. Nonhemorrhagic forms of hypovolemic shock tend to cause hemoconcentration. If the principal abnormality is caused by loss of free water, then hemoconcentration will be accompanied by hyponatremia. Acutely following hemorrhage there may be no alteration in the hemoglobin or hematocrit values until compensatory fluid shifts have occurred or exogenous red cell-free resuscitation fluid is administered.

In situations in which the underlying shock state is not clear, the most critical distinction is to ensure that one is not treating cardiogenic shock, as the appropriate therapy differs dramatically. The findings of jugular venous distension, rales, and the presence of an S_3 gallop in cardiogenic shock may assist in their differentiation. Both forms of shock, however, are associated with a reduction in cardiac output and a compensatory sympathetic-mediated response. Further, both types of shock may be treated with, and respond to, volume resuscitation. If the diagnosis is in doubt or the clinical situation suggests both as a possibility, then invasive monitoring using a pulmonary artery catheter may be helpful to further assess ongoing therapy.

Treatment of hypovolemic shock involves achieving two primary goals concurrently: to reexpand the circulating blood volume and to proceed with any necessary interventions to control ongoing volume loss. Adequate repletion of the circulating volume reexpands capacitance vessels, restores venous return, and reestablishes ventricular filling. As a result of improved left-ventricular end-diastolic volume, contractile function, stroke volume, and cardiac output respond positively; as cardiac output improves, the systemic vascular resistance returns to normal and tissue perfusion is restored.

Intravenous Access

Resuscitation of hemorrhagic shock or severe hypovolemia irrespective of the cause requires two large-bore (16 gauge or larger) intravenous lines for rapid volume restoration. Access may be achieved by peripheral vein catheterization, cutdowns on the basilic, greater saphenous, or cephalic veins, or percutaneous central venous access via subclavian, internal jugular, or femoral venous puncture.

The most important consideration for vascular access is the choice of catheter and tubing. The rate of flow is proportional to the fourth power of the radius of the cannula and is inversely related to its length (Poiseuille's law). Thus a short, large-bore catheter connected to the widest administration tubing possible or direct insertion of beveled tubing via a cutdown venotomy provides the most rapid flow rates.

Choice of Fluid for Volume Resuscitation

The most efficacious and cost-effective approach is to restore intravascular volume with rapid infusion of isotonic saline or a balanced salt solution. Infusion of 2 to 3 l of crystalloid over 10 to 30 min should restore adequate intravascular volume in most cases as the result of its large volume of distribution. In patients with hemorrhagic shock, final restoration of blood volume with crystalloid usually requires at least three times the estimated blood loss. However, if blood pressure does not improve after rapid administration of 2 l of crystalloid, this

TABLE 9.2. Physical Findings in Hemorrhagic Shock.[a]

	Class I	Class II	Class III	Class IV
Blood loss (ml)	<750	750–1500	1500–2000	>2000
Blood loss	Up to 15%	15%–30%	30%–40%	>40%
Pulse rate	<100	>100	>120	>140
Blood pressure	Normal	Normal	Decreased	Decreased
Pulse pressure (mmHg)	Normal	Decreased	Decreased	Decreased
Respiratory rate	14–20	20–30	30–40	>35
Urine output (ml/h)	>30	20–30	5–15	Negligible
CNS/mental status	Slightly anxious	Mildly anxious	Anxious, confused	Confused, lethargic

[a]Alcohol or drugs (e.g., β-blockers) may alter physical signs.

Source: Adapted from American College of Surgeons. Shock. In: Advanced Trauma Life Support Manual. Chicago: American College of Surgeons, 1997:87–107.

suggests that blood loss is in excess of 1500 ml, there is ongoing active bleeding, or, alternatively, another cause of shock must be considered. Further volume resuscitation should therefore include simultaneous blood transfusion, either as fully cross-matched blood, type-specific blood, or, in dire circumstances, O-positive or O-negative packed cells.

HYPERTONIC SALINE

The primary rationale behind the use of hyperosmotic solutions in patients with hypovolemic shock is relatively simple. The hypertonic component of these solutions draws water out of the intracellular space and acts to replenish the depleted extracellular space. To increase the intravascular oncotic pressure, 6% dextran has been added to the hypertonic saline solution. The colloid component transiently partitions the recruited fluid to the intravascular space and thus, in theory, should prolong the beneficial hemodynamic effects of the solutions. Still, based on published data, hypertonic saline with or without dextran probably offers little benefit to standard resuscitation regimens. In the subset of patients with shock and traumatic brain injury, hypertonic saline may offer some survival benefit. Hypertonic saline as a method of small-volume resuscitation may also offer certain advantages in less controlled medical environments where prolonged transport or evacuation times require longer periods of resuscitation with limited supplies. Additionally, the small weights and volumes of hypertonic saline required for resuscitation may prove advantageous in the battlefield.

FLUID RESUSCITATION USING COLLOID

It is unclear whether the use of colloid solutions confers any benefit over the use of crystalloid solutions. Meta-analysis of randomized controlled trials comparing albumin to crystalloid have suggested that use of colloid solutions in resuscitation may in fact increase mortality. It is thought that albumin, for instance, may increase edema, impair sodium and water excretion, and worsen renal failure. There are two forms of synthetic colloid in use. Hetastarch, a 6% hydroxyethyl starch solution, has a significant volume-expanding effect that lasts as long as 24 h. Potential disadvantages with the use of hetastarch include rare anaphylactic reactions and the development of a coagulopathy when given in excess of 1000 ml/day.[5] Clinical trials with this agent have shown improvements in tissue perfusion without any difference in clinical outcomes.

Pentastarch is another synthetic colloid with several advantages over hetastarch. Its structure allows for a more concentrated solution and therefore higher oncotic pressures for plasma expansion and faster plasma clearance and renal excretion. Further, this new solution has proved to be less allergenic and is associated with fewer renal or anaphylactic complications. Pentastarch has a significant volume-expanding effect that lasts approximately 12 h in comparison to hetastarch (24 h). Approximately 90% of the pentastarch dose is eliminated from the intravascular space within 24 h. Pentastarch induces plasma volume expansion of about 1.5 times the administered volume, whereas hetastarch produces expansion approximately equal to the volume administered. Thus, pentastarch may be a more potent volume expander with a shorter duration of action than either hetastarch or albumin.

ALTERNATIVES TO BLOOD TRANSFUSION

AUTOTRANSFUSION

Transfusion of shed blood has several advantages over homologous blood. In the acutely injured patient in need of immediate blood, autotransfusion is readily available. Autotransfusion is safe without risk of hemolytic, febrile, or allergic reactions or transmissible disease. Further, salvaged blood is already warm and has better oxygen-transport properties because of preservation of normal levels of 2,3-diphosphoglycerol. Despite reductions in platelet count and function, labile clotting factors are present in greater concentration than in banked blood, although fibrinogen levels drop significantly in salvaged blood.[6]

Regardless, the use of autotransfusion devices is cost-effective and reduces the use of banked blood.[7] Its use should be considered in any operative patient with hemorrhagic shock who does not immediately respond to crystalloid resuscitation in the emergency room.[8]

RED BLOOD CELL SUBSTITUTES

There are several potential benefits to using a red blood cell substitute, including immediate availability, no need for compatibility testing, freedom from disease transmission, and long-term storage. The only red blood cell substitute currently available for clinical use in humans is a polymerized stroma-free hemoglobin.[9]

Traumatic Shock

The major contributor to shock following trauma is hypovolemia, and acute hemorrhage is a frequent cause of death after injury.[4] Once hemorrhage ceases or is controlled, patients can continue to suffer loss of plasma volume into the interstitium of injured tissues and develop progressive hypovolemic shock. Additionally, hypovolemia coupled with tissue injury evokes a greater systemic inflammatory response and a potentially more devastating degree of shock than hypovolemia alone. Specific injuries can also produce superimposed cardiogenic or neurogenic shock. Pericardial tamponade or tension pneumothorax can produce hemodynamically significant compression of the heart, and myocardial contusion can cause cardiogenic shock. Neurogenic shock can accompany spinal cord injury.

The management of traumatic shock is similar to that of hypovolemic shock. Apart from prompt reversal of perfusion defects, efforts must be focused on limiting the inflammatory response to other stimuli. For example, maneuvers directed toward aggressive early reestablishment of the circulation to ischemic tissues, prompt debridement of devitalized or necrotic tissues, and early fracture fixation[10,11] might all play a role in limiting the inflammatory response.

Cardiogenic Shock

The syndrome of cardiogenic shock has been defined as the inability of the heart—as a result of impairment of its pumping function—to deliver sufficient blood flow to the tissues to meet resting metabolic demands.[12] Thus, the purest clinical definition of cardiogenic shock requires a low cardiac output and evidence of tissue hypoxia in the presence of an adequate intravascular volume. If hemodynamic monitoring is available, the diagnosis is confirmed by the combination of a low systolic blood pressure and a depressed cardiac index (<2.2 l/min/m^2) in the presence of an elevated pulmonary capillary wedge pressure (>15 mmHg).

The mechanisms leading to the development of cardiogenic shock reflect a complex interplay between the heart, the peripheral circulation, and maladaptive compensatory responses. The progressive deterioration that occurs in the absence of intervention can be seen as a vicious cycle in which normal physiological compensatory mechanisms in response to reduced cardiac output tend to propagate a downward spiral, ultimately leading to death (Fig. 9.1). A reduction in blood pressure activates the sympathetic nervous system through the stimulation of baroreceptors. The adrenergic response leads to an increase in heart rate, myocardial contractility, and arterial and venous vasoconstriction. The renin-angiotensin system is activated by inadequate renal perfusion and sympathetic stimulation, leading to additional vasoconstriction and salt and water retention. Finally, hypotension potentiates the secretion of antidiuretic hormone, which further increases water retention. The reduction in blood pressure in conjunction with an elevated left-ventricular end-diastolic pressure resulting from fluid retention and impaired left-ventricular function reduces coronary perfusion pressure and thus myocardial oxygen delivery. Meanwhile, the increase in heart rate, systemic vascular resistance, and contractility all increase myocardial oxygen consumption and demand. The discrepancy between myocardial oxygen demand and oxygen delivery further impairs left-ventricular function and will lead to circulatory collapse unless appropriate and timely intervention interrupts the cycle.

The clinical features of cardiogenic shock are remarkably similar to those of hypovolemic shock. If right-sided failure predominates, the predominant clinical features are those of accumulation of blood in the systemic veins and capacitance vessels. By contrast, the principal features of left-sided fail-

ure are related to an increase in extravascular lung water. With normal pulmonary capillary permeability, pulmonary interstitial fluid flow overwhelms the capacity of pulmonary lymphatics, and edema develops at capillary pressures higher than 20 mmHg. Overt pulmonary edema develops at pressures of more than 24 mmHg.

In making the diagnosis of cardiogenic shock, any history of cardiac disease may be of diagnostic value. Physical exam may demonstrate evidence of inadequate tissue perfusion in conjunction with an elevated jugular venous pressure, an S$_3$ gallop, and pulmonary edema. An electrocardiogram may indicate myocardial damage. A chest radiograph provides valuable diagnostic information regarding the presence of pulmonary edema, pleural effusion, or cardiac chamber enlargement. Cardiac enzymes may provide evidence of acute myocardial infarction, and arterial blood gas analysis provides information regarding the adequacy of gas exchange. Severe hypoxia in the presence of a normal chest radiograph may support the diagnosis of massive pulmonary embolus rather than a primary cardiac cause of shock. Urinary indices may demonstrate decreased urinary sodium and elevated urine osmolarity, a function of renal conservation of sodium and water in response to a drop in renal perfusion. Transthoracic or transesophageal echocardiography are excellent noninvasive aids in sorting through the differential diagnosis of cardiogenic shock; they may provide information on regional and global ventricular wall function, valvular integrity, and the presence or absence of pericardial fluid. In confusing or complicated cases use of a pulmonary artery catheter may provide additional diagnostic information.

Management of cardiogenic shock is geared toward immediate therapeutic interventions that interrupt the vicious cycle leading to progressive myocardial dysfunction. Critical elements include assuring adequate oxygenation and ventilation, correction of electrolyte and acid–base abnormalities, and restoration of sinus rhythm. Interventions may include cardioversion, administration of crystalloid, or infusion of inotropic or vasopressor drugs. Inotropic support should only

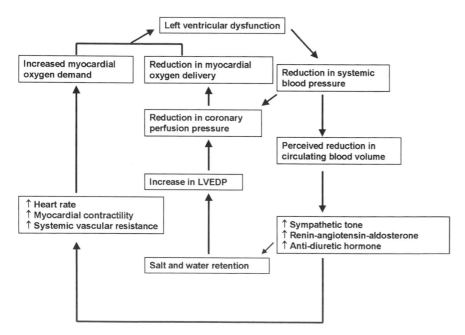

FIGURE 9.1. The reduction in cardiac output associated with left-ventricular dysfunction results in a series of compensatory responses that function to maintain blood pressure at the expense of aggravating any disparity in myocardial oxygen demand and supply. This imbalance increases left-ventricular dysfunction and sets up a vicious cycle.

be considered a temporizing measure; it has never been demonstrated to improve survival in patients with cardiogenic shock.[13]

Afterload reduction through the use of vasodilators may be beneficial for patients in cardiogenic shock, but caution must be exercised because of the risk of exacerbating hypotension. Either intravenous nitroglycerin or sodium nitroprusside may be used.

Patients with right-ventricular infarction leading to cardiogenic shock deserve special mention. The marked reduction in right-ventricular compliance causes these patients to be extremely sensitive to volume depletion. The focus of therapy in such patients should be the immediate restoration of adequate left-ventricular filling pressure while accepting significantly elevated central venous pressures. If volume resuscitation fails to resolve hypotension, then dobutamine should be used in an attempt to improve the contractility of the dysfunctional right ventricle.[12]

One adjunctive approach to patients with severe cardiac dysfunction is the use of intraaortic balloon counterpulsation (IABC), which is achieved by placing a counterpulsation balloon catheter in the descending thoracic aorta via the femoral artery.[14] Inflation of the balloon during diastole augments diastolic pressure at the aortic root and thus improves coronary blood flow; deflation during systole then provides some degree of afterload reduction. The net effect is a reduction in myocardial oxygen requirements. IABC is generally used as a means of temporary support for patients in cardiogenic shock, either with the hope of recovering myocardial function or while preparations are made for other interventions, whether they be percutaneous or operative attempts at myocardial revascularization, correction of other anatomical defects, or cardiac transplantation. There is some evidence that use of the IABC in patients subsequently undergoing revascularization may offer a significant survival benefit.

Compressive (or obstructive) cardiogenic shock is a discrete entity that occurs as a result of extrinsic compression of the heart. The extrinsic compression limits diastolic filling, effectively reducing preload, which adversely affects stroke volume and cardiac output. Blood or fluid within the poorly distensible pericardial sac may cause pericardial tamponade, which is the most frequently cited cause of extrinsic cardiogenic shock. However, any cause of increased intrathoracic pressure—such as tension pneumothorax, herniation of abdominal viscera through a diaphragmatic hernia, mediastinal hematomas (rarely pneumomediastinum), and in some instances excessive positive pressure ventilation or intraabdominal compartment pressure—can cause cardiogenic shock.

The classic clinical findings of pericardial tamponade include jugular venous distension, muffled heart sounds, and hypotension (Beck's triad). A drop in blood pressure with inspiration of more than 10 mmHg, known as pulsus paradoxus, may be demonstrated. Placement of a central venous catheter confirms the elevation in right-sided filling pressures despite persistent hypotension. In the patient at risk, echocardiography is the most sensitive and specific modality to demonstrate pericardial fluid and need for operation. Pericardiocentesis as a diagnostic maneuver is not ideal because of the likelihood of inadvertent ventricular puncture causing a false-positive diagnosis, risk of significant iatrogenic injury, and the inability to withdraw clotted blood that has not yet lysed.

Septic Shock

Septic shock is the second most frequent cause of shock in the surgical patient. Invasive bacterial infection represents the most common cause of septic shock, with the most likely sites of infection being the lungs, abdomen, and urinary tract.

The pathophysiological alterations in septic shock are a result of the local and systemic response to bacteria and their products. Bacterial products stimulate the release of endothelial and macrophage-derived proinflammatory cytokines, the most potent of which are tumor necrosis factor-alpha (TNF-α) and IL-1. TNF-α and IL-1 may stimulate the release of IL-6 and IL-8 and other mediators, including thromboxanes, leukotrienes, platelet-activating factor, prostaglandins, complement, and nitric oxide (NO).

The inflammatory milieu induces several circulatory changes that impair tissue perfusion. First, myocardial depression is often evident despite an increase in cardiac index. Several factors contribute to cardiac dysfunction, including biventricular dilatation,[15] myocardial hyporesponsiveness to catecholamines,[16] and diastolic dysfunction.[17] Together, these phenomena result in a significant reduction in ejection fraction and a suboptimal response to volume infusion that persists for as long as 10 days.

The increase in cardiac index despite a reduction in myocardial contractility occurs as a result of a profound reduction in vasomotor tone, the principal cause of hypotension in septic shock. The reduction in venous tone leads to pooling in large capacitance vessels, effectively reducing circulating blood volume.

Several microcirculatory changes distinct from changes in vasomotor tone also play a role in the manifestations of septic shock. The mediator environment of sepsis results in activation of the coagulation cascade leading to microthrombus formation and marked decreases in deformability of neutrophils and erythrocytes, leading to capillary plugging.[18] This microvascular occlusive phenomenon induces the opening of arteriovenous shunts, effectively depriving tissues of adequate perfusion. Several proinflammatory mediators also increase neutrophil-endothelial adherence and subsequent extravasation of activated inflammatory cells into the interstitium where they induce tissue injury. Increased vascular permeability results in edema which effectively increases the diffusion distance required for cellular oxygen delivery and may, in concert with opening of arteriovenous shunts, induce cellular hypoxia.

Early manifestations of severe sepsis include tachypnea, tachycardia, oliguria, and changes in mental status. These clinical features may precede the onset of fever and leukocytosis, particularly in immunocompromised patients. Thus, these simple clinical features should be considered evidence of impending shock in those at risk.

Early, aggressive management is critical to minimizing the morbidity and mortality of septic shock. Because of the systemic vasodilation and increase in microvascular permeability, it is not unusual for patients to require large amounts of intravenous fluid to restore a normal blood pressure. Vasopressor support with dopamine, epinephrine, or norepinephrine may be necessary if there is an inadequate blood pressure response to fluid resuscitation. In patients not responding to fluid infusion or those with underlying cardiac or renal disease, the use of a pulmonary artery catheter is indicated.

During the resuscitation process, it is imperative that all

measures be taken to reverse the infectious process as expediently as possible. If the organism or site is unknown, treatment may require empiric broad-spectrum antimicrobial agents, based in part on known bacterial patterns in the institution, until further information is available. The correct choice of antibiotic or antibiotic combination is critical as there is a significantly higher case-fatality rate if inappropriate antimicrobials are administered.[19] If the infection source is an abscess or there is ongoing soiling of the pleural or peritoneal cavities, then either drainage or control of contamination is mandatory. Similarly, necrotic, infected tissue requires aggressive debridement.

Neurogenic Shock

Hypotension and bradycardia may occur following acute cervical or high thoracic spinal cord injury as a result of disruption of sympathetic outflow in conjunction with unopposed vagal tone. This constellation of clinical features is referred to as neurogenic shock, a syndrome that must be considered separately from the inappropriate term spinal shock, which refers to loss of spinal cord reflexes below the level of spinal cord injury. Any patient with a spinal cord injury above the level of L-1 is potentially at risk.

The diagnosis should be suspected in any patient with hypotension and bradycardia following injury. In some cases, these findings may represent the first suggestion of a spinal cord injury in a comatose patient. The patient with neurogenic shock is typically warm and well perfused. If a pulmonary artery catheter is in situ, the cardiac index may be elevated while the systemic vascular resistance is markedly reduced.[20] It is critical to remember that hemorrhage remains the most common cause of shock in patients with spinal cord injury. Thus, occult hemorrhage should be ruled out before attributing spinal cord injury as the exclusive cause of hypotension.

Hypoadrenal Shock

Shock secondary to adrenal insufficiency occurs quite infrequently and usually within the context of a concomitant critical illness. In North America, adrenal insufficiency most commonly arises as a consequence of the chronic therapeutic administration of high-dose exogenous corticosteroids with resultant suppression of the hypothalamic-pituitary-adrenal axis. Once the patient is severely stressed, typically following major infection, operation, or trauma, adrenocortical function may be insufficient to support the necessary physiological response and the clinical picture of shock due to adrenal insufficiency will become manifest.

Diagnosis of shock secondary to hypocortisolism requires a high level of suspicion. Findings associated with adrenal insufficiency include weakness, fatigue, anorexia, abdominal pain, fever, nausea, vomiting, and weight loss. If long standing (i.e., Addison's disease), there may be hyperpigmentation of the skin and mucous membranes. Hyponatremia, hypochloremia, and hyperkalemia are consistent with decreased mineralocorticoid activity. Adrenal insufficiency may also present acutely with fever, shock, and an acute abdomen. More typically, surgical patients with adrenal insufficiency present with refractory shock in the course of injury or ill-

ness. There may be no other findings other than the failure to respond to standard shock therapy.

The hemodynamic changes associated with acute adrenal insufficiency tend to occur in two predictable patterns. In the relatively hypovolemic patient, the appearance is one of cardiogenic shock with decreased preload, depressed myocardial contractility, and high systemic vascular resistance. By contrast, if the patient had been adequately volume resuscitated, the cardiac output is usually high with a low systemic vascular resistance. This latter shock state is particularly difficult to differentiate from sepsis because fever and leukocytosis are not unusual in patients with shock secondary to adrenal insufficiency. The diagnosis of acute adrenal insufficiency should therefore be suspected in patients with hemodynamic and clinical findings of septic shock whose infectious origin is not readily apparent. Plasma cortisol and corticotrophin levels should be obtained to assist in diagnosis.

Emergency treatment of hypoadrenal shock requires immediate treatment with high-dose hydrocortisone (100 mg intravenously every 8 h) with a rapid taper to an appropriate maintenance dose.

Diagnostic and Therapeutic Adjuncts in the Management of Shock

Pulmonary Artery Catheter

The differential diagnosis of the shock state is usually relatively straightforward. The clinical setting in conjunction with physical examination is often sufficient to guide diagnosis and therapy. However, occasionally the cause of the shock state is unclear, in which case hemodynamic parameters derived from a pulmonary artery catheter may provide valuable insight into the principal mechanism underlying the shock state (Table 9.3).

Resuscitative Thoracotomy

Resuscitative thoracotomy (also referred to as emergency room thoracotomy) represents an adjunctive measure to manage patients in extremis or profound shock following trauma. This approach involves performing a left anterolateral thoracotomy in the emergency room while the rest of the resuscitation team continues with managing the airway, intravenous access, and fluid resuscitation. After entry into the left chest, the pericardium is inspected for evidence of tamponade and a pericardiotomy performed to decompress the

TABLE 9.3. Differential Diagnosis of Shock States Based on Hemodynamic Parameters.

Type of shock	CVP or PCWP	Cardiac output	Systemic vascular resistance	Venous O$_2$ saturation
Hypovolemic	↓	↓	↑	↓
Cardiogenic	↑	↓	↑	↓
Septic	↓ ↑	↑	↓	↑
Traumatic	↓	↓ ↑	↓ ↑	↓
Neurogenic	↓	↓	↓	↓
Hypoadrenal	↓ ↑	↓ ↑	↑ ↓	↓

CVP, central venous pressure; PCWP, pulmonary capillary wedge pressure.

pericardial space and/or allow for open cardiac massage. Major pulmonary hemorrhage or hilar injury can be managed by cross-clamping the pulmonary hilum. The descending thoracic aorta can be occluded, thus optimizing perfusion to the coronary and cerebral circulation while limiting intraabdominal hemorrhage.

It is quite clear that survival is negligible in patients without signs of life in the prehospital phase of care.[21] Thus, resuscitative thoracotomy is recommended for patients with signs of life at the scene in patients with penetrating trauma and in blunt trauma patients who present with vital signs but decompensate in the emergency department.[22]

Inotropes

Management of shock requires manipulation of intravascular volume (preload), systemic vascular resistance (afterload), and myocardial contractility. Optimal volume resuscitation should precede pharmacological intervention. The use of inotropic agents should be considered when tissue perfusion remains inadequate despite adequate fluid administration.

DOPAMINE

Dopamine is an endogenous sympathetic amine that is a biosynthetic precursor of epinephrine which also functions as a central and peripheral neurotransmitter. At low doses (1–3 μg/kg/min) dopamine may increase renal blood flow and diuresis. At moderate doses (5 μg/kg/min), stimulation of cardiac β-receptors produces increases in contractility and cardiac output with little effect on heart rate or blood pressure. With increasing doses (5–10 μg/kg/min), β-adrenergic effects still predominate, but further increases in cardiac output are accompanied by increases in heart rate and blood pressure. At higher doses (more than 10 μg/kg/min), peripheral vasoconstriction from increasing α-activity becomes more prominent, resulting in elevation of systemic vascular resistance, blood pressure, and myocardial oxygen consumption.

DOBUTAMINE

Dobutamine is a synthetic catecholamine that has been used for its β-adrenergic effects and the absence of significant α-activity. The predominant effect is an increase in cardiac contractility with little increase in heart rate. Dobutamine also has a peripheral vasodilating effect resulting from β_2-receptor activation that is independent of any increase in cardiac output. The combination of increased contractility and reduction in afterload contribute to improved left-ventricular emptying and a reduction in pulmonary capillary wedge pressure. As a result of these properties, dobutamine is an ideal agent when the therapeutic goal is to improve cardiac output rather than to improve blood pressure.

NOREPINEPHRINE

The sympathetic neurotransmitter norepinephrine exerts both α- and β-adrenergic effects. The β-adrenergic effects are most prominent at lower infusion rates, leading to increases in heart rate and contractility. With increasing doses, the α-mediated effects become evident and are responsible for increases in systemic vascular resistance and blood pressure. Norepinephrine is used mainly in patients with hypotension refractory to volume resuscitation and other inotropic agents.

EPINEPHRINE

Epinephrine has a broad spectrum of systemic actions. At lower rates of infusion, β-adrenergic responses predominate, leading to an increase in heart rate and contractility (β_1 effect) in conjunction with peripheral vasodilation (β_2 effect). These effects result in an increase in stroke volume and cardiac output with a variable effect on blood pressure. At a higher rate of infusion, α effects predominate, leading to an increase in systemic vascular resistance and blood pressure.

AMRINONE

Amrinone is a synthetic bipyridine with inotropic and vasodilator effects. Its principal mechanism of action involves phosphodiesterase inhibition, through which it raises the intracellular concentration of cyclic AMP. It appears to be a useful agent in cardiogenic shock complicating myocardial infarction as it may significantly increase cardiac contractility and cardiac output without increasing myocardial oxygen requirement due to concomitant vasodilation and afterload reduction. Drawbacks to the use of amrinone are the variability of the individual response, its relatively long half-life (3.6 h), and the potential for acute significant hypotension if intravascular volume is inadequate. In addition, its use is not infrequently accompanied by the development of thrombocytopenia.

Complications of Shock and Resuscitation

Multiple Organ Dysfunction Syndrome

The syndrome associated with multiple organ dysfunction (MODS) has evolved only recently as a result of advances in our ability to salvage patients who would have otherwise died as a result of their shock state. Shock in all its forms represents the most common predisposing factor leading to the development of MODS. There is no specific treatment for MODS. Efforts should be directed toward minimizing the duration of shock and rapidly ensuring adequate organ perfusion.

Immunosuppression

In a large series of trauma patients with hemorrhagic shock, almost 40% of patients surviving the first 24 h developed infectious complications.[4] The mechanism of the apparent immunosuppression is unclear. It may be related to allogeneic blood transfusion and/or to the marked depression of both macrophage and lymphocytic functional capacities that has been observed following hemorrhagic shock.

Hypothermia

Hypothermia invokes a variety of systemic responses, including a reduction in heart rate and cardiac output, while temperatures below 32°C may induce supraventricular or ventricular arrhythmias.[23] Most importantly, at temperatures less than 35°C hypothermia induces a coagulopathy due to effects on both coagulation factors and platelet function. The combination of coagulopathy and hypothermia produces a vicious cycle; the coagulopathy leads to more blood loss, requiring more replacement with cool fluids or blood products, leading to further hypothermia and aggravation of the coagulopathy.

Prevention of hypothermia should be considered in all patients with shock. Methods to achieve this include the use of fluid warmers, warming blankets, warmed ventilator circuits, and continous arteriovenous rewarming.

Abdominal Compartment Syndrome

The abdominal compartment syndrome (ACS) is a sequela of massive resuscitation following shock or visceral ischemia. Aggressive fluid resuscitation in concert with alterations in microvascular permeability result in marked visceral edema. Similarly, increasing soft tissue edema results in a reduction in abdominal wall compliance. The combination of an increase in the volume of intraabdominal contents in concert with a stiff abdominal wall significantly increases the pressure in the abdominal cavity.

A progressive increase in intraabdominal pressure produces a graded decrease in cardiac output, an effect mediated by a reduction in venous return and an increase in systemic vascular resistance due to caval compression and mechanical compression of capillary beds, respectively.[24] Left and right atrial filling pressures obtained using a pulmonary artery catheter may be spuriously elevated because of the increase in intrathoracic pressure.[25]

Passive elevation of the diaphragm allows the transmission of high intraabdominal pressure into the pleural cavity, reducing both static and dynamic lung compliance.[25,26] This reduction in compliance results in the need for very high inspiratory airway pressures to maintain effective ventilation. Intraabdominal hypertension may also result in significant increases in intracranial pressure due to impaired cerebral venous outflow secondary to an increase in intrathoracic pressure.[27,28]

Diagnosis of the abdominal compartment syndrome requires recognizing the clinical syndrome and, ultimately, some objective measurement of intraabdominal pressure. The classic clinical clues to the presence of ACS are (1) a tense or distended abdomen, (2) massive intravenous fluid requirements, (3) elevated central venous and pulmonary capillary wedge pressures, (4) decreased cardiac output, (5) elevated peak airway pressures, and (6) oliguria.

Physical exam is unreliable, however, and objective measurement of intraabdominal pressure (IAP) may be required.

The most widely used method of measuring IAP involves transurethral measurement of urinary bladder pressure using a Foley catheter.[29,30] In the supine position the normal intraabdominal pressure is less than 10 mmHg. Following abdominal surgery, pressures are typically in the range of 3 to 15 mmHg.[29] Treatment should be considered if intraabdominal pressures exceed 25 to 30 mmHg.[30,31] Optimally, management involves either reopening a prior laparotomy incision or, in patients without a recent laparotomy, opening the peritoneal cavity via a midline incision. Some form of temporary abdominal closure is then necessary to bridge the fascial defect and prevent evisceration. There are no studies demonstrating a survival benefit with decompressive celiotomy.

References

1. Rangel-Frausto MS, Pittet D, Costigan M, Hwang T, Davis CS, Wenzel RP. The natural history of the systemic inflammatory response syndrome. JAMA 1995;273:117–123.

2. Muckart DJJ, Bhagwanjee S. American College of Chest Physicians/Society of Critical Care Medicine consensus conference definitions of the systemic inflammatory response syndrome and allied disorders in relation to critically injured patients. Crit Care Med 1997;25:1789–1795.

3. American College of Chest Physicians—Society of Critical Care Medicine Consensus Conference. Definitions for sepsis and organ failure and guidelines for the use of innovative therapies in sepsis. Crit Care Med 1992;20:864–875.

4. Heckbert SR, Vedder NB, Hoffman W, et al. Outcome after hemorrhagic shock in trauma patients. J Trauma 1998;45:545–549.

5. Stump DC, Strauss RG, Henriksen RA, et al. Effects of hydroxyethyl starch on blood coagulation, particularly factor VIII. Transfusion 1985;25:349.

6. Jacobs LM, Hsieh JW. A clinical review of autotransfusion and its role in trauma. JAMA 1984;251:3283.

7. Huth JF, Maier RV, Pavlin EG, et al. Utilization of blood recycling in nonelective surgery. Arch Surg 1983;118:626–629.

8. Jurkovich GJ, Moore EE, Mediana G. Autotransfusion in trauma: a pragmatic analysis. Am J Surg 1984;148:782.

9. Gould SA, Moss GS. Clinical development of human polymerized hemoglobin as a blood substitute. World J Surg 1996;20:1200–1207.

10. Broos PL, Stappaerts KH, Luite EJ, Gruwez JA. The importance of early internal fixation in multiply injured patients to prevent late deaths and sepsis. Injury 1987;18:235–237.

11. Lozman J, Deno DC, Feustel PJ, et al. Pulmonary and cardiovascular consequences of immediate fixation or conservative management of long-bone fractures. Arch Surg 1986;121:992–999.

12. Kinch JW, Ryan TJ. Right ventricular infarction. N Engl J Med 1994;330:1211–1217.

13. Moscucci M, Bates ER. Cardiogenic shock. Cardiol Clin 1995;13:391–406.

14. Freed PS, Wasfre T, Zado B, Kentrowitz A. Intraaortic balloon pumping for prolonged circulatory support. Am J Cardiol 1988;61:554.

15. Parker MM, Shelhamer JH, Bacharach SL, et al. Profound but reversible myocardial depression in patients with septic shock. Ann Intern Med 1984;100:483–490.

16. Silverman HJ, Penaranda R, Orens JB, Lee NH. Impaired beta-adrenergic receptor stimulation of cyclic adenosine monophosphate in human septic shock: association with myocardial hyporesponsiveness to catecholamines. Crit Care Med 1993;21:31–39.

17. Jafri SM, Lavine S, Field BE, Bahorozian MT, Carlson RW. Left ventricular diastolic function in sepsis. Crit Care Med 1990;18:709–713.

18. Hinshaw LB. Sepsis/septic shock: participation of the microcirculation: an abbreviated review. Crit Care Med 1996;24:1072–1078.

19. Leibovici L, Drucker M, Konigsberger H, et al. Septic shock in bacteremic patients: risk factors, features and prognosis. Scand J Infect Dis 1997;29:71–75.

20. Levi L, Wolf A, Belzberg H. Hemodynamic parameters in patients with acute cervical cord trauma: description, intervention, and prediction of outcome. Neurosurgery (Baltim) 1993;33:1007–1017.

21. Ivatury RR, Kazigo J, Rohman M, Gaudino J, Simon R, Stahl WM. "Directed" emergency room thoracotomy: a prognostic prerequisite for survival. J Trauma 1991;31:1076–1081.

22. Boyd M, Vanek VW, Bourguet CC. Emergency room resuscitative thoracotomy? when is it indicated. J Trauma 1992;33:714–721.

23. Paton BC. Cardiac function during accidental hypothermia. In: Pozos RE, Wittmer LE, eds. The Nature and Treatment of Hypothermia. Minneapolis: University of Minnesota Press, 1983:133–142.

24. Ivatury RR, Diebel L, Porter JM, Simon RJ. Intra-abdominal hy-

pertension and the abdominal compartment syndrome. Surg Clin North Am 1997;77:783–800.

25. Cullen DJ, Coyle JP, Teplick R, Long MC. Cardiovascular, pulmonary, and renal effects of massively increased intra-abdominal pressure in critically ill patients. Crit Care Med 1989;17:118–121.

26. Meldrum DR, Moore FA, Moore EE, Haenel JB, Cosgriff N, Burch JM. Cardiopulmonary hazards of perihepatic packing for major liver injuries. Am J Surg 1995;170:537–542.

27. Bloomfield GL, Ridings PC, Blocher CR, Marmarou A, Sugerman HJ. A proposed relationship between increased intra-abdominal, intrathoracic and intracranial pressure. Crit Care Med 1997;25:496–503.

28. Bloomfield GL, Ridings PC, Blocher CR, Marmarou A, Suger-

man H. Effects of increased intra-abdominal pressure upon intracranial and cerebral perfusion pressure before and after volume expansion. J Trauma 1996;40:936–943.

29. Kron IL, Harman PK, Nolan SP. The measurement of intra-abdominal pressure as a criterion for abdominal re-exploration. Ann Surg 1984;199:28–30.

30. Iberti TJ, Kelly KM, Gentili DR, Hirsch S, Benjamin E. A simple technique to accurately determine intra-abdominal pressure. Crit Care Med 1987;15:1140–1142.

31. Burch JM, Moore EE, Moore FA, Franciose R. The abdominal compartment syndrome. Surg Clin North Am 1996;76:833–842.

32. Meldrum DR, Moore FA, Moore EE, Franciose RJ, Sauia A, Burch JM. Prospective characterization and selective management of the abdominal compartment syndrome. Am J Surg 1997;174:667–672.

Critical Care: A System-Oriented Approach

J. Perren Cobb

Neurological Dysfunction

Etiology and Diagnosis

Brain dysfunction presents as an alteration in mental function (altered mental status) that spans the spectrum from delirium to coma. The most common manifestations are disorientation and agitation, characterized by disorganized thinking, deficits in short-term memory, and auditory hallucinations. The etiology is usually listed as multifactorial (potential contributing factors are listed in Table 10.1). Establishing a diagnosis is difficult (often made by exclusion) and requires a careful history and focused neurological examination.[1] Computed tomography of the head to establish an anatomical abnormality is indicated in patients with focal neurological findings, in patients at risk for stroke or intracranial hemorrhage, or in those with a history of trauma. Lumbar puncture to obtain cerebral spinal fluid should be reserved for patients with a history and physical exam suggestive of meningitis.

Treatment

It is helpful to objectively document neurological status with a simple scoring system. One example is the modified Ramsay sedation scale (Table 10.2).[2] Regular use of this scale minimizes interobserver variance and facilitates communication regarding neurological status and titration of sedatives.

The treatment of brain dysfunction is supportive. Anxiolytics, typically benzodiazepines given intravenously, are used to treat agitation. In a randomized, prospective multicenter study comparing intermittent i.v. lorazepam to continuous i.v. midazolam,[3] the two agents were found to be equally safe and effective and without significant differences in their effects on hemodynamic profiles. A prospective, randomized, multicenter trial found that an infusion of continuous i.v. propofol was equally safe and effective but had a significantly shorter duration of action when compared to continuous i.v. midazolam.[4] As neither benzodiazepines nor propofol offer analgesia, the additional use of a narcotic (morphine or fentanyl) is particularly helpful in those patients experiencing postoperative pain or discomfort from invasive devices (e.g., an endotracheal tube). Another type of agent used to treat agitation is i.v. haloperidol, especially in combination with benzodiazepines, for the treatment of delirium, hypervigilance, and paranoia ("ICU psychosis").[5]

Prognosis

The prognosis for brain dysfunction in the critically ill is usually excellent. In the absence of acquired anatomical abnormalities (e.g., stroke or trauma), the mental status changes associated with critical illness almost always improve as MODS resolves and neuroactive drugs are discontinued.

Cardiovascular Dysfunction

Etiology and Diagnosis

Failure of the cardiovascular system presents as hypotension, variably defined. Widely accepted criteria include systolic blood pressure (SBP) less than 90 mmHg or mean arterial blood pressure (MAP) less than 60 mmHg. The pathophysiology of hypotension can be easily understood by analyzing the determinants of blood pressure. If Ohm's law, pressure = flow × resistance, is applied to blood flow, one approximation is

$$MAP \approx CO \times SVR$$

That is, MAP is proportional to cardiac output (CO) and some measure of systemic vascular resistance (SVR). As CO is determined by heart rate (HR) and stroke volume (SV), then

$$MAP \approx HR \times SV \times SVR$$

TABLE 10.1. Etiology of Brain Dysfunction in the ICU.

Neuroactive drugs (H$_2$-blockers, acyclovir)

Neurotoxin accumulation secondary to renal dysfunction

Hepatic encephalopathy

Septic encephalopathy

Ethanol or drug (benzodiazepine) withdrawal

Catecholamine excess associated with the neurohumoral response to stress

"Sundowning" (nighttime psychomotor agitation)

Cerebrovascular event (stroke)

Meningitis

As SV is determined by myocardial preload, afterload, and contractility, then

$$MAP \approx HR \times preload \times afterload \times contractility$$

In other words, MAP is proportional to heart rate and some measure of myocardial preload, afterload, and contractility. The conclusion is that hypotension can only result from a decrease in one of these four determinants: heart rate, preload, afterload, or contractility.

The clinical (bedside) assessment of patients who present with shock is notoriously unreliable. Of the four determinants of blood pressure—preload, afterload, contractility, and heart rate—only the latter can be determined at the bedside with a reliable degree of accuracy.

Because of ambiguities and the critically ill, unstable nature of patients in shock, hemodynamic data obtained from invasive indwelling monitors can be particularly useful, both diagnostically and therapeutically (Chapter 17). Indwelling arterial catheters permit continuous real-time measurement of systemic arterial pressures and easy access to the arterial circulation for blood gas measurements. Venous catheters placed in a central vein permit assessment of central venous and right atrial pressures, two measures of right-ventricular preload. The balloon-tipped, thermodilution pulmonary artery (PA) catheter provides access to mixed venous blood, permits an estimation of left ventricular preload in the "wedged" position, and provides data allowing the clinician to estimate right- and left-ventricular contractility (cardiac index, stroke volume, right ventricular ejection fraction). Cardiac rhythm, conduction, and perfusion abnormalities are assessed routinely on a 12-lead ECG tracing. Transthoracic and, more re-

TABLE 10.2. Modified Ramsay Sedation Scale.

Level	Findings
1	Awake, anxious, agitated, or restless
2	Awake, cooperative, oriented, and tranquil
3	Awake, responds to commands only
4	Asleep or drowsy, responds to loud auditory stimulus or light glabellar tap
5	Asleep, unresponsive to loud auditory stimulus or glabellar tap, but responds when prodded
6	Asleep, unresponsive to loud auditory stimulus, glabellar tap, or prodding
UTO	Chemically paralyzed

cently, transesophageal echocardiography can be used to determine valvular and regional myocardial function and an estimation of filling pressures in patients with evidence of primary heart dysfunction or endocarditis.

Treatment

The goals of pharmacological therapy for shock mirror those of the endogenous response to stress, that is, optimization of myocardial preload, contractility, afterload, and heart rate.

As the most frequent etiology of shock in the perioperative period is hypovolemic or septic shock, administration of i.v. fluids to increase preload is a safe, logical first step. The goal is to "load" the ventricles to optimize stroke volume and thereby cardiac output (Starling relationship); this can be attained typically by increasing filling pressures to 12 to 18 mmHg. The usual initial bolus dose of i.v. fluids (IVF) is 10 to 20 ml/kg. Both crystalloid and colloid (hetastarch, albumin) solutions are effective, but balanced salt solutions are the most cost-effective initial choice because of their low cost and physiological concentrations of salts (large volumes can be infused with minimal changes in serum electrolytes).[6] Infusion of blood products is reserved for specific therapy of anemia or coagulopathy (see Chapter 10).

Once preload has been optimized, distributive forms of shock are treated with agents that increase afterload (Table 10.3). Doses of the alpha-adrenergic receptor agonists norepinephrine, epinephrine, phenylephrine, or dopamine are titrated to maintain blood pressure at an arbitrary level, typically a mean arterial pressure (MAP) of 60 to 65 mmHg.

For shock secondary to myocardial failure, a number of pharmacological agents are available to increase cardiac contractility (see Table 10.3). The drugs used most commonly are dobutamine, dopamine, and phosphodiesterase inhibitors such as amrinone.

A heart rate of approximately 90 bpm is regarded as optimal in patients with shock. Lower heart rates decrease oxygen demand (thereby protecting the myocardium) but do so at the expense of cardiac output. Dopamine and dobutamine can be titrated to increase heart rate and cardiac index; atropine and isoproteronol are used in the setting of bradycardiac emergencies. When preload is adequate, heart rates higher than 90 bpm may increase cardiac index but also increase oxygen demand and the possibility of myocardial ischemia. Heart rates greater than approximately 140 bpm in adults are associated with inadequate diastolic filling and resultant decreased cardiac index.

Historically, resuscitation endpoints have include normalization of vital signs and indicators of organ perfusion (resolution of oliguria, hyperlactatemia, and acidemia). Other endpoints such as supranormal oxygen activity, subcutaneous tissue oximetry, and gastric tonometry remain controversial or investigational.

Prognosis

Shock, especially refractory shock requiring vasopressor therapy, is a robust predictor of increased mortality. Persistent hyperlactatemia is also accurate,[7,8] suggesting that prolonged tissue hypoperfusion may play a role in determining outcome.

TABLE 10.3. Vasoactive Drugs and Receptor Activities for the Treatment of Shock.

Class and drug	Blood pressure	Systemic vascular resistance	Cardiac output	Heart rate	Isotrope Low-dose	Isotrope High-dose	Renal blood flow	Coronary blood flow	MvO$_2$
Alpha only									
Phenylephrine	↑↑↑	↑↑↑↑	↓↓↓	↓↓↓	±	±	↓↓↓↓	±↑↑	↑
Alpha and beta									
Norepinephrine	↑↑	↑↑↑	↓↓	↓↓±	↑	↑	↓↓↓↓	↑↑	↑↑
Epinephrine	↑±	↑±	↑↑	↑↑↑	↑	↑↑↑	↓±	↑↑	↑↑↑
Dopamine	↑↑	↑↑	↑↑	↑	±	↑↑	↑↑↑	↑↑	↑↑
Beta only									
Isoproterenol	↑±	↓↓	↑↑↑↑	↑↑↑↑	↑↑↑	↑↑↑↑	±	↑↑↑	↑↑↑↑
Dobutamine	↓↓	↓↓↓	↑↑↑	↑↑	↑↑↑	↑↑↑	±	↑↑↑	↑↑↑
Beta-blocker									
Propanolol	+↓	±	↓↓↓	↓↓↓↓	↓↓	↓↓↓	↓	↓↓	↓↓↓
Metoprolol	↓↓↓	↓	↓↓	↓↓↓	↓↓	↓↓↓	±	↓↓	↓↓
Other									
Nitroglycerine	±↓	↓↓	↑↑	±	±	±	±↑	↓	↓↓
Hydralazine	↓↓↓	↓↓↓	↑↑	↑↑	±	±	±↑	↓	↓↓
Prazosin	↓↓↓	↓↓	↑↑	±	±	±	±↑	↓	↓↓
Nitroprusside	↓↓	↓↓↓	↑↑↑	±↑	±	±	↑↑	±	↓↓

Source: T.W. Pettitt and J.P. Cobb. Critical care. In: The Washington Manual of Surgery, edited by G.M. Doherty, D.S. Bauman, L.L. Creswell, J.A. Goss, and T.C. Lairmore. Philadelphia: Lippincott-Williams & Wilkins, 1996:166 with permission.

Pulmonary Dysfunction

Definitions

The patient with respiratory (pulmonary) insufficiency is able to compensate, through increased minute ventilation, for pulmonary dysfunction (normal minute ventilation is approximately 60–80 ml/kg/min). Respiratory failure describes the patient who requires exogenous support (mechanical ventilation) because increased ventilatory requirements outstrip their ability to compensate (minute ventilation typically in excess of 150 ml/kg/min). A consensus conference of investigators in Europe and America identified two grades of respiratory failure secondary to injury: acute lung injury (ALI) and acute respiratory distress syndrome (ARDS, previously known as adult respiratory distress syndrome).[9]

Etiology and Pathophysiology

Pulmonary insufficiency results from impaired diffusion of oxygen or carbon dioxide at the alveolar–capillary (respiratory) interface. Although there are myriad causes (Table 10.4), the underlying adaptive response is similar. Worsening diffusion at the respiratory interface decreases the efficiency of alveolar ventilation, and hypoxia or hypercapnia ensue. As a consequence, respiratory drive increases, manifested clinically as tachypnea and dyspnea. This condition is often exacerbated by decreased pulmonary compliance, a consequence of disease-induced decreased lung elasticity and surfactant production. So long as the increased work of breathing can be met, pulmonary insufficiency remains compensated. As the degree of respiratory efficiency worsens or the patient tires, compensated respiratory insufficiency evolves into uncompensated insufficiency and frank respiratory failure. Therapy is aimed at reversing hypoxemia by increasing the fraction of inspired oxygen (F$_i$O$_2$) or supporting the work of breathing by initiating mechanical ventilation.

Diagnosis

The signs and symptoms of respiratory insufficiency include dyspnea, tachypnea, cyanosis, and use of accessory respiratory muscles. Blood gases and oximetry typically indicate relative hypoxemia (oxyhemoglobin saturation of 90%–92%) concomitant with respiratory alkalosis. As compensatory efforts fail with progressive hypoxemia and hypercapnia, respiratory efforts weaken and an agonal (gasping) respiratory pattern is observed; this is manifested by profound hypoxemia and respiratory acidosis. Respiratory failure due to interstitial or alveolar disease (see Table 10.4) is accompanied by infiltrates seen on plain chest radiographs. The differential of pulmonary infiltrates includes increased lung water secondary to transudate (e.g., congestive heart failure), exudate (e.g., acute lung injury or ARDS), pus (e.g., pneumonia), blood (e.g., intraparenchymal hemorrhage), or gastric fluid (e.g., aspiration).

TABLE 10.4. Common Causes of Respiratory Insufficiency and Failure.

Inadequate ventilation
  Airway obstruction
  Atelectasis
  Reactive airway disease (e.g., asthma)
  Drug overdose
  Nerve injury (e.g., spinal cord, phrenic nerve)
  Respiratory muscle weakness (e.g., Guillian–Barre syndrome)

Inadequate perfusion
  Pulmonary embolism
  Right-to-left cardiac shunt

Inadequate ventilation and perfusion
  Chronic obstructive pulmonary disease (COPD)
  Adult respiratory distress syndrome (ARDS)
  Pneumonia
  Pulmonary venous hypertension (e.g., congestive heart failure)
  Tension pneumothorax

Treatment

The goal of supportive therapy for acute respiratory failure is to improve gas exchange while allowing the lungs to heal. Several devices are available to increase (supplement) F_iO_2, ranging from nasal cannula (F_iO_2, 0.24–0.30) to reservoir masks (F_iO_2, 0.80–1.0). Short-term (<24-h) mechanical support can be provided noninvasively (i.e., without use of an endotracheal airway) using a bag-mask apparatus or a nasal mask connected to a small, specialized ventilator (bilevel positive airway pressure, BiPAP®).

The mainstay of ventilatory support is invasive ventilation through an entodotracheal tube placed via the nose, mouth, or neck (tracheostomy). "Conventional" modes of ventilation are compared in Table 10.5 and depicted graphically in Fig. 10.1.

INITIATING VENTILATOR SUPPORT

Because volume-limited modes are used most commonly, the first order is to determine the size of V_T. The goal is to optimize lung expansion (thus decreasing the risk of atelectasis) while minimizing the risk of barotrauma. Current opinion suggests that a V_T that creates a peak inspiratory pressure (PIP) of 20 to 25 cm H_2O is ideal; this is typically produced by a V_T of 5 to 8 ml/kg body weight.[10,11] PEEP is used also to prevent atelectasis; it is typically set at 5 cm H_2O ("physiological" PEEP). The ventilator rate is then set to deliver a minute ventilation ($V_E = V_T \times$ rate) that keeps the P_aCO_2 normal (35–45 mmHg). The F_iO_2 is titrated down from 1.0 to 0.4 to keep the S_aO_2 greater than or equal to 92% to 95%.[12]

OPTIONS FOR SEVERE RESPIRATORY FAILURE

Collapsed lung units characteristic of severe lung injury and ARDS can be recruited to improve alveolar ventilation by increasing PEEP as needed up to 15 to 20 cm H_2O.[13] As the condition of the lungs deteriorates and pulmonary compliance decreases, the PIP for a typical 5 to 7 ml/kg V_T may reach a level (>60 cm H_2O) consistent with severe barotrauma (e.g., tension pneumothoraces). In these instances, resistance to gas flow can be minimized by relief of increased intraabdominal pressure if present (see abdominal compartment syndrome) and the use of sedatives and muscle relaxants. Pressure-limited ventilator modes (e.g., pressure control ventilation) may be useful in these instances because they allow the clinician to limit (control) the PIP and thereby minimize the risk of barotrauma. Other potential ventilator manipulations are listed in Table 10.6.

DISCONTINUATION OF MECHANICAL VENTILATION

Several strategies for discontinuation of ventilation ("weaning" the patient off the ventilator) have been compared recently. The time-honored approach consists of gradually decreasing the minute ventilation supported by or initiated by the machine, allowing the patient to supply the difference. This strategy is aimed at strengthening the respiratory muscles that are presumably made weak by disease or by days to weeks of ventilator support. The tactic usually involves switching the patient to a mode that combines IMV plus PSV, and then decreasing the rate of machine-initiated breaths while supporting patient-initiated breaths with enough pressure to generate adequate V_T. This strategy of weaning is frequently operated most efficiently by protocol.[14] The results of

prospective, randomized controlled clinical trials, however, do not support the concept that the diaphragm needs conditioning or strengthening during prolonged mechanical ventilation. Instead, it appears that more or less complete support with prompt recognition of the absence of respiratory failure by a once-daily trial of spontaneous breathing (T-piece trial) is significantly better than traditional IMV weaning.[15,16] The most important part of weaning, therefore, may be simply recognizing when the patient is capable of unassisted breathing.

EXTUBATION

Currently, the ratio of respiratory frequency to $V_T/(f/V_T)$ is regarded as a reliable indicator of successful extubation, based upon a prospective, blinded comparative trial of extubation criteria in critically ill medical patients that indicated a sensitivity of 81% and a specificity of 89% for an f/V_T less than 80.[17,18] Patients who are unsuccessfully extubated, especially if prolonged respiratory insufficiency is anticipated, may benefit from tracheostomy.

Prognosis

The outcome for patients with severe respiratory failure and ARDS has improved over the last decade. Abnormalities of gas exchange may persist long term, but lung mechanics in survivors return to normal values within 1 year of hospital discharge.[10]

Gastrointestinal Dysfunction

Nutrition

Most experimental models indicate that perfusion to the intestinal tract decreases as a result of the adaptive response to severe injury and that intestinal secretions and motility decrease. This change is manifested clinically as intestinal ileus and food intolerance. Loss of mucosal integrity can be demonstrated endoscopically, the result of intestinal villus and epithelial cell loss.

Gastrointestinal Hemorrhage

As a result of loss of intestinal mucosal integrity, critically ill patients are at increased risk for GI hemorrhage, particularly those who are coagulopathic and require mechanical ventilation. Strong data exist to support the use of drugs to maintain gastric and duodenal mucosal integrity in patients at risk. The best available evidence supports the use of H_2-blockers (ranitidine) in critically ill patients with respiratory failure requiring mechanical ventilation for more than 48 h or in those with coagulopathy.[19]

Renal Dysfunction

Definitions and Pathophysiology

The kidney resorbs more than 99% of the plasma filtered by the glomerulus (normally about 120 ml/min or 7.2 l/h). This matching of glomerular filtration and tubular resorption is

TABLE 10.5. "Conventional" Ventilator Modes.

Mode	Description	Advantages	Disadvantages	Uses
A. Volume-limited	Set tidal volume; peak inspiratory pressure varies	Ensures adequate tidal volume	Barotrauma in those with very poor lung compliance	
1. Assist/control (A/C)	Both spontaneous (patient-initiated, "assisted") and ("controlled") breaths have same tidal volume	Minimal work of breathing	Easy for patient to hyperventilate, Makes assessment of ventilatory muscle strength difficult to evaluate	Weak, heavily sedated, or paralyzed
2. Intermittent mandatory ventilation (IMV)	Tidal volume of machine-initiated ("mandatory") breaths set; no ventilator support for spontaneous breaths	Allows gradual decrease of support by decreasing rate of mandatory breaths	No support for spontaneous breaths	Often used in combination with PSV for weaning
B. Pressure-limited	Set peak inspiratory pressure; tidal volume varies	Decreased risk of barotrauma	Does not ensure tidal volume	
1. Pressure control ventilation (PCV)	Inspiratory pressure and rate set	Inverse ratio ventilation (IRV); increased alveolar "recruitment"	Requires heavy sedation and/or paralytics	Patients with very poor lung compliance
2. Pressure support ventilation (PSV)	Inspiratory pressure set; no rate	Most comfortable of the conventional modes	Increased risk of hypoventilation	Awake patients; often used in combination with IMV for weaning

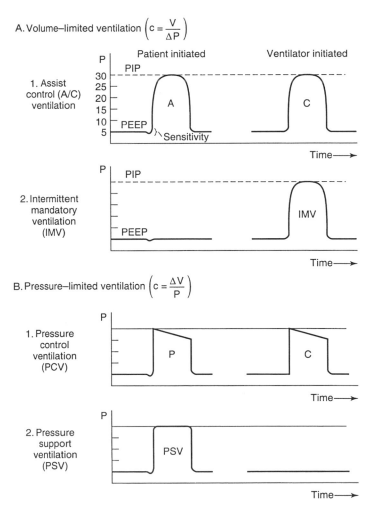

FIGURE 10.1. Conventional ventilator modes. Shown *above* are the pressure versus time graphs for the four most common modes. The curves are divided into two general groups, based upon whether the tidal volume (V_T) or peak inspiratory pressure (PIP) is set (volume-limited and pressure-limited modes, respectively). For volume-limited modes (A), the V_T is set and the PIP varies from breath to breath. For pressure-limited modes, the PIP is set and the V_T varies. The four curves on the *left* correspond to typical patient-initiated breaths and those on the *right* to machine-initiated breaths. Inspiration for each of the eight breaths shown begins at 5 cm H_2O PEEP (peak end-expiratory pressure). During patient-initiated breaths, the pressure drops in the circuit as the ventilatory muscle contract; this change in pressure is calibrated (the "sensitivity") to trigger opening of the inspiratory valve on the ventilator. Thereafter, pressure increases until the V_T is delivered (for volume-limited modes) or the PIP is reached (for pressure-limited modes). The pressure in the circuit decreases when the inspiratory valve closes and the expiratory valve opens, allowing passive exhalation (triggered in pressure limited modes by a predetermined threshold decrease in inspiratory flow). Note that the patient-initiated and ventilator-initiated curves are similar during A/C and PCV, resulting in a low work of breathing (useful for ventilating heavily sedated patients or those with weak respiratory efforts). On the other hand, intermittent mandatory ventilation (IMV) provides no inspiratory support for patient-initiated breaths, while pressure support ventilation (PSV) has no set respiratory rate to provide machine-initiated backup should the patient stop making respiratory efforts. The most commonly used mode is a combination IMV plus PSV.

A. Volume–limited ventilation $\left(c = \dfrac{V}{\Delta P}\right)$

1. Assist control (A/C) ventilation

Patient initiated   Ventilator initiated

P
30
25
20
15
10
5

PIP
PEEP
Sensitivity
A
C
Time →

2. Intermittent mandatory ventilation (IMV)

P   PIP
PEEP
IMV
Time →

B. Pressure–limited ventilation $\left(c = \dfrac{\Delta V}{P}\right)$

1. Pressure control ventilation (PCV)

P
P
C
Time →

2. Pressure support ventilation (PSV)

P
PSV
Time →

TABLE 10.6. Options for Support of Severe Respiratory Failure.

Increase extrinsic PEEP
Increase MAWP using PCV
Create intrinsic PEEP using IRV
Inhaled nitric oxide
"Open lung" approach
Oscillatory ventilation
Permissive hypercapnia
Prone positioning
Partial liquid ventilation
ECMO

PEEP, positive end-expiratory pressure; MAWP, mean airway pressure; PCV, pressure control ventilation; IRV, inverse ratio ventilation; ECMO, extracorporeal membrane oxygenators.

essential to maintenance of normal fluid balance. If this did not occur, for example, then decreased resorption in the face of normal filtration would very quickly result in profound hypovolemia and shock. The most common presentation of renal dysfunction is decreased urine output (oliguria), usually accompanied by increased levels of compounds cleared by the kidney, that is, blood urea nitrogen (BUN) and serum creatinine (Cr). Anuria is defined as urine output less than 100 ml/day and requires renal replacement therapy (approximately 5% of all ICU admissions). Renal dysfunction can also present as polyuria when decreased fluid resorption is not coupled with decreased glomerular filtration (high-output renal dysfunction). When renal insufficiency progresses to the point that renal replacement therapy is indicated, the term renal failure is used.

Etiology and Diagnosis

Traditionally, the etiology of renal failure has been divided into three categories: prerenal, intrarenal, and postrenal causes.[20] A careful history and review of the medical record are essential to making the correct diagnosis. Prerenal renal failure is a common cause (40%–70%) of renal insufficiency in the ICU, frequently as a result of perioperative hypovolemia, hypotension, decreased cardiac output, or intraoperative vascular manipulation (e.g., placement of a suprarenal aortic cross-clamp). The rise in BUN is typically greater than the rise in the serum creatinine, and the ratio of BUN to Cr is greater than 20. The tubular concentrating ability of the nephrons is normal and thus the urine osmolality and fractional excretion of sodium remain normal (>500 mOsm and $FE_{Na} > 1$, respectively).

Intrarenal failure is caused by tubular injury resulting from ischemia or toxins. Nephrotoxins frequently encountered by surgical ICU patients include aminoglycoside antibiotics, i.v. radiocontrast agents, amphotericin, chemotherapeutic drugs (e.g., cisplatin), and myoglobin. Patients with preexisting renal disease or with diabetes are particularly vulnerable. Because the ability of the tubules to concentrate is compromised, urine osmolality is typically low (<350 mOsm) and the FE_{Na} is greater than 1.

Postrenal dysfunction is caused by tubular pressure-induced injury secondary to obstruction of flow, which may be caused by direct intraoperative injury or manipulation, prostate disease (hypertrophy or cancer), clot in the urinary system, or extrinsic compression from pelvic tumors (e.g., cervical cancer). Urinary catheter obstruction must always be ruled out, typically by flushing and aspirating the catheter with a sterile saline to confirm the absence of resistance to flow. Ultrasound examination of the urinary system can be used to rule out hydronephrosis as a consequence of distal urinary obstruction.

Abdominal Compartment Syndrome

Increased intraabdominal pressure results from massive tissue or bowel edema within the abdominal compartment, frequently but not always accompanied by abdominal packing and retroperitoneal hemorrhage as a complication of severe trauma. Intraabdominal hypertension (pressure >20 cm H_2O) progressively decreases renal perfusion while retarding renal venous and urinary outflow, thereby inducing renal injury by a poorly understood combination of pre-, intra-, and postrenal insults. Assessment of urinary bladder pressure via an indwelling (Foley) catheter serves as an indirect but accurate measure of intraabdominal pressure.[21] Pressures greater than 25 cm H_2O demand intervention, typically release of pressure by reexploration of the abdomen, evacuation of blood clots, removal of abdominal packs, and closure of the abdomen with absorbable mesh. The kidneys usually respond to the relief of intraabdominal hypertension with a brisk diuresis.

Treatment

The initial therapy of renal dysfunction is supportive, aimed at minimizing ongoing injury by optimizing perfusion and discontinuing potentially nephrotoxic agents. Measurement of left- or right-sided cardiac filling pressures (CVP or PCWP, respectively) can be used to guide fluid management and optimization of cardiac output. The use of low-dose dopamine or diuretics (e.g., furosemide, mannitol) to increase urine output per se has not been shown to improve either renal function or outcome.[22] The dosages of medications that are excreted predominantly by the kidneys should be adjusted for the degree of renal dysfunction.

Indications for renal replacement therapy (dialysis) include hypervolemia-induced congestive heart failure, uremia manifested by pericarditis or encephalopathy, acidemia with a pH below 7.20, hyperkalemia unresponsive to medical management, and hemorrhage associated with uremia-induced platelet dysfunction.

Intermittent hemodialysis[23] is the method of choice for renal replacement therapy. The disadvantage of this technique is that some degree of hemodynamic impairment usually results as a consequence of rapid, large fluid shifts from the intravascular compartment to the dialysis machine.

For hemodynamically unstable patients, however, continuous hemodialysis by vein (continuous venovenous hemodialysis, CVVHD) may be more appropriate.[24] CVVHD decreases the rate of fluid redistribution and thus may be associated with more stability, with the added benefit of permitting more precise control of fluid and electrolyte balance. The disadvantage of this type of dialysis is that CVVHD usually requires systemic anticoagulation to prevent blood from clotting in the dialysis filter and requires sophisticated nursing surveillance.

Hematological and Immunological Dysfunction

Coagulopathy

Major trauma significantly increases the risk of venous thrombosis and thromboembolism. However, the adaptive hypercoagulable response to stop trauma-induced hemorrhage may be limited then by a counterregulatory response that results in some of the abnormalities measured.[25] Factors commonly predisposing to coagulopathy in the ICU include hemodilution, malnutrition (vitamin K deficiency), hepatic insufficiency, consumption of factors by disseminated coagulation, and hypothermia. Measured abnormalities in lab tests, however, are usually not clinically significant as manifested by overt hemorrhage, a tribute to the redundancy of the coagulation system. The clinician should resist therefore the temptation to correct mild to moderate coagulopathy and thrombocytopenia in otherwise stable, nonbleeding patients.

Anemia

Perioperative anemia is tolerated without evidence of significant organ failure or mortality down to a hemoglobin of approximately 7 g/dl (hematocrit, 20%). Conventional clinical wisdom thus supported the use of red cell transfusion to keep hemoglobin values in the "safe" range of 9 to 10 g/dl (hematocrit, 27%–30%),[26] particularly in critically ill patients with preexisting cardiopulmonary disease. The effectiveness of this approach, however, has recently been called into question, and the results of several ongoing randomized studies on this strategy are eagerly awaited.

Immunosuppression and Nosocomial Infection

The systemic inflammatory response to severe injury leads to aberrations in adaptive immunity, resulting in immunosuppression. Coupled with the use of invasive devices (e.g., vascular catheters and endotracheal tubes) that bypass normal immune barriers such as the skin and respiratory epithelium, these changes put the ICU patients at very high risk for developing nosocomial infections.

References

1. Samuels MA. The evaluation of the comatose patient. Hosp Pract 1993;23:165–182.
2. Hansen-Flaschen J, Cowen J, Polomano RC. Beyond the Ramsay scale: need for a validated measure of sedating drug efficacy in the intensive care unit. Crit Care Med 1994;22:732–733.
3. Cernaianu AC, DelRossi AJ, Flum DR, et al. Lorazepam and midazolam in the intensive care unit: a randomized, prospective, multicenter study of hemodynamics, oxygen transport, efficacy, and cost. Crit Care Med 1996;24:222–228.
4. Chamorro C, de Latorre FJ, Montero A, et al. Comparative study of propofol versus midazolam in the sedation of critically ill patients: results of a prospective, randomized, multicenter trial. Crit Care Med 1996;24:932–939.
5. Crippen DW. Pharmacologic treatment of brain failure and delerium. In: Critical Care Clinics. Philadelphia: Saunders, 1994: 733–766.
6. Vermeulen LCJ, Ratko TA, Erstad BL, Brecher ME, Matuszewski KA. A paradigm for consensus. The University Hospital Consortium guidelines for the use of albumin, nonprotein colloid, and crystalloid solutions. Arch Intern Med 1995;155:373–379.
7. Duke TD, Butt W, South M. Predictors of mortality and multiple organ failure in children with sepsis. Intensive Care Med 1997;23:684–692.
8. Bakker J, Gris P, Coffernils M, Kahn RJ, Vincent JL. Serial blood lactate levels can predict the development of multiple organ failure following septic shock. Am J Surg 1996;171:221–226.
9. Bernard GR, Artigas A, Brigham KL, et al. Report of the American-European consensus conference on ARDS: definitions, mechanisms, relevant outcomes and clinical trial coordination. The Consensus Committee. Intensive Care Med 1994;20:225–232.
10. Luce JM. Acute lung injury and the acute respiratory distress syndrome. Crit Care Med 1998;26:369–376.
11. Kollef MH, Schuster DP. The acute respiratory distress syndrome. N Engl J Med 1995;332:27–37.
12. Jubran A, Tobin MJ. Reliability of pulse oximetry in titrating supplemental oxygen therapy in ventilator-dependent patients. Chest 1990;97:1420–1425.
13. Gattinoni L, D'Andrea L, Pelosi P, Vitale G, Presenti A, Fumagalli R. Regional effects and mechanism of positive end-expiratory pressure in early adult respiratory distress syndrome. JAMA 1993;269:2122–2127.
14. Kollef MH, Shapiro SD, Silver P, et al. A randomized, controlled trial of protocol-directed versus physician-directed weaning from mechanical ventilation. Crit Care Med 1997;25:567–574.
15. Esteban A, Frutos F, Tobin MJ, et al. A comparison of four methods of weaning patients from mechanical ventilation. Spanish Lung Failure Collaborative Group. N Engl J Med 1995;332:345–350.
16. Ely EW, Baker AM, Dunagan DP, et al. Effect on the duration of mechanical ventilation of identifying patients capable of breathing spontaneously. N Engl J Med 1996;335:1864–1869.
17. Yang KL, Tobin MJ. A prospective study of indexes predicting the outcome of trials of weaning from mechanical ventilation. N Engl J Med 1991;324:1445–1450.
18. Jaeschke RZ, Meade MO, Guyatt GH, Keenan SP, Cook DJ. How to use diagnostic test articles in the intensive care unit: diagnosing weanability using f/Vt. Crit Care Med 1997;25:1514–1521.
19. Cook D, Guyatt G, Marshall J, et al. A comparison of sucralfate and ranitidine for the prevention of upper gastrointestinal bleeding in patients requiring mechanical ventilation. Canadian Critical Care Trials Group. N Engl J Med 1998;338:791–797.
20. Thadhani R, Pascual M, Bonventre JV. Acute renal failure. N Engl J Med 1996;334:1448–1460.
21. Saggi BH, Sugerman HJ, Ivatury RR, Bloomfield GL. Abdominal compartment syndrome. J Trauma 1998;45:597–609.
22. Perdue PW, Balsar JR, Lipsett PA, Breslow MJ. "Renal dose" dopamine in surgical patients: dogma or science? Ann Surg 1998; 227:470–473.
23. Pastan S, Bailey J. Dialysis therapy. N Engl J Med 1998;338: 1428–1437.
24. Forni LG, Hilton PJ. Continuous hemofiltration in the treatment of acute renal failure. N Engl J Med 1997;336:1303–1309.
25. Dries DJ. Activation of the clotting system and complement after trauma. New Horiz 1996;4:276–288.
26. Thurer RL. Evaluating transfusion triggers [editorial; comment]. JAMA 1998;279:238–239.

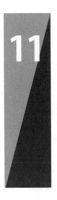

Monitoring Techniques and Complications in Critical Care

Mitchell P. Fink

Ideally, patients are monitored to provide advanced warning of impending deterioration in the status of one or more organ systems so that appropriate steps can be taken in a timely way to prevent or ameliorate the physiological derangement. This chapter focuses on the hemodynamic monitoring of the critically ill patient.

Systemic Arterial Pressure

The pressure exerted by blood in the systemic arterial system is commonly referred to simply as blood pressure and is a cardinal parameter measured as part of the hemodynamic monitoring of patients. Although we now know that arterial blood pressure is a complex function of both cardiac output and vascular input impedance, clinicians, especially inexperienced ones, tend to assume that the presence of a normal blood pressure is evidence that cardiac output and tissue perfusion are adequate. This assumption, while often valid, is frequently incorrect, and is the reason why some critically ill patients may benefit from forms of hemodynamic monitoring in addition to measurement of arterial pressure.

Noninvasive Measurement of Arterial Pressure

Both manual and automated means for the noninvasive determination of blood pressure use an inflatable cuff to increase pressure around an extremity. If the cuff is too narrow (relative to the extremity), the measured pressure will be artifactually elevated. Therefore, the width of the cuff should be about 40% of its circumference.

Methods for detection of blood pressure include oscillometry—detection of pressure oscillations in the inflatable bladder encircling the extremity, use of a piezoelectric crystal positioned over the brachial artery as a pulse detector, and a technique called photoplethysmography, which can provide continuous information because systolic and diastolic blood pressure are recorded on a beat-to-beat basis. A recent clinical study suggests that the most accurate are the oscillometric devices.[1]

Direct Measurement

Direct monitoring of arterial pressure is almost always performed by using fluid-filled tubing to connect an intraarterial catheter to an external strain gauge transducer. The signal generated by the transducer is electronically amplified and displayed as a continuous waveform by an oscilloscope. Digital values for systolic and diastolic pressure are also displayed. Mean pressure, calculated by electronically averaging the amplitude of the pressure waveform, also can be displayed.

The radial artery at the wrist is the site most commonly used for intraarterial pressure monitoring. It is important to recognize, however, that measured arterial pressure is determined in part by the site at which the pressure is monitored. Typically, systolic pressures are higher and diastolic pressures are lower in the periphery, whereas mean pressure is approximately the same in the aorta and more distal sites. In certain circumstances femoral arterial monitoring may be preferable to radial arterial monitoring.

Distal ischemia is an uncommon complication of intraarterial catheterization. The incidence of thrombosis is increased when larger-caliber catheters are employed and when catheters are left in place for an extended period of time. The incidence of thrombosis can be minimized by using a 20-gauge (or smaller) catheter in the radial position and leaving the catheter in place for as short a duration as feasible, preferably less than 4 days. The risk of distal ischemic injury can be minimized by ensuring that adequate collateral flow is present. At the wrist, adequate collateral flow can be documented by performing a modified version of Allen's test.

Cardiac Output and Related Parameters

Clearly, many clinicians must believe that information valuable for the management of critically ill patients is afforded by having a pulmonary artery catheter (PAC) in place. Remarkably, however, unambiguous data in support of this view are scarce. Indeed, quite the opposite seems to be true; several studies suggest that bedside pulmonary artery catheterization is associated with poorer outcomes in selected populations of patients. The controversy regarding the value of pulmonary artery catheterization is reviewed next.

Placement of Central Venous or Swan–Ganz Catheters

Placement of a PAC requires access to the central venous circulation. Such access can be obtained at a variety of sites, including the antecubital, femoral, jugular, and subclavian veins. In general, percutaneous placement through either the jugular or subclavian vein is preferred. Right internal jugular vein cannulation carries the lowest risk of complications, and the path of the catheter from this site into the right atrium is straight. Moreover, in the event of inadvertent arterial puncture, local pressure is much more effective in controlling bleeding from the carotid as compared to the subclavian artery. Nevertheless, it is more difficult to keep occlusive dressings in place on the neck than in the subclavian fossa. Furthermore, the anatomical landmarks in the subclavian position are quite constant, even in patients with anasarca or massive obesity; the subclavian vein is always attached to the deep (concave) surface of the clavicle. In contrast, the appropriate landmarks to guide jugular venous cannulation are sometimes difficult to discern in obese or very edematous patients. However, ultrasonic imaging can facilitate jugular venipuncture.[2]

Cannulation of the vein is normally performed percutaneously, using the Seldinger technique. A small-bore needle is inserted through the skin and subcutaneous tissue into the vein. After documenting return of nonpulsatile, venous blood, a guidewire with a flexible tip is inserted through the needle into the vein and the needle is withdrawn. If central venous catheterization is all that is required, then a dilator is passed over the wire to enlarge the subcutaneous tract and the hole in the vein. After the dilator is removed, a single- or multiple-lumen catheter (which has been previously flushed with saline solution) is passed over the wire into the vein. The wire is removed, and the catheter is connected through low fluid-filled low-compliance tubing to a strain gauge transducer.

In its simplest form, the PAC has four channels. One channel terminates in a balloon at the tip of the catheter. The proximal end of this channel is connected to a syringe to permit inflation of the balloon with air. Before insertion of the PAC, the integrity of the balloon should be verified by inflating it. To minimize the risk of vascular or ventricular perforation by the relatively inflexible catheter, it also is important to verify that the inflated balloon extends just beyond the tip of the device. A second channel in the catheter contains wires that are connected to a thermistor located near the tip of the catheter. At the proximal end of the PAC, the wires terminate in an appropriate fitting that permits connection to appropriate hardware for the calculation of cardiac output using the thermodilution technique (see following). The final two channels are used for pressure monitoring and the injection of the thermal indicator for determinations of cardiac output. One of these channels terminates at the tip of the catheter; the other terminates 20 cm proximal to the tip.

To insert a Swan–Ganz catheter, a guidewire is inserted into a central vein as previously described. A dilator/introducer sheath is passed over the wire, and the wire and the dilator are removed. The introducer sheath is equipped with a side port, which can be used for administering fluid. The introducer sheath also is equipped with a diaphragm that permits insertion of the PAC while preventing the backflow of venous blood. The proximal terminus of the distal port of the PAC is connected through low-compliance tubing to a strain gauge transducer, and the tubing-catheter system is flushed with fluid. While one is constantly observing the pressure tracing on an oscilloscope, the PAC is advanced with the balloon deflated until respiratory excursions are observed. The balloon is then inflated, and the catheter advanced further, taking care to record pressures sequentially in the right atrium and right ventricle en route to the pulmonary artery. The pressure waveforms for the right atrium, right ventricle, and pulmonary artery are each very characteristic and easy to recognize (Fig. 11.1). The catheter is advanced out the pulmonary artery until a damped tracing, indicative of the wedged position, is obtained. The balloon is then deflated, taking care to ensure that a normal pulmonary arterial tracing is again observed on the monitor; leaving the balloon inflated can increase the risk of pulmonary infarction or perforation of the pulmonary artery.

Hemodynamic Measurements

By combining data obtained through use of the PAC with results obtained by other means (blood hemoglobin concentration and saturation), derived estimates of systemic oxygen transport and utilization can be calculated. Direct and derived parameters obtainable by bedside pulmonary arterial catheterization are summarized in Table 11.1. The equations used to calculate the derived parameters are summarized in Table 11.2. The approximate normal ranges for a number of these hemodynamic parameters (in adults) are shown in Table 11.3.

Measurement of Cardiac Output by Thermodilution

The principle underlying the thermodilution method is straightforward. If a bolus of an indicator is rapidly and thoroughly mixed with a moving fluid upstream from a detector, then the concentration of the indicator at the detector will increase sharply and then exponentially diminish back to zero. The area under the resulting time–concentration curve is a function of the volume of indicator injected and the flow rate of the moving stream of fluid; larger volumes of indicator result in greater areas under the curve, and faster flow rates of the mixing fluid result in smaller areas under the curve. When Q_T is measured by theromodilution, the indicator is heat and the detector is a temperature-sensing thermistor at the distal end of the PAC. The relationship used for calculating Q_T is called the Stewart–Hamilton equation:

$$Q_T = [V \times (T_B - T_I) \times K_1 \times K_2] \div \int T_B(t)\,dt$$

where V is the volume of the indicator injected, T_B is the temperature of blood (i.e., core body temperature), T_I is the temperature of the indicator, K_1 is a constant that is a function of the specific heats of blood and the indicator, K_2 is an empirically derived constant that accounts for several factors (the dead space volume of the catheter, heat lost from the indicator as it traverses the catheter, and the injection rate of the

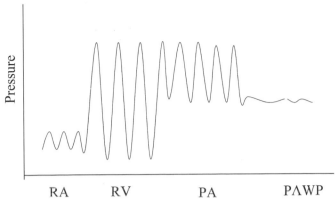

FIGURE 11.1. Stylized representation of the characteristic pressure tracings recorded during passage of a balloon-tipped (Swan-Ganz) pulmonary artery catheter as the tip of the device transverses in turn the right atrium (RA), right ventricle (RV), and pulmonary artery (PA). The final part of the tracing depicts the small pressure changes typically observed when the device is in the wedge or occlusion position (PAWP).

TABLE 11.1. Directly Measured and Derived Hemodynamic Data Obtainable by Bedside Pulmonary Artery Catheterization (PAC).

Standard PAC	PAC with additional feature(s)	Derived parameters
CVP	Svo_2 (continuous)	SV
Ppa	Q_T or Q_T^* (continuous)	SVR (or SVRI)
$Ppao$	RVEF	PVR (or PVRI)
Svo_2 (intermittent)		RVEDV
Q_T or Q_T^* (intermittent)		Do_2
		Vo_2
		ER
		Qs/Q_T

CVP, mean central venous pressure; Ppa, pulmonary artery pressure; $Ppao$, pulmonary artery occlusion ("wedge") pressure; Svo_2, fractional mixed venous (pulmonary artery) hemoglobin saturation; Q_T, cardiac output; Q_T^*, cardiac output indexed to body surface area ("cardiac index"); RVEF, right ventricular ejection fraction; SV, stroke volume; SVR, systemic vascular resistance; SVRI, systemic vascular resistance index; RVEDV, right ventricular end-diastolic volume; Do_2, systemic oxygen delivery; Vo_2, systemic oxygen utilization; ER, systemic oxygen extraction ratio; Qs/Q_T, fractional pulmonary venous admixture ("shunt fraction").

indicator), and $\int T_B(t)\,s$ is the area under the time–temperature curve. In clinical practice, the Stewart–Hamilton equation is solved by a microprocessor.

The thermodilution method is generally quite accurate, although Q_T tends to be systematically overestimated at very low values.[3] Changes in blood temperature and Q_T during the respiratory cycle can influence the measurement. Therefore, results generally should be recorded as the mean of two or three determinations obtained at random points in the respiratory cycle. Most authorities recommend using room temperature injectate (normal saline or 5% dextrose in water) to minimize errors resulting from warming of the fluid as it is transferred from its reservoir to a syringe for injection.

Mixed Venous Oximetry

The Fick equation, $Q_T = Vo_2/(Cao_2 - Cvo_2)$, can be rearranged as follows: $Cvo_2 = Cao_2 - Vo_2/Q_T$. If the small contribution of dissolved oxygen to Cvo_2 and Cao_2 is ignored, the rearranged equation can be rewritten: $Svo_2 = Sao_2 - Vo_2/(Q_T \times Hgb \times 1.36)$. Thus, it can be seen that Svo_2 is a function of Vo_2 (i.e., metabolic rate), Q_T, Sao_2, and Hgb. Accordingly, subnormal values of Svo_2 can be caused by a decrease in Q_T (due, for example, to heart failure or hypovolemia), a decrease in Sao_2 (due, for example, to intrinsic pulmonary disease), a decrease in Hgb (i.e., anemia), or an increase in metabolic rate (due, for example, to seizures or

TABLE 11.2. Formulas for Calculation of Hemodynamic Parameters, Which Can Be Derived by Using Data Obtained by Pulmonary Artery Catheterization.

Q_T^* ($L \cdot min^{-1} \cdot M^{-2}$) = Q_T/BSA, where BSA is body surface area (M^2)

SV (ml) = Q_T/HR, where HR is heart rate (min^{-1})

SVR (dyne·sec·cm^{-5}) = $[(MAP - CVP) \times 80]/Q_T$, where MAP is mean arterial pressure (mmHg)

SVRI (dyne·sec·cm^{-5}·M^{-2}) = $[(MAP - CVP) \times 80]/Q_T^*$

PVR (dyne·sec·cm^{-5}) = $[(Ppa - Ppao) \times 80]/Q_T$, where Ppa is mean pulmonary artery pressure

PVRI (dyne·sec·cm^{-5}·M^{-2}) = $[(Ppa - Ppao) \times 80]/Q_T^*$

RVEDV (ml) = SV/RVEF

Do_2 (ml·min^{-1}·M^{-2}) = $Q_T^* \times Cao_2 \times 10$, where Cao_2 is arterial oxygen content (ml/dl)

Vo_2 (ml·min^{-1}·M^{-2}) = $Q_T^* \times (Cao_2 - Cvo_2) \times 10$, where Cvo_2 is mixed venous oxygen content (ml/dl)

Cao_2 = $1.36 \times Hgb \times Sao_2) + (0.003 + Pao_2)$, where Hgb is hemoglobin concentration (g/dl), Sao_2 is fractional arterial hemoglobin saturation, and Pao_2 is the partial pressure of oxygen in arterial blood

Cvo_2 = $(1.36 \times Hgb \times Svo_2) + (0.003 + Pvo_2)$, where Pao_2 is the partial pressure of oxygen in pulmonary arterial (mixed venous) blood

Qs/Q_T = $(Cco_2 - Cao_2)/(Cco_2 - Cvo_2)$, where Cco_2 (ml/dl) is the content of oxygen in pulmonary end capillary blood

Cco_2 = $(1.36 \times Hgb) + (0.003 + Pao_2)$, where Pao_2 is the alveolar partial pressure of oxygen

Pao_2 = $[Fio_2 \times (P_B - Ph_2o)] - Paco_2/RQ$, where Fio_2 is the fractional concentration of inspired oxygen, P_B is the barometric pressure (mmHg), Ph_2o is the water vapor pressure [usually 40 is the partial pressure of carbon dioxide in arterial blood (mmHg)], and RQ is respiratory quotient (usually assumed to be 0.8)

TABLE 11.3. Approximate Normal Ranges for Selected Hemodynamic Parameters in Adults.

Parameter	Normal range
CVP	0–6 mmHg
Right ventricular systolic pressure	20–30 mmHg
Right ventricular diastolic pressure	0–6 mmHg
PAOP	6–12 mmHg
Systolic arterial pressure	100–130 mmHg
Diastolic arterial pressure	60–90 mmHg
MAP	75–100 mmHg
Q_T	4–6 l/min
Q_T*	2.5–3.5 $l \cdot min^{-1} \cdot M^{-2}$
SV	40–80 ml
SVR	800–1400 $dyne \cdot sec \cdot cm^{-5}$
SVRI	1500–2400 $dyne \cdot sec \cdot cm^{-5} \cdot M^{-2}$
PVR	100–150 $dyne \cdot sec \cdot cm^{-5}$
PVRI	200–400 $dyne \cdot sec \cdot cm^{-5} \cdot M^{-2}$
Ca_{O_2}	16–22 ml/dl
Cv_{O_2}	12–17 ml/dl
D_{O_2}	400–660 $ml \cdot min^{-1} \cdot M^{-2}$
V_{O_2}	115–165 $ml \cdot min^{-1} \cdot M^{-2}$

fever). With a conventional PAC, measurements of Sv_{O_2} require aspirating a sample of blood from the distal (i.e., pulmonary arterial) port of the catheter and injecting the sample into a blood gas analyzer. On practical grounds, therefore, measurements of Sv_{O_2} can be performed only intermittently. By adding a fifth channel to the PAC, it has become possible to monitor Sv_{O_2} continuously, but data are lacking to show that this capability favorably improves outcome.[4–7]

Right Ventricular Ejection Fraction

Ejection fraction (EF) is the fraction of the end-diastolic volume of blood in the ventricle remaining in the chamber at the end of systole, and is an ejection-phase measure of myocardial contractility. By equipping a PAC with a thermistor with a short time constant, the thermodilution method can be used to estimate RVEF. Data are lacking to show that outcomes are improved by making measurements of RVEF in addition to Q_T and other parameters measured by the conventional PAC.

Effect of Pulmonary Artery Catheterization on Outcome

In a recent study, two groups of patients, those who did and those who did not undergo placement of a PAC during their first 24 h of ICU care, were compared. The investigators concluded that placement of a pulmonary artery catheter during the first 24 h of stay in an ICU is associated with a significant increase in the risk of mortality, even when statistical methods are used to account for severity of illness.

These results actually confirmed those of two prior observational studies, although in neither of these earlier reports did the authors conclude that placement of a PAC was truly the cause of worsened survival after myocardial infarction.

Relatively few prospective, randomized controlled trials

of pulmonary artery catheterization have been performed.[8–13] The limitations of these studies notwithstanding, the weight of current evidence suggests that routine pulmonary artery catheterization is not necessary for patients undergoing cardiac or major peripheral vascular surgical procedures. Based upon the exclusion criteria used in two recent prospective randomized trials, reasonable criteria for perioperative monitoring without use of a PAC are presented in Table 11.4.

One of the reasons for using a PAC to monitor critically ill patients is to optimize cardiac output and systemic oxygen delivery. Defining what constitutes the optimum cardiac output, however, has proven to be difficult.

It has been suggested that failure of PAC-directed monitoring to demonstrate a clear benefit may be due to adverse events related to catheter placement, inaccurate date generation, or clinical misinterpretation of obtained measurements. In any case, PAC use remains controversial and judicious application is warranted.

Doppler Ultrasonography

When ultrasonic sound waves are reflected by moving erythrocytes in the bloodstream, the frequency of the reflected signal is increased or decreased, depending on whether the cells are moving toward or away from the ultrasonic source (Doppler shift). Measurements of the Doppler shift can be used to calculate red blood cell velocity. With knowledge of both the cross-sectional area of a vessel and the mean red blood cell velocity of the blood flowing through it, one can calculate blood flow rate.

Transesophageal transducers utilizing these properties appear to provide sufficiently accurate measurements of Q_T and may be clinically useful because of their ability to provide a continuous readout.

Impedance Cardiography

Because of insufficient reliability, impedence cardiography cannot be recommended at the present time for hemodynamic monitoring of critically ill patients.

Other Noninvasive Methods

The pressure waveform obtained by photoplethysmography can be used to estimate the aortic flow waveform and thereby estimate Q_T. Unfortunately, the results obtained are not sufficiently accurate to be used clinically.[14]

TABLE 11.4. Suggested Exclusion Criteria for Perioperative Monitoring Without Use of a PAC in Patients Undergoing Cardiac or Major Vascular Surgical Procedures.

Anticipated need for suprarenal or supraceliac aortic cross-clamping

History of myocardial infarction during 3 months before operation

History of poorly compensated congestive heart failure

History of coronary artery bypass graft surgery during 6 weeks before operation

History of ongoing symptomatic mitral or aortic valvular heart disease

History of ongoing unstable angina pectoris

Tissue Capnometry

In theory, knowing that tissue pH is not in the acid range should be enough information to conclude that perfusion (and, for that matter, arterial oxygen content) are sufficient to meet the metabolic demands of the cells. By the same token, the detection of tissue acidosis should alert the clinician to the possibility that perfusion is inadequate.

Unfortunately, the notion of using tonometric estimates of gastrointestinal mucosal pH_i for monitoring perfusion is predicated by a number of assumptions, some of which may be partially or completely invalid. Furthermore, currently available methods for performing measurements of gastric mucosal PCO_2 in the clinical setting remain rather cumbersome and expensive. Perhaps for these reasons, gastric tonometry for monitoring critically ill patients remains largely a research tool and is far from being adopted as a standard of practice. Nevertheless, some recent developments in the field may be changing this situation, and monitoring tissue PCO_2 seems likely to become common in emergency departments, intensive care units, and operating rooms in the relatively near future.

References

1. Lehmann KG, Gelman JA, Weber MA, Lafrades A. Comparative accuracy of three automated techniques in the noninvasive measurement of central blood pressure in men. Am J Cardiol 1998; 81:1004–1012.
2. Mallory DL, McGee WT, Shawker TH, et al. Ultrasound guidance improves the success rate of internal jugular vein cannulation. A prospective, randomized trial. Chest 1990;98:157–160.
3. van Grondelle A, Ditchey RV, Groves BM, Wagner WW, Reeves JT. Thermodilution method overestimates low cardiac output in humans. Am J Physiol 1983;245:H690–H692.
4. Boutros AR, Lee C. Value of continuous monitoring of mixed venous blood oxygen saturation in the management of critically ill patients. Crit Care Med 1986;14:132–134.
5. Jastremski MS, Chelluri L, Beney KM, Bailly RT. Analysis of the effects of continuous on-line monitoring of mixed venous oxygen saturation on patient outcomes and cost-effectiveness. Crit Care Med 1989;17:148–153.
6. Kyff JV, Vaughn S, Yang SC, Raheja R, Puri VK. Continuous monitoring of mixed venous oxygen saturation in patients with acute myocardial infarction. Chest 1989;95:607–611.
7. Gattinoni L, Brazzi L, Pelosi P, et al. A trial of goal-oriented hemodynamic therapy in critically ill patients. N Engl J Med 1995;333:1025–1032.
8. Pearson KS, Gomez MN, Moyers JR, Carter JG, Tinker JH. A cost/benefit analysis of randomized invasive monitoring for patients undergoing cardiac surgery. Anesth Analg 1989;69:336–341.
9. Tuman KJ, McCarthy RJ, Spiess BD, et al. Effect of pulmonary artery catheterization on outcome in patients undergoing coronary artery surgery. Anesthesiology 1989;70:199–206.
10. Isaakson IJ, Lowdon JD, Berry AJ, et al. The value of pulmonary artery and central venous monitoring in patients undergoing abdominal aortic reconstructive surgery: a comparative study of two selected, randomized groups. J Vasc Surg 1990;12:754–760.
11. Joyce WP, Provan JL, Ameli FM, McEwan MM, Jelenich S, Jones DP. The role of central haemodynamic monitoring in abdominal aortic surgery. A prospective randomised study. Eur J Vasc Surg 1990;4:633–636.
12. Bender JS, Smith-Meek MA, Jones CE. Routine pulmonary artery catheterization does not reduce morbidity and mortality of elective vascular surgery: results of a prospective, randomized trial. Ann Surg 1997;226:229–236.
13. Valentine RJ, Duke ML, Inman MH, et al. Effectiveness of pulmonary artery catheters in aortic surgery: a randomized trial. J Vasc Surg 1998;27:203–211.
14. Hirschl MM, Binder M, Gwechenberger M, et al. Noninvasive assessment of cardiac output in critically ill patients by analysis of the finger blood pressure waveform. Crit Care Med 1997;25:1909–1914.

12

Burns

Roger W. Yurt

The magnitude of the problem of burn injury and the need for all physicians to be prepared to care for these patients is demonstrated by the fact that in the United States alone 1.25 million people each year sustain burn injury with 51,000 requiring hospitalization.[1] The impact on society is not just measured in the annual mortality rate of 5,500 persons, but by the long-term morbidity arising from organ dysfunction and mechanical, psychological, and cosmetic disability.

Evaluation of the Patient

The initial evaluation of the patient with burn injury is the same as with all victims of traumatic injury and should proceed as recommended in the Advanced Trauma Life Support course of the American College of Surgeons.[2] First, attention is turned to maintenance of airway, breathing, and circulation. Although some aspects of the evaluation are specific with regard to burns, for example, inhalation injury, it should always be remembered that a burn-injured patient may have multiple system injury. Only the aspects of evaluation that are peculiar to the burn-injured patient are emphasized in this chapter.

Extent of Burn Injury

The extent of injury sustained from tissue damage by burning is more easily quantified than in most other types of trauma. A knowledge of the surface area involved and the depth of injury assists in determining a prognosis for the patient and is used to guide fluid resuscitation and to develop a plan of care. The area of the body surface that has been injured can be estimated in adults by using the rule of nines, which divides the surface area into sections or multiples of 9% (Fig. 12.1). Although the use of this estimate is helpful in initial assessment and triage of patients, a more exact measurement should be made using a Lund & Browder chart or Berkow's formula.[3] A

section taken from the patient chart used at the Burn Center of the New York Presbyterian Hospital (Fig. 12.1) shows the distribution of surface area at several different ages. It is essential that such a chart be used when children are evaluated because the distribution of body surface area varies with age.

The determination of the depth of injury presents a greater challenge because the clinical findings are not exact except in the extremes and the wound is dynamic. A partial-thickness burn involves the outer layer of the skin and may extend into the dermis. This wound, commonly termed a second-degree burn, is characterized by blistering of the skin and is red, moist, and painful; sensation is intact. This depth of injury is further subdivided into superficial and deep partial-thickness injury. The clinical differentiation of these different depths of injury is challenging as evidenced by the fact that even experienced burn surgeons are able to accurately determine depth of injury only 64% of the time.[4] The only absolute way to confirm the depth of injury is by the length of time it takes these injuries to heal. A superficial partial-thickness burn should heal within 2 weeks, whereas a deep partial-thickness wound takes 3 weeks to reepithelialize. Figure 12.2 depicts a cross section of skin with indication of the various depths of injury. As shown, the superficial burn wound involves the epidermis, but spares islands of epidermis that provide the source of new epidermal covering. The deep partial-thickness injury can only resurface from residual epidermis from the organelles of the skin.

The clinical importance of differentiating between these depths of injury lies in the recognition that a superficial wound heals with minimal cosmetic or functional consequence. The deep partial-thickness wound, although it will heal given enough time, results in both cosmetic deformity and disturbance of function. In this case skin grafting will improve the outcome and is the preferred approach in this depth of injury. Complicating the evaluation of depth of injury is the fact that the wound evolves over a 3-day period and that external influences such as adequacy of resuscitation, exposure of the wound to noxious agents, and infection modify

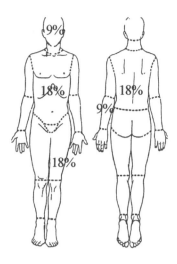

AREA	0-1 YEAR	5-9 YEARS	ADULT
Head	19	11	7
Neck	2	2	2
Ant. Trunk	13	13	13
Post. Trunk	13	13	13
R. Buttock	2 ½	2 ½	2 ½
L. Buttock	2 ½	2 ½	2 ½
Genitalia	1	1	1
R.U. Arm	4	4	4
L.U. Arm	4	4	4
R.L. Arm	3	3	3
L.L. Arm	3	3	3
R. Hand	2 ½	2 ½	2 ½
L. Hand	2 ½	2 ½	2 ½
R. Thigh	5 ½	8	9 ½
L. Thigh	5 ½	8	9 ½
R. Leg	5	5 ½	7
L. Leg	5	5 ½	7
R. Leg	3 ½	3 ½	3 ½
L. Foot	3 ½	3 ½	3 ½

FIGURE 12.1. Distribution of body surface area at different ages.

the progression of the wound. Furthermore, wounds often are of mixed depth such that evaluation of discrete areas may not reflect the depth of the overall wound.

Full-thickness wounds are leathery, white or charred, dry, and insensate. Because all the epidermis is destroyed (Fig. 12.2), these wounds can only heal by migration of epidermis from the margins of the wound. During the process of healing, contraction occurs; this decreases the area that must be epithelialized but leads to a poor cosmetic result and a wound that is less resistant to trauma. Further, if the wound is adjacent to or involves a joint, the function of the joint will be impaired. Except for small surface area wounds, full-thickness wounds should be either excised and closed primarily or grafted with the patient's skin.

Types of Injury

The pathophysiology involved in the wounds of a patient with a burn injury is basically the same regardless of the cause. In the superficial area of injury, coagulative necrosis occurs. In this zone protein is irreversibly denatured and cellular integrity is lost.[5] Adjacent to this zone is the zone of stasis in which tissue is viable but subject to further necrosis as the wound evolves. A third zone has been recognized below the zone of stasis and is characterized as a zone of hyperemia. The zones of stasis and hyperemia are the areas where the inflammatory response of the patient is initiated.

The depth of the coagulative necrosis that occurs in burns which are caused by scalding, flame, or contact with a hot object is directly related to the temperature, duration of exposure, thickness of the tissue, and state of the blood supply in the tissue.

Chemical burns cause denaturation of protein and disruption of cellular integrity. The degree of injury is dependent on the time of exposure, the strength of the agent, and the solubility of the agent in tissue. Alkali tends to penetrate deeper into tissues than does an acid. One exception to this is hydrofluoric acid, which penetrates lipid membranes very readily. Table 12.1 provides a list of common agents that cause burn injury.[6]

The major concern in evaluating patients who sustain electrical injuries is that the surface injury, which may appear similar to other burn injuries, is often not indicative of the extent of injury. In the local area of injury subcutaneous tissue, muscle, and bone may be injured. Electrical current follows the path of least resistance and therefore will pass through nerve and blood vessels preferentially[7] and cause injury to these tissues. If the current passes through the torso of the patient, organ injury may result. Injury of the heart is primarily associated with arrhythmia.[8] Injury of other viscera including the pancreas[9] and gastrointestinal tract have been reported.[10] Late sequelae of electrical injury include the development of cataracts and transverse myelitis of the spinal cord. These sequelae have been reported to occur months or even years after electrical injury.[11]

Injury caused by exposure to ionizing radiation may be limited to the skin but often is deeper. Because these wounds do not heal well, care must be taken to avoid additional damage of the tissue. The vasculitis that is associated with these injuries is usually a lifelong problem.[12]

Inhalation Injury

Inhalation injury is often inappropriately attributed to heat-related damage to the airway or lung. Thermal injury to the airway is very rare because the upper airway can dissipate heat effectively,[13] but upper airway injury may occasionally be associated with a direct inhalation of superheated steam.[14] The majority of injuries to the lung are caused by inhalation

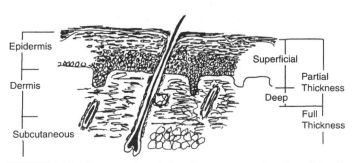

FIGURE 12.2. Cross-section of skin showing tissue levels and depth of injury.

TABLE 12.1. Common Agents that Cause Burn Injury to the Skin by Category.

Agent	Site of injury	Treatment
Acids		
Hydrochloric	Superficial	Irrigate with water
Nitric, sulfuric		
Hydrofluoric	Deep	Initial irrigation with water, then calcium gluconate
Phenol	Deep	Irrigate with 50:50 water and polyethelene glycol
Alkali		
Ammonia, sodium hydroxide	Deep	Irrigate with water
Cement	Superficial	Irrigate with water
Tar	Superficial/deep	Cool, then vasoline

of toxic chemical products of combustion. The deleterious components of smoke are primarily aldehydes.[15] In addition, carbon monoxide and cyanide may be inhaled. Similar to a chemical burn of the skin, these agents cause erythema and edema of the airway and can lead to blistering, ulceration, erosions, and sloughing of the airways. The local edema, infiltration of the tissue with polymorphonuclear leukocytes, and sloughing of bronchial mucosa lead to the formation of an endobronchial cast and obstruction of terminal bronchioles. Pulmonary edema occurs from increases in pulmonary lymph flow and microvascular permeability.[16] The debris in the airway cannot be cleared because of the injury to the mucosa and disruption of the mucociliary transport mechanism. The obstruction of the small airways and the accumulation of carbonaceous material and necrotic debris provide a fertile ground for the development of infection. Some authors have reported that the incidence of pneumonia in these patients is as high as 70%[17] within a week of injury.

Because the diagnosis of inhalation injury is difficult to make, a presumptive diagnosis is made based on a history that is consistent and signs and symptoms that are associated with injury to the airway. Any patient who sustains injury in a closed space and has burns above the clavicle, singeing of nasal vibrissae, hoarseness, or carbonaceous sputum should be assumed to have sustained an inhalation injury. Elevated carboxyhemoglobin levels will confirm exposure to carbon monoxide, but are not diagnostic for injury to the lung. Because the primary concern early after inhalation injury is obstruction of the airway, the upper airway should be evaluated immediately, usually in the emergency department. Flexible bronchoscopy provides the opportunity to confirm the diagnosis and initiate therapy. An endotracheal tube is passed over the bronchoscope before the endoscopy, and if injury is identified in the airway the tube is passed over the scope into the trachea.

Injury to the parenchyma of the lung is subtle in presentation in the early period after injury except in the most severe injuries such as those found in patients who sustained cardiac or respiratory arrest in the field. Findings on chest X-ray, arterial blood gases, and physical exam are frequently not helpful in the first 48 to 72 h post injury.[18] Xenon ventilation/perfusion scans are of value in detecting parenchymal injury to the lung; however, the extent of injury cannot be determined with this test. Consequently, treatment is often empiric. Therapy consists of aggressive pulmonary toilet, use of mucolytics, and early identification and treatment of infection. Prophylaxis with antibiotics is not used, and steroids are of no benefit and are potentially harmful.[19]

Decision to Transfer to Specialized Care

The resources required to care for patients with significant burn injury are not available at many medical centers. For this reason, a regionalized system for care of the burn-injured patient has been developed. Although travel time and distance to a burn center are of concern, transfer of burn-injured patients after initial evaluation has been shown to be safe especially if initiated early after injury.[20] Patients with burns over more than 30% of their body surface area, those at the extremes of age, and those with significant preexisting disease should be cared for in a burn center.

Resuscitation

General Principles

Because intravascular fluid loss begins to occur immediately after burn injury, initial resuscitative efforts are oriented toward volume replacement. If transport of the patient to an emergency care facility can be accomplished within 30 min of injury, intravenous access can be delayed until arrival at the receiving institution. Peripheral venous cannulation is preferred over central venous access and may be performed through burn-injured tissue if access through noninjured sites is not available. Patients with greater than 20% total body surface area injury (15% in children) require intravenous fluid resuscitation and should have a catheter placed in the urinary bladder. In addition, patients who have sustained a major injury should have a nasogastric tube placed to decompress the dilated stomach. During transport and resuscitation every effort should be made to maintain body temperature. Patients are wrapped in clean sheets or blankets and in the initial phase in the emergency care area the room is warmed. Behr hugger blankets are also of use. Resuscitation fluids should be warmed when fluids are given at rates of greater than 200 ml/h. Burn-injured extremities should be elevated above the level of the heart.

Fluid Resuscitation

During the first 24 h after injury there is fluid loss into and through the burn injury. In addition there is a shift of intravascular fluid into noninjured tissues. There is general agreement that during this period crystalloid solutions should be used.[21–23] As the fluid losses are large, formulae have been developed to provide an estimate of the fluid requirements.

Every guideline that has been developed carries with it the mandate that the patient's response to resuscitation be used as the actual determinant of fluid administration, not the formula! The goal of resuscitation is to maintain adequate tissue perfusion and therefore preserve organ function. The traditional assessment of adequacy of resuscitation in burn injury has been based on observation of blood pressure, heart rate, and urine output.[24,25] In this approach the patient is "titrated" with fluid to maintain a normal blood pressure and heart rate and a urine output of 1 ml/kg per hour[24] or 30 to 50 ml/h[26] in an adult patient. Other resuscitation endpoints are controversial.

The Parkland formula[24] was the crystalloid-based formula that provided the foundation for current methods of resuscitation (Table 12.2). This formula calls for the initiation of resuscitation with Ringer's lactate solution at a rate based on the body surface area of burn injury and the patient's body weight. The calculated resuscitation volume for the first 24 h is 4 ml times weight in kilograms times the percent of the body surface area that is burned. One-half of this volume is given in the first 8 h after injury and the other half is given in the following 16 h. Resuscitation of children is based on this volume plus a volume equal to the estimated daily maintenance fluid requirements. Goodwin et al.[27] at the U.S. Army Institute of Surgical Research have suggested that the same success can be obtained by using a formula that estimates requirements as 3 ml/kg per percent of the body surface area that is burned. The use of hypertonic saline to minimize fluid volume has not shown a clear benefit.

Most authors continue to suggest that administration of colloid-containing solutions be reserved for the second 24 h after injury when the capillary leak is assumed to have resolved.[24] Thereafter, daily maintenance fluids are given with a recognition of ongoing evaporative losses and the knowledge that total body sodium content is high. Evaporative fluid loss from the burn-injured tissue has been estimated to occur at an hourly rate equal to the sum of 25 and the percent of the body surface area that is injured multiplied by the total body surface area.

Wound Care

General Principles

Small (quarter size or less) blisters are often left intact whereas larger blisters and full-thickness wounds should be debrided and covered with a topical agent. This step can be accom-

TABLE 12.2. Intravenous Fluid Resuscitation of the Burn-Injured Patient.

First 24 h:
   Total milliliters of ringer's lactate solution[a] = 4 × weight in kg × % BSA injury (1/2 given in first 8 h)
Second 24 h:
   5% dextrose in water[b] estimated based on evaporative loss
   Evaporative loss from injury = (25 + % BSA injury) × TBSA
   Colloid (as necessary in >40% burn injury) estimated as 0.3–0.5 ml × weight in kg × % BSA injury

[a]In children, add daily maintenance fluid to calculated amount.

[b]In children, use 5% dextrose in ¼ NS.

plished in the office or the emergency room environment for patients who are to be treated as outpatients. Inpatient wound care is provided in a warm environment at the bedside or more often in an area reserved for wound care in a burn center. The objective of wound care is to avoid infection and protect the wound from further injury. Agents that may cause additional tissue damage are avoided, and the circulation of the wound is protected by avoiding hypotension and excluding the use of alpha-adrenergic agents, which will lead to additional tissue ischemia. Sterile gloves should be worn at all times when a wound is manipulated.

Chemical injury of tissue is treated with irrigation with copious amounts of either normal saline or tap water for as long as 6 h. Neutralizing agents are not used because they can lead to additional tissue damage caused by heat generated in an exothermic reaction between the chemicals. Hydrofluoric acid injuries can lead to systemic hypocalcemia, and therefore brief irrigation should be followed by topical application of calcium gluconate gel. If pain persists, clysis of the wound with calcium gluconate is used except in digits. For injury to distal extremities intraarterial infusion of calcium gluconate has been recommended.[28]

Prophylaxis Against Wound Infection

Because there is concern for inducing microbial resistance to antibiotics, systemic antimicrobial prophylaxis is not used in patients admitted to the hospital. The wounds are closely observed for infection and treatment is initiated if this occurs. There is no clear consensus on the use of antibiotics in the outpatient setting.

The advent of effective topical antimicrobial agents has substantially reduced the mortality associated with burn wound infection.[29] The commonly used agents and their advantages and disadvantages are listed in Table 12.3. The ideal topical regimen rests on the use of an agent with good prophylactic antimicrobial activity that also provides an opportunity to easily evaluate the wound and to perform regular physical therapy.

Surgical Care

Excision and closure of wounds has the advantage of reducing the extent of injury and eliminating the risk of wound infection. Tangential excision, which is the sequential removal of necrotic tissue until viable tissue is identified, is the most commonly used method of excision of burn-injured tissue. The advantage of this method is that it yields the best cosmetic and functional result; however, it also is associated with considerable blood loss. Tourniquets have been shown to minimize blood loss when they are applied during excision of extremities.[30] This approach presents a challenge to even the experienced burn surgeon because the identification of the depth to excise to viable tissue is difficult to ascertain in the absence of capillary bleeding. Excision of the wound to the level of the fascia is associated with minimal blood loss and is used when wounds are deep full thickness, are infected, or when large areas are excised. The cosmetic results are poor and lymphatic drainage is impaired after this type of excision.

At the present time the ultimate closure of the excised wound requires the use of autograft. If sufficient donor sites are available, the preferred skin graft is a split-thickness au-

TABLE 12.3. Commonly Used Topical Antimicrobial Agents.

Agent	Wound dressing	Advantages	Disadvantages
Silver sulfadiazine	Open or light gauze	Soothing, optimal physical therapy, good antimicrobial	Does not penetrate eschar, possible neutropenia
Mafenide acetate cream	Open or light gauze	Penetrates eschar, optimal physical therapy, good antimicrobial activity	Painful, metabolic acidosis caused by inhibition of carbonic anhydrase
Mafenide acetate (5% solution)	Continuous moist bulky dressing	Good antimicrobial, use over skin grafts	Restricts physical therapy
Aqueous silver nitrate (0.5%)	Continuous moist bulky dressing	Good antimicrobial	Restricts physical therapy, stains wound, hyponatremia, docs not penetrate

tograft (0.008–0.01 in. thick). A thicker, full-thickness graft is preferred for cosmetic reconstruction and in areas where scarring would lead to functional compromise. However, this thickness of donor skin requires that the donor site be grafted. When donor sites are limited, autograft can be expanded by passing it through a mechanical meshing device that allows it to be enlarged up to six times the surface area of the original donor skin. For practical purposes the skin is not usually meshed to a size greater than three times the initial area.

Closure of the excised wound may be staged by temporary coverage with biological or manufactured dressings. Allograft provides for closure of the wound and also is often used as a test graft in areas where there is a concern for infection or when the adequacy of the excised wound bed is suspect. If an allograft is left in place for longer than 10 to 14 days, it becomes incorporated into the wound to the extent that the wound must be excised to remove it. In recent years a number of skin substitutes have been developed that replace the function of some or all layers of the skin. The advantage that these products offer for patients with large surface areas of injury is that donor sites are available in shorter time frames for recropping of epidermis for further grafting.

Circumferential Burns

A full-thickness circumferential burn injury carries with it the risk of compression of structures underneath the wound. In the extremities the combination of increased extravascular fluid in the wound and underlying tissues and the lack of elasticity of the burn wound can lead to subeschar pressures that compromise blood flow to viable tissue. All extremities with circumferential full-thickness burns should be elevated to minimize edema formation and should be evaluated hourly for signs of vascular compromise. The classic signs of pallor, pain, parasthesia, paralysis, and poikilothermia should be assessed. Because these signs are often difficult to evaluate in a burn-injured extremity, additional assessment of Doppler-measured blood flow in the distal extremity should be performed. Loss of Doppler signals may not be seen until after damage has occurred,[31] and therefore one should have a low threshold for performing an escharotomy to release subeschar pressure. An escharotomy is performed by making an incision through the eschar on the lateral surface of the extremity. An additional escharotomy may need to be performed on the medial surface as well. The preferred sites for escharotomy are indicated in Figure 12.3. Decompression of the hand should be performed when full-thickness burn injury of the hand leads to compromise of blood flow and function. Escharotomies are performed in fingers in the midaxial line on the ulnar side and on the radial side of the thumb so as to preserve tactile sensation of the surfaces of opposition of the fingers and thumb.

A circumferential full-thickness burn of the chest can compromise chest wall motion and cause a decrease in lung compliance. When this occurs, escharotomy of the chest in the anterior axillary line will often decrease the inspiratory pressures required to maintain tidal volume. If in addition there are circumferential full-thickness burns of the abdomen and back, an escharotomy following the costal margin may be necessary. Incision of the eschar may be performed with a scalpel but is often done with electrocautery so that minor bleeding can be controlled. Because full-thickness wounds are insensate and avascular, anesthesia is not necessary and these procedures may be performed under sterile conditions at the bedside.

Infection

General Aspects in Burn Injury

The systemic inflammatory response that is associated with a major burn ignites a cascade of events that presents a clinical syndrome which is difficult to distinguish from infection. These patients often have core body temperatures of 39° to 39.5°C, often develop an intestinal ileus, become disoriented, develop hyperglycemia, and sustain changes in fluid balance.

An increased susceptibility to infection related to the ex-

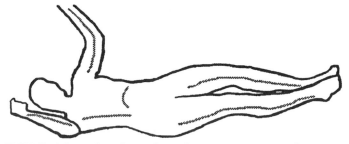

FIGURE 12.3. Preferred sites for escharotomy incisions. The patient should be in the anatomical position as depicted. The incisions are made in the lateral or medial aspect of the extremities.

tent of burn injury that has been noted clinically has been confirmed in animal models.[32] Polymorphonuclear leukocytes (PMNs) are activated and cytokines such as inteleukin-1-beta (IL-1-β), interleukin-6 (IL-6), and tumor necrosis factor-alpha (TNF-α) are elevated. The net result of activation of cells and mediator pathways appears to be indiscriminant recruitment of the normal pathways that maintain homeostasis, which leads to susceptibility of infection and distant organ and further local tissue injury.

Burn Wound Infection

In an attempt to standardize the evaluation and classification of infection in the wounds of the burn-injured patient, a subcommittee of the American Burn Association has recently provided a proposal for categorization of these infections.[33] Although these guidelines are open for comment at this time, they provide a foundation for describing the four categories of wound-related infection and are used here as a basis for describing the infections that occur in the patient with burn injury.

IMPETIGO

This infection "involves the loss of epithelium from a previously reepitheialized surface such as a grafted burn, a partial thickness burn allowed to heal by secondary intention, or a healed donor site."[33] This definition assumes that no other cause for epithelial loss is present such as mechanical damage, hematoma formation, or ischemia of the tissue. This infection, which has also been termed melting graft syndrome,[34] is not necessarily associated with systemic signs of fever or elevated white blood cell count. Although it is often caused by streptococcal or staphylococcal species, it may be caused by other organisms as well. In distinction to burn wound surface cultures, which give no insight into what is occurring in the wound, surface cultures are helpful in determining the organism that is the agent of these infections. Treatment consists of local care of the wound and systemic antibiotics.

OPEN SURGICAL WOUND INFECTION

These infections occur in wounds associated with surgical intervention that are not healed. As defined by the committee they may occur in an ungrafted excised burn or donor sites that have not healed and are associated with culture-positive purulent exudate. In addition, at least one of the following conditions is present:

1. Loss of synthetic or biological covering of the wound
2. Changes in wound appearance, such as hyperemia
3. Erythema in the uninjured skin surrounding the wound
4. Systemic signs, such as fever or leukocytosis

These infections require a change in local wound care, usually the addition of a topical antimicrobial, more frequent dressing changes, and the administration of systemic antibiotics.

CELLULITIS

The local inflammatory response to a burn injury is manifest at the margin of the wound as erythema. This finding is differentiated from cellulitis by its localized nature, usually less than 1 to 2 cm from the margin of the wound, and by its lack of extension beyond that zone. The guidelines suggest that in

addition to a requirement for antibiotic treatment the definition of cellulitis requires at least one of the following:

1. Localized pain, tenderness, swelling, or heat at the affected site
2. Systemic signs of infection, such as hyperemia, leukocytosis, or septicemia
3. Progression of erythema and swelling
4. Signs of lymphangitis, lymphadenitis, or both

INVASIVE INFECTION

The diagnosis of invasive burn wound infection rests on the recognition of changes in the wound, which include discoloration of the wound, maceration, or early separation of eschar and systemic manifestations of infection. In addition to the clinical assessment of the wound, biopsy may be performed for quantitative culture or histological evaluation. When more than 100,000 organisms are cultured from a gram of tissue it has been held that invasive wound infection is present.[35] Histological evaluation, although not readily available at most institutions, is diagnostic for invasive infection when organisms are identified in viable tissue.[36] Invasive wound infection requires surgical excision of the wound to the level of viable tissue and administration of systemic antibiotics. The topical antimicrobials, with the exception of Sulfamylon, which may be used in preparation for excision, are not used for therapy for invasive burn wound infection because they do not penetrate eschar.

The criteria for definition of invasive infection as outlined in the guidelines may be associated with these conditions:

1. Inflammation of the surrounding uninjured skin
2. Histological examination that shows invasion of the infectious organism into adjacent viable tissue
3. An organism that can be isolated from a blood culture in the absence of other infection
4. Systemic infection such as hyperthermia, hypothermia, leukocytosis, tachypnea, hypotension, oliguria, or hyperglycemia at a previously tolerated level of dietary carbohydrate, or mental confusion

Pneumonia

The advent of effective topical antimicrobials for prevention and therapy of wound infection along with earlier surgical intervention in wound care has led to a decrease in the incidence of wound infection, and respiratory failure is now the leading cause of death in the patient with thermal injury.[37] The presence of white blood cells and bacteria in the sputum associated with other signs of infection should prompt the initiation of systemic antimicrobials that will address the organisms which predominate in the flora of the unit at the time. Specific antimicrobials are then selected when culture reports are available.

Suppurative Thrombophlebitis

Bacterial colonization of venous catheters in patients in intensive care units[38] and in particular of central catheters in the burn-injured patient has been reported to be as high as 25%.[39]

The reason for concern especially in burn-injured individuals is that suppurative thrombophlebitis can be an insidious and life-threatening infection.[40] The only findings may be persistent fever and a bacteremia that continues during appropriate antibiotic treatment. The classic findings of edema, erythema, pain, and a palpable cord at an intravenous site that are associated with phlebitis may not be identifiable. Diagnosis is confirmed by aspiration of purulent material from the affected vein, and treatment consists of excision of the involved vein to the point that the vessel is normal where bleeding is encountered.[41,42]

Suppurative Chondritis

Infection of the external ear that has sustained a partial- or full-thickness injury can lead to loss of integrity of the entire ear.[43,44] The cartilage of the ear has minimal protection and blood supply and is highly susceptible to infection when the overlying tissue is damaged. Dressings should not be applied to the ear, and pillows should not be used. Auricular burns should be treated with twice-daily open wound care and gently debrided. The topical of choice is mefanide acetate because it penetrates eschar and avascular cartilage. When suppurative chondritis occurs, systemic antibiotics are of little value due to the avascular nature of the tissue,[45] and the ear must be surgically drained under anesthesia by bivalving of the ear with excision of infected and necrotic tissue.

Bacteremia Associated with Wound Manipulation

It is anticipated that debridement and surgical excision of the burn wound will lead to bacteremia; however, the data to support such an occurrence are not consistent. Nevertheless, bacteremia related to burn care, especially in patients with a large burn injury who have colonization of or infection in their wounds, may seed distant sites such as cardiac valves or the brain,[46] and it is likely that in this population of patients perioperative administration of antibiotics which will treat the flora of the wound will be of benefit.

Other Infections

Just as in any seriously injured patient, the associated immunocompromise may set the stage for infection at any site. These patients have a high incidence of urinary tract infections and pneumonia.[47] They also develop other infections such as appendicitis acute calculus cholecystitis, and diverticulitis but often do not present with classic features due to the lack of the normal inflammatory response. A high index of suspicion is necessary to detect these infections. Additional infections of concern in the burn-injured patient include sinusitis and bacterial endocarditis.

Hypermetabolism and Nutrition

The classic description of the metabolic response to injury includes an early ebb phase that is characterized by low cardiac output and a decreased metabolic rate followed by a hypermetabolic phase that starts at 24 to 36 h after injury. In the patient with thermal injury, the increase in metabolic rate may often exceed the resting energy expenditure (REE) by twofold.[48] Studies indicate that there is a wide variation in metabolic rate among patients and that the hypermetabolism associated with thermal injury may persist well beyond wound closure. Patients with large burns often do not return to a normal metabolic rate until weeks or months after the burn wound is closed.[49] Most clinicians advocate the use of a formula such as that of Curreri or the Harris–Benedict equation adjusted with a stress factor, but in patients with large injury or who sustain complications the metabolic rate should be measured by indirect calorimetry.

Because of losses in the wound, muscle breakdown, and increased demands for healing of the wound, the patient with thermal injury has a requirement for protein replacement that is proportionately greater than that for calories. Protein administration should be two to three times greater than the normal requirement of 0.8 g/kg/day or 2.0 to 2.5 g/kg/day. This amount can be provided in relation to the estimated or measured calorie needs by providing a nonprotein calorie to nitrogen ratio of 100 to 150:1.[50]

Prognosis

Survival after burn injury has improved significantly during the past 20 years[51] and appears to have reached a plateau over the past 10 years. Multiple studies have confirmed that patient age and extent of injury are the two most powerful predictors of outcome.[51–53] Studies from the current decade suggest that the overall mortality rate in burn centers is approximately 4%.[54] These data also confirm the significant contribution of inhalation injury in that the mortality rate was 25% to 35% in the presence of this injury and only 0.5% to 4% in its absence.

Rehabilitation

Advances in medical care leading to increased survival from thermal injury have led to a renewed emphasis on quality of life after these injuries. Rehabilitation of the patient with a burn injury begins from the time of initial medical care, requires intense care in the first year after injury, and often is lifelong. Splinting of injured extremities begins as soon as the patient is stabilized, and range-of-motion exercises begin within the first day. The team approach is important to coordinate therapy, surgical intervention, and medical care. As soon as wounds have a stable epidermal closure, usually within 2 weeks after grafting or primary healing has occurred, attention is turned to wound and scar management. Garments that apply pressure to the wounds are tailormade for the patient and worn 24 h per day. Surgical intervention for cosmetic deformity is usually delayed until the wound is mature, as is intervention for functional restriction, unless a surgical procedure is necessary to allow for physical therapy.

References

1. Brigham PA, McLoughlin E. Burn incidence and medical care use in the United States: estimates, trends, and data sources. J Burn Care Rehabil 1996;17:95–107.
2. Advanced Trauma Life Support Manual. Chicago: American College of Surgeons, 1997.
3. Miller SF, Finley RK, Waltman M, et al. Burn size estimate reliability: a study. J Burn Care Rehabil 1991;12:546–559.

4. Heimbach DM, Afromowitz MA, Engrav LH, et al. Burn depth estimation—man or machine. J Trauma 1984;24:373–377.

5. Jackson D. The diagnosis of the depth of burning. Br J Surg 1953;40:588–596.

6. Goodwin CW, Finkelstein JL, Madden MR. Burns. In: Schwartz SI, Shires GT, Spencer FC, et al., eds. Principles of Surgery. New York: McGraw-Hill, 1994:265–268.

7. Lee RC. Injury by electrical forces: pathophysiology, manifestations, and therapy. Curr Probl Surg 1997;34:677–764.

8. Arrowsmith J, Usgaocar RP, Dickson WA. Electrical injury and the frequency of cardiac complications. Burns 1997;23:576–578.

9. Goodwin CW. Electrical injury. In: Wyngaarden JB, Smith LH Jr, Bennet JC, eds. Cecil Textbook of Medicine. Philadelphia: Saunders, 1992:2356.

10. Haberal M, Bayraktar U, Oner Z, et al. Visceral injuries, wound infection and sepsis following electrical injuries. Burns 1996;22:158–161.

11. Ratnayake B, Emmanuel ER, Walker CC. Neurologic sequelae following a high voltage electrical burn. Burns 1996;22:574–577.

12. Mathes SJ, Alexander J. Radiation injury. Surg Oncol Clin N Am 1996;5:809–824.

13. Madden MR, Finkelstein JL, Goodwin CW. Respiratory care of the burn patient. Clin Plast Surg 1986;13:29–38.

14. Pruitt BA Jr, Cioffi WG, Shimazu T, et al. Evaluation and management of patients with inhalation injury. J Trauma 1990;30:S63–S68.

15. Zikria BA, Ferrer JM, Floch HF. The chemical factors contributing to pulmonary damage in "smoke poisoning." Surgery (St. Louis) 1972;71:704–709.

16. Kramer GC, Herndon DN, Linares HA, et al. Effects of inhalation injury on airway blood flow and edema. J Burn Care Rehabil 1989;10:45–51.

17. Shirani KZ, Pruitt BA Jr, Mason AD. The influence of inhalation injury and pneumonia on burn mortality. Ann Surg 1986;205:82–87.

18. Agee RN, Long JM III, Hunt JL, et al. Use of 133 xenon in early diagnosis of inhalation injury. J Trauma 1976;16:218–224.

19. Levine BA, Petroff PA, Slade CL, et al. Prospective trials of dexamethasone and aerosolized gentamycin in the treatment of inhalation injury in the burned patient. J Trauma 1978;18:188–193.

20. Treat RC, Sirinek KR, Levine BA, et al. Air evacuation of thermally injured patients: principles of treatment and results. J Trauma 1980;20:275–279.

21. Goodwin CW, Dorethy J, Lam V, et al. Randomized trial of efficacy of crystalloid and colloid resuscitation on hemodynamic response and lung water following thermal injury. Ann Surg 1983;197:520–531.

22. Shirani KZ, Vaughan GM, Mason AD, et al. Update on current therapeutic approaches in burns. Shock 1996;5:4–16.

23. Morehouse JD, Finkelstein JL, Marano MA, et al. Resuscitation of the thermally injured patient. Crit Care Clin 1992;8:355–365.

24. Baxter CR, Shires T. Physiologic response to crystalloid resuscitation of severe burns. Ann NY Acad Sci 1968;150:874–894.

25. Baxter CR. Fluid volume and electrolyte changes in the early postburn period. Clin Plast Surg 1974;1:693–703.

26. Pruitt BA Jr. The effectiveness of fluid resuscitation. J Trauma 1979;19:868–870.

27. Graves TA, Cioffi WG, McManus WF, et al. Fluid resuscitation of infants and children with massive thermal injury. J Trauma 1988;28:1656–1659.

28. Graudins A, Burns MJ, Aaron CK. Regional intravenous infusion of calcium gluconate for hyrofluoric acid burns of the upper extremity. Ann Emerg Med 1997;30:604–607.

29. Pruitt BA Jr, McManus AT. The changing epidemiology of infections in burn patients. World J Surg 1992;16:57–67.

30. Marano MA, O'Sullivan G, Madden M, et al. Tourniquet technique for reduced blood loss and wound assessment during excisions of burn wounds of the extremity. Surg Gynecol Obstet 1990;171:249–250.

31. Clayton JM, Russell HE, Hartford CE, et al. Sequential circulatory changes in the circumferentially burned limb. Ann Surg 1977;185:391–396.

32. Yurt RW, McManus AT, Mason AD Jr, et al. Increased susceptibility to infection related to extent of injury. Arch Surg 1984;119:183–188.

33. Peck MD, Weber J, McManus A, et al. Surveillance of burn wound infections: a proposal for definitions. J Burn Care Rehabil 1998;19:386–389.

34. Matsumura H, Meyer NA, Mann R, et al. Melting graft-wound syndrome. J Burn Care Rehabil 1998;19:292–295.

35. Teplitz C. The pathology of burns and the fundamentals of burn wound sepsis. In: Artz CP, Moncrief JA, Pruitt BA Jr, eds. Burns: A Team Approach. Philadelphia: Saunders, 1979.

36. Pruitt BA Jr, Foley DF. The use of biopsies in burn patient care. Surgery (St. Louis) 1973;73:887–897.

37. Pruitt BA Jr, Flemma RJ, DiVencenti FC, et al. Pulmonary complications in burn patients. J Thorac Cardiovasc Surg 1970;59:7–20.

38. Samsoondar W, Freeman JB, Coultish I, et al. Colonization of intravascular catheters in the intensive care unit. Am J Surg 1985;149:730–732.

39. Still JM, Law E, Thiruvaiyaru D, Belcher K, et al. Central line-related sepsis in acute burn patients. Am Surg 1998;64(2):165–170.

40. Pruitt BA Jr, McManus WF, Kim SH, et al. Diagnosis and treatment of cannula-related intravenous sepsis in burn patients. Ann Surg 1980;191:546–554.

41. Graham C, Hair A. Suppurative thrombophlebitis. Br J Hosp Med 1995;54(2–3):115.

42. Khan EA, Correa AG, Baker CJ. Suppurative thrombophlebitis in children: a ten-year experience. Pediatr Infect Dis J 1997;16(1):63–67.

43. Bentrem DJ, Bill TJ, Himel HN, et al. Chondritis of the ear: a late sequelae of deep partial thickness burns of the face. J Emerg Med 1996;14:469–471.

44. Skedros DG, Goldfard IW, Slater H, Rocco J. Chondritis of the burned ear: a review. Ear Nose Throat J 1992;71(8):359–362.

45. Mills DC II, Roberts LW, Mason AD Jr, et al. Suppurative chondritis: its incidence, prevention, and treatment in burn patients. Plas Reconstr Surg 1988;82(2):267–276.

46. Suzuki T, Ueki I, Isago T, et al. Multiple brain abscesses complicating treatment of a severe burn injury: an unusual case report. J Burn Care Rehabil 1992;13(4):446–450.

47. Weber JM, Sheridan RL, Pasternack MS, et al. Nosocomial infections in pediatric patients with burns. Am J Infect Control 1997;25:195–201.

48. Wilmore DW, Long JM, Mason AD, et al. Catecholamines: mediator of the hypermetabolic response to thermal injury. Ann Surg 1974;180:653–669.

49. Saffle JR, Medina E, Raymond J, et al. Use of indirect calorimetry in the nutritional management of burned patients. J Trauma 1985;25:32–39.

50. Rodriguez DJ. Nutrition in major burn patients: state of the art. J Burn Care Rehabil 1996;17:62–70.

51. Tompkins RG, Burke JF, Schoenfeld DA, et al. Prompt eschar excision: a treatment system contributing to reduced burn mortality: a statistical evaluation of burn care at the Massachusetts General Hospital (1974–1984). Ann Surg 1986;204:272–281.

52. Pruitt BA Jr, Tumbusch WT, Mason AD Jr, et al. Mortality in 1,100 consecutive burns treated at a burns unit. Ann Surg 1964;159:396–401.

53. Curreri PW, Luterman A, Braun DW, et al. Burn injury: analysis of survival and hospitalization time for 937 patients. Ann Surg 1980;192:472–476.

54. Monafo WW. Initial management of burns. N Engl J Med 1996;335:1581–1586.

13

Perioperative Management

Philip S. Barie

Defining the Perioperative Period

The preoperative period begins when it is decided that a patient needs surgery. This period may extend for the few minutes that it takes to get a trauma patient to the operating room, or for several weeks if multiple or complex comorbid factors must be addressed in preparation. The postoperative period is more defined, albeit arbitrarily. Traditionally, the postoperative period has extended for 30 days after surgery, and operative mortality and complication rates are generally reported using that criterion.

Who Should Provide Perioperative Care?

Traditionally, perioperative care was provided by the patient's surgeon with consultative assistance by the primary care physician. The primacy of the surgeon in directing perioperative care was emphasized. Nowadays, nontraditional practitioners such as hospitalists, advanced practice nurses, physician assistants and critical care intensivists have largely assumed the role of "primary" caregiver.

In a true open ICU model, all patient care decisions are made by the primary team. Continuity of care is assured, and surgical residents receive the direct patient care experience requisite to their training. In a true closed ICU model, decisions regarding triage and therapy become the responsibility of the ICU service. In academic centers, the ICU team is most often composed of surgeons and sometimes anesthesiologists, but in other circumstances it becomes a nonsurgical team in charge. In effect, the operating surgeon becomes a consultant on his or her own patient, but involved subspecialty consultants are fewer. This model is effective for cost-containment initiatives[2,3] and highly concentrated educational activities. Communication is often facilitated, which is a positive attribute of high-quality units.[4,5] Data indicate that the closed ICU model may provide superior and cost-effective patient care.[6–8]

The status of perioperative care is in flux, as is the even thornier issue of whether complex or rarely performed operations should be undertaken outside specialized centers.[9,10] For surgeons to maintain a central role in perioperative care, they are well advised to exert leadership rather than to assert ownership.

Outcomes Assessment

Increasingly, a good surgical outcome is defined by the quality of life enjoyed by the patient after surgery.[11] Surgical results reporting must extend beyond the hospital portal. These types of quality endpoints will be incorporated increasingly into clinical research and quality audits, and therefore clinicians must be familiar with the administration and interpretation of these types of studies.

Preoperative Cardiovascular Assessment

More than 3 million patients with coronary artery disease undergo surgery each year in the United States. Among them, 50,000 patients sustain a perioperative myocardial infarction (MI). The incidence may be increasing because of an aging population. Overall mortality for perioperative MI remains nearly 40%. Aortic and peripheral vascular surgery, orthopedic surgery, and major intrathoracic and intraperitoneal procedures are more frequently associated with perioperative cardiac mortality than are other types of surgery. Absent a history of heart disease, men are at increased risk above 35 years of age, whereas women are at increased risk after age 40. Cardiac mortality risk increases markedly in patients over age 70. Cigarette smoking also confers increased risk.

A recent MI is the single most important risk factor for perioperative infarction (Table 13.1). The risk is greatest within the early aftermath following an infarction, probably the first 30 days. Estimates of the risk of anesthesia following an MI range as high as a 27% reinfarction rate within 3 months, 11% between 3 and 6 months, and 5% after a 6-month interval. Patients who suffer subendocardial (non-Q-wave) infarctions appear to be at identical risk. However, cardiac risk management strategies may be succeeding. With intraoperative invasive hemodynamic monitoring, the risk may be reduced to as low as 6% within 3 months of the first MI, and only 2% incidence within 3 to 6 months. Elective surgery should be postponed for 6 months following an acute MI. When major emergency surgery is necessary, it should be performed with full hemodynamic monitoring. When operation is urgent, as for a potentially resectable malignant tumor, it can be undertaken from 4 to 6 weeks after infarction if the patient has had an uncomplicated recent course and the results of noninvasive stress testing are favorable.

The cardiac risk index system (CRIS) is an accepted system that was developed from a cohort of patients aged 40 years or more who underwent noncardiac surgery.[12] Risk classes (I–IV) are assigned on the basis of accumulated points (Table 13.2). According to CRIS, any elective operation is contraindicated if the patient falls within class IV. One benefit of CRIS is that more than one-half of the total points are potentially controllable (treating CHF reduces the score by 11 points, delaying surgery for a recent MI, 10 points, and so on) for the avoidance of emergency surgery or improvement of the overall medical status. Further study of coronary artery disease (CAD) serves primarily to quantify risk in patients with identified risk factors. Whether patients with no cardiac risk factors should undergo additional preoperative testing is still debated. Algorithms from the American College of Cardiology/American Heart Association Task Force on Practice Guidelines can be used to guide the evaluation (Fig. 13.1–13.3).[13]

Adjustment of Cardiovascular Medications

Congestive heart failure, poorly controlled hypertension (diastolic blood pressure >110 mmHg), and diabetes must be stabilized before an elective procedure is undertaken. In general, cardiovascular medications should be continued through the perioperative period. Continuation of antihypertensive therapy throughout the perioperative period does not contribute to hemodynamic instability, although the data are conflicting as to whether continuation of antihypertensive therapy actually decreases morbidity. Discontinuation of antihypertensive therapy does pose potential hazards. Rebound hypertension may be precipitated when centrally acting α_2-adrenergic agonists (e.g., clonidine) are withheld abruptly. Congestive heart failure may recur if angiotensin-converting enzyme inhibitors are withheld. Diuretic therapy may cause hypovolemia or hypokalemia, but neither problem poses major difficulties if recognized and treated. There is widespread agreement that β-adrenergic blockade should not be discon-

TABLE 13.1. Risk Stratification Parameters and Criteria for Cardiac Events Following Noncardiac Surgery.

Parameter	Low risk	Intermediate risk	High risk
Clinical characteristic	Advanced age	Mild angina	Myocardial infarction within previous 7–30 days
	Abnormal ECG (LVH, LBBB, ST-T abnormalities)	Prior myocardial infarction	Unstable or severe angina
	Atrial fibrillation or other nonsinus rhythm	Previous or compensated congestive heart failure	
	Low functional capacity (climb <1 flight stairs with bag of groceries)	Diabetes mellitus	
	Hypertension		
	History of stroke		
Type of operation (partial list) Low: <1% cardiac risk; High: >5% cardiac risk.	Endoscopic procedures	Carotid endarterectomy	Emergent major surgery
	Skin or skin structure operation (i.e., groin hernia, breast procedure)	Head and neck procedure	Aortic and other major vascular procedures, including peripheral procedures
	Cataract excision	Intraabdominal procedures	Long procedures/major fluid shifts or blood loss
		Intrathoracic procedures	
		Orthopedic surgery	
		Prostate surgery	
Characteristics of ECG stress test (i.e., treadmill)	No ischemia	Ischemia at moderate-level exercise (heart rate 100–130)	Ischemia at low-level exercise (heart rate <100)
	Ischemia only at high-level exercise (heart rate >130)		
	ST depression >0.1 mV	ST depression >0.1 mV	ST depression >0.1 mV
	Typical angina	Typical angina	Typical angina
	One or two abnormal leads	Three or four abnormal leads	Five or more abnormal leads
		Persistent ischemia 1–3 min after exercise	Persistent ischemia >3 min after exercise

TABLE 13.2. Cardiac Risk Index System (CRIS).

Factors	Points
History	
Age >70 years	5
Myocardial infarction <6 months ago	10
Aortic stenosis	3
Physical examination	
S_3 gallop, jugular venous distension, or congestive heart failure	11
Bedridden	3
Laboratory	
PO_2 <60 mmHg	3
PCO_2 >50 mmHg	3
Potassium <3 mEq/dl	3
Blood urine nitrogen >50 mg/dl	3
Creatinine >3 mg/dl	3
Operation	
Emergency	4
Intrathoracic	3
Intraabdominal	3
Aortic	3

Approximate cardiac risk (percent incidence of major complications):

	Class[a]				
	Baseline	I	II	III	IV
Minor surgery	1	0.3	1	3	19
Major noncardiac surgery, age >40 years	4	1	4	12	48
Abdominal aortic surgery, or age >40 with other characteristics	10	3	10	30	75

[a]CRIS class I, 0–5 points; class II, 6–12 points; class III, 13–25 points; class IV, ≥26 points.

Source: Adapted from Goldman et al.[12]

tinued abruptly. Abrupt discontinuation may be associated with a hyperadrenergic withdrawal syndrome characterized by unstable angina, tachyarrhythmias, MI, or sudden death.

Current ACC/AHA recommendations are to screen for MI in patients without evidence of CAD only if signs of cardiovascular dysfunction develop. For patients with CAD undergoing high-risk operations, an ECG at baseline, immediately postoperatively, and daily for the first 2 postoperative days (POD) should be obtained. Measurements of cardiac enzymes are best reserved for patients at high risk or those who demonstrate ECG or hemodynamic evidence of myocardial dysfunction.[13] Two recent studies suggested that both short- and long-term survival can be improved by β-adrenergic blockade for patients who undergo noncardiac surgery.[14,15]

Continuation of calcium channel antagonists in the perioperative period has been controversial. Rebound phenomena associated with abrupt drug discontinuance are less common than with β-blockers, but patients receiving combined therapy with β-adrenergic and calcium channel blockers are at increased risk of conduction abnormalities and depressed ventricular function. Digoxin therapy for chronic CHF, particularly with complicating supraventricular tachyarrhythmias, should be continued through the perioperative period.

Preoperative Preparation in the Intensive Care Unit

The practice of preoperative admission to the ICU for final preparation for surgery is falling out of favor and is infrequently done.

Preoperative Pulmonary Evaluation

In patients with a history of lung disease or those for whom a pulmonary resection is contemplated, preoperative assessment of pulmonary function is of value. Late postoperative pulmonary complications are leading causes of morbidity and mortality after surgery, second only to cardiac complications as im-

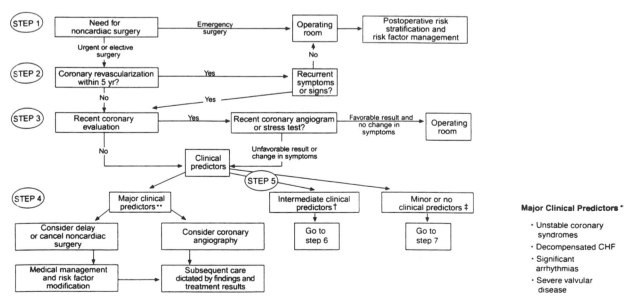

FIGURE 13.1. American College of Cardiology/American Heart Association Guideline algorithm for evaluation of cardiac risk before noncardiac surgery. Patients with major clinical predictors of risk may have to have surgery postponed or cancelled, or undergo an invasive evaluation. See Table 19.3 for additional information. (Reprinted from Eagle KA, Brundage BH, Chaitman BR, et al. Guide-

lines for perioperative cardiovascular evaluation for noncardiac surgery. Report of the American College of Cardiology/American Heart Association Task Force on Practice Guidelines (Committee on Perioperative Cardiovascular Evaluation for Noncardiac Surgery). J Am Coll Cardiol 1996;27:910–948, with permission.[13])

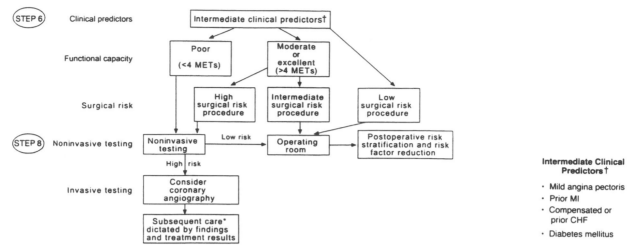

FIGURE 13.2. American College of Cardiology/American Heart Association Guideline algorithm for evaluation of cardiac risk before noncardiac surgery. Patients with intermediate clinical predictors of risk or who are about to undergo high-risk surgery may have to have noninvasive testing before surgery. See Table 13.3 for additional information. Four metabolic equivalents (METs) are equivalent to climbing one flight of stairs with a bag of groceries. (Reprinted from Eagle KA, Brundage BH, Chaitman BR, et al. Guidelines for perioperative cardiovascular evaluation for noncardiac surgery. Report of the American College of Cardiology/American Heart Association Task Force on Practice Guidelines (Committee on Perioperative Cardiovascular Evaluation for Noncardiac Surgery). J Am Coll Cardiol 1996;27:910–948, with permission.[13])

mediate causes of death. Prolonged postoperative decreases in functional residual capacity (FRC) and forced vital capacity (FVC) are associated with atelectasis, decreased pulmonary compliance, increased work of breathing, and tachypnea at low tidal volumes. Poor cough effort and impaired airway reflexes increase the susceptibility of postoperative patients to retained secretions, bacterial invasion, and pneumonia. Upper abdominal and thoracic incisions, increased operative time, increased severity of underlying pulmonary disease (COPD or chronic bronchitis), cigarette smoking, and poor preoperative nutrition are independent risk factors for major pulmonary morbidity.

Although the value of the routine, perioperative chest radiograph has been discounted, it may be of value for dyspneic patients with underlying lung disease or to serve as a basis for comparison. Radiographic indicators of possible airflow obstruction include depression of the right hemidiaphragm at or below the seventh rib anteriorly on a conventional posteroanterior view, a cardiac silhouette with a transverse dimension less than 11.5 cm, and a retrosternal air space greater than 4.4 cm on a lateral view. Substantive airflow obstruction may be associated with a normal X-ray.

Most laboratory studies are of little benefit for prediction in chronic lung disease. A room air arterial oxygen tension (PaO$_2$) less than 60 mmHg correlates with pulmonary hyper-

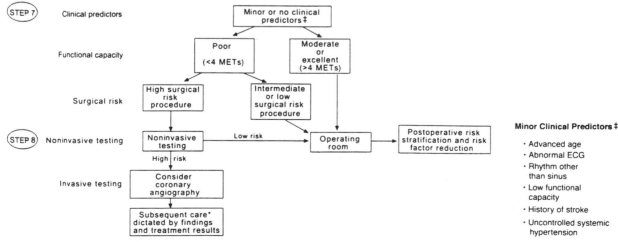

FIGURE 13.3. American College of Cardiology/American Heart Association Guideline algorithm for evaluation of cardiac risk before noncardiac surgery. Patients with minor or no clinical who are about to undergo high-risk surgery may have to have noninvasive testing before surgery. See Table 19.3 for additional information. Four metabolic equivalents (METs) are equivalent to climbing one flight of stairs with a bag of groceries. (Reprinted from Eagle KA, Brundage BH, Chaitman BR, et al. Guidelines for perioperative cardiovascular evaluation for noncardiac surgery. Report of the American College of Cardiology/American Heart Association Task Force on Practice Guidelines (Committee on Perioperative Cardiovascular Evaluation for Noncardiac Surgery). J Am Coll Cardiol 1996;27:910–948, with permission.[13])

tension, whereas a $PaCO_2$ greater than 45 mmHg is associated with increased perioperative morbidity. Spirometry before and after bronchodilators is simple and safe to obtain. Analysis of forced expiratory volume in 1 s (FEV_1) and FVC usually provides sufficient information for clinical decision making. Dyspnea is assumed to occur when FEV_1 is less than 2 l, whereas an FEV_1 less than 50% of the predicted value correlates with exertional dyspnea. For abdominal surgery, there is no indication for evaluation beyond spirometry and arterial blood gas analysis.

Objective data of good quality that document improved outcome from the provision of preoperative pulmonary toilet are scant. Pulmonary toilet probably accomplishes more by educating the patient about perioperative care and engendering a cooperative attitude about chest physiotherapy than by actually improving gas exchange. Chronic bronchodilator therapy should be continued through the perioperative period. Cessation of cigarette smoking is very important for those who smoke more than 10 cigarettes per day. Short-term abstinence (48 h) decreases the carboxyhemoglobin concentration to that of a nonsmoker, abolishes the effects of nicotine on the cardiovascular system, and improves mucosal ciliary function. Sputum volume decreases after 1 to 2 weeks of abstinence, and spirometry improves after about 6 weeks of abstinence.

Prophylaxis of Venous Thromboembolism

The morbidity and mortality of venous thromboembolism make consideration of prophylaxis mandatory for every major operation. A number of risk factors have been identified (Table 13.3). The risk of a venous thromboembolic complication is increased by the number of defined risk factors that the patient has (Table 13.4).[16] Many prophylactic regimens have proven efficacy for patients at moderate to high risk, and the morbidity is acceptable[17]; therefore, standard regimens are employed increasingly for virtually all patients (Tables 13.4, 13.5). Table 13.6 compares the effectiveness of these different modalities.

Evaluation of the Risk of Bleeding

Evaluation of the patient's risk of bleeding requires a careful history and physical assessment if the evaluation is to be cost-effective, because the yield of positive findings from routine screening tests of hemostasis is low. Historical information of importance includes whether the patient or a family member has had a prior episode of bleeding or a thromboembolic event, and whether the patient has a history of prior transfusions, prior surgery, heavy menstrual bleeding, easy bruising, frequent nosebleeds, or bleeding gums after brushing the teeth. Coexistent liver or kidney disease, poor dietary habits, excessive ingestion of alcohol, ingestion of aspirin, other nonsteroidal antiinflammatory drugs, or lipid-lowering drugs (possible vitamin K deficiency), and anticoagulant therapy (usually warfarin) must be ascertained. Answers to these questions should uncover most potential problems with hemostasis. If the history is completely negative and the patient has had a previous hemostatic challenge from surgery or trauma, then an important hemostatic defect is extremely unlikely. A mild coagulopathy in the previously unchallenged patient is not excluded; however, the consequences once such a mild defect is unmasked can be managed readily. If a clinically important coagulopathy is identified, therapeutic strategies for management of various coagulation disorders in preparation for surgery are listed in Table 13.7.

Management of the Therapeutically Anticoagulated Patient

It is often necessary to perform elective or emergency surgery on an anticoagulated patient. In such circumstances

TABLE 13.3. Risk Factors[a] for the Development of Venous Thromboembolism in the Perioperative Period.

General	Hematological
Age	Activated protein C resistance (factor V Leiden mutation)
Cancer	Antiphospholipid antibody
Congestive heart failure	Antithrombin III deficiency
Estrogen therapy	Disorders of plasminogen/plasminogen activation
Fracture of pelvis, hip, or leg	Dysfibrinogenemia
Indwelling femoral vein catheter	Heparin-associated thrombocytopenia
Inflammatory bowel disease	Hyperviscosity syndromes
Major surgery (abdomen, pelvis, lower extremity)	Homocysteinemia
Myocardial infarction	Lupus anticoagulant
Nephrotic syndrome	Myeloproliferative disorders
Obesity	Protein C deficiency
Prior venous thromboembolic disease	Thrombocytosis
Prolonged immobility; paralysis	
Stroke	
Varicose veins	

[a]Patients may have multiple risk factors. If multiple factors are present, the risk is cumulative.

Source: Adapted from Clagett et al.[16]

TABLE 13.4. Risk Stratification Scheme and Incidence of Venous Thromboembolic Events.

Event	Low (no risk factors)	Moderate (any surgery, age 40–60; major surgery age <40; no other risks)	High (major surgery, age >60, no risk factors; major surgery age >40 with risk)	Very high (Major surgery at age >40 with major risk factors [VTE, cancer, coagulopathy, elective lower-extremity surgery, hip fracture, stroke, multiple trauma, spinal cord injury])
			Level of risk (% incidence)	
Calf vein thrombosis	2	10–20	20–40	40–80
Proximal deep venous thrombosis	0.4	2–4	4–8	10–20
Clinical pulmonary embolism	0.2	1–2	2–4	4–10
Fatal pulmonary embolism	0.002	0.1–0.4	0.4–1.0	1–5
Prevention strategies	None needed	LDUH q 12 h LMWH IPC	LDUH q 8 h LMWH IPC	LMWH Warfarin IPC plus a heparinoid Intravenous adjusted-dose heparin Vena cava interruption

VTE, venous thromboembolism; LDUH, low-dose unfractionated heparin; LMWH, low molecular weight heparin; IPC, intermittent pneumatic compression device.

Source: Adapted from Clagett et al.[16] and Palmer et al.[17]

TABLE 13.5.

Summary of Evidence-Based Guidelines for Prevention of Venous Thromboembolic Disease in Surgical Patients from Fifth American College of Chest Physicians Consensus Conference on Antithrombotic Therapy, 1998.

General Surgery

Level I: In moderate-risk patients, it is recommended that low-dose unfractionated heparin, low molecular weight heparin, an intermittent pneumatic compression device, or graded-compression elastic stockings be used.

In high-risk patients, it is recommended that low-dose unfractionated heparin in higher dosage or low molecular weight heparin be used for prophylaxis. For patients at high risk for wound complications such as hematoma or infection, an intermittent pneumatic compression device is a good alternative.

Aspirin is not recommended for prophylaxis because other measures are more efficacious.

Level II: In very high risk patients, it is recommended that low-dose unfractionated heparin or low molecular weight heparin be combined with an intermittent pneumatic compression device. For selected patients, warfarin (international normalized ratio 2.0–3.0) may be used.

Level III: For low-risk patients, no specific prophylaxis is recommended other than early ambulation.

Total Hip Replacement

Level I: In patients undergoing hip replacement surgery, prophylaxis with low molecular weight heparin should begin 12–24 h before surgery, or warfarin (international normalized ratio, 2.0–3.0) should be started preoperatively or immediately after surgery, or adjusted-dose heparin should be started preoperatively. Adjuvant prophylaxis with intermittent pneumatic compression or graded-compression elastic stockings may provide additional protection. Low-dose unfractionated heparin, aspirin, dextran, and intermittent pneumatic compression alone are less effective and are not recommended.

In patients undergoing elective knee replacement surgery, low molecular weight heparin, warfarin, or intermittent pneumatic compression should be used for prophylaxis.

The optimal duration of prophylaxis is uncertain. Abundant data suggest that a 7- to 10-day duration of prophylaxis is appropriate. Emerging data suggest that a 29- to 35-day duration of prophylaxis may confer additional protection, but additional data are needed.

Routine screening with duplex ultrasonography is not recommended after hip or knee replacement surgery in asymptomatic patients.

Source: Adapted from Clagett et al.[16]

TABLE 13.6. Effectiveness of Various Modalities for Risk Reduction in Prophylaxis of Perioperative Deep Venous Thrombosis.

Modality	General surgery			Total hip replacement		
	n	Incidence (%)	Risk reduction (%)	n	Incidence (%)	Risk reduction (%)
Controls	54	25		13	51	
LDUH	53	8	−68	10	31	−39
LMWH	17	7	−72	20	11	−78
Warfarin	2	10	−60	7	22	−57
Dextran	11	18	−28	5	30	−41
Aspirin	5	10	−60	7	52	None
IPC device	5	10	−64	4	22	−57

LDUH, low-dose unfractionated heparin; LMWH, low molecular weight heparin; IPC, intermittent pneumatic compression device; n, number of studies reviewed; 95% CI, 95% confidence intervals for the incidence.

Source: Data extracted from Claggett et al.[16]

it is desirable to reverse the patient's anticoagulation temporarily so that hemostasis can be optimized. Most patients who take warfarin and who are to undergo ambulatory or same-day admission elective surgery can be managed simply by having them discontinue their warfarin for several days before surgery. The timing of the medication adjustment depends on the degree of anticoagulation determined by preoperative testing, which in turn depends on the indication for the anticoagulation. For example, a patient with a valve prosthesis can be maintained chronically at an international normalized ratio (INR) of 2.5 to 3.0. If there is concern that the patient should not be without anticoagulation, the patient can be heparinized systemically with an infusion of unfractionated heparin or placed on LMWH. The heparin infusion is discontinued approximately 4 h preoperatively (the half-life of heparin is about 90 min), and surgery proceeds with good hemostasis. However, data are insufficient to provide a definitive recommendation in the circumstance of LMWH.

TABLE 13.7. Preoperative Management of Selected Coagulation Disorders.

Diagnosis		Treatment
Factor deficiencies		
Hemophilia A:	Mild, factor VIII >10%	Desmopressin, 0.3 mg/kg i.v. q 12–24 h × 5–7 days for minor surgery.
	Severe	Factor VIII concentrate (level 50%–75% for mild–moderate injury, 75%–100% for severe insults). Dose: 1 U will increase F VIII level by 2% in a 70-kg patient; give one-half i.v. q 12 h or 1/24 dose i.v. q 1 h by infusion after the initial bolus. Levels should be maintained for 5–7 (moderate injury) or 7–14 days (severe injury), as delayed bleeding is typical. Levels of 25%–30% are adequate for a minor operation.
Hemophilia B:	Mild	Desmopressin, 0.3 mg/kg i.v. q 12–24 h.
	Severe	Factor IX concentrate (level 50%–75% for mild–moderate injury, 75%–100% for severe insults). Dose: 1 U will increase F IX level by 2% in a 70-kg patient; give one-half i.v. q 18–24 h after the initial bolus. Levels should be maintained for 5–7 (moderate injury) or 7–14 days (severe injury), as delayed bleeding is typical. Levels of 10%–25% are adequate for a minor operation.
von Willebrand's disease:	Type 1	Desmopressin, 0.3 mg/kg i.v. q 12–24 h × 5–7 days. Tachyphylaxis can be restored by a 24-h drug holiday to allow repletion of endothelial stores. Keep VIII:vWF 60% for 24–72 h for minor surgery, 80% for 5–7 days for major surgery.
	Type 2	Trial of desmopressin (unpredictable effect). Cryoprecipitate (contains 80–100 units vWF/10 units).
Liver disease (multifactorial)		Based on specific defect. Fresh-frozen plasma to keep PT/aPTT <1.3 × control (difficult to correct factor VII deficiency). Vitamin K, 10 mg i.m., if vitamin K deficiency suspected. Platelet count >50,000–100,000. Cryoprecipitate if low fibrinogen (<100–150 mg/dl), factor VIII. Warfarin (vitamin K deficiency, factor II, VII, IX, X). Fresh frozen plasma to keep PT <1.3 × control. Vitamin K, 10 mg i.m., if the patient does not require immediate correction (<12–48 h) or short-term anticoagulation.
Platelet Abnormalities		
Thrombocytopenia		Transfuse platelets <50,000 if bleeding or invasive procedure is anticipated; <20,000 otherwise.
Idiopathic thrombocytopenic purpura		Intravenous immunoglobulin, 2 g/kg over 2–4 days (VERY expensive). Platelet infusion after ligation of the splenic artery during splenectomy if the response to immune globulin is poor.
Drug-induced		Discontinue all noncritical medications. Transfuse platelets only if surgery cannot be delayed to allow spontaneous recovery.
Uremia		Aggressive hemodialysis? Transfuse to hematocrit ~30% to allow improved adhesion? Desmopressin, 0.3 mg/kg i.v. q 12–24 h (rapid effect of short duration). Cryoprecipitate, 10 units (rapid effect but short duration). Conjugated estrogens, 25 mg i.v./day for 3 days (slow onset of action but effective for up to 2 weeks).

In most circumstances, there is probably less urgency for reanticoagulation than is generally appreciated. Protection of a cardiac valve prosthesis is the most urgent indication, but a metallic valve can be left without anticoagulation for at least 72 h and perhaps as long as 1 week (especially in the aortic position), although such a long interval is seldom necessary. High-risk patients or those who will be unable to take warfarin by mouth for several days can be heparinized with safety as early as 12 h after almost any operation in which operative hemostasis was secure, except neurosurgical procedures and some operations for major trauma.

Antibiotic Prophylaxis

Surgery unquestionably induces systemic and local changes in immune function, including suppression of neutrophil function. The interaction between bacteria inoculated into the surgical wound and prophylactic antibiotic administration is a critical determinant of the fate of the wound. The efficacy of perioperative antibiotic prophylaxis for many surgical procedures is unquestioned. According to the National Nosocomial Infections Surveillance System (NNIS) of the Centers for Disease Control and Prevention (CDC), the risk of any operation for a surgical site infection is composed of three factors: the medical condition of the patient according to the American Association of Anesthesiologists (ASA) classification system, the status of the wound in the Altemeier classification (i.e., only clean wounds pose no additional risk), and if the duration of the procedure exceeds the predefined 75th percentile for duration. As the number of risk factors increases, the risk of surgical site infection increases for virtually every type of operation, even those considered clean (Table 13.8). Obesity, protein-calorie malnutrition, diabetes, hypocholesterolemia, and hypothermia are believed to increase the risk of surgical site infection, along with a host of environmental factors. Tables 13.9 and 13.10 describe some common guidelines for prophylaxis.[18]

Examples of "clean" operations for which antibiotic prophylaxis is of benefit include open heart operations, operations on the aorta or vessels in the groin (regardless of the type of vascular graft to be used, if any), craniotomy, and open reduction of closed fractures. The administration of antibiotic prophylaxis may be considered optional for breast surgery and groin hernia surgery.

Studies indicate clearly that antibiotic prophylaxis is most effective when the antibiotic is present in tissue before the skin incision is made. Antibiotics are ineffective when administration is delayed for 3 h, and effectiveness is intermediate when antibiotics are administered within that interval. Administration is ideally complete, or at least under way, when the patient arrives in the operating room.

Current trends are toward a limited duration of prophylaxis. A regimen consisting of only a single preoperative dose of antibiotic appears to be as effective as a longer regimen. A second dose may be beneficial after 3 to 4 h (1–2 half-lives of the drug used) if the operation lasts longer. No data exist to support prophylactic use beyond that point, although many surgeons still prefer to continue the regimen for 24 h. Regimens that extend beyond 24 h are unsupportable. In particular, there is no rationale for longer courses of antibiotics because an operation was subjectively more difficult or because of inadvertent contamination of the operative field.

Steroid Prophylaxis

It is traditional that patients who are on a maintenence glucocorticoid regimen, or who have received corticosteroids within the last 6 months, should receive supplemental "stress-dose" steroid prophylaxis from concern that a hypophyseal–pituitary–adrenal axis suppressed by exogenous steroids may not respond to surgical stress. However, this

TABLE 13.8. Surgical Site Infection Rates (%) For Selected Operations, Stratified by Risk Category.[a]

Operation	Zero risk factors	One risk factor	Two risk factors	Three risk factors
Coronary artery bypass graft, chest and leg (combined)	0.84	3.29	5.56	17.86
Cholecystectomy	0.54	0.81	2.25	3.98
Colectomy	4.32	6.51	10.53	13.90
Exploratory laparotomy	1.94	3.32	6.92	9.89
Vascular surgery	1.34	2.01	5.15	8.83
			Two or three risk factors	
Thoracic surgery	0.50	1.59	3.49	
Appendectomy	1.30	3.11	6.25	
Hepatic/pancreatic surgery	2.80	6.10	10.20	
Gastric surgery	2.79	5.57	12.37	
Small-bowel surgery	5.28	7.70	10.65	
Herniorraphy	0.93	2.06	3.10	
Open reduction of fracture	0.81	1.44	2.91	

[a]Risk factors are outlined in text.
National Nosocomial Infection Surveillance System, Centers for Disease Control and Prevention 1992–1997.

TABLE 13.9.

Summary of Consensus-Based Guideline Recommendations for Endocarditis Prophylaxis for Nondental Procedures by the American Heart Association, 1997.

High-Risk Cardiac Lesions		Previous endocarditis Prosthetic heart valve Complex cyanotic congenital heart disease Surgical systemic–pulmonary shunt or conduit
Moderate-Risk Cardiac Lesions		Other forms of congenital heart disease (but not uncomplicated secundum atrial septal defect) Acquired valvular disease (e.g., rheumatic) Hypertrophic cardiomyopathy Mitral valve prolapse with documented regurgitation or thickened leaflets.
Cardiac Lesions Not at Risk		Prior coronary artery bypass Pacemaker Implanted automatic defibrillator
Surgical Procedures with Endocarditis Risk		Incision of any gastrointestinal, lower respiratory tract, or genitourinary tract mucosa Tonsillectomy/adenoidectomy Rigid bronchoscopy Biliary tract surgery, ERCP with sphincterotomy Cystoscopy Esophageal sclerotherapy or dilation of stricture
Surgical Procedures with No Endocarditis Risk		Clean operations, especially of skin or skin structures (e.g., inguinal herniorraphy, breast surgery) Percutaneous vascular catheter placement Endotracheal, gastrointestinal, or urinary catheterization (intubation) Bronchoscopy or gastrointestinal endoscopy without biopsy Cardiac catheterization Vaginal delivery or hysterectomy
Route of Administration for Dosing in Adults	Low/Moderate Endocarditis Risk	High Endocarditis Risk
Oral	Amoxicillin 2 g, 1 h preop	Oral prophylaxis not recommended primarily. If ampicillin is given parenterally to a high-risk patient, a single 1-g dose of ampicillin i.m./i.v. or amoxicillin p.o. should be given 6 h afterward.
Parenteral	Ampicillin 2 g i.v./i.m., 30 min preop	Ampicillin 2 g i.v./i.m., 30 min preop, plus gentamicin 1.5 mg/kg i.v./i.m., 30 min preop (120 mg max). A postoperative dose of ampicillin or amoxicillin is given as noted above.
Penicillin allergy	Vancomycin 1 g i.v. over 1 h, beginning 1 h before procedure	Vancomycin 1 g i.v. over 1 h beginning 1 h before procedure, plus gentamicin 1.5 mg/kg i.v./i.m., 30 min preop (120 mg max). No postoperative dose is necessary.

conventional wisdom is being revisited. A consensus-based guideline (there being virtually no class I data) has suggested that traditional doses are far too high and are given for too long.[19] A minor surgical stress (e.g., inguinal herniorraphy) may not need steroid supplementation at all, whereas a major stress (e.g., esophagogastrectomy) may need only 150 to 200 mg hydrocortisone/day for 1 to 2 days.

Of course, there must be a high index of suspicion for adrenal insufficiency in such patients, which can be precipitated by postoperative events, such as infection. The diagnosis is best made by a stimulation test using cosyntropin. A baseline cortisol concentration is drawn and 0.01 or 0.25 mg cosyntropin is administered intravenously; it is believed that the lower dose is more sensitive. The serum cortisol concentration is repeated 30 to 60 min after the challenge. Glucocorticoids can be given immediately thereafter as indicated, pending the results. The diagnosis is confirmed if none of the values exceeds 20 ng/ml and the stimulated cortisol concentration does not increase by at least 7 ng/ml. Patients respond hemodynamically within 12 to 24 h of starting glucocorticoid (hydrocortisone, 75 mg q 8 h or equivalent), but it may take several days to correct the electrolyte abnormalities.

Resuscitation: The Interface Between Pre- and Postoperative Care

Patients may require resuscitation to prepare for surgery (e.g., small-bowel obstruction, penetrating trauma to the torso), or resuscitation may be the primary therapeutic modality (e.g., acute alcoholic pancreatitis, stable pelvic fracture with no associated injuries). Postoperative patients often require fluid resuscitation, especially if intraoperative fluid requirements have been underestimated, evaporative losses are high because a body cavity (especially both chest and abdomen) is open for a prolonged period, the patient is hypothermic, or there has been an osmotic diuresis from hyperglycemia or the administration of mannitol.

Blood Tests and Monitoring Technology as Guides to Resuscitation

Several blood tests are available to guide resuscitation. Either a lactate concentration can be measured or the base deficit can be calculated. Either, in the absence of another cause of metabolic acidosis, can be used to estimate the adequacy of global tissue perfusion.

TABLE 13.10. Appropriate Cephalosporin Prophylaxis for Selected Operations.[a]

Operation	Alternative prophylaxis in serious penicillin allergy
First-generation cephalosporin (i.e., cefazolin) Cardiovascular and thoracic	Vancomycin (for all cases herein except amputation)[b]
Median sternotomy	
Pacemaker insertion	
Vascular reconstruction involving the abdominal aorta, insertion of a prosthesis, or a groin incision (except carotid endarterectomy, which requires no prophylaxis)	
Implantable defibrillator	
Pulmonary resection	
Lower limb amputation	Gentamicin and metronidazole
General	
Cholecystectomy (High risk only: age >60, jaundice, acute, prior biliary procedure)	Gentamicin
Gastrectomy (High risk only: not uncomplicated chronic duodenal ulcer)	Gentamicin and metronidazole
Hepatobiliary	Gentamicin and metronidazole
Major debridement of traumatic wound	Gentamicin
Genitourinary	
Ampicillin plus gentamicin	Ciprofloxacin
Gynecological	
Cesarean section (STAT)	Metronidazole (after cord clamping)
Hysterectomy	Doxycycline
Head and neck/oral cavity	
Major procedures entering oral cavity or pharynx	Gentamicin and metronidazole
Neurosurgery	
Craniotomy	Clindamycin, vancomycin
Orthopedics	
Major joint arthroplasty	Vancomycin[b]
Open reduction of closed fracture	Vancomycin[b]
Second-generation (i.e., cefoxitin)[c]	
Appendectomy	Metronidazole with or without gentamicin (for all cases herein)
Colon surgery[d]	
Surgery for penetrating abdominal trauma	

[a]Should be given as a single intravenous dose just before the operation. Consider an additional dose if the operation is prolonged.

[b]Primary prophylaxis with vancomycin (i.e., for the non-penicillin-allergic patient) may be appropriate for cardiac valve replacement, placement of a nontissue peripheral vascular prosthesis, or total joint replacement in institutions where a high rate of infections with methicillin-resistant *Staphylococcus aureus* or *Staphylococcus epidermidis* has occurred. A single dose administered immediately before surgery is sufficient unless operation lasts for more than 6 h, in which case the dose should be repeated. Prophylaxis should be discontinued after a maximum of two doses.

[c]An intraoperative dose should be given if cefoxitin is used and the duration of surgery exceeds 3–4 h, because of the short half-life of the drug. A postoperative dose is not necessary.

[d]Benefit beyond that provided by bowel preparation with mechanical cleansing and oral neomycin and erythromycin base is debatable.

Hemodynamic monitoring is usually instituted at some point if the clinician is disconcerted by the volume of fluid required by a high-risk patient, or if there is persistent acidosis or hemodynamic instability. Vascular access is usually obtained via percutaneous cannulation of a subclavian or internal jugular vein. Central venous pressure (CVP) can be measured from the superior vena cava; the access is more reliable than that provided by peripheral vein cannulas, and prodigious volumes of fluid (several liters/hour) can be administered through a multilumen catheter. Central venous pressure is only tangentially related to intravascular volume or myocardial function; it can provide an estimate of right ventricular preload, but right ventricular function is more a function of right ventricular end-diastolic volume than any

right-sided pressure. Only in the setting of left ventricular function that is known to be normal can any inference be drawn from CVP data. Valvular heart disease (especially mitral stenosis and tricuspid insufficiency) and pulmonary hypertension (common in acute lung injury and acute hydrostatic pulmonary edema and occasionally present in chronic obstructive pulmonary disease) can make CVP readings very difficult to interpret.

Even more invasive is placement of a balloon-tipped pulmonary artery flotation (PA) catheter, but there is scant evidence to suggest that its use improves outcomes. See the chapter on critical care for further discussion of the use of PA catheters and use of oxygen delivery/consumption monitoring techniques.

TABLE 13.11. Indications for Blood and Blood Component Therapies.

Leukocyte-reduced red blood cell units
    Congental hemolytic anemias
    Hypoproliferative anemias likely to need multiple transfusions
    Recurrent severe febrile hemolytic transfusion reactions
    Known HLA alloimmunization
Irradiated cellular blood components
    Bone marrow/stem cell transplants
    Intrauterine/postuterine transfusions
    Directed donations (HLA-matched or blood-relative donors)
    Hodgkin disease
    Acute lymphocytic leukemia
    Solid-organ transplant recipients
    Antineoplastic chemo- or radiotherapy
    Exchange transfusion/extracorporeal membrane oxygenation
    HIV opportunistic infections

TABLE 13.12.

Summary of Evidence-Based Guidelines for Red Blood Cell Transfusions for Acute Blood Loss.[a]

Evaluate for risk of ischemia
Estimate/anticipate degree of blood loss
    <30% rapid volume loss probably does not require transfusion in a previously healthy person
Measure hemoglobin concentration
    <6 g/dl: transfusion usually needed
    6–10 g/dl: transfusion dictated by clinical circumstance
    >10 g/dl: transfusion rarely needed
Measure vital signs/tissue oxygenation when Hb 6–10 g/dl and extent of blood loss is unknown
    Tachycardia hypotension refractory to volume: transfusion needed
    PvO$_2$, O$_2$ extraction ratio >50%, VO$_2$ <50% of baseline: transfusion usually needed

[a]Practice Parameter of the College of American Pathologists, 1997.

Transfusion of Blood and Blood Products

The decision to transfuse a patient with blood or blood products must be predicated on several factors, such as the underlying diagnosis (Tables 13.11–13.13),[20,21] the availability of blood, the "optimal" hematocrit for oxygen transport, and alternatives to transfusion itself. Several recent studies indicate that higher transfusion targets (hemoglobin, 8–10 g/dl) may lead to higher mortality than the more parsimonious strategy of transfusion for a hemoglobin concentration of about 7–8 g/dl.[22,23]

Predonation Strategies

Acute preoperative hemodilution with reinfusion and perioperative autologous blood salvage ("cell saver") techniques are essentially autologous transfusion practices. However, from the standpoint of patient preparation for elective surgery, preoperative autologous blood donation is the popular approach. Directed blood transfusions are no safer than transfusions from anonymous volunteer donors, but are encouraged in select circumstances in which the likelihood of transfusion is high. Such a strategy, employed rationally, can decrease the likelihood of allogeneic transfusion by up to 80% in elective surgery. Successful donation of the requested number of units of blood, based on established maximal surgical blood-ordering schedules maintained by the blood bank, requires attention to the mechanics of the donation process (Table 13.14). Patients who are not anemic (hematocrit ≥40%) can donate approximately one unit of blood per week, although the final donation can be as few as 3 days before surgery. Anemic patients are less likely to complete the scheduled donations and to receive allogeneic blood, and therefore may benefit from aggressive and innovative blood procurement strategies. All patients accepted by the blood bank are placed on oral iron supplementation (325 mg p.o. tid) before the first scheduled donation. Concomitant ingestion of 500 mg vitamin C with each dose of iron optimizes absorption of iron from the duo-

TABLE 13.13.

Summary of Evidence-Based Guidelines for Red Blood Cell and Plasma Transfusions.[a]

Red Blood Cell Transfusions
    Level I: No recommendations.
    Level II: Transfusions should be given to alleviate symptoms or mortality.
                No single transfusion trigger is appropriate for all patients or situations.
                Red blood cell concentrates should not be used to expand intravascular volume when oxygen carrying capacity is adequate.
                Red blood cell concentrates should not be used to treat anemia if less risky alternatives are available.

Fresh Frozen Plasma Transfusions
    Level I: FFP is indicated for adult thrombotic thrombocytopenic purpura, followed by plasmapheresis.
    Level II: FFP is indicated for bleeding in patients with abnormal PT, aPTT, or INR. FFP is not indicated prophylactically for INR <2.0.
                FFP is indicated for therapy of disseminated intravascular coagulation, provided the precipitant can be treated effectively.
                FFP is indicated for massive transfusion with microvascular bleeding and abnormal tests of coagulation.

[a]Canadian Medical Association Expert Working Group; level III guidelines excluded.
Source: Adapted from Innes.[21]

TABLE 13.14. Selected Surgical Procedures and Likelihood of Blood Transfusion.

Low (<25%) risk: no likely benefit from preoperative autologous donation
   Childbirth
   Cesarean section
   Cholecystectomy
   Transurethral prostatectomy
   Vaginal delivery
   Vaginal hysterectomy
High (>5%) risk: likely benefit from preoperative autologous donation
   Abdominal hysterectomy
   Cardiac surgery
   Colorectal surgery
   Craniotomy
   Mastectomy
   Radical prostatectomy
   Spinal surgery
   Total joint replacement
   Vascular graft surgery

denum. A unit of blood can usually be collected twice a week so long as the hematocrit is 33% or higher.

Gastrointestinal Prophylaxis

Most gastrointestinal prophylactic efforts are directed against stress-related gastric mucosal hemorrhage, which has decreased in incidence and importance in the aftermath of the introduction of effective prophylactic methods and improved nutritional therapy. Historically, "stress gastritis," as it is popularly but inaccurately known, affected about 20% of critically ill patients, but the incidence has been reduced by about 90% with the introduction of antacid prophylaxis, and parenteral H_2-histamine receptor antagonists.

Nutritional Support

Total Parenteral Nutrition

Total parenteral nutrition (TPN) is standard therapy for many hospitalized patients when clinical conditions preclude enteral or oral feeding. However, clear evidence that this administration improves outcome is lacking. Long-term nutritional support is possible by administration of vitamins and minerals along with amino acids and dextrose and the periodic supplementation of 10% lipid emulsion. The concentration of amino acids and dextrose can be modified to tailor therapy to specific conditions (e.g., 40% dextrose rather than 25% for patients whose fluid intake must be minimized).

Parenteral nutrition has numerous complications that limit its use. Although dilute solutions are sometimes administered peripherally, TPN therapy usually requires administration into a central vein. Complications associated with central vein administration include those related to catheter placement (e.g., arterial puncture, dysrhythmias, mediastinal hematoma, pneumothorax, extravascular placement) or the indwelling state (e.g., infection, especially bactermia), central vein thrombosis, and the rare complications of air embolism or erosion of the catheter tip into the mediastinum).

Potential metabolic complications include fluid overload, electrolyte abnormalities, hyperglycemia or hypoglycemia, and overfeeding. Hyperglycemia is common because of the large number of diabetic patients who require major surgery, and because of the insulin resistance that is characteristic of sepsis and surgical stress (see following). Regular insulin is most conveniently added to the solution directly, but can also be administered either by subcutaneous injection, intravenous bolus, or supplemental infusion. In the event of an abrupt cessation of TPN therapy, the infusion of even a 5% dextrose solution should be sufficient to prevent hypoglycemia. In unusual cases, hepatic dysfunction (usually resulting from ischemia/reperfusion injury or cholestasis, but to which TPN may contribute) may become so severe that gluconeogenesis is impaired.

Patients who are fed intravenously with TPN sustain small-bowel mucosal atrophy and may have impaired immune function. Whether this translates into a clinically important injury in most patients remains a matter of speculation. Patients fed with TPN may develop cholestasis with or without the formation of sludge or stones in the gallbladder. It has been hypothesized that the administration of even small amounts of enteral feedings to TPN-dependent patients may protect the gut, but proof is lacking.

Enteral Nutrition

At least 18 randomized, controlled prospective trials have examined the effects of early enteral feedings (usually defined as feedings within 24 h vs. 3–5 days), mostly in clinical settings of trauma of various types, burns, and major elective abdominal surgery.[24] The principal endpoints involved have been mortality, length of stay, and the incidence of infection. Significant benefit was demonstrated in 5 of 7 studies of major abdominal surgery, without a predominant type of benefit. In contrast, an improved outcome was demonstrated in 6 of 7 studies of trauma patients, manifested notably by a reduced length of hospital stay of patients with a femur fracture. An improved outcome was noted in all 3 studies of burn patients as well.

Regarding nasoenteric tubes, it is not clear that the catheter tip must be in the duodenum before the initiation of feedings. Many clinicians now have few reservations about feeding into the stomach so long as caution is exercised (head of bed up 30°, frequent checks for residuals that may reflect ileus or intolerance, meticulous pulmonary toilet, and use of promotility agents).

The most common complication of enteral nutrition is diarrhea, which causes loss of nutrients as well as fluid and electrolyte abnormalities. Diarrhea can occur even when feeding with an iso-osmotic solution. Once a diagnosis of *Clostridium difficile* colitis has been excluded, diarrhea may be controlled by the addition of opioids (e.g., dilute tincture of opium), or discontinuance of any promotility agents. Hyperglycemia is less of a problem than with TPN, but is managed in a similar fashion. The clinician must also be alert to the possibility of the late complications of sinusitis and tracheoesophageal fistula, especially in patients with endotracheal or tracheostomy tubes.

Diabetes Management

Carbohydrate metabolism is inherently unstable surrounding periods of surgical stress, yet there are relatively few studies available to inform management. The perceived need to keep patients NPO for several hours before elective endotracheal intubation will decrease caloric intake, as will mechanical bowel preparation before colon surgery. For those patients who require insulin and inject small amounts frequently according to current recommended protocols, fluctuations in blood glucose can be smoothed. For these patients who take long-acting insulin or oral hypoglycemic agents, the potential danger of hypoglycemia before surgery often leads to a recommendation to reduce the drug dosages. In the case of metformin, cessation of therapy 48 h before surgery is mandatory to preclude the development of severe lactic acidosis.

Hyperglycemia is common in the immediate postoperative period owing to the metabolic stress and counterregulatory hormone responses. Concentrated feeding, especially parenterally, can aggravate hyperglycemia. Hyperglycemia begets glycosuria, which in turn is associated with osmotic diuresis. Impaired wound healing and impaired leukocyte function are additional consequences of diabetes.

Exogenous insulin can reverse or overcome many of the metabolic disturbances, but blood glucose is not always checked during surgery, and insulin is not always administered, despite the widespread availability of accurate hand-held glucometers. In the immediate postoperative period, short-acting insulin is administered on a titrated "sliding-scale" unless administered as a continuous infusion, usually with TPN. Longer-acting agents, whether oral or parenteral, are usually reserved until the patient is metabolically stable with reliable oral intake. It may take 3 to 5 days after a major surgical intervention to restore metabolic homeostasis,[25,26] regardless of the type of surgery.

Diabetic Ketoacidosis

Insulin deficiency and a synergistic increase in "stress" hormone secretion (epinephrine, cortisol, glucagon) produce a volume-depleted, acidemic, hyperglycemic, and ketonemic state with severe electrolyte abnormalities. Acutely decompensated type I diabetes mellitus is the most common underlying problem, and the cause of the destabilization is usually infection. Frequently, diabetic ketoacidosis (DKA) is the presenting manifestation of previously undiagnosed diabetes. Other precipitants may include pregnancy, acute myocardial infarction, trauma, acute psychiatric illness, or major surgery. Endocrine precipitants include thyrotoxicosis and pheochromocytoma.

The massive hyperglycemia is caused primarily by accelerated gluconeogenesis in the face of reduced peripheral glucose utilization and catabolism of lean tissue and lipid stores. Serum hyperosmolarity precipitates an osmotic diuresis with subsequent volume depletion and paradoxical dilutional hyponatremia. Ketonemia results from the inability to metabolize mobilized long-chain fatty acids via lipogenic pathways. A high index of suspicion for DKA is indicated in patients with dehydration, vomiting, tachypnea, severe abdominal pain, obtundation, or a combination of those findings. Diagnostic criteria for DKA include blood glucose above 700 mg/dl, serum osmolarity above 340 mOsm/l, arterial pH below 7.30 with $PaCO_2$

40 mm Hg or less, ketonemia, and ketonuria. The differential diagnosis includes lactic acidosis, uremia, various intoxicants (including ethanol), sepsis syndrome, cerebrovascular accident, and intraabdominal catastrophe. Patients with hyperosmolar nonketotic coma (HHNC; see following) by definition do not have ketonemia, although HHNC and DKA may coexist.

Effective treatment for DKA requires simultaneous metabolic management and a search for the precipitant. An electrocardiogram must always be obtained to rule out the "silent" myocardial infarction typical of diabetic patients. Patients with DKA may have a volume deficit as great as 10 l, and therefore vigorous fluid replacement is essential. Hypotonic saline is the treatment of choice. When the blood glucose decreases below 250 mg/dl, resuscitation continues with 5% dextrose in water (D5W) to prevent hypoglycemia and cerebral edema. Central hemodynamic monitoring is used as indicated.

All patients in DKA require prompt insulin treatment. After a bolus dose of 10 to 30 units, a continuous infusion of short-acting (regular) insulin, 5 to 10 units per hour, is effective and safe if monitored closely. Longer-acting insulin preparations should not be used until the patient's condition has stabilized and oral intake is possible.

Bicarbonate therapy in DKA is seldom necessary, because metabolism of acetoacetate and β-hydroxybutyrate generates bicarbonate. Indications for bicarbonate therapy in DKA include arterial pH below 7.1 or HCO_3 level below 10 mEq/dl, or to relieve the discomfort of Kussmaul respirations. In contrast, potassium supplementation is invariably required. Ketonuria, diuresis, and frequent vomiting can produce marked potassium depletion, which may be masked initially as intracellular stores shift to the extracellular space in response to acidosis. Correction of acidosis will unmask marked hypokalemia.

Hyperglycemic Hyperosmolar Nonketotic Coma

Patients with HHNC present with very high blood glucose concentrations (sometimes >1000 mg/dl), depressed sensorium, marked dehydration, and prerenal azotemia. By definition, acidosis, ketonemia, and ketonuria are absent unless there is coexistent DKA. Precipitants include many stresses typical of the surgical patient, including burns, severe infections, pancreatitis, and major surgery.

As with DKA, therapy consists of rehydration, intravenous insulin, electrolyte replacement, and correction of the precipitant. Isotonic saline is the fluid of choice except for the hypernatremic patient. As much as 10 l may be required in the first 24 h. Potassium supplementation up to 20 mEq/h may be necessary. Fluid administration is then adjusted based upon the response to resuscitation. Intravenous insulin is given as an infusion of 6–10 U/h until blood glucose is below 250 mg/dl, when a change is also made to dextrose-containing fluid to prevent hypoglycemia and cerebral edema.

The Approach to the Febrile Surgical Patient

Fever is common in surgical patients. The list of potential causes of fever is long, and includes many noninfectious etiologies (Table 13.15). Any fever in a surgical patient is a potential cause for concern. Current guidelines for the evalua-

TABLE 13.15. Noninfectious Causes of Fever of Importance in Surgical Patients.

Cardiovascular
  Myocardial infarction
  Aortic dissection
  Pericarditis
Central nervous system disease
  Cavernous sinus thrombosis
  Hypothalamic dysfunction
  Nonhemorrhagic infarction/stroke
  Seizures
  Subarachnoid hemorrhage
  Traumatic brain injury
Gastroenterological
  Acalculous cholecystitis
  Gastrointestinal hemorrhage
  Hepatitis (toxic/ischemic)
  Inflammatory bowel disease
  Ischemic colitis
  Pancreatitis (early)
Hematological
  Venous thrombosis (superficial or deep)
  Retroperitoneal/pelvic hemorrhage/hematoma
  Transfusion reaction
Inflammatory
  Gout/pseudogout
  Intramuscular injections
  Transplant rejection
  Vasculitis
Endocrine/metabolic
  Adrenal insufficiency
  Alcohol/drug withdrawal
  Hyperthyroidism
Miscellaneous
  Allergic drug reaction
  Drug fever
  Tissue ischemia/infarction
Neoplastic
  Febrile neutropenia
  Metastatic disease
  Primary tumors
Pulmonary/airway
  Acute respiratory distress syndrome (fibroproliferative phase)
  Atelectasis
  Aspiration pneumonitis
  Pulmonary embolism/infarction

tion of fever in critically ill adults suggest that fever mandates a history and physical examination (Table 13.16).[27] Subsequent testing should be based on the findings of the clinical evaluation; in some instances, no further evaluation will be necessary.

What Constitutes a Fever?

The magnitude of elevation in temperature necessary to constitute a fever may simply be the particular temperature at which the clinician believes that investigation is necessary, most commonly in the range of 38.0° to 38.5°C. Elevated body temperature increases basal metabolic rate 7%–15%/°C, but aside from increased insensible fluid losses and some discomfort, fever is usually not the primary source of morbidity. Tachycardia or increased oxygen demand may make it desirable to suppress fever in select patients with coronary ischemia or critical acute respiratory failure. However, most adults with a temperature of 40°C or less do not specifically require a reduction in temperature (if the temperature is ≥41°C, there is a risk of neurological injury). If antipyretic therapy is chosen, cyclooxygenase inhibition is most effective, bearing in mind that deleterious effects upon renal function and the gastric mucosa are possible with nonspecific COX inhibitors. The new COX-2 selective inhibitors are effective antipyretics, but at this time they are only available orally, and the risk of gastric injury is not entirely eliminated. Topical cooling is ineffective, although core cooling (e.g., iced fluid lavage of the stomach) can be effective.

Noninfectious Causes of Fever

A nosocomial infection is a less likely cause of postoperative fever than a noninfectious cause in the first 48 h after surgery.

The most common cause of postoperative fever is atelectasis. If early postoperative atelectasis is present, pulmonary physiotherapy and early ambulation (if possible) should be undertaken immediately; cultures are generally not useful in the immediate postoperative period. It is unusual for a fresh postoperative patient to have been admitted with a community-acquired pneumonia, but the clinician must remain alert to the possibility. After the third postoperative day, nosocomial pneumonia is possible. In addition to atelectasis, aspiration pneumonitis (which is usually noninfectious), tissue ischemia or infarction, acute vasculitis, gout or pseudogout, intracerebral hemorrhage, retroperitoneal hematoma, pericarditis, and transfusion reactions can cause fever. There are several miscellaneous causes of fever that are not caused by infection. Withdrawal of alcohol, benzodiazepines, or opioids can all cause fever.

Endocrine emergencies, including acute adrenal insufficiency or thyroid storm, can be very challenging to diagnose because they can be precipitated by infection. Adrenal insufficiency and thyrotoxicosis can create extremely high fevers with a constellation of systemic signs. These endocrinopathies can be precipitated by infection, compounding the diagnostic confusion. Two types of patients are at high risk for adrenal insufficiency, including those patients with a history of corticosteroid use and those with a acute condition that ablates adrenal function. Patients with adrenal insufficiency present with variable degrees of temperature elevation, hypotension, hyponatremia, hyperkalemia, or hypoglycemia. Severe thyrotoxicosis or thyroid storm can cause fevers above 39.0°C with a variety of other systemic signs including tachyarrhythmias, atrial fibrillation, diaphoresis, palpitations, congestive heart failure, gastrointestinal symptoms (abdominal pain, nausea, vomiting, and diarrhea), neurological symptoms (tremors, seizures, anxiety), and heat intolerance. Treatment is supportive and includes propranolol, fluids, iodine, and possibly antithyroidal agents such as methimazole or propylthiouracil.

DRUG FEVER

Fever coincident with administration of a drug that disappears after discontinuance, when no other cause of fever is apparent, characterizes the disorder. The diagnosis is therefore one of exclusion, and skepticism is always in order for fear of overlooking another treatable cause of fever. True drug-related fever probably accounts for no more than 2% to 3% of episodes of fever in hospitalized patients. As a group,

TABLE 13.16.

Evidence-Based Practice Management Guideline for the Evaluation of Fever in Critically Ill Adult Patients.[a]

Temperature Measurement

Level I: Record the temperature and the site of measurement in the patient's medical record.
The nosocomial spread of pathogens must be avoided when using temperature measurement devices.

Level II: Temperature is measured most accurately by indwelling vascular or bladder thermistors, but most other sites are acceptable. Axillary measurements should not be used.
Laboratory testing for the evaluation of fever should be individualized for each patient.

Blood Cultures

Level I: For skin preparation, povidone-iodine should be allowed to try for 2 min, or tincture of iodine for 30 s. Alcohol skin preparation, an acceptable alternative for iodine-allergic patients, need not be allowed to dry.

Level II: Obtain a single pair of blood cultures after appropriate skin disinfection after the initial temperature elevation, and another pair within 24 h thereafter from a second peripheral site. Additional cultures should be based on high clinical suspicion of bacteremia or fungemia, and not instituted automatically for each temperature elevation.
If two peripheral sites are not available, one pair of cultures may be drawn through the most recently inserted catheter, but the diagnostic accuracy is reduced.
Draw at least 10–15 ml blood/culture.

Suspected Intravascular Catheter Infection

Level II: Examine the catheter insertion site for purulence, and distally on the extremity for signs of vascular compromise or embolization.
Any expressed purulence from an insertion site should be collected for culture and Gram stain.
The catheter should be removed and cultured for evidence of a tunnel infection, embolic phenomena, vascular compromise, or sepsis.
Two blood cultures should be drawn peripherally, or one may be drawn from the most proximal port (if a multilumen catheter).
Both the introducer and the catheter itself should be cultured for suspected pulmonary artery catheter infection.
It is not routinely necessary to culture the intravenous fluid infusate.

Suspected ICU-Acquired Pneumonia

Level I: A chest X-ray should be obtained to evaluate for suspected pneumonia. Postero-anterior and lateral films or computed tomography of the chest can offer more information.

Level II: Lower respiratory tract secretions should be sampled for direct examination and culture. Bronchoscopy may be considered.
Respiratory secretions should be transported to the laboratory within 2 h of collection
Pleural fluid should be obtained for culture and Gram stain if there is an adjacent infiltrate or another reason to suspect infection.

Evaluation of the Febrile Patient with Diarrhea

Level II: If more than two diarrheal stools occur, a single stool sample should be sent for *Clostridium difficile* evaluation. A second sample should be sent if the first is negative and suspicion remains high.
If illness is severe and rapid testing is unavailable or nondiagnostic, consider flexible sigmoidoscopy.
If illness is severe, consider empiric therapy with metronidazole until the results of studies are available. Empiric therapy (especially with vancomycin) is not recommended if two stool evaluations have been negative for *C. difficile*, and is discouraged because of the risk of producing resistant pathogens.
Stool cultures are rarely indicated for other enteric pathogens if the patient is HIV-negative or did not present to the hospital with diarrhea.

Suspected Urinary Tract Infection

Level II: Obtain urine for culture and to evaluate for pyuria. If the patient has an indwelling Foley catheter, urine should be collected from the urine port and not the drainage bag.
The specimen should be transported rapidly to the laboratory, or refrigerated if transport will exceed 1 h.

Suspected Sinusitis

Level I: Aspirate should be Gram stained and cultured.

Level II: Computed tomography of the facial sinuses is the imaging modality of choice for the diagnosis of sinusitis.
Puncture and aspiration of the sinuses should be performed using sterile technique if mucosal thickening or an air–fluid level is present in the sinus.

Postoperative Fever

Level II: Examine the surgical wound for erythema, fluctuance, tenderness, or purulent drainage.
Open the wound for suspicion of infection.
Culture and Gram stain should be obtained from purulent material if from deep within the wound.

Suspected Central Nervous System Infection

Level II: Gram stain and culture of cerebrospinal fluid should be performed in cases of suspected infection. Other tests should be predicated on the clinical situation.
A computed tomographic study is usually required before lumbar puncture, which may need to be deferred if a mass lesion is present.
Consider lumbar puncture for new fever with unexplained alteration of consciousness or focal neurological signs.
In febrile patients with an intracranial device, cerebrospinal fluid should be sent for culture and Gram stain.

Noninfectious Causes of Fever

Level II   Reevaluate all recent medications and blood products the patient has received.
Stop all nonessential medications, or substitute medications for treatments that cannot be stopped.

---

[a]Summary of clinical recommendations, Society of Critical Care Medicine, 1998; level III guidelines excluded.
Source: Adapted from O'Grady et al.[27]

antimicrobial agents are the most common cause of fever. Penicillins, cephalosporins, tetracyclines, and vancomycin are commonly prescribed culprits. Fever usually abates within 72 h of discontinuance of the offending drug unless its half-life is prolonged (e.g., phenytoin), so additional therapy is usually unwarranted.

Malignant hyperthermia sundrome can occur when certain anesthetics and adjuncts (e.g., succinylcholine, volatile hydrocarbons) produce a rapid uncoupling of oxidative phosphorylation in susceptible patients, which is often fatal (30%–70% mortality). Medication for both prophylaxis and the overt syndrome includes the administration of freshly prepared dantrolene (1–2 mg/kg every 10 min), along with supportive care. Malignant hyperthermia usually does not respond to antipyretic therapy.

Another form of hyperthermia, neuroleptic malignant syndrome (NMS), occurs in patients taking neuroleptic drugs, typically phenothiazines or butyrophenones, although metoclopramide therapy has been implicated. Both malignant hyperthermia and NMS present with similar symptoms and have similar therapies, except that the magnitude of the core temperature response is somewhat lower, and signs of muscle damage (tenderness, immobility, and elevated serum creatinine phosphokinase) are absent in NMS.

Hematological Causes of Fever

Several hematological causes of fever exist (see Table 13.15). One of the most common causes of fever in the inpatient setting is a transfusion reaction. Almost any neoplasm itself may manifest fever. The postchemotherapeutic state may lead to the "tumor lysis syndrome," which is a common source of fever in hospitalized cancer patients. Febrile neutropenia is common on oncology wards and bone marrow transplant units, and the initiation of therapy with any of the colony-stimulating factors or cytokines (e.g., IL-2 therapy) may also cause fever.

Almost any intracranial pathology can lead to centrally mediated fevers. Any traumatic or infectious condition of the brain can stimulate a hyperpyrexic response, but most common is subarachnoid hemorrhage. In actuality, a blood clot anywhere in the body can cause fever. For lower-extremity deep venous thrombosis, the diagnostic approach includes lower-extremity duplex ultrasound studies, or, in some institutions, magnetic resonance imaging of the pelvic veins.[28] Although ICU patients are at high risk for venous thromboembolism, routine screening does not appear to be cost-effective. Many authorities believe that helical CT has now supplanted venography/pulmonary angiography for the diagnosis of venous thromboembolism.[29]

If a central catheter-related venous thrombosis occurs, the therapy includes the removal of the catheter and the possible institution of anticoagulant or thrombolytic therapy. If thrombolysis is chosen, it must be accomplished before the catheter is removed to avoid the possibility of hemorrhage. With arterial thrombosis, it is often the resulting tissue ischemia that causes fever.

Infectious Causes of Fever: Nosocomial Infection

Many emergency operations are performed for control of an infection. Even under optimal circumstances (definitive surgical source control, timely administration of appropriate broad-spectrum antibiotics), it may take 72 h or more for the patient to defervesce. New or persistent fever more than 3 days after surgery should raise a strong suspicion of persistent illness or a new complication.

Device-Related Infections, Catheter-Related Infections, and Ventilator-Associated Pneumonia

Nosocomial infections often arise in association with indwelling devices. Examples of indwelling devices include intravascular catheters, endotracheal or tracheostomy tubes, or other devices that breach or degrade a natural epithelial barrier to infection. The presence of such catheters may suppress local host defenses (e.g., endotracheal tubes), impede drainage (e.g., nasotracheal tube), or increase the risk of aspiration (e.g., transesophageal or percutaneous gastric tubes; any artificial airway).

The patients most at risk for pneumonia are those who require prolonged mechanical ventilation ventilator-associated pneumonia, (VAP). Although the presence of (1) purulent sputum, (2) fever, (3) leukocytosis, and (4) a new or changed radiographic infiltrate may suggest pneumonia, the diagnosis of pneumonia may not always be straightforward, as critically ill patients may have abnormal studies from nonpneumonic processes. Only about 40% of patients with the four typical findings just enumerated are found to have pneumonia when evaluated with a consistent and systematic protocol that includes bronchoscopic sputum collection.[30]

Any oropharyngeal or nasopharyngeal apparatus can promote the development of sinusitis.[31] Patients with maxillofacial or skull fractures or traumatic brain injury are at particularly increased risk. The optimal test for the diagnosis of sinusitis is a CT scan with thin cuts of the facial bones, followed by guided sinus aspiration and drainage for culture and lavage in any patient with mucosal thickening or an air–fluid level. The yield for such an approach is low and the evaluation is laborious.

Peripheral or central venous catheters may become infected. The notion that central catheters may be left unchanged in situ is increasing. However, central lines are accessed frequently, may be used to infuse concentrated solutions of dextrose or lipid formulas, and usually possess multiple ports. Central venous catheters are therefore more likely to lead to infection than peripheral catheters, although new central venous catheters impregnated with antimicrobial agents can decrease the risk.[32] If the catheter has been placed percutaneously, it should be removed.

Urinary tract infection is commonplace because of the ubiquitous use of urinary catheters but is seldom destabilizing. The duration of catheterization is the most important risk factor for the development of nosocomial bacterial cystitis. Most episodes of bacteriuria are asymptomatic, but symptoms, including fever and leukocytosis, can develop in 10% to 30% of patients. The indications for catheterization should be reviewed daily. The best prevention and therapy is removal of the catheter at the earliest opportunity.

Nosocomial Infections Not Related to Devices

Surgical site infection (SSI) or infection of a traumatic wound is rare in the first few days after operation, because effective methods of prevention are recognized. The only important exceptions to this rule are the development of erysipelas, a necrotizing soft tissue infection caused by pyogenic streptococci, and clostridial fasciitis. Thus, it is important to take down the surgical dressing to inspect the wound for a fever in the early postoperative period. Other wound infections, either of the incision or deeper tissues, generally manifest themselves after the fourth postoperative day in the absence of a gross break in technique.

ANTIBIOTIC-ASSOCIATED COLITIS

One complication to which every surgical patient who receives antibiotics is potentially subject is antibiotic-associated colitis (AAC). The most distinguishable of these syndromes, pseudomembranous colitis, results from *Clostridium difficile* overgrowth and toxin production after antibiotic use, even a single dose of a cephalosporin used appropriately for surgical wound prophylaxis. Practically every antibiotic has been implicated in the pathogenesis. The diagnosis of AAC usually depends on isolation of exotoxin A or B from a fresh stool sample. Treatment for AAC includes supportive care, the exclusion of peritonitis or an indication for laparotomy, and metronidazole (intravenous or oral), which is comparable to oral vancomycin at about 80% effectiveness, even for clinically severe cases. Oral vancomycin can be used for patients who are intolerant of metronidazole or who fail therapy with metronidazole, but vancomycin use is discouraged for infection control reasons. Vancomycin can be administered by gavage or enema if necessary, because intravenous vancomycin is ineffective.

ACUTE ACALCULOUS CHOLECYSTITIS

Acalculous cholecystitis is sufficiently common that the diagnosis should be considered in every critically ill or injured patient with a clinical picture of sepsis and no other obvious source. Fever is generally present but other physical findings are less reliable. Leukocytosis and hyperbilirubinemia are nonspecific, and biochemical assays of hepatic enzymes are of little help. The diagnosis of AAC thus often rests on radiologic studies. Ultrasound of the gallbladder is the most accurate modality to diagnose AAC.

The mainstay of therapy for AAC has been cholecystectomy. Cholecystostomy can be a lifesaving alternative in the unstable patient. Percutaneous cholecystostomy is gaining acceptance as an alternative to open procedures.[33] The advantages of percutaneous cholecystostomy are bedside applicability, local anesthesia, and avoidance of an open procedure. The technique controls the acute syndrome in about 85% of patients.

Diagnostic Approach to Fever

An individual approach is essential, both for evaluation and for therapy. Two major problems to resolve are distinguishing sterile systemic inflammation from systemic infection and distinguishing bacterial colonization from tissue invasion. Many patients with sterile inflammation (early pancreatitis, major trauma, burns) develop an inflammatory host response characterized by elaboration of the very cytokines implicated in the febrile response. The clinical picture may be indistinguishable from clinical infection. The distinction is critical because these patients are at high risk to develop antibiotic-resistant infections if unnecessary antibiotics are administered.[34]

A careful history and physical examination should direct further diagnostic tests. The most commonly ordered initial tests are cultures of blood, sputum, and urine. These tests may be helpful in many patients, especially if the patient is believed to have an infection, although the yield of blood cultures is low in the postoperative period and in patients already on broad-spectrum antibiotics.[35]

Other frequently utilized tests include radiologic studies. The most commonly performed is chest radiography to help detect pneumonia. However, a CT scan can be often quite helpful, especially after abdominal surgery. Because of the earlier presence of various nonspecific changes, the best yield for CT scan for suspected intraabdominal abscess is at least 7 days after operation.

Empiric Antibiotic Therapy

Many courses of antibiotic therapy are inappropriate, either because an amenable infection is not present or the chosen drug is not effective against the likely pathogens, or because the duration of treatment is too long.

In the absence of definitive data, the decision to start antibiotics is based upon the likelihood of infection, its likely source and the likely pathogens, and whether the patient's condition is sufficiently precarious that a delay will be detrimental. Outcome from many serious infections is improved if antibiotics are started promptly, but on the other hand, only about 40% of fever episodes in hospitalized patients are caused by infection. Culture yields are highest before antibiotics have been administered, which for certain types of specimens (e.g., blood, cerebrospinal fluid) can be crucial. However, for many infections (e.g., bacteremia, intraabdominal infection, pneumonia), data indicate that early therapy with an appropriate antibiotic in adequate dosage improves outcome.

Likely pathogens and corresponding choice of antimicrobial agent(s) must bve determined. It may be desirable to use more than one antibiotic to treat an infection. This approach is most common with empiric therapy, where the pathogen (or even the source of the infection) is assumed (or guessed at), and the potentialities are so broad and the consequences of inaccurate initial therapy so deleterious that more than one drug must be chosen. Two-drug empiric therapy is commonplace for presumed polymicrobial infections such as nosocomial pneumonia or recurrent or persistent abdominal sepsis, or for sepsis of unknown origin in the hospital. It is recommended strongly that triple-antibiotic regimens (e.g., ampicillin *or* vancomycin, *plus* gram-negative coverage, *plus* metronidazole) should be avoided, because administration costs are high and there is no added benefit.

DURATION OF THERAPY

The endpoint of antibiotic therapy is difficult to define. Unfortunately, duration of therapy is not well established in the literature, and new studies are seldom designed with duration of therapy as a primary endpoint. Much depends on expertise and clinical judgment, which is accumulating in favor of shorter courses of therapy.

Every decision to start antibiotics must be accompanied by a decision regarding the duration of therapy. A reason to continue therapy beyond the predetermined endpoint must be compelling.

Among the many reasons to limit therapy to only that which is needed is that antibiotic therapy has adverse consequences. Adverse consequences of antibiotics include allergic reactions; development of nosocomial superinfections, including fungal infections, enterococcal infections, and *Clostridium difficile*-related disease; organ toxicity; promotion of antibiotic resistance; reduced yield from subsequent cultures; and vitamin K deficiency. The worldwide emergence of multidrug-resistant bacteria, superinfections in immunosuppressed patients, and the increased mortality associated with nosocomial infections in general make it important that adequate therapy is provided rapidly and for the shortest possible duration.

References

1. Trunkey DD. An unacceptable concept. Ann Surg 1999;229:172–173.
2. Barie PS, Hydo LJ. Learning to not know: results of a program for ancillary cost reduction in surgical critical care. J Trauma 1996;41:714–720.
3. Barie PS, Hydo LJ. Lessons learned: durability and progress of a program for ancillary cost reduction in surgical critical care. J Trauma 1997;43:590–596.
4. Knaus WA, Draper EA, Wagner DP, Zimmerman JE. A evaluation of outcome from intensive care in major medical centers. Ann Intern Med 1986;104:410–418.
5. Daley J, Forbes MG, Young GJ, et al. Validating risk-adjusted surgical outcomes: site visit assessment of process and structure. J Am Coll Surg 1997;185:341–351.
6. Ghorra S, Reinert SE, Cioffi W, et al. Analysis of the effect of conversion from open to closed surgical invensive care unit. Ann Surg 1999;229:163–171.
7. Hanson CW III, Deutschman CS, Anderson HL III, et al. Effects of an organized critical care service on outcomes and resource utilization: a cohort study. Crit Care Med 1999;27:270–274.
8. Pronovost PJ, Jenckes MW, Durman T, et al. Organizational characteristics of intensive care units related to outcomes of abdominal aortic surgery. JAMA 1999;281:1310–1317.
9. Gordon TA, Burleyson GP, Tielsch JM, Cameron JL. The effects of regionalization on cost and outcome for one general high-risk surgical procedure. Ann Surg 1995;221:43–49.
10. Glasgow RE, Showstack JA, Katz PP, et al. The relationship between hospital volume and outcomes of hepatic resection for hepatocellular carcinoma. Arch Surg 1999;134:30–35.
11. Velanovich V. Using quality-of-life instruments to assess surgical outcomes. Surgery 1999;126:1–4.
12. Goldman L, Caldera DL, Nussbaum SR, et al. Multifactorial index of cardiac risk in noncardiac surgical procedures. N Engl J Med 1977;297:845–850.
13. Eagle KA, Brundage BH, Chaitman BR, et al. Guidelines for perioperative cardiovascular evaluation for noncardiac surgery. Report of the American College of Cardiology/American Heart Association Task Force on Practice Guidelines (Committee on Perioperative Cardiovascular Evaluation for Noncardiac Surgery). J Am Coll Cardiol 1996;27:910–948.
14. Mangano DT, Layug EL, Wallace A, Tateo I. Effect of atenolol on mortality and cardiovascular morbidity after noncardiac surgery. Multicenter Study of Perioperative Ischemia Research Group. N Engl J Med 1996;335:1713–1720.
15. Poldermans D, Boersma E, Bax JJ, et al. The effect of bisoprolol on perioperative mortality and myocardial infarction in high-risk patients undergoing vascular surgery. N Engl J Med 1999;341:1789–1794.
16. Clagett GP, Anderson FA Jr, Geerts W, et al. Prevention of venous thromboembolism. Chest 1998;114(suppl 5):531S–560S.
17. Palmer AJ, Schramm W, Kirchhof B, Bergemann R. Low molecular weight heparin and unfractionated heparin for prevention of thrombo-embolism in general surgery: a meta-analysis of randomised clinical trials. Haemostasis 1997;27:65–74.
18. Mangram AJ, Horan TC, Pearson ML, et al. Guideline for prevention of surgical site infection, 1999. Hospital Infection Control Practices Advisory Committee. Infect Control Hosp Epidemiol 1999;20:250–278.
19. Salem M, Tainsh RE Jr, Bromberg J, et al. Perioperative glucocorticoid coverage. A reassessment 42 years after emergence of a problem. Ann Surg 1994;219:416–425.
20. Simon TL, Alverson DC, Au Buchon J, et al. Practice parameter for the use of red blood cell transfusions: developed by the Red Blood Cell Administration Practice Guideline Development Task Force of the College of American Pathologists. Arch Pathol Lab Med 1998;122:130–138.
21. Innes G. Guidelines for red blood cells and plasma transfusion for adults and children: an emergency physician's overview of the 1997 Canadian blood transfusion guidelines. Part 1: Red blood cell transfusion. Canadian Medical Association Expert Working Group. J Emerg Med 1998;16:129–131.
22. Spiess BD, Let C, Body SC, et al. Hematocrit value on intensive care unit entry influences the frequency of Q-wave myocardial infarction after coronary artery bypass grafting. J Thorac Cardiovasc Surg 1998;116:460–467.
23. Hebert PC, Wells G, Blajchman MA, et al. A multicenter, randomized, controlled clinical trial of transfusion requirements in critical care. N Engl J Med 1999;340:409–417.
24. Zaloga GP. Early enteral nutritional support improves outcome: fact or fancy? Crit Care Med 1999;27:259–261.
25. Kaufman FR, Devgan S, Roe TF, Costin G. Perioperative management with prolonged intravenous insulin infusion versus subcutaneous insulin in children with type I diabetes mellitus. J Diabetes Complications 1996;10:6–11.
26. Thorell A, Efendic S, Gutmak M, et al. Insulin resistance after abdominal surgery. Br J Surg 1994;81:59–63.
27. O'Grady NP, Barie PS, Bartlett JG, et al. Practice guidelines for evaluating new fever in critically ill adult patients. Task Force of the Society of Critical Care Medicine and the Infectious Diseases Society of America. Clin Infect Dis 1998;26:1042–1059.
28. Montgomery KD, Potter HG, Helfet DL. Magnetic resonance venography to evaluate the deep venous system of the pelvis in patients who have an acetabular fracture. J Bone Joint Surg [Am] 1995;77:1639–1649.
29. Ferretti GR, Bosson JL, Buffaz PD, et al. Acute pulmonary embolism: role of helical CT in 164 patients with intermediate probability at ventilation-perfusion scintigraphy and normal results at duplex US of the legs. Radiology 1997;205:453–458.
30. Meduri GU, Mauldin GL, Wunderink RG, et al. Causes of fever and pulmonary densities in patients with clinical manifestations of ventilator-associated pneumonia. Chest 1994;106:221–235.
31. Talmor M, Li P, Barie PS. Acute paranasal sinusitis in critically ill patients: Guidelines for prevention, diagnosis and treatment. Clin Infect Dis 1997;25:1441–1446.
32. Veenstra DL, Saint S, Saha S, et al. Efficacy of antiseptic-impregnated central venous catheters in preventing catheter-related bloodstream infection: a meta-analysis. JAMA 1999;281:261–267.
33. Barie PS, Fischer E, Eachempati SR. Acute acalculous cholecystitis. Curr Opin Crit Care 1999;5:144–150.
34. Kollef MH. Antibiotic use and antibiotic resistance in the intensive care unit: are we curing or creating disease? Heart Lung 1994;23:363–367.
35. Darby JM, Linden P, Pasculle W, Saul M. Utilization and diagnostic yield of blood cultures in a surgical intensive care unit. Crit Care Med 1997;25:989–994.

Gastrointestinal and Abdominal Disease

Peritoneum and Acute Abdomen

William P. Schecter

Anatomy of the Peritoneal Cavity

The peritoneum is composed of a layer of polyhedral-shaped squamous cells approximately 3 mm thick and may be viewed anatomically as a closed sac that allows for the free movement of abdominal viscera.[1] Adherent to the anterior and lateral abdominal walls, the peritoneum invests the intraabdominal viscera in such a way as to form the mesentery for the small and large bowel, a peritoneal diverticulum posterior to the stomach (the lesser sac) and a number of spaces or recesses in which blood, fluid, or pus can localize in response to various disease processes (Fig. 14.1).

Fluid can therefore collect in (1) the right and left subphrenic spaces (left more commonly than right), (2) the subhepatic space (posterior to the left lobe of the liver), (3) Morrison's pouch (adjacent to the gallbladder), (4) the lesser sac (usually in response to pancreatitis or pancreatic injury), (5) the left and right gutters (lateral to the left and right colon respectively), (6) the pelvis, and (7) the interloop spaces (between the loops of intestine).

The Omentum

The omentum is a membranous adipose tissue within the peritoneal cavity forming (1) the roof of the lesser sac between the greater curvature of the stomach and the transverse colon (lesser omentum) and (2) a veil-like structure suspended from the transverse colon covering the small intestine (the greater omentum).

Surgeons have referred to the omentum as "the policeman of the abdomen" because of its role in walling off intraabdominal abscesses and preventing free peritonitis. However, there is no evidence that there is any intrinsic omental movement.[2,3] The precise mechanism by which the intraabdominal viscera and the omentum wall off collections of pus is not known. The omentum also contains areas with high concentrations of macrophages called "milky spots" which play a major role in the immune response to peritoneal infection.

The Retroperitoneum

The liver, duodenum, and the right and left colon are all partially invested by the peritoneal membrane so that portions of these structures are actually located in the retroperitoneum. The pancreas, kidneys, ureters, and bladder are located entirely in the retroperitoneum. A long retrocecal appendix may be considered as a retroperitoneal structure. These anatomical considerations are important because injuries, diseases, or perforations of these structures in their retroperitoneal location usually produce subtle early symptoms and signs that are often more difficult to diagnose than intraperitoneal infections owing to delay in the onset of peritoneal irritation.

Innervation of the Abdomen

Pain is transmitted from the abdomen to the central nervous system by both the visceral and somatic sensory pathways (Fig. 14.2). Visceral pain (dull, crampy, poorly localized pain) is caused by ischemia, stretching, compression, traction, or chemical irritation of the peritoneum investing the intraabdominal viscera (visceral peritoneum) and transmitted via the slow C fibers running with the sympathetic nerves. Somatic pain (sharp, well-localized pain) is caused by irritation of the peritoneum investing the abdominal wall (parietal peritoneum) and transmitted via the A-∂ fibers of the somatic sensory nerves (T7–L1 anteriorly and L2–L5 posteriorly). Shifting pain is an important historical finding during evaluation of patients with acute abdominal pain. The usual mechanism is the initial development of poorly localized visceral pain caused by distension and ischemia of the abdominal viscera with subsequent irritation of the somatically innervated pari-

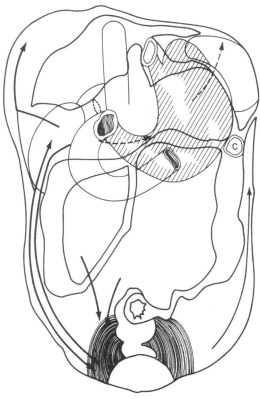

FIGURE 14.1. Diagram of the pathways of flow of intraperitoneal exudates. Broken arrows indicate spread anterior to the stomach to the left subphrenic area. C = splenic flexure of colon. (Modified from Meyers. MA. The spread and localization of acute intraperitoneal effusions. Radiology 95:547–554, 1970, with permission.

etal peritoneum as the inflammatory process progresses, thereby causing localization of the pain.

Physiology of the Peritoneum

The major function of the peritoneal membrane is the maintenance of peritoneal fluid balance.[4] The bidirectional semipermeable membrane has an exchange surface area of 1 m^2.[1,5] Normally the peritoneal cavity contains less than 100 ml of serous fluid.[6] Although the parietal peritoneum of the anterolateral abdominal wall behaves as a passive semipermeable membrane, the diaphragmatic peritoneum is capable of absorbing bacteria.[1,4] Von Recklinghausen in 1863 described intercellular gaps called stomata in the diaphragmatic peritoneum that serve as portals to the diaphragmatic lymphatic pools, called lacunae.[7] Lymph flows from the lacunae via subpleural lymphatics to the regional lymph nodes and then to the thoracic duct.[8,9] As the diaphragm relaxes during exhalation, the stomata open and a negative pressure develops, drawing bacteria into the stomata, which vary in size from 4 to 23 μm.[7] When the diaphragm contracts on inhalation, the stomata close and the increased pressure propels the lymph through the mediastinal lymphatic channels.[4]

Peritoneal fluid travels cephalad toward the diaphragm by action of the "diaphragmatic pump".[10] The concept of the diaphragmatic pump is useful in explaining several clinical phenomena observed in patients with peritoneal infection. Septicemia in patients with peritonitis may in part be explained by the rapid clearance of bacteria from the peritoneum by the diaphragmatic lymphatics. The propensity for the development of subphrenic abscess after peritonitis and the perihepatitis of the Fitz–Hugh–Curtis syndrome related to pelvic inflammatory disease is probably related to the cephalad flow of peritoneal fluid.

Peritoneal Response to Infection

The peritoneum responds to infection in three ways: (1) rapid absorption of bacteria via the diaphragmatic stomata and lymphatics; (2) opsonization and destruction of bacteria via the complement cascade; and (3) localization of bacteria within fibrin to promote abscess formation.[1] Two intraabdominal organs, the liver and spleen, filter bacteria and serve to isolate the infected peritoneal cavity from the rest of the body. The liver filters the portal circulation draining the gastrointestinal tract. This function explains the development of polymicrobial liver abscesses in patients with severe cases of diverticulitis and appendicitis. The spleen filters the systemic circulation and plays an important adjuvant role in bacterial opsonization during bacteremia.

The Bacteriology and Antibiotic Therapy of Peritonitis

The classification of peritonitis as primary peritonitis, secondary peritonitis, or tertiary peritonitis is useful when considering its bacteriology and antibiotic therapy. Primary peritonitis refers to an extraabdominal source of hematogenously transmitted bacterial infection such as spontaneous bacterial peritonitis (SBP), tuberculosis peritonitis, or peritonitis associated with chronic ambulatory peritoneal dialysis (CAPD). SBP occurring in children is usually associated with nephrogenic or hepatogenic ascites. Group A *Streptococcus*, *Staphylococcus aureus*, and *Streptococcus pneumoniae* are the most common organisms.[11] In adults, SBP is most often associated with liver cirrhosis. Aerobic enteric flora such as *Escherichia coli* and *Klebsiella pneumoniae* are the most common organisms.

Secondary bacterial peritonitis refers to infections arising as a result of intraperitoneal processes such as hollow viscus perforation, biliary tract disease, bowel ischemia, and pelvic inflammatory disease. There is a gradient of bacterial concentration (organisms/ml) within the gastrointestinal tract ranging from 10^0 to 10^2 for the stomach, 10^4 to 10^6 for the distal small bowel, and 10^5 to 10^8 for the colon.[12] The consequences of perforation of different parts of the gastrointestinal tract relate, in part, to these differences in bacterial concentration.

The primary treatment of secondary bacterial peritonitis is surgical correction of the anatomical pathology and peritoneal toilet. Empiric antibiotic therapy for established secondary bacterial peritonitis plays an important supplemental role.

The goals of antibiotic therapy are the prevention and treatment of both the systemic inflammatory response syndrome (caused predominantly by facultative gram-negative bacteria) and intraabdominal abscesses (caused predominantly by anaerobes). For community-acquired infections of mild to moderate severity, single drug therapy with a second-generation ceph-

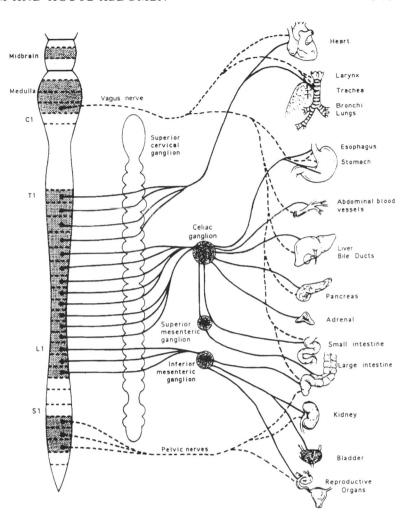

FIGURE 14.2. Pathways of visceral innervation. The visceral afferent fibers mediating pain travel with autonomic nerves to communicate with the central nervous system; in the abdomen, these include both vagal and pelvic parasympathetic nerves and thoracolumbar sympathetic nerves. *Solid lines*, sympathetic fibers. *Dashed lines*, parasympathetic fibers. (From Feldman, Sleisenger, and Scharschmidt, eds. Sleisenger & Fordtran's Gastrointestinal and Liver Disease, 6th ed. Philadelphia: Saunders, © 1998, with permission.)

alosporin with activity against anaerobes (e.g., cefotetan, cefoxitin) or a semisynthetic penicillin in combination with a β-lactamase inhibitor (e.g., ticarcillin-clavulinic acid, ampicillin-sulbactan, or piperacillin-tazobactan) is reasonable. For severe infections, coverage with an aminoglycoside (e.g., gentamicin, tobramycin) and an antibiotic with anaerobic coverage (e.g., metronidazole, clindamycin) is an excellent choice. Adjustments may be made for concerns about nephrotoxicity or penicillin allergy. The newer quinolones (e.g., levofloxacin) will probably assume an increasingly important role in the management of intraabdominal infection because of their anaerobic coverage. Antibiotics are recommended for 5 to 7 days for generalized peritonitis,[13] although therapy up to 14 days is reasonable for patients with severe fecal peritonitis.[14] Antibiotics should be stopped if the patient becomes afebrile and leukocytosis resolves. If signs of infection persist despite a course of antibiotics, a search for an intraabdominal abscess or other source of infection is necessary.

Ill-advised prolonged use of antibiotics, particularly in patients with persistent sources of intraabdominal infection, can lead to so-called tertiary peritonitis, opportunistic infection with normally nonpathogenic gut flora such as *Candida albicans*, *Enterococcus*, and even *Staphylococcus*.[15] The development of tertiary peritonitis is a serious occurrence and a poor prognostic sign.[16]

The Acute Abdomen (Fig. 14.3)

History

A careful, complete history is essential to avoid serious mistakes. The time course, nature, location, and radiation of pain are important clues. The sudden onset of severe pain (the patient can often state the precise time of onset) is associated with hollow viscus perforation. The gradual progression of intermittent spasmodic pain is characteristically associated with hollow viscus obstruction. Epigastric pain radiating to the back is a common complaint in patients with pancreatitis. Colicky flank pain radiating to the groin is typical in patients with renal colic. Ask the patient specifically about a change in the location of the pain (shifting pain). Generalized abdominal pain shifting to a specific location is an important finding as it may indicate the onset of local inflammation of the parietal (somatically innervated) peritoneum as often occurs in appendicitis.

Ask about nausea, vomiting, and hematemesis. What color is the vomitus? Clear vomitus may indicate gastric outlet obstruction. Feculent emesis, on the other hand, often indicates a distal bowel obstruction. What is the relationship of the vomiting to the other symptoms and signs? Early extensive vomiting associated with a scaphoid abdomen indi-

Acute Abdomen

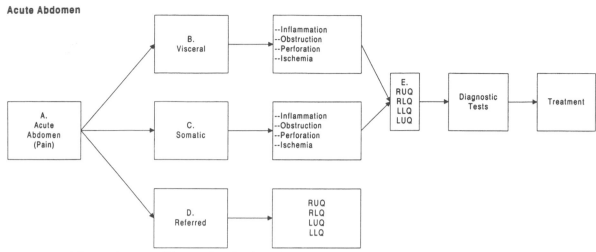

FIGURE 14.3. Acute abdomen. (From Millikan and Saclarides, eds. Common Surgical Diseases: An Algorithmic Approach to Problem Solving. New York: Springer-Verlag, © 1998, with permission.)

cates high small-bowel obstruction. Late or absent vomiting associated with abdominal distension indicates distal small-bowel or colonic obstruction.

Are the bowel movements regular? What is their color and consistency? Inquire about symptoms of dysuria, frequency, or hematuria. Has the urine changed color (possibly indicating excretion of metabolites of bilirubin)? In women, a careful menstrual and obstetric history is essential. What is the relationship of the pain to the menstrual cycle? Could the patient be pregnant? Inquire about alcohol and drug use and recent injuries or accidents. Finally, a careful cardiac and respiratory history can help to identify nonsurgical causes of abdominal pain.

Physical Examination

The patient with acute abdominal pain requires a complete physical examination. General assessment may reveal a rapid, thready pulse and a "worried look" or glazed disinterested response to questions, which should raise the suspicion of serious illness.

Deep palpation has little or no role in the initial assessment of the patient with peritonitis. The goal of the examination is to move the peritoneum with minimum force to see if the patient experiences pain. First, inspect the abdomen and note whether it is scaphoid or distended. Ask the patient to cough before touching the abdomen. Cough tenderness, particularly cough tenderness that localizes to a specific abdominal location, is an important sign of peritoneal irritation.

If the patient has an umbilical hernia, the peritoneum is lying adjacent to the skin of the umbilicus. Gently tap over the umbilical hernia to see if pain is elicited. Gently scratch the skin of the four abdominal quadrants. Rarely, hyperesthesia of the skin is present over the area of peritoneal irritation. Next, apply graded stimuli to the four abdominal quadrants. "Guarding" or rigidity of the abdomen wall musculature may result from peritonitis. Start by "jiggling" the skin with your fingers, gently palpate, and then percuss to apply a firmer controlled stimulus. Finally, deep palpation should be done followed by quick release to assess direct and referred rebound tenderness, two very important signs of peritoneal irritation akin to cough tenderness.

Examine the patient for flank and costovertebral angle tenderness indicative of renal colic or pyelonephritis. Search for abdominal wall hernias and examine the scrotum and testicles in men. Sometimes torsion of the testicle or epididymitis can present as lower abdominal pain in embarrassed and frightened young men.

Auscultation can be useful in patients with suspected bowel obstruction. The characteristic high-pitched "auscultatory rush" of a peristaltic wave vainly attempting to propel intestinal chyme beyond a point of obstruction supports the diagnosis of mechanical obstruction. Although bowel sounds are said to be absent in diffuse peritonitis, I do not find abdominal auscultation helpful in assessing most cases because a "quiet" abdomen can be normal and a patient with "active bowel sounds" can have abdominal pathology requiring emergency surgery. The digital rectal exam usually identifies rectal and pelvic masses. The presence of blood or edema and air in the rectal ampulla are also important diagnostic clues.

In women, a vaginal speculum and bimanual and pelvic examination are important to evaluate the possibility of pregnancy, tubal pregnancy, endometriosis, and pelvic inflammatory disease. The diagnosis of pelvic inflammatory disease may be subtle. Not all patients have exquisite cervical motion tenderness when examined. Adnexal masses can be difficult to palpate in patients who are guarding or who are obese. Pelvic ultrasonography, an abdominal CT scan, or diagnostic laparoscopy may be necessary to make the diagnosis in patients with subtle signs of gynecological disease causing acute abdominal pain.

Laboratory Evaluation

Routine laboratory evaluation for the patient with an acute abdomen should include a complete blood count, a urinalysis, and an assessment of renal function (measurement of the blood urea nitrogen [BUN] and serum creatinine). The serum electrolytes are usually measured along with the BUN and creatinine. Measurement of the electrolytes is mandatory if there has been a prolonged period of vomiting. The serum amylase should be measured if there is any question of pancreatitis. Measure serum alkaline phosphatase, bilirubin, and serum transaminase levels if liver or biliary tract disease is a possibility. Women in their reproductive years should have a pregnancy test.

Radiology of the Acute Abdomen

The traditional radiologic evaluation begins with an upright chest film and flat plate and upright abdominal films. The chest film can rule out pneumonia and pleural effusion as a cause of upper abdominal pain. Occasionally a dehydrated patient with pneumonia and upper abdominal pain will have a clear chest X-ray. The pulmonary infiltrate becomes apparent only after rehydration with intravenous fluids. The upright chest film is also an excellent test for demonstrating free intraperitoneal air (Fig. 14.4). Search the X-ray carefully below the diaphragm for the characteristic radiolucent line indicating extraluminal air, easiest to see between the liver and the right hemidiaphragm. If an upright chest film is impossible to obtain because of the severity of the patient's illness, free air may be demonstrated by turning the patient to the left lateral decubitus position and waiting a few minutes. The extraluminal air will rise and be evident as a radiolucent line between the abdominal wall and the right lobe of the liver after shooting a cross-table lateral X-ray.[17]

Pelvic ultrasonography is an important imaging test in the evaluation of women with lower abdominal pain. Using the distended urinary bladder as an acoustic window, the uterus and adnexae can usually be accurately examined, permitting diagnosis of intrauterine pregnancy, tubal pregnancy, tuboovarian abscess, and pelvic inflammatory disease. Often, the pelvic ultrasound is most useful in distinguishing appendicitis from gynecological diseases causing right lower quadrant pain in women.[18]

Ultrasonography is the initial imaging test of choice in the evaluation of right upper quadrant pain.[19] The exam usually provides accurate information about the gallbladder and the common bile duct. The kidney can be visualized to look for nephrolithiasis or hydronephrosis in patients with flank pain. Ultrasonography by surgeons in the trauma resuscitation room is rapidly becoming a standard test to diagnose the presence of intraabdominal hemorrhage and hemopericardium after blunt and penetrating torso trauma.[20]

The CT scan provides the best anatomical information about the acute abdomen. The introduction of the helical (spiral) abdominal CT scan has reduced the time of the scan to less than 5 min and vastly improved the quality of the im-

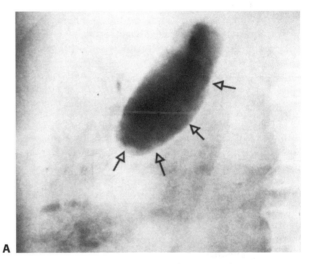

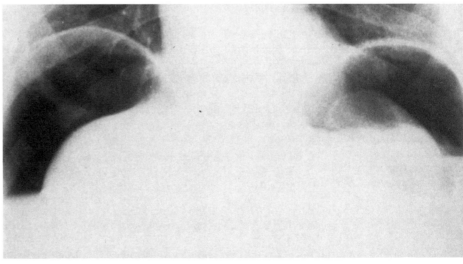

FIGURE 14.4. Free intraperitoneal air. (A) Supine. Although no increased lucency is directly apparent, it is revealed by the visualized density of the wall of a small bowel loop. This presents as a subtle white line around the gas-containing lumen (arrows). (B) Erect film documents considerable free air. At surgery, a perforated duodenal ulcer was found. (Reproduced with permission from Meyers and Oliphant, Current Problems in Radiology, vol. IV, no. 2, pp. 1–37. © 1974 Year Book Medical Publishers.)

ages by reducing respiratory misregistration.[17] The CT scan provides highly accurate anatomical information about the liver, spleen, kidney, ureter, and bladder (if a retrograde cystogram is performed during the CT scan). It is an excellent test for the identification of intraabdominal abscesses.[21] It is a useful test in diagnosing pancreatitis and pancreatic injury after trauma. Further, the spiral abdominal CT, can detect small amounts of intraperitoneal fluid associated with a hollow viscus injury[22] and has improved the accuracy of this preoperative diagnosis.

A recent study showed that spiral CT scans of the appendix improved patient care by reducing the number of unnecessary appendectomies and reducing the delay to operation in patients without a definitive diagnosis.[23] Hospital costs were also lowered in this study. Still, it is important to use this technology judiciously, since the routine use of the abdominal CT scan in all patients with an acute abdomen will expose many patients who obviously need surgery, based on clinical criteria, to unnecessary irradiation and could potentially delay required surgery due to scheduling difficulties.

The Differential Diagnosis of the Acute Abdomen

After reviewing the history, physical exam, and appropriate laboratory and radiologic data, the surgeon must develop a differential diagnosis and decide whether or not the patient requires surgery. Serial abdominal examinations searching for evolving peritoneal signs and repeat measurements of the WBC are critical if the diagnosis is uncertain. Several variables determine the speed of the diagnostic evaluation, the diagnoses to be considered, and the necessity for exploratory laparotomy in the absence of a definitive diagnosis. These variables are (1) the hemodynamic stability of the patient, (2) the presence or absence of a rigid abdomen on physical examination, (3) the character and anatomical location of the abdominal pain, and (4) the deterioration or improvement in symptoms, signs, and laboratory data during the period of observation.[24]

The hemodynamically unstable patient with acute abdominal pain is a surgical emergency and requires rapid evaluation and treatment. The first priority is to consider the diagnosis of a leaking abdominal aortic aneurysm (AAA). Patients with intraperitoneal or retroperitoneal hemorrhage require resuscitation and control of hemorrhage in the operating room, in the interventional radiology suite, or in the intensive care unit depending upon the source of the bleeding and the response to fluid resuscitation. The emergency department is not the appropriate place for a prolonged evaluation of the unstable patient. These patients should be transported to the OR or the ICU as soon as feasible for assessment and treatment.

In general, hemodynamic instability caused by peritonitis is a late development occurring in patients with hollow viscus perforation, prolonged obstruction, or intestinal ischemia. Urosepsis should always be considered as it is a common cause of hemodynamic instability, particularly in the elderly patient, and does not require laparotomy. Patients with pyelonephritis usually have costovertebral angle tenderness or flank pain. Elderly septic men with lower abdominal pain may have massive distension of the bladder from prostatic hypertrophy, which can be diagnosed by dullness to percussion of the lower abdomen. A Foley catheter, antibiotics, and fluids will usually solve the acute problem.

Another relatively common cause of hemodynamic instability in the septic elderly patient is cholangitis. The first line of treatment is antibiotics and biliary drainage. The patient should be resuscitated and undergo elective biliary surgery when completely stable. The hemodynamically stable patient with a rigid abdomen and peritoneal signs should be studied with an upright chest X-ray and plain and upright abdominal X-rays. Patients with evidence of hollow viscus perforation or obstruction should undergo immediate abdominal exploration.

If the abdomen is soft without generalized peritoneal signs, a reasonable differential diagnosis can be developed based on the nature and the location of the abdominal pain. Poorly localized abdominal pain, particularly severe abdominal pain out of proportion to the findings on physical examination, suggests the diagnosis of bowel ischemia. Pain caused by obstructive processes (bowel obstruction and appendicitis), visceral inflammation (inflammatory bowel disease, enteritis, or colitis), and retroperitoneal disease (pancreatitis) may initially present as poorly localized abdominal pain transmitted by the visceral C fibers. Localization occurs when the somatically innervated parietal peritoneum becomes inflamed.

Abdominal pain can localize to the (1) epigastrium, (2) right upper quadrant, (3) left upper quadrant, (4) right lower quadrant, (5) left lower quadrant, and (6) the right and left flanks. The location of the pain is an important clue to the diagnosis.

Upper abdominal pain localizing to either the epigastrium or the right or the left upper quadrant may be caused by diseases of the myocardium (infarction, pericarditis), lungs (pneumonia, pleuritis, pleural effusion, empyema, pulmonary infarction), peptic ulcer disease, and pancreatitis. Subphrenic abscesses may also cause left or right upper abdominal pain and are frequently associated with sympathetic pleural effusions and occasionally associated with hiccups. Pain localizing to the right upper quadrant is classically associated with hepatobiliary disease (cholangitis, biliary colic, cholangitis, hepatitis). Appendicitis, particularly a long retrocecal inflamed appendix, can present with right upper quadrant pain. Right-sided pyelonephritis or nephrolithiasis can also cause right upper quadrant pain. A careful physical examination, however, will usually elicit more tenderness in the right flank than the right upper quadrant in these cases.

Splenomegaly, ruptured spleen, pancreatitis, and pancreatic pseudocysts are diagnoses that should be considered in patients with left upper quadrant pain. Patients with irritation of the left hemidiaphragm may also have referred pain to the left shoulder.

Lower abdominal pain can be caused by musculoskeletal injury, rectus sheath hematoma (particularly in patients receiving anticoagulation medication), ileopsoas muscle abscess (the ipsilateral hip is usually held in flexion[25]), and ureterolithiasis. Appendicitis commonly presents with a history of generalized abdominal pain subsequently localizing to the right lower quadrant. Meckel's diverticulitis, diverticulitis of the right colon, mesenteric adenitis, and regional enteritis (Crohn's disease) must be considered in the differential diagnosis. A history of diarrhea with mucus or blood in the stool is usually present with active Crohn's disease causing right lower quadrant pain. Occasionally, the surgeon can be fooled by a patient with a perforated duodenal ulcer who presents with right lower quadrant pain. In such cases, the duodenal contents pool in the right gutter adjacent to the cecum, causing irritation of the parietal peritoneum. At laparotomy, bile-stained fluid is found without evidence of appendicitis or Meckel's diverticulitis.

The distinction between appendicitis and right lower quadrant pain caused by gynecological disease in women, is often difficult. Pelvic inflammatory disease, tuboovarian abscesses, ectopic pregnancy, endometriosis, and even mittelschmerz should be considered on the differential diagnosis. The pelvic ultrasound examination is currently the most important test for diagnosing gynecological disease in patients with acute abdominal pain. However, the role of the helical CT scan is becoming increasingly important in the evaluation of patients with right lower quadrant pain. The differential diagnosis of left lower quadrant pain is similar to right lower quadrant pain except that diverticulitis replaces appendicitis as the most common diagnosis in the differential. Neoplasm and bowel obstruction should also be considered.

Abdominal distension and obstipation suggest the diagnosis of bowel obstruction. The obstruction may be located in the small or large intestine. Patients with large-bowel obstruction have a dilated colon usually visible on the plain film of the abdomen. The goals of the evaluation are determination of the precise location of the obstruction, assessment of whether the obstruction is partial or complete, determination of whether emergency surgery or conservative management is required, and ultimately diagnosis of the precise cause of the obstruction.

The history elicits the duration of symptoms, the presence of nausea or vomiting, and whether the patient has recently passed flatus. A careful review of previous operations, weight loss, or previous diagnoses of malignancy or endometriosis may reveal important clues. The physical examination should include a careful search for incarcerated hernias, peritoneal signs, or localized abdominal pain and fever. The absence of air in the rectal ampulla is an important sign of complete obstruction. Leukocytosis may indicate ischemia resulting from closed loop obstruction.

Examine the abdominal plain films carefully for signs of air in the colon or colonic distention. A large air-filled loop of colon located between the left lower and right upper quadrants suggests the diagnosis of sigmoid volvulus. Conversely, a dilated loop of colon between the right lower and left upper quadrants suggests cecal volvulus. Volvulus can often be treated by sigmoidoscopic or colonoscopic decompression. However, extreme caution must be exercised to avoid colon perforation. It is far better to achieve safe surgical decompression than to unwisely persist with a prolonged difficult endoscopy that may result in massive fecal contamination of the peritoneal cavity due to perforation. A gentle water-soluble contrast enema can be used to identify the point of obstruction. Barium should **never** be used in this clinical situation because of the risk of perforation.

Small-bowel obstruction is suggested by a plain film with multiple air–fluid levels and the absence of air in the colon. Peritoneal signs, localized abdominal pain, fever, and leukocytosis are absolute indications for exploration. A patient with a distended abdomen who has recently passed flatus may be only partially obstructed. If the patient appears to be partially obstructed, nasogastric decompression, fluid resuscitation, and serial abdominal examinations are appropriate initial therapy.

Unusual Nonoperative Causes of Abdominal Pain

NEUROLOGICAL CAUSES OF ABDOMINAL PAIN

Varicella zoster viral infections can cause radiating pain and hyperesthesia along the dermatome of an intercostal nerve followed by a typical vesicular rash 5 to 7 days after the onset of symptoms. "Shingles" is usually a self-limited disease treated by analgesics. Treatment with acyclovir is indicated in severe cases. Occasionally, a herniating disk producing compression radiculopathy causes confusing symptoms of abdominal wall pain. A CT or MRI will make the definitive diagnosis.

PAIN CAUSED BY TOXIC SUBSTANCE INGESTION

Ingestion of toxic substances such as iron, lead, poisonous mushrooms, and alcohol (ethanol, isopropanol, and methanol) all cause crampy abdominal pain often associated with diarrhea. Patients withdrawing from opiates (heroin) have abdominal pain as a characteristic part of the withdrawal symptoms.

ENDOCRINE CAUSES OF ABDOMINAL PAIN

Endocrine and metabolic diseases can cause abdominal pain. Glucocorticoid deficiency (Addison's disease) presents with hypotension, tachycardia, weakness, fatigue, and crampy abdominal pain (50% of cases). Glucocorticoid therapy results in resolution of the abdominal pain.

Hypercalcemia can cause diffuse symptoms including crampy abdominal pain. Hypercalcemia is also associated with other causes of abdominal pain including peptic ulcer disease, pancreatitis, and nephrolithiasis.

Diabetic ketoacidosis sometimes presents with acute abdominal pain. The mechanism is poorly understood. More often, the patient develops ketoacidosis as a consequence of pulmonary, intraabdominal (urinary tract, biliary tract), or soft tissue infection. Treatment consists of restoration of intravascular volume, correction of hyperglycemia and the electrolyte imbalance, and identification and treatment of the source of infection.

GENETIC DISORDERS CAUSING ABDOMINAL PAIN

Familial Mediterranean fever is an autosomal recessive genetic disease characterized by recurrent episodes of abdominal pain, peritoneal inflammation, and fever. Other serosal membranes such as the pleura, pericardium, and meninges also become intermittently inflamed.

Porphyria is a term referring to a group of autosomal dominant disorders caused by defective heme synthesis. Neurotoxic intermediates of heme metabolism (porphyrins) accumulate that cause abdominal pain, ileus, changes in mental status, psychiatric disturbance, muscle weakness, and skin photosensitivity.

Sickle cell anemia is an autosomal recessive disease of the hemoglobin molecule resulting in red cell deformation and clotting in the microcirculation under hypoxic conditions. Abdominal pain is a frequent symptom. Treatment includes volume expansion, oxygenation, and analgesics followed by serial abdominal examinations. Pain that fails to resolve should raise the suspicion of bowel infarction. Sickle cell anemia is also associated with cholecystitis caused by bilirubin stones, splenomegaly caused by sequestration of damaged red cells, and splenic infarction.

Vasculitis: a number of immune-mediated diseases causing mesenteric vasculitis can cause acute abdominal pain, the most classic of which is Henoch–Schonlein purpura (HSP).

Special Situations

THE ACUTE ABDOMEN IN THE ELDERLY

Some geriatric patients are poor historians because of either confusion accompanying serious illness or senile dementia. The abdominal examination can also be misleading. The signs of peritoneal irritation that are so important in the evaluation of the younger patient are often absent in geriatric patients. A "surgical abdomen" should be suspected in all elderly patients who present with abdominal pain and distension or obtundation and sepsis regardless of the absence of peritoneal signs. Bowel ischemia, biliary and urosepsis, bowel obstruction, and occult appendicitis are all common diagnoses that should be considered (Table 14.1).

THE ACUTE ABDOMEN IN THE ICU

The evaluation of the sedated, intubated ICU patient is challenging. There are four situations in which acute abdomen presents in the ICU patient.

1. Patient "found down": These patients are usually septic, acidotic, and often hypothermic. Bowel ischemia, either as a cause of the problem or a consequence of the low flow state, should be considered. Abdominal CT scan and diagnostic laparoscopy are assuming an increasingly important role in the workup of this clinical situation.
2. Missed injury: If a multiple trauma patient is behaving in a manner unanticipated by the extent of the known injuries (e.g., hemodynamic instability, large intravenous volume requirement, progressive hypoxemia, unexplained blood requirement), the possibility of a missed injury should be considered. Prolonged delay in laparotomy in these cases will lead to a significant increase in morbidity and mortality.
3. Postoperative surgical complications: Postoperative hemorrhage, obstruction, anastomotic leak, and intraabdominal abscess formation are all potential complications of abdominal surgery. The abdominal CT scan is a critical tool in this situation as it permits accurate identification and often drainage of localized collections of intraabdominal pus without resorting to repeat laparotomy.
4. Abdominal complications of intensive care: Acalculous cholecystitis and perforation or hemorrhage due to stress ulceration of the stomach or duodenum are the most common causes of the acute abdomen as a consequence of the ICU experience.

Planned Abdominal Reexploration

Planned abdominal reexploration is assuming an increasingly important role in the management of selected patients. There are four situations in which planned reexploration is helpful:

1. Second-look laparotomy for bowel ischemia: Intestinal ischemia is a disease process in evolution. Despite a careful inspection and Wood's lamp ultraviolet examination of the bowel after intravenous fluorescein to assess intestinal viability, the surgeon often cannot be completely sure of the viability of the remaining intestine after resection for ischemia. In this situation, a "second-look" laparotomy 24 to 48 h after the first operation is prudent.[26]
2. Peritoneal toilet: Patients with severe fecal peritonitis of long-standing duration may benefit from repeated trips to the OR every 24 to 48 h for peritoneal irrigation until the effluent becomes clear.[27] Usually a relatively clean peritoneal cavity can be achieved after two or three trips to the OR.
3. Reexploration after "damage-control" laparotomy: Hemodynamically unstable, acidotic, hypothermic, coagulopathic patients with major intraabdominal injuries require rapid control of hemorrhage (often with intraabdominal packing) and closure and/or resection of hollow viscus injuries. Temporary abdominal closure before intestinal reconstruction allows time for continued resuscitation, patient rewarming, and correction of the coagulopathy in the ICU. The patient can then be returned to the operating room in 12 to 24 h for reexploration and appropriate intestinal reconstruction under stable conditions.
4. Abdominal compartment syndrome: The abdominal compartment syndrome occurs when intraabdominal pressure increases to a level resulting in oliguria, hypoperfusion of the intraabdominal viscera, inadequate mechanical ventilation despite high peak inspiratory pressures, and collapse of the vena cava and renal veins (as seen on abdominal CT scan). Clinically, the abdomen is rigid. The urinary bladder pressure measured by transducing the pressure in the Foley catheter approximates the intraabdominal pressure. An elevated urinary bladder pressure (>30 mmHg) is an objective sign of abdominal compartment syndrome. Loose abdominal closure with a temporary nonadherent prosthetic material decompresses the high intraabdominal pressure.

TABLE 14.1. Common Locations and Corresponding Diagnosis in Elderly Abdominal Pain.

Epigastrium	**Right upper quadrant and flank**
Abdominal aortic aneurysm	Cholecystitis
Colon carcinoma	Choledocholithiasis
Duodenal ulcer	Gastric ulcer
Early appendicitis	Intestinal obstruction
Gastritis	Pancreatitis
Mesenteric ischemia	Penetrating ulcer
Pancreatitis	Pyelonephritis
Penetrating ulcer	Renal colic
	Retrocecal appendicitis
Left upper quadrant and flank	**Right lower quadrant**
Bowel obstruction	Appendicitis
Diverticulitis	Bowel obstruction
Pyelonephritis	Cholecystitis
Renal colic	Diverticulitis
Splenic enlargement	Hernia
	Leaking aneurysm
	Psoas abscess
	Pyelonephritis
Left lower quadrant	
Abdominal wall hematoma	
Bowel obstruction	
Diverticulitis	
Hernia	
Leaking aneurysm	
Pyelonephritis	
Geriatric abdominal pain	
Mesenteric ischemia	

Source: Modified with permission from Caesar, Emerg Med Rep 1994;3(20):191–202.

The Acute Abdomen in the Tropics

A variety of bacterial and parasitic diseases endemic to tropical regions are potential causes of an acute surgical abdomen. Typhoid fever, amebiasis, and ascariasis are the most likely to be encountered by surgeons practicing in the United States and Western Europe.

The Acute Abdomen in the HIV-Infected Patient

An increasing number of patients presenting with acute abdominal pain have concommitant HIV infection because of the increasing prevalence of HIV. In the absence of obvious peritoneal signs, a CT scan is advisable in most HIV-infected patients before surgery to rule out a nonoperative cause of the pain. Approximately 40% of HIV-infected patients with acute surgical abdomens have diagnoses directly related to their immunocompromised state (e.g., perforated colon from CMV [cytomegalovirus] colitis, CMV cholecystitis, bowel obstruction from lymphoma, etc.).[28] The remaining diagnoses result from common causes of the acute abdomen.

The Acute Abdomen in Pregnancy

The enlarging uterus alters the intraabdominal location of adjacent organs. The cecum is pushed into the right upper quadrant, making assessment of the physical findings more difficult. If appendicitis is suspected, the incision should be centered over the point of maximum tenderness rather than over McBurney's point to optimize exposure.

The surgeon has two patients, the mother and the fetus. If laparotomy is indicated, the surgeon should work in concert with the obstetrician and the anesthesiologist to monitor the fetus and provide tocolytic therapy to prevent premature labor and delivery.[29]

Laparotomy or Laparoscopy

The recent expansion of both diagnostic and therapeutic laparoscopy has added a new tool to the surgical armamentarium. Unfortunately, laparoscopic technology has not yet developed to the point where the average surgeon can adequately examine the entire bowel. At the present time, the choice of diagnostic laparoscopy versus exploratory laparotomy when the diagnosis is unknown depends on the experience and judgment of the individual surgeon.[30]

References

1. Hall JC, Heel KA, Papadimitrou JM, Palytell C. The pathophysiology of peritonitis. Gastroenterology 1998;114:185–196.
2. Rothenberg RE, Rosenblatt P. Motility and response of the great omentum: fluoroscopic observations on the omental activity of dogs. Arch Surg 1942;44:764–771.
3. Florey H, Walker JL, Carleton HM. The nature of the movement of the omentum. J Pathol Bacteriol 1926;29:97–106.
4. Maddaus MA, Ahrenholz D, Simmons R. The biology of peritonitis and implications for treatment. Surg Clin North Am 1988;68:431–443.
5. Henderson LW, Nolph KD. Altered permeability of the peritoneal membrane using hypertonic peritoneal dialysis fluid. J Clin Invest 1969;48:992–1001.
6. Robinson SC. Observations on the peritoneum as an absorbing surface. Am J Obstet Gynecol 1962;83:446–452.
7. Tsilbary EC, Wissig SL. Lymphatic absorption from the peritoneal cavity: regulation of the patency of the mesothelial stomata. Microvasc Res 1983;25:22.
8. Abu-Hijleh MF, Habbal OA, Moqattash ST. The role of the diaphragm in lymphatic absorption from the peritoneal cavity. J Anat 1995;186:453–467.
9. Li J, Jiang B. A scanning electron microscopic study on three-dimensional organization of human diaphragmatic lymphatics. Fimet Dev Morphol 1993;3:129–132.
10. Last M, Kurtz L, Stein TA, Wise L. Effect of PEEP on the rate of thoracic duct lymph flow and clearance of bacteria from the peritoneal cavity. Am J Surg 1983;145:126–130.
11. Conn HV. Spontaneous bacterial peritonitis: variant syndromes. South Med J 1987;80:1343–1346.
12. Di Piro JT, Mansberger JA, Davis JB Jr. Current concepts in clinical therapeutic intraabdominal infections. Clin Pharm 1986;5:34–50.
13. Bohner JMA, Solomkin JS, Dellinger EP, et al. Guidelines for clinical care: antiinfective agents for intra-abdominal infection. A Surgical Society Policy Statement. Arch Surg 1992;127:83–89.
14. Bartlett JG. Intra-abdominal sepsis. Med Clin North Am 1995;79:599–617.
15. Rotstein OD, Pruett TL, Simmons RL. Microbiologic features and treatment of persistent peritonitis in the intensive care unit. Can J Surg 1986;29:247–250.
16. Nathan AB, Rotstein OD, Marshall JC. Tertiary peritonitis: clinical features of a complex nosocomial infection. World J Surg 1998;22:158–163.
17. Gypta H, Dupuy DE. Advances in imaging the acute abdomen. Surg Clin North Am 1997;77:1245–1283.
18. Fa EM, Cronan EJ. Compression ultrasonography as an aid in the differential diagnosis of appendicitis. Surg Gynecol Obstet 1989;169:290–298.
19. Carroll BA. Preferred imaging techniques for the diagnosis of cholecystitis and cholelithiasis. Ann Surg 1989;210:1–12.
20. Healey MA, Simons RK, Winchell RJ, et al. A prospective evaluation of abdominal ultrasound in blunt trauma: is it useful? J Trauma 1996;40:875–883.
21. Goletti O, Lippolis PV, Chiarugi M, et al. Percutaneous ultrasound guided drainage of intra-abdominal abscesses. Br J Surg 1993;80:336–339.
22. Livingston DH, Lavery RF, Passannante MR, et al. Admission or observation is not necessary after a negative abdominal computed tomography scan in patients with blunt abdominal trauma: results of a prospective multi-institutional trial. J Trauma 1998;44:273–280.
23. Rao PM, Rhea JT, Novelline RA, et al. Effect of computed tomography of the appendix on treatment of patients and use of hospital resources. N Engl J Med 1998;338:141–146.
24. Martin RF, Ross RL. The acute abdomen: an overview and algorithm. Surg Clin North Am 1997;77:1227.
25. Schecter W, Rintel T, Slutkin G, et al. Tropical pyomyositis of the iliacus muscle. Am J Trop Med Hyg 1983;34:809–811.
26. Montgomery RA, Venbrux AC, Bulkley GB. Mesenteric vascular insufficiency. Curr Probl Surg 1997;34:941–1028.
27. Butler JA, Huang J, Wilson SE. Repeated laparotomy for postoperative intra-abdominal sepsis: an analysis of outcome predictors. Arch Surg 1987;122:702–706.
28. Whitney TM, Brunell W, Russell TR, et al. Emergent abdominal surgery in AIDS: experience in San Francisco. Am J Surg 1994;168:239–243.
29. Fallon WF, Newman JS, Fallon GL, Malangoni MA. The surgical management of intraabdominal inflammatory conditions during pregnancy. Surg Clin North Am 1995;75:15–31.
30. Memon MA, Fitzgibbons RJ. The role of minimal access surgery in the acute abdomen. Surg Clin North Am 1997;77:1333–1353.

General Principles of Minimally Invasive Surgery

Edward G. Chekan and Theodore N. Pappas

Equipment

The equipment required for basic laparoscopy can be grouped into three categories: image production, peritoneal access devices, and instrumentation. Because functional equipment is available in both disposable and reusable forms, most decisions regarding these issues have been based on a cost analysis.

Access Devices

Access to the peritoneal cavity is gained using the closed, Veress needle technique or the open, Hasson technique. The open technique first calls for the Veress needle (fashioned with a safety shield) to be placed through a small cutaneous incision. Next, the abdominal wall is grasped and lifted as the needle is placed through the abdominal fascia and into the peritoneal cavity. Proponents of this technique claim that it is safer, easier, and quicker than alternatives. The open technique, similar to that used for open diagnostic peritoneal lavage, provides peritoneal access under direct visualization. Although the open technique is often claimed to be safer,[1] both techniques have been associated with complications and serious injuries. However, most would agree that the open technique is superior in patients who have undergone previous abdominal surgery.

GASES

Once access has been gained to the peritoneal cavity, a working space is created through insufflation or by mechanical lifting. In most centers, CO_2 is the insufflation gas of choice. Advantages of CO_2 include its noncombustible nature (allowing for the use of electrocautery) and its high solubility (allowing for easy expiration via the lungs). However, because the absorbed CO_2 is converted to H_2CO_3 in the bloodstream, the extra hydrogen ion is responsible for lowering the plasma pH, which can lead to several physiological consequences. Conse-quently, other gases with varying properties, such as nitrous oxide, air, argon, helium and oxygen, have been used.

TROCARS

Following insufflation, additional trocars are placed under direct visualization. In general, the trocars should be arranged in a triangle so that the instruments are moving toward the operative field in the same direction as the laparoscope. The trocars should be placed far enough apart (8–10 cm) to allow for easy external access and to avoid unnecessary internal interactions or "swordfighting." In general, three to five trocars are adequate to accomplish most laparoscopic procedures, with the exact number being dictated by the individual procedure.

Image Production

Laparoscopic surgery is dependent on adequate visualization of the operative field. The standard 0° Hopkins rod-lens laparoscope ranges in size between 5 and 10 mm in outer diameter with oblique viewing scopes (30° and 45°) also available. The light originates from a high-intensity external source and is transmitted in a zigzag pattern along a fiberoptic cable to an attachment on the laparoscope with subsequent transmission through the laparoscope to the operative field. The illuminated image is then interpreted by a camera that is mounted on the extracorporeal end on the laparoscope. The inherent disadvantage of such a system is the creation of a two-dimensional image and subsequent loss of depth perception. Systems for three-dimensional imaging are available, but remain under development.[2]

Instrumentation

There are now two separate, distinct groups of laparoscopic instruments: the more accepted 5- to 12-mm instrumentation and the miniature version or small-caliber instrumentation. The latter are often referred to as mini-instruments. A basic laparoscopic instrument set should include graspers, dissectors, scissors, and a needle holder. Additionally, most procedures also require a clip applier, stapling or suturing device, and the suction/irrigator. Advanced procedures employ more specialized instrumentation.

Physiology of Pneumoperitoneum

Within this section, the term pneumoperitoneum (PNP) refers to the physiological changes associated with intraperitoneal carbon dioxide insufflation.

Circulatory Effects

CARDIOVASCULAR

Pneumoperitoneum significantly and reproducibly affects the venous and arterial systems. These hemodynamic alterations result from increased intraabdominal pressure and volume and, to a lesser extent, systemic hypercarbia. In the supine patient, the main pressure–volume effect of intraperitoneal insufflation to approximately 10 to 20 mmHg is to simultaneously decrease preload and increase afterload. In turn, several authors have reported a subsequent decrease in cardiac output (CO).

PRELOAD
Studies have shown that PNP causes an increase in central venous pressure (CVP) and pulmonary capillary wedge pressure (PCWP), both traditional markers of cardiac filling, but a concurrent decrease in stroke volume (SV). The rise in measured CVP is the result of an increase in intraabdominal pressure (IAP) that directly compresses the low-pressure vasculature such as the abdominal vena cava.[3] Paradoxically, the increase in CVP and PCWP actually results in decreased cardiac filling pressures or preload.

AFTERLOAD
Most of the reported studies have shown an increase in both mean arterial pressure (MAP) and systemic vascular resistance (SVR) with moderate degrees of PNP. Most authors believe that the increase in afterload in conjunction with PNP is the result of two factors: the release of humoral factors (catecholamines and vasopressin) soon after commencing insufflation, and from direct aortic compression due to increased IAP.[4,5]

Although there is a mild decrease in CO, most agree that the effects of PNP on CO are clinically insignificant.

Patient positioning and duration of insufflation are additional factors influencing various hemodynamic parameters measured during PNP. Reverse-Trendelenberg (head-up) positioning combined with PNP, as in LC, counteracts the effects of PNP by causing a decrease in CVP and PCWP in comparison to the supine patient. Likewise, Trendelenberg (head-down) positioning combined with PNP, as in gynecological procedures, causes an increase in measured CVP and PCWP when compared to supine positioning.[6] Although some warn that head-up positioning may compromise CO by decreasing preload,[7] the incidence of documented clinically significant sequelae in such patients is low.

SPLANCHNIC/HEPATIC/RENAL

Just as PNP has been shown to decrease cardiac venous return, studies have also illustrated that an increase in IAP similarly effects the perfusion of many abdominal organs. These effects may occur locally before the recognition of the aforementioned systemic hemodynamic effects. For instance, both hepatic and renal perfusions are decreased with increasing IAP. The clinical implications of this are unclear, however, since there is no convincing evidence to suggest lasting significant organ dysfunction as a result.

Coagulation Effects

Virchow's triad of hypercoagulability, venous stasis, and trauma are the three main factors responsible for venous thromboembolism. Laparoscopic surgery entails the same risks of thromboembolism as the traditional approach; however, some have postulated that certain risk factors, namely venous stasis caused by PNP and hypercoagulability, pose a greater threat to the patient undergoing a laparoscopic procedure.

The increase in IAP causes compression on the abdominal IVC, a subsequent rise in CVP, and a decrease in lower extremity venous return. As a result, venous stasis, a known risk factor for deep vein thrombosis (DVT), occurs in the lower extremities. In addition, it has been shown that laparoscopic surgical intervention induces a postoperative hypercoagulable state, which may be due in part to the body's response to general anesthesia and indirectly to venous stasis.[8] Despite a low reported rate of DVT/PE, the theoretical risk of thromboembolism during laparoscopy, coupled with measured decreased femoral venous flow without SCDs, make it prudent to recommend DVT prophylaxis for all patients who are approached laparoscopically. In patients at high risk for thrombosis, the benefits of laparoscopy must be weighed against the risks of thromboembolism.

Pulmonary Effects

The pulmonary system is influenced by PNP both mechanically and chemically (Table 15.1).

From a mechanical standpoint, as IAP is increased intraoperatively the diaphragm is shifted in the cephalad direction, which increases intrathoracic pressure. This reduced, paradoxical diaphragmatic movement in the face of increased intrathoracic pressure leads to an increase in peak airway pressure[9] and the collapse of alveoli. As a result, forced residual capacity (FRC) is decreased.[10] Concurrently, there is also a decrease in tidal volume[11] as well as a decrease in compliance of both the lung and chest wall,[9,12] leading to an overall increase in the work of breathing to maintain constant minute ventilation volume.[13] The addition of positive endexpiratory pressure (PEEP) is a helpful ventilatory adjunct during conventional surgery to help recruit alveoli and to prevent further alveolar collapse. However, the hemodynamic implications of additional PEEP during PNP are complex. Although the direct implications of additional PEEP during PNP are controversial, there is clearly more hemodynamic instability with increasing levels of PEEP.

Hypercapnia is another pulmonary concern requiring the attention of anesthesiologists during laparoscopic cases. Hypercapnia is defined as an increase in the plasma CO_2

TABLE 15.1.

Prospective Clinical Studies (Level II Evidence) of the Postoperative Effects of Laparoscopy Versus Open Procedures on Pulmonary Function in Healthy Adults.

Author	Year	n	Procedure	Time	Study groups	FVC	FEV1	PEFR	P_aCO_2	P_aO_2	Author's conclusions
Chung et al.	1996	22	Urological	POD 3	Retroperitoneoscopic / Flank incision	↓	↓				Retroperitoneoscopy caused less postoperative pulmonary dysfunction than open surgery on POD 3
Eden et al.	1994	16	Nephrectomy	POD 2	Laparoscopic / Open	↓	↓	↓	NC / NC		—
Gunnarsson et al.	1995	36	Cholecystectomy	POD 1	Laparoscopic / Open	↓	↓		NC / NC	↓	Cholecystectomy irrespective of whether it was performed by open or laparoscopic technique was followed by deterioration in ventilatory function and gas exchange; the magnitude of impairment was less pronounced in LC
Joris et al.	1992	30	Cholecystectomy	POD2	Laparoscopic / Open	↓	↓		NC / NC	↓	LC results in less respiratory dysfunction than OC
McMahon et al.	1994	107	Cholecystectomy	POD 2	Laparoscopic / Mini-lap	↓	↓				Pulmonary changes associated with upper abdominal surgery are significantly reduced with the laparoscopic approach
Mealy et al.	1992	21	Cholecystectomy	POD 1	Laparoscopic / Open	↓	↓	↓	↑	NC / NC	Improved respiratory responses to laparoscopic surgery
Peters et al.	1993	40	Cholecystectomy	POD 1	Laparoscopic / Open	↓	↓				LC provides less decrement in pulmonary function than OC
Putensen-Himmer et al.	1992	20	Cholecystectomy	POD 1	Laparoscopic / Open	↓	↓		NC / NC	NC / NC	Respiratory function is less impaired and its recovery improved after LC compared to OC
Rademaker et al.	1992	30	Cholecystectomy	POD 1	Laparoscopic / Laparoscopic with epidural / Open	↓	↓	↓	NC / NC	NC / NC	Pulmonary function is significantly better after LC than after OC via subcostal incision
Schauer et al.	1993	40	Cholecystectomy	POD 1	Laparoscopic / Open	↓	↓	↓			Compared to OC, LC results in a significantly reduced compromise in pulmonary function

↓↑ Arrows: the direction of change was the same for all groups compared. Arrow marks the group with the more significant effect. POD, postoperative day; LC, laparoscopic cholecystectomy; OC, open cholecystectomy; FVC, forced vital capacity; FEV1, forced expiratory volume in 1 min; PEFR, peak expiratory flow rate; P_aCO_2, arterial partial pressure of CO_2; P_aO_2, arterial partial pressure of O_2; NC, no change.

concentration and may occur intraoperatively because CO_2 can easily diffuse across the peritoneal lining.[14] In healthy patients, as CO_2 is absorbed (i.e., P_aCO_2 increases), the respiratory rate increases and CO_2 is expired through the lungs (i.e., P_aCO_2 increases). In unhealthy patients, or in patients unable to spontaneously increase their respiratory rate (i.e., anesthetized, intubated patients), the dissolved CO_2 in the blood is not effectively eliminated and this can lead to systemic acidosis. Mild hypercapnia has very few significant hemodynamic effects. However, severe hypercapnia (50–70 mmHg) can result in systemic hypotension by decreasing CO and SV, given that hypercarbia is both a myocardial depressant and a vasodilator.[15] Because end-tidal CO_2 underestimates P_aCO_2 during PNP and is increasingly unreliable as P_aCO_2 increases,[16] invasive blood gas analysis is imperative in patients in whom minimal hypercarbia could be detrimental.

Effects on Intestinal Function

Many studies have documented an earlier return of bowel function after laparoscopic procedures compared to open procedures.[17a] However, although laparoscopic colon resection may afford the patient less postoperative pain[18] and shorter hospitalization,[19] there seems to be no improvement in myoelectric activity.[20]

Effects on Neurological Function

Cerebral blood flow depends on cerebral perfusion pressure, which is calculated as MAP minus intracranial pressure (ICP). Mortality is increased with elevated, uncontrolled levels of ICP.[21] Chemically, as P_aCO_2 levels rise during PNP, concomitant reflex cerebral vasodilatation occurs that allows for an increase in cerebral blood flow and ICP. There are limited reports of neurological deterioration with PNP[22]; however, laparoscopic intervention should be discouraged in patients in whom a marginal increase in ICP could be devastating (i.e., patients with head trauma).

Metabolic and Immune Effects

It is well known that the extent of surgical intervention or trauma leads to a proportional acute-phase inflammatory response and postoperative immunosuppression. In general, laparoscopy causes a blunted acute-phase and catabolic response compared to open surgery. Moreover, delayed-type hypersensitivity (DTH), a marker for cell-mediated immunity, is less depressed following laparoscopic procedures.

Special Circumstances Concerning Pneumoperitoneum

Pneumoperitoneum and Cancer

Host immunity and cancer should be considered simultaneously. The systemic immune system seems to be better preserved following laparoscopy; however, some studies demonstrate that CO_2 PNP actually encourages tumor growth intraperitoneally. The initial reports documenting an increased risk of trocar site tumor recurrence following laparoscopic cancer procedures led some investigators to question

the safety of CO_2 PNP in oncological patients. Should laparoscopy be performed for cancer? A discussion of PNP and cancer can be divided into systemic and local oncological effects of PNP.

Systemic Oncological Effects

Both laparotomy and laparoscopy encourage tumor growth. However, in several animal studies, it appears that full laparotomy encourages systemic postoperative tumor growth more than CO_2 PNP.

Port Site Metastasis

Several early reports claimed an increase in the incidence of port site tumor recurrences following laparoscopic tumor resection as compared to incisional tumor recurrences following traditional surgery.[23–26] In fact, these initial efforts of laparoscopic colon cancer resection reported an incidence of port site metastases as high as 21%,[27] as compared to a 0.69% to 3.3% incidence of abdominal wound recurrence following traditional resection for colorectal cancer.[28]

However, with an increase in experience with laparoscopic colon resection, more recent reports claim that these rates of trocar site recurrences were largely overestimated. As the true incidence of port site tumor recurrence becomes increasingly defined, experimental studies have provided insight into the pathophysiology behind this phenomenon (Fig. 15.1). Most researchers agree that because systemic immunological and antioncological effects appear to be well preserved with laparoscopy, the increased port site tumor implantation demonstrated in these studies is most likely caused by a direct effect of PNP on the peritoneum, an effect that allows for the implantation of tumor.

Clearly, tumor recurrence requires the presence of tumor cells at the trocar site, and direct contact between the solid tumor and the port site enhances port site tumor growth[29]; this contact could occur by removing the pathological specimen through an unprotected trocar site. A specimen containing or potentially containing cancer should be carefully manipulated and removed through a protected wound.

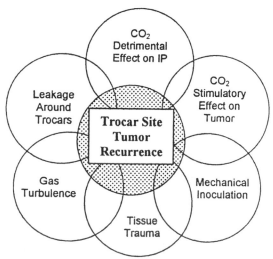

FIGURE 15.1. Factors influencing trocar site tumor recurrence.[88] IP, intraperitoneal immunity.

Pneumoperitoneum and Pregnancy

If surgery during pregnancy is unavoidable, the optimal time period for such intervention is during the second trimester. Second-trimester operative intervention avoids the potential disruption of organogenesis during the first trimester and possible labor induction during the third. For the safety of both mother and fetus, operative time should be kept to a minimum and the fetus should be monitored intraoperatively. The typical indications for laparoscopic surgical intervention during pregnancy include acute appendicitis, acute cholecystitis, ectopic pregnancy, and ovarian torsion.[30] When operating on the pregnant patient, three unique physiological factors must be considered: maternal physiological alterations with pregnancy, uteroplacental blood flow, and the overall well-being of the fetus[30] (Fig. 15.2). There are very few studies presently available to delineate the effects of PNP on the developing fetus or the pregnant mother. The limited evidence that is available supports the safety of laparoscopy during pregnancy.

COMPLICATIONS OF LAPAROSCOPY

Fortunately, major complications occur in well under 1% of laparoscopic procedures, with an overall mortality of 4 to 8 deaths per 100,000 procedures.[31] However, the minimally invasive nature of laparoscopy does not eliminate the potential for serious surgical complications. Several categories of complications unique to laparoscopy include complications related to needle and trocar site insertion, those specific to insufflation, and the establishment of PNP, and those related to the use or misuse of specialized laparoscopic equipment. Most of the data illustrating the complications during laparoscopy have been accumulated during LC (Table 15.2).

The overall morbidity rate for needle and trocar complications is between 0.2% and 0.5%, with mortality rates of 0.0033% to 0.1%.[32–35] The placement of the first trocar or Veress needle accounts for the majority of these injuries.[36] The organ most likely injured is the small bowel (52%), followed by colon, duodenum, and stomach (32%, 11%, and 4.5%, respectively).[37] Bladder perforation can occur any time; however, this complication occurs most frequently during laparoscopic procedures in patients who have had previous surgery. Bladder perforation can be recognized by bubbling within the urine collection bag. Vascular injuries are reported less frequently[38,39] but if unrecognized can be devastating.[33] The

TABLE 15.2.

Vascular and Bowel Injuries During 77,604 Laparoscopic Cholecystectomies (Level III Evidence).

Injury site	No. of patients (%)	No. of patients requiring laparotomy
Vascular		
Retroperitoneal vessels		
Aorta	13	12
Inferior vena cava	5	3
Iliac artery	11	10
Iliac vein	7	6
Total	36 (0.05)	31
Portal vessels		
Hepatic artery	44	36
Cystic artery	73	63
Portal vein	5	4
Total	122 (0.16)	103
Other intraabdominal vessels	35 (0.05)	24
Total vascular	193 (0.25)	158
Bowel		
Small intestine	57	42
Colon	35	26
Duodenum	12	12
Stomach	5	5
Total	109 (0.14)	85

Source: Deziel D, Millikan K, Economou S. Complications of laparoscopic cholecystectomy: a national survey of 4,292 hospitals and an analysis of 77,604 cases. Am J Surg 1992;165:9–14, by permission.

placement of additional trocars can lead to bleeding from abdominal wall vessels, especially the epigastric vessels. The reported incidence of hemorrhage caused by injury of the epigastric vessels during trocar insertion ranges between 0.25% and 6.0%.[39,40] These injuries can be controlled with electrocautery, by tamponade using a balloon-tipped catheter that is pulled against the abdominal wall, or by enlargement of the incision for suture ligation. Port site infection occurs in less than 1% of patients. The risk factors for port site infection are the same as for any incision, including poor nutrition, obesity, and diabetes mellitus. Port site infection can lead to hernia development. The overall incidence of port site herniation is relatively low with larger trocar sites posing the highest risk. The umbilical trocar is the most common site of herniation,

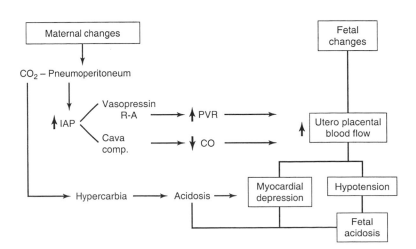

FIGURE 15.2. Maternal and fetal changes in pneumoperitoneum during pregnancy. (From Silva JK, Platt LD. Laparoscopic surgery in pregnancy. In: Rosenthal RJ, Friedman RL, Phillips EH, eds. The Physiology of Pneumoperitoneum. New York: Springer-Verlag, 1998, by permission.)

TABLE 15.3.

Clinical Studies Comparing Laparoscopic and Open Approaches.

Procedure	Type of study	Level of evidence	Author	Year	Country	Study design
Appendectomy	RAN, PRO	I	Heikkinen et al.[64]	1998	Finland	Open vs. LAP
	RAN, PRO	I	Macarulla et al.[65]	1997	Spain	Open vs. LAP
	RAN, PRO	I	Minne et al.[67]	1997	USA	Open vs. LAP
Inguinal herniorrhaphy	RAN, PRO	I	Heikkinen et al.[64]	1998	Finland	Lichtenstein mesh vs. transabdominal LAP
	PRO	II	Wilson et al.	1995	UK	Lichtenstein mesh vs. transabdominal LAP
	RAN, CON	II	Tanphiphat et al.	1998	Thailand	Modified Bassini vs. preperitoneal LAP
Splenectomy	PRO	II	Gigot	1995	Belgium	Multicenter, consecutive (ITP)
	RET	II	Delaitre and Pitre[86]	1997	France	Open vs. LAP (ITP)
Fundoplication	OBS, PRO	II	Blomqvist et al.[87]	1998	Sweden	Open vs. LAP
	RET	I	Hunter et al.[76]	1996	USA	Consecutive
Adrenalectomy	RET	III	Brunt et al.[77]	1996	USA	Open anterior vs. open posterior vs. LAP transabdominal flank
	RET	III	Linos et al.[78]	1997	Greece	Open anterior vs. open posterior vs. LAP posterior extraperitoneal

Open Appendectomy

Author	n	Mean operative time (min)	Mean LOS (days)	Postoperative morbidity (n)	Global costs ($)
Heikkinen et al.[64]	21	41	4	1	949*
Macarulla et al.[65]	104	44.68*	4.75*	8	508.32*
Minne et al.[67]	23	66.8*	1.2 (median)	1	3673*

Laparoscopic Appendectomy

n	Mean operative time (min)	Mean LOS (days)	Postoperative morbidity (n)	Global costs ($)
18	31.5	2	2	1197*
106	55.20*	3.42*	6	394.19*
27	81.7*	1.1 (median)	5	5430*

Inguinal Herniorrhaphy

Author	n	Mean operative time (min)	Mean LOS (days)	Postoperative morbidity (n)	Patient satisfaction (%)
Heikkinen et al.[64]	20	65	3.5 hours	8	Very satisfied 70 satisfied 30
Wilson et al.[65]	121	40 (median)	2 (median)	36	—
Tanphiphat et al.	60	67*	3	30	—

Inguinal Herniorrhaphy

n	Mean operative time (mins)	Mean LOS (days)	Postoperative morbidity (n)	Patient satisfaction (%)
20	62	6.5 hours	5	Very satisfied 55 Satisfied 45
121	35 (median)	24 (median)	23	—
60	95*	2.6	25	—

Splenectomy

Author	n	Mean operative time (min)	Mean LOS (days)	Postoperative morbidity (n)	Recurrence
Gigot					
Delaitre and Pitre[86]	28	127*	8.6*	9	4

Splenectomy

n	Mean operative time (mins)	Mean LOS (days)	Postoperative morbidity (n)	Recurrence
50	203	4.7	11	8 (27%)
28	183*	5.1*	3	2

(continued)

Open Funduplication

Author	n	Mean operative time (min)	Mean LOS (days)	Postoperative sick leave (days)	Post-operative % time ph < 4
Blomqvist et al.[87]	19	129	8*	29.9*	1
Hunter et al.[76]					

Laparoscopic Funduplication

n	Mean operative time (min)	Mean LOS (days)	Postoperative sick leave (days)	Post operative % time ph < 4
12	125	2*	9.9*	1
300	185	2.2	—	3.6

Open anterior Adrenalectomy

Author	n	Mean operative time (min)	Mean LOS (days)
Brunt et al.[77]	25	142	8.7
Linos et al.[77]	81	155[A]	8

Open posterior Adrenalectomy

n	Mean operative time (min)	Mean LOS (days)
24	136	6.2
61	106	4.5

Laparoscopic Adrenalectomy

n	Mean operative time (min)	Mean LOS (days)
24	183[A]	2.2[A]
18	116	2.2[A]

RAN, randomized; PRO, prospective; RET, retrospective; OBS, observational; CON, controlled; ITP, idiopathic thrombocytopenic purpura; LAP, laparoscopic; LOS, postoperative length of hospital stay; *$p < 0.05$ LAP vs. open; A, $p < 0.05$ as compared independently to other groups; $ = US dollars.

occurring in 0.1% of patients undergoing LC.[32] Inappropriate closure of a trocar site can lead to the development of a trocar site hernia. All trocar sites measuring 10 mm or greater should be sutured closed. Mechanical factors (wound infections, abdominal distention, and coughing) are more often responsible for causing wound disruption than systemic factors (malnutrition, increased age, and chronic treatment with steroids).[41]

Abdominal gas insufflation has been implicated as the cause of unusual laparoscopic complications. The diffusion of CO_2 into the bloodstream or its direct introduction into the vascular system can lead to cardiac dysrythmias or embolization.[42–50] Large volumes of intravascular CO_2 can lead to sudden cardiac collapse by forming a gas lock in the right ventricular outflow tract. The signs of CO_2 embolization include hypotension, cyanosis, arrhythmia, and "millwheel" murmur that can be heard through an esophageal stethoscope. Fortunately, CO_2 embolization during laparoscopy is rare, with an incidence of 0.002% to 0.016%.[45,51] When it occurs, treatment entails release of the PNP and repositioning the patient in the left lateral decubitus position, head down, to float the gas bubble into the right atrium, thus avoiding obstruction of the pulmonary outflow tract.

Inappropriate patient positioning and misuse of the specialized laparoscopic equipment can also lead to complications. The lithotomy position, often used during antireflux procedures or colon resections, can cause nerve stretching and ischemia that can lead to femoral neuropathy.[52] As previously discussed, head-up and head-down positioning can each have cardiovascular implications. Proper functioning of all laparoscopic equipment should be assured before beginning the operation. Unless on standby, the laparoscopic light source should be immediately attached to the laparoscope. If left unattached, surgical drape combustion is possible. Instrumentation should be periodically inspected for proper functioning and intact insulation. To avoid intestinal perforation, only smooth graspers should be used for intestinal manipulation. Bowel injuries have also been reported by careless application of the suction[53] and irrigation stream. Because these devices

are deployed with considerable force, the suction or irrigator should not be directed toward recently applied clips (i.e., cystic duct). Finally, thermal injuries from electrocautery can result from careless application, defective insulation, or improper grounding. It is safest to use properly insulated electrocautery instruments and short bursts of current to avoid thermal injuries. Attention to detail in laparoscopy, just as in all surgical procedures, avoids most complications.[54]

Laparoscopy Today

Laparoscopic cholecystectomy has replaced the traditional approach to calculous gallbladder disease as the new gold standard.[55] Strong scientific clinical evidence supports the superiority of LC over OC. Laparoscopic cholecystectomy results in shorter length of hospital stay, less postoperative pain, less postoperative pulmonary embarrassment, faster return of bowel function, and greater patient satisfaction than its open counterpart. Recently, several other laparoscopic procedures have challenged the position of well-described open techniques. In fact, most general surgery procedures have been performed laparoscopically. However, demonstrating feasibility of a certain procedure does not illustrate practicality. Data have accumulated examining relative benefits of laparoscopic and open procedures (Table 15.3). A complete discussion of the indications for each of these procedures is not possible in this introductory section, but most agree that there is a place for each of the following procedures in the general surgeon's armamentarium.

Diagnostic Laparoscopy

Diagnostic laparoscopy has long been used in gynecology and has more recently been employed in general surgery and intensive care unit patients. In appropriately chosen, hemodynamically stable patients, laparoscopy is both helpful and cost effective.[56,57]

Appendectomy

Several randomized, prospective clinical studies comparing laparoscopic appendectomy (LA) to open appendectomy (OA) clearly show the feasibility and safety of the laparoscopic procedure.[60-69] The laparoscopic approach allows for comparable, or shorter,[64,67] length of postoperative hospital stay[65] and complication rates when compared to OA. The indications for LA that seem most clear include patients with right lower quadrant pain with an atypical presentation, women of childbearing age, obese patients, and those patients that routinely participate in strenuous activity.

Inguinal Herniorrhaphy

There are presently two well-studied approaches to laparoscopic herniorrhaphy, the transabdominal preperitoneal (TAPP) repair and the totally extraperioneal (TEPP) approach. The repair fashioned with each of these approaches is nearly identical, with the difference lying merely in the manner in which the preperitoneal space is accessed. Both laparoscopic repairs require the positioning and attachment of mesh over the hernia defect. Currently, there remains considerable debate as to the specific indications for laparoscopic herniorrhaphy versus open herniorrhaphy. The position of laparoscopic herniorrhaphy will become clarified only after long-term follow-up data for hernia recurrence become available.

Splenectomy

Several available studies report that laparoscopic splenectomy (LS) is both feasible and safe.[70-74] For patients with disorders not requiring intact splenic architecture for pathological processing (i.e., idiopathic thrombocytopenic purpura), some claim LS has already replaced open splenectomy (OS) as the new gold standard.[75] However, it must be recognized that LS remains a technically challenging procedure requiring significantly longer operative time to complete. Laparoscopic splenectomy should be reserved for surgeons with significant laparoscopic experience and skill.

Esophagogastric Surgery

The approach to patients with gastroesophageal reflux disease (GERD) has undergone dramatic change over the last several years. Several studies show that laparoscopic fundoplication has indeed replaced open fundoplication as the procedure of choice for patients with severe GERD. Laparoscopic fundoplication provides excellent control of reflux symptoms (both subjectively and objectively), shorter postoperative hospital stay, and few complaints of late postoperative dysphagia. For patients with achalasia, laparoscopic longitudinal myotomy (Heller myotomy) has also been shown to be a feasible, acceptable, and often preferable alternative to a traditional open approach to such patients.[76]

Adrenalectomy

As with other laparoscopic procedures, the advantage of laparoscopic adrenalectomy (LAD) lies with significantly shorter postoperative hospital stays and less patient discomfort as compared to open adrenalectomy (OAD).[77,78] The laparoscopic approach is advised for patients with benign and/or bilateral adrenal disease. In addition, LAD has been shown to be safe in patients with pheochromocytoma, provided that adequate anesthetic monitoring is employed.[79] In the hands of an experienced laparoscopist, LAD has replaced OAD for most patients requiring adrenalectomy.

Other Procedures

Laparoscopic colon and vascular procedures are clearly feasible but have not yet gained widespread acceptance. Laparoscopic colon resection is well suited for patients with benign diseases (e.g., diverticular disease, colonic inertia) as well as patients with dysplastic or suspicious polyps. The concept of endovascular stenting of abdominal aortic aneurysms currently is the most provocative alternative to conventional aneurysmectomy,[80] while laparoscopic-assisted vascular procedures remains in their infancy.[81] In carefully chosen patients, laparoscopic small-bowel resection, biliary-enteric bypass for pancreatic malignancy, and operations for peptic ulcer disease are also indicated. In patients with intervertebral disk disease, laparoscopic anterior exposure is both possible and practical. Laparoscopic ventral hernia repair has shown promising preliminary results but still awaits long-term follow-up.[82,83] Finally, bedside laparoscopy for the evaluation of mesenteric ischemia has been performed safely and is feasible in centers dedicated to its use.[84,85]

References

1. McKernan JB, Champion JK. Access techniques: Veress needle—initial blind trocar insertion versus open laparoscopy with the Hasson trocar. Endosc Surg Allied Technol 1995;3:35–38.
2. Dion Y, Gaillard F. Visual integration of data and basic motor skills under laparoscopy: influence of 2-D and 3-D video-camera systems. Surg Endosc 1997;11:995–1000.
3. Ishizaki Y, Bandai Y, Shimomura K, Abe H, Ohtomo Y, Idezuki Y. Changes in splanchnic blood flow and cardiovascular effects following peritoneal insufflation of carbon dioxide. Surg Endosc 1993;7:420–423.
4. Joris JL, Noirot DP, Legrand MJ, Jacquet NJ, Lamy ML. Hemodynamic changes during laparoscopic cholecystectomy. Anesth Analg 1993;76:1067–1071.
5. Safran DB, Orlando R. Physiologic effects of pneumoperitoneum. Am J Surg 1994;167:281.
6. Gannedahl P, Odeberg S, Brodin LA, Sollevi A. Effects of posture and pneumoperitoneum during anaesthesia on the indices of left ventricular filling. Acta Anaesthesiol Scand 1996;40:160–166.
7. Odeberg S, Ljungqvist O, Svenberg T, et al. Haemodynamic effects of pneumoperitoneum and the influence of posture during anaesthesia for laparoscopic surgery. Acta Anaesthesiol Scand 1994;38:276–283.
8. Caprini JA, Arcelus JI. Prevention of postoperative venous thromboembolism following laparoscopic cholecystectomy. Surg Endosc 1994;8:741.
9. Volpino P, Cangemi V, Da N, Cangemi B, Piat G. Hemodynamic and pulmonary changes during and after laparoscopic. Surg Endosc 1998;12:119–123.
10. Drummond GB, Martin LV. Pressure-volume relationships in the lung during laparoscopy. Br J Anaesth 1978;50:261–270.
11. Simmonneau G, Vivien A, Sartene R, et al. Diaphragm dysfunction induced by upper abdominal surgery: role of postoperative pain. Am Rev Respir Dis 1983;128:899–903.
12. Fahy BG, Barnas GM, Flowers JL, Nagle SE, Njoku MJ. The effects of increased abdominal pressure on lung and chest wall

mechanics during laparoscopic surgery. Anesth Analg 1995;81: 744–750.

13. Sharma KC, Brandstetter RD, Brensilver JM, Jung LD. Cardiopulmonary physiology and pathophysiology as a consequence of laparoscopic surgery (see comments). Chest 1996;110:810–815.

14. Fitzgerald S, Andrus C, Baudendistel L, Dahms T, Kaminski D. Hypercapnia during carbon dioxide pneumoperitoneum. Am J Surg 1992;163:186–190.

15. Smith I, Benzie RJ, Gordon NL, Kelman GR, Swapp GH. Cardiovascular effects of peritoneal insufflation of carbon dioxide for laparoscopy. Br Med J 1971;3:410–411.

16. Wahba R, Mamazza J. Ventilatory requirements during laparoscopic cholecystectomy. Can J Anaesth 1993;40:206–210.

17. Litwin DEM, Girotti MJ, Poulin EC, Mamazza J, Nagy AG. Laparoscopic cholecystectomy: trans-Canada experience with 2201 cases. Can J Surg 1992;35:291.

17a. S.A.G.E.S. Integrating advanced laparoscopy into surgical residency. Surg Endosc 1998;12:374–376.

18. Ballantyne G. Laparoscopic assisted colorectal surgery: review of results in 752 patients. Gastroenterology 1995;3:75–89.

19. Liberman M, Phillips E, Carroll B, Fallas M, Rosenthal R. Laparoscopic colectomy versus traditional colectomy for diverticulitis. Surg Endosc 1996;10:15–18.

20. Garcia-Caballero M, Vara-Thorbeck C. The evolution of postoperative ileus after laparoscopic cholecystectomy. Surg Endosc 1993;7:416.

21. Pitts L, Martin N. Head injuries. Surg Clin North Am 1982;62: 47–60.

22. Paulson GW, DeVoe K Jr. Neurological complications of laparoscopy. Am J Obstet Gynecol 1981;140:468–469.

23. Cirocco WC, Schwartzman A, Golub RW. Abdominal wall recurrence after laparoscopic colectomy for colon cancer (see comments). Surgery (St. Louis) 1994;116:842–846.

24. Fodera M, Pello MJ, Atabek U, Spence RK, Alexander JB, Camishion RC. Trocar site recurrence after laparoscopic-assisted colectomy. J Laparoendosc Surg 1995;5:259–262.

25. Jacquet P, Averbach AM, Jacquet N. Abdominal wall metastasis and peritoneal carcinomatosis after laparoscopic-assisted colectomy for colon cancer. Eur J Surg Oncol 1995;21:568–570.

26. Jones DB, Guo LW, Reinhard MK, et al. Impact of pneumoperitoneum on trocar site implantation of colon cancer in hamster model. Dis Colon Rectum 1995;38:1182–1188.

27. Wexner S, Cohen S. Port-site metastases after laparoscopic colorectal surgery for cure of malignancy. Br J Surg 1995;82:295–298.

28. Hughes E, McDermott F, Polglase A, Johnson W. Tumor recurrence in the abdominal wall scar tissue after large bowel cancer surgery. Dis Colon Rectum 1983;26(9):571–572.

29. Bouvy ND, Marquet RL, Jeekel H, Bonjer HJ. Impact of gas(less) laparoscopy and laparotomy on peritoneal tumor growth and abdominal wall metastases. Ann Surg 1996;224:694–700; discussion 700–701.

30. Silva J, Platt L. Laparoscopic surgery during pregnancy. In: Rosenthal R, Friedman R, Phillips E, eds. The Pathophysiology of Pneumoperitoneum. New York: Springer, 1998:168–180.

31. Phillips K, Hulka J, Peterson H. American Association of Gynecologic Laparoscopist's 1982 Membership Survey. J Reprod Med 1982;29:592–594.

32. Larson G, Vitale G, Casey J. Multipractice analysis of laparoscopic cholecystectomy in 1,983 patients. Am J Surg 1992;163: 221–226.

33. Peterson H, Greenspan J, Ory W. Death following puncture of the aorta during laparoscopic sterilization. Am J Obstet Gynecol 1982;59:133–134.

34. Frenkel Y, Oelsner G, Baruch B. Major surgical complications of laparoscopy. Eur J Obstet Gynecol Reprod Biol 1981;12:107–111.

35. Yuzpe A. Pneumoperitoneum needle and trocar injuries in laparoscopy—a survey of possible contributing factors and prevention. J Reprod Med 1990;35:485–490.

36. Oshinsky GS, Smith AD. Laparoscopic needles and trocars: an overview of designs and complications. J Laparoendosc Surg 1992;2:117–125.

37. Deziel D, Millikan K, Economou S. Complications of laparoscopic cholecystectomy: a national survey of 4,292 hospitals and an analysis of 77,604 cases. Am J Surg 1992;165:9–14.

38. Nordestgaard AG, Bodily KC, Osborne RW Jr, Buttorff JD. Major vascular injuries during laparoscopic procedures. Am J Surg 1995;169:543–545.

39. Youkey Y, Clagett G, Rich N. Vascular trauma secondary to diagnostic and therapeutic procedures: 1974 through 1982. A comparative review. Am J Surg 1983;1446:788–791.

40. Loffer FD, Pent D. Indications, contraindications and complications of laparoscopy. Obstet Gynecol Surv 1975;30:407–427.

41. Poole G. Mechanical factors in abdominal wound closure: the prevention of fascial dehisscence. Surgery (St. Louis) 1985;97: 631–640.

42. Brooks PG. Venous air embolism during operative hysteroscopy (see comments). J Am Assoc Gynecol Laparosc 1997;4:399–402.

43. Cottin V, Delafosse B, Viale JP. Gas embolism during laparoscopy: a report of seven cases in patients. Surg Endosc 1996;10:166–169.

44. Gillart T, Bazin JE, Bonnard M, Schoeffler P. Pulmonary interstitial edema after probable carbon dioxide embolism. Surg Laparosc Endosc 1995;5:327–329.

45. Gomar C, Fernandez C, Villalonga A, Nalda MA. Carbon dioxide embolism during laparoscopy and hysteroscopy. Ann Fr Anesth Reanim 1985;4:380–382.

46. Wadhwa RK, McKenzie R, Wadhwa SR, Katz DL, Byers JF. Gas embolism during laparoscopy. Anesthesiology 1978;48:74–76.

47. Yacoub OF, Cardona I Jr, Coveler LA, Dodson MG. Carbon dioxide embolism during laparoscopy. Anesthesiology 1982;57:533–535.

48. Wolf JS Jr, Carrier S, Stoller ML. Gas embolism: helium is more lethal than carbon dioxide. J Laparoendosc Surg 1994;4:173–177.

49. Ostman PL, Pantle-Fisher FH, Faure EA, Glosten B. Circulatory collapse during laparoscopy. J Clin Anesth 1990;2:129–132.

50. Li TC, Saravelos H, Richmond M, Cooke ID. Complications of laparoscopic pelvic surgery: recognition, management and prevention. Hum Reprod Update 1997;3:505–515.

51. Hodgson R, McClelland, Newton J. Some effects of peritoneal insufflation of carbon dioxide at laparoscopy. Anaesthesia 1970; 25:382–390.

52. Herschlag A, Loy R, Lavy G. Femoral neuropathy after laparoscopy. J Reprod Med 1990;35:575–576.

53. Riedel H, Lehmann-Willenbrock E, Mecke H. The frequency distribution of various peliscopic (laparoscopic) operations, including complication rates—statistics of the Federal Republic of Germany in the years 1983–1985. Zentralbl Gynecol 1989;66:78–91.

54. Levinson C, Qattiez A. Complications and safety of laparoscopy. In: Martin D, ed. Manual of Endoscopy. Santa Fe Springs: American Society of Gynecologic Laparoscopists, 1990:35.

55. Soper N, Stockmann P, Dunnegan D, Ashley S. Laparoscopic cholecystectomy: the new "gold standard"? Arch Surg 1992;127: 917.

56. Hallfeldt K, Trupka A, Erhard J, Waldner J, Schweiberer L. Emergency laparoscopy for abdominal stab wounds. Surg Endosc 1998;12:907–910.

57. Smith R, Tsoi E, Fry W. Laparoscopy is cost effective in the evaluation of abdominal trauma. Surg Endosc 1993;7:137.

58. Salky B, Edye M. The role of laparoscopy in the diagnosis and treatment of abdominal pain syndromes. Surg Endosc 1998;12:911–914.

59. Cuesta M, Eijsbouts Q, Gordijn R, Borgstein P, de Jong D. Diagnostic laparoscopy in patients with an acute abdomen. Surg Endosc 1998;12:915–917.

60. Attwood SE, Hill AD, Murphy PG, Thornton J, Stephens RB. A prospective randomized trial of laparoscopic versus open appendectomy. Surgery (St. Louis) 1992;112:497–501.

61. Cox MR, McCall JL, Toouli J, et al. Prospective randomized comparison of open versus laparoscopic. World J Surg 1996;20:263–266.

62. Frazee RC, Roberts JW, Symmonds RE, et al. A prospective randomized trial comparing open versus laparoscopic. Ann Surg 1994;219:725–728; discussion 728–731.
63. Hansen JB, Smithers BM, Schache D, Wall DR, Miller BJ, Menzies BL. Laparoscopic versus open appendectomy: prospective randomized trial. World J Surg 1996;20:17–20; discussion 21.
64. Heikkinen T, Haukipuro K, Hulkko A. Cost-effective appendectomy; open or laparoscopic? a prospective randomized study. Surg Endosc 1998;12:1204–1208.
65. Macarulla E, Vallet J, Abad JM, Hussein H, Fernandez E, Nieto B. Laparoscopic versus open appendectomy: a prospective randomized. Surg Laparosc Endosc 1997;7;335–339.
66. Martin LC, Puente I, Sosa JL, et al. Open versus laparoscopic appendectomy. A prospective randomized. Ann Surg 1995;222:256–261; discussion 261–262.
67. Minne L, Varner D, Burnell A, Ratzer E, Clark J, Haun W. Laparoscopic vs open appendectomy. Prospective randomized study. Arch Surg 1997;132:708–711; discussion 712.
68. Ortega AE, Hunter JG, Peters JH, Swanstrom LL, Schirmer B. A prospective, randomized comparison of laparoscopic appendectomy. Am J Surg 1995;169:208–212; discussion 212–213.
69. Tate JJ, Dawson JW, Chung SC, Lau WY, Li AK. Laparoscopic versus open appendicectomy: prospective randomised. Lancet 1993;342:633–637.
70. Hashizume M, Ohta M, Kishihara F, et al. Laparoscopic splenectomy for idiopathic thrombocytopenic purpura: comparison of laparoscopic surgery and conventional open surgery. Surg Laparosc Endosc 1996;6:129–135.
71. Smith CD, Meyer TA, Goretsky MJ, et al. Laparoscopic splenectomy by the lateral approach: a safe and effective alternative to open splenectomy for hematologic diseases. Surgery (St. Louis) 1996;120:789–794.
72. Stephens BJ, Justice JL, Sloan DA, Yoder JA. Elective laparoscopic splenectomy for hematologic disorders. Am Surg 1997;63:700–703.
73. Watson DI, Coventry BJ, Chin T, Gill PG, Malycha P. Laparoscopic versus open splenectomy for immune thrombocytopenic purpura. Surgery (St. Louis) 1997;121:18–22.
74. Brunt LM, Langer JC, Quasebarth MA, Whitman ED. Comparative analysis of laparoscopic versus open splenectomy. Am J Surg 1996;172:596–599; discussion 599–601.
75. Friedman RL, Fallas MJ, Carroll BJ, Hiatt JR, Phillips EH. Laparoscopic splenectomy for ITP. The gold standard. Surg Endosc 1996;10:991–995.
76. Hunter J, Trus T, Branum G. Waring P. Laparoscopic Heller myotomy and fundoplication for achalasia. Ann Surg 1997;225(6):655–664; discussion 644–665.
77. Brunt LM, Doherty GM, Norton JA, Soper NJ, Quasebarth MA, Moley JF. Laparoscopic adrenalectomy compared to open adrenalectomy for benign adrenal neoplasms (see comments). J Am Coll Surg 1996;183:1–10.
78. Linos DA, Stylopoulos N, Boukis M, Souvatzoglou A, Raptis S, Papadimitriou J. Anterior, posterior, or laparoscopic approach for the management of adrenal diseases? Am J Surg 1997;173:120–125.
79. Gagner M, Pomp A, Heniford BT, Pharand D, Lacroix A. Laparoscopic adrenalectomy: lessons learned from 100 consecutive procedures. Ann Surg 1997;226:238–246; discussion 246–247.
80. Moore W, Rutherford R. Transfemoral endovascular repair of abdominal aortic aneurysms: results of the North American EVT phase I trial. J Vasc Surg 1996;23:543–552.
81. Dion Y, Katkhouda N, Rouleau CAA. Laparoscopy-assisted aortobifemoral bypass. Surg Laparosc Endosc 1993;3:425–429.
82. Holzman M, Purut C, Reintgen K, Pappas T. Laparoscopic ventral and incisional hernioplasty. Surg Endosc 1997;11:32–35.
83. Toy F, Bailey R, Carey S, et al. Prospective, multicenter study of laparoscopic ventral hernia hernioplasty: preliminary results. Surg Endosc 1998;12:955–959.
84. Walsh R, Popovich M, Hoadley J. Bedside diagnostic laparoscopy and peritoneal lavage in the intensive care unit. Surg Endosc 1998;12:1405–1409.
85. Zamir G, Reissman P. Diagnostic laparoscopy in mesenteric ischemia. Surg Endosc 1998;12:390–393.
86. Delaitre B, Pitre J. Laparoscopic splenectomy versus open splenectomy: a comparative study. Hepatogastroenterology 1997;44:45–49.
87. Blomqvist A, Lonroth H, Dalenback J, Lundell L. Laparoscopic or open fundoplication? a complete cost analysis. Surg Endosc 1998;12:1209–1212.
88. Bonjer H, Gutt C, Hubens G, et al. Port site metastases in laparoscopic surgery: first workshop on experimental laparoscopic surgery, Frankfurt, 1997. Surg Endosc 1998;12:1102–1103.

Esophagus

C. Daniel Smith

Anatomy

General

The esophagus is a muscular tube lined with nonkeratinizing squamous epithelium that starts as a continuation of the pharynx and ends as the cardia of the stomach. The esophagus is fixed only at its upper and lower ends, the upper end being firmly attached to the cricoid cartilage and the lower end to the diaphragm. This lack of fixation throughout its length allows the esophagus both transverse and longitudinal mobility. This mobility is important in normal esophageal function, as well as pathological states that can easily displace the esophagus or require extensive surgical mobilization for correction.

Course

Although the esophagus lies in the midline, it does not follow a straight vertical course from pharynx to stomach, but rather deviates to the left of midline as it courses through the neck and upper thorax and slightly to the right of midline in the midportion of the thorax near the tracheal bifurcation. It is this deflection to the right of midline that dictates a right thoracotomy when transthoracic esophagointestinal anastomosis is necessary. In the lower portion of the thorax, the esophagus again deviates to the left of midline as it passes behind the heart and through the diaphragmatic hiatus. Overall, the esophageal axis through the chest is vertical. Any distortion of this vertical axis strongly suggests malignancy with mediastinal invasion and retraction. Additionally, the esophagus has anteroposterior deflections that correspond to the curvatures of the cervical and thoracic spine. At its distal end, the esophagus leaves the normal curvature of the spine and deviates anteriorly to pass through the diaphragmatic hiatus.

In its course from the pharynx to the stomach, the esophagus passes through three compartments, the neck, thorax, and abdomen. The cervical portion of the esophagus is approximately 5 cm in length and courses between the trachea and the vertebral column, passing into the chest at the level of the sternal notch. The thoracic esophagus is approximately 20 cm long and courses behind the tracheal bifurcation and heart before entering the abdominal cavity at about the level of the xiphoid process of the sternum. The abdominal portion of the esophagus is approximately 2 cm in length and is surrounded by the phrenoesophageal ligament. This phrenoesophageal membrane provides an airtight seal between the thoracic and abdominal cavities, and must be strong enough to resist abdominal pressure, yet flexible enough to move with the pressure changes and movements incidental to breathing and swallowing. The phrenoesophageal ligament is comprised of pleura, subpleural (endothoracic) fascia, phrenoesophageal fascia, transversalis fascia, and peritoneum (Fig. 16.1).

Length

The length of the esophagus is defined anatomically as the distance from the cricoid cartilage to the gastric orifice. In the adult male, this length is from 22 to 28 cm and averages 2 cm shorter in the female; esophageal length varies more with individual height than sex. Because the precise location of the cricoid cartilage is difficult to determine, the length of the esophagus is more commonly measured as the distance from the incisors to the gastric inlet. This distance is easily determined during esophagoscopy and averages 40 cm. Finally, the length of the esophagus as measured manometrically is the distance from the cricopharyngeus to the lower esophageal sphincter (LES).

Normal Constrictions

At rest, the esophagus is collapsed and in its proximal two-thirds is flat with a diameter of 2.3×1.9 cm. At its lower end, the esophagus is rounded with a diameter of 2.2×2.2 cm. Compression by adjacent structures or muscles causes normal constrictions that are evident on a barium esophagogram or during esophagoscopy. The most proximal constriction represents the narrowest portion of the entire gastrointestinal tract and

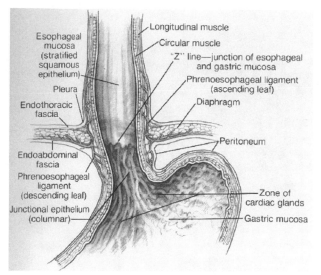

FIGURE 16.1. Anatomical relationships of the distal esophagus and phrenoesophageal ligament. (From Gray SW, Skandalakis JE, McClusky DA. Atlas of Surgical Anatomy for General Surgeons. Baltimore: Williams & Wilkins, 1985, with permission.)

occurs at the beginning of the esophagus where the cricopharyngeal musculature is located. The next constriction is located 20 cm from the incisors and is the result of indention of the esophagus by the aortic arch and the left mainstem bronchus. The lowermost narrowing, which is not constant, is located at about 44 cm from the incisors and is caused by the gastroesophageal sphincter mechanism. Ingested foreign bodies tend to lodge at these points of normal constriction; also, the transit of swallowed corrosives slows at these narrowings, leading to prominent mucosal injury at these sites.

Structure

The esophagus consists primarily of three layers (Fig. 16.2). The outer layer, the muscularis externa, comprises the chief muscles of the esophagus and is made up of an internal circular muscle layer and an external longitudinal muscle layer. In the upper third of the esophagus, both layers are primarily striated (voluntary) muscle fibers. In the middle third of the esophagus, striated and smooth (involuntary) muscle fibers are intermingled, and in the lower third, smooth muscle fibers predominate. Most of the clinically significant esophageal motility disorders involve only the smooth muscle portion of the esophagus; thus, esophageal myotomy for the management of most esophageal motor disorders needs to only extend along the lower esophagus. Two bundles of longitudinal muscle fibers diverge and meet in the midline of the posterior esophageal wall 3 cm below the cricoid cartilage. This V-shaped area along the posterior wall of the proximal esophagus covered only with circular muscle fibers represents a potential weak area for subsequent diverticula formation (see section on Esophageal Diverticula). The squamous epithelium of the esophagus meets the junctional columnar epithelium of the gastric cardia in a sharp transition called the Z-line, typically located at or near the physiological LES. The submucosa contains elastic and fibrous tissue and is the strongest part of the esophageal wall. It is this layer that contains the lamina propria which the surgeon relies on for a sound esophageal anastomosis. Meissner's plexus of nerves also resides within the submucosal layer.

Vessels

ARTERIAL

The arterial blood supply to the esophagus is segmental with three main sources supplying the upper, middle, and lower sections of the esophagus (Fig. 16.3). The cervical esophagus receives blood from the superior thyroidal artery as well as the inferior thyroidal artery of the thyrocervical trunk, and both sides communicate through a rich collateral network. The thoracic portion of the esophagus is supplied proximally by two to three bronchial arteries, and distally from esophageal arteries arising directly from the aorta. The abdominal esopha-

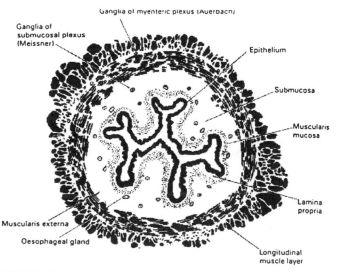

FIGURE 16.2. Cross section of the esophagus showing the layers of the wall. (From Jamieson GG, ed. Surgery of the Esophagus. Edinburgh: Churchill Livingstone, 1988:19–35, with permission.)

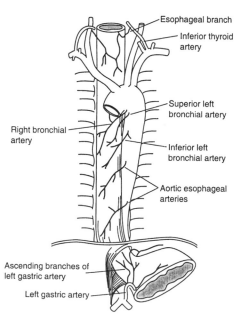

FIGURE 16.3. Arterial blood supply of the esophagus. (From Shields TW, ed. General Thoracic Surgery, 3rd Ed. Philadelphia: Lea & Febiger, 1989:84, with permission.)

gus receives blood from branches of the left gastric and inferior phrenic arteries.

VENOUS

The venous drainage of the esophagus follows the arterial capillary network. Longitudinally oriented periesophageal venous plexi return blood in the cervical esophagus to the inferior thyroid vein, in the thoracic esophagus to the bronchial, azygous, and hemiazygous veins, and in the abdominal esophagus to the coronary vein.

LYMPHATIC

The lymphatic drainage of the esophagus is abundant and forms a dense submucosal plexus. Flow of lymph runs longitudinally, coursing cephalad in the upper two-thirds of the esophagus and caudad in the lower third. Because this lymphatic system is not segmental, lymph can travel a long distance in this plexus before traversing the muscle layer and entering the regional lymph nodes. As a consequence, free tumor cells of the upper esophagus can metastasize to superior gastric nodes, or conversely, a cancer of the lower esophagus can metastasize to superior mediastinal nodes. More commonly, the lymphatic drainage from the upper esophagus courses primarily into the cervical and peritracheal lymph nodes, while that from the lower thoracic and abdominal esophagus drains into the retrocardiac and celiac nodes.

Innervation

The esophageal neural branches are secretomotor to glands and motor to muscular layers. The esophagus has both sympathetic and parasympathetic innervation. The sympathetic nerve supply is through the cervical and thoracic sympathetic chain and from the celiac plexus and ganglia. The parasympathetic innervation of the pharynx and esophagus is primarily through the vagus nerve. In the neck, the superior laryngeal nerves arise from the vagus nerve and divide into the external and internal laryngeal branches. The external laryngeal nerve innervates the cricothyroid muscle and in part the inferior pharyngeal constrictor, while the internal laryngeal nerve provides sensation to the pharyngeal surface of the larynx and base of the tongue. Injury to the recurrent laryngeal nerve may cause both hoarseness and upper esophageal sphincter dysfunction with secondary aspiration during swallowing. Distally, the vagal trunks contribute to the anterior and posterior esophageal plexi, and at the diaphragmatic hiatus, these plexi fuse to form the anterior and posterior vagus nerves. Finally, a rich intrinsic nervous supply called the myenteric plexus exists between the longitudinal and circular muscle layers (Auerbach's plexus) and in the submucosa (Meissner's plexus).

Physiology

Once initiated, swallowing is entirely a reflex. The tongue acts like a piston propelling the bolus into the posterior oral pharynx and forcing it into the cylinder of the hypopharynx. With this piston-like movement of the tongue posteriorly, the soft palate is elevated, sealing the passage between the oral pharynx and the nasopharynx. The closing of the valve of the soft palate prevents dissipation of the pressure generated within the pharyngeal cylinder through the nasopharynx and nose. Nearly

concomitant with this, the hyoid bone and larynx move upward and anteriorly, bringing the epiglottis under the tongue and sealing the opening of the larynx to prevent aspiration (Fig. 16.4). This sequence, the pharyngeal phase of swallowing, occurs within 1.5 s of initiation of a swallow. Dysfunction or paralysis of any of these interrelated actions, as following a cerebrovascular accident, leads to discoordinated movements and regurgitation of food into the nasopharynx or aspiration.

During the *pharyngeal phase* of swallowing, the pressure in the hypopharynx quickly rises to at least 60 mmHg, creating a sizable pressure difference between the hypopharyngeal and the less than atmospheric midesophageal or intrathoracic pressure. With this pressure gradient, when the cricopharyngeus or upper esophageal sphincter relaxes, food is quickly moved from the hypopharynx into the esophagus. In this way, the bolus is both pushed through peristaltic contraction of the posterior pharyngeal constrictors and sucked into the thoracic esophagus. Immediately after the bolus clears the upper esophageal sphincter (UES), the UES closes to an immediate closing pressure of approximately twice its resting level of 30 mmHg. This post-UES contraction initiates a migrating contraction that continues down the esophagus as a primary peristaltic wave (Fig. 16.5). The high closing pressure and progression of the peristaltic wave prevents reflux of the bolus back into the pharynx. Shortly after the peristaltic wave has migrated down the esophagus, the pressure of the UES quickly returns to its resting level.

The *esophageal phase* of swallowing requires well-coordinated motor activity to propel the food from the negative-pressure environment of the chest (−6 mmHg) to the positive-pressure environment of the stomach (+6 mmHg). Peaks of a *primary* peristaltic contraction result in an occlusive pressure wave varying from 30 to 100 mmHg, with this primary peristaltic contraction moving down the esophagus at 2 to 4 cm per second (see Fig. 16.5). The transit time from initiation of a swallow to the bolus reaching the distal esophagus is about 9 s.

A second type of peristaltic wave (*secondary* peristalsis)

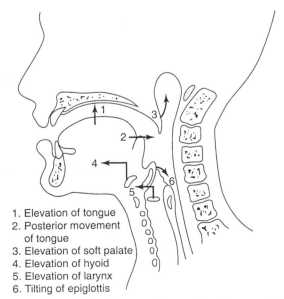

1. Elevation of tongue
2. Posterior movement of tongue
3. Elevation of soft palate
4. Elevation of hyoid
5. Elevation of larynx
6. Tilting of epiglottis

FIGURE 16.4. Sequence of events during the pharyngeal phase of swallowing. (From Zuidema GD, Orringer MD, eds. Shackelford's Surgery of the Alimentary Tract, Vol. 1, 3rd Ed. Philadelphia: Saunders, 1991:95, with permission.)

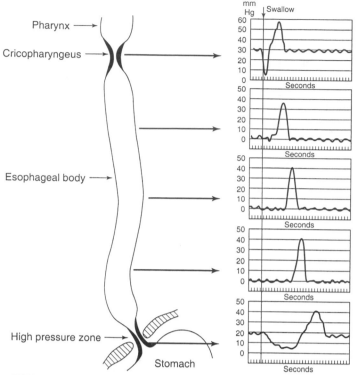

FIGURE 16.5. Intraluminal esophageal pressures in response to swallowing. (From Waters PF, Demeester TR. Foregut motor disorders and their surgical management. Med Clin North Am 1981;65:1238, with permission.)

is not triggered by voluntary swallowing, but rather refers to peristaltic waves that usually appear after esophageal dilation either from a retained bolus or from active distention of the esophagus. These secondary contractions occur without any movements of the mouth or pharynx, and can occur as independent local reflexes to clear the esophagus of ingested material left behind after the passage of the primary wave. A third pattern of contractile activity, *tertiary* contractions, occurs after voluntary swallows or spontaneously between swallows. Tertiary contractions are nonpropulsive, generate peak pressures in the range of 10 to 13 mmHg, and follow 3% to 4% of all swallows.

The lower esophageal sphincter (LES) acts as the valve at the end of the esophageal body and provides a pressure barrier between the esophagus and stomach. Although an anatomical lower esophageal sphincter does not exist, the architecture of the muscle fiber at the junction of the esophagus and the stomach helps explain some of the sphincter-like activity of the LES. The resting tone of the LES is approximately 20 mmHg and resists reflux of gastric content into the lower esophagus. With initiation of a pharyngeal swallow, the lower esophageal sphincter pressure decreases to allow the primary peristaltic wave to propel the bolus into the stomach.

Assessment of Esophageal Function

Several diagnostic tests are available to evaluate patients with esophageal disease. Remembering the anatomical and physiological features of the esophagus, these tests can be di-

TABLE 16.1. Assessment of Esophageal Function.

Condition	Diagnostic test
Structural abnormalities	Barium swallow Endoscopy Chest X-ray CT scan Cine fluoroscopy Endoscopic ultrasound
Functional abnormalities	Manometry (stationary and 24 hour) Transit studies
Esophageal exposure to gastric content	24-hour pH monitoring
Provoke esophageal symptoms	Acid perfusion (Berstein) Edrophonium (tensilon) Balloon distension
Others	Gastric analysis Gastric emptying study Gallbladder ultrasound

vided into (1) tests to detect structural abnormalities, (2) tests to detect functional abnormalities, (3) tests to assess esophageal exposure to gastric content, and (4) tests to provoke esophageal symptoms (Table 16.1).

Assessment of Structural Abnormalities

RADIOLOGIC STUDIES

CONTRAST ESOPHAGOGRAM
The simplest and often first diagnostic test for esophageal disease is a contrast esophagogram, most commonly a barium swallow. Structural abnormalities including diverticula, narrowing or stricture, ulcers, and hiatal or para-esophageal hernias can all be nicely demonstrated with an esophagogram.

OTHER RADIOLOGIC STUDIES
Plain chest X-ray films may reveal changes in cardiac silhouette or tracheobronchial location suggesting esophageal disorders. CT scan of the chest or magnetic resonance imaging (MRI) may also be useful in assessing lesions identified with barium swallow or endoscopy thought to be malignancies. Finally, a modified barium study in the lateral projection under ciné fluoroscopy may be especially useful in identifying mechanical disorders of the pharyngeal swallowing mechanism.

ENDOSCOPY

Most patients with esophageal symptomatology should undergo esophagoscopy. All patients with dysphagia should undergo esophagoscopy, even in the presence of a normal barium swallow. A barium swallow performed before esophagoscopy helps the endoscopist to focus on any subtle radiographic findings and helps to prevent endoscopic misadventures with anatomic abnormalities such as esophageal diverticula.

For the initial assessment, the flexible esophagoscope allows a safe, thorough assessment, which can be performed quickly in an outpatient setting with high patient tolerance and acceptance. Rigid esophagoscopy is rarely indicated and remains a tool used primarily in the operating room when cricopharyngeal or cervical esophageal lesions prevent passage of a flexible scope, or when biopsies deeper than those obtainable with flexible endoscopy are needed to stage disease and plan resective therapy for malignancy.

More recently, endoscopic ultrasound (EUS) allows characterization and staging of esophageal lesions by imaging the layers of the esophageal wall and surrounding structures to identify depth of tumor invasion, periesophageal lymphadenopathy, and EUS-guided fine-needle aspiration of lymph nodes.

Assessing Functional Abnormalities

ESOPHAGEAL MANOMETRY

Manometry is indicated when a motor abnormality is suspected on the basis of symptoms of dysphagia or odynophagia and the barium swallow and esophagoscopy do not show an obvious structural abnormality. Manometry is essential to confirm the diagnosis of primary esophageal motility disorders of achalasia, diffuse esophageal spasm, nutcracker esophagus, and hypertensive lower esophageal sphincter. It may be useful in identifying nonspecific esophageal motility disorders and motility abnormalities secondary to systemic diseases of scleroderma, dermatomyositis, polymyositis, or mixed connective tissue disease. Finally, in patients with symptomatic gastroesophageal reflux, manometry is particularly useful in assessing preoperative esophageal clearance mechanisms and competency and function of the distal esophageal sphincter.

Assessing Esophageal Exposure to Gastric Content

AMBULATORY 24-HOUR pH MONITORING

Ambulatory 24-h pH monitoring in the distal esophagus has become the gold standard for quantitating esophageal exposure to acidic gastric content. A pH electrode is positioned 5 cm proximal to the manometrically identified distal esophageal sphincter. The esophageal pH at this location is then recorded continuously throughout a 24-h cycle while the patient continues his or her normal routine including eating and usual activities. During the test, the patient maintains a diary recording body positions, meals, and symptoms so that esophageal exposure to acid can be correlated with symptoms. At the completion of the test, the results are tallied and compared to normal values for esophageal exposure to acid. An episode of acid reflux is defined as pH less than 4 in the distal esophagus.

Twenty-four-hour ambulatory pH monitoring is indicated for patients who have typical symptoms of gastroesophageal reflux for whom other diagnostic tests are equivocal, atypical symptoms of gastroesophageal reflux such as noncardiac chest pain, persistent cough, wheezing, or unexplained laryngitis, or previously failed esophageal or gastric surgery with recurrent symptoms.

Provocation of Esophageal Symptoms

The acid perfusion test (Bernstein test), edrophonium (Tensilon) test, and balloon distension test to identify a relationship between symptoms and esophageal exposure to acid or motor abnormalities have been virtually replaced by 24-h ambulatory pH monitoring and esophageal manometry. These tests are primarily of historical and academic interest only.

Assessment of Esophageal Symptoms

Table 16.2 lists patient symptoms that may be attributable to esophageal disorders.

Motor Disorders of the Esophagus

Disordered Pharyngeal Swallowing

Diseases affecting pharyngoesophageal function produce a characteristic type of dysphagia. Patients experience the more

TABLE 16.2. **Patient Symptoms and Likely Etiologies.**

Symptom	Definition	Likely etiology
Heartburn	Burning discomfort behind breast bone Bitter acidic fluid in mouth Sudden filling of mouth with clear/salty fluid	Gastroesophageal reflux (GER)
Dysphagia	Sensation of food being hindered in passage from mouth to stomach	Motor disorders Inflammatory process Diverticula Tumors
Odynophagia	Pain with swallowing	Severe inflammatory process
Globus sensation	Lump in throat unrelated to swallowing	
Chest pain	Mimics angina pectoris	GER Motor disorders Tumors
Respiratory symptoms	Asthma/wheezing, bronchitis, hemoptysis, stridor	GER Diverticula Tumors
ENT symptoms	Chronic sore throat, laryngitis, halitosis, chronic cough	GER Diverticula
Rumination	Regurgitation of recently ingested food into mouth	Achalasia Inflammatory process Diverticula Tumors

universally understood symptom of "difficulty in swallowing," with difficulty propelling food out of the mouth and through the hypopharyngeal region into the esophageal body. Aspiration or nasopharyngeal regurgitation are frequent outcomes.

Disorders of the pharyngoesophageal phase of swallowing are rare and are usually a consequence of (1) inadequate oral pharyngeal bolus transit, (2) inability to pressurize the pharynx, (3) inability to elevate the larynx, or (4) discoordination of the cricopharyngeus.

DIAGNOSIS

The diagnosis of disordered pharyngoesophageal swallowing relies on a strong suspicion of disordered swallowing based on a carefully taken history. Dysphagia immediately following initiation of a swallow, associated with coughing or nasopharyngeal regurgitation, will predominate. The single most objective measure in assessing oropharyngeal dysfunction is the modified barium swallow in which the barium is thickened, and during swallowing a fluoroscopic recording in the lateral projection is made to document bolus passage from the mouth, through the oral pharynx, and into the esophageal body. Careful slow motion review of this study allows identification of abnormalities in any of the previously listed steps of oropharyngeal swallowing. Additionally, all patients should undergo an endoscopic evaluation to rule out structural abnormalities or malignancy.

TREATMENT

Once identified, most disorders of pharyngoesophageal swallowing are managed with diet modification and swallowing retraining.

Disordered Esophageal Body and LES

ACHALASIA

Achalasia is characterized by an absence of esophageal peristalsis and failure of the lower esophageal sphincter (LES) to completely relax upon swallowing. Primary achalasia is the result of one or more neural defects, with the most common neuroanatomical change being a decrease or loss of myenteric ganglion cells.[1,2]

Achalasia has an incidence of 0.4 to 0.6 per 100,000 and a prevalence of 8 per 100,000.[3,4] It has been described from infancy to the elderly with the majority of patients presenting between the ages of 20 and 40 years. There is no sex predilection. Familial cases have been identified,[5,6] primarily in the pediatric population, with the role of genetic factors remaining unclear. Achalasia is considered a risk factor for esophageal malignancy.[7,8]

DIAGNOSIS

Patients typically present with solid food dysphagia and varying degrees of liquid dysphagia. Often, exacerbation of their dysphagia is brought on with ingestion of cold liquids or emotional stress. Symptoms onset is gradual with the average duration of dysphagia before presentation being 2 years.

The typical symptoms of dysphagia and regurgitation prompt the performance of a barium swallow, revealing the typical bird's-beak deformity in the distal esophagus with more proximal esophageal dilatation; 90% of patients with achalasia have this typical radiographic finding.[9] This typical esophagogram may also be found with "pseudo-achalasia," a condition in which compression by intrinsic or extrinsic masses may mimic the classic radiographic findings of achalasia.[10] Pseudoachalasia is typically seen with gastroesophageal malignancies or as part of a paraneoplastic syndrome.[11,12] Finally, vigorous achalasia, a very early stage of achalasia, may present with strong tertiary esophageal contractions resulting in a radiographic appearance similar to diffuse esophageal spasm.[13]

The classic endoscopic picture is that of a dilated, patulous esophageal body tapering down to a puckered LES which fails to open with air insufflation. However, the endoscope usually passes the LES easily with minimal force or pressure.

Esophageal manometry remains the gold standard for diagnosing achalasia, characterized by absent peristalsis in the distal smooth muscle segment of the esophagus with incomplete LES relaxation.[14] While an elevated LES pressure (greater than 35 mmHg) may be seen, it is the incomplete sphincter relaxation that is characteristic, occurring in more than 80% of patients with achalasia. The manometric finding of normal esophageal motility should prompt an aggressive search for a tumor that may be causing pseudoachalasia.

TREATMENT

PHARMACOTHERAPY

The agents traditionally used to treat patients with achalasia have been smooth muscle relaxants aimed at decreasing LES tone, including calcium channel blockers (nifedipine, verapamil), opioids (loperamide), nitrates (isorsorbide dinitrate), and anticholinergics (cimetropium bromide).[15–23] These drugs, while effective in reducing LES pressure, either fail to alter symptoms[23] and are poorly tolerated due to side effects,[17,22] or have no sustainable effects.[18,21] Given these results and the excellent results obtained with other modes of therapy, pharmacotherapy is best reserved as an adjunct to the other therapies or for those patients not candidates for other more effective treatments.

BOTULINUM TOXIN

Botulinum toxin (BoTox) is a potent inhibitor of acetylcholine release from presynaptic nerve terminals. Recently, BoTox endoscopically injected into the LES has been used in the management of achalasia to decrease resting LES tone. The exact role of BoTox injection in the overall management of achalasia remains to be defined.

ESOPHAGEAL DILATION

Pneumatic dilatation is considered the standard nonoperative therapy for achalasia. In many institutions it is considered the overall treatment of choice. The objective of forced dilation of the esophagus is to break the muscle fibers of the LES and thereby decrease LES tone. Response to pneumatic dilatation is variable with most studies documenting response rates between 60% and 80%.[24–28] However, a decrease in LES pressure does not always correspond to improvement in clinical symptoms,[29] and up to 50% of patients with initial good response to dilation have recurrence of their symptoms within 5 years of treatment.[30] Fortunately, patients who respond to dilatation appear to respond equally well to a sec-

TABLE 16.3.

Review of Cited Experience Using Balloon Dilatation versus Operative Myotomy for Treatment of Achalasia.

Author	No. patients	Results
Felix 1998[78] (pr)	40	Myotomy, lower LESP, less GER; otherwise no difference
Csendes 1989[79] (pr)	81	Myotomy, 95% improved at 65 months Dilatation, 65% improved at 58 months
Moreno-Gonzalez 1988[80] (ret, multi)	1416 320	Myotomy, 82% improved Dilatation, 65% improved
Okike 1979[28] (ret)	468 431	Myotomy, 85% improved Dilatation, 65% improved

pr, prospective randomized; ret, retrospective; multi, multi-institutional.

ond session. Pneumatic balloon dilatation is considered by many to be the most effective nonoperative therapy for achalasia. Dilatation carries a risk of esophageal perforation with devastating effects, and the long-term effectiveness of dilatation falls short of the long-term results following operative myotomy (Table 16.3).

OPERATIVE MYOTOMY

Operative myotomy involves dividing the muscle layers of the LES while preserving the integrity of the esophageal mucosa. A dissection plane is usually easily developed in the submucosa where the overlying muscle fibers can be transected. An antireflux procedure often accompanies the esophageal myotomy. Esophageal myotomy has been performed either through the chest or abdomen, using traditional open techniques or laparoscopy or thoracoscopy. Overall results with operative myotomy are excellent with low complication rates.

Who should be offered operative myotomy? A careful review of the data does not answer this question. Generally, there are four groups for whom one should consider myotomy. The first is young patients for whom a single intervention with the best long-term result is the most effective overall. Pneumatic dilatation is clearly less effective in younger patients, and because of the short duration of its effect, treatment with BoTox is less desirable for young patients. The second group is those who have failed either BoTox or pneumatic dilatation. It is not clear what constitutes a failure of these therapies because they can be repeated with some increase in response with successive treatments. It seems reasonable to offer an operative myotomy to a patient who is an operative candidate and has failed two trials of either nonoperative therapy. The third group is patients who are at excessive risk for esophageal perforation with pneumatic dilatation, including patients with a tortuous esophagus, esophageal diverticula, or previous gastroesophageal junction surgery. These same conditions will also limit endoscopic access for BoTox injection. Finally, there is an increasing number of patients who are looking for more lasting therapy and wish to avoid multiple interventions. The success of laparoscopic approaches to GER and hiatal hernia is now prompting patients to seek out "minimally invasive" therapies for achalasia that have a low complication rate and lasting results.

What technique of operative myotomy should be used? Recent success with laparoscopic myotomy has shown the laparoscopic approach to be comparable to open myotomy, with enhanced postoperative recovery and shorter hospital stay.[31] The data do not clearly support any technique over another, although the laparoscopic technique of operative myotomy currently appears to be the most widely applied and reproducible.

Should an antireflux procedure accompany myotomy? The two most common reasons for a poor outcome following operative myotomy are persistent dysphagia or GER. The occurrence of each of these may reflect differences in operative approach or technique. In cases where a shorter distal myotomy is performed, GER rates are less, and dysphagia rates are increased. The answer to whether to perform an antireflux procedure may lie in the extent of distal myotomy performed, although there are no solid data to substantiate this claim.

Spastic Disorders of the Esophagus

Spastic disorders of the esophagus are primarily disorders defined by manometric abnormalities in the smooth muscle segment of the esophagus. These smooth muscle "spasms" typically consist of tertiary contractions that are simultaneous, repetitive, nonperistaltic, and often of prolonged duration and increased power. Spastic disorders of the esophagus are classically discussed as four distinct entities (diffuse esophageal spasm, nutcracker esophagus, hypertensive LES, and nonspecific esophageal motility dysfunction), but reports of evolution of one motility pattern into another suggest that these separate disorders may be within a single spectrum of motor dysfunction.

DIAGNOSIS

Dysphagia and chest pain are the dominant presenting symptoms. Esophageal manometry remains the gold standard for diagnosing spastic esophageal disorders (Table 16.4).

TREATMENT

Approaches to the treatment of esophageal spastic disorders are aimed at ameliorating symptoms. Strategies have included those same therapies applied to achalasia and include pharmacotherapy, botulinum toxin injection into the LES, balloon dilation, or operative myotomy. Due to the rarity of these

TABLE 16.4. Manometric Criteria for Spastic Motor Disorders of the Esophagus.

Diffuse esophageal spasm	Simultaneous contractions (>10% of wet swallows)
	Intermittent *normal* peristalsis
Nutcracker esophagus	High-amplitude contractions (>180 mmHg)
	Normal peristalsis
Hypertensive LES	High resting LES pressure (>45 mmHg)
	Normal LES relaxation
	Normal peristalsis
Nonspecific motor dysfunction	Frequent nonpropagated or retrograde contractions
	Low-amplitude contractions (<30 mmHg)
	Abnormal waveforms
	Body aperistalsis with normal LES

LES, lower esophageal sphincter.

conditions and the difficulty in their diagnosis, no data exist on which to base definitive statements regarding treatment.

Esophageal Diverticula

An esophageal diverticulum is an epithelial-lined mucosal pouch that protrudes from the esophageal lumen. Most esophageal diverticula are acquired and occur in adults. Esophageal diverticula are classified according to their location (pharyngoesophageal, midesophageal, or epiphrenic), the layers of the esophagus that accompany them (true diverticulum, which contain all layers, or false diverticulum, containing only mucosa and submucosa), or mechanism of formation (pulsion or traction) (Table 16.5). Most esophageal diverticula are pulsion diverticula.

Pharyngoesophageal Diverticulum (Zenker's)

This is the most common of the esophageal diverticula, with a prevalence between 0.01% and 0.11%. It is a condition of the elderly, with 50% of cases occurring during the seventh and eighth decades of life. Pharyngoesophageal diverticula consistently arise within the inferior pharyngeal constrictor, between the oblique fibers of the thyropharyngeus muscle and through or above the more horizontal fibers of the cricopharyngeus muscle (the upper esophageal sphincter). The point of transition in the direction of these muscle fibers represents an area of potential weakness in the posterior pharynx (Killian's triangle). Pharyngoesophageal diverticula appear to be acquired, as evidenced by the predominance in the elderly.

DIAGNOSIS

The presenting symptoms of pharyngoesophageal diverticulum are usually characteristic and consist of cervical esophageal dysphagia, regurgitation of bland undigested food, frequent aspiration, noisy deglutition (gurgling), halitosis, and voice changes. Dysphagia is present in 98% of patients, and

pulmonary aspiration is a serious consequence, occurring in up to one-third of patients. Cancer has been reported in a pharyngoesophageal diverticulum, but the frequency of this occurrence is no higher than that in the general population.

The diagnosis of pharyngoesophageal diverticulum is easily made with a barium esophagogram. Endoscopy, 24-h pH monitoring, and esophageal manometry are not indicated unless some feature of the symptoms or the esophagogram raise suspicion of other conditions (malignancy or GER).

TREATMENT

As is the case with all pulsion diverticula, the proper treatment must be directed at relieving the underlying neuromotor abnormality responsible for the increased intraluminal pressure and then managing the diverticulum. Most techniques described have employed division of the cricopharyngeus muscle followed by resection, imbrication, obliteration, or fenestration of the diverticulum. Most approaches to management agree that relief of the relative obstruction distal to the pouch through cricopharyngeal myotomy is the most important aspect of treatment.

Midesophageal Diverticulum

Midesophageal diverticula are rare and most commonly associated with mediastinal granulomatous disease (histoplasmosis or tuberculosis). They are thought to arise because of adhesions between inflamed mediastinal lymph nodes and the esophagus. By contraction, the adhesions exert "traction" on the esophagus with eventual localized diverticulum development. These are true diverticula with all layers of the esophagus present in the diverticulum. Some midesophageal diverticula are related to motility disorders and represent more classic pulsion features (typically larger, false diverticulum).

DIAGNOSIS/TREATMENT

A midesophageal diverticulum is typically asymptomatic and diagnosed incidentally on a barium esophagogram for other reasons. When such an asymptomatic diverticulum is found, no treatment is necessary. In patients with symptoms, esophageal manometry is indicated to search for an esophageal motor disorder. Symptomatic diverticula require treatment. When associated with an esophageal motility disorder, a small diverticulum may be treated with esophageal myotomy only. Larger diverticula usually require an accompanying resection or diverticulopexy. In the absence of a motor abnormality, diverticulectomy alone is indicated. Diverticulectomy with or

TABLE 16.5. Classification of Esophageal Diverticula.

Diverticulum	Location	Mechanism	Type
Pharyngoesophageal	UES	Pulsion	False
Midesophageal	Tracheal bifurcation	Traction	True
Epiphrenic	Distal esophagus	Pulsion	False

UES, upper esophageal sphincter.

without myotomy usually requires a transthoracic approach, either open or thoracoscopic.

Epiphrenic (Pulsion) Diverticulum

A fairly rare condition, an epiphrenic diverticulum typically occurs within the distal 10 cm of the esophagus and is a pulsion type. It is most commonly associated with esophageal motor abnormalities (achalasia, hypertensive LES, diffuse esophageal spasm, nonspecific motor disorders), but may be the result of other causes of increased esophageal pressure.

DIAGNOSIS/TREATMENT

Most epiphrenic diverticula are symptomatic because of the underlying esophageal motor disorder. Diagnosis of the diverticulum is made during barium esophagogram. Manometry, esophagoscopy, and 24-h pH testing may be necessary to diagnose associated conditions and direct specific treatments. Most epiphrenic diverticula require esophageal myotomy extending from the neck of the diverticulum onto the gastric cardia for a distance of 1.5 to 3.0 cm (see section on myotomy for achalasia). Diverticulectomy, fundoplication, or repair of hiatal hernia may also be necessary depending on the size of the diverticulum or associated conditions.

Gastroesophageal Reflux

Definition

Gastroesophageal reflux (GER) is defined as the failure of the antireflux barrier, allowing abnormal reflux of gastric contents into the esophagus.[32,33] It is a mechanical disorder that is caused by a defective lower esophageal sphincter (LES), a gastric emptying disorder, or failed esophageal peristalsis. These abnormalities result in a spectrum of disease ranging from the symptom of "heartburn" to esophageal tissue damage with subsequent complications. GER is an extremely common condition accounting for nearly 75% of all esophageal pathology.

Pathophysiology

ANTIREFLUX MECHANISM

Although the exact nature of the antireflux barrier is incompletely understood, the current view is that the lower esophageal sphincter (LES), the diaphragmatic crura, and the phrenoesophageal ligament are key components.[34,35] LES dysfunction is the most common cause of GER. A popular model proposed by DeMeester details three factors that determine the competence of the LES: (1) resting LES pressure, (2) resting LES length, and (3) abdominal length of the LES (Table 16.6).

LES dysfunction may be either physiological and transient, or pathological and permanent. Postprandial gastric distension results in pressure against the LES, stretching and pulling the sphincter open while shortening the LES length. The resulting incompetence of the LES leads to transient periods of reflux.

Permanent failure of the LES occurs when there is structural damage to the components of the LES (resting pressure, overall length, and intraabdominal length). Any or all of these

TABLE 16.6. Features of an Incompetent Lower Esophageal Sphincter (LES).

LES characteristics	Incompetent if:
Resting LES pressure	<6 mmHg
Resting LES length	<2 cm
Length intraabdominal LES	<1 cm

components of LES function interrelate to provide a structural barrier against reflux. If one component is abnormal, the probability of GER is 73%. If two components are abnormal this increases to 74%, and if all three are abnormal, 92%. Because the probability of GER does not reach 100% with complete LES dysfunction, there are clearly other components of the antireflux barrier.

CONSEQUENCES OF REFLUX

Gastroesophageal reflux may lead to symptoms related to the reflux of gastric content into the esophagus, lungs, or oropharynx, or to damage to the esophageal mucosa and respiratory epithelium with subsequent changes related to repair, fibrosis, and reinjury. Manifestations of GER are typically classified as esophageal and extraesophageal. Esophageal manifestations of GER include heartburn, chest pain, water brash, or dysphagia (see Table 16.2). Dysphagia often suggests a complication of GER such as esophagitis and ulceration, stricture, or Barrett's metaplastic changes. Extraesophageal manifestations are generally pulmonary, resulting from pulmonary aspiration of refluxate, or a vagally mediated reflex that induces bronchospasm when refluxate stimulates the distal esophagus. Other extraesophageal manifestations include chronic cough, laryngitis, dental damage, and chronic sinusitis.

DIAGNOSIS

The clinical diagnosis of GER is fairly straightforward if the patient reports the classic symptom of heartburn that is readily relieved after ingesting antacids. Other typical symptoms of GER include regurgitation or dysphagia. Recently it has been appreciated that chest pain, asthma, laryngitis, recurrent pulmonary infections, chronic cough, and hoarseness may be associated with reflux, and this association is leading to increasing numbers of patients with these *atypical* GER symptoms to be evaluated for reflux.

In a patient with typical symptoms, endoscopic findings of esophageal erosions, ulcers, or columnar-lined esophagus is fairly specific for GER. During esophagogastroduodenoscopy (EGD), esophageal mucosal biopsy should be obtained to confirm esophagitis, and esophageal length and the presence of a hiatal hernia or stricture can be assessed and may eliminate the need for a confirmatory barium swallow. With these findings, no other tests beyond EGD are necessary to diagnose GER. However, in many patients the EGD will be normal due to empiric treatment of symptoms by primary care physicians. In this setting, 24-h pH testing is necessary to objectively establish the diagnosis of GER.

TREATMENT

MEDICAL

The principles of nonoperative management of GER include lifestyle modifications, medical therapy to control symptoms, and identification of those patients who would be best served with an antireflux operation. Although lifestyle modifications have always been the initial step in therapy, only those patients with mild and intermittent symptoms seem to benefit from lifestyle changes alone. Most patients who seek medical advice will be best treated either medically or surgically.

Numerous trials have shown that short-term treatment of GER with acid suppression regimens can effectively relieve symptomatic GER and heal reflux esophagitis; however, levels of success depend on the type, duration, and dosage of antisecretory therapy. Recurrence of esophagitis and symptoms is frequently observed. Proton pump inhibitors (PPI) have profoundly changed the medical treatment of GER. Rates of healing of esophagitis have dramatically improved with PPIs when compared to H_2 receptor antagonists (H_2RA). However, the cost of PPI has lead many to recommend their use in only complicated or refractory GER.

There are no contemporary prospective studies from which to make definitive recommendations regarding medical management of GER or medical versus surgical management. Treatment algorithms based on endoscopic findings are shown in Figs. 16.6 and 16.7.

SURGICAL

Medical therapy is the first line of management for GER. Esophagitis heals in approximately 90% of cases with intensive medical therapy. However, medical management does

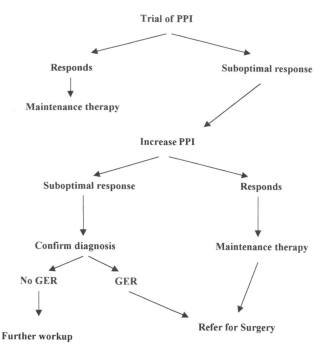

FIGURE 16.7. Management algorithm for treatment of complicated gastroesophageal reflux (based on endoscopic findings). PPI, proton pump inhibitor; GER, gastroesophageal reflux. (After Fennerty MB, Castell D, Fendrick AM, et al. The diagnosis and treatment of gastroesophageal reflux disease in a managed care environment. Suggested disease management guidelines. Arch Intern Med 1996;156: 477–484, with permission.)

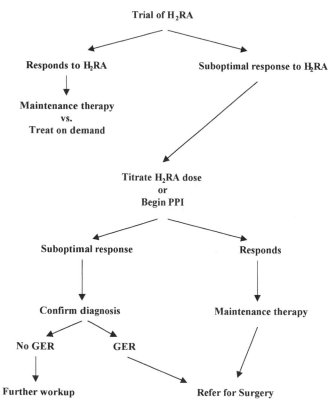

FIGURE 16.6. Management algorithm for treatment of uncomplicated gastroesophageal reflux (based on endoscopic findings). H_2RA, H_2 receptor antagonist; PPI, proton pump inhibitor; GER, gastroesophageal reflux. (After Fennerty MB, Castell D, Fendrick AM, et al. The diagnosis and treatment of gastroesophageal reflux disease in a managed care environment. Suggested disease management guidelines. Arch Intern Med 1996;156:477–484 with permission.)

not address the condition's mechanical etiology; thus, symptoms recur in more than 80% of cases within 1 year of drug withdrawal.[36] In addition, although medical therapy may effectively treat the acid-induced symptoms of GER, esophageal mucosal injury may continue because of ongoing alkaline reflux.[37] Because GER is a chronic condition, medical therapy involving acid suppression or promotility agents may be required for the rest of a patient's life. Surgical therapy, which addresses the mechanical nature of this condition, is curative in 85% to 93% of patients.[38–41] Chronic medical management may be most appropriate for patients with limited life expectancy or comorbid conditions that would prohibit safe surgical intervention.

Who should be considered for antireflux surgery? There remain two clear indications. First, antireflux surgery should be considered in patients who have failed intensive medical therapy; with the advent of proton pump inhibitors, true medical failures are unusual. Second, and more commonly, antireflux surgery should be offered to patients whose symptoms recur immediately after stopping medications and thus require long-term daily medication. Antireflux surgery effectively relieves symptoms in 93% of patients, returning an individual's quality of life to normal.[42]

What preoperative workup is necessary? At a minimum, all patients being considered for surgery should undergo a thorough history and physical exam, EGD, and esophageal manometry.[43]

Esophageal manometry allows evaluation of the lower esophageal sphincter and is diagnostic in differentiating GER from achalasia. Equally important is its use in assessing esophageal body pressures and identifying individuals with impaired esophageal clearance who may not do as well with a 360° fundoplication. In those patients who have impaired peristalsis, as evidenced by mean distal esophageal pressures of 30 mmHg or less, or esophageal peristalsis in 60% or less of wet swallows, many advocate modifying the surgical approach by performing a partial fundoplication (270° wrap).

What antireflux procedure should be performed? The goal of antireflux surgery is to establish effective LES pressure. To realize this goal, most surgeons believe it necessary to position the LES within the abdomen where the sphincter is under positive (intraabdominal) pressure and to close any associated hiatal defect.[44] To accomplish this, various safe and effective surgical techniques have been developed.

The laparoscopic Nissen fundoplication has emerged as the most widely accepted and applied antireflux operation.[42,45–50] In many centers, it is the antireflux procedure of choice in patients with normal esophageal body peristalsis. Key elements of the procedure include the complete dissection of the esophageal hiatus and both crura, mobilization of the gastric fundus by dividing the short gastric vessels, closure of the associated hiatal defect, creation of a tensionless 360° gastric wrap at the distal esophagus around a 50- to 60-French intraesophageal dilator, limiting the length of the wrap to 1.5 to 2.0 cm, and stabilizing the wrap to the esophagus by partial thickness bites of the esophagus during creation of the wrap.

Overall, 97% of patients undergoing this procedure are satisfied with their results.

The Toupet fundoplication is identical to the Nissen except that the fundoplication is a 270° wrap rather than a 360° wrap. The gastric fundus is brought posterior to the esophagus and sutured to either side of the esophagus leaving the anterior surface bare. This 270° fundoplication has the theoretical advantage of limiting postoperative bloating and dysphagia, especially in those with impaired esophageal body peristalsis.

Barrett's Esophagus

In 1950 Norman Barrett described the condition in which the tubular esophagus becomes lined with metaplastic columnar epithelium that is at risk for adenocarcinoma, rather than the normal squamous epithelium. Most recently, it has been recognized that the specialized intestinal metaplasia (not gastric-type columnar changes) constitutes true Barrett's esophagus, with a risk of progression to dysplasia and adenocarcinoma.

This abnormality occurs in 7% to 10% of people with GER and may represent the end stage of the natural history of GER. Clearly, Barrett's esophagus is associated with a more profound mechanical deficiency of the LES, severe impairment of esophageal body function, and marked esophageal acid exposure.[51] The endoscopic feature most strongly associated with intestinal metaplasia is the finding of long segments of esophageal columnar lining, with more than 90% of patients with greater than 3 cm of esophageal columnar lining have intestinal metaplasia.

Endoscopically obvious Barrett's esophagus with intestinal metaplasia is a major risk factor for adenocarcinoma of the esophagus, with the annual incidence of adenocarcinoma in this condition estimated at approximately 0.8%, 40 times higher than in the general population. Once high-grade dysplasia is identified in more than one biopsy from columnar-lined esophagus, nearly 50% of patients already harbor a focus of invasive cancer. This frequency is the basis for recommending careful endoscopic surveillance in patients with Barrett's esophagus with intestinal metaplasia and esophagectomy when high-grade dysplasia is identified.[52,53]

Treatment goals for patients with Barrett's esophagus are similar to those for patients with GER, that is, relief of symptoms and arrest of ongoing reflux-mediated epithelial damage. Additionally, those with Barrett's esophagus, regardless of type of treatment (surgical or medical), require long-term endoscopic surveillance with biopsy of columnar segments to identify progressive metaplastic changes or progression to dysplasia.[54,55]

Several studies have compared medical and surgical therapy in patients with Barrett's esophagus (Table 16.7). These data support the notion that Barrett's esophagus is associated with more severe and refractory GER, and antireflux surgery is effective at alleviating these symptoms in 75% to 92% of patients.[56,57] However, many patients are asymptomatic (perhaps explaining why they have such advanced sequelae of GER), and there is mounting evidence to suggest that an alkaline refluxate may be as damaging as acid reflux.[58] For these reasons, correction of the mechanically defective antireflux barrier may be especially important in these patients. Although symptom control in these patients suggests control of ongoing damage, the ultimate goal in therapy is to change the natural history in Barrett's of progression to adenocarcinoma. With this goal, several questions arise:

TABLE 16.7.
Medical versus Surgical Treatment of Barrett's Esophagus.

	No. patients		Symptom control		Stricture/esophagitis	
Author	Medical	Surgical	Medical	Surgical	Medical	Surgical
Attwood 1992[81] (p)[a]	26	19	22%	81%	38%	21%
Oritz 1996[82] (pr)	27	32	85%	89%	53%/45%	5%/15%
Sampliner 1994[83] (p)	27	—	70%	—	50%	—
Csendes 1998[84] (pr)	—	152	—	46%	—	64%

pr, prospective randomized; p, prospective; ret, retrospective.

[a]Before availability of proton pump inhibitors.

(1) Does antireflux surgery result in regression of Barrett's epithelium? Operative therapy corrects the mechanically defective antireflux barrier and therefore might be expected to have a higher likelihood than medical therapy alone of inducing regression of Barrett's epithelium. However, current evidence suggests that neither medical nor surgical therapy result in regression of Barrett's epithelium.[59]

(2) Does antireflux surgery prevent progression of metaplastic changes? There is growing evidence suggesting that antireflux surgery may prevent progression of Barrett's changes and thereby protect against dysplasia and malignancy.

(3) Is there a role for antireflux surgery accompanied by other therapies for metaplastic or dysplastic epithelium? Combination therapy, that is, pharmacological or operative control of acid reflux plus endoscopic ablation of Barrett's mucosa, is having encouraging preliminary results.[60,61] These early experiences suggest that the ablated areas reepithelialize with more normal squamous mucosa. Ablative therapies have included laser ablation, photodynamic therapy, and cryotherapy.

Diaphragmatic Hernia

To complete its course from mouth to stomach, the esophagus must traverse the diaphragm. The site of transit of the esophagus from chest into the abdomen, the esophageal hiatus, is the site of a variety of defects (Fig. 16.8).

A type I hiatal hernia, also known as a sliding hiatal hernia, consists of a simple herniation of the gastroesophageal junction into the chest. The phrenoesophageal ligament is attenu-

ated and there is no true hernia sac. This, the most common of the hiatal hernias, is more common in women and in the fifth and sixth decades of life. With a type II hiatal hernia, commonly referred to as a paraesophageal hernia, the gastroesophageal junction remains at the esophageal hiatus while the gastric fundus herniates alongside the esophagus into the chest. The type III hiatal hernia is a combination of type I and type II hernias, with the esophagogastric junction being displaced into the chest along with the gastric fundus and body. Paraesophageal hernias (types II and III) have a true hernia sac accompanying the herniated stomach. Finally, some have characterized a type IV hernia as an advanced stage of paraesophageal hernia in which the entire stomach and other intraabdominal content (e.g., colon, spleen) are herniated into the chest, although use of this fourth classification is not widely accepted.

Diagnosis

Most type I and III hiatal hernias are diagnosed incidentally during a contrast upper GI or during upper endoscopy performed for other reasons. Type II hernias can be similarly diagnosed, but are also frequently found on a radiograph of the chest showing an air–fluid level in the mediastinum or the left chest.

When symptoms are present, sliding hernias have a different presentation than paraesophageal hernias. Paraesophageal hernias tend to produce more dysphagia, chest pain, bloating, and respiratory problems than do sliding hernias. Symptoms associated with a sliding hernia are more often related to LES dysfunction and include heartburn, regurgitation, and dysphagia.

TREATMENT

Because hiatal hernia is a purely mechanical abnormality, there is no nonoperative treatment. The risk of bleeding, incarceration, strangulation, perforation, and death with paraesophageal hernias is such that when a type II or type III hernia is identified, operative repair should be performed.[62] In contrast, a significant number of patients with type I hiatal hernias are asymptomatic, and remain so throughout the remainder of their life. Therefore, the presence of a sliding hiatal hernia alone does not mandate intervention.

Operative correction of esophageal hiatal hernia should (1) return the herniated content to its anatomically correct position below the diaphragm, (2) repair the hernia defect, and (3) prevent recurrence while minimizing associated morbidity. There are a number of proven operations that can be performed through the chest or abdomen to accomplish these goals. Questions remain regarding the need for an accompanying antireflux procedure and the method of abdominal or thoracic access.

Are hiatal hernia and gastroesophageal reflux associated? Sliding hiatal hernia alone presently appears to be not causative of GER, but the presence of a hiatal hernia in patients with GER magnifies this condition and its sequelae.

Should an antireflux procedure accompany all hiatal hernia repairs? Whether to include an antireflux procedure with all hiatal hernia repairs remains controversial, especially when dealing with a type II paraesophageal hernia. Because most sliding type hernias are repaired on the basis of symptoms, adding an antireflux procedure seems more straightforward because of the prevalence of reflux symptoms in type I and III hernias. In contrast, most patients who have type II hernias

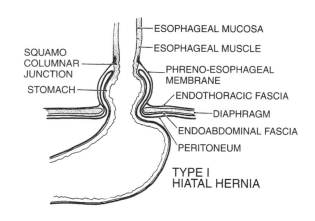

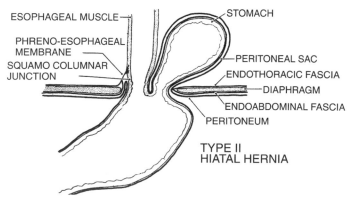

FIGURE 16.8. Classification of hiatal hernia.

do not have reflux symptoms, and an antireflux operation for these patients may add little benefit to the outcome. Few studies have objectively evaluated addition of an antireflux procedure to hiatal hernia repair, and there are limited data available to definitively answer this question.

Should hiatal hernias be repaired laparoscopically? Anecdotal data suggest that hernia recurrence is higher following laparoscopic repair than after traditional open hiatal hernia repair. The proposed basis for this is the relative absence of intraabdominal adhesions that accompanies laparoscopic hernia repair as compared to open operations. These anecdotal experiences need further investigation before any conclusions regarding route of abdominal access for repair of hiatal hernia can be made.

Tumors

The vast majority of esophageal tumors are malignant, with less than 1% of neoplasms being benign. The majority of malignant esophageal tumors are either squamous cell carcinomas or adenocarcinomas.

Benign Tumors

Benign tumors of the esophagus are uncommon, with three histological types accounting for 87% of benign esophageal tumors (leiomyomas, cysts, and polyps). These three tumors have distinct locations in the esophagus that reflect their cells of origin. Polyps occur almost exclusively in the cervical esophagus, while leiomyomas and cysts tend to occur in the distal two-thirds of the esophagus.

LEIOMYOMAS

Leiomyomas constitute 50% of benign tumors of the esophagus with an average patient age at presentation of 38 years, in contrast to esophageal malignancy, which typically presents at a more advanced age. There is a distinct male predominance, and 90% of lesions are located in the lower two-thirds of the esophagus. Leiomyomas are typical solitary, although they can be multiple 3% to 10% of the time.

Most patients present with dysphagia and pain, but asymptomatic lesions are increasingly being identified during imaging studies for other reasons. Weight loss is uncommon, and bleeding is rare. Barium swallow reveals the classic smooth, oval-shaped filling defect of the esophageal lumen. Endoscopy is necessary to rule out malignancy, and usually reveals a mass protruding into the lumen with uninvolved overlying mucosa.

The natural history of leiomyomas suggests slow growth and low malignant potential, but those that are symptomatic or bothersome to the patient should be removed. Asymptomatic leiomyomas can be observed with serial esophagograms and follow-up. Operative removal involves simple enucleation without entering the esophageal lumen, followed by reconstruction of the outer esophageal wall.

CYSTS

Esophageal cysts are most commonly congenital and are lined by columnar epithelium of the respiratory type, glandular epithelium of the gastric type, squamous epithelium, or transitional epithelium. Enteric and bronchogenic cysts are the most common.

The resulting symptoms are very similar to those of other benign tumors of the esophagus, and the radiographic and endoscopic appearance is identical to leiomyoma. A softer, more compressible lesion during endoscopy, and presence of fluid within the mass found with ultrasound or CT scan, confirm the diagnosis of esophageal cyst.

Treatment is similar to that for leiomyoma, with resection for large or symptomatic lesions. During removal, all the cyst wall should be removed and a search for a fistulous tract to the respiratory tract should be carried out, especially in patients who have had recurrent respiratory tract infections.

Malignant Esophageal Tumors

Esophageal cancer is among the top 10 leading causes of cancer-related deaths in the United States and its incidence is increasing. Its late presentation and early spread lead to a poor prognosis and an overall 5-year survival rate of less than 10%.

Squamous cell carcinomas account for 60% of esophageal cancers and are equally distributed among the upper, middle, and lower thirds of the esophagus. The remaining 40% are adenocarcinomas, which are most commonly found in the lower third of the esophagus. Most adenocarcinomas are thought to arise in columnar cell-lined Barrett's mucosa.

Alcohol consumption and tobacco use are well-established etiological factors for the development of esophageal carcinoma. Additionally, premalignant esophageal abnormalities include achalasia, reflux esophagitis with Barrett's mucosa, radiation esophagitis, caustic esophageal injury, Plummer–Vinson syndrome, leukoplakia, esophageal diverticula, ectopic gastric mucosa, and the inherited condition of familial keratosis palmaris et plantaris (tylosis).

DIAGNOSIS

The vast majority of esophageal carcinomas are clinically occult, and present well after disease progression prevents cure. Common presenting symptoms are listed in Table 16.8.[63]

The initial study should be a barium swallow; this most frequently reveals distinct mucosal irregularity, stricture, a shelf in the lower esophagus, or rigidity. Upper esophageal endoscopy allows visualization of the affected area and biopsy to confirm the diagnosis.

STAGING

The stage of esophageal cancer is determined by the depth of penetration of the primary tumor and the presence of lymph node and distant organ metastasis (Table 16.9), and preoperative staging determines the intent of subsequent treatment, curative or palliative. Initial staging includes a careful phys-

TABLE 16.8. Presenting Symptoms of Esophageal Carcinoma.

Symptom	Incidence (%)
Dysphagia	87
Weight loss	71
Substernal or epigastric pain/burning	46
Vomiting or regurgitation	28
Aspiration pneumonia	14
Palpable cervical nodes	14
Hoarseness	7
Coughing and choking	3

ical examination looking for the sequelae of esophageal cancer (weight loss, supraclavicular adenopathy, pleural effusion, etc.), routine blood tests, and CT scan of the chest and abdomen. Bronchoscopy is indicated for midesophageal tumors because of their propensity to invade the trachea and left mainstem bronchus. The more recent development of endoscopic ultrasonography (EUS) has improved staging by allowing the depth of invasion into the esophageal wall to be accurately determined and surrounding lymph node involvement to be identified and even biopsied.

Beyond TNM staging, weight loss greater than 10% has been shown to be associated with a significantly poorer outcome in patients with operable esophageal cancer. Staging groups patients into two groups: those with potentially curable disease, and those with metastatic disease (disease outside of the local or regional area) in whom palliation is currently the only treatment option.

TREATMENT

Based on preoperative staging, treatment of esophageal cancer aims at either cure or effective palliation. To effect these results, there are a variety of therapies available, with optimal outcomes often utilizing a combination of therapies. These options include surgery, irradiation, chemotherapy, or a combination of these.

SURGERY

Surgery is the treatment of choice for small tumors confined to the esophageal mucosa or submucosa. Surgical treatment for resectable esophageal cancers results in 5% to 20% 5-year survival rates and an operative mortality of 2% to 7%. Once symptoms appear, most esophageal cancers have invaded adjacent structures or spread to distant organs. In these cases where significant obstructive symptoms exist, operative management often is the most effective means of relieving dysphagia and long-term palliation.

In all procedures, a laparotomy is done first to assess for celiac nodal disease and to mobilize the gastric conduit for esophageal replacement. In the subtotal thoracic esophagectomy (the Ivor–Lewis esophagectomy), the esophagus is resected through a right thoracotomy with an intrathoracic esophagogastric anastomosis at the level of the azygous vein. With the total thoracic esophagectomy, the esophagus is resected into the neck and the gastric conduit is brought through the chest, with a cervical esophagogastric anastomosis completed in the neck through a left cervical neck incision. A transhiatal esophagectomy (also known as blunt esophagectomy) consists of resection of the intrathoracic esophagus through the esophageal hiatus without an open thoracotomy. The esophagus is dissected bluntly from both the abdominal and cervical incisions and an esophagogastric anastomosis is performed in the neck. The transhiatal esophagectomy has the potential disadvantages of inadequate resection, understaging of disease because of incomplete lymph node resection, and risk of tracheobronchial or vascular injury. Advantages include the avoidance of a thoracotomy and its associated respiratory compromise and complications.

No controlled clinical trials have directly compared these various techniques, and few series have substantial data from which to make conclusions regarding choosing any one of these techniques over another (Table 16.10). In general, because esophageal cancer can have extensive and unpredictable spread longitudinally, it seems prudent to perform total esophagectomy, especially for those proximal- and middle-third lesions. Distal small lesions may be approached through the abdomen only, or resection for palliation alone can avoid total esophagectomy and its associated morbidity.

IRRADIATION

There is substantial experience with external beam radiation for esophageal carcinoma with appropriate doses (50–65 Gy).

TABLE 16.9. AJCC TNM Definitions for Esophageal Cancer.

Primary Tumor (T)	Regional Lymph Nodes (N)	Distant Metastasis (M)	Survival groupings
TX: Primary tumor cannot be assessed	NX: Regional lymph nodes cannot be assessed	MX: Presence of distant metastasis cannot be assessed	Stage 0: TisN0M0 5-year survival: EXCELLENT
T0: No evidence of primary tumor	N0: No regional lymph node metastasis	M0: No distant metastasis	Stage I: T1N0M0 5-year survival: >50%
Tis: Carcinoma in situ	N1: Regional lymph node metastasis	M1: Distant metastasis	Stage IIA: T2N0M0; T3N0M0 5-year survival: 15%
T1: Tumor invades lamina propria or submucosa			Stage IIB: T1N1M0; T2N1M0 5-year survival: 10%
T2: Tumor invades muscularis propria			Stage III: T3N1M0; T4, any N,M0 5-year survival: <10%
T3: Tumor invades adventitia			Stage IV: Any T, any N, M1 5-year survival: rare
T4: Tumor invades adjacent structures			

Source: Used with the permission of the American Joint Committee on Cancer (AJCC), Chicago, IL. The original source for this material is the AJCC Cancer Staging Manual, Sixth Edition (2002) published by Springer-Verlag New York, www.springer-ny.com. The above TNM classification will be implemented in January 2003.

TABLE 16.10. Comparison of Outcomes for Various Techniques of Esophagectomy for Cancer.

Author	Technique	Mortality (%)	Survival[a]
Lanouis 1983[85]	Lt. thoracotomy	26/147 (17.7)	6
Lanouis 1983[85]	Rt. thoracotomy	10/58 (17.2)	14
Hankins 1972[86]	Rt. thoracotomy	0/11 (0)	—
Hankins 1972[86]	Lt. thoracotomy	0/6 (0)	—
Carey 1972[87]	Rt. thoracotomy	0/37 (0)	13
Roth 1994[88]	Rt. thoracotomy	1/34 (2.9)	9
Katlic 1990[89]	Rt. thoracotomy	7/67 (10.4)	18
Putnam 1994[90]	Rt. thoracotomy	10/134 (9.6)	24
Putnam 1994[90]	Transhiatal	2/42 (4.8)	24
Orringer 1984[91]	Transhiatal	6/100 (6)	17
Yonezawa 1984[92]	Transhiatal	0/31 (0)	—

[a]Actuarial 5-year survival (months).

Cure is possible in selected cases. Most applications of radiotherapy are for palliation, because radiation often fails to control local disease, and relief of dysphagia is brief in duration, ranging from 3 to 6 months.

CHEMOTHERAPY

Chemotherapy (typically, platinum +5Fu) as a single modality has limited use, even in palliation. Only a few patients realize a modest and short-lived response.

Esophageal Perforation/Injury

The most common cause of esophageal injury or perforation is instrumentation of the esophagus during diagnostic or therapeutic procedures. Esophageal injury may also result from ingestion of a caustic substance (either accidental or intentional), ingestion of a foreign body, profound retching, progression of disease (malignancy), or external trauma.

Perforation

DIAGNOSIS

Regardless of the cause, esophageal perforation is a true emergency requiring immediate recognition and treatment. A high index of suspicion, especially when an iatrogenic cause is suspected, allows early diagnosis of esophageal perforation. Early diagnosis is the key to obtaining the most favorable outcome of treatment.

Abnormalities on chest radiography are variable and should not be relied upon to diagnose esophageal perforation. Air within the soft tissues of the mediastinum or neck indicates perforation but fails to localize the site and magnitude of perforation. The diagnosis is best made with a contrast esophagogram. Water-soluble contrast is initially administered, followed by dilute barium if the initial swallow fails to reveal a perforation.[64] Barium provides much better mucosal detail than water-soluble contrast, and the risk of missing a perforation far outweighs the risks of barium extravasation in the neck or mediastinum. If a perforation is demonstrated with water-soluble contrast, barium is unnecessary and should be avoided. Chest CT may be helpful. The risks of further injury or increased spillage and soiling mean

there is virtually no role for esophagoscopy in diagnosing esophageal perforation.

TREATMENT

When esophageal perforation occurs intraoperatively, immediate primary closure should be performed, with drainage of the operative field over closed suction drains. In this setting, outcomes are excellent, with 98% survival and success.[65–69] Otherwise, immediate treatment is first aimed at minimizing bacterial and chemical contamination of the neck or mediastinum and restoring intravascular volume. Oral intake is withheld, and broad-spectrum intravenous antibiotics are given.

The best outcome is obtained when the perforation has occurred less than 24 h previously and can be closed primarily (80% to 90% survival). Critical to this success is the viability of the tissue for closure, debridement of any necrotic or stained tissue, and drainage of the field. Occasionally, cervical esophageal perforations can be managed with drainage alone, especially when the perforation is small, making intraoperative localization difficult or hazardous. When the perforation has been present more than 24 h, survival decreases to less than 50%, regardless of whether the perforation is managed by closure and drainage or by drainage alone.

In select circumstances, nonoperative management is appropriate: (1) contrast esophagogram demonstrates a perforation that is contained within the mediastinum and drains well back into the esophagus, (2) associated symptoms are mild, and (3) there is no clinical evidence of sepsis.[70] In this setting, oral intake is withheld for 7 to 14 days, hyperalimentation is given, and gastric antisecretory medication is administered. Any decline in clinical course mandates immediate operative management. Free perforation into the pleural cavity contraindicates nonoperative management.

Injury

CAUSTIC INGESTION

Although acid is occasionally ingested, the immediate mucosal burn with acids minimizes its ingestion. In contrast, alkalies result in a slower and delayed mucosal burn, allowing ingestion of larger amounts of substance before pain prevents swallowing.[71]

DIAGNOSIS

Because a history of caustic ingestion is usually known at initial presentation, diagnostic maneuvers center on assessing the extent and magnitude of injury. Pain in the mouth and sternal region, hypersalivation, odynophagia, and dysphagia suggest ingestion rather than attempted ingestion. Contrast esophagogram is not a reliable way to assess acute esophageal injury, but is necessary in later follow-up to identify strictures. Esophagogastroscopy is the single best maneuver when performed early after presentation, allowing confirmation of significant caustic ingestion and grading of the severity of the injury.[72]

TREATMENT

Treatment must address both the immediate and long-term consequences of caustic ingestion. The immediate treatment focuses on fluid resuscitation and initiation of broad-spectrum antibiotics.[73] Early intubation may be necessary because loss of the airway can rapidly develop after significant laryngeal or epiglottic injury. Neutralization of the corrosive risks causes exacerbation of the mucosal injury and should be avoided. Emetics reexpose the esophagus to the corrosive agent and are contraindicated, and nasogastric intubation is not recommended because of the risk of perforating the friable esophagus. During this acute phase, operative treatment is based on endoscopic grading of injury and intraoperative assessment of extent of injury and tissue viability.

Once the acute phase has passed, management focuses on prevention and treatment of strictures. Occasionally, optimal management of strictures requires operative resection or esophagoplasty. Operative intervention is indicated when (1) there is complete stenosis in which all attempts have failed to establish a lumen, (2) there is marked irregularity and pocketing on esophagogram, (3) severe periesophageal reaction or mediastinitis develops with dilation, (4) a fistula forms, (5) a lumen cannot be maintained with repeated dilation, or (6) the patient is unable to undergo repeated dilation for a prolonged period of time.[74,75] The ideal conduit for esophageal replacement, in order of preference, is (1) colon, (2) stomach, and (3) jejunum.

Mallory–Weiss

During vomiting, significant intragastric pressures are generated. Fortunately, the extragastric pressure usually equals intragastric pressure, thereby minimizing the stretching of the gastric wall. When there is a paraesophageal hernia and the LES is fixed within the abdomen, these intragastric pressures are transmitted to the supradiaphragmatic portion of the gastric wall, resulting in a mucosal tear with subsequent bleeding. Bleeding can be profuse and mimic a bleeding duodenal ulcer or varices. A history of retching immediately before an upper gastrointestinal bleed should raise the suspicion of a Mallory–Weiss tear.[76]

Immediate esophagogastroscopy is usually diagnostic, showing a proximal source of bleeding and no esophageal varices.[77] Treatment is supportive with gastric lavage and decompression, maintenance of intravascular volume, and transfusion to replace blood loss. Bleeding is usually self-limited. Rarely, laparotomy is indicated for ongoing blood loss and hemodynamic instability. At laparotomy, a gastrotomy and oversewing of mucosal tears arrests bleeding.

Miscellaneous

Schatzki's Ring

Schatzki's ring is a thin submucosal circumferential ring in the lower esophagus at the squamocolumnar junction. It is often associated with a hiatal hernia. The etiology of a Schatzki's ring remains unclear.

Clinical symptoms associated with Schatzki's ring are self-limited episodes of dysphagia during hurried ingestion of dry and solid foods. The best treatment of Schatzki's ring in patients who do not have gastroesophageal reflux is dilation.

Scleroderma

Scleroderma is a systemic collagen-vascular disease with 80% of patients having some degree of esophageal involvement. In the gastrointestinal tract, the predominant feature is smooth muscle atrophy with resulting sphincter and motor dysfunction. Most commonly, the lower esophageal sphincter mechanism is weakened, and esophageal peristalsis in the smooth muscle-lined distal esophagus is impaired. The result is reflux esophagitis with subsequent stricture formation and esophageal shortening.

Heartburn and dysphagia are frequent presenting complaints. Endoscopy confirms esophagitis, and esophageal manometry typically shows preservation of the motor activity of the striated muscle-lined proximal esophagus, absence of motor activity in the distal esophagus, and a hypotensive lower esophageal sphincter. When planning management, a gastric emptying study should be performed to assess the magnitude of gastric dysfunction.

Medical treatment with antacids and prokinetics frequently fails. An antireflux procedure may be the best method to arrest reflux, but may eventually lead to worsening dysphagia as the disease progresses. Esophageal shortening requires a Collis esophageal lengthening accompanied by an antireflux procedure.

Plummer–Vinson Syndrome

This clinical syndrome is very uncommon and is characterized by dysphagia associated with atrophic oral mucosa, spoon-shaped fingers with brittle nails, and chronic iron deficiency anemia. It characteristically occurs in middle-aged edentulous women, and is more common in Scandinavian countries. Radiographic and endoscopic studies reveal a fibrous web just below the cricopharyngeus muscle as the cause of their dysphagia.

Treatment of the dysphagia is dilation of the web. Careful long-term follow-up is necessary because 100% of these patients will eventually develop malignant lesions of the oral mucosa, hypopharynx, and esophagus.

References

1. Csendes A, Smok G, Braghetto I, et al. Gastroesophageal sphincter pressure and histological changes in distal esophagus in patients with achalasia of the esophagus. Dig Dis Sci 1985;30:941–945.
2. Goldblum JR, Whyte RI, Orringer MB, et al. Achalasia. A morphologic study of 42 resected specimens. Am J Surg Pathol 1994; 18:327–337.

3. Mayberry JF, Atkinson M. Studies of incidence and prevalence of achalasia in the Nottingham area. Q J Med 1985;56:451–456.

4. Mayberry JF, Probert CS, Sher KS, et al. Some epidemiological and aetiological aspects of achalasia. Dig Dis 1991;9:1–8.

5. Nihoul-Fekete C, Bawab F, Lortat-Jacob S, et al. Achalasia of the esophagus in childhood. Surgical treatment in 35 cases, with special reference to familial cases and glucocorticoid deficiency association. Hepatogastroenterology 1991;38:510–513.

6. Chawla K, Chawla SK, Alexander LL. Familiar achalasia of the esophagus in mother and son: a possible pathogenetic relationship. J Am Geriatr Soc 1979;27:519–521.

7. Streitz JM Jr, Ellis FH Jr, Gibb SP, et al. Achalasia and squamous cell carcinoma of the esophagus: analysis of 241 patients. Ann Thorac Surg 1995;59:1604–1609.

8. Meijssen MA, Tilanus HW, van Blankenstein M, et al. Achalasia complicated by oesophageal squamous cell carcinoma: a prospective study in 195 patients. Gut 1992;33:155–158.

9. Schima W, Stacher G, Pokieser P, et al. Esophageal motor disorders: videofluoroscopic and manometric evaluation—prospective study in 88 symptomatic patients. Radiology 1992;185:487–491.

10. Tracey JP, Traube M. Difficulties in the diagnosis of pseudoachalasia. Am J Gastroenterol 1994;89:2014–2018.

11. Rozman RW Jr, Achkar E. Features distinguishing secondary achalasia from primary achalasia. Am J Gastroenterol 1990;85:1327–1330.

12. Campos CT, Ellis FH Jr, LoCicero J III. Pseudoachalasia: a report of two cases with comments on possible causes and diagnosis. Dis Esophagus 1997;10:220–224.

13. Goldenberg SP, Burrell M, Fette GG, et al. Classic and vigorous achalasia: a comparison of manometric, radiographic, and clinical findings. Gastroenterology 1991;101:743–748.

14. Couturier D, Samama J. Clinical aspects and manometric criteria in achalasia. Hepatogastroenterology 1991;38:481–487.

15. Bortolotti M, Labo G. Clinical and manometric effects of nifedipine in patients with esophageal achalasia. Gastroenterology 1981;30:39–44.

16. Bortolotti M, Coccia G, Brunelli F, et al. Isosorbide dinitrate or nifedipine: which is preferable in the medical therapy of achalasia? Ital J Gastroenterol 1994;26:379–382.

17. Ferreira-Filho LP, Patto RJ, Troncon LE, et al. Use of isosorbide dinitrate for the symptomatic treatment of patients with Chagas' disease achalasia. A double-blind, crossover trial. Braz J Med Biol Res 1991;24:1093–1098.

18. Marzio L, Grossi L, DeLaurentiis MF, et al. Effect of cimetropium bromide on esophageal motility and transit in patients affected by primary achalasia. Dig Dis Sci 1994;39:1389–1394.

19. Nasrallah SM, Tommaso CL, Singleton RT, et al. Primary esophageal motor disorders: clinical response to nifedipine. South Med J 1985;78:312–315.

20. Penagini R, Bartesaghi B, Zannini P, et al. Lower oesophageal sphincter hypersensitivity to opioid receptor stimulation in patients with idiopathic achalasia. Gut 1993;34:16–20.

21. Penagini R, Bartesaghi B, Negri G, et al. Effect of loperamide on lower oesophageal sphincter pressure in idiopathic achalasia. Scand J Gastroenterol 1994;29:1057–1060.

22. Traube M, Dubovik S, Lange RC, et al. The role of nifedipine therapy in achalasia: results of a randomized, double-blind, placebo-controlled study. Am J Gastroenterol 1989;84:1259–1262.

23. Triadafilopoulos G, Aaronson M, Sackel S, et al. Medical treatment of esophageal achalasia. Double-blind crossover study with oral nifedipine, verapamil, and placebo. Dig Dis Sci 1991;36:260–267.

24. Nair LA, Reynolds JC, Parkman HP, et al. Complications during pneumatic dilation for achalasia or diffuse esophageal spasm. Analysis of risk factors, early clinical characteristics, and outcome. Dig Dis Sci 1993;38:1893–1904.

25. Parkman HP, Reynolds JC, Ouyang A, et al. Pneumatic dilatation or esophagomyotomy treatment for idiopathic achalasia: clinical outcomes and cost analysis. Dig Dis Sci 1993;38:75–85.

26. Kadakia SC, Wong RK. Graded pneumatic dilation using Rigiflex achalasia dilators in patients with primary esophageal achalasia. Am J Gastroenterol 1993;88:34–38.

27. Barnett JL, Eisenman R, Nostrant TT, et al. Witzel pneumatic dilation for achalasia: safety- and long-term efficacy. Gastrointest Endosc 1990;36:482–485.

28. Okike N, Payne WS, Neufeld DM, et al. Esophagomyotomy versus forceful dilation for achalasia of the esophagus: results in 899 patients. Ann Thorac Surg 1979;28:119–125.

29. Kim CH, Cameron AJ, Hsu JJ, et al. Achalasia: prospective evaluation of relationship between lower esophageal sphincter pressure, esophageal transit, and esophageal diameter and symptoms in response to pneumatic dilation. Mayo Clin Proc 1993;68:1067–1073.

30. Eckardt VF, Aignherr C, Bernhard G. Predictors of outcome in patients with achalasia treated by pneumatic dilation. Gastroenterology 1992;103:1732–1738.

31. Ancona E, Anselmino M, Zaninotto G, et al. Esophageal achalasia: laparoscopic versus conventional open Heller-Dor operation. Am J Surg 1995;170:265–270.

32. Patti MG, Bresadola V. Gastroesophageal reflux disease: basic considerations. Probl Gen Surg 1996;13:1–8.

33. Wetscher GJ, Redmond EJ, Vititi LMH. Pathophysiology of gastroesophageal reflux disease. In: Hinder RA, ed. Gastroesophageal Reflux Disease. Austin: Landes, 1993:7–29.

34. Ireland AC, Holloway RH, Toouli J, et al. Mechanisms underlying the antireflux action of fundoplication. Gut 1993;34:303–308.

35. Little AG. Mechanisms of action of antireflux surgery: theory and fact. World J Surg 1992;16:320–325.

36. Klingman RR, Stein HJ, DeMeester TR. The current management of gastroesophageal reflux. Adv Surg 1991;24:259–291.

37. Vaezi MF, Richter JE. Synergism of acid and duodenogastroesophageal reflux in complicated Barrett's esophagus. Surgery (St. Louis) 1995;117:699–704.

38. Hill LD. An effective operation for hiatal hernia: an eight year appraisal. Ann Surg 1967;166:681.

39. Lerut T, Coosemans W, Christiaens R, et al. The Belsey Mark IV antireflux procedure: indications and long-term results. Acta Gastroenterol Belg 1990;53:585–590.

40. Luostarinen M. Nissen fundoplication for reflux esophagitis. Long-term clinical and endoscopic results in 109 of 127 consecutive patients. Ann Surg 1993;217:329–337.

41. Shirazi SS, Schulze K, Soper RT. Long-term follow-up for treatment of complicated chronic reflux esophagitis. Arch Surg 1987;122:548–552.

42. Hunter JG, Trus TL, Branum DG, et al. A physiologic approach to laparoscopic fundoplication for gastroesophageal reflux disease. Ann Surg 1996;223:673–687.

43. Waring JP, Hunter JG, Oddsdottir M, et al. The preoperative evaluation of patients considered for laparoscopic antireflux surgery. Am J Gastroenterol 1995;90:35–38.

44. Smith CD, Fink AS, Applegren K. Guidelines for surgical treatment of gastroesophageal reflux disease (GERD). Society of American Gastrointestinal Endoscopic Surgeons (SAGES). Surg Endosc 1998;12:186–188.

45. Anvari M, Allen C, Borm A. Laparoscopic Nissen fundoplication is a satisfactory alternative to long-term omeprazole therapy. Br J Surg 1995;82:938–942.

46. Champault G. Gastroesophageal reflux. Treatment by laparoscopy: 940 cases—French experience. Ann Chir 1994;48:159–164.

47. Hinder RA, Filipi CJ, Wetscher G, et al. Laparoscopic Nissen fundoplication is an effective treatment for gastroesophageal reflux disease. Ann Surg 1994;220:472–481; discussion 481–483.

48. Anvari M, Allen C. Laparoscopic Nissen fundoplication: two-year comprehensive follow-up of a technique of minimal paraesophageal dissection. Ann Surg 1998;227:25–32.

49. Bloomston M, Zervos E, Gonzalez R, et al. Quality of life and antireflux medication use following laparoscopic Nissen fundoplication. Am Surg 1998;64:509–513; discussion 513–514.

50. McKernan JB, Champion JK. Minimally invasive antireflux surgery. Am J Surg 1998;175:271–276.

51. Peters JH. The surgical management of Barrett's esophagus. Gastroenterol Clin North Am 1997;26:647–668.

52. Edwards MJ, Gable DR, Lentsch AB, et al. The rationale for esophagectomy as the optimal therapy for Barrett's esophagus with high-grade dysplasia. Ann Surg 1996;223:585–589; discussion 589–591.

53. Heitmiller RF, Redmond M, Hamilton SR. Barrett's esophagus with high-grade dysplasia. An indication for prophylactic esophagectomy. Ann Surg 1996;224:66–71.

54. Sampliner RE. Practice guidelines on the diagnosis, surveillance, and therapy of Barrett's esophagus. The Practice Parameters Committee of the American College of Gastroenterology. Am J Gastroenterol 1998;93:1028–1032.

55. Spechler SJ. Esophageal columnar metaplasia (Barrett's esophagus). Gastrointest Endosc Clin North Am 1997;7:1–18.

56. McDonald ML, Trastek VF, Allen MS, et al. Barretts's esophagus: does an antireflux procedure reduce the need for endoscopic surveillance? J Thorac Cardiovasc Surg 1996;111:1135–1138; discussion 1139–1140.

57. DeMeester TR, Attwood SE, Smyrk TC, et al. Surgical therapy in Barrett's esophagus. Ann Surg 1990;212:528–540; discussion 540–542.

58. Csendes A, Braghetto I, Burdiles P, et al. A new physiologic approach for the surgical treatment of patients with Barrett's esophagus: technical considerations and results in 65 patients. Ann Surg 1997;226:123–133.

59. Wetscher GJ, Profanter C, Gadenstatter M, et al. Medical treatment of gastroesophageal reflux disease does not prevent the development of Barrett's metaplasia and poor esophageal body motility. Langenbecks Arch Chir 1997;382:95–99.

60. Sampliner RE. Ablation of Barrett's mucosa. Gastroenterologist 1997;5:185–188.

61. Sampliner RE. New treatments for Barrett's esophagus. Semin Gastrointest Dis 1997;8:68–74.

62. Skinner DB, Belsey RHR. Surgical management of esophageal reflux and hiatus hernia: long-term results with 1030 patients. J Thorac Cardiovasc Surg 1967;53:33.

63. Gore RM. Esophageal cancer: clinical and pathologic features. Radiol Clin North Am 1997;35:243–263.

64. Buecker A, Wein BB, Neuerburg JM, et al. Esophageal perforation: comparison of use of aqueous and barium-containing contrast media. Radiology 1997;202:683–686.

65. Enns R, Branch MS. Management of esophageal perforation after therapeutic upper gastrointestinal endoscopy. Gastrointest Endosc 1998;47:318–320.

66. Wetstein L, Duerr A, Wagner RB. Esophageal perforation. Ann Thorac Surg 1998;65:875–876.

67. Bufkin BL, Miller JI Jr, Mansour KA. Esophageal perforation: emphasis on management. Ann Thorac Surg 1996;61:1447–1451; discussion 1451–1452.

68. Reeder LB, DeFilippi VJ, Ferguson MK. Current results of therapy for esophageal perforation. Am J Surg 1995;169:615–617.

69. Whyte RI, Iannettoni MD, Orringer MB. Intrathoracic esophageal perforation. The merit of primary repair. J Thorac Cardiovasc Surg 1995;109:140–144; discussion 144–146.

70. Altorjay A, Kiss J, Voros A, et al. Nonoperative management of esophageal perforations. Is it justified? Ann Surg 1997;225:415–421.

71. Zargar SA, Kochhar R, Nagi B, et al. Ingestion of strong corrosive alkalis: spectrum of injury to upper gastrointestinal tract and natural history. Am J Gastroenterol 1992;87:337–341.

72. Zargar SA, Kochhar R, Mehta S, et al. The role of fiberoptic endoscopy in the management of corrosive ingestion and modified endoscopic classification of burns. Gastrointest Endosc 1991;37:165–169.

73. Andreoni B, Farina ML, Biffi R, et al. Esophageal perforation and caustic injury: emergency management of caustic ingestion. Dis Esophagus 1997;10:95–100.

74. Altorjay A, Kiss J, Voros A, et al. The role of esophagectomy in the management of esophageal perforations. Ann Thorac Surg 1998;65:1433–1436.

75. Berthet B, Castellani P, Brioche MI, et al. Early operation for severe corrosive injury of the upper gastrointestinal tract. Eur J Surg 1996;162:951–955.

76. Pate JW, Walker WA, Cole FH Jr, et al. Spontaneous rupture of the esophagus: a 30-year experience. Ann Thorac Surg 1989;47:689–692.

77. Bharucha AE, Gostout CJ, Balm RK. Clinical and endoscopic risk factors in the Mallory-Weiss syndrome. Am J Gastroenterol 1997;92:805–808.

78. Felix VN, Cecconello I, Zilberstein B, et al. Achalasia: a prospective study comparing the results of dilatation and myotomy. Hepatogastroenterology 1998;45:97–108.

79. Csendes A, Braghetto I, Henriquez A, et al. Late results of a prospective randomised study comparing forceful dilatation and oesophagomyotomy in patients with achalasia. Gut 1989;30:299–304.

80. Moreno-Gonzalez E, Garcia Alvarez A, Landa Garcia I, et al. Results of surgical treatment of esophageal achalasia. Multicenter retrospective study of 1,856 cases. GEEMO (Groupe Europeen Etude Maladies Oesophageennes) Multicentric Retrospective Study. Int Surg 1988;73:69–77.

81. Attwood SE, Barlow AP, Norris TL, et al. Barrett's oesophagus: effect of antireflux surgery on symptom control and development of complications. Br J Surg 1992;79:1050–1053.

82. Ortiz A, Martinez de Haro LF, Parrilla P, et al. Conservative treatment versus antireflux surgery in Barrett's oesophagus: long-term results of a prospective study. Br J Surg 1996;83:274–278.

83. Sampliner RE. Effect of up to 3 years of high-dose lansoprazole on Barrett's esophagus. Am J Gastroenterol 1994;89:1844–1848.

84. Csendes A, Braghetto I, Burdiles P, et al. Long-term results of classic antireflux surgery in 152 patients with Barrett's esophagus: clinical, radiologic, endoscopic, manometric, and acid reflux test analysis before and late after operation. Surgery (St. Louis) 1998;126:645–657.

85. Launois P, Lygidakis C, Malledant G. Results of the surgical treatment of carcinoma of the esophagus. Surg Gynecol Obstet 1983;156:753–760.

86. Hankins JR, Colen EN, Ward A. Carcinoma of the esophagus: the philosophy for palliation. Ann Thorac Surg 1972;14:189–197.

87. Carey JS, Plestad WG, Hughes RK. Esophagogastrectomy. Ann Thorac Surg 1972;14:59–68.

88. Roth JA, Putnam JBJ. Surgery for cancer of the esophagus. Semin Surg Oncol 1994;21:453–461.

89. Katlic MR, Wilkins EW, Grillo HC. Three decades of treatment of esophageal squamous carcinoma at the Massachusetts General Hospital. J Thorac Cardiovasc Surg 1990;99:929–938.

90. Putnam JBJ, Suell DA, Natarajan G. A comparison of three techniques of esophagectomy for carcinoma of the esophagus from one institution with a residency training program. Ann Thorac Surg 1994;57:319–325.

91. Orringer MB. Transhiatal esophagectomy without thoracotomy for carcinoma of the thoracic esophagus. Ann Surg 1984;200:282–288.

92. Yonezawa T, Tsuchiya S, Ogoshi S. Resection of cancer of the thoracic esophagus without thoracotomy. J Thorac Cardiovasc Surg 1984;88:146–149.

17

Stomach and Duodenum

Edward H. Livingston

Anatomy

Gross Anatomy

The stomach lies in the left upper quadrant crossing the midline at the pylorus. Proximally it is attached to the esophagus and distally to the duodenum. The most proximal portion of the stomach is the gastric cardia, which is a small area just distal to the gastroesophageal junction. Mucus gland cells populate this area. The largest portion of the stomach is the corpus. It lies between the cardia and antrum, and in addition to mucous cells contains parietal and chief cells. The parietal cells secrete acid and the chief cells make pepsin. The surgical boundary between the corpus and antrum is the line between the incisura along the lesser curve and the point where the gastroepiploic artery enters the stomach along the greater curve. The pylorus has strong muscles that contract powerfully to pump food into the duodenum. Pyloric G-cells secrete gastrin, a hormone of great importance for the regulation of gastric acid secretion.

Blood Supply

The left gastric artery is a branch of the celiac axis and is the largest artery supplying the stomach (Fig. 17.1). It courses along the lesser curve of the stomach and is continuous with the right gastric artery, a branch of the common hepatic artery. The gastroduodenal artery gives off the right gastroepiploic artery, which courses along the greater curvature of the stomach. The left gastroepiploic artery branches from the splenic artery supplying the greater curvature of the fundus. An anatomical misconception is that these two gastroepiploic arteries are contiguous. They are not, and the point where the right gastroepiploic artery enters the greater curvature marks the border between the fundus and antrum in that location. The superior aspect of the duodenum is supplied by the superior pancreaticoduodenal artery, a branch of the gastroduodenal artery. The inferior duodenum is supplied by the inferior pancreaticoduodenal artery, a branch of the superior mesenteric artery. Both the stomach and duodenum have extensive submucosal channels that ensure a rich blood supply to the mucosa. This rich vascular submucosal plexus ensures an adequate blood supply for the stomach even if only one of the four major vessels is intact. Additionally, the gastroduodenal artery receives blood from the superior mesenteric artery such that the gastric vasculature receives blood from two of the major aortic branches. The venous drainage of the stomach is via the coronary, gastroepiploic, and splenic veins that drain into the portal vein. Lymph channels draining the stomach parallel the arterial supply, having major nodal collections at the celiac axis and superior mesenteric artery.

Nerve Supply

Knowledge of vagal anatomy is crucially important in gastric surgery. There are two major vagal trunks that innervate the stomach (see Fig. 17.1). The largest is the anterior vagus, which is closely adherent to the intraabdominal esophagus slightly left of the midline. This is a very large nerve, easily identified during surgery. The posterior vagus resides slightly behind and to the right of the intraabdominal esophagus. It is much smaller than the anterior nerve. Placing one's finger behind the esophagus and feeling the thin cord of tissue behind the esophagus identifies the nerve.

The anterior nerve is frequently referred to as the left nerve and the posterior the right. During embryogenesis, the stomach rotates 90° to the right such that the left branch becomes anterior and the right posterior. However, functionally the anterior and posterior branches have fibers deriving from both the true left and right nerves.

The nerve of Grassi is a branch of the posterior vagus that innervates the fundus. Failure to divide this branch may result in ulcer recurrence following vagotomy. The crow's foot

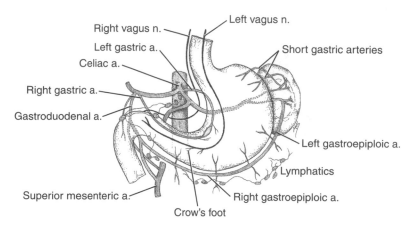

FIGURE 17.1. Neurovascular supply of the stomach. The stomach is richly vascularized by a highly redundant blood supply. Based on the celiac axis, the left and right gastric arteries supply the lesser curvature. The gastroepiploics supply the greater curvature. The gastroduodenal artery passes immediately behind the duodenum and may result in formidable bleeding should a duodenal ulcer perforate it. The lymphatics follow the arterial blood supply. The left (anterior) and right (posterior) vagi are depicted.

is a tangle of nerves that branch from the main trunks at the incisura which marks the border between the fundus and antrum. The crow's foot innervates the antrum and must be spared when performing a highly selective vagotomy.

Sympathetic nerves emanate from the celiac ganglion and follow the course of the arteries into the stomach. Although important physiologically, they have little importance to surgery of the stomach.

Physiology

Acid Secretion

Acid secretion occurs in the gastric corpus and fundus by the parietal cells.[1] These cells can secrete acid against a very large concentration gradient by virtue of the ATP-expending proton pump. The maximal luminal acid concentration is 0.15 N. Thus, the pump is capable of concentrating acid more than 10 million times the concentration of hydrogen in blood. Acid of this strength is highly corrosive and would disintegrate any tissue in the body if it came into contact with it. However, gastric epithelium has characteristic tight intercellular junctions that not only facilitate protective function but also enable the concentration gradient to exist, in contradistinction to the duodenum and small bowel, which are permeable and easily absorb luminal substances. Additional protection of the gastric surface is provided by luminal bicarbonate secretion across the gastric epithelial layer. For each acid molecule generated by H-K-ATPase, a molecule of bicarbonate ion is created.

A thick, alkaline mucous gel lies immediately adjacent to the gastric epithelium. This layer assists in protecting the gastric epithelium against injury. Acid is secreted through pits that transiently perforate the mucous layer, facilitating movement of acid away from the gastric surface without acidifying the mucous gel layer.[2] Because the stomach is constantly exposed to very high concentrations of acid, gastric ulceration is unrelated to acid production. Loss of gastric epithelial protective mechanisms are primarily responsible for gastric ulceration.

There are numerous signals for gastric acid secretion. The vagus nerve is critically important. Vagal activation potently stimulates acid secretion by several mechanisms. The vagus enters the gastric wall closely approximating arterial perfo-

rators and has end terminals in the myenteric plexus. Vagal fibers activate myenteric plexus interneurons that in turn release acetylcholine in the immediate vicinity of parietal cells. Cholinergic stimulation results in increased parietal cell intracellular calcium, which leads to acid secretion (Fig. 17.2). The vagus also stimulates antral interneurons to release gastrin-releasing peptide (GRP or bombesin); GRP stimulates antral G-cell release of gastrin into the bloodstream. This hormone circulates until it reaches the parietal cells, stimulating them to secrete acid. Both vagal simulation and gastrin cause gastric mucosal mast cells to release histamine immediately adjacent to the parietal cells. Histamine is a very potent stimulus for acid secretion. Gastrin is also released when the antral surface pH falls below 3.0. From a surgical standpoint, division of the vagus is highly effective in reducing acid secretion because it simultaneously reduces all three acid secretory stimulatory systems. However, gastrin can still be secreted in the absence of vagus activity, which is why both vagotomy and antrectomy, that removes the antral G-cell mass, are needed to ensure that acid secretion is eliminated when operating for peptic ulcer disease.

Gastric parietal cells have receptors to acetylcholine, gastrin, and histamine. Histamine is probably the most important receptor because its inhibition results in marked reduction in acid secretion. However, the other receptors play a role because acid secretion cannot be totally suppressed by histamine inhibition. Proton pump inhibitors completely block acid secretion, making them very potent medications for the treatment of peptic disorders. Prostaglandins inhibit acid secretion by reducing adenylate cyclase activity (Fig. 17.2).

Motility

Contractile activity of the GI tract initiates in the stomach. The gastric pacemaker is located along the greater curve in the upper third of the stomach. This pacemaker cycles at 3 cycles per minute. Not all pacemaker activity is translated to muscular contractions. The migrating motor complexes are complexes of muscular contractions that are highly coordinated and sweep down the GI tract during fasting. These powerful contractions serve as the "housekeeper" of the gut, clearing the luminal contents between feedings. Contractions associated with feeding are less powerful but more numerous, and the period of contractile activity is prolonged.

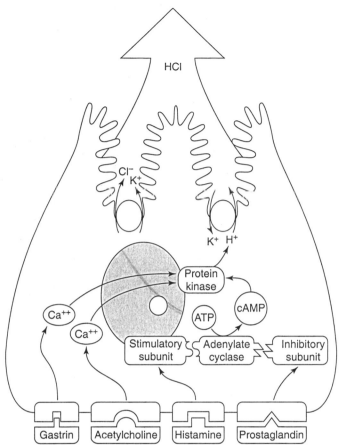

FIGURE 17.2. Parietal cell molecular signals regulating acid secretion. Both acetylcholine and gastrin bind to receptors on the basal surface of the parietal cell, raising intracellular calcium levels. The higher calcium stimulates protein kinase, which in turn activates the proton pump. Histamine binds its receptor, resulting in increased adenylate cyclase activity. The higher cAMP levels stimulate protein kinase, which causes increased proton pump activity. Prostaglandins act to inhibit acid secretion by adenylate cyclase inhibition.

As is the case with acid secretion, the vagus nerve plays a crucial role in regulating gut contractile activity. As food enters the stomach, the fundus gradually stretches. This "receptive relaxation" is mediated by the vagus. Vagotomy abolishes this mechanism, contributing to the dumping syndrome (see below).

The antrum is a powerful pump that drives the gastric contents against the pylorus, serving to pump out small amounts of gastric material into the duodenum. Particles greater than 1 mm in size reflect back into the pylorus until they are mashed into a smaller size by the antral contractions. The vagus mediates this activity.

Peptic Ulcer

Duodenal Ulcer

Duodenal ulceration principally results from increased acid load in the duodenum. Consequently, the mainstay therapy is acid reduction. Antacids provide transient symptomatic relief but fail to definitively treat ulcers. A major therapeutic ad-

vance for duodenal ulcer treatment was the advent of histamine-II (H_2) receptor antagonists. As discussed for acid secretion, histamine receptor antagonism at the parietal cell results in profoundly reduced acid secretion. Mast cell histamine release in response to both vagal simulation and gastrin potentiates histamine effect on acid secretion. Consequently, histamine blockade substantially reduces acid secretion. Thus, H_2-blockers have been highly effective in controlling the symptoms of duodenal ulcer and accelerating ulcer healing.[3,4]

Proton pump inhibitors (PPI) are more effective than H_2-blockers in treating duodenal ulcers and accelerating healing.[5] Because there are multiple signals that can initiate parietal cell acid secretion, H_2-blockers cannot completely eliminate acid secretion. PPIs act to block the proton pump and, therefore, can totally stop acid secretion. The greater degree of acid secretion inhibition results in highly effective pain control, improved ulcer healing, and lower recurrence rates than for ulcers treated with H_2-blockers.

Ulcer operations are now uncommon and are limited primarily to the treatment of life-threatening complications such as bleeding, perforation, and obstruction.

Prepyloric and pyloric channel ulcers resemble duodenal ulceration, all resulting from excessive acid secretion. Although technically located in the stomach, these lesions are treated identically to duodenal ulcers.

Perforation

Deep, penetrating ulcers on the anterior duodenal surface may perforate into the abdominal cavity. Lesions on the posterior surface penetrate into the pancreas and present as bleeding lesions rather than free perforations. During the past decade, a slightly increased peptic ulcer incidence has been attributed to widespread use of nonsteroidal antiinflammatory drugs (NSAIDs). These agents damage the gastroduodenal barrier by a variety of mechanisms. NSAID use invariably results in peptic ulcers.

Gastroduodenal ulcer perforations have two major presentations. Young patients present with acute onset of severe, intolerable abdominal pain. Generally, patients can precisely identify the exact time the pain began because of the sudden onset and its severe intensity. The pain is unremitting and exacerbated by any movement. Nausea and vomiting may be present. Abdominal wall rigidity with diffuse tenderness can be expected. Posterior perforations present with substantial bleeding and not very much pain. Posterior perforations induce pancreatitis, manifested by acute abdominal pain. Elevated amylase occurs with both anterior and posterior perforations and, therefore, is not reliable for the differentiation between these two. Free air is common with anterior perforations, but may be absent in as many as 20% of cases. Thus, the absence of free air does not reliably exclude a duodenal perforation. When the suspicion is high for duodenal perforation, the best approach is immediate exploration.

Chronically ill, elderly patients have a more subtle presentation. Abdominal pain is vague and poorly localized. The pain may develop over the course of days to weeks. Patients typically present with fever and leukocytosis, the etiology of which is very difficult to discern. Free air in the peritoneum is unusual, and CT scanning of the abdomen often makes the diagnosis.

TREATMENT

Because of the extensive peritonitis, patients require vigorous resuscitation. A vertical midline incision is made. Typically one finds a pinpoint hole on the anterior surface of the duodenum, pylorus, or distal antrum. Extensive inflammation of the duodenal or gastric wall adjacent to the perforation makes simple closure unreliable. For this reason the omentum is sutured over the closure to reinforce it, a procedure known as the Graham patch. Patients who have had a prior ulcer history should have a definitive antiulcer operation such as a highly selective vagotomy or truncal vagotomy and pyloroplasty, provided that there is little peritonitis. If extensive peritonitis is found, only the patch procedure may be performed. Patients without an ulcer history can undergo the patch procedure alone. However, longitudinal studies have demonstrated that recurrence rates following patch alone might be very high even in patients without prior history. Thus, because of its low morbidity, highly selective vagotomy can be advocated for all patients who present with perforation and do not have extensive peritonitis.

Gastric Ulcer

Gastric ulcers differ from duodenal lesions in that they result more from a defect in mucosal defense rather than acid hypersecretion. Acid worsens gastric ulcers but is not required for their development because ulcers occur in achlorhydric patients. Consequently, acid-blocking agents are less effective for the treatment of gastric than duodenal ulcers. Gastric ulcers develop along the lesser curve (type I ulcers) or high on the lesser curve below the gastroesophageal junction (type IV ulcers). Exceptions to this general concept are the midbody gastric ulcers (type II) that coexist with duodenal lesions and prepyloric channel ulcers (type III). In contrast to type I and IV lesions, type II and III ulcers result from acid-induced epithelial injury and are treated similarly to duodenal ulcers.

Malignant gastric ulcerations are indistinguishable from benign ones. For this reason, all gastric ulcers must be biopsied. Following biopsy, if the lesion is confirmed to be benign, gastric ulcers should be treated with a course of mucosal protective agents such as sucralfate. Although hyperacidity is usually not the cause of gastric ulcers, a trial of proton pump inhibitors should be given before consideration of aggressive resectional therapy. The first line of therapy is removal of ulcerogenic conditions such as use of NSAIDs, corticosteroids, and tobacco. Giant gastric ulcers are those greater than 5 cm in diameter. These rarely respond to conservative treatment and present a high risk for complications of perforations or bleeding. In general, these should be resected but if treated nonoperatively the patient must be closely monitored.

Surgical treatment for gastric ulcers involves wedge resection of the lesion. This treatment is the same irrespective of the indications, that is, whether the operation is performed for a nonhealing lesion, perforation, or bleeding. For perforations, resection is preferred but if this is not technically possible or the risk is too high, the perforation can be patched[6] but must be biopsied because of the risk of gastric carcinoma.

Helicobacter pylori

H. pylori is a microaerophilic gram-negative rod well adapted for growth in the gastric acidic environment. Infection occurs by the fecal–oral route such that contaminated water is a major source for the organism. The organism swims freely in the gastric mucus, secreting urease that catalyzes ammonia synthesis. The ammonia protects the bacteria from acid-induced injury but also is damaging to the gastric epithelium, resulting in gastritis.

Acute *H. pylori* infection is manifested by nausea, vomiting, abdominal pain, and fever lasting 3 to 14 days. Several weeks following the initial infection, gastritis results in achlorhydria that may persist for several months.[7,8] Chronic infection is often asymptomatic. Gastric and duodenal ulcer disease have been attributed to *H. pylori* because 95% of patients with duodenal and 50% to 80% with gastric ulcers have this organism. Eradication is associated with fewer relapses,[9] but recurrences continue to occur despite eradication of the organism.[10] Nonulcer dyspepsia is not related to *H. pylori*, and eradication under these circumstances resulted in delayed healing of gastric ulcers.[11]

NSAID-Induced Ulcerations

The widespread use of NSAIDs has resulted in an increase in the incidence of ulcer disease. Bleeding and perforation are more common now than a decade ago. Gastric epithelium contains cyclooxygenase-1 (COX-1), an enzyme essential for prostaglandin synthesis. Prostaglandins preserve gastric mucosal blood flow,[12] and increase mucus production[13] and bicarbonate secretion.[14] Each of these is essential for maintaining gastric epithelial protective systems. NSAIDs act by inhibiting COX. NSAID ulcerations do improve with antacid therapy such that patients requiring long-term NSAID use should receive concurrent H_2-blockers or PPIs.

Operations for Peptic Ulcer Disease

Exposure

Exposure for the stomach is best achieved through an upper midline incision. The Bookwalter retractor provides excellent exposure for the left upper quadrant. Placement of the patient in steep reverse Trendelenburg position assists in retracting the small bowel away from the field.

Placement of a nasogastric tube facilitates identification of the esophagus, although recent meta-analyses of all published trials revealed that nasogastric tubes were not necessary and caused significant complications.

Parietal Cell Vagotomy

The parietal cell vagotomy, also known as the highly selective vagotomy, was devised to minimize the side effects of acid reduction operations. The operation "selects" the nerves to the parietal cell mass of the gastric fundus and body. Innervation to the antrum, pylorus, and remaining gastrointestinal tract is spared. The operation is performed by devascularizing the gastric lesser curve. The distal 5 cm of esophagus should be mobilized and also devascularized to ensure that small vagal branches traveling along the esophagus are divided as is the "criminal nerve of Grassi." It is important not to divide branches of the crow's foot that supply the antrum and pylorus to ensure that gastric emptying is preserved following this operation.

Obstructing ulcers should not be treated by parietal cell vagotomy. Because operative relief of obstruction is required, patients with obstruction should undergo vagotomy and antrectomy. The most common indication for parietal cell vagotomy is peptic ulcer perforation, although it may be used in stable, bleeding patients or in those with intractable ulcer disease. This operation does not have the side effects of diarrhea or dumping associated with truncal vagotomy procedures. Gastric emptying is not affected by parietal cell vagotomy.[15]

Vagotomy and Pyloroplasty

For many years, this operation was considered a second choice after vagotomy and antrectomy because of a 10% to 15% recurrence rate. Improved management of recurrences make this less of a problem so that vagotomy and pyloroplasty is probably the best procedure to perform in emergency circumstances.

Dividing the main vagus branch anterior to the esophagus is the first step when performing a truncal vagotomy. The cut nerve ends are ligated. The posterior nerve is more difficult to find lying posterior, to the right and somewhat removed from the esophageal surface. That nerve is divided in the same manner as with the anterior nerve. Failure to completely divide the posterior vagus probably is the main reason truncal vagotomy without antrectomy results in a high ulcer recurrence rate.

If not already made, a full-thickness incision is made in the pylorus, extending 2 cm into the antrum and 1 cm into the duodenum. The incision is closed by approximating the proximal and distal ends of the incision together in what is now the middle of the closure. Dumping syndrome and diarrhea are the main long-term complications of vagotomy and pyloroplasty.

Vagotomy and Antrectomy

Vagotomy and antrectomy eliminate two of the three major stimuli for acid secretion. Acetylcholine from the vagus nerve and gastrin from the antrum are eliminated, making this a very effective procedure for the treatment of peptic ulceration of the prepyloric region and duodenum. When pyloric ulcers or obstructing lesions are present, vagotomy and antrectomy is the operation of choice. This operation has the most consistent results, with recurrence rates invariably being less than 2%. However, it has the highest complication rate and the most significant long-term side effects.

Truncal vagotomy as just described in "Vagotomy and Pyloroplasty" is performed. The antrum is divided along a line connecting the incisura to the point along the greater curvature where the gastroepiploic artery enters the stomach (Fig. 17.3A). The duodenum is resected approximately 1 cm distal to the pylorus. Because scarring may have distorted the anatomy, a frozen section of the distal margin of the resected specimen is useful to ensure that the antrum has been completely resected.

There are two major reconstructive options following antrectomy. The Billroth I involves anastomosing the duodenum to the gastric remnant (Fig. 17.3B). This method has the major advantage of avoiding the presence of a duodenal stump or the afferent limb of a gastrojejunostomy. The operation has greater long-term morbidity than the Billroth II from alkaline reflux. The Billroth II is performed by closing the duodenum as a stump and anastomosing a loop of jejunum to the gastric remnant (Fig. 17.3C). The duodenal stump is at risk for perforation with subsequent duodenal stump leak, a complication associated with 50% mortality. The risk of this complication is minimized by providing adequate decompression of the duodenum by placing a nasogastric tube into the duodenum through the gastrojejunostomy.[16]

Laparoscopic Vagotomy

Laparoscopic vagotomy techniques have received increasing acceptance. The reduced morbidity associated with large incisions is advantageous. A modification of the highly selective vagotomy is performed.

Complications of Ulcer Operations

JAUNDICE

This complication can be a vexing problem in the postoperative phase. Most patients undergoing emergent gastric surgery for bleeding have had multiple blood transfusions as well as periods of shock. Thus, jaundice may be from transfusion reaction or hepatic dysfunction. The most worrisome and difficult problem to evaluate is bile duct injury occurring following suture ligation of a posterior duodenal lesion or following antrectomy.

Differentiating the bilirubin into conjugated and unconjugated fractions is usually not helpful. Other tests such as the Coomb's test and red cell smear for hemolytic reactions or ultrasound for bile duct obstruction will establish the diagnosis.

If bile duct injury is suspected and the patient has had a Billroth I reconstruction, ERCP should be performed. Generally this can be done 1 week following surgery. For patients with Billroth II reconstruction, the evaluation is more difficult. An ultrasound should be performed looking for bile duct dilation. However, this may take a week to occur. When the bile duct in dilated, transhepatic cholangiography should be performed with the catheter left in place. If drainage is achieved from above, then bile duct reconstructive surgery may be delayed several months until inflammation of the upper quadrants and bowel have subsided such that a reconstruction is technically feasible. If bile duct injury is suspected during the ulcer operation, a cholangiogram should be obtained during the operation through the cystic duct following cholecystectomy or through a needle inserted into the bile duct. Failure of the contrast to enter the duodenum confirms bile duct injury such that the bile duct can be reconstructed during the initial operation.

REBLEEDING

Ongoing bleeding immediately following surgery generally occurs because an ulcer was oversewn without addition of an antiulcer operation. Prospective trials of differing ulcer operations have demonstrated that gastric resection was superior to vagotomy and oversew of the ulcer in preventing rebleeding.[17] When bleeding occurs following vagotomy and pyloroplasty, the patient should be returned to the operating room for conversion to a vagotomy and antrectomy.

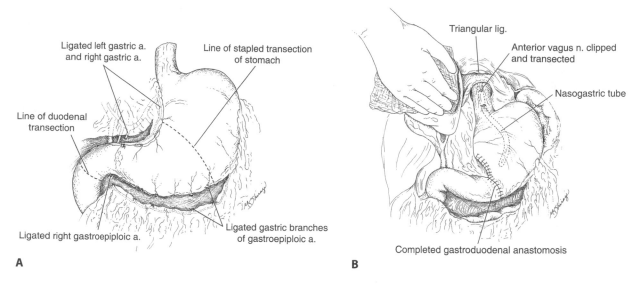

A

Ligated left gastric a.
and right gastric a.

Line of stapled transection
of stomach

Line of duodenal
transection

Ligated right gastroepiploic a.

Ligated gastric branches
of gastroepiploic a.

B

Triangular lig.

Anterior vagus n. clipped
and transected

Nasogastric tube

Completed gastroduodenal anastomosis

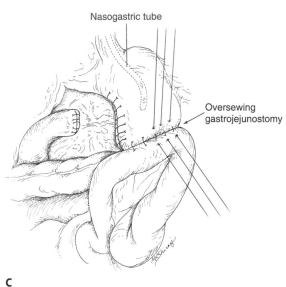

Nasogastric tube

Oversewing
gastrojejunostomy

C

FIGURE 17.3. Vagotomy and antrectomy. **A.** The vagal
trunks are identified and divided. The stomach is resected
along a line from just above the incisura to the point along
the greater curvature where the gastroepiploic vessels disappear or are at their closest approximation to the gastric wall.
The duodenum is divided approximately 2 cm distal to the
pylorus. **B.** The Billroth I reconstruction entails creation of a
gastroduodenostomy. **C.** The Billroth II reconstruction is accomplished by closing the duodenal stump and the gastric
remnant. The stomach is anastomosed to a loop of jejunum.

DELAYED GASTRIC EMPTYING

Gastroparesis following gastric surgery is common. Patients
should be treated with nasogastric suction if they are vomiting or experiencing severe nausea, but the tube should be removed as soon as possible and bowel rest continued until nausea resolves. Total parental nutrition should be initiated as
soon as possible. When food is resumed it should be in the
form of liquids that contain minimal sugar; sugar will elicit
the dumping syndrome, which can be especially severe during the immediate postoperative period. The patient should
remain on liquids for 2 to 3 weeks following initiation of the
diet because gastric emptying for solids is severely compromised following vagotomy. Once begun, solids should be only
slowly introduced.

Gastroparesis may be an early sign of an anastomotic leak
or intraabdominal abscess. A variety of electrolyte disorders
may result in gastroparesis such that electrolytes, calcium,
and magnesium levels should be checked and corrected if abnormal. If gastrograffin studies suggest anastomotic stricture,
nasogastric decompression should be continued for a week

following the initial surgery. If the nasogastric output remains
high, suggestive of continued obstruction, endoscopy should
be performed with the intent to dilate the anastomosis. Prokinetic agents are often tried, but clinical outcomes from
these agents are discouraging.

ANASTOMOTIC LEAKS AND ABSCESSES

Gastrograffin upper GI studies are helpful for identifying anastomotic leaks or strictures. Computed tomography scans may
diagnose abscesses, which generally will not be visualized on
CT scans until at least a week after surgery. Once an abscess
or fluid collection associated with a leaking anastomosis is
identified, percutaneous drainage should be performed. Failure to improve clinically after percutaneous drainage mandates laparotomy with placement of large sump drains into
areas of fluid collections.

DUODENAL STUMP DISRUPTION

This complication occurs following Billroth II reconstruction
of an antrectomy. Oftentimes the duodenum is scarred, mak-

ing secure closure difficult. Additionally, obstruction of the afferent jejunal limb may blow out the stump. This complication may be prevented by duodenal decompression with a nasogastric tube placed through the gastrojejunostomy.[16] When the duodenal stump closure is questionable, placement of a left upper quadrant drain is indicated. Presentation, workup, and management are similar to that for anastamotic leak. Tube duodenostomy for fistula control may sometimes be necessary.

RECURRENT ULCERATION

Ulcer recurrence is not common but may occur. When recurrence occurs, treatment with H$_2$-blockers or proton pump inhibitors is often adequate. If medical therapy fails, then conversion to vagotomy and antrectomy is indicated.

Recurrent ulcers caused by excessive acid secretion may be due to excessive gastrin; this may result from retained antrum in the duodenal closure or from a gastrinoma. Elevated gastrin levels suggest these diagnoses.

DUMPING SYNDROME

Dumping syndrome is manifested by abdominal pain, vertigo, hypotension, and tachycardia. The syndrome occurs in any patient who has had a pyloroplasty or gastrojejunostomy. Rapid entry of food into the small bowel is clearly related to the underlying dumping syndrome pathogenesis, but underlying mechanism for this syndrome remains unknown.

Patients are very sensitive to carbohydrate ingestion following creation of any gastrojejunostomy. The most useful intervention is intense dietary counseling. Only rarely will dumping remain problematic for patients if they comply with dietary advice. Surgical interventions for dumping have had discouraging results.

ALKALINE REFLUX/POSTVAGOTOMY GASTROPARESIS

The presentation of these two entities differs only by the presence of gastritis on biopsy present in alkaline reflux gastritis and delayed emptying seen with radionuclide scanning in postvagotomy gastroparesis. Because revisional gastric surgery is technically difficult and incurs significant morbidity, it is generally best to resect the gastric remnant and create a Roux-en-Y gastrojejunostomy in patients with either of these syndromes.

POSTVAGOTOMY DIARRHEA

Watery diarrhea occurring approximately 30 min following eating may occur following vagotomy. The cause for this is unknown, and fortunately this is a self-limiting problem for most patients that resolves spontaneously. For patients with persistent symptoms, conventional antidiarrheal agents should be administered. This problem should be treated symptomatically and the various operations described for its treatment should be avoided.

PERNICIOUS ANEMIA

This disorder occurs following gastric resection. Intrinsic factor secreted by the parietal cells is required for vitamin B$_{12}$ absorption. Intrinsic factor binds vitamin B$_{12}$ so that the complex may be absorbed in the ileum. Very little unbound B$_{12}$

is absorbed. Vitamin B$_{12}$ injection should be given periodically to these patients. Patients also require iron supplementation following ulcer surgery to avoid anemia.

Upper Gastrointestinal Tract Hemorrhage

Peptic Ulcer Bleeding

Bleeding from peptic ulcer disease occurs frequently and is generally a self-limited process. Advances in endoscopic therapy have made surgery for this problem uncommon. Patients usually present with melena or, if the bleeding is severe enough, hematemesis will be present.

Patients who have evidence for massive blood loss should be immediately resuscitated. The airway is assessed to ensure there is no obstruction, and oxygen administration is required for all patients. Obtunded patients, those who cannot protect their airway, or those with massive emesis that presents an aspiration risk should be endotracheally intubated. Large-bore intravenous access with 18 gauge or larger catheters should be placed. A nasogastric tube should be placed. The nasogastric tube should be lavaged until clear. Foley catheter placement and administration of large volumes of intravenous fluids are essential. Normal saline or Ringer's lactate are the fluids of choice. Patients presenting with massive hemorrhage are given O negative or type-specific blood until cross-matched blood is available.[18] The mortality for upper gastrointestinal hemorrhage is approximately 10%.

Endoscopy is essential for managing patients with upper gastrointestinal tract hemorrhage. Only 10% to 20% of patients presenting with upper GI bleeding have peptic ulcers as the cause for the bleed. Other sources for GI bleeding include varices, esophagitis, Dieulafoy's lesions, Mallory–Weiss tears, and gastritis. Most of these are nonsurgical entities and are diagnosed by endoscopy.

The National Institutes of Health convened a consensus conference examining the role of endoscopy for upper gastrointestinal hemorrhage.[19] The panel assessed clinical features predicting the need for intervention because of continued bleeding. Table 17.1 summarized these features.

Although 60% to 70% of all patients presenting with gastrointestinal bleeding will stop bleeding spontaneously, those presenting with the clinical scenarios listed in Table 17.1 should be considered for endoscopic therapy. Of the therapies available, the heater probe and bipolar electrocoagulation device are the most useful.

TABLE 17.1. Predictors of Peptic Ulcer Rebleeding.

Magnitude of bleeding
  Hemodynamic instability
  Bloody emesis or nasogastric lavage that fails to clear
  Blood-red stools
Host factors
  Anticoagulated patient
  Patient hospitalized for a related or unrelated condition
Endoscopic features
  Visible vessel
  Arterial spurting or oozing
  Raised pigmented discoloration on ulcer base
  Adherent clot on ulcer base

Source: Anonymous (1989).[19]

Once bleeding has been controlled, the need for subsequent therapy has not been clearly established. Consideration must be given to the facilities available as well as to the skills of the surgeons and endoscopists in managing bleeding ulcers.

Surgery must be considered when endoscopic treatment has failed or is impractical. In general, when a patient has required more than six units of blood to be transfused they should be considered for surgery. When surgery is performed, the preferred operations are the vagotomy and antrectomy or the vagotomy and pyloroplasty. Endoscopic localization of the bleeding lesion is helpful before exploration.

Infrequently, patients present with continued blood loss whose surgical risk for morbidity or mortality are excessive. These patients may be considered for angiographic embolization. Angiographic techniques may control the bleeding, but the risk of necrosis at the embolization site is high. This complication will almost certainly result in mortality and must be considered before this approach is taken.

Mallory–Weiss Syndrome

Mallory–Weiss tears of the proximal stomach commonly occur following emesis. Classically associated with alcoholics,[20] the syndrome is manifested by hematemesis that follows episodes of intense vomiting.[21] More recently the syndrome has been observed following endoscopy, childbirth, coughing, and cardiopulmonary resuscitation. The diagnosis is suggested by a history of vomiting before the onset of the hematemesis. Endoscopy reveals liner tears below the gastroesophageal junction, occasionally extending proximally into the esophagus. Initial management includes resuscitation and correction of any coagulopathy. Bleeding is usually self-limited.[22–25] Endoscopic sclerotherapy of the bleeding vessel is effective.[26] Rarely is surgical intervention required. If so, an anterior gastronomy is made and the tear oversewn.

Gastric Outlet Obstruction

Gastric outlet obstruction is manifest by nausea and vomiting. Generally, it develops over weeks to months but occasionally an acute obstruction develops from a pyloric channel ulcer. The patient must be treated by nasogastric suction with vigorous fluid resuscitation. Often patients will have hypochloremic, hypokalemic metabolic alkalosis from chronic vomiting. These patients require large volumes of intravenous saline and potassium. Because this condition is often chronic, malnutrition is frequently present. Malnutrition is the most significant predictor of postoperative complications.[27] Almost all patients presenting with gastric outlet obstruction will require surgery; thus, to minimize the risk of complications total parenteral nutrition should be initiated. As an overall strategy it is best to place a nasogastric tube when these patients present, initiate fluid resuscitation, and begin TPN. Delaying surgery for about a week is reasonable to allow the stomach proximal to the obstruction to decompress and gastric wall edema to subside. Operating acutely on an obstructed stomach is technically difficult, secondary to edema and thickening of the gastric wall increasing the complication risk.

Peptic ulcer disease or carcinoma can cause gastric outlet obstruction. Barium upper GI tests will demonstrate the obstruction. Endoscopy may be helpful for diagnostic purposes, especially when a malignancy is visualized and biopsied. CT scans may be helpful when malignancy is suspected to demonstrate a mass distal to the obstruction or the presence of metastatic disease. Obstruction caused by peptic ulcer disease may transiently respond to medical therapy; however, 92% of patients presenting this way will require surgery within 3 years of initial diagnosis.[28] These patients require vagotomy and antrectomy. Patients with malignant obstruction always require resection. If metastatic disease is present, the resection should be limited to removing enough stomach for palliative purposes. In rare cases the tumor is confined to the gastric antrum, in which case total gastrectomy is indicated. In cases in which resection is not possible, a gastrojejunostomy can be created to bypass the obstructed stomach.

Stress Ulcer

Gastroduodenal ulcers are generally associated with stress. However, *stress ulcers* are a distinct clinical entity characterized by superficial gastric fundic lesions having a tendency to bleed but not perforate. In contrast, classical gastroduodenal ulcers are deep, penetrating all layers of the gastric or duodenal epithelium, which may result in bleeding, perforation, or obstruction. Head injury, burns, shock, and sepsis are some of the major diseases that result in stress ulceration. Apart from stress, there is no common etiological mechanism to explain why these lesions develop. Special variants occur, such as the Curling ulcers, which are associated with burns and are distributed along the entire GI tract. Singular, deep duodenal or gastric ulcers associated with head trauma are known as Cushings ulcers.

Pathophysiology

Stress ulcers are small, numerous lesions occurring in the superficial gastric mucosa. Their major clinical consequence is bleeding, which potentially compromises already very ill patients. The pathogenesis of these lesions remains unclear. Like most gastric ulcers, the major defect appears to be in the mucosal defense system. However, acid may play a role, the extent of which remains unknown.

Prophylaxis and Treatment for Stress Ulcer Bleeding

The American Society of Hospital Pharmacists (ASHP) performed an extensive analysis of the available clinical trials and meta-analyses. They concluded that stress ulcer prophylaxis should be administered to patients who will remain on a ventilator for more than 48 h or any ICU patient with a coagulopathy. Prophylaxis was also recommended for patients with a history of gastrointestinal ulceration or bleeding within 1 year before admission and in patients with at least two of the following risk factors: sepsis, ICU stay of more than 1 week, occult bleeding lasting 6 days or more, and use of high-dose corticosteroids (>250 mg/day of hydrocortisone or the equivalent).

A variety of special circumstances were considered with recommendations for prophylaxis. ICU patients with a Glasgow Coma Score less than or equal to 10 (or the inability to obey simple commands) or thermal injuries to more than 35% of their BSA (body surface area) should be treated. Prophylaxis is beneficial for patients following partial hepatectomy or in those with hepatic failure. Severely injured multiple trauma patients and spinal cord–injured patients also benefit from stress ulcer prophylaxis. Organ transplant patients should also be considered for prophylaxis. Patients not in ICUs do not benefit from prophylaxis.[29]

The studies supporting these recommendations demonstrated reduced clinically important bleeding with the use of H_2-blockers and sucralfate. Insufficient data exist showing the efficacy of proton pump inhibitors or misoprostol. The major complication of prophylaxis is pneumonia, but clinical data fail to convincingly demonstrate this as a significant event.

Gastric Carcinoma

The incidence of gastric carcinoma is declining, yet it remains a significant disease because of a high mortality. The median age of gastric cancer patients is 65 with 60% of cases in men and 40% in women.

There are two major histological types of gastric cancer. The *intestinal* histology consists of cell groupings organized into glands. Grossly these lesions appear as ulcerations. Intestinal-type tumors occur most frequently in the distal stomach. The decline in gastric cancer is attributable primarily to fewer intestinal-type lesions. Cancer cells that have no specific organization characterize the *diffuse* histology. They tend to infiltrate the gastric wall forming a thickened gastric wall but not a discrete mass. These lesions occur anywhere in the stomach but predominately occur at the cardia. The incidence of diffuse tumors has been relatively constant over the years. Diffuse lesions occur in younger patients and are more clinically aggressive than intestinal-type lesions.[30]

Several gastric conditions appear to be associated with the development of gastric cancer. Gastric atrophy or atrophic gastritis may result in intestinal metaplasia. Once present, metaplastic tissue may progress to dysplastic and ultimately carcinomatous histologies.[31] There have been studies demonstrating associations with *H. pylori* infection and gastric cancer[32,33]; however, the prevalence of *H. pylori* is very high and most patients with this infection do not develop gastric carcinoma. Gastric polyps do present an increased risk for the development of gastric carcinomas per se; however, as with any other polyp, the risk is associated with the degree of dysplasia in the polyp.[34] An association between Menetrier's disease (hypertrophic gastropathy) and gastric carcinoma has been proposed, but there are too few cases of these two entities coexisting to allow any conclusions to be drawn.[35] Although pernicious anemia results in two- to threefold excess risk for the development of gastric carcinoma,[36] the reason for this association remains unknown. Achlorhydria resulting from acid suppression has not led to increased cancer risk.[37] Benign gastric ulcers also do not result in increased cancer risk.[38]

The tumors can grow to considerable size before any symptoms develop. For this reason, patients often present with advanced-stage disease. Frequently, patients will present with anorexia, early satiety, weight loss, or other vague symptoms. Not uncommonly, patients with the most minimal symptoms will present with very large, metastatic tumors. A review of 18,365 gastric cancer patients by the American College of Surgeons revealed that weight loss and abdominal pain were the most frequent presenting symptoms (Table 17.2).[39] Gastric cancers bleed or obstruct, requiring operation for palliation irrespective of curative intent. For this reason, extensive preoperative evaluation is not necessary because the in-

TABLE 17.2. Presenting Symptoms for 18,265 Patients Surveyed by the American College of Surgeons.

Symptom	Frequency (%)
Weight loss	61.6
Abdominal pain	51.6
Nausea	34.3
Anorexia	32.0
Dysphagia	26.1
Melena	20.1
Early satiety	17.5
Ulcer-type pain	17.1
Lower-extremity edema	5.9

Source: Wanebo et al. (1993).[39]

traabdominal cavity can be assessed at the time of laparotomy. Patients should be explored irrespective of the presence of metastatic disease because of the need to palliate for obstruction or bleeding.

Approximately one-fourth of gastric carcinomas present as an ulcerating lesion. The radiographic or gross appearance at endoscopy or laparotomy is indistinguishable from a benign gastric ulcer. For this reason, it is essential to biopsy all gastric ulcers to ensure that a malignancy is not missed. Another 25% of lesions present as large polyps. Superficial spreading carcinoma is an early lesion that is manifested by tumor confinement to the gastric mucosa and submucosa. These lesions have a very favorable prognosis but only 15% of the tumors present this way. Linitis plastica is a condition in which the entire stomach is indurated secondary to a desmoplastic reaction to the cancer. Linitis has a very poor prognosis and fortunately only occurs in about 10% of gastric carcinoma cases.

Gastric remnant carcinoma is a clinical entity in which cancer develops in the remaining stomach following gastric resection. However, the specific risk of carcinoma development in gastric remnants is low and only becomes slightly significant more than 25 years following gastric resection.

Extent of Resection

Gastric carcinoma invades adjacent organs, spreads via lymphatics, and can metastasize by hematogenous spread. Before surgery, patients should be examined for the presence of a Virchow's node. These nodes are in the left supraclavicular fossa and represent spread of the cancer via the thoracic duct. Physical exam findings suggestive of metastatic disease include a Sister Mary Joseph's node (periumbilical nodule suggestive of tumor of the peritoneal surface) and a Blumer's shelf (tumor mass in the cul-de-sac). Hematogenous spread of the cancer to the liver occurs in 30% of patients. Gastric cancer may also metastasize to the ovary, resulting in a Krukenberg tumor. These lesions are easily identified at surgery. Less frequently metastases are found in the lungs or brain, mandating chest radiography and head CT scanning before surgery. A systematic approach for metastatic disease should be performed. Identification of metastatic lesions preoperatively is important because a planned curative resection will be downgraded to a palliative one.

During surgery the tumor should be assessed for resectability by ensuring that the cancer has not spread into the adjacent pancreas, colon, or liver. Peritoneal metastases are obvious and preclude any type of surgery. Knowledge of the ma-

TABLE 17.3. Location for the Major Nodal Groups Relevant to Gastric Resection for Cancer.

Nodal group	Location
N1	Perigastric along the greater and lesser curves
N2	Adjacent to the celiac axis and its major branches: the common hepatic, splenic and left gastric arteries
N3	Hepatoduodenal ligament; retropancreatic region; celiac plexus; superior mesenteric artery
N4	Paraaortic area

jor nodal groups is essential. Table 17.3 presents the location for the major lymph node locations relevant for gastric resection. Resection extent is classified as in Table 17.3. An R0 resection is one in which all the examined lymph nodes are free of tumor. R1 resections include the entire N1 nodal group and the omentum. An R2 resection is one that includes the entire stomach with the N2 nodes, an R3 with the N3 nodes, etc. Survival is predicted on the basis of the tumor stage. The TNM classification for gastric cancer (to be implemented in January 2003) is presented in Table 17.4.[40]

Surgical resection of gastric cancer provides the only chance for cure. Because gastric carcinomas will eventually obstruct or bleed, palliation is required so that all patients should be explored unless there is clear evidence of distant metastases or other contraindications to surgery.[41] Patients with distal lesions should undergo distal gastrectomy. For proximal lesions, or distal lesions where less than 5 cm of proximal margin can be obtained or lesions are diffusely distributed in the stomach, total gastrectomy is indicated. Previously, it was thought that splenectomy was necessary to ensure adequate tumor clearance. Splenectomy results in substantially increased perioperative morbidity without any clear survival benefit and is not recommended.[42–44]

Reconstruction Techniques

Several reconstructive options are available that attempt to minimize functional problems associated with gastric resection. Following gastric resection, early satiety and anorexia result in less caloric intake with subsequent weight loss. Malabsorption following gastric resection occurs in part because of rapid food transit time through the small bowel and less

TABLE 17.4. AJCC Definition of TNM and Stage Groupings for Gastric Carcinoma.

Primary Tumor (T)
TX	Primary tumor cannot be assessed
T0	No evidence of primary tumor
Tis	Carcinoma *in situ*: intraepithelial tumor without invasion of lamina propria
T1	Tumor invades lamina propria or submucosa
T2	Tumor invades muscularis propria or subserosa*
T2a	Tumor invades muscularis propria
T2b	Tumor invades subserosa
T3	Tumor penetrates serosa (visceral peritoneum) without invasion of adjacent structures**,***
T4	Tumor invades adjacent structures**,***

Regional Lymph Nodes (N)
NX	Regional lymph node(s) cannot be assessed
N0	No regional lymph node metastasis
N1	Metastasis in 1 to 6 regional lymph nodes
N2	Metastasis in 7 to 15 regional lymph nodes
N3	Metastasis in more than 15 regional lymph nodes

Distant Metastasis (M)
MX	Distant metastasis cannot be assessed
M0	No distant metastasis
M1	Distant metastasis

Stage
0	Tis	N0	M0
IA	T1	N0	M0
IB	T1	N1	M0
	T2a/b	N0	M0
II	T1	N2	M0
	T2a/b	N1	M0
	T3	N0	M0
IIIA	T2	N2	M0
	T3	N1	M0
	T4	N0	M0
IIIB	T3	N2	M0
IV	T4	N1-3	M0
	T1-3	N3	M0
	Any T	Any N	M1

Source: Used with permission of the American Joint Committee on Cancer (AJCC), Chicago, IL. The original source for this material is the AJCC Cancer Staging Manual, Sixth Edition (2002) published by Springer-Verlag, www.springer-ny.com. The above TNM classification will be implemented in January 2003.
*A tumor may penetrate the muscularis propria with extension into the gastrocolic or gastrohepatic ligaments or into the greater or lesser omentum without perforation of the visceral peritoneum coveirng these structures. In this case, the tumor is classified T2. If there is perforation of the visceral peritoneum covering the gastric ligaments or the omentum, the tumor should be classified T3.
**The adjacent structures of the stomach include the spleen, transverse colon, liver, diaphragm, pancreas, abdominal wall, adrenal gland, kidney, small intestine, and retroperitoneum.
***Intramural extension to the duodenum or esophagus is classified by the depth of greatest invasion in any of these sites, including stomach.

TABLE 17.5.
Reconstructive Options Following Distal Gastrectomy (Level I Evidence).

Reconstruction type	Outcome measurement	Results	Reference
BI (n = 30) vs. BII (n = 32)	M&M, 5-year survival, digestive comfort	Same	Chareton[47]
RY to gastric remnant (n = 13) vs. total gastrectomy with RYEJ[a]	M&M, QOL	Mostly the same, except slightly less diarrhea following subtotal gastrectomy	Svedlund[46]

BI, BII, Billroth I, II; Ry, Roux-en-Y; RYEJ, Roux-en-Y esophagojejunostomy.
[a]Not explicitly stated.
This study had three arms. Thirteen patients underwent subtotal gastrectomy with Roux-en-Y esophagojejunostomy for distal lesions and 20 underwent jejunal pouch interposition following total gastrectomy for proximal gastric lesions. Thirty-one had a Roux-en-Y reconstruction following total gastrectomy, some for proximal and others for distal lesions, the exact number of each was not specified.

contact with digestive enzymes. Dyspepsia, reflux, and bloating might also contribute to diminished food ingestion. Many of these symptoms result from the loss of gastric reservoir function. The standard operation for gastric cancer has been total gastrectomy with Roux-en-Y esophagojejunostomy. Newer reconstructive techniques attempt to recreate the gastric reservoir function. Studies have been performed to determine if better functional results are obtained with subtotal gastrectomy without compromising survival.

Subtotal gastrectomy has the theoretical disadvantage of less tumor clearance with potentially greater recurrence rate. For proximal and gastric midbody lesions, subtotal gastrectomy is impractical because the tumor cannot be adequately cleared and the remaining gastric remnant would be too small to be of any functional value. For distal gastric lesions, subtotal gastrectomy is preferred. Cure rates are equivalent to total gastrectomy with better functional results.[45,46] Table 17.5 summarizes results of randomized trials comparing various reconstructions following distal gastrectomy. Billroth II reconstruction has been thought to be associated with better function results than Billroth I. A randomized trial comparing these two reconstructions following distal gastric resection for cancer found that the morbidity, perioperative mortality, and 5-year survival were equivalent. Most notably, the functional results for these two reconstructions were the same, dispelling the notion that the Billroth II is superior.[47] Distal gastrectomy with Roux-en-Y gastrojejunostomy reconstruction has been compared to total gastrectomy with Roux-en-Y reconstruction. Theoretically, leaving a gastric remnant improves eating because of retention of some degree of gastric storage capacity. When these operations, which differed only by preservation of a gastric remnant, were compared there was little functional difference.[46]

Regarding creation of a reservoir, studies suggest that standard Roux-en-Y esophagojejunostomy provides equivalent results to any other reservoir-forming pouch. Thus, the pouches are an unnecessary addition to the reconstruction following total gastrectomy.

Chemotherapy and Radiotherapy

Gastric cancers are highly radioresistant. Radiation-induced injury to the spine and other organs adjacent to the stomach preclude utilization of high radiation doses. For this reason, radiation can only be recommended for palliative purposes.[48] Intraoperative radiation may result in somewhat better local control of gastric cancer but does not result in improved survival.[49]

Numerous trials investigating the value of postoperative chemotherapy have been performed. These have been assessed by meta-analysis concluding that there is no benefit.[50] For advanced-stage gastric cancers, chemotherapy may transiently reduce the tumor size. However, there has not been any demonstrable improvement in survival irrespective of the agents or combinations of drugs investigated.[51]

Gastric Surgery for Obesity

Obesity surgery was thoroughly evaluated by a consensus panel assembled by the National Institutes of Health in 1990. The panel recommended[52] that a multidisciplinary team of

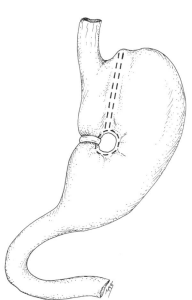

FIGURE 17.4. Vertical banded gastroplasty (VBG). A vertical staple line is placed parallel to the lesser curve, 1 cm away from its edge. Approximately 5 cm distal to the gastroesophageal junction, an EEA stapler is used to create a hole in the stomach. A piece of mesh is wrapped around the edge of the stomach and the EEA hole, creating a 1-cm outlet. The pouch has a 15- to 30-ml volume. The silastic ring gastroplasty is performed similar to the VBG except that the EEA hole is not created. A piece of silastic tubing is wrapped from the anterior surface of the staple line, around the medial edge of the stomach, and fixed to the posterior surface of the staple line, creating a 1-cm outlet.

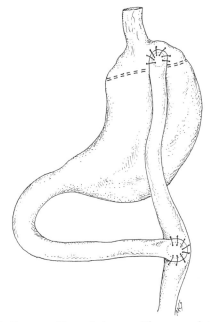

FIGURE 17.5. Roux-en-Y gastric bypass. The stomach is stapled shut horizontally, creating a 30-ml gastric pouch. The small bowel is divided beyond the ligament of Treitz. The distal cut end is brought through the transverse mesocolon, anterior to the stomach, and anastomosed to the pouch. This anastomosis is performed over a 32-French Bougie catheter to ensure the anastomosis is 1 cm in diameter. The proximal end of the small bowel is anastomosed 40 cm distal to the gastrojejunostomy for the standard Roux-en-Y and 150 cm for the long-limb gastric bypass.

providers evaluate surgical candidates. All aspects of medical, surgical, psychological, and nutritional issues must be adequately addressed before recommending surgery. Patients must commit to compliance with diets postoperatively. They must also ensure that they comply with lifelong follow-up for their medical conditions.

Body mass index (BMI) is the preferred means for assessing obesity. BMI is calculated by dividing the weight in kilograms by the height squared. Alternatively, the weight in pounds is divided by the height in inches squared times 705. The normal range of BMI is 25 to 28. Any BMI greater than 28 is considered overweight: obesity is defined as having a BMI greater than 30, morbid obesity a BMI greater than 40, and superobesity a BMI greater than 50. Above a BMI of 40, all-cause mortality sharply increases. Thus, the threshold for obesity surgery was set at a BMI of 40 by the NIH panel. The panel also included criteria for surgery when the BMI was in the range of 35 to 40 but only if the comorbid conditions were severe and life threatening.

The panel also reviewed the available weight loss operations. They found insufficient scientific evidence to support any of the malabsorptive surgeries. They concluded that only the vertical band gastroplasty (VBG) (Figure 17.4) and Roux-en-Y gastric bypass (RYGB) (Figure 17.5) could be recommended. Subsequent to publication of the statement, several high-quality reports demonstrated that the RYGB is a superior operation to the VBG.

References

1. Livingston EH, Guth PH. Peptic ulcer disease. Am Sci 1992;80: 592–598.
2. Holm L, Flemstreom G. Microscopy of acid transport at the gastric surface in vivo. J Intern Med (Suppl) 1990;732:91–95.
3. Feldman M, Burton ME. Histamine-2-receptor antagonists. Standard therapy for acid-peptic diseases. 1. N Engl J Med 1990;323: 1672–1680.
4. Feldman M, Burton ME. Histamine-2-receptor antagonists. Standard therapy for acid-peptic diseases (2) [see comments]. N Engl J Med 1990;323:1749–1755.
5. Maton PN. Omeprazole. N Engl J Med 1991;324:965–975.
6. Turner WJ, Thompson WJ, Thal ER. Perforated gastric ulcers. A plea for management by simple closures. Arch Surg 1988;123: 960–964.
7. Blaser MJ. *Helicobacter pylori* and the pathogenesis of gastroduodenal inflammation. J Infect Dis 1990;161:626–633.
8. Parsonnet J. *Helicobacter pylori.* Infect Dis Clin North Am 1998;12:185–197.
9. Hopkins RJ, Girardi LS, Turney EA. Relationship between *Helicobacter pylori* eradication and reduced duodenal and gastric ulcer recurrence: a review. Gastroenterology 1996;110:1244–1252.
10. Lainc L, Hopkins RJ, Girardi LS. Has the impact of *Helicobacter pylori* therapy on ulcer recurrence in the United States been overstated? A meta-analysis of rigorously designed trials. Am J Gastroenterol 1998;93:1409–1415.
11. Hawkey CJ, Tulassay Z, Szczepanski L, et al. Randomised controlled trial of *Helicobacter pylori* eradication in patients on non-steroidal anti-inflammatory drugs: HELP NSAIDs study. Helicobacter Eradication for Lesion Prevention [see comments]. Lancet 1998;352:1016–1021.
12. Leung FW, Robert A, Guth PH. Gastric mucosal blood flow in rats after 16,16-dimethyl PGE$_2$ given at a cytoprotective dose. Gastroenterology 1985;88:1948–1953.
13. Bickel M, Kauffman GL. Gastric gel mucus: effect of distention, 16,16-dimethyl prostaglandin E$_2$ and carbenoxolone. Gastroenterology 1981;80:770–775.
14. Isenberg JI, Smedfors B, Johansson C. Effect of graded doses of intraluminal H$^+$, prostaglandin E$_2$, and inhibition of endogenous prostaglandin synthesis on proximal duodenal bicarbonate secretion in unanesthetized rat. Gastroenterology 1985;88:303–307.
15. Mistiaen W, Van Hee R, Blockx P, Hubens A. Gastric emptying for solids in patients with duodenal ulcer before and after highly selective vagotomy. Dig Dis Sci 1990;35:310–316.
16. Passaro EJ, Bircoll M. Internal duodenal decompression. J Surg Res 1972;13:97–101.
17. Millat B, Hay JM, Valleur P, Fingerhut A, Fagniez PL. Emergency surgical treatment for bleeding duodenal ulcer: oversewing plus vagotomy versus gastric resection, a controlled randomized trial. French Associations for Surgical Research. World J Surg 1993;17: 568–573.
18. Livingston EH, Passaro EJ. Resuscitation. Revival should be the first priority. Postgrad Med 1991;89:117–120, 122.
19. Anonymous Consensus conference: therapeutic endoscopy and bleeding ulcers. JAMA 1989;262:1369–1372.
20. Bubrick MP, Lundeen JW, Onstad GR, Hitchcock CR. Mallory-Weiss syndrome: analysis of fifty-nine cases. Surgery (St. Louis) 1980;88:400–405.
21. Montalvo RD, Lee M. Retrospective analysis of iatrogenic Mallory-Weiss tears occurring during upper gastrointestinal endoscopy. Hepatogastroenterology 1996;43:174–177.
22. Graham DY, Schwartz JT. The spectrum of the Mallory-Weiss tear. Medicine (Baltimore) 1978;57:307–318.
23. Sugawa C, Benishek D, Walt AJ. Mallory-Weiss syndrome. A study of 224 patients. Am J Surg 1983;145:30–33.
24. Bharucha AE, Gostout CJ, Balm RK. Clinical and endoscopic risk factors in the Mallory-Weiss syndrome. Am J Gastroenterol 1997;92:805–808.
25. Todd GJ, Zikria BA, Mallory-Weiss syndrome. A changing clinical picture. Ann Surg 1977;186:146–148.
26. Bataller R, Llach J, Salmeraon JM, et al. Endoscopic sclerotherapy in upper gastrointestinal bleeding due to the Mallory-Weiss syndrome [see comments]. Am J Gastroenterol 1994;89:2147–2150.
27. Khuri SF, Daley J, Henderson W, et al. Risk adjustment of the postoperative mortality rate for the comparative assessment of the quality of surgical care: results of the National Veterans Affairs Surgical Risk Study. J Am Coll Surg 1997;185:315–327.
28. Jaffin BW, Kaye MD. The prognosis of gastric outlet obstruction. Ann Surg 1985;201:176–179.
29. Erstad BL, Grant KL, Boucher BA, et al. ASHP therapeutic guidelines on stress ulcer prophylaxis. Am J Health Syst Pharm 1999;56:347–379.
30. Lauren P. The two histological main types of gastric carcinoma: diffuse and so-called intestinal-type carcinoma. Acta Pathol Microbiol Scand 1965;64:31–49.
31. Correa P. Human gastric carcinogenesis: a multistep and multifactorial process—First American Cancer Society Award Lecture on Cancer Epidemiology and Prevention. Cancer Res 1992;52:6735–6740.
32. Parsonnet J, Friedman GD, Vandersteen DP, et al. *Helicobacter pylori* infection and the risk of gastric carcinoma [see comments]. N Engl J Med 1991;325:1127–1131.
33. Nomura A, Stemmermann GN, Chyou PH, Kato I, Perez-Perez GI, Blaser MJ. *Helicobacter pylori* infection and gastric carcinoma among Japanese Americans in Hawaii [see comments]. N Engl J Med 1991;325:1132–1136.
34. Nakamura T, Nakano G. Histopathological classification and malignant change in gastric polyps. J Clin Pathol 1985;38:754–764.
35. Matzner MJ, Raab AP, Spear PW. Benign gastric giant rugae complicated by submucosal gastric carcinoma: report of a case. Gastroenterology 1951;18:296–302.

36. Hsing AW, Hansson LE, McLaughlin JK, et al. Pernicious anemia and subsequent cancer. A population-based cohort study. Cancer (Phila) 1993;71:745–750.

37. Klinkenberg-Knol EC, Festen HP, Jansen JB, et al. Long-term treatment with omeprazole for refractory reflux esophagitis: efficacy and safety [see comments]. Ann Intern Med 1994;121:161–167.

38. Hole DJ, Quigley EM, Gillis CR, Watkinson G. Peptic ulcer and cancer: an examination of the relationship between chronic peptic ulcer and gastric carcinoma. Scand J Gastroenterol 1987;22: 17–23.

39. Wanebo HJ, Kennedy BJ, Chmiel J, Steele GJ, Winchester D, Osteen R. Cancer of the stomach. A patient care study by the American College of Surgeons. Ann Surg 1993;218:583–592.

40. Evans DB, et al. Part III: Digestive System. In: Greene, FL, Page DL, Fleming ID, et al, editors. AJCC Cancer Staging Manual, Sixth Edition. New York: Springer-Verlag, 2002.

41. Douglass HJ, Nava HR. Gastric adenocarcinoma—management of the primary disease. Semin Oncol 1985;12:32–45.

42. Brady MS, Rogatko A, Dent LL, Shiu MH. Effect of splenectomy on morbidity and survival following curative gastrectomy for carcinoma. Arch Surg 1991;126:359–364.

43. Sugimachi K, Kodama Y, Kumashiro R, Kanematsu T, Noda S, Inokuchi K. Critical evaluation of prophylactic splenectomy in total gastrectomy for the stomach cancer. Gann 1980;71:704–709.

44. Suehiro S, Nagasue N, Ogawa Y, Sasaki Y, Hirose S, Yukaya H. The negative effect of splenectomy on the prognosis of gastric cancer. Am J Surg 1984;148:645–648.

45. Gouzi JL, Huguier M, Fagniez PL, et al. Total versus subtotal gastrectomy for adenocarcinoma of the gastric antrum. A French prospective controlled study. Ann Surg 1989;209:162–166.

46. Svedlund J, Sullivan M, Liedman B, Lundell L, Sjeodin I. Quality of life after gastrectomy for gastric carcinoma: controlled study of reconstructive procedures. World J Surg 1997;21:422–433.

47. Chareton B, Landen S, Manganas D, Meunier B, Launois B. Prospective randomized trial comparing Billroth I and Billroth II procedures for carcinoma of the gastric antrum [see comments]. J Am Coll Surg 1996;183:190–194.

48. Moertel CG, Childs DJ, Reitemeier RJ, Colby MJ, Holbrook MA. Combined 5-fluorouracil and supervoltage radiation therapy of locally unresectable gastrointestinal cancer. Lancet 1969;2:865–867.

49. Sindelar WF, Kinsella TJ, Tepper JE, et al. Randomized trial of intraoperative radiotherapy in carcinoma of the stomach. Am J Surg 1993;165:178–186.

50. Hermans J, Bonenkamp JJ, Boon MC, et al. Adjuvant therapy after curative resection for gastric cancer: meta-analysis of randomized trials [see comments]. J Clin Oncol 1993;11:1441–1447.

51. Fuchs CS, Mayer RJ. Gastric carcinoma [see comments]. N Engl J Med 1995;333:32–41.

52. Anonymous. NIH Conference. Gastrointestinal surgery for severe obesity. Consensus Development Conference Panel. Ann Intern Med 1991;115:956–961.

18

Pancreas

Sean J. Mulvihill

Anatomy of the Pancreas

Embryology

The pancreas is derived as an outpouching of the primitive foregut endoderm in the region of the duodenum.[1] It has two main embryological components: (1) a dorsal bud, first identifiable at 4 weeks gestation, which goes on to become the body and tail of the gland, and (2) a ventral bud producing the head of the gland and the extrahepatic biliary system. As these outpouchings grow, the ventral aspect rotates to fuse with the dorsal aspect by about the seventh week of gestation. The ductal system of the pancreas is derived from these two anlages. The embryonic ventral duct arises from the bile duct, drains with it into the duodenum at the major papilla, and fuses with the dorsal duct to drain the body of the gland as the main pancreatic duct of Wirsung. The embryonic dorsal duct persists as a separate structure in its proximal portion (duct of Santorini), draining into the duodenum at the minor papilla on the medial duodenal wall about 1 to 2 cm cephalad to the major papilla. In 5% to 10% of people, the ventral and dorsal ducts fail to fuse, resulting in a condition known as pancreas divisum.[2,3] In this anatomical arrangement, the majority of pancreatic secretions are carried to the duodenum through the duct of Santorini and the minor papillae.

The neurons innervating the pancreas, and the rest of the gastrointestinal tract, are part of the enteric nervous system (ENS), best thought of as the third component of the autonomic nervous system.[4] The ENS plays an important role in the regulation of secretion, motility, blood flow, and immune function in the gut.

Developmental abnormalities of the pancreas are rare, but can occasionally come to attention clinically. The risk of development of acute pancreatitis was shown to be increased in patients with pancreas divisum in some studies, but not others.[3,5–8] Congenital pancreatic cysts are uncommon and usually solitary. Multiple congenital cysts can occur in the setting of polycystic kidney disease, von Hippel–Lindau syndrome, or cystic fibrosis. Annular pancreas occurs when the ventral pancreas encircles the duodenum, usually just proximal to the ampulla of Vater. Annular pancreas may be an incidental finding, or it may cause obstruction, in which case it is treated by duodenojejunostomy.

Anatomical Relationships

The normal pancreas is about 15 cm in length, weighs approximately 120 g, and is located in the retroperitoneum, covered by a thin peritoneum (Fig. 18.1).[1] The head of the gland lies nestled in the C-loop of the second part of the duodenum, and the tail of the gland extends obliquely into the hilum of the spleen. The superior mesenteric vein passes from the small-bowel mesentery toward the liver behind the neck of the pancreas, where it joins the spenic vein to become the portal vein. The inferior mesenteric vein similarly runs in a cephalad direction from the left colon mesentery behind the body of the pancreas near the ligament of Treitz to join the superior mesenteric and portal vein confluence. The splenic vein courses posterior to the body of the pancreas, and the splenic artery runs from its celiac origin to the spleen along the cephalad aspect of the pancreatic body. The body of the pancreas lies anterior to the left kidney and adrenal gland. The head of the pancreas lies anterior to the inferior vena cava, which can be exposed with the Kocher maneuver. The neck of the pancreas overlies the spine, where it is susceptible to injury in blunt abdominal trauma.

Blood Supply, Lymphatic Drainage, and Innervation

The pancreas has a redundant arterial blood supply. The head of the gland is supplied by paired (anterior and posterior) pancreaticoduodenal arteries, which course along the interface between the duodenum and the head of the pancreas.[9] The celiac artery branches supply the right cephalic portion of the pancreatic head (dorsal anlag), the region around the intra-

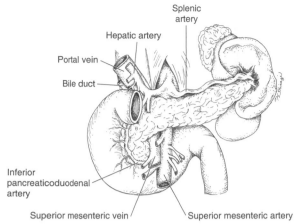

FIGURE 18.1. An anterior view of the pancreas, showing the major relationships with the duodenum, spleen, splenic artery, superior mesenteric artery, and superior mesenteric vein.

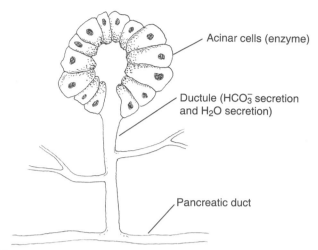

FIGURE 18.2. Microscopic anatomy of the pancreatic acinus. In the pancreatic acinus, the cells are arranged around a central ductule. The apical region of the acinar cells contains the machinery necessary for exocytosis of secretory granules. The basolateral surface of the acinar cell is exposed to a rich capillary bed. This region of the cell contains specific receptors for secretagogues such as cholecystokinin.

pancreatic portion of the bile duct, and the first and second portions of the duodenum.[10] The superior mesenteric artery branches supply the left caudal portion of the pancreatic head (ventral anlag) and the third and fourth portions of the duodenum. The body of the gland is supplied by small branches from the splenic artery. The venous drainage of the pancreas is entirely into the portal vein.

The pancreas is drained by an extensive network of lymphatic channels, which coalesce into lymph nodes.[11] These nodal drainage basins have importance in the treatment of patients with pancreatic cancer, where nodal metastasis is common. In the head of the gland, the initial drainage is to pancreaticoduodenal nodes, located near the groove between the pancreas and duodenum. Additional drainage is to nodes along the hepatoduodenal ligament, including those along the right lateral aspect of the portal vein and also along the hepatic artery. Secondary drainage is seen to celiac and periaortic lymph nodes from the hepatic and gastroduodenal regions. From the uncinate process, drainage is toward the superior mesenteric arterial nodes and from there to the periaortic chain. From the body of the pancreas, drainage is mainly to nodes along the splenic artery and splenic hilum, and from there to the celiac and periaortic nodes.

The pancreas is innervated extrinsically by parasympathetic fibers from the vagus nerve and sympathetic fibers from the splanchnic nerves. Visceral afferent fibers largely pass via spinal nerves to the dorsal root ganglia, although the vagus nerves also contain afferent fibers. These sensory fibers are likely involved in pain perception in disorders such as chronic pancreatitis and pancreatic cancer.

Microscopic Anatomy

The pancreas is a finely nodular gland composed of exocrine tissue (80% of the total mass), ducts, vessels, nerves, and connective tissue (18% of the total mass), and endocrine tissue, the islets of Langerhans (2% of the total mass). The exocrine portion of the gland is made up of pancreatic acinar cells, arranged in spherical masses termed acini, which in turn are grouped as lobules. Pancreatic exocrine secretions are drained via small ductules originating in the acini, becoming pro-

gressively larger in the lobules and eventually emptying into the main pancreatic duct.

Pancreatic acinar cells are large and pyramidal shaped. Their basolateral aspect is in contact with nerves, blood vessels, and a connective tissue stroma, and their apical aspect converges on the central lumen of the acinus (Fig. 18.2). With stimulation, the zymogen granules in the apex of the cell are depleted as they empty enzymes into the ductule lumen.

The islets of Langerhans are small islands of endocrine cells within a sea of exocrine tissue (Fig. 18.3). The pancreas contains approximately 1 million islets, distributed throughout the gland. The islets contain four endocrine cell types: (1) *B cells* account for 50% to 80% of the total islet volume and

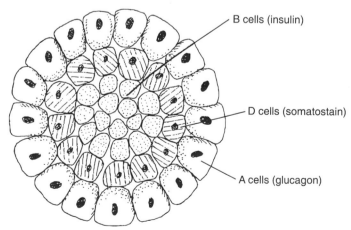

FIGURE 18.3. Microscopic appearance of the islets of Langerhans. The islets of Langerhans contain hormones, including insulin, glucagon, and somatostatin, involved in regulation of blood glucose levels. The islets are scattered throughout the pancreas within a sea of exocrine tissue. The islets can be well seen through the use of special immunoreactive stains, such as this one to chromogranin.

contain insulin; (2) *PP cells* account for 10% to 35% of the islet volume and contain pancreatic polypeptide; (3) *A cells* account for 5% to 20% of the islet volume and contain glucagon; and (4) *D cells* account for less than 5% of the islet volume and contain somatostatin.

Physiology of the Pancreas

Exocrine Function

The pancreas has a major exocrine function in the production of digestive enzymes. These include (1) amylase, which functions in the breakdown of starches, (2) lipase, which functions to hydrolyze fatty acids, (3) trypsin and chymotrypsin, which function to degrade proteins in the meal, and (4) nucleases such as deoxyribonuclease and ribonuclease, which function to break down DNA and RNA, respectively. These enzymes are largely made and stored in the pancreas in an inactive form, and are activated after secretion by the duodenal epithelial brush border enzyme, enterokinase. Enterokinase hydrolyzes trypsinogen to its active form, trypsin; the latter molecule, in turn, activates other proenzymes. To prevent damage from inadvertent intrapancreatic activation of digestive enzymes, a trypsin inhibitor is also secreted by the pancreas. The other components of pancreatic juice and their normal concentrations are summarized in Table 18.1.

Pancreatic juice is clear, colorless, and alkaline. In addition to its organic constituents, pancreatic juice contains a number of inorganic salts, including Na^+, K^+, Cl^-, and HCO_3^-. The concentrations of Cl^- and HCO_3^- are reciprocally linked, according to the volume of secretion. The daily total volume of secretion of pancreatic juice is approximately 2.5 l. The hormone secretin, found in duodenal epithelium, is released in response to duodenal acidification and stimulates pancreatic water and bicarbonate secretion from pancreatic ductal and centroacinar cells.

In the basal state, pancreatic enzyme secretion is minimal, due to the tonic inhibition by the peptide hormone and neurocrine agent somatostatin. With ingestion of a meal, the presence of fat or amino acids in the duodenum stimulates release of a trypsin-sensitive peptide termed cholecystokinin-releasing factor (CCK-RF).[12] CCK-RF acts in the duodenum to stimulate the release of cholecystokinin (CCK), which in turn stimulates enzyme secretion from pancreatic acinar cells as well as gallbladder contraction. The presence of activated trypsin in the duodenal lumen inactivates CCK-RF, thus reducing further stimulation of secretion.

Cholecystokinin is the major stimulant of pancreatic exocrine secretion, but a number of other neurocrine agents are also involved, including acetylcholine, vasoactive intestinal polypeptide, gastrin-releasing peptide, and substance P.[13] The main inhibitor of pancreatic exocrine secretion is somatostatin.[14]

Endocrine Function

Besides secretion of digestive enzymes, a second major function of the pancreas is in regulation of blood glucose levels. The islets of Langerhans, which contain the endocrine cells of the pancreas, are distributed widely throughout the gland. Three main cell types make up the islets: (1) alpha cells, which produce glucagon, (2) beta cells, which produce insulin, and (3) delta cells, which produce somatostatin. The organization of these cells within the islet follows a specific pattern, with the alpha cells rimming the outer part of the islet, beta cells making up the core, and delta cells distributed at the interface between the alpha and beta cells. The islet has a special venous drainage that bathes the acinar (exocrine) glands before entering the portal vein. These two features, the anatomical distribution of cells within the islet and the special islet venous drainage, likely contribute to regulation of islet hormone secretion and islet–acinar interaction in regulation of exocrine enzymes, respectively.

Acute Pancreatitis

Acute pancreatitis is an inflammatory disorder of the pancreas with local and systemic manifestations. About 5,000 new cases per year are seen in the United States, with an overall mortality rate of 10%, making pancreatitis a significant health problem.[15] An international symposium on pancreatitis held in Atlanta (GA, USA) in 1992 reached consensus on terminology to describe various conditions related to pancreatitis (Table 18.2).[16] Acute pancreatitis is best defined as an acute inflammatory disease of the pancreas with variable involvement of distant organs such as the lung, kidney, and heart. Two main pathological forms of acute pancreatitis are recognizable: (1) a mild, interstitial or edematous pancreatitis, characterized by interstitial edema and infiltration of polymorphonuclear cells, and (2) a more severe necrotizing pancreatitis, characterized by focal or diffuse necrosis of both the pancreatic parenchyma and adjacent soft tissue. The former is usually a self-limited process that rarely results in local complications, organ failure, or death, whereas the latter commonly results in infection, systemic manifestations such as pulmonary, renal, or cardiac failure, and death.

Pathophysiology

Acute pancreatitis has many and varied underlying causes, which remarkably produce a relatively uniform clinical picture. Common causes of pancreatitis are listed in Table 18.3. The mechanisms by which these various factors cause pancreatitis are an ongoing subject of study.

Clinical Presentation

The most prominent symptom in patients with acute pancreatitis is abdominal pain. Typically, the pain is located diffusely across the upper abdomen and radiates through to the

TABLE 18.1. Inorganic Components of Pancreatic Juice During Secretion.

Component	Amount or concentration
Water	1500–3000 ml/day
Sodium	140 mmol/l
Potassium	10 mmol/l
Chloride	20 mmol/l
Bicarbonate	110 mmol/l

TABLE 18.2. Definitions of Terminology in Pancreatitis.

Acute interstitial pancreatitis:
  A mild, self-limited form of pancreatitis characterized by interstitial edema and an acute inflammatory response without necrosis, local complications, or systemic manifestations such as organ failure.

Necrotizing pancreatitis:
  A severe form of acute pancreatitis characterized by locoregional tissue necrosis and systemic manifestations such as pulmonary, renal, or cardiac failure.

Sterile necrosis:
  Acute pancreatitis leading to tissue necrosis without supervening infection.

Infected necrosis:
  Acute pancreatitis with locoregional tissue necrosis complicated by bacterial or fungal infection.

Acute fluid collections:
  A fluid collection occuring early in the course of acute pancreatitis, located in or near the pancreas, and lacking an epithelial lining or a defined wall of granulation or fibrous tissue.

Pancreatic pseudocyst:
  A pancreatic or peripancreatic fluid collection with a well-defined wall of granulation tissue and fibrosis, absence of an epithelial lining. Pancreatic pseudocysts can arise in the setting of chronic pancreatitis, without as a sequela of an episode of necrotizing pancreatitis. One of the common complications of pseudocyst is the development of infection.

Pancreatic cysts:
  A fluid-filled pancreatic mass with an epithelial lining. These may be neoplastic lesions, such as serous cystadenomas or mucinous cystic tumors, or congenital cysts.

Pancreatic abscess:
  A circumscribed intraabdominal collection of pus, usually in proximity to the pancreas, containing little or no pancreatic necrosis, arising as a consequence of necrotizing pancreatitis or pancreatic trauma.

Suppurative cholangitis:
  Bacterial infection within the biliary tree, associated with ductal obstruction, usually from a stone or stricture.

Source: Adapted from the Atlanta classification.[16]

TABLE 18.3. Causes of Acute Pancreatitis.

Cause	Relative frequency in the United States
Gallstones	40%
Alcohol	30%
Idiopathic	15%

Metabolic
  Hyperlipidemia
  Hypercalcemia
  Cystic fibrosis
	5%

Anatomical and functional lesions
  Pancreas divisum
  Pancreatic duct strictures or tumors
  Ampullary stenosis or obstruction
  Sphincter of Oddi dysfunction
	<5%

Mechanical insults
  Blunt abdominal trauma
  Intraoperative injury
  Endoscopic retrograde cholangiopancreatography (ERCP)
	<5%

Drugs Azathioprine, thiazide diuretics, pentamidine, dideoxyinosine (ddI), sulfonamides, corticosteroids, furosemide	<5%
Infections and toxins Mumps, viral hepatitis, cytomegalovirus, ascariasis, scorpion venom, anticholinesterase insecticides	<5%

Ischemia
  Cardiac surgery
  Vasculitis
	Rare

Hereditary	Rare

Miscellaneous
  Burn injury
  Long-distance running
	Case reports

back. In most patients, the onset of pain is relatively sudden, and may mimic other intraabdominal catastrophes such as perforated ulcer. The pain is usually severe and steady in nature, without the cramping characteristic of bowel obstruction or the waxing and waning course of renal colic. Nausea and vomiting frequently accompany the pain. Vomiting does not alleviate the pain.

On physical examination, the patient is usually found lying still in bed, as movement exacerbates the discomfort. Low-grade fever is typically present at the outset of illness, and high fevers to 39°C may be present within 2 or 3 days in severely afflicted patients. Tachycardia is commonly present, along with other signs of intravascular volume depletion. The abdomen is mildly distended, with tenderness and guarding in the upper quadrants. A picture of diffuse peritonitis can be seen in severe cases, but usually without the boardlike quality of perforated duodenal ulcer. Although not commonly seen today, occasional patients presenting with hemorrhagic pancreatitis have ecchymoses in the flanks (Grey Turner sign) or the periumbilical area (Cullen sign).

Associated physical signs include diminished breath sounds with dullness at the lung bases from consolidation or effusion. In patients with gallstone pancreatitis, jaundice may be present, reflecting biliary obstruction from a gallstone. Pancreatitis related to alcohol ingestion may be accompanied by stigmata of chronic liver disease, such as spider angiomata, gynecomastia in males, and parotid enlargement.

Diagnostic Evaluation

The most useful single test in the diagnosis of pancreatitis is the serum amylase level. Hyperamylasemia occurs early in the course of acute pancreatitis, and its return to normal levels generally follows the improving clinical course of uncomplicated patients. Hyperamylasemia is not specific for pancreatitis, however, as it has been described in a number of unrelated conditions (Table 18.4). The level of amylase elevation does not correlate with the severity of the illness. In the presence of hypertriglyceridemia, serum amylase levels may be falsely low.

Other blood tests useful in the diagnosis of pancreatitis include the white blood cell count, which is usually moderately elevated. In the presence of pancreatic necrosis, the white blood cell count may rise markedly. Hyperglycemia is common in acute pancreatitis but is nonspecific. Liver function tests are commonly transiently elevated in pancreatitis. Serum lipase measurements are roughly as sensitive as amylase measurements in the diagnosis of acute pancreatitis. Lipase remains elevated somewhat longer in the course of illness than amylase and is somewhat more specific, because lipase is not

TABLE 18.4. Causes of Hyperamylasemia.

Causes associated with acute abdominal pain	Miscellaneous causes
Acute pancreatitis	Mumps
Pancreatic ascites	Acute parotitis
Perforated viscus	Scorpion stings
Pancreatic pseudocyst	Ovarian cysts and tumors
Acute cholecystitis	Lung cancer
Small-bowel obstruction	Renal failure
Acute appendicitis	Macroamylasemia
Ruptured ectopic pregnancy	Endoscopic retrograde cholangiopancreatography
Acute salpingitis	Diabetic ketoacidosis Intracranial hemorrhage HIV infection

found in organs such as the salivary glands and ovaries. Serum calcium levels often fall in the course of pancreatitis, mainly because of a concomitant fall in serum albumin, as serum ionized calcium levels remain normal in most patients.[17]

Radiographic assessment of patients with pancreatitis should include right upper quadrant ultrasonography in those suspected of gallstones as the cause. The positive predictive value of ultrasound has been reported to be as high as 100% in this situation, with a negative predictive value of about 75%.[18] In severely ill patients, computed tomography (CT) should be performed to assess the degree of necrosis present and to identify fluid collections. Endoscopic retrograde cholangiopancreatography (ERCP) plays a diagnostic role in identifying certain causes of pancreatitis, such as pancreas divisum, ductal strictures, and tumors, and a therapeutic role in selected patients with gallstone pancreatitis complicated by cholangitis.[2]

Measures of Severity of Pancreatitis

The severity of pancreatitis can be estimated with both clinical and radiographic criteria. Ranson's criteria for estimating severity is one of the most commonly used clinical systems (Table 18.5). These 11 criteria were found, in multivariate analysis, to predict survival in patients with acute pancreatitis.[19,20] These criteria include 5 measured at the time of presentation and 6 others during the initial 48 h of treatment. Patients with fewer than 3 of these criteria present were found to have uniformly good outcomes, whereas the mortality rate increased substantially in the presence of greater numbers of criteria (3–4 criteria: 20% mortality; 5–6 criteria: 40% mortality; 7 or greater criteria: 100% mortality).

The recognition of the importance of necrosis in determining outcome was recognized by the development of computed tomographic staging systems to estimate severity of pancreatitis.[21–23] Necrosis in more than 50% of the gland, the presence of extensive peripancreatic fluid collections, and the presence of gas within the pancreas or adjacent soft tissue are all markers predicting poor outcome.[22]

Treatment of Pancreatitis

MILD TO MODERATE ACUTE PANCREATITIS

Most patients with pancreatitis have a relatively mild, self-limited disease.[24] The average patient with pancreatitis of mild to moderate severity should be initially supported with intravenous hydration and pain medications. Nasogastric tube suction, when used routinely, appears to have no benefit,[25] but should be considered for patients with significant vomiting. In patients with gallstone pancreatitis, a laparoscopic cholecystectomy should be performed at a convenient time before discharge.[26,27] An intraoperative cholangiogram should be obtained during cholecystectomy and, if common bile duct stones are found, a laparoscopic common bile duct exploration or postoperative endoscopic sphincterotomy with stone extraction should be performed.[28,29] The outcome with this strategy is excellent.

SEVERE ACUTE PANCREATITIS

The patient with severe acute pancreatitis from any cause is at risk for the development of complications for which surgical decision making plays a central role. A small group of patients with severe acute pancreatitis may benefit from an early approach to clearing the common bile duct. This group is critically ill at presentation and fails to improve in the first 12 to 24 h of treatment. If gallstones are confirmed by ultrasonography, then ERCP, spincterotomy, and stone extraction within the first 48 h decrease mortality (Table 18.6). Laparoscopic cholecystectomy is delayed until recovery from the pancreatitis, but during the same hospitalization.[27] For many of these patients, additional procedures such as pseudocyst drainage are required.

STERILE NECROSIS

Necrotizing pancreatitis can produce necrotic areas of pancreas and retroperitoneal tissue without becoming infected. The clinical course of some of these patients is relatively benign, but in others, the clinical course mimics that of patients with necrosis complicated by infection.[30] If the patient is improv-

TABLE 18.5. Ranson Criteria for Assessing Severity of Acute Pancreatitis.

Criteria at admission	Criteria within the first 48 h
Age >55 years	Drop in hematocrit >10%
White blood cell count >16,000/μl	Fluid deficit >4000 ml
Serum glucose >200 mg/dl (11 mmol/l)	Serum calcium <8.0 mg/dl (<1.9 mmol/l)
Serum LDH >400 IU/l	Hypoxemia (PO$_2$ <60 mmHg)
Serum AST >250 IU/l	Rise in BUN >5 mg/dl (>1.8 mmol/l)
	Drop in albumin <3.2 g/dl

Source: Ranson et al. (1976).[19]

TABLE 18.6.

Early Endoscopic Sphincterotomy in Gallstone Pancreatitis: Results from Randomized, Controlled Clinical Trials (Level I Evidence).

Reference	Patient groups	Mortality rate	Biliary sepsis rate	Comments
Neoptolemos, England, 1988[114]	Early ERCP/ES ($n = 59$)	1.7% ($p < 0.05$)	6 of 25 severe pancreatitis patients ($p < 0.05$)	Benefit confined to patients with severe pancreatitis. LOS also shortened by routine ERCP/ES
	Selective ERCP ($n = 62$)	8.0%	17 of 28 severe pancreatitis patients	
Fan, Hong Kong, 1993[115]	Early ERCP/ES ($n = 97$)	5% (p = 0.4, ns)	0% ($p = 0.001$)	Benefit limited to patients with severe pancreatitis
	Selective ERCP ($n = 98$)	9%	12%	
Nitsche, European multicenter trial, 1995[116]	Early ERCP/ES ($n = 48$)	1% (ns)	Cholangitis (odds ratio = 3.3) and sepsis (odds ratio = 3.5) slightly more frequent in selective group (ns)	No benefit observed with early, routine endoscopic sphincterotomy
	Selective ERCP ($n = 52$)	2%		
Neoptolemos, England, 1988[114]	Early ERCP/ES ($n = 59$)	1.7% ($p < 0.05$)	6 of 25 severe pancreatitis patients ($p < 0.05$)	Benefit confined to patients with severe pancreatitis. LOS also shortened by routine ERCP/ES
	Selective ERCP ($n = 62$)	8.0%	17 of 28 severe pancreatitis patients	

ns, not significant.

ing clinically, conservative therapy is appropriate. If fever, leukocytosis, abdominal pain, ileus, or organ dysfunction is present, CT-guided percutaneous aspiration of necrotic areas should be performed to rule out infection.[31] If the Gram stain and culture of this material are sterile, bowel rest, total parenteral nutrition, analgesics, and intravenous antibiotics are appropriate treatment.[32,33] In general, a worsening clinical course or failure to improve within 3 to 4 weeks is a reasonable indication for debridement in the absence of infection. Persistent fever or stable organ system failure are not absolute indications for surgery, although a search for infection with fine-needle aspiration biopsy is warranted.

NECROTIZING PANCREATITIS WITH INFECTION

Infection can complicate severe acute pancreatitis as (1) infected pancreatic necrosis, (2) pancreatic abscess, (3) infected pseudocyst, and (4) acute suppurative cholangitis; these terms are defined in Table 18.2. Infected pancreatic necrosis is a fulminant infection occurring within the first 2 weeks of the onset of necrotizing pancreatitis. The reported incidence is 17% in a large series of patients with acute pancreatitis.[34] The usual pathogens are gram-negative rods from the gut, and in three-quarters of cases the infection is monomicrobial. Animal data[35] and randomized, controlled clinical data suggest that early, empiric antibiotic treatment (i.e. cefuroxime or imipenem) in patients with severe acute (necrotizing) pancreatitis decreases infectious complications and mortality (Table 18.7).[36] Mortality rates in infected necrosis as high as 32% have been reported in recent series.[37] In contrast, pancreatic abscess is less common, with an incidence of 2%, and generally does not develop until an average of 5 weeks following onset of pancreatitis.[16,34,38] Although the spectrum of responsible organisms is similar to that seen in infected pancreatic necosis, multimicrobial involvement is far more common. Pancreatic abscess has a somewhat less fulminant course and lesser mortality rate than infected necrosis. Infection developing in preexisting pancreatic pseudocysts is a

different problem and should be distinguished from infected necrosis or pancreatic abscess. These patients may develop a septic picture late in the course of pancreatitis. Infected pseudocysts generally are more indolent than infected necrosis or pancreatic abscess and commonly respond to external tube drainage and intravenous antibiotics. Finally, cholangitis may complicate the course of acute pancreatitis if common bile duct obstruction occurs; this usually occurs in the setting of gallstone pancreatitis and may be fulminant. Relief of biliary obstruction by endoscopic papillotomy and stone extraction is the preferred management.

Patients with severe pancreatitis should undergo contrast enhanced CT examination (CE-CT). If hypoperfused areas suggestive of necrosis are identified, CT-guided fine-needle aspiration is performed for Gram stain and culture to detect infection. Infection occurs as a complication of pancreatic necrosis in up to 70% of patients.[39,40]

If infected pancreatic necrosis is identified, the appropriate management is broad-spectrum intravenous antibiotics and immediate operative debridement. Techniques for subsequent management include closed passive (Penrose) drainage, closed suction drainage, open packing (marsupialization), and peritoneal lavage. Multiple operative procedures are often required to debride the ongoing necrosis. Nonoperative drainage techniques are generally insufficient to adequately evacuate this necrotic tissue. No randomized data exist comparing these various treatment strategies, but good results have been reported in retrospective reviews with each technique.[34,41–44] Peritoneal lavage is popular in some centers as an adjunctive therapy in patients with severe acute pancreatitis.

PANCREATITIS COMPLICATED BY BLEEDING

Bleeding associated with acute necrotizing pancreatitis is a serious problem, with mortality rates in excess of 50%.[45] Bleeding may arise from extension of the necrotizing process into nearby major vessels, such as the gastroduodenal or splenic arteries, or from the gastrointestinal tract. This latter

TABLE 18.7.

Randomized, Controlled Clinical Trials of Prophylactic Antibiotic Therapy in Necrotizing Pancreatitis (Level I Evidence).

Reference	Patient groups	Infectious complications	Mortality rate	Comment
Trials of intravenous antibiotics				
Sainio, 1995, Helsinki University[117]	Cefuroxime (n = 30)	1.0 infections per patient (p < 0.01) 30% with pancreatic infection (ns)	3.3% (p = 0.03)	Enrollment of patients with necrotizing pancreatitis only. Penetration data of cefuroxime unclear. Good activity against expected pathogens.
	Control (n = 30)	1.8 infections per patient 40% with pancreatic infection	23.3%	Randomized, but not double-blind or placebo controlled Only study to show improved mortality with i.v. antibiotics but no improvement in pancreatic infection rate.
Pederzoli, 1993, Italian multicenter trial[118]	Imepenem (n = 41)	Pancreatic sepsis in 12.2% (p < 0.01) Nonpancreatic sepsis in 14.6% (p < 0.01)	7.3% (ns)	Necrotizing pancreatitis only. Imepenem has good penetration into pancreatic tissue. Randomized, but not placebo controlled. Significant improvement in pancreatic and other infection rates.
	Control (n = 33)	Pancreatic sepsis in 30.3% Nonpancreatic sepsis in 48.5%	12.1%	
Howes, 1975, Johns Hopkins University[119]	Ampicillin (n = 48)	10.4% (ns)	0%	Mild pancreatitis included. Ampicillin has poor pentration into pancreatic tissue and secretion.
	Control (n = 47)	12.8%	0%	
Finch, 1976[120]	Ampicillin (n = 31)	Infectious complications not specifically reported. No significant differences in length of stay or duration of fever.	3.2% (ns)	Mild pancreatitis included Ampicillin has poor penetration into pancreatic tissue and secretion.
	Control (n = 27)		0%	
Trials of selective gut decontamination				
Luiten, 1995, Netherlands multicenter trial[121]	Selective decontamination (n = 50)	Pancreatic infection in 18% (p = 0.03)	11 of 50, 22% (p = 0.048)	Enrollment criteria: Imrie score ≥3, Balthazar grade D or E. Randomized, but not placebo controlled.
	Control (n = 52)	Pancreatic infection in 38%	18 of 52, 35%	

is usually secondary to severe stress gastritis or varices related to splenic vein thrombosis. Initial management of bleeding in this setting is by angiographic identification and embolization of the involved artery. Surgery is required if angiography is unsuccessful.

MANAGEMENT OF PANCREATITIS ASSOCIATED WITH PANCREAS DIVISUM

The incidence of pancreas divisum is about three- to fourfold higher in patients with recurring bouts of idiopathic pancreatitis than in unaffected controls. Several small series of patients have suggested benefit from endoscopic minor papillotomy or pancreatic duct stent placement to reduce the incidence of recurrent pancreatitis.[3]

MANAGEMENT OF PATIENTS WITH PANCREATITIS AND NO CLEAR CAUSE

Occasional patients present with acute pancreatitis and no clear underlying cause (see Table 18.3). This disorder has been called idiopathic pancreatitis, but this term should be reserved for those patients in whom the cause remains obscure after a thorough evaluation. If these efforts are unrevealing, empiric laparoscopic cholecystectomy should be considered, especially if (1) the clinical course has been consistent with gallstone pancreatitis, (2) there is a family history of gallstones, or (3) if the patient's liver function tests were transiently abnormal. Under these circumstances, it is likely that occult cholelithiasis is the cause of the patient's symptoms. A common mistake is to assume that a negative ultrasound examination excludes gallstones, when in fact the false-negative rate is about 5%.[46]

Chronic Pancreatitis

Chronic pancreatitis affects about 8 new patients per 100,000 population per year in the United States, with a prevalence of 26.4 cases per 100,000 population.[47] Autopsy series, however, suggest a higher prevalence, 0.04% to 5%. Chronic pancreatitis is characterized pathologically by parenchymal fibrosis, ductal strictures, and atrophy of acinar and islet tissue.[48] Three subgroups of chronic pancreatitis have been described, including (1) *chronic calcific pancreatitis*, (2) *chronic obstructive pancreatitis*, and (3) *chronic inflammatory pancreatitis*. The most common pattern is chronic calcific pancreatitis, usually related to alcohol ingestion, and characterized by fibrosis, calcification in small ducts, and intraductal protein plugging. Chronic obstructive pancreatitis is commonly observed in the setting of pancreatic cancer, where ductal obstruction by the tumor leads to dilation, acinar atrophy, and fibrosis. The least common type is chronic inflammatory pancreatitis, usually associated with autoimmune diseases such as Sjögren's syndrome and sclerosing cholangitis.

Etiology

The underlying pathophysiology of alcohol-related chronic pancreatitis remains unclear, but probably involves ductal plugging and calcification related to abnormalities in pancreatic juice.[49,50] In tropical countries, chronic pancreatitis occurs in young individuals in the absence of alcohol ingestion, perhaps from dietary factors or micronutrient deficiency. A small number of patients have chronic pancreatitis with a genetic basis.[51] Gallstone disease does not result in chronic pancreatitis.

Clinical Presentation

There is no simple, accurate way to confirm the diagnosis of chronic pancreatitis. Clinical criteria for diagnosis include unrelenting epigastric abdominal pain that radiates through to the back, accompanied by nausea, poor appetite, and weight loss. Pancreatic exocrine insufficiency, resulting in steatorrhea, does not occur until about 90% of function is lost. Endocrine insufficiency, resulting in diabetes, does not occur until greater than 80% of the gland is destroyed. Because both insulin and glucagon secretion are lost with islet atrophy, the diabetes in chronic pancreatitis tends to be brittle and difficult to control.

The physical examination in patients with chronic pancreatitis is often unrevealing. Weight loss and malnutrition may be evident. Occasional patients may have concomitant chronic liver disease evident on examination. Epigastric tenderness is common.

Diagnostic Evaluation

Routine laboratory investigation is not generally revealing in chronic pancreatitis. Serum amylase and lipase levels may be mildly elevated but are usually normal. Liver function tests are normal unless there is underlying liver disease or bile duct obstruction. Malnutrition may be revealed by decreased serum albumin levels. In patients with steatorrhea, fat malabsorption can be confirmed by Sudan staining of the stool of 72-h stool collection while the patient consumes a diet containing 100 g fat per day. Stool fat excretion greater 7 g/day is abnormal.

Imaging studies are performed to provide an assessment of the extent of disease. A plain film of the abdomen may detect calcification in the gland. An abdominal CT scan is useful to identify pancreatic calcification, masses suspicious for carcinoma, dilated ducts, and pseudocysts. Reported sensitivity of CT in the diagnosis of chronic pancreatitis ranges from 75% to 90% with a specificity of 85% to 100%.[52] Pancreatic calcification is a hallmark of the diagnosis of chronic pancreatitis, but the degree of calcification does not correlate well with the degree of exocrine insufficiency.[53] Magnetic resonance cholangiopancreatography[54,55] (MRCP) or endoscopic retrograde cholangiopancreatography[56] (ERCP) is necessary to determine the size and anatomy of the pancreatic duct, as well as unsuspected pathology such as biliary stricture and cancer. These studies allow patients to be categorized into those with "small duct" disease and those with "large ducts." This differentiation is important in that those with large ducts are far more amenable to surgical correction.

Treatment

Surgery for chronic pancreatitis is indicated for disabling pain and obstruction of adjacent hollow viscera, commonly the bile duct or duodenum. For surgery to be effective, an identifiable anatomical lesion amenable to correction must be present. Options in surgical management broadly include drainage procedures, resective procedures, and nerve blocks. Successful treatment in terms of pain relief is improved in patients who cease alcohol and nicotine consumption.[57]

DISABLING PAIN

Pain is the usual reason for a patient with chronic pancreatitis to seek medical attention, and most treatment strategies are oriented around its relief. The severity of pain is a major factor in determining the advisability of surgery. In general, surgery is indicated if the pain interferes with the patient's ability to work, is refractory to pancreatic enzyme therapy, requires high doses of oral narcotics for control, and other possible causes for pain have been excluded.

If the preoperative assessment has demonstrated a dilated pancreatic duct (>6 mm diameter) with or without associated strictures, a drainage procedure of the duct is indicated. Conversely, if the duct is small (<6 mm diameter), resectional surgery should be considered. Because of the relatively poor results in this latter group of patients and the morbidity of pancreatic resection, it should be considered only as a last resort.

PANCREATIC DUCTAL DRAINAGE

In patients with disabling pain and ERCP evidence of a dilated pancreatic duct, pancreatic ductal drainage is the procedure of choice. The best operation is longitudinal pancreaticojejunostomy, also known as the modified Puestow procedure (Fig. 18.4).[58,59] In this operation, the anterior surface of the pancreas is exposed, and the location of the duct identified. The duct is opened longitudinally for most of its length. Stones and debris are removed as possible. An anastamosis is constructed between a Roux-en-Y limb of proxi-

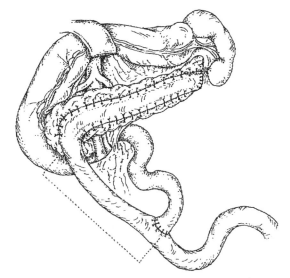

FIGURE 18.4. Longitudinal pancreaticojejunostomy (Puestow procedure). A 45-cm-long Roux-en-Y limb of jejunum is brought through the mesocolon for a side-to-side anastamosis with the dilated pancreatic duct. This technique is useful in patients with chronic pancreatitis, pain, and a dilated ductal system. Results are poorer in nondilated (<6-mm) ducts.

mal jejunum and the pancreatic duct, usually in two layers. Operative mortality rates for this operation are low, ranging from 0% to 4%. Relief of pain occurs in 80% to 90% of patients when assessed within the first year, and in most series this is maintained at 5-year follow-up. Patients who cease consuming alcohol clearly do better than those who persist. Ductal drainage may prevent or delay further loss of exocrine or endocrine function.[60] Results from recent published series with long-term (>5-year) follow-up are shown in Table 18.8.

Recent enthusiasm has been expressed for endoscopic pancreatic ductal stent placement to relieve pain in chronic pancreatitis. In early series, about 50% of patients experienced clinical improvement in short-term follow-up.[61,62] To date, no randomized data exist to document a benefit of endoscopic stenting over standard therapy.

RESECTIONAL SURGERY FOR CHRONIC PANCREATITIS

In a subset of patients with disabling pain and chronic pancreatitis, resection is appropriate. In general, resection is favored only for those patients with small ducts in whom all nonoperative measures have failed. Enthusiasm for resectional surgery is tempered by the significant complication rates and relatively poor long-term results.

TABLE 18.8.

Results of Longitudinal Pancreaticojejunostomy for Chronic Pancreatitis (Level III Evidence).

Reference	Number of patients	Operative mortality rate (%)	Pain relief	Comment
Partington, Cleveland, 1960[58]	7	0	Excellent in 4 of 7 patients	Partington and Rochelle modified the Puestow procedure by creating a longitudinal anastamosis between the pancreas and jejunum
Warshaw, Massachusetts General Hospital, 1980[122]	10	0	8 of 10 with substantial relief	Diabetes in 3 of 10 preoperatively and 5 of 10 postoperatively
Prinz, Chicago, 1981[123]	100	4	80%	Diabetes present preoperatively in 30% and developed postoperatively in another 14%
Holmberg, Sweden, 1985[124]	51	0	Good to excellent in 65% of drinkers and 88% of abstinent patients	Mean 8-yr follow-up
Munn, Chicago, 1987[125]	61	2	84% of patients obtained pain relief	39% of patients had pseudocysts
Bradley, Emory, 1987[126]	46	0	Good 28% Fair 38% Poor 34%	8 late deaths at mean follow-up of 69 months
Nealon, Galveston, 1988[127]	41	0	Pain relief in 93%	87% of patients had postoperative weight gain; 16% had progression of pancreatitis
Greenlee, Chicago, 1990[128]	50	2	Complete in 42% Substantial in 40%	Follow-up, 7.9 years
Adams, South Carolina, 1994[129]	85	0	"Good" in 24% "Fair" in 31% "Poor" in 45% Narcotic dependence in 35%	Diabetes requiring insulin in 23% of patients 42% continued to drink
Rios, Charleston, 1988[130]	17	0	Poor 76%	All with small duct disease
Lucas, Detroit, 1999[131]	124	2/124	Substantial in 39% Complete in 61%	Diabetes in 13/124 preop and 16/124 postop

SPLANCHNICECTOMY, CELIAC GANGLIONECTOMY, AND PERCUTANEOUS CELIAC PLEXUS BLOCK

Nerve block or ablation procedures have had limited success in the management of patients with chronic pancreatitis.

OBSTRUCTION OF ADJACENT HOLLOW VISCERA

The most common adjacent hollow viscus affected by chronic pancreatitis is the intrapancreatic portion of the common bile duct, which occurs in 5% to 10% of patients.[47] The usual cause is fibrosis of the pancreatic parenchyma in the head of the gland, although on occasion the obstruction is due to pseudocyst. ERCP or MRCP examinations reveal the abnormality. CT or MRI is helpful to exclude an underlying carcinoma. Endoscopic papillotomy or stenting is seldom curative. Jaundiced patients should be treated with choledochoduodenostomy. Thought should be given to the possibility of carcinoma, and brushings and biopsies are obtained as warranted.

Pancreatic Pseudocysts

Pseudocysts are among the most common complications of acute and chronic pancreatitis, occurring in 2% to 10% of patients.

Terminology

Pancreatic pseudocysts are abnormal collections of fluid arising in the setting of acute or chronic pancreatitis, or trauma; they can be located within the substance of the pancreas, adjacent to the gland, or even some distance away. An occasional pseudocyst is found extending through the pelvis into the groin or cephalad into the mediastinum. They contain fluid rich in pancreatic secretions from a duct system disrupted by inflammation or trauma, or obstructed by a stricture or stone. Pseudocysts differ from true cysts in that they lack an epithelial lining and have walls composed of adjacent organs, fibrosis, and inflammatory granulation tissue.

Clinical Presentation

The most common symptom associated with pseudocysts is abdominal pain, which is present in 80% to 90% of patients. The pain can be associated with chronic pancreatitis, or can persist or recur after a bout of acute pancreatitis. Nausea, vomiting, early satiety, and weight loss are also common. Physical examination may reveal abdominal tenderness, a palpable epigastric mass (found in about 50% of patients), fever, jaundice, and ascites. The presenting signs and symptoms can be related to the mass effect of the pseudocyst itself, or from a complication of the pseudocyst. Complications arising from pseudocysts include hemorrhage, rupture, infection, or obstruction. Decisions regarding the advisability of treating a pseudocyst must balance the possibility of spontaneous resolution with observation against the risk of development of one of these potentially life-threatening complications.

Treatment of Pseudocysts

Today, intervention for pseudocysts includes four main treatment options: percutaneous drainage, endoscopic drainage, laparotomy with internal drainage, or laparoscopic internal drainage. Occasionally, external drainage may be required via laparotomy. Resection is rarely indicated.

Pancreatic Cancer

Background

Carcinoma of the pancreas is an uncommon tumor, constituting only 2% of newly reported malignancies in the United States in 1995, but it accounts for 5% of cancer deaths.[63] This rate makes pancreatic cancer the fourth leading cause of cancer death in males and the fifth leading cause in females in the United States, behind lung, breast, prostate, colorectal, and ovarian cancer. Surgery remains the only curative treatment.

The cause of pancreatic cancer is unknown.[64] Only a handful of epidemiological factors have been associated with pancreatic cancer, and they play a role in a minority of patients. Cigarette smoking, for example, is associated with a statistically significant increase in risk of pancreatic cancer, about fourfold above nonsmokers.[65] Chronic pancreatitis similarly is associated with an increased risk.[64,66] The relationship of diabetes to pancreas cancer is complex, as it may either be a primary risk factor or arise as a result of the cancer. Prior gastrectomy is a minor risk factor for pancreatic cancer.[67]

Progress in our understanding of the molecular basis of cancer has helped define genetic abnormalities underlying these tumors in some patients.[68] Mutations in K-ras oncogene have been described in as many as 75% of patients.[69,70] Other oncogenes, such as C-erb B-12, HER2/neu, and Bcl-2, are also overexpressed in patients with pancreatic cancer.[71,72] Loss of p53 tumor suppressor function may be present in one-half of cases.[70,71] Similarly, mutations of the p16[73,74] and DPC4[75] tumor suppressor genes have been described.

Clinical Presentation

Pancreatic cancer unfortunately develops insidiously, and the majority of patients have advanced disease at the time of diagnosis. About 70% of tumors develop in the head of the gland, a location that often leads to stricture of the intrapancreatic portion of the common bile duct and the development of jaundice. The typical yellow discoloration of the sclera and skin is accompanied by dark, cola-colored urine and pale, clay-colored stools. Pruritis is a common and troubling symptom. In small, early tumors, the jaundice is painless, but larger, advanced lesions invade retroperitoneal nerves and cause abdominal and back pain. Weight loss is common, particularly in advanced lesions. Diabetes occurs in association with pancreatic cancer in about 20% of cases.[76] In about 15% of cases, the tumor produces distortion of the duodenum, causing symptoms suggestive of gastric outlet obstruction. Rarely, acute pancreatitis caused by pancreatic duct obstruction is the first sign of the presence of the tumor. Thus, in patients with acute pancreatitis and no clear underlying inciting event such as gallstones or alcohol ingestion, ERCP is useful to exclude an anatomical lesion.[77] Tumors of the body and tail do not typically involve the bile duct and seldom present with jaundice. These tumors grow until they involve splanchnic nerves, at which time the patient experiences a dull, visceral pain in the epigastrium radiating into the back.

Physical examination of the patient with pancreatic cancer typically reveals jaundice. The tumor itself is rarely palpable. Weight loss is often evident on examination. In body and tail lesions, splenic vein thrombosis is common and splenomegaly may be detected on examination. Advanced lesions may present with lymphadenopathy palpable in the left supraclavicular fossa (Virchow's node) or periumbilical area (Sister Mary Joseph's node). Carcinomatosis may reveal itself by the presence of ascites, palpable tumor in the omentum, or pelvic tumor palpable on rectal examination (Blumer's shelf). Extra-abdominal signs of pancreatic cancer include deep venous thrombosis and migratory thrombophlebitis.

Diagnostic Evaluation

In the typical patient with painless jaundice, the initial goal is to differentiate obstructive jaundice from disorders of hepatocyte function, such as hepatitis. Evaluation of the liver function tests is helpful (Table 18.9). When the clinical picture and pattern of blood test abnormality suggest obstructive jaundice, an imaging study of the biliary tree should be obtained. The two most commonly used screening studies today are ultrasound and computed tomography (CT). Ultrasound has the advantages of being easily obtainable, inexpensive, and highly accurate for the diagnosis of gallstones. If the clinical suspicion is of obstructive jaundice related to gallstone passage, a right upper quadrant ultrasound is the best approach. On the other hand, if the clinical picture is more suggestive of malignancy, such as the elderly patient with a prolonged duration of symptoms, associated weight loss, and markedly elevated bilirubin, CT has advantages over ultrasound.

If the CT does not clearly identify the obstructing lesion, ERCP usually identifies its location and extent in the bile duct.[78,79] Classically, pancreatic cancer is recognized at ERCP by the "double duct sign" where the tumor, arising in the pancreatic duct, eventually grows to also obstruct the bile duct in

its intrapancreatic portion.[80] The sensitivity of ERCP in the diagnosis of pancreatic cancer is greater than 90%, but it should be recognized that small tumors and lesions in the uncinate process may be difficult to identify.

Today, magnetic resonance cholangiopancreatography (MRCP) is finding a role in hepatopancreaticobiliary imaging.[48,55] As the quality of the images improves, MRCP has the potential to replace diagnostic ERCP, as it is cheaper, safer, and less invasive.

Endoscopic ultrasonography has high reported sensitivity in the diagnosis of pancreatic cancer and can also help in staging, particularly in the assessment of the relationship of the tumor to the superior mesenteric and portal veins.[2,81] Directed biopsies of the pancreatic head lesions for cytological analysis can be obtained with an endoscopic needle, using endoscopic ultrasonography for guidance.

Additional staging studies may be warranted before treatment is begun. All patients should have a chest X-ray to exclude pulmonary metastases and occult cardiopulmonary disease that may affect the risk of operation. Nuclear medicine bone scans are appropriate for patients with new onset of bone pain. The frequency of bony metastases in the absence of advanced intraabdominal disease is low, however, making bone scans unnecessary as a routine preoperative measure. Similarly, head CT examinations to exclude brain metastases are indicated in patients with new onset of neurological symptoms, but are unnecessary as a routine screening test.

Positon emission tomography (PET scanning) using labeled fluorodeoxyglucose-18 (^{18}FDG) has a potential role in identifying occult metastatic disease before treatment in patients with pancreatic cancer.

Treatment of Patients with Pancreatic Cancer

PREOPERATIVE BILIARY DRAINAGE

The development of transhepatic and endoscopic techniques for biliary drainage in the 1980s led to the hypothesis that

TABLE 18.9. Evaluation of Liver Function Tests in Jaundice.

Test	Source	Pattern in gallstone obstruction of the biliary tree	Pattern in malignant obstruction of the biliary tree	Pattern in acute hepatitis
Total bilirubin	Red blood cell destruction, hepatocyte processing	Elevated, but typically less than 10 mg/dl	Elevated, commonly more than 10 mg/dl	Elevated
Direct bilirubin	Conjugation by hepatocytes	Elevated	Markedly elevated	Mildly elevated
Indirect bilirubin	Red blood cell turnover, hepatocyte processing	Minimally elevated	Elevated	Elevated
Alkaline phosphatase	Biliary epithelial cells and bone	Elevated	Markedly elevated	Minimally elevated
Transaminases	Hepatocytes	Minimally elevated	Minimally elevated	Markedly elevated
Gamma glutamyl transferase	Biliary epithelial cells	Elevated	Markedly elevated	Minimally elevated

preoperative drainage would improve the outcome of major biliary surgery. Results of those trials were disappointing, in that in general no reduction in operative morbidity or mortality was achieved with preoperative drainage (Table 18.10). These data suggest that, as a routine, preoperative drainage is not advisable.

RESECTION WITH CURATIVE INTENT

Surgical resection is the only potentially curative treatment for pancreatic cancer. For lesions arising in the head of the gland, the four main surgical options are the standard Whipple pancreaticoduodenectomy, pylorus-preserving pancreati-

TABLE 18.10.

Studies Examining Preoperative Biliary Decompression before Resective Surgery for Periampullary Cancer.

Reference	Patient group	Morbidity	Operative mortality rate	Comment
Level I Evidence (Randomized, controlled trials)				
Hatfield, 1982[132]	Preop transhepatic drainage (n = 29) No drainage (n = 28)	Similar postoperative complication rates in the two groups. Substantial complications associated with drain placement.	14% 15%	Mean 12 days of preop drainage. No significant improvement in outcome.
McPherson, Royal Postgraduate Medical School, 1984[133]	Preop transhepatic drainage (n = 34) No drainage (n = 31)	5 patients required surgery for complications of preop drainage	32% 19%	Mean 18 days of drainage. No significant improvement in outcome.
Pitt, UCLA, 1985[134]	Preop transhepatic drainage (n = 37) No drainage (n = 38)	Overall morbidity 57% Overall morbidity 53%	8.1% 5.3%	Hospital stay = 31 days Hospital stay = 23 days (p < 0.005)
Lygidakis, 1987[135]	Preop endoscopic drainage (n = 19) No drainage (n = 19)	Decreased biliary pressure, biliary infection, bacteremia, and blood loss in preop drainage group	0% 10%	Mean delay in surgery of 11 days with preop drainage. This trial suggests benefit of drainage.
Lai, Hong Kong, 1994[136]	Preop endoscopic drainage (n = 43) Surgery alone (n = 44)	37% 41% (ns)	13.9% 13.6% (ns)	Stent insertion successful in 37 and effective in 25 patients No apparent benefit of preop drainage
Level III Evidence (Large, prospective, uncontrolled case series)				
Trede, Mannhein, 1988[137]	Resection in 285 patients Preoperative drainage in 82 patients	Relaparotomy for complications in 15% Pancreatic fistula in 9%. Postop hemorrhage in 5.6%	3.1%	No improvement with preop drainage
Bakkevold, Norway, 1993[138]	Total patients = 472 Resection = 108 Palliative surgery = 252 Preop drainage = 35	43% in patients undergoing resection 23% in patients after palliative surgery	11% in patients undergoing resection 14% in patients after palliative surgery	Prospective study. Preoperative drainage had no impact on the outcome of surgery
Karsten, Amsterdam, 1996[139]	Total patients = 241 Preop drainage = 184	Overall complication rate 57%, 56% with and 61% without preop drainage (p = 0.4)	6%	Bacterial contamination of bile increased with preop drainage
Povoski, Memorial Sloan-Kettering, 1999[140]	Preoperative biliary drainage (n = 126) No preoperative drainage (n = 114)	41% (p = 0.014) 25%	8% (p = 0.037) 3%	Retrospective review. Logistic regression showed increased mortality rate with preoperative drainage

codudenectomy, total pancreatectomy, and regional pancreatectomy. No convincing evidence demonstrates a survival advantage of one over another of these options. For lesions in the body and tail of the gland, distal pancreatectomy is the preferred approach.

The standard operation for periampullary malignancy, popularly known as the Whipple procedure, involves en bloc resection of the head of the pancreas to the neck overlying the portal vein, the duodenum, gallbladder, intrapancreatic portion of bile duct, and antrum with their associated lymph nodes. Reconstruction is via pancreaticojejunostomy, choledochojejunostomy, and gastrojejunostomy (Fig. 18.5). Case series of the pylorus preserving modification of this procedure have now shown survival rates that do not appear inferior to those following standard Whipple resection.[82,83]

The rationale for total pancreatectomy for carcinoma of the head of the pancreas is to eliminate multifocal disease, achieve wider lymphadenectomy, avoid spillage of tumor cells during transection of the pancreas, and avoid postoperative leakage from the pancreatic anastamosis. These theoretical advantages have not translated into improved operative mortality or long-term survival.

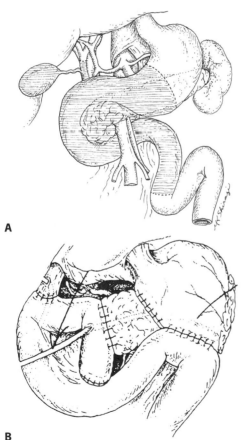

FIGURE 18.5. Pancreaticoduodectomy. **A.** Localized tumors of the head of the pancreas, proximal duodenum, and distal bile duct are treated with pancreaticoduodenectomy. The classic operation includes an en bloc distal gastrectomy, duodenectomy, cholecystectomy, bile duct excision, and pancreatic head resection. Smaller tumors not involving the region of the first part of the duodenum can be treated with a pylorus-preserving resection in which the antrum and pylorus are spared. **B.** Reconstruction following resection typically includes pancreaticojejunostomy, choledochojejunostomy, and duodenojejunostomy.

Regional pancreatectomy for carcinoma of the pancreas, including en bloc total or subtotal pancreatectomy with radical lymph node dissection and portal vein resection have not indicated that survival with this approach is superior to that achieved with standard resection.

It remains unclear whether or not extended lymphadenectomy alone improves survival in pancreatic cancer.

ADJUVANT RADIATION AND CHEMOTHERAPY

The effect of adjuvant therapy on cure rates in pancreatic cancer is controversial.[84] It is known that about half of resected patients recur regionally in the absence of distant metastases, suggesting a potentially important role for postoperative adjuvant radiation therapy.[85] However, no conclusive studies support this approach. Similarly, intraoperative radiation therapy has been examined as an adjunct to resection and postoperative external beam radiation, but no data conclusively show a survival benefit.[86,87] In some trials intraoperative radiotherapy has been associated with high complication rates that may obviate any beneficial effects on tumor growth.[88] In unresectable patients, intraoperative radiation therapy may improve local tumor control and pain management.

Preliminary studies have examined the safety of preoperative (neoadjuvant) radiation and chemotherapy in patients with potentially resectable carcinoma of the pancreas.[89,90] No randomized data have been published. Recent data suggest that locoregional control of tumor is enhanced by preoperative chemoradiation but that the majority of patients still succumb to systemic disease.[90,91]

CANCER OF THE PANCREATIC BODY AND TAIL

Typically, patients with adenocarcinoma of the body and tail of the gland present with advanced disease, oft times unresectable, and have poor prognosis. The resectability rate averages 10%. In general, patients with body and tail lesions should be approached in the same manner as those with the more common lesion of the head of the gland; those without evidence of metastatic disease or vascular invasion should be considered candidates for resection. Preliminary laparoscopy may be useful in identifying occult liver or peritoneal metastases and avoiding unnecessary laparotomy.

PALLIATIVE TREATMENT

The majority of patients with pancreatic cancer present with either locally advanced disease or metastases, making cure impossible at the present time. In this group of patients, the treatment goal is palliative. Palliative treatment has two main goals: first, to improve the quality of the patient's life and, second, to increase lifespan. Quality of life is markedly affected by cancer pain, as well as by complications of the tumor such as biliary or gastric obstruction. Asymptomatic patients cannot be made to feel better by aggressive, ill-advised therapy.

PAIN RELIEF

Careful attention should be paid to pain relief, as evidence suggests that survival is prolonged when pain is well controlled.[92] Nonsteroidal antiinflammatory agents, oral and transdermal narcotics, and celiac plexus blocks are the main strategies.

RELIEF OF BILIARY OBSTRUCTION

Biliary obstruction is a common presentation of pancreatic malignancy. Options in palliation include surgical bypass, endoscopic stenting, and transhepatic stenting. Patients expected to live longer than 6 months, or those requiring gastrojejunostomy for duodenal obstruction, are probably best treated operatively. Those with widespread metastatic disease, and especially those with ascites and carcinomatosis, are best treated with stents.

RELIEF OR PREVENTION OF DUODENAL OBSTRUCTION

Duodenal obstruction occurs in 10% to 20% of patients with pancreatic cancer.[93] The main palliative method is gastrojejunostomy, which can be accomplished laparoscopically or via open laparotomy. Data suggest that prophylactic gastrojejunostomy is indicated in patients with unresectable periampullary malignancy undergoing laparotomy. For patients with known unresectable tumors complicated by gastric outlet obstruction, laparoscopic gastrojejunostomy is a reasonable option. No randomized, controlled data comparing open to laparoscopic bypass are available. Endoscopic duodenal stenting can be considered for patients at high risk for surgery.

PROLONGATION OF SURVIVAL

Palliative radiation and chemotherapy have a limited role in patients with unresectable pancreatic cancer. A number of chemotherapy regimens for patients with advanced pancreatic cancer have been studied, but objective response rates are low.[94,95] The role of radiation therapy in patients with unresectable pancreatic cancer is controversial.

Prognosis

A number of clinical and pathological factors have been shown to significantly predict prognosis. Recent series suggest 5-year survival is possible in about 20% of resected patients (Table 18.11).

CLINICAL FACTORS

SYMPTOMS

Pancreatic cancer tends to grow insidiously, making late presentation common. Features on presentation such as back pain, abdominal pain, and weight loss suggest an advanced lesion, making resection less likely. Deep jaundice is known to increase the operative risk, but does not appear to affect long-term survival if the cancer is resectable.[96–98] Other features, such as abdominal pain, steatorrhea, and thrombophlebitis, have not been shown to influence long-term survival.[97] Weight loss, long duration of symptoms, and the presence of anemia, while implying long-standing disease, were not predictors of long-term survival by univariate analysis if the patient could undergo resection.[96]

BLOOD TRANSFUSION

A significant association between the use of perioperative blood transfusion and poorer survival has been identified. The reason for this relationship is not certain, but it has been proposed that blood transfusion induces immunosuppression, which increases the risk of tumor recurrence.

DEMOGRAPHICS

Patient demographic factors do not play strong roles in predicting prognosis following treatment of pancreatic cancer.

EFFECT OF RESIDUAL DISEASE

In large series of patients with pancreatic cancer, one of the strongest factors predicting survival is complete resection.[83,99] Population studies show that resection offers survival rates approximately twofold greater than palliative bypass procedures.[100]

PATHOLOGICAL FACTORS

HISTOLOGICAL TYPE

Ductal adenocarcinoma is the most common type of pancreatic cancer, accounting for 90% to 95% of cases. Pancreatic

TABLE 18.11.

Survival Following Pancreaticoduodenectomy for Pancreatic Adenocarcinoma: Recent Trials.

Reference	Number of patients	Operative mortality (%)	Median survival	Five-year survival	Comments
Trede, 1990, Mannheim[141]	n = 118	0	Not reported	36% in 76 patients with R0(−) resections; actual survival = 25%	One of the best reports of survival for pancreatic adenocarcinoma
Nitecki, Mayo Clinic, 1995[98]	n = 186	3	17.5 months	6.8% (23% in subgroup with negative nodes)	12 patients initially classified as ductal adenocarcinoma found to have other diagnoses on re-review Mean follow-up = 22 months
Nagakawa, Japan, 1996[142]	n = 53	9.4	13 months	27.4%	Survival for GI cancers tends to be better in Japan than in Western series
Conlon, Memorial Sloan-Kettering, 1996[143]	n = 118	3.4	14.3 months	10.2%	Resection for cure possible in 17% of all patients
Yeo, Johns Hopkins, 1997[144]	n = 174	0.6	19.5 months with adjuvant therapy; 13.5 months without	Five-year survival not reported (36% 2-year survival)	Apparent improvement in survival with adjuvant chemoradiation

ductal adenocarcinoma is thought to arise directly from ductal epithelium, progressing through dysplasia and carcinoma in situ to invasive carcinoma, and its growth pattern typically includes the formation of ductal structures. A number of subtypes of ductal adenocarcinoma have been described, including mucinous noncystic carcinoma, signet ring cell carcinoma, adenosquamous carcinoma, mixed ductalendocrine carcinoma, and anaplastic carcinoma. No significant differences in biological behavior or prognosis among different subtypes of ductal carcinoma have been identified.[101]

Certain other histological types of epithelial tumors of the pancreas are regarded as being both morphologically and biologically distinct from ductal adenocarcinoma. Included in this group are carcinomas with acinar cell differentiation (i.e., acinar cell carcinoma, acinar cell cystadenocarcinoma, and mixed acinar-endocrine carcinoma) and tumors with neuroendocrine differentiation (i.e., tumors formerly known as islet cell tumors and now more commonly termed pancreatic endocrine tumors). Acinar cell carcinomas are typically associated with aggressive biological behavior and poor prognosis. Pancreatic endocrine tumors vary widely in their biological behavior from benign to highly virulent but lack reliable histological indicators of malignancy. Also included in this group of unique epithelial malignancies are intraductal mucinous papillary carcinoma and mucinous cystadenocarcinoma, both of which are associated with a better overall prognosis compared to ductal adenocarcinoma. Intraductal papillary-mucinous carcinoma (known clinically as mucinous ductal ectasia) is a pancreatic ductal neoplasm that displays indolent behavior compared to typical ductal adenocarcinoma. Mucinous cyst-adenocarcinomas also appear to arise in most cases from benign precursor lesions called mucinous cystic neoplasms (mucinous cystadenomas). Arguably, the overall favorable prognosis of mucinous cystadenocarcinomas compared to ductal adenocarcinoma may be related to earlier clinical presentation secondary to symptoms created largely by the precursor lesion.

HISTOLOGICAL GRADE

Grading of ductal adenocarcinomas is somewhat subjective, and reports on the prognostic significance of histological grade in pancreatic cancer often conflict. In most studies, a three- or four-tiered grading system is usually employed, as follows: grade 1 = well differentiated; grade 2 = moderately differentiated; grade 3 = poorly differentiated; and grade 4 = undifferentiated. Histological grade is an expression of the relative degree of structural and functional differentiation of the tumor and is typically based on the amount of gland (duct) formation and mucin production. In one multivariate analysis in which histological grade was found to have independent prognostic significance, the 5-year survival was 50% for well-differentiated carcinomas and 10% for poorly differentiated carcinomas.[102]

PATHOLOGICAL TUMOR STAGE

The stage of disease is currently the most powerful predictor of outcome among all defined prognostic factors in pancreatic cancer. The recognition of the direct strong relationship between stage of disease and outcome led to the development of the TNM staging system (Table 18.12).[103] Currently, the observed postoperative 5-year survival following resection is about 38%, 15%, 10%, and 4% for stages I, II, III, and IV, respectively.[104]

TABLE 18.12. AJCC Definition of TNM and Stage Groupings for Staging of Pancreatic Adenocarcinoma.

Primary Tumor (T)

TX	Primary tumor cannot be assessed
T0	No evidence of primary tumor
Tis	Carcinoma *in situ**
T1	Tumor limited to the pancreas 2 cm or less in greatest dimension
T2	Tumor limited to the pancreas, more than 2 cm in greatest dimension
T3	Tumor extends beyond the pancreas but without involvement of the celiac axis or the superior mesenteric artery
T4	Tumor involves the celiac axis or the superior mesenteric artery

Regional Lymph Nodes (N)

NX	Regional lymph nodes cannot be assessed
N0	No regional lymph node metastasis
N1	Regional lymph node metastasis

Distant Metastasis (M)

MX	Distant metastasis cannot be assessed
M0	No distant metastasis
M1	Distant metastasis

*This also includes the "PanInIII" classification

Stage Grouping

0	Tis	N0	M0
IA	T1	N0	M0
IB	T2	N0	M0
II	T3	N0	M0
IIB	T1	N1	M0
	T2	N1	M0
	T3	N1	M0
III	T4	Any N	M0
IV	Any T	Any N	M1

Source: Used with permission of the American Joint Committee on Cancer (AJCC), Chicago, IL. The original source for this material is the AJCC Cancer Staging Manual, 6th Ed., published by Springer-Verlag, www.springer-ny.com. The above classification will be implemented in January 2003.

Cystic Tumors of the Pancreas

Cystic tumors of the pancreas are relatively uncommon, but are important, both because they generally have a better prognosis than solid pancreatic tumors and because they can be confused with pancreatic pseudocysts. Overall, about 80% of pancreatic cystic lesions are pseudocysts, and the minority, about 20%, are the lesions discussed in this section. Pseudocysts can generally be distinguished from other cystic lesions by the clinical situation in which they arise and by their radiographic appearance. When the clinician is uncertain as to the nature of the lesion, biopsy of the cyst wall with examination of its lining for epithelial elements is useful, as these elements are absent in pseudocysts but present in other cystic lesions. Cyst fluid analysis has limited usefulness in distinguishing among the diagnostic possibilities.[105,106]

Simple (Congenital) Cysts

Simple cysts are thought to be congenital and are usually found in children. They have no malignant potential. In adults, they cannot reliably be differentiated from mucinous cystadenomas radiographically; thus, when identified, they are best treated with excision.

Retention Cysts

Cysts can occur from obstruction of the pancreatic duct, as in pancreatitis, with progressive dilatation of the obstructed segment of duct. Most arise in the setting of chronic pancreatitis with ductal stricture or, less commonly, from an obstructing pancreatic cancer. Communication with the ductal system may be evident on endoscopic retrograde cholangiopancreatography.

Polycystic Disease of the Pancreas

Multiple pancreatic cysts can be present in association with polycystic kidney and liver disease, cystic fibrosis, and von Hippel–Lindau disease. About 10% of patients with polycystic kidney disease have pancreatic cysts, which generally are small, asymptomatic, and do not require specific treatment.

Serous Cystadenoma

Serous cystadenomas are benign cystic tumors, seen most often in middle-aged women, that average about 6 cm in size at the time of presentation. Symptoms commonly include vague abdominal pain. Jaundice and weight loss are rare. Radiographic assessment is key to their diagnosis. By ultrasonography, they generally appear as a complex low-density mass composed of multiple small cysts separated by fine septae. Computed tomography shows a similar appearance and may identify a central stellate calcification in a "sunburst" pattern. Treatment is excision; formal pancreatectomy is generally not required.

Mucinous Cystic Neoplasms

Mucinous cystic neoplasms are important to differentiate from serous cystadenomas because of the potential for malignancy in the former. The clinical presentation is similar to serous cystadenomas, with an apparent female preponderance. Most patients present with nonspecific abdominal pain, bloating, or an incidentally discovered mass. Jaundice is uncommon. Ultrasonography or computed tomography shows a large cystic mass similar in appearance to a pseudocyst. Unlike pseudocysts, however, patients with mucinous cystic neoplasms do not generally have a history of acute or chronic pancreatitis.[107]

Treatment of mucinous cystic neoplasms is resection, including a margin of normal pancreas. The prognosis is generally good. In about 25% of cases, areas of malignancy will be identified in the cyst wall. Overall survival appears to be about 70% at 5 years.

Cystadenocarcinoma

Cystadenocarcinoma is the end stage of mucinous cystic neoplasm. These lesions tend to present as bulky cystic masses with irregular walls in the head or body of the pancreas. These lesions do not tend to be as invasive as typical ductal adenocarcinoma, and even bulky lesions may not invade the portal vein or hepatic artery. Treatment is resection. In the recent French multiinstitutional review of cystic neoplasms, the 5-year survival rate for patients with cystadenocarcinoma of the pancreas was 63%.[108]

Solid and Cystic Papillary Neoplasm of the Pancreas

This papillary neoplasm is a rare lesion, typically arising in young women. The lesions tend to be large, averaging 10 cm in diameter. Most patients present with abdominal pain, and in many cases the lesions are confused with pseudocysts. Jaundice is rare. Computed tomography shows a large mass with heterogeneous solid and cystic components. Treatment is resection.

Intraductal Papillary Mucinous Tumors

This is a rare lesion, but increasingly recognized today. Most patients present with features of pancreatitis, probably from ductal obstruction. Computed tomography demonstrates a cystic pancreatic mass, which may represent either ductal distension or an associated mucinous cystic neoplasm. Endoscopic retrograde cholangiopancreatography is key to the diagnosis, and reveals extrusion of mucous through the papilla, a dilated and irregular ductal system, and filling defects within the duct.

Treatment of intraductal papillary mucinous tumor is with surgical recection. Although some cases have successfully been treated with local excision, because of its malignant potential, formal pancreatectomy is the preferred option. The prognosis is good, with better long-term survival than typical ductal adenocarcinoma.[109,110]

Other Tumors

Pancreatic Lymphoma

Pancreatic lymphomas are rare, especially as an isolated lesion.[111,112] More commonly, the pancreas is involved in non-Hodgkin's lymphoma as an incidental part of advanced intraabdominal and extraabdominal disease. Pancreatic lymphomas tend to present as bulky lesions with nonspecific symptoms, such as abdominal pain. These tumors respond favorably to radiation and chemotherapy. Thus, suspicion of such a lesion warrants percutaneous fine-needle aspiration biopsy, as a diagnosis of lymphoma makes surgical resection unnecessary.

Adenosquamous Carcinoma

These tumors are rare, accounting for about 1% of pancreatic tumors. They are also known as squamous carcinoma of the pancreas, adenoacanthomas, or mucoepidermoid cancers. Generally, these lesions cannot be distinguished from the more common ductal adenocarcinoma on the basis of clinical or radiographic criteria. Treatment is resection, but the prognosis is poor. In a recent review of the reported literature, summarizing 134 patients, the average survival was only 5.7 months.[113] Radiation and chemotherapy appear relatively ineffective.

Pancreatic Sarcomas

Pancreatic sarcomas are rare lesions, usually presenting as a bulky solid lesion in the body of the gland. Metastatic disease is commonly present at the time of diagnosis. Radical distal pancreatectomy and splenectomy is warranted for lesions in the body and tail of the gland. Pancreaticoduodenectomy is indicated for lesions of the head of the gland.

References

1. Skandalakis LJ, Rowe JS, Jr., Gray SW, et al. Surgical embryology and anatomy of the pancreas. Surg Clin North Am 1993; 73(4):661–697.
2. Brugge WR, Van Dam J. Pancreatic and biliary endoscopy. N Engl J Med 1999;341:1808–1816.
3. Cotton PB. Pancreas divisum—curiosity or culprit? Gastroenterology 1985;89(6):1431–1435.
4. Debas HT, Mulvihill SJ. Neuroendocrine design of the gut. Am J Surg 1991;161(2):243–249.
5. Kozarek RA, Ball TJ, Patterson DJ, et al. Endoscopic approach to pancreas divisum. Dig Dis Sci 1995;40(9):1974–1981.
6. Bernard JP, Sahel J, Giovannini M, et al. Pancreas divisum is a probable cause of acute pancreatitis: a report of 137 cases [see comments]. Pancreas 1990;5(3):248–254.
7. Delhaye M, Engelholm L, Cremer M. Pancreas divisum: congenital anatomic variant or anomaly? Contribution of endoscopic retrograde dorsal pancreatography. Gastroenterology 1985;89(5):951–958.
8. Richter JM, Schapiro RH, Mulley AG, et al. Association of pancreas divisum and pancreatitis, and its treatment by sphincteroplasty of the accessory ampulla. Gastroenterology 1981;81(6):1104–1110.
9. Murakami G, Hirata K, Takamuro T, et al. Vascular anatomy of the pancreaticoduodenal region: a review. J Hepato-Biliary-Pancreatic Surg 1999;6(1):55–68.
10. Furukawa H, Iwata R, Moriyama N, et al. Blood supply to the pancreatic head, bile duct, and duodenum. Arch Surg 1999;134: 1086–1090.
11. Pansky B. Anatomy of the pancreas. Emphasis on blood supply and lymphatic drainage. Int J Pancreatol 1990;7(1–3):101–108.
12. Liddle RA. Regulation of cholecystokinin secretion by intraluminal releasing factors. Am J Physiol 1995;269(3):G319–G327.
13. Nelson MT, Debas HT, Mulvihill SJ. Vagal stimulation of rat exocrine pancreatic secretion occurs via multiple mediators. Gastroenterology 1993;105(1):221–218.
14. Mulvihill SJ, Bunnett NW, Goto Y, et al. Somatostatin inhibits pancreatic exocrine secretion via a neural mechanism. Metabolism 1990;39(9 suppl 2):143–148.
15. Bank, PA. Practice guidelines in acute pancreatitis. Am J Gastroenterol 1997;92:377–386.
16. Bradley ELD. A clinically based classification system for acute pancreatitis. Summary of the International Symposium on Acute Pancreatitis, Atlanta, GA, September 11–13, 1992. Arch Surg 1993;128(5):584–590.
17. Allam BF, Imrie CW. Serum ionized calcium in acute pancreatitis. Br J Surg 1977;64(9):665–668.
18. Goodman AJ, Neoptolemos JP, Carr-Locke DL, et al. Detection of gall stones after acute pancreatitis. Gut 1985;26(2):125–132.
19. Ranson JH, Rifkind KM, Turner JW. Prognostic signs and nonoperative peritoneal lavage in acute pancreatitis. Surg Gynecol Obstet 1976;143(2):209–219.
20. Ranson JH, Rifkind KM, Roses DF, et al. Prognostic signs and the role of operative management in acute pancreatitis. Surg Gynecol Obstet 1974;139(1):69–81.
21. De Sanctis JT, Lee MJ, Gazelle GS, et al. Prognostic indicators in acute pancreatitis: CT vs APACHE II. Clin Radiol 1997;52(11): 842–848.
22. Balthazar EJ, Freeny PC, vanSonnenberg E. Imaging and intervention in acute pancreatitis. Radiology 1994;193(2):297–306.
23. Balthazar EJ, Robinson DL, Megibow AJ, et al. Acute pancreatitis: value of CT in establishing prognosis. Radiology 1990;174(2): 331–336.
24. Steinberg W, Tenner S. Acute pancreatitis. N Engl J Med 1994;330(17):1198–1210.
25. Sarr MG, Sanfey H, Cameron JL. Prospective, randomized trial of nasogastric suction in patients with acute pancreatitis. Surgery (St. Louis) 1986;100(3):500–504.
26. Soper NJ, Brunt LM, Callery MP, et al. Role of laparoscopic cholecystectomy in the management of acute gallstone pancreatitis. Am J Surg 1994;167(1):42–50.
27. Tang E, Stain SC, Tang G, et al. Timing of laparoscopic surgery in gallstone pancreatitis. Arch Surg 1995;130(5):496–499.
28. Carr-Locke DL. Role of endoscopy in gallstone pancreatitis. [Review.] Am J Surg 1993;165(4):519–521.
29. Miller RE, Kimmelstiel FM, Winkler WP. Management of common bile duct stones in the era of laparoscopic cholecystectomy. Am J Surg 1995;169(2):273–276.
30. Karimgani I, Porter KA, Langevin RE, et al. Prognostic factors in sterile pancreatic necrosis [see comments]. Gastroenterology 1992;103(5):1636–1640.
31. Gerzof SG, Banks PA, Robbins AH, et al. Early diagnosis of pancreatic infection by computed tomography-guided aspiration. Gastroenterology 1987;93(6):1315–1320.
32. Uomo G, Visconti M, Manes G, et al. Nonsurgical treatment of acute necrotizing pancreatitis. Pancreas 1996;12(2):142–148.
33. Ho HS, Frey CF. Gastrointestinal and pancreatic complications associated with severe pancreatitis. Arch Surg 1995;130(8):817–822; discussion 822–883.
34. Beger HG, Büchler M, Bittner R, et al. Necrosectomy and postoperative local lavage in necrotizing pancreatitis. Br J Surg 1988;75(3):207–212.
35. Mithofer K, Fernandez-del Castillo C, Ferraro MJ, et al. Antibiotic treatment improves survival in experimental acute necrotizing pancreatitis. Gastroenterology 1996;110(1):232–240.
36. Golub R, Siddiqi F, Pohl D. Role of antibiotics in acute pancreatitis: a meta-analysis. J Gastrointest Surg 1998;2(6):496–503.
37. Bittner R, Block S, Büchler M, et al. Pancreatic abscess and infected pancreatic necrosis. Different local septic complications in acute pancreatitis. Dig Dis Sci 1987;32(10):1082–1087.
38. vanSonnenberg E, Wittich GR, Chon KS, et al. Percutaneous radiologic drainage of pancreatic abscesses. AJR 1997;168(4):979–984.
39. Bradley ELD, Allen K. A prospective longitudinal study of observation versus surgical intervention in the management of necrotizing pancreatitis. Am J Surg 1991;161(1):19–24; discussion 24–25.
40. Frey DF. Management of necrotizing pancreatitis [see comments]. West J Med 1993;159(6):675–680.
41. Fernandez-del Castillo C, Rattner DW, Makary MA, et al. Debridement and closed packing for the treatment of necrotizing pancreatitis. Ann Surg 1998;228(5):676–684.
42. Bradley ELD. Mangement of infected pancreatic necrosis by open drainage. Ann Surg 1987;206(4):542–550.
43. Stanten R, Grey CF. Comprehensive management of acute necrotizing pancreatitis and pancreatic abscess. Arch Surg 1990; 125(10):1269–1274; discussion 1274–1275.
44. Tsiotos GG, Luque-de Leon E, Seoreide JA, et al. Management of necrotizing pancreatitis by repeated operative necrosectomy using a zipper technique. Am J Surg 1998;175(2):91–98.
45. Stroud WH, Cullom JW, Anderson MC. Hemorrhagic complications of severe pancreatitis. Surgery (St. Louis) 1981;90(4):657–665.
46. Shea JA, Berlin JA, Escarce JJ, et al. Revised estimates of diagnostic test sensitivity and specificity in suspected biliary tract disease. Arch Intern Med 1994;154(22):2573–2581.
47. Steer ML, Waxman I, Freedman S. Chronic pancreatitis. N Engl J Med 1995;332(22):1482–1490.
48. DiMagno EP. A short, eclectic history of exocrine pancreatic insufficiency and chronic pancreatitis. Gastroenterology 1993;104(5): 1255–1262.
49. Freedman SD, Sakamoto K, Venu RP. GP2, the homologue to the renal cast protein uromodulin, is a major component of intraductal plugs in chronic pancreatitis. J Clin Invest 1993;92(1):83–90.
50. Schmiegel W, Burchert M, Kalthoff H, et al. Immunochemical characterization and quantitative distribution of pancreatic stone protein in sera and pancreatic secretions in pancreatic disorders [see comments]. Gastroenterology 1990;99(5):1421–1430.

51. Sarles H, Camarena J, Bernard JP, et al. Two forms of hereditary chronic pancreatitis. Pancreas 1996;12(2):138–141.

52. Luetmer PH, Stephens DH, Ward EM. Chronic pancreatitis: reassessment with current CT. Radiology 1989;171(2):353–357.

53. Lankisch PG, Otto J, Erkelenz I, et al. Pancreatic calcifications: no indicator of severe exocrine pancreatic insufficiency. Gastroenterology 1986;90(3):617–621.

54. Barish MA, Yucel EK, Ferrucci JT. Magnetic resonance cholangiopancreatography. N Engl J Med 1999;341(4):258–264.

55. Soto JA, Barish MA, Yucel EK, et al. Magnetic resonance cholangiography: comparison with endoscopic retrograde cholangiopancreatography [see comments]. Gastroenterology 1996;110(2):589–597.

56. Axon AT, Classen M, Cotton PB, et al. Pancreatography in chronic pancreatitis: international definitions. Gut 1984;25(10):1107–1112.

57. Talamini G, Bassi C, Falconi M, et al. Pain relapses in the first 10 years of chronic pancreatitis. Am J Surg 1996;171(6):565–659.

58. Partington PF, Rochelle REL. Modified Puestow procedure for retrograde drainage of the pancreatic duct. Ann Surg 1960;152:1037–1043.

59. Puestow CB, Gillesby WJ. Retrograde surgical drainage of pancreas for chronic relapsing pancreatitis. Arch Surg 1958;76:898–907.

60. Nealon WH, Thompson JC. Progressive loss of pancreatic function in chronic pancreatitis is delayed by main pancreatic duct decompression. A longitudinal prospective analysis of the modified puestow procedure. Ann Surg 1993;217(5):458–466; discussion 466–468.

61. Cremer M, Deviere J, Delhaye M, et al. Stenting in severe chronic pancreatitis: results of medium-term follow-up in seventy-six patients. Endoscopy 1991;23(3):171–176.

62. Ponchon T, Bory RM, Hedelius F, et al. Endoscopic stenting for pain relief in chronic pancreatitis. Gastrointest Endosc 1995;42(5):452–456.

63. Wingo PA, Tong T, Bolden S. Cancer statistics, 1995 [published erratum appears in CA Cancer J Clin 1995;45(2):127–128]. CA: Cancer J Clin 1995;45(1):8–30.

64. Haddock G, Carter DC. Aetiology of pancreatic cancer [see comments]. Br J Surg 1990;77(10):1159–1166.

65. Olsen GW, Mandel JS, Gibson RW, et al. A case-control study of pancreatic cancer and cigarettes, alcohol, coffee and diet. Am J Public Health 1989;79(8):1016–1019.

66. Bansal P, Sonnenberg A. Pancreatitis is a risk factor for pancreatic cancer [see comments]. Gastroenterology 1995;109(1):247–251.

67. van Rees BP, Tascilar M, Hruban RH, et al. Remote partial gastrectomy as a risk factor for pancreatic cancer: potential for preventive strategies. Ann Oncol 1999;10(4):204–207.

68. Hilgers W, Kern SE. Molecular genetic basis of pancreatic adenocarcinoma. Genes Chromosomes Cancer 1999;26(1):1–12.

69. Berthelemy P, Bouisson M, Escourrou J, et al. Identification of K-ras mutations in pancreatic juice in the early diagnosis of pancreatic cancer [see comments]. Ann Intern Med 1995;123(3):188–191.

70. Rall CJ, Yan YX, Graeme-Cook F, et al. Ki-ras and p53 mutations in pancreatic ductal adenocarcinoma. Pancreas 1996;12:10–17.

71. Bold RJ, et al. Prognostric factors in resectable pancreatic cancer: p53 and Bcl-2. J Gastrointest Surg 1999;3:263–277.

72. Lei S, Appert HE, Nakata B, et al. Overexpression of HER2-neu oncogene in pancreatic cancer correlates with shortened survival. Int J Pancreatol 1995;17(1):15–21.

73. Schutte M, Hruban RH, Geradts J, et al. Abrogation of the Rb/p16 tumor-suppressive pathway in virtually all pancreatic carcinomas. Cancer Res 1997;57(15):3126–3130.

74. Goldstein AM, Fraser MC, Struewing JP, et al. Increased risk of pancreatic cancer in melanoma-prone kindreds with p16INK4 mutations [see comments]. N Engl J Med 1995;333(15):970–974.

75. Hahn SA, Schutte M, Hoque AT, et al. DPC4, a candidate tumor suppressor gene at human chromosome 18q21.1. Science 1996;271(5247):350–353.

76. Gullo L, Pezzilli R, Morselli-Labate AM. Diabetes and the risk of pancreatic cancer. Italian Pancreatic Cancer Study Group. N Engl J Med 1994;331(2):81–84.

77. Venu RP, Geenen JE, Hogan W, et al. Idiopathic recurrent pancreatitis. An approach to diagnosis and treatment [see comments]. Dig Dis Sci 1989;34(1):56–60.

78. Shimizu S, Kutsumi H, Fujimoto S, et al. Diagnostic endoscopic retrograde cholangio-pancreatography. Endoscopy 1999;31(1):74–79.

79. Freeny PC, Bilbao MK, Katon RM. "Blind" evaluation of endoscopic retrograde cholangiopancreatography (ERCP) in the diagnosis of pancreatic carcinoma: the "double duct" and other signs. Radiology 1976;119(2):271–274.

80. Plumley TF, Rohrmann CA, Freeny PC, et al. Double duct sign: reassessed significance in ERCP. AJR 1982;138(1):31–35.

81. Rosch T, Braig C, Gain T, et al. Staging of pancreatic and ampullary carcinoma by endoscopic ultrasonography. Comparison with conventional sonography, computed tomography, and angiography. Gastroenterology 1992;102(1):188–199.

82. Grace PA, Pitt HA, Longmire WP. Pylorus preserving pancreatoduodenectomy: an overview. Br J Surg 1990;77(9):968–974.

83. Lillemoe KD. Current management of pancreatic carcinoma. Ann Surg 1995;221(2):133–148.

84. Ghaneh P, Kawesha A, Howes N, et al. Adjuvant therapy for pancreatic cancer. World J Surg 1999;23(9):937–945.

85. Tepper J, Nardi G, Suit H. Carcinoma of the pancreas: review of MGH experience from 1963–1973. Analysis of surgical failure and implications for radiation therapy. Cancer (Phila) 1977;37:1519–1524.

86. Evans DB, Termuhlen PM, Byrd DR, et al. Intraoperative radiation therapy following pancreaticoduodenectomy. Ann Surg 1993;218(1):54–60.

87. Zerbi A, Fossati V, Parolini D, et al. Intraoperative radiation therapy adjuvant to resection in the treatment of pancreatic cancer. Cancer (Phila) 1994;73(12):2930–2935.

88. Kasperk R, Klever P, Andreopoulos D, et al. Intraoperative radiotherapy for pancreatic carcinoma. Br J Surg 1995;82(9):1259–1261.

89. Evans DB, Rich TA, Byrd DR, et al. Preoperative chemoradiation and pancreaticoduodenectomy for adenocarcinoma of the pancreas. Arch Surg 1992;127(11):1335–1339.

90. Evans DB, Pisters PW, Lee JE, et al. Preoperative chemoradiation strategies for localized adenocarcinoma of the pancreas. Journal of Hepato-Biliary-Pancreatic Surg 1998;5(3):242–250.

91. Staley CA, Lee JE, Cleary KR, et al. Preoperative chemoradiation, pancreaticoduodenectomy, and intraoperative radiation therapy for adenocarcinoma of the pancreatic head. Am J Surg 1996;171(1):118–124; discussion 124–125.

92. Lillemoe KD, Cameron JL, Kaufman HS, et al. Chemical splanchnicectomy in patients with unresectable pancreatic cancer. A prospective randomized trial. Ann Surg 1993;217(5):447–455; discussion 456–457.

93. Sarr MG, Cameron JL. Surgical management of unresectable carcinoma of the pancreas. Surgery (St. Louis) 1982;91(2):123–133.

94. Glimelius B. Chemotherapy in the treatment of cancer of the pancreas. J Hepato-Biliary-Pancreatic Surg 1998;5(3):235–241.

95. Kelsen D. The use of chemotherapy in the treatment of advanced gastric and pancreas cancer. Semin Oncol 1994;21(4):58–66.

96. Allema JH, Reinders ME, van Gulik TM, et al. Prognostic factors for survival after pancreaticoduodenectomy for patients with carcinoma of the pancreatic head region. Cancer (Phila) 1995;75(8):2069–2076.

97. Mannell A, van Heerden JA, Weiland LH, et al. Factors influencing survival after resection for ductal adenocarcinoma of the pancreas. Ann Surg 1986;203(4):403–407.

98. Nitecki SS, Sarr MG, Colby TV, et al. Long-term survival after resection for ductal adenocarcinoma of the pancreas. Is it really improving? Ann Surg 1995;221(1):59–66.

99. Murr MM, Sarr MG, Oishi AJ, et al. Pancreatic cancer. CA: Cancer J Clin 1994;44(5):304–318.

100. Bramhall SR, Allum WH, Jones AG, et al. Treatment and survival in 13,560 patients with pancreatic cancer, and incidence of the disease, in the West Midlands: an epidemiological study [see comments]. Br J Surg 1995;82(1):111–115.

101. Eskelinen M, Lipponen P. A review of prognostic factors in human pancreatic adenocarcinoma. Cancer Detect Prevent 1992; 16(5–6):287–295.

102. Geer RJ, Brennan MF. Prognostic indicators for survival after resection of pancreatic adenocarcinoma. Am J Surg 1993;165(1): 68–72.

103. Evans DB, et al. Part III Digestive System. In: Greene FL, Page DL, Fleming ID, et al., eds. AJCC Cancer Staging Manual, 6th Ed. New York: Springer-Verlag, 2002.

104. Yamamoto M, Saitoh Y, Hermanek P. Ch. 12, pp. 105–117. Exocrine pancreatic carcinoma. In: Hermanek P, et al. eds. Prognostic Factors in Cancer. Berlin: Springer-Verlag, 1995.

105. Lewandrowski K, Warshaw A, Compton C. Macrocystic serous cystadenoma of the pancreas: a morphologic variant differing from microcystic adenoma. Hum Pathol 1992;23(8):871–875.

106. Hammel P, Levy P, Voitot H, et al. Preoperative cyst fluid analysis is useful for the differential diagnosis of cystic lesions of the pancreas. Gastroenterology 1995;108(4):1230–1235.

107. Martin I, Hammond P, Scott J, et al. Cystic tumours of the pancreas. Br J Surg 1998;85(11):1484–1486.

108. Le Borgne J, de Calan L, Partensky C. Cystadenomas and cystadenocarcinomas of the pancreas: a multiinstitutional retrospective study of 398 cases. French Surgical Association. Ann Surg 1999;230(2):152–161.

109. Rivera JA, Fernandez-del Castillo C, Pins M, et al. Pancreatic mucinous ductal ectasia and intraductal papillary neoplasms. A single malignant clinicopathologic entity. Ann Surg 1997;225(6): 637–644; discussion 644–646.

110. Loftus EV Jr, Olivares-Pakzad BA, Batts KP, et al. Intraductal papillary-mucinous tumors of the pancreas: clinicopathologic features, outcome, and nomenclature. Members of the Pancreas Clinic, and Pancreatic Surgeons of Mayo Clinic. Gastroenterology 1996;110(6):1909–1918.

111. Behrns KE, Sarr MG, Strickler JG. Pancreatic lymphoma: is it a surgical disease? Pancreas 1994;9(5):662–667.

112. Bouvet M, Staerkel GA, Spitz FR, et al. Primary pancreatic lymphoma. Surgery (St. Louis) 1998;123(4):382–390.

113. Madura JA, Jarman BT, Doherty MG, et al. Adenosquamous carcinoma of the pancreas. Arch Surg 1999;134(6):599–603.

114. Neoptolemos JP, Carr-Locke DL, London NJ, et al. Controlled trial of urgent endoscopic retrograde cholangiopancreatography and endoscopic sphincter-otomy versus conservative treatment for acute pancreatitis due to gallstones. Lancet 1988;2(8618):979–983.

115. Fan ST, Lai EC, Mok FP, et al. Early treatment of acute biliary pancreatitis by endoscopic papillotomy [see comments]. N Engl J Med 1993;328(4):228–232.

116. Nitsche R, Fölsch UR, Lüdtke R, et al. Urgent ERCP in all cases of acute biliary pancreatitis? A prospective randomized multicenter study. Eur J Med Res 1995;1(3):127–131.

117. Sainio V, Kemppainen E, Puolakkainen P, et al. Early antibiotic treatment in acute necrotising pancreatitis [see comments]. Lancet 1995;346(8976):663–667.

118. Pederzoli P, Bassi C, Vesentini S, et al. A randomized multicenter clinical trial of antibiotic prophylaxis of septic complications in acute necrotizing pancreatitis with imipenem. Surg Gynecol Obstet 1993;176(5):480–483.

119. Howes R, Zuidema GD, Cameron JL. Evaluation of prophylactic antibiotics in acute pancreatitis. J Surg Res 1975;18(2):197–200.

120. Finch WT, Sawyers JL, Schenker S. A prospective study to determine the efficacy of antibiotics in acute pancreatitis. Ann Surg 1976;183(6):667–671.

121. Luiten EJ, Hop WC, Lange JF, et al. Controlled clinical trial of selective decontamination for the treatment of severe acute pancreatitis. Ann Surg 1995;222(1):57–65.

122. Warshaw AL, Popp JW Jr, Schapiro RH. Long-term patency, pancreatic function, and pain relief after lateral pancreaticoduodenectomy for chronic pancreatitis. Gastroenterology 1980;79(2):289–293.

123. Prinz RA, Greenlee HB. Pancreatic duct drainage in 100 patients with chronic pancreatitis. Ann Surg 1981;194(3):313–320.

124. Holmberg JT. Chronic pancreatitis. Ann Surg 1985;160:3.

125. Munn JS, Aranha GV, Greenlee HB, et al. Simultaneous treatment of chronic pancreatitis and pancreatic pseudocyst. Arch Surg 1987;122(6):662–667.

126. Bradley ELD. Long-term results of pancreatojejunostomy in patients with chronic pancreatitis. Am J Surg 1987;153(2):207–213.

127. Nealon WH, Townsend CM Jr, Thompson JC. Operative drainage of the pancreatic duct delays functional impairment in patients with chronic pancreatitis. A prospective analysis. Ann Surg 1988;208(3):321–329.

128. Greenlee HB, Prinz RA, Aranha GV. Long-term results of side-to-side pancreaticojejunostomy. World J Surg 1990;14(1):70–76.

129. Adams DB, Ford MC, Anderson MC. Outcome after lateral pancreaticojejunostomy for chronic pancreatitis. Ann Surg 1994; 219(5):481–487; discussion 487–489.

130. Rios GA, Adams DB, Yeoh KG, et al. Outcome of lateral pancreaticojejunostomy in the management of chronic pancreatitis with nondilated pancreatic ducts. J Gastrointest Surg 1998; 2(3):223–229.

131. Lucas CE, McIntosh B, Paley D, et al. Chronic pancreatitis. Surgery (St. Louis) 1999;126:790.

132. Hatfield AR, Tobias R, Terblanche J, et al. Preoperative external biliary drainage in obstructive jaundice. A prospective controlled clinical trial. Lancet 1982;2(8304):896–899.

133. McPherson GA, Benjamin IS, Hodgson HJ, et al. Pre-operative percutaneous transhepatic biliary drainage: the results of a controlled trial. Br J Surg 1984;71(5):371–375.

134. Pitt HA, Gomes AS, Lois JF, et al. Does preoperative percutaneous biliary drainage reduce operative risk or increase hospital cost? Ann Surg 1985;201(5):545–553.

135. Lygidakis NJ, van der Heyde MN, Lubbers MJ. Evaluation of preoperative biliary drainage in the surgical management of pancreatic head carcinoma [see comments]. Acta Chir Scand 1987; 153(11–12):665–668.

136. Lai EC, Mok FP, Fan ST, et al. Preoperative endoscopic drainage for malignant obstructive jaundice. Br J Surg 1994;81(8):1195–1198.

137. Trede M, Schwall G. The complications of pancreatectomy. Ann Surg 1988;207(1):39–47.

138. Bakkevold KE, Kambestad B. Morbidity and mortality after radical and palliative pancreatic cancer surgery. Risk factors influencing the short-term results. Ann Surg 1993;217(4):356–368.

139. Karsten TM, Allema JH, Reinders M, et al. Preoperative biliary drainage, colonisation of bile and postoperative complications in patients with tumours of the pancreatic head: a retrospective analysis of 241 consecutive patients. Eur J Surg 1996;162(11): 881–888.

140. Povoski SP, Karpeh MS Jr, Conlon KC, et al. Association of preoperative biliary drainage with postoperative outcome following pancreaticoduodenectomy [see comments]. Ann Surg 1999;230(2): 131–142.

141. Trede M, Schwall G, Saeger HD. Survival after pancreatoduodenectomy. 118 consecutive resections without an operative mortality. Ann Surg 1990;211(4):447–458.

142. Nagakawa T, Nagamori M, Futakami F, et al. Results of extensive surgery for pancreatic carcinoma. Cancer (Phila) 1996;77(4):640–645.

143. Conlon KC, Klimstra DS, Brennan MF. Long-term survival after curative resection for pancreatic ductal adenocarcinoma. Clinicopathologic analysis of 5-year survivors. Ann Surg 1996; 223(3):273–279.

144. Yeo CJ, Abrams RA, Grochow LB, et al. Pancreaticoduodenectomy for pancreatic adenocarcinoma: postoperative adjuvant chemoradiation improves survival. A prospective, single-institution experience. Ann Surg 1997;225(5):621–633; discussion 633–666.

Biliary System

Hobart W. Harris

Anatomy

In the extrahepatic biliary tree, the gallbladder (vesica fellea) is a hollow, piriform (L., pear-shaped) organ, 7 to 10 cm in length, approximately 4 cm in diameter, with a capacity of 30 to 60 ml (Fig. 19.1).

For descriptive purposes the gallbladder is divided into a fundus, body, infundibulum, and neck. Attached to the liver by loose areolar connective tissue, the portion of the gallbladder not embedded within the liver substance is covered by visceral peritoneum. Small veins and lymphatics course between the gallbladder fossa and the gallbladder wall, connecting the lymphatic and venous drainage of the two organs. The shared lymphovascular drainage explains the spread of gallbladder inflammation and carcinoma to the liver. In addition, a small accessory bile duct may drain directly into the gallbladder (cholecystohepatic duct of Luschka) in a similar manner. During a cholecystectomy these accessory ducts should be identified and ligated, if present, to prevent postoperative bile leaks.

The body of the gallbladder narrows toward the neck of the organ known as the infundibulum. Major portions of the body and infundibulum of the gallbladder are in juxtaposition to the first portion of the duodenum and the transverse colon. Inflammation of the gallbladder wall can result in the formation of adhesions between the gallbladder and the adjacent intestines, setting the stage for the creation of cholecystoenteric fistulas (e.g., a cholecystoduodenal fistula). The infundibulum of the gallbladder is attached to the first part of the duodenum by an avascular peritoneal reflection termed the cholecystoduodenal ligament. This ligament is an inferior extension of the hepatoduodenal ligament and can be used during surgery as a landmark for the major vascular structures of the hepatic hilum. The infundibulum joins the cystic duct through the neck of the gallbladder, which is a short S-shaped structure, frequently curved on itself. Protruding from the lateral wall of the neck of the gallbladder, there may be a dilatation termed Hartmann's pouch. Pro-

jecting in an inferoposterior direction toward the duodenum, gallstones frequently become lodged in this outpouching in such a way that if this area becomes inflamed it may adhere to and obstruct the cystic duct.

The cystic duct is a tubular structure attaching the gallbladder neck to the common hepatic duct. Its length varies from 1 to 5 cm and its diameter from 3 to 7 mm. The mucosa that lines the cystic duct is thrown into 4 to 10 spiral folds, the spiral valves of Heister. These valves prevent the ready passage of gallstones and excessive distension or collapse of the cystic duct, despite wide variations in ductal pressure. It is important to keep the cystic duct patent at all times so that bile easily enters the gallbladder when the choledochal sphincter is closed, and so that bile flows in the opposite direction down into the duodenum when the gallbladder contracts. The cystic duct may join the extrahepatic biliary tree in a variety of ways, including an angular, parallel, or spiral configuration.

A single cystic artery usually accomplishes the arterial supply to the gallbladder, but in 12% of cases double cystic arteries exist.[1,2] The origin and course of the cystic artery are highly variable; indeed, the course of this artery is one of the most variable in the body. In the majority of cases (75%) the cystic artery originates from the proximal right hepatic artery and immediately divides into two branches: the superficial branch, which runs along the peritoneal surface of the gallbladder, and the deep branch, which runs along the gallbladder fossa between the gallbladder and liver. The cystic artery usually lies superior to the cystic duct and passes posterior to the common hepatic duct. With this anatomical arrangement, the common hepatic duct, the liver, and the cystic duct define the boundaries of Calot's triangle (see Fig. 19.1). Located within this triangle are some structures of great importance to the surgeon: the cystic artery, the right hepatic artery, and the cystic duct lymph node. Calot's node is often involved with inflammatory or neoplastic disease of the gallbladder because this is one of the primary routes of lymphatic drainage.

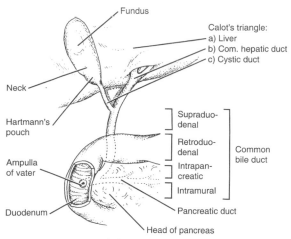

FIGURE 19.1. Anatomy of the gallbladder and bile ducts. (Redrawn with permission from Braasch and Tompkins. Surgical Diseases of the Biliary Tract and Pancreas. Mosby-Yearbook Co., 1994)

Unlike the arterial system, there are no named veins draining the gallbladder. As previously mentioned, some of the organ's venous return passes directly into the liver across the gallbladder fossa. The remaining venous drainage parallels the cystic duct lymphatics forming venous networks along the common bile duct before joining the portal venous system. Occasionally patients with portal hypertension have obvious varices in the area of the gallbladder and extrahepatic biliary tree.

Fibers from the sympathetic and parasympathetic nervous systems innervate the gallbladder. Although the nerves supplying the gallbladder and choledochal sphincter contribute to overall gallbladder function, they are of no major clinical significance and can be sacrificed without consequence. However, afferent sympathetic nerve fibers supplying the extrahepatic bile ducts include some pain fibers that are responsible for the referred epigastric and right upper quadrant abdominal pain characteristic of biliary disease.

As depicted in Figure 19.1, the common bile duct results from the confluence of the common hepatic and cystic ducts, varies in length from 5 to 17 cm, and is normally 3 to 8 mm in diameter, unless obstructed, when it can dilate to a diameter in excess of 2 cm. The common bile duct can be divided into four segments as a function of its anatomical relationship to the duodenum and pancreas: the supraduodenal, retroduodenal, intrapancreatic, and intramural segments. Enveloped within the peritoneal covering of the hepatoduodenal ligament, the common bile duct generally lies anterolateral to the hepatic artery and portal vein, making it readily available for surgical manipulation (e.g., common bile duct exploration). The hepatoduodenal ligament is an important anatomical landmark as it represents the right border of the hepatogastric ligament (lesser omentum) and defines the anterior border of the epiploic foramen of Winslow connecting the greater and lesser peritoneal cavities. In addition to yielding entry to the lesser sac, the foramen of Winslow enables the structures of the portal triad to be easily encircled and compressed (Pringle maneuver). After the common duct descends posterior to the first part of the duodenum, it travels through the head of the pancreas, then for 1 to 2 cm obliquely within the medial wall of the second portion of the duode-

num before forming a common channel with the main pancreatic duct (ampulla of Vater), which empties into the duodenal lumen through a mucosal papilla. The terminal portion of the common bile duct is encircled by a combination of circular and longitudinal smooth muscle, which serve to control the entry of biliopancreatic secretions into the proximal intestinal tract. This muscular structure, termed the choledochalduodenal sphincter of Oddi, has a phasic resting tone ranging from a baseline of approximately 13 mmHg to as high as 200 mmHg. The contractile activity of the sphincter of Oddi demonstrates a cyclical pattern that varies in relationship to the intermittent myoelectric migratory complex (IMMC) of the intestinal tract, with the majority (85%) of peristaltic waves migrating in a caudal direction.

The common bile duct derives its blood supply not from any named blood vessels but rather from a complex network of interwoven small vessels derived predominantly from the cystic and the posterior pancreaticoduodenal arteries. Because there is no specific vessel to identify and preserve during dissections of the common bile duct, this tubular structure is vulnerable to ischemic injury. To avoid disrupting the fragile inconstant blood supply to the duct and thus increase the risk of postoperative bile leakage or stricture formation, it is critically important to not strip the common bile duct of the investing loose areolar tissue during its isolation and manipulation. The nerve supply to the common duct is the same as described for the gallbladder.

Physiology

The biliary tree is designed for the transport and storage of bile produced in the liver by hepatocytes and destined for the duodenal lumen to participate in the digestion of foodstuffs. The pattern of bile flow throughout the biliary tree differs when a person is in the fasted versus the postprandial state. Under fasting conditions, biliary tree motility and thus bile flow are regulated by the IMMC and approximated by the cyclical activity of the duodenum. Observations of the fasting gallbladder over time have shown a predictable pattern of filling, followed by gallbladder contraction and partial (15%–20%) emptying associated with increased plasma levels of motilin. The enterohepatic circulation of bile acids predominantly regulates the overall production rate of bile by the liver. Thus, the rate of hepatic bile synthesis is inversely proportional to the amount of bile acid reclaimed from the terminal ileum and recycled to the liver. Actual filling of the gallbladder results from the continuous production of bile by the liver in the face of a contracted sphincter of Oddi. As the pressure within the common bile duct exceeds that within the gallbladder lumen, hepatic bile enters the gallbladder via retrograde flow through the cystic duct, wherein it is rapidly concentrated.

Following a meal, the gallbladder contracts in response to both a vagally mediated cephalic phase of activity and the release of cholecystokinin (CCK), the major regulator of gallbladder function. During the following 60 to 120 min, approximately 80% to 90% of gallbladder bile is steadily emptied into the intestinal tract. CCK is localized to the proximal small intestine, especially the duodenal epithelial cells, where its release is stimulated by intraluminal fat, amino acids, and gastric acid and inhibited by bile. In addition to stimulating gallbladder contractions, CCK also acts to functionally inhibit the normal phasic motor activity of the sphincter of Oddi. By reducing the frequency and amplitude of the basal contractions, the sphincteric mechanism relaxes in coordination with gallbladder contraction, thus facilitating the delivery of bile into the proximal small intestine. Gallbladder function is also influenced by other hormones, including vasoactive intestinal polypeptide (VIP), somatostatin, substance P, and norepinepherine. Both VIP and somatostatin inhibit contraction of the gallbladder, consistent with their inhibitory effects on gastrointestinal motility. The role of substance P, norepinepherine, and other neuropeptides in the regulation of gallbladder function remains to be elucidated.

Diagnosis

Clinically significant symptoms originating from biliary tract pathology are common, and generally the result of obstruction, infection, or both. As is true with any hollow tubular structure, the source of bile duct obstruction can be either extramural (pancreatic cancer), intramural (cholangiocarcinoma), or intraluminal (choledocholithiasis). Similarly, as with infections elsewhere in the body, for an infection to develop within the biliary tree requires the following three components: a susceptible host, a sufficient inoculum, and stasis. Given these basic principles, the most common symptoms related to biliary tract disease are abdominal pain, jaundice, fever, and a constellation of constitutional complaints, including nausea, anorexia, weight loss, and vomiting.

Abdominal Pain

Gallstones and inflammation of the gallbladder are the most frequent causes of abdominal pain resulting from biliary tract disease. Acute obstruction of the gallbladder by calculi results in *biliary colic*, a misnomer in that the pain is not colicky but rather a constant abdominal pain typically localized to the epigastrium or right upper quadrant. Although the pain is often precipitated by eating fatty foods, it can also be triggered by eating other types of food or even begin spontaneously. Unlike intestinal colic, which presents in episodic waves lasting several minutes each, biliary colic is a more constant pain, which gradually builds in intensity, and can radiate to the back, interscapular region, or right shoulder. Many patients describe the pain as a band- or beltlike constriction of the upper abdomen that may be associated with nausea or vomiting. This recognizable type of abdominal pain results from a normal gallbladder contracting against a luminal obstruction, such as a gallstone impacted in the neck of the organ, the cystic duct, or common bile duct.

The pain of biliary colic is distinct from that associated with acute cholecystitis. Although biliary colic can also be localized to the right upper quadrant, the pain of acute cholecystitis is exacerbated by touch, somatic in nature, and often associated with the systemic findings of fever and leukocytosis. The transmural inflammation of the gallbladder provokes irritation of the adjacent visceral and parietal peritoneal surfaces. Therefore, any increases in wall tension or tactile pressure can stimulate nerve endings within the inflamed tissue, as evidenced by a positive *Murphy's sign*. This physical finding, of a patient abruptly stopping their inspiratory effort because of pain as the examiner palpates under the right costal margin, is indicative of acute cholecystitis. The clinical implication of acute cholecystitis is quite different than that of biliary colic. Although biliary colic is an episodic, even unpredictable functional disorder of the gallbladder that many patients can live with for months to years, acute cholecystitis involves irreversible organ injury and activation of a locoregional inflammatory response, and it invariably requires a definitive therapeutic intervention.

Jaundice

When the serum concentration of bilirubin exceeds approximately 2.5 mg/dl, a yellowish discoloration of the sclera becomes evident (*scleral icterus*). A similar discoloration of the skin (*jaundice*) develops with serum bilirubin levels in excess of 5 mg/dl. Under both circumstances the visible changes in color represent the deposition of bile pigments in the affected tissues. The rise in conjugated bilirubin (direct reacting) is in contrast to the increased levels of unconjugated bilirubin (indirect reacting) observed with hepatocellular injury. Significant elevations of the total serum bilirubin level are indicative of common bile duct obstruction.

Fever

Significant elevations in body temperature ($\geq 38.0°C$) due to biliary tract disease represent a systemic manifestation of an initially localized inflammatory process. Bacterial contamination of the biliary system is a common feature of acute cholecystitis or choledocholithiasis with obstruction, and is to be expected following percutaneous or endoscopic cholangiography. The combination of right upper quadrant abdominal pain, jaundice, and fever, known as *Charcot's triad*, signifies an active infection of the biliary system termed acute cholangitis. Severely afflicted patients may also display an altered mental status and hypotension (*pentad of Reynolds*). Fever should be viewed as a signal that an otherwise localized disease process has progressed to a systemic illness.

Laboratory Tests

Simple biliary colic, in the absence of gallbladder wall pathology or common bile duct obstruction, does not produce abnormal laboratory test values. On the other hand, obstructive choledocholithiasis is commonly associated with an element of both liver dysfunction and acute cellular injury with resultant elevations in liver function tests. In addition to hyperbilirubinemia (see Jaundice, earlier), the magnitude of which directly correlates with the severity and duration of the biliary system blockade, an increased serum alkaline phosphatase level is virtually pathognomonic of bile duct obstruction. Serum transaminase (aspartate and alanine) levels can also be mildly elevated in biliary system disease, either because of direct injury of the liver adjacent to an inflamed gallbladder or from the effect of biliary sepsis on hepatocellular membrane integrity. Leukocytosis with a predominance of neutrophils is often present with acute cholecystitis or cholangitis, but is a nonspecific finding that does not distinguish these conditions from other infectious or inflammatory processes within the abdomen.

Radiographic Studies

ABDOMINAL RADIOGRAPHS

Although frequently obtained during the initial evaluation of abdominal pain, plain radiographs of the abdomen are seldom of significant diagnostic value. Only about 15% of gallstones contain enough calcium to render them radiopaque and thus visible on plain films of the abdomen. The most important value of plain abdominal films is the exclusion of other potential diagnoses, such as a perforated ulcer with free intraabdominal air or an intestinal obstruction with dilated loops of bowel and multiple air–fluid levels.

ULTRASONOGRAPHY

Surface ultrasound of the abdomen is an extremely useful and accurate method for identifying gallstones and pathological changes in the gallbladder consistent with acute cholecystitis. Abdominal ultrasound should be part of the routine evaluation of patients suspected of having gallstone disease, given the high specificity (>98%) and sensitivity (>95%) of this test for the diagnosis of cholelithiasis (Fig. 19.2). In addition to confirming the presence of gallstones within the gallbladder, ultrasound can also detail various signs of acute cholecystitis (thickening of the gallbladder wall, pericholecystic fluid) as well as gallbladder neoplasms.

COMPUTED TOMOGRAPHY (CT)

Although abdominal CT scanning is probably the most informative single radiographic tool for examining intraabdominal pathology, its overall value for the diagnosis of biliary tract disease pales in comparison to ultrasonography. This disadvantage is largely because gallstones and bile appear nearly isodense on CT; that is, it is difficult to distinguish gallstones from bile, unless the stones are heavily calcified. Therefore, CT documents the presence of gallstones within the biliary tree and gallbladder with a sensitivity of approximately 55% to 65%. However, abdominal CT is a

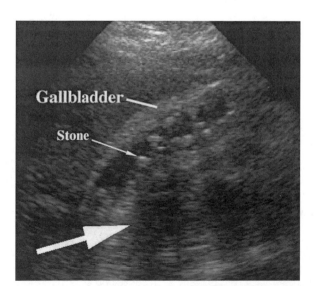

FIGURE 19.2. Ultrasonography of the gallbladder. The sonographic signs of gallstones include visible stones that produce acoustic shadowing (white arrow) and which move with the patient. (Courtesy of the Department of Radiology, UCSF.)

powerful tool for evaluating biliary tract diseases when the differential diagnosis includes a question of hepatobiliary or pancreatic neoplasm, liver abscess, or hepatic parenchymal disease (e.g., biliary cirrhosis, organ atrophy).

CHOLANGIOGRAPHY

Defined as the mapping of bile ducts, cholangiography functionally involves the installation of contrast directly into the biliary tree and is the most accurate and sensitive method available to anatomically delineate the intra- and extrahepatic biliary tree. A cholangiogram is indicated when the diagnosis or therapy depends on a precise knowledge of biliary anatomy. Generally obtained to determine the location and extent of an intraluminal obstruction, diagnostic cholangiograms can be performed percutaneously, endoscopically, transabdominally (e.g., intraoperative cholangiogram), or through the use of intravenous or oral contrast material taken up and excreted by the liver into bile. Magnetic resonance cholangiopancreatography (MRCP) is a recently developed, totally noninvasive imaging technique that can provide detailed anatomical information without the direct injection of contrast into the biliary system.[3] MRCP obviates the need for physically manipulating the patient, and thus promises to combine the convenience of CT with the data quality of traditional cholangiograms. As this imaging method is new and incompletely proven, its overall role in the diagnosis of biliary system disease awaits further experience.

SCINTIGRAPHY

Biliary scintigraphy is useful to visualize the biliary tree, assess liver and gallbladder function, and diagnose several common disorders with a sensitivity and specificity of 90% to 97%.[4] Although an excellent test to decide whether the common bile and cystic ducts are patent, biliary scintigraphy does not identify gallstones or yield detailed anatomical information.

ORAL CHOLECYSTOGRAPHY

Instead of using a radiolabeled pharmaceutical, patients are given oral contrast pills 12 to 16 hours before the exam, during which time the peroral contrast material is absorbed by the small intestine, cleared by the liver, excreted into bile, and concentrated within the gallbladder. Subsequently, the gallbladder and common bile duct are visualized using traditional abdominal radiographs. Oral cholecystography generates images with much greater clarity and resolution than scintigraphy, but requires more planning to perform and yields less dynamic information.

Calculous Disease

Pathogenesis

CLASSIFICATION OF GALLSTONES

There are three types of gallstones: cholesterol, pigment, and mixed cholesterol and pigment stones. The distribution and location of biliary calculi varies throughout the world, undoubtedly reflecting different risk factors for their formation.

In patients in the United States and most westernized countries, approximately 75% of gallstones are of the mixed type, 15% are pigment stones, and the remaining 10% pure cholesterol. The stones are most commonly located within the gallbladder, but can on occasion be found within the common bile duct or the liver or to have migrated into the intestinal tract. These findings are in stark contrast to those in other regions of the world, such as Southeast Asia, where the majority of biliary calculi are of the pigment variety and are most commonly located within the liver itself and not the gallbladder. Such variation also applies to the overall incidence of gallstone disease. In the United States about 12% of the population has cholelithiasis, with more than 950,000 new cases diagnosed each year, while in East Africa and other selected Third World countries the incidence is as low as 2% to 3%. The risk of developing biliary calculi throughout America and Western Europe is directly proportional to a person's age and sex. While children and adolescents rarely have gallstones, by the seventh decade of life 10% of men and 25% of women have documented cholelithiasis.

CHOLESTEROL-ENRICHED GALLSTONE FORMATION

The exact mechanism by which gallstones are formed is not fully understood, but calculi are likely the result of a complex, multifaceted alteration in hepatobiliary function (Table 19.1).

CHOLESTEROL-SUPERSATURATED BILE

An early event in the process of gallstone formation is a change in the composition of bile, specifically a relative increase in the cholesterol content. Normally bile is an isotonic combination of water, electrolytes, and organic macromolecules that is actively secreted by the liver. Designed to aid in the solubilization (emulsification) and subsequent absorption of dietary fats, the solute composition of bile includes bile salts, cholesterol, and phospholipids, predominantly phosphatidylcholine (lecithin). As the molar ratio of cholesterol relative to either bile salts or phospholipid deviates from a relatively narrow range, the cholesterol solubilization capacity of bile is exceeded, resulting in rapid cholesterol crystal formation.

GALLSTONE NUCLEATION

Once bile has become supersaturated with cholesterol, the formation of a cholesterol-enriched gallstone presumably begins with a nucleation event. The precipitation of crystalline cholesterol is thought to occur via either the fusion or implosion of cholesterol-rich vesicles.[5,6] A variety of different crystal shapes have been recently identified in bile samples from numerous patients with gallstones.[7] These distinct cholesterol structures, including arcs/needles, spirals, tubes, and plates, may represent different stages in the nucleation process, as well as the existence of different cholesterol crystallization pathways.

GALLBLADDER AND FOREGUT MOTILITY

Gallbladder stasis has long been associated with the formation of gallstones. Beyond the intuitive sense that a stagnant pool of supersaturated bile must promote nucleation and stone growth, there is a growing body of data to support the concept. Specifically, investigators have demonstrated that the volume of bile flow through the gallbladder during the postprandial period is dramatically reduced and leads to a large, flaccid gallbladder.[8,9] Furthermore, women with gallstones were found to have significantly longer whole-gut transport times with only half the stool output as compared to stone-free patients.

GENDER AND GENES

Gallstone disease is more common in women than in men at virtually all stages of life. Because this gallstone gender gap narrows by the eighth and ninth decades of life, it is likely the result of estrogen-induced changes in biliary lipid metabolism and gallbladder function. In the United States, the typical patient with symptomatic gallstones is "female, forty, fat and fair."

The role of heredity in biliary calculous disease is not well understood, but the importance of genetics as a risk factor for gallstones is evident in studies of family history. A history of cholelithiasis in a first-degree relative doubles a person's risk

TABLE 19.1. Clinical Risk Factors Associated with Cholesterol Gallstones.

Risk factor	Pathogenesis
Age	Gallstone formation is a time-dependent process; 40 is the typical age at clinical diagnosis; possible age-related decrease in the conversion of cholesterol to bile salts
Gender	Female:male ratio = 3:1; estrogens increase the uptake of plasma cholesterol by the liver with subsequent increased bile cholesterol saturation.
Race and ethnicity	High-risk: Pima Indians, other Native Americans, Hispanics, Whites Low-risk: Black Africans and African-Americans
Genetics	Increased relative risks if parents, siblings, or first-degree relatives have gallstones
Obesity	Increased activity of hydroxy-methyl-glutaryl-CoA (HMG) reductase leads to increased cholesterol synthesis and bile cholesterol saturation
Crohn's disease	Decreased ileal resorption of bile salts
Total parenteral nutrition	Gallbladder stasis and distension; risk exacerbated in patients with Crohn's disease
Rapid weight loss	Intestinal bypass surgery and low-calorie, high-protein diets associated with high incidence of gallstones because of decreased bile salt secretion and gallbladder stasis

of developing gallstones, and this genetic risk factor is greatest with a parental history of biliary calculi.[10]

BILE CALCIUM

Calcium was not originally thought to contribute to the formation of cholesterol stones, but recent studies have identified calcium carbonate within the core of these stones. Also, there are data showing that increased biliary calcium can promote cholesterol crystallization and gallstone nucleation via an unknown mechanism.

OBESITY

While the pathogenic mechanism linking obesity to cholelithiasis is unclear, it may involve alterations in lipid biogenesis with increased cholesterol synthesis. Regardless of mechanism, the relative risk of gallstones increases dramatically with morbid obesity.

Pigment Stones

While only about 15% of gallstones in the United States are pigment stones, this type of biliary calculus is the predominant variety throughout the world. The sine qua non of pigment stones is their high concentration of bilirubin combined with low cholesterol content. These stones are usually mixed with a substantial amount of calcium bilirubinate and can be further categorized as either black or brown as a function of their gross appearance. Considerably less is known regarding the pathogenesis of pigment versus cholesterol-enriched gallstones, but some clinical and in vitro studies suggest that biliary infection and stasis play critical roles in their development.

Gallbladder Sludge and Microcalculi

Generally identified via abdominal sonography, sludge appears as echogenic material within the gallbladder that layers in the dependent area of the gallbladder yet does not generate the postacoustic shadows characteristic of gallstones. Commonly seen following prolonged fasting, sludge is thought to represent bile that has become very concentrated within a relative static gallbladder. Although the natural history of gallbladder sludge is not known, it is not considered a pathological finding as it generally resolves with resumption of an oral diet.

Clinical Syndromes

Gallstone disease continues to be a major health care problem in the United States and throughout selected parts of the world. There are more than 26 million Americans with gallstones and, although most of these people are asymptomatic, more than 700,000 cholecystectomies are performed each year. The total annual cost of medical care for patients suffering from biliary calculous disease is estimated at more than 7 billion dollars. Still, not all gallstones require treatment. In fact, in the majority of patients (60%–80%) gallstones are completely asymptomatic. However, once symptoms develop patients are at risk for a wide range of problems, ranging from simple biliary colic to ascending cholangitis and septic shock.

ASYMPTOMATIC GALLSTONES

Data from several longitudinal studies reveal that approximately 10% to 20% of patients with silent gallstones go on to develop symptoms, most commonly biliary colic.[11–14] Serious symptoms or complications such as acute cholecystitis develop in these patients at a rate of 1% to 3% per year. These observations, combined with the fact that only 0.5% to 1.0% of patients die of complications from their silent gallstones, strongly suggest that asymptomatic gallstones generally follow a benign course. Therefore, there is little role for the prophylactic medical or surgical treatment of asymptomatic gallstones. These interventions should be reserved for those patients who have experienced significant clinical symptoms, a calcified (porcelain) gallbladder, or gallbladder polyps.

ACUTE CHOLECYSTITIS

One of the most common complications of symptomatic gallstones that requires surgical intervention is acute cholecystitis. This condition is thought to result from impaction of a gallstone in the cystic duct or neck of the gallbladder, thereby completely obstructing the organ. Consequently, the gallbladder becomes distended and somehow initiates a localized acute inflammatory reaction. The exact pathogenesis of acute cholecystitis is not well delineated, but the clinical syndrome begins with biliary colic-type pain. Biliary colic typically resolves over several hours, but the pain of acute cholecystitis persists and intensifies over days. Initially the pain is vague and visceral in nature, but as the acute inflammation of the gallbladder becomes transmural, the visceral and adjacent parietal peritoneal coverings become irritated. At this point the patient's discomfort is no longer vague and diffuse, but localizes to the right upper quadrant and is associated with guarding and rebound tenderness. As described earlier, the classical physical finding of acute cholecystitis is a positive Murphy's sign (inspiratory arrest on palpation of the right upper quadrant). Patients may also complain of nausea and vomiting, anorexia, and a low-grade fever. In many cases the physical exam reveals a mass in the right upper quadrant. This mass or "phlegmon" represents the body's effort to wall off and compartmentalize the inflamed gallbladder using adjacent organs, including the greater omentum, first portion of the duodenum, and right colon.

Laboratory abnormalities are nonspecific, but may reveal a mild leukocytosis and minor elevations in the liver function tests. The diagnosis is confirmed via abdominal ultrasound, with the findings of gallbladder wall thickening and pericholecystic fluid being virtually pathognomonic. For further confirmation, the ultrasonographer can demonstrate a "sonographic Murphy's sign." With the ultrasound transducer placed directly over the distended gallbladder, the sonographer presses down in an effort to recreate the patient's discomfort. The source of pain from the gallbladder can thus be distinguished from other conditions, such as liver tenderness or hepatitis. Severe forms of acute cholecystitis can result in *gallbladder empyema*, wherein the organ is filled with purulent bile and debris, and *emphysematous cholecystitis*, which is characterized by necrosis and gas within the wall of the gallbladder. The latter condition typically occurs in diabetic patients and demands aggressive decompression of the gallbladder to avoid gallbladder perforation, intraabdominal abscess formation, and progressive sepsis.

Once the diagnosis is confirmed the patient is rehydrated, any metabolic abnormalities corrected, and pain is controlled with analgesics. There is a commonly cited concern regarding the use of morphine and other opiates in the setting of biliary tract disease. These drugs can have a hypertensive effect on the sphincter of Oddi and thus potentially exacerbate a patient's condition. Despite the data in support of this contention, clinical practice suggests that completely avoiding the use of opiates in patients with biliary system disease is generally unnecessary. Definitive treatment involves removal of the inflamed and irreversibly damaged gallbladder and its contents. Historically surgeons recommended that the patient's gallbladder be allowed to "cool down" before performing a cholecystectomy, theoretically allowing the acute inflammation to resolve and thus render the procedure less technically demanding. The results of several randomized, controlled trials comparing early versus delayed surgery for acute cholecystitis in more than 1000 patients is presented in Table 19.2. As a result of these data, it is now generally accepted that early cholecystectomy (within 24–48 h of making the diagnosis) is not only technically feasible but the preferred method of treatment as it effectively short circuits the illness. Although there is an increase in the morbidity rate for early as compared to delayed surgery (21.0% versus 16.5%, respectively), the complications are generally minor and the overall mortality rated is reduced. Furthermore, patients return to normal activities more quickly, they avoid the risk of recurrent gallbladder symptoms while awaiting surgery, and the total cost of the illness is reduced.[15–20] As with open cholecystectomy, several prospective randomized, controlled trials have also confirmed the advantage of early versus delayed laparoscopic surgery for acute cholecystitis provided the surgeon is experienced.[21,22]

CHOLEDOCHOLITHIASIS

Choledocholithiasis represents gallbladder stones that have migrated into the common bile duct via the cystic duct, stones which were left in the common duct following biliary tract surgery (retained stones), or stones that originated within the intra- or extrahepatic bile ducts primarily (Fig. 19.3). The overall incidence of choledocholithiasis is difficult to know, but up to 15% of patients who undergo gallbladder surgery are found to have common duct stones.

Specific clinical syndromes and biochemical tests can suggest the presence of common duct stones, but they are definitively identified by radiographic evaluation of the biliary tree, including cholangiography. Considering the frequency with which calculi are found during cholecystectomy surgery, to avoid exposing every patient to the risks and costs of an intraoperative cholangiogram, a series of relative indications for performing this test have been developed. Indications for cholangiography include palpable choledocholithiasis, a dilated common bile duct, elevated liver function tests, or a recent history of jaundice, cholangitis, or pancreatitis.

CHOLANGITIS

In 1877, Charcot described the triad of abdominal pain, fever, and jaundice in patients suffering from cholangitis. This constellation of findings is most commonly caused by an obstructing stone lodged in the distal common bile duct. Of note, cholangitis is a potentially life-threatening infection that can rapidly progress from mild fever and malaise to full-blown septic shock and multisystem organ failure over a matter of hours. The clinical volatility of this condition results from the relative ease with which bacteria and endotoxin under pressure can reflux from the bile duct lumen, cross the canalicular membrane, and enter the systemic circulation. Beyond supportive measures and antibiotics, the treatment for cholangitis must include decompression of the obstructed biliary system. Recent prospective, randomized trials have shown that endoscopic decompression is associated with lower morbidity and mortality rates than open surgical procedures.[23–26] Another potentially serious clinical consequence of choledocholithiasis is acute (gallstone) pancreatitis. Discussed in greater detail elsewhere in this book, common duct stones can initiate a dysregulated inflammatory reaction in the pancreas by an incompletely understood mechanism.

The appropriate treatment for choledocholithiasis is entirely dependent on the clinical circumstances but generally entails removal of the common duct calculi and the gallbladder. Of note, small common duct stones (<5–6 mm in diameter) will likely spontaneously pass into the intestinal tract and therefore do not require treatment.[27,28] Stones discovered at the time of gallbladder surgery should be removed and a choledochostomy (T-tube) tube placed for 2 to 6 weeks. If common duct stones are identified in the perioperative period (i.e., before or after the cholecystectomy), then they can frequently be removed either endoscopically or percutaneously.

GALLSTONE ILEUS

Biliary calculi can produce many different symptoms, including changes in bowel function and motility. In addition to the nonspecific nausea and vomiting occasionally observed with simple biliary colic and frequently associated with acute cholecystitis, a gallstone ileus represents a unique type of small-bowel obstruction. As previously mentioned, during acute cholecystitis the body attempts to compartmentalize the inflammatory process by surrounding it with adjacent soft tissues. The resultant phlegmon is composed of omentum and nearby bowel, including the duodenum. If the inflammatory process is of sufficient intensity and duration, then the diseased gallbladder can form a fistulous communication with adjacent hollow organs. This process most commonly results in a cholecystoduodenal fistula, but can also involve the colon, stomach, or more distal segments of the small intestine. The gallstones responsible for a gallstone ileus are large, generally greater than 2 to 3 cm in diameter. When a stone of this size enters the intestinal tract through a cholecystoenteric fistula, it migrates distally until either it exits the rectum or becomes lodged in the narrowest segment of the bowel, the terminal ileum. The typical patient is an elderly woman with previous biliary colic who now presents with a "tumbling" bowel obstruction. The diagnosis of gallstone ileus should be suspected in patients presenting with bowel obstruction in the absence of an incarcerated hernia or a history of prior abdominal surgery. Treatment entails an exploratory laparotomy to not only remove the stone causing the obstruction, but to carefully inspect the remainder of the small intestine for additional calculi. Simultaneous removal of the gallbladder is ill advised. The gallbladder rarely (<4% of patients) causes future symptoms, and the morbidity and

TABLE 19.2.

Clinical Trials Comparing Early versus Delayed Surgery for Acute Cholecystitis.

Reference	n	Study design	Level of evidence	Complications	Mortality	Findings/comments
Linden and Sunzel 1970,[15] Sweden	140	Randomized, controlled trial	I	Early: 14.3% Delayed: 3.4%	Early: 0% Delayed: 0%	More than two-thirds of patients randomized to early surgery underwent operation within 10 days of diagnosis Low mortality in part the result of excluding 3 high-risk, elderly patients Noted that 17% of patients randomized to delayed surgery ultimately refused operation once acute symptoms resolved No difference in technical difficulty between early and delayed operations when the surgeon was experienced Early surgery (paradoxically) resulted in a 2-day-longer average length of stay, but fewer extended hospitalizations Concluded that early surgery avoids the hazards of diagnostic error, symptom recurrence during the waiting period, and shortened the convalescence period after early surgery
McArthur et al. 1975[16] England	35	Randomized, controlled trial	I	Early: 40.0% Delayed: 29.4%	Early: 0% Delayed: 0%	Early surgery defined as immediately following confirmation of the diagnosis Reported no overall difference in the technical difficulty of early versus delayed cholecystectomy, but recommended that early surgery take place within 5 days of diagnosis Most complications were minor infections; Concluded that the major benefits of early surgery are the shortened hospitalization and the avoidance of the serious complications of conservative management, including gallbladder perforation and empyema
Lahtinen et al. 1978,[17] Finland	100	Randomized, controlled trial	I	Early: 29.7% Delayed: 47.7%	Early: 0% Delayed: 9%	Noted a technically easier operation, shorter OR time (70 vs. 79 min), reduced wound infection rate (6% vs. 18%), and shorter postoperative hospital LOS (12 vs. 15 days) for early vs. delayed surgery High complication rates in both groups predominantly related to localized or systemic infection Authors recommend early surgery
Norrby et al. 1983,[19] Sweden	192	Randomized, controlled, multicenter, trial	I	Early: 14.9% Delayed: 15.4%	Early: 0% Delayed: 1.1%	Early surgery defined as operation within 7 days of symptoms Studied patients ≤75 years old, randomized by odd vs. even birthdays Complications were similar between the two groups, but early surgery reduced hospital length of stay by >6 days.
Sianesi et al. 1984,[20] Italy	471	Retrospective (1970–77) and prospective (1977–82) data	III	Early: 18.5% Delayed: 15%	Early: 0% Delayed: 1.6%	Study combined retrospective and prospective data, collected over 12 years, during which time patient management evolved Reported low incidence of biliary infection, low morbidity and mortality, and shorter hospitalization period Authors recommend early surgery, within 48–72 h of diagnosis
Ajao et al. 1991, Nigeria	81	Retrospective	III	Early: 41% Delayed: 12.5%	Early: 2.6% Delayed: 0%	Retrospective review over 12 months, compared early (≤48 h) versus delayed (7–14 days) surgery Prohibitive rate of complications reported early surgery including 7 (18%) common bile duct injuries; only complications reported were wound infections (23%) and duct injuries Authors recommend delayed surgery, recommendations seemingly specific to the practice environment and level of surgical experience
Summary/totals	1019	—	—	Early: 21.0% Delayed: 16.5%	Early: 0.2% Delayed: 1.8%	Early surgery was technically more challenging with a higher complication rate, but shorter hospital stay and convalescence, more rapid return to work, and lower overall mortality than delayed surgery for acute cholecystitis

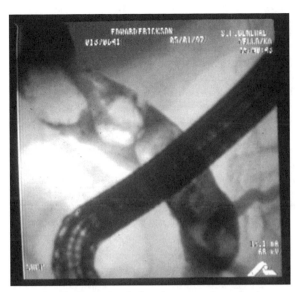

FIGURE 19.3. Endoscopic cholangiopancreatography in a patient with choledocholithiasis as evidenced by multiple filling defects within the common bile duct. (Courtesy of JP Cello, MD, Department of Medicine, UCSF.)

mortality of a frequently difficult prophylactic operation in an elderly patient are greater than that of leaving the organ in place.

ACALCULOUS CHOLECYSTITIS

Acalculous cholecystitis is a rare but potentially lethal condition that involves acute transmural inflammation of the gallbladder in the absence of identifiable gallstones. In contrast to classical acute cholecystitis, its pathogenesis is likely the result of gallbladder ischemia rather than cystic duct obstruction. The typical patient is critically ill or septic, fasting, and found in the intensive care unit. Under these circumstances, bile stasis, activation of factor XII, endotoxins, and distension of the gallbladder can each contribute to the organ's diminished perfusion and predispose to irreversible injury.[29] Gangrene, empyema, and perforation more commonly complicate the course of acalculous cholecystitis than of acute cholecystitis resulting from gallstones, with an incidence approaching 75% and a mortality of approximately 40% in some series.[30] Diagnosis of acalculous cholecystitis can be challenging, as many of the patients are sedated and unable to actively participate in the history and physical examination. Cholecystectomy is the mainstay of therapy for acalculous cholecystitis.

RECURRENT PYOGENIC CHOLANGITIS

This complex biliary system disease, also known as oriental cholangiohepatitis, is endemic to Southeast Asia and seen with increasing frequency in the United States.[31] Characterized by the presence of intrahepatic (i.e., hepatolithiasis) and extrahepatic pigment stones in the absence of disease within the gallbladder, recurrent pyogenic cholangitis has been reported as the number one cause of acute abdominal pain in Hong Kong emergency rooms. As a result of the recent, widespread immigration of Southeast Asians to the United States, the diagnosis of recurrent pyogenic cholangitis must be entertained when evaluating patients with biliary tract disease who were born in a country rimming the South China Sea.

Patients present with complaints of abdominal pain and fever. As there is usually segmental rather than complete bile duct obstruction, frank jaundice is uncommon. Treatment is aimed at decompression of the obstructed bile ducts and removal of as many stones and as much intraluminal debris as possible.

MIRIZZI'S SYNDROME

First reported in 1948, Mirizzi's syndrome entails obstruction of the common bile duct by a stone impacted in the adjacent cystic duct or Hartmann's pouch. Although this condition is more prevalent in the elderly, it can occur in any patient with cholelithiasis. Two types have been described.[32] In type I, the hepatic duct is compressed by a large stone that has become impacted in the cystic duct or Hartmann's pouch. Associated inflammation may contribute to the stricture. In other patients (type II), the calculus has eroded into the hepatic duct, producing a cholecystocholedochal fistula. Patients present with either painless jaundice or cholangitis, depending on the presence of contaminated bile. The treatment for type I lesions is cholecystectomy, but awareness of this syndrome is important because the surgical removal of the gallbladder under these circumstances is associated with an increased incidence of bile duct injury. Management of type II strictures is best accomplished through partial cholecystectomy and bilioenteric anastomosis.

BILIARY COLIC AND PREGNANCY

Gallbladder disease is occasionally first noted or becomes more troublesome during pregnancy. The most common clinical presentations are worsening biliary colic and acute cholecystitis. Jaundice and acute pancreatitis as a result of choledocholithiasis are rare. Radiological evaluation of symptoms suggestive of biliary tract disease can nearly always be limited to ultrasonography. Several series have demonstrated that the laparoscopic removal of the gallbladder during all stages of pregnancy is safe, resulting in minimal fetal and maternal morbidity.[33–35]

Medical Treatments

ORAL DISSOLUTION

In theory, biliary calculi, which specifically result from the cholesterol supersaturation of bile, should dissolve if the ratio of cholesterol to bile salts is reversed. In practice, this therapy (i.e. administration of chenodeoxycholic acid) is most effective for the treatment of small noncalcified cholesterol stones in patients with a functioning gallbladder. Successful therapy in many patients can require upward of 6 to 12 months, and necessitates periodic monitoring until the stones are dissolved. Approximately 50% to 60% of cholesterol stones measuring less than 10 mm in diameter respond; however, the gallstones recur in one-half of these patients within 5 years. Considering the duration, expense, potential side effects, and lack of a durable cure, oral dissolution therapy should be reserved for those patients who either cannot risk or do not want an operation.

CONTACT DISSOLUTION

Another approach to dissolving gallstones is to directly apply an agent that can solubilize cholesterol. While technically feasible, contact dissolution has at present a role limited to the treatment of cholelithiasis in patients who are not suitable for surgery.

EXTRACORPOREAL SHOCK WAVE LITHOTRIPSY

Introduced in the mid-1980s, extracorporeal shock wave lithotripsy (ESWL) utilizes high-energy sound (shock) waves to physically fragment gallstones into pieces small enough to be passed into the intestinal tract via the common bile duct. The potential advantages of ESWL include the noninvasive destruction of biliary calculi, decreased morbidity and mortality, shortened hospitalization, and the ability to treat patients who are poor candidates for a surgical procedure. However, shock wave lithotripsy has remained investigational to this day.

Surgical Treatments

OPEN CHOLECYSTECTOMY

In retrospective studies, 90% to 95% of patients undergoing cholecystectomy are substantially relieved or cured of their symptoms following surgery.[36]

Open cholecystectomy requires a general anesthetic, an incision in the anterior abdominal wall 12 to 20 cm in length, a 4- to 7-day hospitalization, and a 4- to 6-week recuperation period. Under direct vision the surgeon defines the extrahepatic biliary anatomy, resects the gallbladder and cystic duct, and when indicated explores the common bile duct to identify and remove all intraluminal calculi. This procedure is a safe and effective operation, with an overall morbidity of 2% to 8% and mortality of less than 2%. Thus, open cholecystectomy remains the time-honored standard against which newer therapies should be compared.[37–43]

The common postoperative complications following open cholecystectomy can be divided into biliary and nonbiliary complications. The most frequent complications are retained common bile duct stones, a bile leak or fistula, or a bile duct injury. The most feared of all complications during cholecystectomy is a major injury to the hepatic or common bile ducts. Such an injury can subsequently evolve into a benign stricture, and may initiate a sequence of events that includes many corrective surgeries, secondary biliary cirrhosis, and liver failure. Fortunately this complication occurs with an incidence of 0.08% to 0.3% and, as it is generally caused by an inadequate appreciation of the extrahepatic ductal anatomy, can be usually avoided.[44]

POSTCHOLECYSTECTOMY SYNDROME

Patients who return following cholecystectomy complaining of severe, episodic epigastric or right upper quadrant abdominal pain exemplify the postcholecystectomy pain syndrome. Although the majority of patients are symptomatically improved, it is not uncommon for patients to suffer minor gastrointestinal complaints after cholecystectomy. Indeed, following surgery up to 40% of patients may complain of excessive gas, bloating, abdominal pain, or dyspepsia. For the majority of patients, the pain resolves altogether with time; however, for 2% to 5% the pain is of sufficient severity to necessitate further investigation and treatment.[45,46]

The failure of a cholecystectomy to resolve abdominal pain in selected patients may be the result of an initial misdiagnosis. Therefore, the first step in evaluating patients with postcholecystectomy syndrome is to search for a confounding nonbiliary diagnosis. The key issue in treating patients who return after cholecystectomy complaining of pain is the systematic evaluation and accurate diagnosis of their complaint. A thorough history, physical examination, screening laboratory evaluation, and endoscopic intervention as indicated are essential to the successful management of these complex patients.

LAPAROSCOPIC CHOLECYSTECTOMY

Laparoscopic cholecystectomy is usually performed under general anesthesia with special attention paid to muscle relaxation. After induction of anesthesia, bladder and nasogastric tubes are placed for decompression. Intravenous antibiotics are not routinely required for prophylaxis against wound infection in elective cases. Either sequential compression stockings or low-dose subcutaneous heparin are used in patients at high risk for deep venous thrombosis. The operating room setup is shown in Figure 19.4.

A pneumoperitoneum carbon dioxide is created through a small umbilical incision to provide the space necessary to view the abdominal contents and manipulate instruments. After satisfactory development of the pneumoperitoneum, a periumbilical trocar is placed for the lap-aroscope, and three additional trocars are placed in the right upper quadrant for exposure and dissecting instruments (Fig. 19.5). The assistant, standing on the patient's right side, elevates the gallbladder fundus toward the ipsilateral hemidiaphragm and retracts the infundibulum laterally, exposing the triangle of Calot. The surgeon, standing at the patient's left side, dissects the cystic artery and duct from the gallbladder wall down toward porta hepatis. This is a crucial step, and special care must be taken to avoid mistaking the common bile duct for the cystic duct. Once the anatomy is identified, a metallic clip is placed across the cystic duct at its gall-

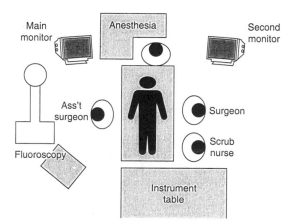

FIGURE 19.4. Operating room setup for laparoscopic cholecystectomy. (Reprinted with permission from Seminars in Gastrointestinal Disease 1994;5:122. WB Saunders Co.)

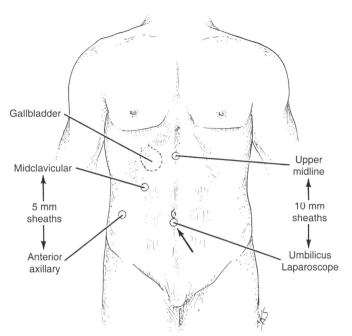

FIGURE 19.5. Trocar placement for performing a laparoscopic cholecystectomy.

bladder origin and a small incision is made in the cystic duct for placement of a cholangiogram catheter.

Cholangiography is performed in selected cases when it is necessary to both confirm the ductal anatomy and exclude the presence of gallstones in the common bile duct. Following completion of the cholangiogram, the cystic duct and artery are secured with metal clips and divided. The gallbladder is then dissected off the liver bed with electrocautery and delivered out the umbilical or epigastric trocar site. Care is taken during the procedure to avoid iatrogenic perforation of the gallbladder, because the resultant spillage of bile or gallstones is associated with an increased risk of postoperative fever and intraabdominal abscess formation.[47,48]

Postoperative management is straightforward. The bladder and nasogastric catheters are removed at the end of the procedure, and a diet of clear liquids is offered the evening of surgery. Most patients require mild oral analgesics for several days; narcotic injections are rarely necessary to control pain. Patients are allowed to resume full physical activity within 1 week after surgery, although patients may return to sedentary employment before this time.

RESULTS OF LAPAROSCOPIC SURGERY

After little more than a decade of experience, many practitioners consider laparoscopic cholecystectomy to have replaced the open approach as the treatment of choice, if not the standard of care. In 14 series reviewed, the cumulative operative morbidity was 7.2%, with an operative mortality of 0.12%. Bile duct injury occurred in 0.35%. Patients spent on average less than 2 days in the hospital, and returned to work or their normal daily activities after 6 days. Laparoscopic cholecystectomy is not only a safe and well-tolerated procedure, but has the attendant benefits of reduced perioperative morbidity and convalescence when compared to the standard open approach.[49–55]

Neoplasms

Cancers of the gallbladder and biliary tree fortunately are uncommon because these malignancies are associated with an extremely poor prognosis. Despite recent advances in imaging technology, biliary cancers are clinically silent tumors that only become symptomatic when they reach an advanced stage of development and are difficult to treat. Surgery is the only curative therapy; chemotherapy and radiation therapies are largely experimental efforts or directed at palliation. Approximately 4000 deaths occur each year in the United States from biliary cancer, with half originating in the gallbladder and 25% in the extrahepatic bile ducts; the remaining tumors arise within the ampulla or arc otherwise indeterminate.

Gallbladder Cancer

EPIDEMIOLOGY

Carcinoma of the gallbladder represents 1% of all cancers, is the most common biliary system malignancy, and is the fifth most common GI tract cancer with an overall incidence of 2 to 3 cases per 100,000 persons in the United States. Women outnumber men almost 3 to 1, with a mean age in the seventh decade of life. Interestingly, high-risk groups around the world for the development of gallbladder cancer include Native Americans (sixfold), Israelis, Chileans, Poles, Japanese, Bolivians, and Mexicans. The etiology of this devastating disease is unknown, but has been associated with cholelithiasis, chronic cholecystitis, exposure to specific industrial carcinogens, gallbladder adenomas, and inflammatory bowel disease.

DIAGNOSIS

Cancer of the gallbladder is a difficult diagnosis to make as only 8% to 10% of these malignancies are diagnosed preoperatively. The diagnostic challenge is largely because there are no signs or symptoms specific to gallbladder cancer. As the condition most often mimics benign biliary disease, with a clinical course reminiscent of anything from biliary colic to chronic cholecystitis, the history and physical examination are insensitive diagnostic tools. Three-quarters of patients have had symptoms for more than 6 months before seeking medical attention. When they do present, the most common complaint is abdominal pain, followed by weight loss, jaundice, nausea, and a host of other nonspecific symptoms. As noted earlier, these tumors are clinically unrecognizable as cancer until the disease is quite advanced, by which time the patient is usually incurable. Of the standard diagnostic studies for biliary tract disease, ultrasound is the most sensitive for detecting early-stage disease. In practical terms, most gallbladder cancers are unexpectedly diagnosed in the operating room during cholecystectomy for gallstones. Thus, the practice of carefully examining the resected gallbladder following its removal is important.

PATHOLOGY AND STAGING

Of gallbladder cancers, 85% are adenocarcinomas (papillary and mucinous variants), with the remaining tumors either squamous cell (3%), adenosquamous (1.5%), or undifferenti-

TABLE 19.3. Gallbladder Cancer Staging Systems.

Nevin classification[56]:

Nevin stage	Depth	5-Year survival (%)
Stage I	Mucosa only	50–97%
Stage II	Muscularis,	57–72%
Stage III	All layers	0–25%
Stage IV	Lymph nodes	0–20%
Stage V	Liver invasion Adjacent organ Distant metastasis	0–15%

AJCC TNM definitions for carcinoma of the gallbladder[68]:

Primary tumor (T)
TX   Primary tumor cannot be assessed
T0   No evidence of primary tumor
Tis   Carcinoma *in situ*
T1   Tumor invades lamina propria or muscle layer (Fig. 15.1)
T1a   Tumor invades lamina propria
T1b   Tumor invades muscle layer
T2   Tumor invades perimuscular connective tissue; no extension beyond serosa or into liver (Fig. 15.2)
T3   Tumor perforates the serosa (visceral peritoneum) and/or directly invades the liver and/or one other adjacent organ or structure, such as the stomach, duodenum, colon, or pancreas, omentum or extrahepatic bile ducts
T4   Tumor invades main portal vein or hepatic artery or invades multiple extrahepatic organs or structures

Reginal Lymph Nodes (N)
NX   Regional lymph nodes cannot be assessed
N0   No regional lymph node metastasis
N1   Regional lymph node metastasis

Distant Metastasis (M)
MX   Distant metastasis cannot be assessed
M0   No distant metastasis
M1   Distant metastasis

Source: Used with permission of the American Joint Committee on Cancer (AJCC), Chicago, IL. The original source for this material is the AJCC Cancer Staging Manual, 6th Edition (2002) published by Springer-Verlag New York, www.springer-ny.com

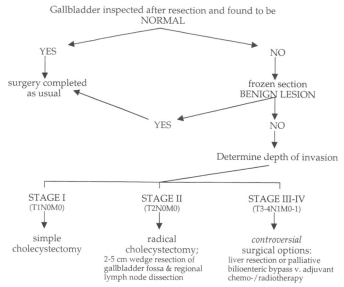

FIGURE 19.6. Treatment algorithm for cancer of the gallbladder.

TREATMENT

Treatment recommendations are dependent on the stage of the disease (Fig. 19.6). When the cancer is limited to the mucosa and muscularis of the gallbladder (stage I), a simple cholecystectomy should prove curative. When the tumor is transmural and found to invade the subserosa (stage II), however, most authors favor a radical cholecystectomy, with resection of the gallbladder fossa and a regional lymphadenectomy. Even though a survival advantage has not been definitively proven, this recommendation reflects concern for an increased risk of lymphovascular spread and locoregional recurrence once the tumor extends beyond the muscular wall of the organ. How to best treat stage III and IV tumors remains controversial, with the treatment recommendations ranging from major surgery (e.g., hepatic lobectomy, and orthotopic liver transplantation) to palliative bilioenteric bypass to adjuvant chemo- or radiotherapy. Opinions aside, at present there is no effective treatment for advanced gallbladder cancer.

Cholangiocarcinoma

EPIDEMIOLOGY

Approximately 2,700 new cases of bile duct cancer are diagnosed annually in the United States. With an overall yearly incidence of 1 per 100,000 population, this tumor occurs less frequently than cancer of the gallbladder.[58] Interestingly, the epidemiology and proposed pathogenesis of cholangiocarcinoma are very similar to that of gallbladder cancer, suggesting that these tumors may represent variants of the same disease process. As with gallbladder cancer, the incidence increases with age. High-risk groups include Native Americans, Israelis, and Japanese. The etiology appears related to chronic inflammation, gallstones, and stasis within the biliary system. In contrast, bile duct tumors occur with equal frequency in men and women, are associated with several biliary tract diseases, and usually present with painless jaundice. Among the etiological risk factors for this cancer are ulcerative colitis, primary scle-

ated (7%). On rare occasions the gallbladder can be the site of a melanoma, sarcoma, or carcinoid tumor. In 1976, Nevin et al. proposed a five-stage classification for cancer of the gallbladder predicated on the depth of tumor invasion into the gallbladder wall, presence of lymph node involvement, and invasion into adjacent or distant organs (Table 19.3).[56] More recently the standard TNM staging system has been applied to this cancer, which principally differs from the Nevin classification by stratifying the depth of direct liver invasion by the tumor. As described here, this stratification dramatically affects the recommended surgical treatment. Regardless of staging classification, once the tumor is transmural, the chances of cure are remote (Table 19.4).[57]

TABLE 19.4. Survival Statistics for Gallbladder Cancer.

Stage of disease	n	Median survival (months)	2-Year survival (%)
0	98	>60	78
I	621	19	45
III	117	7	15
III	678	4	4
IV	936	2	2

Source: Modified from Henson et al.[67]

TABLE 19.5. TNM Staging of Carcinoma of the Extrahepatic Bile Ducts.

Primary Tumor (T)

TX	Primary tumor cannot be assessed
T0	No evidence of primary tumor
Tis	Carcinoma *in situ*
T1	Tumor confined to the bile duct histologically
T2	Tumor invades beyond the wall of the bile duct
T3	Tumor invades the liver, gallbladder, pancreas, and/or ipsilateral branches of the portal vein (right or left) or hepatic artery (right or left)
T4	Tumor invades any of the following: main portal vein or its branches bilaterally, common hepatic artery, or other adjacent structures, such as the colon, stomach, duodenum, or abdominal wall

Regional Lymph Nodes (N)

NX	Regional lymph nodes cannot be assessed
N0	No regional lymph node metastasis
N1	Regional lymph node metastasis

Distant Metastasis (M)

MX	Distant metastasis cannot be assessed
M0	No distant metastasis
M1	Distant metastasis
	Biopsy of metastatic site performed . . . .☐Y . . . .☐N
	Source of pathologic metastatic specimen _____

Stage Grouping

0	Tis	N0	M0
IA	T1	N0	M0
IB	T2	N0	M0
IIA	T3	N0	M0
IIB	T1	N1	M0
	T2	N1	M0
	T3	N1	M0
III	T4	Any N	M0
IV	Any T	Any N	M1

Source: Used with the permission of the American Joint Committee on Cancer (AJCC), Chicago, IL. The original source for this material is the AJCC Cancer Staging Manual, 6th Edition (2002) published by Springer-Verlag New York, www.springer-ny.com.

rosing cholangitis, hepatolithiasis, and choledochal cysts. Common to each of these factors is an element of biliary stasis, infection, and stones. Exactly how these elements yield a cancer are unknown, but as with gallbladder cancer it is thought to involve a sequence of chronic inflammation leading to mucosal dedifferentiation and neoplasia.

DIAGNOSIS

The diagnosis is generally made when evaluating a patient with a case of gradually progressive, painless jaundice. More than 90% of patients present with this complaint, which may be accompanied by pruritus, weight loss, anorexia, fatigue, and other constitutional symptoms consistent with a malignancy. Malignant obstruction of the common bile duct generally produces a marked elevation in the total serum bilirubin of more than 10 mg/dl and an alkaline phosphatase that averages 500 to 600 IU/l.[58] Abdominal ultrasound or CT scan

clearly identify the dilated intrahepatic ducts proximal to the obstruction but rarely visualize the tumor itself. Cholangiography remains the most sensitive and informative method for evaluating obstructing ductal masses. The level and nature of the lesion, along with the patient's overall medical condition, are the primary guidelines that dictate which approach is most appropriate. ERCP does enable one to obtain biopsies and brushings from any abnormal areas; however, these tissue samples are diagnostic in less than half of cases given the fibrotic, relatively acellular nature of this cancer. Angiography can be used to evaluate possible vascular invasion by tumor.

PATHOLOGY AND STAGING

Cholangiocarcinomas are classified according to their location within the biliary ductal system rather than their histology. The simplest classification schema for bile duct cancers divides the lesions into those located in the upper, middle, or lower third of the extrahepatic biliary tree.[59] This method of stratifying cholangiocarcinomas proves very useful with respect to their surgical management. Cancers of the extrahepatic bile ducts are staged according to the TNM classification (Table 19.5).

TREATMENT

As with gallbladder cancer, surgery offers the only chance for cure when confronted with stage I and II tumors. Once there is lymph node, regional, or distant metastasis, the goal of intervention turns from cure to palliation. Therefore, when appropriately staged, resection is the treatment of choice.

HILAR CHOLANGIOCARCINOMAS

Half of extrahepatic bile duct cancers are located within the hilum of the liver and have been classified according to the pattern of right and left hepatic ductal involvement (Fig. 19.7).[60] There is considerable controversy regarding the value of surgical versus nonsurgical treatment for hilar bile duct cancers (Klatskin tumors). Because the determination of resectability often cannot be made preoperatively, all patients who are reasonable candidates for surgery deserve an exploratory operation. The criteria for unresectability are extensive vascular invasion of the portal vein or hepatic arteries, tumor involvement of secondary biliary radicals, evidence of metastatic disease, or carcinomatosis. As with gallbladder cancer, approximately 10% to 20% of patients can be resected for cure because most present with advanced disease.

For those patients with unresectable disease, opinions vary regarding the optimal method of palliation. At one end of the therapeutic spectrum are those who favor resection and intrahepatic bilioenteric bypass to palliate the obstructive jaundice, citing this as a durable and reasonably safe procedure.[61] At the other extreme are those who favor the use of

I II IIIA IIIB IV

FIGURE 19.7. Modified Bismuth–Corlette classification of hilar cholangiocarcinomas. (From Bismuth et al,[69] with permission.)

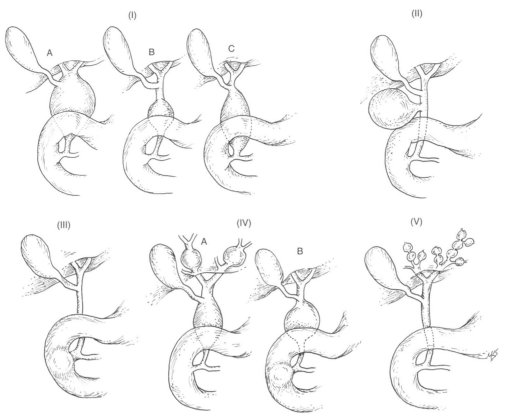

FIGURE 19.8. Todani classification of choledochal cysts. (From Todani et al,[65] with permission.)

percutaneously or endoscopically placed intraductal stents.[62] Stents require more frequent manipulation to maintain ductal patency, but their insertion is associated with significantly lower periprocedural morbidity and mortality rates.

Unfortunately, radiation therapy has had no demonstrable effect on patient survival. The same conclusion currently applies to single and combination adjuvant chemotherapy.

Benign Neoplasms

CHOLEDOCHAL CYSTS

Choledochal cysts are defined as localized or diffuse dilatations of the biliary tract that can be either congenital or acquired in nature and predominantly affect women.[63,64] The etiology of choledochal cysts is unknown. The clinical significance of choledochal cysts results from their propensity for complications, including cholangitis, biliary cirrhosis, portal hypertension, lithiasis, rupture, and malignant degeneration. The signs and symptoms of a choledochal cyst depend on its location, size, and specific consequence. Frequently, they present as a right upper quadrant mass with associated jaundice and fever in up to 60% of patients. Other complaints include weight loss and back pain. The diagnosis can be confirmed through the use of various diagnostic modalities, including ultrasound, abdominal CT, biliary scintigraphy, and endoscopic cholangiography. Choledochal cysts have been classified according to their pattern of extra- and intrahepatic bile duct involvement (Fig. 19.8).[65] Previous attempts to treat these cysts by internal cyst drainage via cystojejunostomy or cystoduodenostomy failed because of an unacceptably high

rate of late complications, including cholangitis and the development of cholangiocarcinoma. Complete surgical excision and bilioenteric reconstruction constitute the current treatment of choice.

BILIARY POLYPS

Polyps can be rarely found in the gallbladder and less frequently in the biliary tree.[66] Rarely themselves symptomatic, gallbladder polyps may represent a risk factor for the subsequent development of gallbladder cancer.

References

1. Lindner HH. Embryology and anatomy of the biliary tree. In: Way LW, Pellegrini CA, eds. Surgery of the Gallbladder and Bile Ducts, 1st Ed. Philadelphia: Saunders, 1987:3–15.
2. Moore KL. Clinically Oriented Anatomy, 2nd Ed. Baltimore: Williams & Wilkins, 1980.
3. Adamek HE, Albert J, Weitz M, Breer H, Schilling D, Riemann JF. A prospective evaluation of magnetic resonance cholangiopancreatography in patients with suspected bile duct obstruction [see comments]. Gut 1998;43:680–683.
4. Davis LP, McCarroll K. Correlative imaging of the liver and hepatobiliary system. Semin Nucl Med 1994;24:208–218.
5. Portincasa P, van de Meeberg P, van Erpecum KJ, Palasciano G, VanBerge-Henegouwen GP. An update on the pathogenesis and treatment of cholesterol gallstones. Scand J Gastroenterol Suppl 1997;223:60–69.
6. Strasberg SM. The pathogenesis of cholesterol gallstones, a review. J Gastrointest Surg 1998;2:109–125.
7. Konikoff FM, Laufer H, Messer G, Gilat T. Monitoring choles-

terol crystallization from lithogenic model bile by time-lapse density gradient ultracentrifugation. J Hepatol 1997;26:703–710.

8. Portincasa P, Di Ciaula A, Baldassarre G, et al. Gallbladder motor function in gallstone patients: sonographic and in vitro studies on the role of gallstones, smooth muscle function and gallbladder wall inflammation. J Hepatol 1994;21:430–440.

9. Pauletzki J, Althaus R, Holl J, Sackmann M, Paumgartner G. Gallbladder emptying and gallstone formation: a prospective study on gallstone recurrence [see comments]. Gastroenterology 1996;111:765–771.

10. Diehl AK. Epidemiology and natural history of gallstone disease. Gastroenterol Clin North Am 1991;20:1–19.

11. Lund J. Surgical indications in cholithiasis: prophylactic cholecystectomy elucidated on the basis of long-term follow up on 526 nonoperated cases. Ann Surg 1960;151:153–161.

12. Gracie WA, Ransohoff DF. The natural history of silent gallstones: the innocent gallstone is not a myth. N Engl J Med 1982;307:798–800.

13. McSherry CK, Ferstenberg H, Calhoun WF, Lahman E, Virshup M. The natural history of diagnosed gallstone disease in symptomatic and asymptomatic patients. Ann Surg 1985;202:59–63.

14. Friedman GD. Natural history of asymptomatic and symptomatic gallstones. Am J Surg 1993;165:399–404.

15. Linden WVD, Sunzel H. Early versus delayed operation for acute cholecystitis. A controlled clinical trial. Am J Surg 1970;120:7–13.

16. McArthur P, Cuschieri A, Sells RA, Shields R. Controlled clinical trial comparing early with interval cholecystectomy for acute cholecystitis. Br J Surg 1975;62:850–852.

17. Lahtinen J, Alhava EM, Aukee S. Acute cholecystitis treated by early and delayed surgery. A controlled clinical trial. Scand J Gastroenterol 1978;13:673–678.

18. Jarvinen IIJ, Hastbacka J. Early cholecystectomy for acute cholecystitis: a prospective randomized study. Ann Surg 1980;191:501–505.

19. Norrby S, Herlin P, Holmin T, Sjodahl R, Tagesson C. Early or delayed cholecystectomy in acute cholecystitis? A clinical trial. Br J Surg 1983;70:163–165.

20. Sianesi M, Ghirarduzzi A, Percudani M, Dell'Anna B. Cholecystectomy for acute cholecystitis: timing of operation, bacteriologic aspects, and postoperative course. Am J Surg 1984;148:609–612.

21. Lo CM, Liu CL, Fan ST, Lai EC, Wong J. Prospective randomized study of early versus delayed laparoscopic cholecystectomy for acute cholecystitis [see comments]. Ann Surg 1998;227:461–467.

22. Lai PB, Kwong KH, Leung KL, et al. Randomized trial of early versus delayed laparoscopic cholecystectomy for acute cholecystitis. Br J Surg 1998;85:764–767.

23. Leese T, Neoptolemos JP, Baker AR, Carr-Locke DL. Management of acute cholangitis and the impact of endoscopic sphincterotomy. Br J Surg 1986;73:988–992.

24. Lai EC, Mok FP, Tan ES, et al. Endoscopic biliary drainage for severe acute cholangitis [see comments]. N Engl J Med 1992;326:1582–1586.

25. Chijiiwa K, Kozaki N, Naito T, Kameoka N, Tanaka M. Treatment of choice for choledocholithiasis in patients with acute obstructive suppurative cholangitis and liver cirrhosis. Am J Surg 1995;170:356–360.

26. Sugiyama M, Atomi Y. Treatment of acute cholangitis due to choledocholithiasis in elderly and younger patients. Arch Surg 1997;132:1129–1133.

27. Acosta JM, Ledesma CL. Gallstone migration as a cause of acute pancreatitis. N Engl J Med 1974;290:484–487.

28. Kelly TR. Gallstone pancreatitis: pathophysiology. Surgery (St. Louis) 1976;80:488–492.

29. Barie P, Fischer E. Acute acalculous cholecystitis. J Am Coll Surg 1995;180:232–244.

30. Kalliafas S, Ziegler DW, Flancbaum L, Choban PS. Acute acal-

culous cholecystitis: incidence, risk factors, diagnosis, and outcome. Am Surg 1998;64:471–475.

31. Harris H, Kumwenda Z, Sheen-Chen S, Shah A, Schecter W. Recurrent pyogenic cholangitis. Am J Surg 1998;176:34–37.

32. Csendes A, Diaz JC, Burdiles P, Maluenda F, Nava O. Mirizzi syndrome and cholecystobiliary fistula: a unifying classification. Br J Surg 1989;76:1139–1143.

33. Glasgow RE, Visser BC, Harris HW, Patti MG, Kilpatrick SJ, Mulvihill SJ. Changing management of gallstone disease during pregnancy. Surg Endosc 1998;12:241–246.

34. Gouldman JW, Sticca RP, Rippon MB, McAlhany JC Jr. Laparoscopic cholecystectomy in pregnancy. Am Surg 1998;64:93–97; discussion 97–98.

35. Barone JE, Bears S, Chen S, Tsai J, Russell JC. Outcome study of cholecystectomy during pregnancy. Am J Surg 1999;177:232–236.

36. Gilliland TM, Traverso LW. Modern standards for comparison of cholecystectomy with alternative treatments for symptomatic cholelithiasis with emphasis on long-term relief of symptoms. Surg Gynecol Obstet 1990;170:39–44.

37. Glenn F, McSherry CK, Dineen P. Morbidity of surgical treatment for nonmalignant biliary tract disease. Surg Gynecol Obstet 1968;126:15–26.

38. Magee RB, MacDuffee RC. One thousand consecutive cholecystectomies. Arch Surg 1968;96:858–862.

39. Haff RC, Butcher HR Jr, Ballinger WFD. Biliary tract operations. A review of 1,000 patients. Arch Surg 1969;98:428–434.

40. Arnold DJ. 28,621 cholecystectomies in Ohio. Results of a survey in Ohio hospitals by the Gallbladder Survey Committee, Ohio Chapter, American College of Surgeons. Am J Surg 1970;119:714–717.

41. McSherry CK, Glenn F. The incidence and causes of death following surgery for nonmalignant biliary tract disease. Ann Surg 1980;191:271–275.

42. Morgenstern L, Wong L, Berci G. Twelve hundred open cholecystectomies before the laparoscopic era. A standard for comparison. Arch Surg 1992;127:400–403.

43. Roslyn JJ, Binns GS, Hughes EF, Saunders-Kirkwood K, Zinner MJ, Cates JA. Open cholecystectomy. A contemporary analysis of 42,474 patients. Ann Surg 193;218:129–137.

44. Strasberg SM, Hertl M, Soper NJ. An analysis of the problem of biliary injury during laparoscopic cholecystectomy [see comments]. J Am Coll Surg 1995;180:101–125.

45. Lasson A. The postcholecystectomy syndrome: diagnostic and therapeutic strategy. Scand J Gastroenterol 1987;22:897–902.

46. Moody FG. Postcholecystectomy syndromes. Surg Annu 1987;19:205–220.

47. Rice DC, Memon MA, Jamison RL, et al. Long-term consequences of intraoperative spillage of bile and gallstones during laparoscopic cholecystectomy. J Gastrointest Surg 1997;1:85–91.

48. Schafer M, Suter C, Klaiber C, Wehrli H, Frei E, Krahenbuhl L. Spilled gallstones after laparoscopic cholecystectomy. A relevant problem? A retrospective analysis of 10,174 laparoscopic cholecystectomies [see comments]. Surg Endosc 1998;12:305–309.

49. Attwood SE, Hill AD, Mealy K, Stephens RB. A prospective comparison of laparoscopic versus open cholecystectomy [see comments]. Ann R Coll Surg Engl 1992;74:397–400.

50. Farrow HC, Fletcher DR, Jones RM. The morbidity of surgical access: a study of open versus laparoscopic cholecystectomy. Aust N Z J Surg 1993;63:952–954.

51. Sanabria JR, Clavien PA, Cywes R, Strasberg SM. Laparoscopic versus open cholecystectomy: a matched study [see comments]. Can J Surg 193;36:330–336.

52. Barkun JS, Barkun AN, Meakins JL. Laparoscopic versus open cholecystectomy: the Canadian experience. The McGill Gallstone Treatment Group. Am J Surg 1993;165:455–458.

53. Williams LF Jr, Chapman WC, Bonau RA, McGee EC Jr, Boyd RW, Jacobs JK. Comparison of laparoscopic cholecystectomy

with open cholecystectomy in a single center. Am J Surg 193;165:459–465.

54. Berggren U, Gordh T, Grama D, Haglund U, Rastad J, Arvidsson D. Laparoscopic versus open cholecystectomy: hospitalization, sick leave, analgesia and trauma responses [see comments]. Br J Surg 1994;81:1362–1365.

55. Stevens HP, van de Berg M, Ruseler CH, Wereldsma JC. Clinical and financial aspects of cholecystectomy: laparoscopic versus open technique. World J Surg 1997;21:91–96, discussion 96–97.

56. Nevin JE, Moran TJ, Kay S, King R. Carcinoma of the gallbladder: staging, treatment, and prognosis. Cancer (Phila) 1976;37:141–148.

57. Donohue JH, Stewart AK, Menck HR. The National Cancer Data Base report on carcinoma of the gallbladder, 1989–1995. Cancer (Phila) 1998;83:2618–2628.

58. Henson DE, Albores-Saavedra J, Corle D. Carcinoma of the extrahepatic bile ducts. Histologic types, stage of disease, grade, and survival rates. Cancer (Phila) 1992;70:1498–1501.

59. Langer JC, Langer B, Taylor BR, Zeldin R, Cummings B. Carcinoma of the extrahepatic bile ducts: results of an aggressive surgical approach. Surgery (St. Louis) 1985;98:752–759.

60. Nakeeb A, Pitt HA, Sohn TA, et al. Cholangiocarcinoma. A spectrum of intrahepatic, perihilar, and distal tumors. Ann Surg 1996;224:463–473; discussion 473–475.

61. Jarnagin WR, Burke E, Powers C, Fong Y, Blumgart LH. Intrahepatic biliary enteric bypass provides effective palliation in selected patients with malignant obstruction at the hepatic duct confluence. Am J Surg 1998;175:453–460.

62. England RE, Martin DF. Endoscopic and percutaneous intervention in malignant obstructive jaundice. Cardiovasc Intervent Radiol 1996;19:381–387.

63. Fieber SS, Nance FC., Choledochal cyst and neoplasm: a comprehensive review of 106 cases and presentation of two original cases. Am Surg 1997;63:982–987.

64. Miyano T, Yamataka A. Choledochal cysts. Curr Opin Pediatr 1997;9:283–288.

65. Todani T, Watanabe Y, Narusue M, Tabuchi K, Okajima K. Congenital bile duct cysts: classification, operative procedures, and review of thirty-seven cases including cancer arising from choledochal cyst. Am J Surg 1977;134:263–269.

66. Furukawa H, Kosuge T, Shimada K, et al. Small polypoid lesions of the gallbladder: differential diagnosis and surgical indications by helical computed tomography. Arch Surg 1998;133:735–739.

67. Henson DE, Albores-Saavedra J, Corle D. Carcinoma of the gallbladder. Histologic types, stage of disease, grade, and survival rates. Cancer (Phila) 1992;70:1493–1497.

68. Evans DB, et al. Part III. Digestive system. In: Greene FL, Page DL, Fleming ID, et al., editors. AJCC Cancer Staging Manual, 6th ed. New York: Springer-Verlag, 2002.

69. Bismuth H, Nakache R, Diamond T. Management strategies in resection for hilar cholangiocarcinoma. Ann Surg 1992;215:31–38.

20

Liver

Alan Hemming and Steven Gallinger

Anatomy

The liver is approximately 4% to 5% of the total body weight and has multiple complex functions. The anatomy of the liver (Fig. 20.1) has been described using various methods[1–5]; however, surgical anatomy is based on the segmental nature of vascular and bile duct distribution. The liver receives a dual blood supply from both the portal vein and the hepatic artery, which run, along with the bile duct, within the Glissonian sheath or main portal pedicle. The portal pedicle divides into right and left branches and then supplies the liver in a segmental fashion. Venous drainage is via the hepatic veins, which drain directly into the inferior vena cava. Hepatic segmentation is based on the distribution of the portal pedicles and their relation to the hepatic veins (Fig. 20.1). The right hemiliver is divided into segments V, VI, VII and VIII; the left hemiliver into segments I, II, III and IV. Segment I is the caudate lobe, which lies between the inferior vena cava and the hepatic veins. The caudate lobe has variable portal venous, hepatic arterial, and biliary anatomy and is essentially independent of the portal pedicle divisions and hepatic venous drainage. Segmental anatomy becomes important in considering surgical resection when essentially any segment or combination of segments can be resected if attention is paid to maintaining vascular and biliary continuity to remaining segments.

Physiology

The liver performs many functions, including uptake, storage, and eventual distribution of nutrients from the blood or GI tract, synthesis, metabolism, and elimination of a variety of endogenous and exogenous substrates and toxins. It is responsible for 20% to 25% of body oxygen consumption and 20% of total energy expenditure.[6] The liver receives a dual blood supply with 75% of flow from the portal vein and 25% from the hepatic artery. Total blood flow to the liver is approximately $1.5 \ l/min/1.73 \ m^2$.[7] There is autoregulation of hepatic arterial flow but not the portal venous system. Por-

tal flow is increased by food intake, bile salts, secretin, pentagastrin, vasoactive intestinal polypeptide (VIP), glucagon, isoproterenol, prostaglandin E_1 and E_2, and papaverine. Portal flow is decreased by serotonin, angiotensin, vasopressin, nitrates, and somatostatin.

Bile is formed at the canalicular membrane of the hepatocyte as well as in the bile ductules and is secreted by an active process that is relatively independent of blood flow.[8] The major organic components of bile are the conjugated bile acids, cholesterol, phospholipid, bile pigments, and protein. Under normal conditions, 600 to 1000 ml of bile is produced per day.[9]

Bilirubin, a degradation product of heme, is eliminated almost entirely in the bile. Bilirubin circulates bound to albumin and is removed from plasma by the liver via a carrier-mediated transport system. In the hepatocyte, bilirubin is bound to glucuronic acid before being secreted in bile.

The liver synthesizes many of the major human plasma proteins, including albumin, γ-globulin, and many of the coagulation proteins. Liver dysfunction can have a profound effect on coagulation by decreased production of coagulation proteins or, in the case of obstructive jaundice, there is a decreased activity of factors II, V, VII, IX, and X secondary to a lack of vitamin K–dependent posttranslational modification. Reversal of coagulation abnormalities by exogenous administration of vitamin K differentiates between synthetic dysfunction and lack of vitamin K absorption secondary to obstructive jaundice.

Benign Noncystic Liver Lesions

A variety of benign and usually innocuous lesions are found quite commonly in the liver. Unless the clinical context raises suspicion of a malignant process, the differential diagnosis of solid liver lesions usually includes hemangioma, focal nodular hyperplasia, and hepatic adenoma. Judicious use of hepatic imaging procedures usually provides enough information to differentiate these three pathological entities.

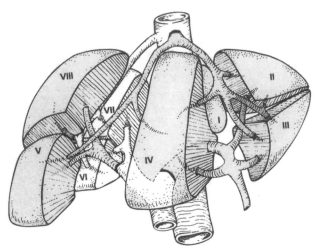

FIGURE 20.1. Diagrammatic representation of segmental liver anatomy. (From Blumgart LH, ed. Surgery of the Liver and Biliary Tract. New York: Churchill Livingstone, 1994, with permission.)

Hemangioma

Hepatic hemangiomas are extremely common with incidences as high as 20% in autopsy series. The great majority of hemangiomas are small, and often multiple. A fairly arbitrary cut-off of 6 to 10 cm has been suggested to differentiate typically small hemangiomas from giant hemangiomas. Nevertheless, the great majority of all hepatic hemangiomas, even giant lesions, remain asymptomatic throughout life. In rare instances, larger hemangiomas may become symptomatic secondary to pressure effects, thrombosis, necrosis, or bleeding.[10–12]

Diagnostic certainty can usually be achieved with appropriate radiologic imaging studies such that percutaneous biopsy and resection are almost never necessary (Table 20.1). Liver resection or enucleation is reserved for the very unusual case where symptoms are disabling.

Focal Nodular Hyperplasia

Focal nodular hyperplasia (FNH) is a typically well-circumscribed lesion with a classical central stellate "scar" with radiating fibrous septae. Although found in both males and females, FNH are more common in females of reproductive age. The etiology of this lesion is not entirely clear. FNH are usually solitary, although at least 20% of individuals with FNH have multiple lesions.[10–12] In some of these latter subjects with multiple FNH, other extrahepatic vascular abnormalities are found, including astrocytoma, neuroendocrine tumors, von Recklinghausen's disease, and multiple hepatic hemangiomas.[13]

Differentiation of FNH from hepatic adenoma and malignant liver tumors is important and can be difficult, as outlined in Table 20.1 and in the following section on adenoma. Once malignancy is excluded, most FNH can be safely observed without the need for biopsy or resection.

Hepatic Adenoma

Liver cell adenomas consist of sheets of hepatocytes with no portal triads. They are usually solitary but may be multiple, in up to 30% of cases.[14] These lesions are typically round but

not encapsulated. Adenomas arise in otherwise normal livers and appear as a focal abnormality or mass ranging in size from 3 mm to 30 cm. Although these are benign tumors, there are isolated case reports of primary hepatocellular carcinomas developing within adenomas.[15] The true incidence of hepatic adenoma is unknown, but there appears to be little doubt that the incidence increased with the introduction of oral contraceptives. Although adenomas may develop in children or adult males, more than 90% develop in women between the ages of 30 and 50 years.

PRESENTATION AND DIAGNOSIS

Abdominal pain, or the sensation of a mass, is the presenting symptom in approximately 50% of patients. Free intraperitoneal rupture occurs in 10% to 20% of cases while the remainder are found incidentally, either through imaging or at laparotomy. Diagnosis of adenoma is based on accurate imaging in the appropriate clinical setting. Although both CT and US will demonstrate a hypervascular mass lesion, neither technique differentiates liver cell adenoma from malignant tumors. Although percutaneous needle biopsy has been used to differentiate between liver cell adenoma and malignant tumors of the liver, the utility of biopsy remains in question because even experienced hepatopathologists have difficulty differentiating between a well-differentiated hepatocellular carcinoma and a liver cell adenoma.

MANAGEMENT

Patients who present with free intraperitoneal rupture or a large intraparenchymal bleed should undergo urgent operation after adequate resuscitation. Patients who present with a liver mass that, on imaging and in the appropriate clinical setting, is suspected to be an adenoma should stop use of oral contraceptives or exogenous steroids because regression of lesions has been reported.[16] Women with lesions that persist after withdrawal of oral contraceptives should be considered for elective resection because of the potential risk of bleeding or progression to hepatocellular carcinoma. Alternatives to resection have been reported, including arterial embolization and local ablation techniques such as cryosurgery and radiofrequency ablation. At present these alternative approaches should be considered investigational.

Liver Cysts

Liver cysts are frequently identified at laparotomy and during the course of investigations of unrelated abdominal symptoms. In most cases, the unexpected finding of a liver cyst, or multiple cysts, is of no clinical importance, although hepatic cysts are occasionally associated with serious pathological processes.

Congenital Liver Cysts

SOLITARY AND MULTIPLE SPORADIC SIMPLE LIVER CYSTS

Solitary unilocular or multilocular simple hepatic cysts appear grossly as variably sized, smooth, shiny, grey-blue cysts more common in the right lobe. The wall usually consists of three layers: an inner lining resembling bile duct epithelium,

TABLE 20.1. Imaging Characteristics of Solid, Benign Liver Lesions.

	Ultrasound	Helical CT	Nuclear medicine	MRI
Hemangioma	≤3 cm, well defined, homogeneous, hyperechoic ± acoustic enhancement, may be hypoechoic in background fatty liver, little or no flow on Doppler	Attenuation value of vascular channels always equal to blood, peripheral globular enhancement with centripetal filling in, larger atypical lesions may not "fill in" completely due to fibrosis or hemorrhage, may contain foci of calcification	Tc-99m pertechnetate-labeled RBC scan highly sensitive and specific for lesions >2 cm, "blind spot" in segments 2 & 3 near the heart, photopenic on early phase, fills in centripetally on delayed (30–50 min) scan, "cold" on Tc-99m sulfur colloid or HIDA scan	T_1 signal: low compared with liver T_2 signal: higher than spleen on intermediate and long TE images (very bright); this finding is strongly suggestive, but overlaps with hyper-vascular metastases and cysts) **Gd-chelate contrast enhancement:** like CT **Comment:** >95% accuracy when all findings present.
Hepatic adenoma	Nonspecific hypo-, iso-, or hyperechoic, may be similar to focal nodular hyperplasia (FNH) on Doppler, ±fluid in or adjacent if hemorrhage	Identification of intralesional or surrounding blood on unenhanced scan very suggestive, typically demonstrate enhancement but findings on arterial and venous phases are nonspecific and overlap with other lesions	80% "cold" on Tc 99m sulfur colloid scan, 20% show uptake, may demonstrate uptake on HIDA scan, early uptake with Tc-99m pertechnetate-labeled RBC scan, "cold" on delayed scan	T_1 signal: variable, often isointense to liver, portions may be black or very bright if contains blood products **Chemical shift imaging:** may see some changes suggestive of fat content (signal goes from bright to dark on comparative pulse sequences) T_2 signal: variable, usually slightly hyperintense to liver, if hemorrhagic may see very bright or dark areas **Gd-chelate contrast enhancement:** like CT. **Comment:** can overlap with HCC in imaging characteristics
FNH	Often subtle, near isoechoic, ± hypoechoic linear or stellate scar, peripheral and central vessels on Doppler	Densely enhancing uniform mass on arterial phase becoming isodense with normal liver on venous phase, usually low attenuation on unenhanced images, central low-attenuation "vascular scar"	80% show uptake on Tc-99m sulfur colloid scan (½ with uptake similar or greater than normal liver, ½ with less uptake than normal liver)	T_1 signal: variable, often isointense or hypointense to liver, may see low-intensity central stellate scar T_2 signal: often only slightly hyperintense to liver, may see central scar, which is hyperintense compared with rest of lesion **Gd-chelate contrast enhancement:** like CT, scar may enhance **Comment:** when all the findings above are present, strongly suggestive of FNH but some overlap with fibrolamellar HCC, and HCC with necrosis or scar

Source: Courtesy of Drs. M. Asch, M. Haider, and M. Margolis, Department of Radiology, University of Toronto.

a middle layer of compact connective tissue, and an outer layer containing looser connective tissue and compressed bile ducts and blood vessels.[17,18] Several theories have been proposed to explain the development of congenital hepatic cysts, but no consensus exists.

POLYCYSTIC DISEASE

The true incidence of congenital cystic disease of the liver is difficult to determine because most individuals with these lesions are asymptomatic. Large, congenital, solitary liver cysts appear to occur in a sporadic, nonhereditary fashion, whereas polycystic disease has a definite genetic component to its presentation. Polycystic disease is often subclassified into childhood and adult variants based on different modes of inheritance, presentation, and clinical consequences.

Childhood polycystic disease is inherited in an autosomal recessive pattern with four general subtypes: perinatal, neonatal, infantile, and juvenile.[19] All four variants of childhood polycystic disease affect both the liver and kidneys uniformly with an absolute increase in the number of intrahepatic bile ducts. Biliary microhamartomas may be found in both childhood and adult polycystic disease. There is an overlap between patients with polycystic liver disease and those with other congenital liver diseases, such as congenital hepatic fibrosis and cystic biliary abnormalities (e.g., Caroli's disease).

Adult polycystic liver disease is inherited in an autosomal dominant pattern. The liver is macroscopically diffusely cystic, although different patterns of disease, including unilobar cysts and different-sized cysts, are typical of the variable expression of polycystic liver disease. Considerable variability in patterns of disease are common even within families. Cysts may be found in the spleen, pancreas, ovaries, lungs, and kidneys. Depending on the imaging technique being used, liver cysts have been found in 29% to 75% of patients with polycystic kidneys.[20] The incidence increases with age and is higher in women than in men.[21]

CLINICAL MANIFESTATIONS

Hepatic cysts in childhood polycystic disease are usually asymptomatic, and the renal manifestations are of greater significance. Liver function is usually preserved throughout life, although fibrosis and portal hypertension can occur.[22,23]

The clinical presentation and complications of both adult polycystic liver disease and sporadic congenital cysts are similar.[24-26] Fewer than 15% of patients are symptomatic, and most series suggest a preponderance of women presenting with symptomatic cysts. Symptoms are usually related to a mass effect. A sensation of upper abdominal fullness and mild pain is the most common presentation, with occasional obstructive complaints or early satiety. Complications of solitary and multiple hepatic cysts are uncommon.

IMAGING

Ultrasound is the most cost-effective imaging modality because it can distinguish between solid and cystic liver lesions as well as give information about the nature of the cyst wall, fluid content, and surrounding liver tissue. Ultrasound and CT are also useful for imaging the kidneys and demonstrating coincidental renal cysts. CT scans show congenital hepatic cysts as nonenhancing, low-attenuation, smooth-contoured, fluid-filled lesions (Fig. 20.2). Atypical features such as septations, solid elements, irregularity, thickening, or calcification of the cyst wall seen on either ultrasound or CT should suggest some other process and prompt additional investigation.

TREATMENT

The great majority of congenital hepatic cysts, either simple or polycystic, never cause symptoms and therefore never require treatment. Serial imaging is only necessary when there is diagnostic uncertainty.

Simple aspiration of hepatic cysts is only of use for diagnostic purposes and occasionally as a provocative test before more definitive therapy. Recurrence rates following percutaneous aspiration alone approach 100%. Percutaneous aspiration under ultrasound control, followed by injection of 95% ethanol or other sclerosants, is now a well-accepted therapeutic modality, although recurrence rates vary widely.[27-29] Surgical unroofing and decompression of large hepatic cysts are an excellent and highly effective treatment in cases of sclerotherapy failures, or as primary treatment in the opinion of some authors.[30,31] Laparoscopic approaches, in which the cyst is decompressed and a large portion of the cyst wall is excised, are currently an attractive strategy because of low morbidity and high efficacy.

Polycystic liver disease in adults produces slow progressive enlargement of the liver with minimal interference with liver function until at a late stage in the disease.[21] Only patients who are clearly disabled should be offered surgery. Surgical methods to reduce symptoms related to size alone include multiple cyst unroofing and fenestration of cysts.[30-34] Laparoscopic unroofing procedures have been reported as variably successful, although long-term symptomatic recurrence rates are quite high because new cysts will grow to replace decompressed cysts.[35,36] Occasional patients develop manifestations of chronic liver disease including portal hypertension, ascites, and variceal bleeding. These cases, as well as the rare patient with intractable symptoms who has failed previous surgical procedures, will benefit from liver transplantation.

Traumatic Cysts

Hemorrhage into the liver parenchyma may occur with blunt or penetrating abdominal trauma. Bleeding is contained within the liver if the capsule is intact and traumatic cysts contain blood, bile, and necrotic liver tissue. Lack of a true epithelial lining denotes that traumatic cysts are in fact pseudocysts. Unless a traumatic cyst becomes infected secondarily, it is best treated expectantly.

Cystadenoma and Cystadenocarcinoma

True neoplastic cysts of the liver are rare compared with congenital cysts. As with congenital cysts, benign cystadenomas occur most often in middle-aged women. Grossly, the tumors are usually large, in the right lobe, and multilocular, and they contain a clear, mucinous fluid. Bloody fluid occurs more often in malignant cysts. Microscopically, the diagnostic features include a multiloculated lesion lined by benign or malignant mucin-producing cells often showing polypoid papillary projections into the cyst. The surrounding stroma is typically dense. The tumors are thought to be congenital in origin and slow growing. It is believed that cystadenocarcinomas are derived from benign cystadenomas, because most of the malignant tumors contain a considerable amount of benign epithelium.[37]

Clinical and radiologic differentiation of neoplastic cysts from congenital cysts may be difficult. Features suggestive of neoplastic cysts on ultrasound and CT include papillary projections or irregularities in the cyst wall, complex multiloc-

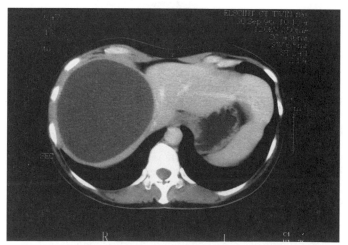

FIGURE 20.2. Large, symptomatic simple liver cyst in 48-year-old woman. Note uniform, low-density fluid, and thin wall without calcifications, septations, or intracystic projections. This cyst was treated successfully by laparoscopic unroofing.

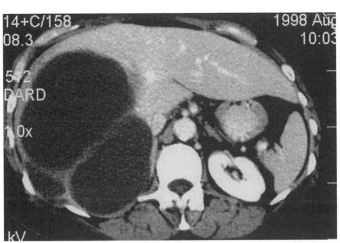

FIGURE 20.3. CT scan demonstrating large, complex, thick-walled cystadenoma in right lobe of liver.

ular cysts, and the presence of cyst contents of different densities in different parts of a multilocular cyst (Fig. 20.3). Cystadenoma, especially when unilocular, may be very difficult to distinguish from congenital cyst. Any cyst suspected of being a cystadenoma should be explored and completely excised either by the technique of enucleation[38] or by liver resection. The long-term results after complete excision of cystadenoma are excellent, but if the excision is incomplete, recurrence is virtually guaranteed. Cyst-adenocarcinoma requires liver resection and, if it is nonmetastatic, results are very good.[39,40]

A number of metastatic tumors occurring in the liver, such as adenocarcinoma from the gastrointestinal tract, sarcomas, and renal cell carcinomas, may undergo cystic change.

Parasitic (Hydatid) Liver Cysts

Hydatid disease in humans is caused by the larval form of parasites of the genus *Echinococcus*. The most common form is cystic hydatid disease resulting from infection with *E. granulosus*. The life cycle of *E. granulosus* requires two hosts: a primary host harboring the adult worm and an intermediate host harboring the larval stage. The adult parasite resides in the intestine of canines. Humans become an accidental intermediate host when contaminated unwashed vegetables are ingested or through contact (usually in childhood) with infected animals who may carry ova on their fur or shed ova onto soil in which children play.[41] Growth is often slow, and it may be many years before the hydatid cyst becomes symptomatic.

Distribution of Hydatid Disease

Hydatid disease is known worldwide, particularly in rural areas where dogs are kept and used for herding livestock.

Pathology

Following entry into the portal circulation, the embryo begins to grow into a larva in the liver and forms a cystic structure that develops three layers in its wall. The outer layer is formed of host tissue as a result of a reaction to the parasite. As the surrounding liver tissue collapses gradually with the expansion of the hydatid cyst, vessels and ductal structures in the liver become incorporated in the wall or in the adjacent compressed liver. This process causes the appearance of a central avascular area (the cyst) with a hypervascular rim or halo on CT scans and angiograms.[42,43] Calcification often occurs in the wall of the mature hydatid cyst, and about half these cysts can be seen on plain films of the abdomen. The parasite itself makes up the two internal layers of the cyst wall. The innermost germinal layer is the living parasite. The cyst fluid is secreted by the germinal lining and is normally clear in color. The high secretion pressure is responsible for the progressive enlargement of the cyst. In the case of dead or infected cysts, the fluid may become turbid or frankly purulent. Bile-stained cyst fluid is an indicator of communication of the cyst with the biliary tract.

CLINICAL PRESENTATION

Hydatid cysts of the liver are often asymptomatic and may remain so until they reach a large size. With recent refinements in noninvasive imaging techniques, they are found frequently as an incidental finding on ultrasound or CT studies (Fig. 20.4).

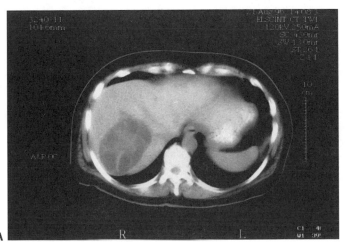
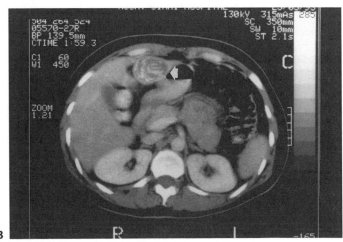

FIGURE 20.4. Hydatid cysts in right lobe (**A**), and in left lateral segment (**B**, *arrow*). Note thick-walled septations of daughter cysts in **A** and whorled calcifications in **B**.

Expansion of cysts in the liver may cause localized pain. If organisms enter the cyst, it may become infected and produce pain and fever and behave clinically as a liver abscess. If frankly infected material enters the biliary tract, the patient may present with jaundice as well as fever.

ALLERGIC REACTIONS

Hydatid cyst fluid is antigenic and, when released into the circulation either directly by a leak into the liver or secondarily as a result of rupture into the peritoneal cavity, acute allergic reactions may occur. These range from mild urticaria to severe acute anaphylaxis.

DIAGNOSIS

Hydatid disease of the liver should be high on the list of diagnostic possibilities in patients who come from an endemic area, especially if they spent their childhood in a rural environment and if they present with abdominal mass, pain, fever, jaundice, or anaphylaxis. Imaging tests are very accurate because ultrasound will demonstrate the cystic nature of the lesion, the presence of daughter cysts, and collections of hydatid sand. CT scanning is as reliable for making the diagnosis and is complementary to ultrasound. In the jaundiced patient with hepatic hydatid disease, endoscopic retrograde cholangiopancreatography (ERCP) should be performed to determine if the jaundice is the result of extrusion of cyst material into the bile duct or is merely a manifestation of cholangitis from the spill of infected fluid into the biliary tract. Routine blood analysis is of little help in making the diagnosis of hydatid disease. Serological studies are currently the most reliable adjunct to imaging tests in confirming the diagnosis of echinococcosis of the liver.[41,44] The complement fixation test is positive in approximately 65% of patients and the indirect hemagglutination test in 85%.

Treatment of Hydatid Disease

DRUG THERAPY

Systemic antihelminthic agents are generally not effective against human *Echinococcus* and are generally considered adjuvants to surgery. However, the group of drugs known as benzimidazolecarbamates have shown promise as parasitocidal and parasitostatic agents. Drug therapy is indicated in patients in whom accidental spillage of cyst fluid has occurred at operation, in patients with active disease who are unfit for surgery, and in patients who rupture hydatid cysts spontaneously into the peritoneal or pleural cavities.[45,46]

PERCUTANEOUS ASPIRATION AND SCOLICIDAL THERAPY

Percutaneous fine-needle aspiration may be necessary as a diagnostic test in the workup of the occasional complex liver cyst for which serology and imaging are nondiagnostic of hydatid disease.[47,48] A number of groups have extended this approach to aspirate unilocular hydatid cysts and instill a variety of scolicidal agents. The long-term value of this method is still unproven.

SURGICAL TREATMENT

Surgery remains the standard approach for hydatid disease of the liver and is indicated in all patients with symptomatic disease. Although hydatid disease tends to advance slowly, it may produce life-threatening complications, and therefore surgical treatment should be considered even in patients with asymptomatic disease discovered accidentally, especially if the cyst is large (>5 cm) and accessible.

There are numerous strategies for handling hepatic hydatid cysts, and opinions vary from conservative to radical. To be curative, surgical therapy must remove all the living parasite and leave no viable daughter cysts or protoscolices either in the residual cavity or elsewhere in the host, while still preserving liver function. Controversies include the role of cyst aspiration, the choice between resection and cyst evacuation, and the management of the residual cavity, including the use of scolicidal agents and the advisability of external drainage.

Complete surgical removal is required for cure, and can be accomplished (1) by removal of all laminated membrane and attached germinal lining, daughter cysts, fluid, and scolices, leaving the pericyst; or (2) by resection of the intact cyst, including the pericyst. Because of the risk of spillage of infective material into the peritoneal or pleural cavity, some favor excision either by formal liver resection or by meticulous separation of the entire cyst, including the pericyst, from surrounding liver. Formal liver resection is used sparingly and is usually needed only for peripherally located cysts.[49–52]

SCOLICIDAL AGENTS

Because large cysts contain thousands of barely visible protoscolices, each of which can implant in its host and create a new cyst, mechanical removal is usually supplemented by some type of scolicidal agent to ensure that overlooked protoscolices are killed. These agents include hydrogen peroxide, cetrimide, hypertonic saline, chlorhexidine, 20% ethyl alcohol, and 0.5% silver nitrate.[53,54] Great care must be taken when scolicidal agents are used to complete sterilization of the surgically evacuated hydatid cavity to avoid spillage into the peritoneum or entry of fluid into the bile ducts.

MANAGEMENT OF THE RESIDUAL CAVITY

There remains controversy regarding the management of the residual cavity after evacuation of the living cysts and treatment with scolicidal agents. Techniques have been described to obliterate the cavity, such as filling with omentum or suturing the walls together from within (the so-called capitonnage technique).[55–57] Our own method of management of the cyst cavity depends on size, depth, and amount of pericyst exposed at the liver surface, as well as the presence or absence of infection or communication with the biliary tract. If either or both of the latter conditions exist, closed suction drainage is used.

COMPLICATIONS OF HYDATID DISEASE

Anaphylaxis may occur with rupture and spillage of hydatid fluid into the peritoneal cavity. Mild symptoms resolve spontaneously but may be helped by antihistamines or steroids. Adrenaline is necessary for severe anaphylaxis. Emergency operation is rarely required, because the leakage is usually only a small amount of fluid. A course of systemic mebendazole or albendazole may be helpful in preventing peritoneal hydatosis with either minor or major rupture of a liver cyst.

Infection is seen in about one-quarter of hydatid cysts in adults.[50,55] Communication with the biliary tract is common in infected hydatids and should be sought carefully.

Biliary tract obstruction occurs when a hydatid cyst ruptures into a bile duct and extrudes daughter cysts or portions of laminated membrane down the common duct. This diagnosis should be made preoperatively by ERCP, and endoscopic sphincterotomy and clearance of the bile duct should be carried out before surgery for the cyst itself.[58]

Associated extrahepatic hydatid disease from previous spontaneous rupture or surgery should be dealt with at the same time as hepatic cysts are treated.

FOLLOW-UP

Recurrence rates are low (about 2%) following surgical management of uncomplicated hydatid disease. Nevertheless, long-term follow-up is advisable, including periodic imaging studies and serology. Serological tests may remain abnormal for a couple of years.

Hepatocellular Carcinoma

Hepatocellular carcinoma (HCC) is one of the commonest malignancies worldwide, causing more than 1 million deaths every year.[59] The annual incidence varies from a high of 30 per 100,000 in Southeast Asia and Africa to around 2 per 100,000 in Northern Europe and North America.[60] A recent report suggested a rising incidence of HCC in the United States over the past two decades.[61]

Tumor Biology

A large number of risk factors have been identified for HCC (Table 20.2); however, most patients have tumors that have occurred on a background of chronic liver disease secondary to hepatitis B or C infection or alcohol abuse. Only 10% of patients with HCC have neither cirrhosis nor chronic viral hepatitis.[62] Hepatocellular carcinoma rarely occurs in the normal liver.[63]

Regenerating nodules are part of the reparative process in the evolution of cirrhosis. Other nodules, termed adenomatous hyperplasia, or dysplastic nodules may also develop; these result from genetic alterations, are monoclonal, and are believed to be the first step in the evolution of malignancy.[64] Subsequent genetic changes lead to dedifferentiation to a well-differentiated HCC, and subsequently to poorly differentiated HCC, over a period of months to years.[62,65]

TABLE 20.2. Risk Factors for Primary Hepatocellular Carcinoma.

Hepatitis B
Hepatitis C
Alcoholic cirrhosis
Others:
Hemochromatosis
Alpha-1 antitrypsin deficiency
Wilson's disease
Tyrosinemia
Glycogen storage disease

Natural History

The survival of a patient with HCC is determined in part by the stage of the malignancy, and in part by the severity of the underlying liver disease. The latter is also an important factor in determining suitability for any treatment. Studies of patients with small asymptomatic untreated HCC show 1-, 2-, and 3-year survival rates of 91%, 55%, and 13%, respectively.[66,67] Symptomatic patients usually have advanced disease and commonly present with abdominal pain, distension, weight loss, and malaise.[68] Symptomatic patients have a much shorter survival, usually measured in months, with most dying of metastatic disease or complications of their underlying liver disease.[68,69]

Diagnosis and Staging

TUMOR MARKERS

Serum concentrations of α-fetoprotein (AFP) are elevated in about 75% of patients with HCC.[70] AFP can also be elevated in a variety of benign diseases, especially acute and chronic hepatitis and cirrhosis. A single elevated AFP level may therefore not be diagnostic, and interpretation must take into account the absolute level, change with time, and presence or absence of chronic hepatitis.

IMAGING

Ultrasound is the least expensive and most widely available imaging technique. In expert hands, it is extremely useful, and some lesions less than 1 cm in diameter can be detected. A major problem in screening is distinguishing regenerating nodules from early HCC. Color Doppler may be helpful if increased vascularity can be demonstrated in a suspicious nodule. Correlation with other imaging modalities is often complementary in making a diagnosis of HCC.[71,72]

CT scanning allows rapid volumetric acquisition of data during separate arterial and portal venous phases of contrast enhancement. Identification of lesions as small as 1 cm in diameter is usually possible, and excellent demonstration of relationships with vessels can also be obtained. Spiral CT is similar to CT angioportography in its sensitivity and specificity, and is probably the imaging method of choice for identifying HCC[73] (Fig. 20.5).

MRI

The limits of detection of MRI, comparable to those of CT, and current high-speed MR software allow high-definition, three-dimensional reconstructions to be carried out that are useful in planning resectional surgery. MRI is also very useful in differentiating other small mass lesions from HCC in a nodular cirrhotic liver, particularly hemangioma and regenerative nodules as small as 1 cm.[74]

BIOPSY

Preoperative histological confirmation of HCC is not required in most cases, particularly if AFP levels are very high or if the clinical setting is highly suggestive in a patient with a new nodule. Biopsy poses significant risks of hemorrhage and tumor rupture, as well as the possibility of tumor implantation, notably in tumors close to the liver surface.[72] In the rare

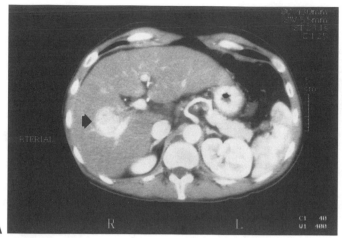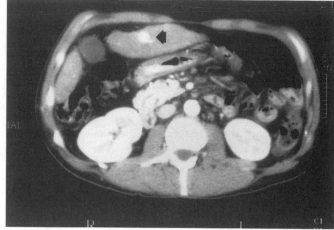

FIGURE 20.5. Early arterial phase helical CT scans demonstrate hypervascular hepatocellular carcinomas (*arrows*). Note nodular cirrhotic liver in **B**.

instance where histological evaluation may alter management, fine-needle aspiration biopsy should be performed through a nontumorous area of liver that will be included in any planned resection.

STAGING

Although a variety of staging systems have been described for HCC, the UICC/AJCC standardized TNM approach has been adopted by most centers and allows for comparison of results.[75]

SCREENING

The heightened awareness of cancer risk in patients with chronic hepatitis B and C has resulted in widespread informal screening, which has probably led to earlier identification of tumors in many patients. Whether the recent improvement in survival rates can be attributed to better surgical outcomes because of earlier diagnosis or to lead-time bias has not yet been determined.

Resection

PREOPERATIVE ASSESSMENT OF RESECTABILITY

Considerations in determining resectability of a primary liver cancer include general health of the patient, tumor stage, and functional capacity of the underlying liver. Most authors would consider stage IIIB or IV disease to be incurable by resection. Other factors that are believed to be relative predictors of poor outcome include multiple tumors,[76,77] large tumor size,[78,79] and vascular invasion.[80,81] There is evidence that each of these variables decreases the likelihood of long-term cure, but no one factor alone is considered an absolute contraindication for resection. The anatomical location of a lesion may result in unresectability for technical reasons, even if staging were favorable.

One of the most difficult aspects of assessment of resectability is determining functional reserve of the liver, that is, the ability of the liver to not only tolerate an anaesthetic and operative procedure but to regenerate after removal of

functional hepatic mass. Exact quantitative predictors are not available, but most surgeons would only consider resection for those patients classified as Child–Pugh A or early B with coagulation function correctable to normal, and without complications of cirrhosis such as ascites, bleeding, or marked portal hypertension.

Some studies suggest that the use of indocyanine green (ICG) clearance or the redox tolerance test can improve patient selection, but experience is limited with these functional studies.[82,83]

INTRAOPERATIVE ASSESSMENT AND THE ROLE OF INTRAOPERATIVE ULTRASOUND

Approximately 12% of patients who are explored for resection of HCC are found to be unresectable at laparotomy because of peritoneal spread, nodal involvement, or additional tumors in the liver found by intraoperative ultrasound. Laparoscopic ultrasound before laparotomy is becoming more widely used and may be able to identify approximately half of those patients who would be deemed unresectable at laparotomy.[84]

EXTENT OF RESECTION

The ideal margin for curative resection in HCC is not yet defined. In the cirrhotic patient, however, preservation of liver function and wide surgical clearance of the tumor are the two main, but frequently contradictory, principles of resection. A disease-free margin of 1 cm is believed to be adequate by most groups but others have advocated a margin of 2 to 3 cm.[85] The frequency of intrahepatic metastases further than 1 cm away from the tumor increases with tumors larger than 4 to 5 cm, and a larger resection margin should be considered.[86,87]

Results of Resection

Both operative mortality and long-term survival rates have improved substantially since the 1970s as a result of better patient selection, operative techniques, and perioperative care. Operative mortality rates in large centers are now less than 5%, although rates are considerably lower in noncirrhotic than cirrhotic patients.

Tumor recurrence rates within the liver are high and increase progressively with time. They range from 38% to 68%[76,88–90] in various reports, and recurrences occur in sites distant from the resection margin, suggesting that most are new tumors rather than recurrences of the resected tumor. A number of adjuvant therapy approaches have been used to decrease the recurrence rate following resection. Repeat resection is another option for patients with isolated intrahepatic recurrence of HCC. Few patients are suitable for treatment, but the reported data suggest that survival figures for reresection are similar to those for primary resection.[91]

Liver Transplantation

Recent 3-month perioperative mortality rates for transplantation are generally in the 10% range.[90,92,93] The incidence of tumor recurrence in these reports ranges from 8% to 37% and may reflect differences in selection criteria. Selection may also have resulted in the wide differences in survival. There are promising new data, however, showing that survival rates (55–87% at 1 year, 20–45% at 5 years) can be achieved similar to those for patients transplanted for nonmalignant disease.[92,94]

Preoperative factors that appear to be important predictors of disease-free and overall survival are absence of tumor-associated symptoms,[95] hepatitis B virus (HBV) negativity,[90,96] early TNM stage,[97–99] small size (less than 2–5 cm),[97–100] single tumor (or fewer than three tumors),[92,95,97,99] low AFP,[97] tumor encapsulation,[97,99] and absence of vascular invasion.[97,99] These factors are generally similar to those reported to be associated with better results following partial hepatectomy for HCC.

The survival of HBV-negative early-stage cancer patients is approaching that achieved for other groups of transplant patients, and raises the question whether transplantation should be considered the preferred treatment for early HCC, rather than resection. A critical limitation to the application of liver transplantation as primary oncotherapy in patients with HCC remains the severe shortage of donor livers. Until organ availability improves, transplantation for HCC can only be offered to patients whose survival rates are predicted to be similar to those of patients transplanted for benign disease. Whether transplantation can be recommended for higher-risk patients (those with larger, multiple, or more advanced tumors, or with HBV) in combination with effective antitumor or antiviral therapy remains to be proven.

Nonsurgical Options

Many nonsurgical approaches to the treatment of HCC have been undertaken for both early and advanced disease. Recent results of percutaneous ethanol injection (PEI) of HCCs less than 3 cm show complete necrosis of the tumor in up to 90% of patients. For small tumors, the recurrence rates and pattern are similar to those for surgical resection. Other methods of local destruction including cryotherapy and radiofrequency ablation have also been reported, with similar results. In patients with good liver function and absence of portal hypertension, surgery still offers the advantage of complete tumor removal along with a surrounding margin that may contain possible satellites.[101] A number of palliative modalities have been advocated including arterial embolization, chemo-embolization, systemic chemotherapy, radiotherapy (either external beam or yttrium microspheres), immunotherapy, and hormonal manipulation.[102] Although there are occasional encouraging reports, these treatment methods should be considered investigational and used only as part of standardized study protocols.

Authors' Approach

All new patients with HCC are reviewed by a multidisciplinary team of hepatobiliary and liver transplant surgeons, hepatologists, interventional radiologists, and oncologists. Surgical resection is considered first-line therapy in patients who meet the previously described selection criteria. Patients who are not resectable and are HBV negative are considered transplant candidates if their tumors are less than 5 cm in diameter and they meet the other criteria for transplantation. If not transplantable, they are considered for one of our study protocols. Patients who have unresectable tumors and are HBV positive are treated with PEI if their tumors are less than 5 cm in diameter; those with larger tumors are considered for one of our experimental protocols.

Liver Metastases

Colorectal Cancer

NATURAL HISTORY AND RESULTS OF RESECTION OF COLORECTAL CANCER HEPATIC METASTASES

The natural history of unresected hepatic metastases is difficult to predict because of the heterogeneity of clinical progression of different malignancies and even considerable variability among patients with the same primary cancer. For reasons that are not clear, approximately 5% to 10% of stage IV colorectal cancer patients present with a synchronous or metachronous "limited hepatic-only" pattern of disease. These individuals are those most frequently referred for consideration of an aggressive surgical approach for their metastatic disease. It is well accepted that hepatic resection for selected patients with colorectal cancer liver metastases is beneficial although the degree of benefit is unclear because a randomized trial with a "no treatment" arm has never been performed. Overall 5-year survival data following hepatic resection of colorectal cancer metastases vary between 20% and 40%.

IMAGING BEFORE LIVER RESECTION OF METASTATIC DISEASE

The goals of radiologic studies for the liver resection candidate include (1) detection of extrahepatic disease and (2) accurate characterization of the number, size, and location of hepatic metastases. Because the results of liver resection for metastatic colorectal cancer are so poor in patients with extrahepatic disease, common sites for recurrent disease and metastatic spread should be studied. Of all the various diagnostic maneuvers performed before liver resection for metastatic disease, careful intraoperative palpation and handheld intraoperative ultrasound should be considered essential in all cases[103–108] (Fig. 20.6).

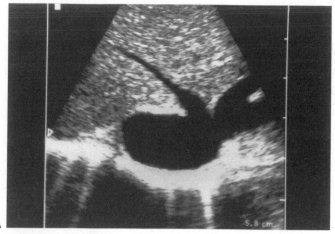 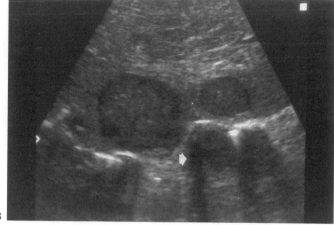

FIGURE 20.6. Intraoperative ultrasound shows excellent view of the main hepatic veins (**A**) and two typical-appearing small colorectal cancer liver metastases (**B**). Note surgeon's fingers in B (*arrow*).

PREOPERATIVE AND INTRAOPERATIVE FACTORS THAT INFLUENCE PROGNOSIS

Because not all patients with colorectal cancer hepatic metastases will benefit from an aggressive operative approach, patient selection, based on well-proven prognostic markers, is important. Numerous case series provide fairly good evidence that various patient and tumor factors are predictive of long-term survival following liver resection. Variables for which data are available are listed below:

Stage of primary colorectal cancer

Interval from resection of primary colorectal cancer

Extent of liver involvement; bilobar versus unilobar, size of metastases, number of metastases

Extrahepatic disease

Preoperative carcinoembryonic antigen (CEA) level

Resection margin

Blood transfusions

Molecular markers

Although there is little doubt that many of these variables affect patient survival, there is strong evidence for only a few, and only weak and occasionally conflicting evidence for the others. Nevertheless, a number of fairly dogmatic statements can be made from the available data. First, although "primary tumor" factors such as prior stage of the primary colorectal cancer, synchronous versus metachronous liver metastases, and interval from resection of the primary might be predicted to be important prognostic variables, published data only partly support this notion. Second, specific "metastasis" factors just listed appear to be fairly important in determining outcome. There appear to be adequate data, and little disagreement, on the positive benefit derived from resecting solitary tumors and perhaps up to four metastases. However, arguments both in favor and against very radical resections of more than four bilobar metastases can be made on the basis of current evidence. Results of liver resection in patients with extrahepatic, noncontiguous disease are so poor that this approach seems rarely justified. Third, the importance of a negative resection margin should be stressed because this is perhaps the only prognostic factor over which the surgeon has any definite control.[109]

NONRESECTIONAL ABLATIVE THERAPIES

Although hepatic resection is considered standard treatment for selected patients with colorectal cancer liver metastases, both patient and tumor factors occasionally preclude a resectional approach. In particular, patients with bilobar disease or situations in which even small metastases are close to major inflow or outflow vessels may preclude resection due to resultant insufficient hepatic parenchyma for survival. These problems have provided impetus for the development and application of locally ablative strategies whereby metastases can be destroyed, with a satisfactory margin, with enough uninvolved liver remaining to provide adequate hepatic function while regeneration proceeds in the postoperative period.

HEPATIC CRYOTHERAPY

Hepatic cryotherapy is now a fairly common procedure in most cancer centers although indications and applications of the technique vary among surgeons in the field. In general, cryotherapy involves the in situ destruction of tumor masses with subsequent resorption of necrotic tumor cells. Current cryotherapy machines and probes are able to destroy tumors as large as 4 to 6 cm. Peripheral lesions are easier to cryoblate because more central lesions are often close to major vessels, which act as heat sinks and prevent complete cryoablation. In addition, large central lesions close to major biliary radicals are difficult to treat with cryotherapy because bile ducts are susceptible to damage by extreme cold (−196°C). Dedicated radiologists with advanced skills in interventional techniques and intraoperative hepatic ultrasound are critical members of our cryotherapy team. Laparoscopic and percutaneous cryotherapeutic approaches have been reported,[110–112] but adequate access and monitoring to achieve thorough cryoablation are usually not possible without a laparotomy.

There is considerable controversy whether hepatic cryotherapy could potentially replace resection as an equivalent or superior curative modality for patients with hepatic metastases. Despite continued enthusiasm for this technique, it is apparent that published cryotherapy series are very heterogeneous with respect to inclusion criteria, use of adjuvant therapy, combining resection with cryotherapy, and use of cryotherapy as a palliative procedure.[113] Therefore, it is very difficult to conclude with certainty that hepatic cryotherapy is better, equivalent, or poorer than liver resection as surgical treatment for liver tumors.

REPEAT HEPATIC RESECTION FOR METASTATIC COLORECTAL CANCER

Despite thorough preoperative and intraoperative imaging studies, a large fraction of patients with colorectal cancer liver metastases have occult microscopic residual disease and will recur in the liver following resection. Based on fairly good overall survival results of first liver resection, many groups will offer repeat resection for selected patients with localized hepatic rerecurrences. five year survival is reported at 16% to 25%.[114]

Liver Resection for Noncolorectal Cancer Hepatic Metastases

Strong evidence in favor of or against hepatic resection of non-colorectal metastases is lacking, primarily due to limited experiences. Nevertheless, most agree that hepatic resection results in improved 5-year survival rates for selected patients with isolated and resectable disease.[115,116] Specifically, results for liver resection for metastases from genitourinary sites (kidney, adrenal, cervix, uterus) were better than those for soft tissue tumor (breast, melanoma, and sarcoma) metastases or liver metastases from other GI sites.[117] Palliative liver resection of hepatic metastases from neuroendocrine tumors is also worthwhile, particularly in cases in which uncontrollable symptoms from elevated hormone levels are a problem.[118]

Portal Hypertension

Portal venous pressure is normally 5 to 10 mmHg. A variety of conditions lead to increased resistance to portal blood flow, which in turn causes a rise in portal venous pressure. When portal venous pressure rises above 10 mmHg, portal hypertension is present with the development of characteristic pathophysiological features. Portal hypertension is characterized by the development of venous collaterals around the area of increased resistance and systemic hemodynamic changes including an increase in splanchnic flow and a hyperdynamic circulation. The major complications of portal hypertension are variceal bleeding, ascites, and liver failure.

Anatomy

The portal vein is the termination of the splanchnic venous outflow and is formed by the junction of the splenic and superior mesenteric veins behind the neck of the pancreas. The inferior mesenteric vein enters into either the superior mesenteric vein or the splenic vein while the coronary (left gastric) vein may enter into either the portal vein or the splenic vein behind the pancreas. The umbilical vein, which runs in the edge of the falciform ligament, consistently enters into the left portal vein and with portal hypertension may become quite large, acting as a collateral pathway. Gastroesophageal varices are the classic collateral pathway that develop from

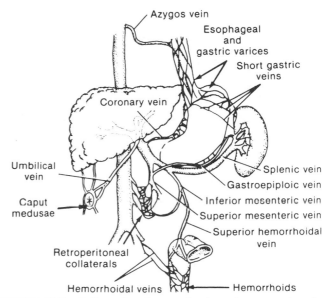

FIGURE 20.7. Collateral pathways develop where portal and systemic venous pathways are in apposition (*large arrows*). (Reproduced from Sabiston DC, ed. Textbook of Surgery, 14th ed. Philadelphia: WB Saunders, 1991, with permission.)

the left gastric and short gastric veins to the lesser and greater curves of the stomach. These veins run submucosally across the gastroesophageal junction up the esophagus. Additional collateral pathways are found in the periumbilical area communicating with the umbilical vein, the retroperitoneum, and between the inferior mesenteric vein and the hemorrhoidal venous plexus of the anal canal (Fig. 20.7).

Etiology

Portal hypertension is classified by the site of obstruction as presinusoidal, sinusoidal, and postsinusoidal hypertension. Presinusoidal portal hypertension is either extrahepatic or intrahepatic. Thrombosis of the extrahepatic portal vein or one of its major branches causes extrahepatic portal hypertension. Schistosomiasis and congenital hepatic fibrosis cause intrahepatic presinusoidal portal hypertension. In general, hepatocellular function is preserved in presinusoidal portal hypertension, which has implications for both prognosis and management. Cirrhosis causes sinusoidal portal hypertension, which is the most common cause of portal hypertension in North Americans. Postsinusoidal portal hypertension is caused by hepatic venous outflow obstruction either at the terminal hepatic venule level (venoocclusive disease) or at the major hepatic vein/suprahepatic inferior vena cava level (Budd–Chiari syndrome).

Natural History

Approximately one-third of patients with compensated cirrhosis will have varices at the time of their initial diagnosis. The risk of initial bleeding from varices can be predicted by variceal size,[119] portal pressure greater than 12 mmHg, and advanced-stage liver disease.[120,121] Acute variceal bleeding is associated with a mortality of approximately 30%. Patients with advanced liver disease (Child's C) are at the highest risk of death usually from progressive liver failure.

Management

Management of varices depends whether the intent is to prevent initial bleeding, to manage an acute variceal bleed, or prevent recurrent variceal bleeding.

PREVENTION OF INITIAL BLEEDING

The high mortality associated with first variceal bleeding episodes has led to the investigation of a variety of methods of prophylaxis. Initial enthusiasm for prophylactic portacaval shunts waned after several studies demonstrated high mortality rates, and thus operative prophylaxis has essentially been abandoned.[122,123] The role of transjugular intrahepatic portasystemic shunting (TIPS) has not been assessed in the prophylactic setting to date but is presently considered in patients awaiting transplantation who have both large high-risk varices and intractable ascites.

Sclerotherapy is not presently considered as primary prophylactic strategy for prevention of first bleeding.[124]

Beta blockers have been demonstrated to lower portal pressure by approximately 20%.[125] Ideally the dose of beta blockade is titrated to lower the portal pressure below 12 mmHg or to achieve a reduction of 20% from baseline. A meta-analysis of nine primary prophylaxis trials using propranolol or nadolol demonstrated a significant decrease in the risk of first bleeding in patients receiving beta blockade. These studies suggest that screening of cirrhotic patients should be performed and that patients with medium to large varices should be started on beta blockade.

MANAGEMENT OF ACUTE VARICEAL BLEEDING

Initial management of the patient with acute variceal bleeding includes intravascular volume replacement, general supportive care, and arresting the bleeding. Intravascular volume resuscitation should be performed using blood products because the use of crystalloid solutions in patients with cirrhosis results in the rapid development of ascites and edema. Patients with active bleeding should be managed in an intensive care unit setting with appropriate hemodynamic monitoring and airway protection. Blood in the GI tract is not tolerated by cirrhotics, with increased risk of bacterial translocation and sepsis as well as inducing encephalopathy. Lactulose should be given orally or via NG tube or enemas in the comatose patient.

The use of octreotide has supplanted vasopressin as pharmacological intervention to prevent bleeding (Table 20.3). Somatostatin and its synthetic analogue octreotide are potent vasoconstrictors at supraphysiological doses. Octreotide is given initially as a 50-μg bolus followed by an infusion of 50 μg/h; this is continued through endoscopic intervention and usually for the subsequent 24 h.

Endoscopy plays a role in both the diagnosis and treatment of acute variceal bleeding. It should be remembered that up to 60% of GI bleeding in alcoholic cirrhotics is of nonvariceal origin. The goal of endoscopy is to identify active bleeding, detect signs of recent bleeding, and exclude other sources of upper GI bleeding. Acute bleeding can be stopped in approximately 90% of patients with an endoscopic approach. Patients who have bleeding that cannot be controlled by endoscopic management should be managed with the insertion of a Sengstaken–Blakemore tube. The goal is to use

TABLE 20.3.

Randomized Controlled Clinical Trials of Vasopressin versus Octreotide and Their Relative Efficacy at Arresting Variceal Bleeding (Level I Evidence).

Reference	Year	Patients (n)	Octreotide efficacy (%)	Vasopressin efficacy (%)
Kravetz et al.[131]	1984	61	53	58
Jenkins et al.[132]	1985	22	100	33
Bagarani et al.[133]	1987	50	67	32
Saari et al.[134]	1990	54	66	52
Hsia et al.[138]	1990	46	55	38
Walker et al.[136]	1992	50	68	80 (glypressin)
Hwang et al.[137]	1992	48	63	46

tamponade as a temporizing maneuver only while definitive management is being arranged.

Definitive management strategies for patients who fail endoscopic management and require balloon placement include TIPS and emergency portacaval shunting. As emergency portacaval shunts are associated with a mortality of at least 50%, there is currently greater enthusiasm for the use of TIPS in the emergency setting. TIPS is an interventional radiologic procedure that creates a communication through the hepatic parenchyma between the hepatic and portal veins (Fig. 20.8). Given the results of recent studies, surgical decompression in the emergency setting is reserved for situations in which TIPS cannot be performed.[126]

PREVENTION OF RECURRENT BLEEDING

First-line management for the prevention of rebleeding from varices requires thorough endoscopic obliteration of varices. In addition beta blockade alone has been used.

Patients who fail first-line management should be considered for portal decompression or devascularization procedures. An exact definition of failure of management does not exist, but patients who generally rebleed after initial obliter-

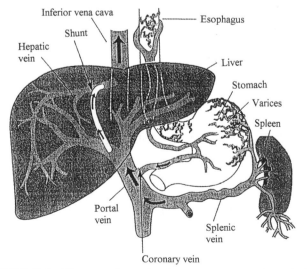

FIGURE 20.8. Diagram of transjugular portasystemic shunt (TIPS) demonstrates the usual placement from an intrahepatic right portal vein to the right hepatic vein. (Reproduced from Henderson et al.,[138] with permission.)

ation of their varices, patients for whom it is not possible to obliterate their varices that rebleed, or patients who develop bleeding gastric varices should be considered for surgical or radiologic intervention.

Options for portal decompression include operative shunts or TIPS. TIPS is effective in the short term in reducing bleeding, but stent stenosis or thrombosis has been reported in 30% to 60% of cases.[127,128] Current recommendations are that patients with poor hepatocellular function who are liver transplant candidates should undergo TIPS, while patients who have preserved hepatocellular function and are unlikely to go on to transplant within the next several years should undergo operative shunting because of the reported higher patency rate with surgical shunts.

Operative shunts are classified as total or partial, and selective or nonselective, depending on their effects on portal flow. Total shunts have a diameter of 1 cm or greater and divert all portal flow into the systemic circulation via the inferior vena cava or one of its major branches. Because portal venous diversion is total, the overall effect on hepatocyte function tends to be detrimental with resultant higher rates of encephalopathy.

Partial portosystemic shunts have limited diameters, between 8 and 10 mm, and can be placed in the mesocaval or, more commonly, portacaval position. The goal of partial shunts is to lower portal pressure to approximately 12 mmHg while maintaining portal venous flow toward the liver with a lesser effect on hepatocellular function compared to total shunts.

A variety of nonshunt or devascularization operations have been described. The most successful and widely adopted procedure has been the Sugiura procedure, which consists of splenectomy, proximal gastric devascularization, selective vagotomy, pyloroplasty, esophageal devascularization, and esophageal transection.[129] The goal of devascularization procedures is to reduce inflow to the esophageal varices and therefore reduce or eliminate bleeding. Devascularization procedures have the advantage of maintaining portal flow and therefore minimizing encephalopathy.

Liver Transplantation

Portal hypertension alone is not considered an indication for liver transplantation but is reserved for patients with variceal bleeding with decompensated cirrhosis. Patients with advanced liver disease and variceal bleeding should undergo either endoscopic control or TIPS as a stabilizing maneuver, with subsequent workup for transplantation. One-year mortality rates for Child's C patients have been reduced from approximately 80% following shunt procedures to 20% with transplantation.

Budd–Chiari Syndrome

Obstruction of hepatic venous outflow by thrombosis of hepatic veins secondary to hematological disorders, trauma, tumor, or venacaval webs leads to congestion of the sinusoids and hepatocellular necrosis. Depending on the acuity and degree of obstruction, patients can present with wide-ranging symptomatology from slowly progressive liver dysfunction to fulminant hepatic failure. Early accurate diagnosis by radiologic imaging and biopsy is essential because early portal de-

compression allows liver function to return to normal.[130] Portal decompression via a side-to-side portacaval or mesocaval shunt allows the portal vein to become the hepatic venous outflow tract. Occasionally inferior vena cava (IVC) obstruction occurs and a mesoatrial or combined portacaval/cavoatrial shunt is required to decompress the liver. Liver transplantation has also been used successfully in Budd–Chiari syndrome; however, it is generally reserved for patients with decompensated liver function.

Ascites

Ascites frequently accompanies portal hypertension, particularly with sinusoidal or postsinusoidal obstruction. Elevated hepatic sinusoidal pressure leads to a transudate of high-protein fluid from the liver into the peritoneal cavity. Ascites accumulation causes decreased intravascular volume, increased aldosterone secretion, redistribution of renal blood flow, and salt retention. Standard management of ascites includes salt (20 mEq/day) and water restriction and diuretic therapy. Ascites that is refractory to diuretics can be managed by repeated paracentesis; however, this is an indication of decompensated cirrhosis and liver transplantation should be considered. In the past, peritoneojugular or LeVeen shunts have been placed for the management of refractory ascites, but this now is largely of historical interest. TIPS has recently become an option for the management of refractory ascites although experience is limited.

References

1. Bismuth H. Surgical anatomy and anatomical surgery of the liver. World J Surg 1982;6:3–9.
2. Botero AC, Strasberg SM. Division of the left hemiliver in man: segments, sectors or sections. Liver Transplant Surg 1998;4:226–231.
3. McCluskey DA III, Skandalakis LJ, Colburn GL, et al. Hepatic surgery and hepatic surgical anatomy: historical partners in progress. World J Surg 1997;21:330–342.
4. Strasberg SM. Terminology of liver anatomy and liver resections: coming to grips with hepatic Babel. J Am Coll Surg 1997;184:413–434.
5. Couinaud C. Surgical anatomy of the liver. Several new aspects. Chirurgie 1986;112:337–342.
6. Baldwin RL, Smith NE. Molecular control of energy metabolism. In: Sink JD, ed. The Control of Metabolism. University Park: Pennsylvania State University Press, 1974:17.
7. Bradley EL III. Measurement of hepatic bloodflow in man. Surgery (St. Louis) 1974;75:783.
8. Brauer RW. Hepatic blood supply and the secretion of bile. In: Taylor RW, ed. The Biliary System. Oxford: Blackwell, 1965:41.
9. Prandi D, Erlinger S, Glasinovic JC, et al. Cannilicular bile production in man. Eur J Clin Invest 1975;5:1.
10. Vauthey JN. Liver imaging: a surgeon's perspective. Radiol Clin North Am 1998;36:445–457.
11. Mergo PJ, Ros PR. Benign lesions of the liver. Radiol Clin North Am 1998;36:319–331.
12. Colle I, Op de Beeck B, Hoorens A, et al. Multiple focal nodular hyperplasia. J Gastroenterol 1998;33:904–908.
13. Wanless JR, Mawdsley C, Adams R. On the pathogenesis of focal nodular hyperplasia of the liver. Hepatology 1985;5:1194–1200.
14. Ishak KG, Rabin L. Benign tumors of the liver: Med Clin North Am 1975;59:995–1013.
15. Janes CH, McGill DB, Luudwig J, et al. Liver cell adenoma at

the age of 3 years and transplantation 19 years later after development of carcinoma: a case report. Hepatology 1993;17:583–585.

16. Edmundson HA, Reynolds TB, Henderson B, et al. Regression of liver cell adenomas associated with oral contraceptives. Ann Intern Med 1977;86:180–182.

17. Coutsoftides T, Hermann RE. Nonparasitic cysts of the liver. Surg Gynecol Obstet 1974;138:906.

18. Henson SW, Gray HK, Dockerty MB. Benign tumors of the liver. III. Solitary cysts. Surg Gynecol Obstet 1956;103:607.

19. Dardik H, Glotzer P, Silver C. Congenital hepatic cyst causing jaundice. Ann Surg 1964;159:585.

20. Milutinovic J, Fialkow PJ, Rudd TG, et al. Liver cysts in patients with autosomal dominant polycystic kidney disease. Am J Med 1980;68:741.

21. Grunfeld J-P, Albouze G, Jungers P, et al. Liver changes and complications in adult polycystic kidney disease. Adv Nephrol 1985;14:1.

22. Campbell GS, Bick HD, Paulsen EP, et al. Bleeding esophageal varices with polycystic liver. N Engl J Med 1958;259:904.

23. Landing BH, Wells TR, Claireaux AE. Morphometric analysis of liver lesions in cystic diseases of childhood. Hum Pathol 1980;11(suppl):549.

24. Fernadez M, Cacioppo JC, Davis RP, et al. Management of solitary nonparasitic liver cyst. Am Surg 1984;50:205.

25. Jones WL, Mountain JC, Warren KW. Symptomatic non-parasitic cysts of the liver. Br J Surg 1974;61:118.

26. Sanfelippo PM, Beahrs OH, Weiland LH. Cystic disease of the liver. Ann Surg 1974;179:922.

27. Kairaluoma M, Leinonen A, Ståhlberg M, et al. Percutaneous aspiration and alcohol sclerotherapy for symptomatic hepatic cysts. Ann Surg 1989;210:208–215.

28. Montorsi M, Torzilli G, Fumagalli U, et al. Percutaneous alcohol sclerotherapy of simple hepatic cysts. Results from a multicentre survey in Italy. Hepatopancreatobiliary Surg 1994;8:89.

29. Hagiwara H, Kasahara A, Hayashi N, et al. Successful treatment of a hepatic cyst by one-shot instillation of minocycline chloride. Gastroenterology 1992;103:675–677.

30. Sanchez H, Gagner M, Rossi RL, et al. Surgical management of nonparasitic cystic liver disease. Am J Surg 1991;161:113–119.

31. Martin IJ, McKinley AJ, Currie EJ, et al. Tailoring the management of nonparasitic liver cysts. Ann Surg 1998;228:167.

32. Lin T-Y, Chen CC, Wang SM. Treatment of non-parasitic cystic disease of the liver: a new approach to therapy with polycystic liver. Ann Surg 1968;168:921.

33. Newman KD, Torres VE, Rakela J, et al. Treatment of highly symptomatic polycystic liver disease. Ann Surg 1990;212:30.

34. Vauthey J-N, Maddern GJ, Kolbinger P, et al. Clinical experience with adult polycystic liver disease. Br J Surg 1992;79:562.

35. Hansen P, Bhoyrul S, Legha P, et al. Laparoscopic treatment of liver cysts. J Gastrointest Surg 1997;1:53–60.

36. Morino M, De Biuli M, Festa V, et al. Laparoscopic management of symptomatic nonparasitic cysts of the liver. Ann Surg 1994;219:157–164.

37. Devine P, Ucci AA. Biliary cystadenocarcinoma arising in a congenital cyst. Hum Pathol 1985;16:92.

38. Pinson CW, Munson JL, Rossi RL, et al. Enucleation of intrahepatic biliary cystadenomas. Surg Gynecol Obstet 1989;168:535.

39. Akwari OE, Tucker A, Seigler HF, et al. Hepatobiliary cystadenoma with mesenchymal stroma. Ann Surg 1990;211:18.

40. Devine P, Ucci AA. Biliary cystadenocarcinoma arising in a congenital cyst. Hum Pathol 1985;16:92.

41. Weller PF. Case records of the Massachusetts General Hospital: case 45-1987. N Engl J Med 1987;317:1209.

42. Lewall DB. Hydatid disease: biology, pathology, imaging and classification. Clin Radiol 1998;53:863.

43. Garti I, Deutsch V. The angiographic diagnosis of echinococcosis of the liver and spleen. Clin Radiol 1971;22:466.

44. Chemtai AK, Bowry TR, Ahmad Z. Evaluation of five immunodiagnostic techniques in echinococcosis patients. Bull WHO 1981;59:767.

45. Nahmias J, Goldsmith R, Soibelman M, et al. Three- to 7-year follow-up after albendazole treatment of 68 patients with cystic echinococcosis (hydatid disease). Ann Trop Med Parasitol 1994;88:295.

46. Morris DL, Sykes PW, Marriner S, et al. Albendazole—objective evidence of response in human hydatid disease. JAMA 1985;253:2053.

47. von Sinner WN, Nyman R, Linjawi T, et al. Fine needle aspiration biopsy of hydatid cysts. Acta Radiol 1995;36:168.

48. Hira PR, Shweiki H, Lindberg LG, et al. Diagnosis of cystic hydatid disease—role of aspiration cytology. Lancet 1988;2:655.

49. Langer B. Surgical treatment of hydatid disease of the liver. Br J Surg 1987;74:237.

50. Langer JC, Rose DB, Keystone JS, et al. Diagnosis and management of hydatid disease of the liver. Ann Surg 1984;199:412.

51. Alfieri S, Doglietto GB, Pacelli F, et al. Radical surgery for liver hydatid disease: a study of 89 consecutive patients. Hepatogastroenterology 1997;44:496.

52. Xynos E, Pechlivanides G, Tzortzinis A, et al. Hydatid disease of the liver: diagnosis and surgical treatment. Hepatopancreatobiliary Surg 1991;4:59.

53. Meymerian E, Luttermoser GW, Frayha GJ, et al. Host-parasite relationships in echinoccosis X: laboratory evaluation of chemical scolicides as adjuncts to hydatid surgery. Ann Surg 1963;158:211.

54. Taylor RB, Langer B. Current surgical management of hepatic cyst disease. Adv Surg 1997;31:127.

55. Akinoglu A, Bilgin I, Erkocak EU. Surgical management of hydatid disease of the liver. Can J Surg 1985;28:171.

56. Karavias DD, Vagianos CE, Bouboulis N, et al. Improved techniques in the surgical treatment of hepatic hydatidosis. Surg Gynecol Obstet 1992;174:176.

57. Romero-Torres R, Campbell JR. An interpretive review of the surgical treatment of hydatid disease. Surg Gynecol Obstet 1965;121:851.

58. Magistrelli P, Masetti R, Coppola R, et al. Value of ERCP in the diagnosis and management of pre- and postoperative biliary complications in hydatid disease of the liver. Gastrointest Radiol 1989;14:315.

59. Wanebo HJ, Falkson G, Order SE. Cancer of the hepatobiliary system. In: DeVita V, Hellman S, Rosenberg SA, eds. Cancer: Principles and Practice of Oncology. Philadelphia: Lippincott, 1989:836–874.

60. Colombo M. Hepatocellular carcinoma. J Hepatol 1992;15:225–236.

61. El-Serag HB, Mason AC. Rising incidence of hepatocellular carcinoma in the United States. N Engl J Med 1999;340:745–750.

62. Okuda K. Hepatocellular carcinoma: recent progress. Hepatology 1992;15:948–953.

63. Melia WM, Wilkinson ML, Portmann BC, et al. Hepatocellular carcinoma in the noncirrhotic liver; a comparison with that complicating cirrhosis. Q J Med 1984;211:391.

64. Kew M, Popper H. Relationship between hepatocellular carcinoma and cirrhosis. Semin Liver Dis 1984;4:136–146.

65. Arakawa M, Kage M, Sugihara S, et al. Emergence of malignant lesions within an adenomatous hyperplastic nodule in a cirrhotic liver. Observations in five cases. Gastroenterology 1986;91:198–208.

66. Ebara M, Ohto M, Shinagawa T, et al. Natural history of minute hepatocellular carcinoma smaller than 3 cm complicating cirrhosis. Gastroenterology 1986;90:289.

67. Cottone M, Virdone R, Fusco G, et al. Asymptomatic hepatocellular carcinoma in Child's A cirrhosis; a comparison of natural history and surgical treatment. Gastroenterology 1988;96:1566–1571.

68. Nagasue N, Yukaya H, Hamada T, et al. The natural history of hepatocellular carcinoma; a study of 100 untreated cases. Cancer (Phila) 1984;54:1561.

69. Okuda K, Ohtsuki T, Obata H, et al. Natural history of hepatocellular carcinoma and prognosis in relation to treatment. Study of 850 patients. Cancer (Phila) 1985;56:918.

70. Kew MC. Tumor markers in hepatocellular carcinoma. J Gastroenterol Hepatol 1989;4:373–384.

71. Rizzi PM, Kane PA, Ryder SD, et al. Accuracy of radiology in detection of hepatocellular carcinoma before liver transplantation. Gastroenterology 1994;107:1425–1429.

72. Chu YS, Metreweli C, Lau WY, et al. Safety of biopsy of hepatocellular carcinoma with an 18 gauge automated needle. Clin Radiol 1997;52:907–911.

73. Jacobs JE, Birnbaum BA. Computed tomography imaging of focal hepatic lesions. Semin Roentgenol 1995;30:308–323.

74. Ebara E. MRI diagnosis of hepatocellular carcinoma. In: Okuda K, Tabor E, eds. Liver Cancer. New York: Churchill Livingstone, 1997:361–369.

75. TNM: American Joint Committee for Staging of Cancer, 4th Ed. Philadelphia: Lippincott, 1992:89–91.

76. Vauthey JN, Klimstra D, Franceschi D, et al. Factors affecting long term outcome after hepatic resection for hepatocellular carcinoma. Am J Surg 1995;169:28–34.

77. Molmenti EP, Marsh JW, Dvorchik I, et al. Hepatobiliary malignancies. Primary hepatic malignant neoplasms. Surg Clin North Am 1999;79:43–57.

78. Ng IO, Lai ECS, Fan ST, et al. Prognosis significance of pathological features of hepatocellular carcinoma. Cancer (Phila) 1995;176:2443–2448.

79. Izume R, Shimizu K, Li T, et al. Prognosis factors of hepatocellular carcinoma in patients undergoing hepatic resection. Gastroenterology 1994;106:720–727.

80. Lee NH, Chau GY, Lui WY, et al. Surgical treatment and outcome in patients with a hepatocellular carcinoma greater than 10 cm in diameter. Br J Surg 1998;85:1654–1657.

81. Nagasue N, Yukaya H, Ogawa Y, et al. Clinical experience with 118 hepatic resections for hepatocellular carcinoma. Surgery (St. Louis) 1986;99:694–701.

82. Hemming AW, Scudamore CH, Shackleton CR, et al. Indocyanine green clearance as a predictor of successful hepatic resection in the cirrhotic patient. Am J Surg 1992;163:515–518.

83. Mori K, Ozawa K, Yamamoto Y, et al. Response of hepatic mitochondrial redox state to oral glucose load redox tolerance test as a new predictor of surgical risk in hepatectomy. Ann Surg 1990;211:438.

84. Tandan V, Asch M, Margolis M, et al. Laparoscopic vs. open intraoperative ultrasound of the liver—a controlled study. J Gastrointestinal Surg 1997;1:146–151.

85. Lai ECS, Ng IOL, You KT, et al. Hepatic resection for small hepatocellular carcinoma: the Queen Mary Hospital experience. World J Surg 1991;15:654–659.

86. Mastutani S, Sasaki Y, Imaoka S, et al. The prognostic significance of surgical margin in liver resection of patients with hepatocellular carcinoma. Arch Surg 1994;129:1025–1030.

87. Yoshida Y, Kanematsu T, Matsumata T, et al. Surgical margin and recurrence after resection of hepatocellular carcinoma in patients with cirrhosis. Further evaluation of limited hepatic resection. Ann Surg 1989;209:297–301.

88. Lai ECS, Fan ST, Lo CM, et al. Hepatic resection for hepatocellular carcinoma: an audit of 343 patients. Ann Surg 1995;221:291–298.

89. Takenaka K, Kawahara N, Yamamoto K, et al. Results of 280 liver resections for hepatocellular carcinoma. Arch Surg 1996;131:71–76.

90. Philisophe B, Greig P, Hemming AW, et al. Surgical management of hepatocellular carcinoma; resection or transplantation. J Gastrointest Surg 1998;2:21–27.

91. Hu R-H, Lee P-H, Yu S-C, et al. Surgical resection for recurrent hepatocellular carcinoma; prognosis and analysis of risk factors. Surgery (St. Louis) 1996;120:23–29.

92. Mazzaferro V, Regalia E, Doci R, et al. Liver transplantation for the treatment of small hepatocellular carcinomas in patients with cirrhosis. N Engl J Med 1996;14:728–729.

93. Hemming AW, Cattral MS, Greig PD, et al. The University of Toronto Liver Transplant Program. In: Cecka JM, Terasaki PI, eds. Clinical Transplants 1996. Los Angeles: UCLA Tissue Typing Laboratory, 1997:P177–P185.

94. Figueras J, Jaurrieta E, Valls C, et al. Survival after liver transplantation in cirrhotic patients with and without hepatocellular carcinoma: a comparative study. Hepatology 1997;25:1485–1489.

95. Bismuth H, Chiche L, Adam R, et al. Liver resection vs. transplantation for hepatocellular carcinoma in cirrhotic patients. Ann Surg 1993;218:145–151.

96. Wong PY, McPeake JR, Potmann B, et al. Clinical course and survival after liver transplantation for hepatitis B virus complicated by hepatocellular carcinoma. Am J Gastroenterol 1995;90:29–34.

97. Collela G, DeCarlis L, Rondinara GF. Is hepatocellular carcinoma in cirrhotics an actual indication for liver transplantation? Transplant Proc 1997;29:492–494.

98. Otto G, Heuschen U, Hofmann WT, et al. Is transplantation really superior to resection in the treatment of small hepatocellular carcinoma? Transplant Proc 1997;29:489–491.

99. Iwatsuki S, Starzl TE, Sheahan DG, et al. Hepatic resection vs. transplantation for hepatocellular carcinoma. Ann Surg 1991;214:221–229.

100. Farmer D, Rosove M, Shaked A, et al. Current treatment modalities for hepatocellular carcinoma. Ann Surg 1994;219:236–247.

101. Bruix J. Treatment of hepatocellular carcinoma. Hepatology 1997;25:259–262.

102. Liu C, Fan S. Non-resectional therapies for hepatocellular carcinoma. Am J Surg 1997;173:358–365.

103. Browser ST, Dumitrescu O, Rubinoff S, et al. Operative ultrasound establishes resectability of metastases by major hepatic resection. World J Surg 1989;13:649–657.

104. Charnley RM, Morris DL, Dennison AR, et al. Detection of colorectal liver metastases using intraoperative ultrasonography. Br J Surg 1991;78:45–48.

105. Gozzetti G, Mazziotti A, Bolondi L, et al. Intraoperative ultrasonography in surgery for liver tumors. Surgery (St. Louis) 1986;90:523–530.

106. Parker GA, Lawrence W, Horsley III JS, et al. Intraoperative ultrasound of the liver affects operative decision making. Ann Surg 1989;209:569–577.

107. Leen E, Angerson WJ, Wotherspoon H, et al. Comparison of the doppler perfusion index and intraoperative ultrasonography in diagnosing colorectal liver metastases. Ann Surg 1994;220:663–667.

108. Machi J, Isomoto H, Kurohiji T, et al. Accuracy of intraoperative ultrasonography in diagnosing liver metastasis from colorectal cancer: evaluation with postoperative follow-up results. World J Surg 1991;15:551–557.

109. Langer B, Gallinger S. The management of metastatic carcinoma in the liver. Adv Surg 1995;28:113–132.

110. Tandan VR, Litwin D, Asch M, et al. Laparoscopic cryosurgery for hepatic tumors. Surg Endosc 1997;11:1115–1117.

111. Adam R, Majno P, Castaing D, et al. Treatment of irresectable liver tumours by percutaneous cryosurgery. Br J Surg 1998;85:1493–1494.

112. Iannitti DA, Heniford BT, Hale J, et al. Laparoscopic cryoablation of hepatic metastases. Arch Surg 1998;133:1011–1015.

113. Tandan VR, Harmantas A, Gallinger S. Long-term survival after hepatic cryosurgery versus surgical resection for metastatic colorectal carcinoma: a critical review of the literature. CJS (Can J Surg) 1997;40:175–181.

114. Wanebo HJ, Chu QD, Avradopoulos KA, et al. Current perspectives on repeat hepatic resection for colorectal carcinoma: a review. Surgery (St. Louis) 1996;119:361–371.

115. Chen H, Pruitt A, Nicol TL, et al. Complete hepatic resection of metastases from leiomyosarcoma prolongs survival. J Gastrointest Surg 1998;2:151–155.

116. Schwartz SI. Hepatic resection for noncolorectal nonneuroendocrine metastases. World J Surg 1995;19:72–75.

117. Harrison LE, Brennan MF, Newman E, et al. Hepatic resection for noncolorectal, nonneuroendocrine metastases: a fifteen-year experience with ninety-six patients. Surgery (St. Louis) 1997;121:625–632.

118. Que FG, Nagorney DM, Batts KP, et al. Hepatic resection for metastatic neuroendocrine carcinomas. Am J Surg 1995;169:36–43.

119. Lebrec D, Fleury P, Rueff B, Nahum H, Benhamou JP. Portal hypertension, size of esophageal varices and risk of gastrointestinal bleeding in alcoholic cirrhosis. Gastroenterology 1980;79:1139–1144.

120. North Italian Endoscopic Club for the Study and Treatment of Esophageal Varices. Prediction of the first variceal hemorrhage in patients with cirrhosis of the liver and esophageal varices. New Engl J Med 1988;319:983–989.

121. Lebrec D, De Fluery P, Bueff B, et al. Portal hypertension, size of esophageal varices and risk of esophageal bleeding in alcoholic cirrhosis. Gastroenterology 1980;79:1139–1140.

122. Jackson FC, Perrin EB, Smith AG, Dagradi AE, Nadal HM. A clinical investigation of the portacaval shunt. II. Survival analysis of the prophylactic operation. Am J Surg 1968;115:22–42.

123. Resnick RH, Chalmers TC, Ishihara AM, et al. A controlled trial of the prophylactic portacaval shunt: a final report. Ann Intern Med 1969;70:675–688.

124. D'Amico G, Pagliano L, Bosch J. The treatment of portal hypertension: a meta-analytic review. Hepatology 1995;22:332–354.

125. Lebrec D, Nouel O, Corbic M, Benhamou JP. Propanolol, a medical treatment for portal hypertension? Lancet 1980;2:180–182.

126. Encarcion CE, Palmaz JC, Rivera FJ, et al. Transjugular intrahepatic portosystemic shunt placement for variceal bleeding: predictors of mortality. J Vasc Interventional Radiol 1995;6:687–694.

127. Rosle M, Haag K, Ochs A, et al. The transjugular portosystemic stent-shunt procedure for variceal bleeding. N Engl J Med 1994;330:165–171.

128. Fillmore DJ, Miller FJ, Fox LF, Disario JA, Tietze CC. Transjugular intrahepatic portosystemic shunt: midterm clinical and angiographic followup. J Vasc Interventional Radiol 1996;7:255–261.

129. Smadja C, Mariette D. Devascularization—modified surgical procedure. In: Blumgart LH, ed. Surgery of the Liver and Biliary Tract. New York: Churchill Livingstone, 1994:1675–1679.

130. Hemming AW, Langer B, Greig P, et al. Treatment of Budd-Chiari syndrome with portosystemic shunt or liver transplantation. Am J Surg 1996;171:176–181.

131. Kravetz D, Bosch J, Teres J, Bruix J, Rimola A, Rodes S. Comparison of intravenous somatostatin and vasopressin infusions in the treatment of variceal hemorrhage. Hepatology 1984;4:422–426.

132. Jenkins SA, Baxter JN, Corbett W, Devitt P, Ware J, Sheilds R. A prospective controlled trial comparing vasopressin and somatostatin. Br Med J 1985;290:275–278.

133. Bagarani M, Albertini V, Anza M, et al. Effect of somatostatin in controlling bleeding from esophageal varices. Ital J Surg Sci 1987;1:121–126.

134. Saari A, Elvilaakso E, Inberg M, et al. Comparison of somatostatin and vasopressin in bleeding esophageal varices. Am J Gastroenterol 1990;85:804–807.

135. Hsia HC, Lee FY, Tsai YE, et al. Comparison of somatostatin and vasopressin in the control of acute esophageal variceal hemorrhage—a randomised controlled study. Clin J Gastroenterol 1990;7:71–78.

136. Walker S, Kreichgauer HP, Bode JC. Terlipressin vs somatostatin in bleeding esophageal varices: a controlled double blind study. Hepatology 1992;15:1023–1030.

137. Hwang SJ, Lin HC, Chang CF, et al. A randomised controlled trial comparing octreotide and vasopressin in the control of acute variceal bleeding. J Hepatol 1992;16:320–325.

138. Henderson M, Barnes DS, Geisinger MA. Portal hypertension. Curr Probl Surg 1998;35:381–452.

Small Intestine

Richard A. Hodin and Jeffrey B. Matthews

Anatomy and Physiology

Gross and Histological Anatomy

GENERAL CONSIDERATIONS

The small bowel measures 12 to 20 feet in length from pylorus to ileocecal valve. The duodenum is mostly retroperitoneal and wraps in a C-shape around the head of the pancreas. Its first and second portions lie adjacent to the gallbladder and liver, and thus duodenal pathology may extend to involve these organs and vice versa. Pathology at the ampulla of Vater may produce obstructive jaundice or pancreatitis. The jejunum begins at the ligament of Treitz. The jejunum and ileum are suspended on a mobile mesentery covered by a visceral peritoneal lining that extends onto the external surface of the bowel to form the serosa. Adhesions caused by surgery or inflammation may limit the mobility of the loops and lead to obstruction or internal hernia. The jejunum and ileum comprise about two-fifths and three-fifths of the mobile portion of the small intestine, respectively. Circumferential mucosal folds (*plicae circularis*) are abundant in the jejunum but absent in proximal duodenum and distal ileum.

BLOOD SUPPLY AND LYMPHATIC DRAINAGE

The proximal duodenum receives its blood supply from the celiac axis, but the remainder of the small intestine is supplied by the superior mesenteric artery (SMA). Although mesenteric arcades form a rich collateral network, occlusion of a major branch of the SMA may result in segmental intestinal infarction. Venous drainage is via the superior mesenteric vein, which then joins the splenic vein behind the neck of the pancreas to form the portal vein. Elliptical, approximately 2 cm, lymphoid aggregates (Peyer's patches) are present on the antimesenteric border along the distal ileum, and

smaller follicles are evident throughout the remainder of the small intestine. Lymphatic drainage of the intestine is abundant. Regional lymph nodes follow vascular arcades and drain toward the *cysterna chyli*.

LAYERS OF THE BOWEL WALL

The small bowel wall consists of the outermost *serosa*, followed by the *muscularis*, *submucosa*, and, innermost, the *mucosa* (Fig. 21.1). The serosa is a single layer of flattened mesothelial cells that covers the jejunum and ileum but only the anterior surface of the duodenum. The muscularis consists of two layers of smooth muscle, a thicker inner circular layer and a thinner outer longitudinal layer. Specialized intercellular junctional structures called gap junctions electrically couple adjacent smooth muscle cells and allow efficient propagation of peristaltic signals. Ganglion cells and nerve fibers of Auerbach's myenteric plexus interdigitate between layers and communicate with smaller neural elements between cells. The submucosa is a dense connective tissue layer populated by diverse cell types, including fibroblasts, mast cells, lymphocytes, macrophages, eosinophils, and plasma cells. The submucosa is the strongest layer of the bowel wall, which should be taken into account when performing sutured anastomoses. Networks of arterioles, lymphatic and venous plexuses, and nerves crisscross through the submucosa. Meissner's submucosal neural plexus interconnects with neural elements from Auerbach's plexus in this region.

The mucosa is characterized by a villus architecture that, combined with circular folds, amplifies potential absorptive surface area 20-fold. The mucosa is subdivided into three layers. The *muscularis mucosae* consists of a thin sheet of smooth muscle cells. The *lamina propria* consists of connective tissue that extends from the base of the crypts up into the core of the intestinal villi. The innermost layer is made up of a continuous sheet of columnar epithelial cells composed of multiple cell types.

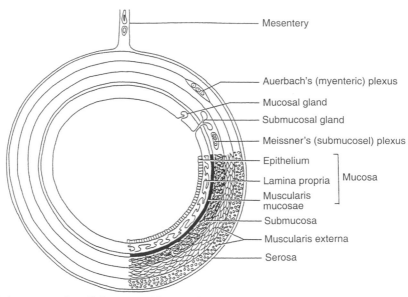

FIGURE 21.1. Layers of the intestinal wall. (From Dodd EE. Atlas of Histology, New York: McGraw-Hill, 1979, with permission.)

The Intestinal Epithelium and Its Functions

GENERAL CONSIDERATIONS

The intestinal epithelium is extraordinarily complex, composed of heterogenous cell types that reside within a highly organized supporting tissue structure containing multiple regulatory elements (Fig. 21.2). Intestinal epithelial cells rest on a thin basement membrane overlying the lamina propria (Fig. 21.3). A central arteriole within the villus core is surrounded by a fenestrated capillary network that optimizes countercurrent exchange of oxygen and plasma solutes while providing an efficient pathway for absorption of nutrients. Mononuclear cells and neutrophils reside in or traffic into the lamina propria during normal or disease states.

There are two major compartments to the intestinal epithelium, the crypt and the villus, each with distinct function and cellular composition. The majority of crypt cells are undifferentiated; some mature into mucus-secreting goblet cells and enteroendocrine cells, but most take on functional characteristics of absorptive enterocytes.[1,2] The lifespan of the enterocyte is 3 to 5 days. The villus compartment is nonproliferative, and senescent enterocytes undergo apoptosis and are extruded.[3]

BARRIER FUNCTION

The intestinal epithelium selectively limits the permeation of potentially harmful luminal substances. The anatomical locus of this "barrier" is the intercellular junctional complex,[4,5] a three-level structure that forms a circumferential seal between adjacent cells. The tight junction (*zonula occludens*) faces the lumen and is the site of membrane-to-membrane "kisses". The intermediate or adherens junction (*zonula adherens*) lies deep to the tight junction, at which site the transmembrane protein E-cadherin interacts with cytoskeletally linked signaling elements. The desmosome is the innermost element of the junctional complex.

DIGESTION AND ABSORPTION

The small intestine receives about 1 to 1.5 l/day of ingested fluid plus about 8 l of salivary, gastric, and pancreaticobiliary secretions. Most of this fluid is reabsorbed before reaching the colon. Water movement is driven by the active transcellular absorption of Na^+ and Cl^- and by the absorption of nutrients such as glucose and amino acids. The energy for many of these transport processes derives from the activity of a basolateral Na^+-K^+ ATPase, which maintains the low Na^+ internal environment that drives uptake via coupled ion ex-

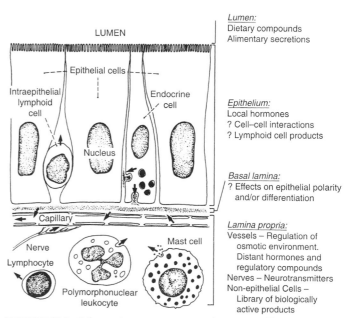

FIGURE 21.2. Schematic representation of various cell types and factors that may affect intestinal epithelial cell function. (From Schultz SG, ed. Handbook of Physiology: IV. The Gastrointestinal System. New York: Oxford University Press, Inc., 1991, with permission.)

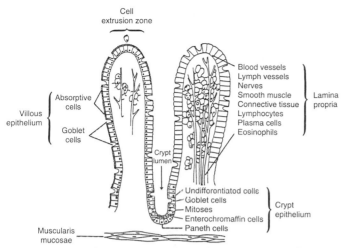

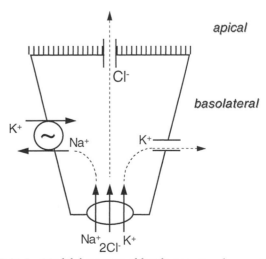

FIGURE 21.3. Schematic cross-sectional representation of two intestinal villi and an intervening crypt, illustrating the structural architecture and relationship to supporting tissue structure. (From Sleisinger MH, Fordtran JS, eds. Gastrointestinal Disease, Philadelphia: WB Saunders Co., 1993, with permission.)

changers (Na^+/H^+ and Cl^-/HCO_3^-) and Na^+-coupled nutrient transporters.

Digestion begins in the stomach with the action of gastric acid and pepsin. In the proximal duodenum, ingested foodstuffs are broken down by pancreatic proteases such as trypsin, elastase, chymotrypsin, and carboxypeptidases. The activity of brush border hydrolases and oligopeptidases then accomplishes terminal protein and carbohydrate digestion, and the resulting monosaccharides, amino acids, or di- and tripeptides then serve as substrates for Na^+- or H^+-coupled transporters in the apical membrane of absorptive enterocytes (Fig. 21.4). The apical membrane of these cells is well suited to the task of absorption by virtue of a microvillus brush border that amplifies absorptive area 30-fold. Fat digestion and absorption occur in the proximal small intestine, where pancreatic lipase partially hydrolyzes triglycerides into two fatty acids plus a central fatty acid linked to glycerol (monoglyceride). These substances are solubilized by bile salts to form micelles or mixed micelles (which additionally contain phospholipids, cholesterol, and fat-soluble vitamins). Micelles diffuse into enterocytes through the overlying mucus and apical plasma membrane, releasing fatty acid and monoglyceride into the cell along the way. Triglycerides are reformed intracellularly and are incorporated along with cellular protein, phospholipid, and cholesterol to form chylomicrons. Chylomicrons, which consist of an inner core of triglycerides and an outer coat of phospholipid and apoproteins, then exit the cell to be absorbed by the lymphatic system. Bile salts are resorbed into the enterohepatic circulation in the distal ileum by an ileal Na^+-coupled bile acid transporter.[6,7]

SECRETION

Intestinal crypt cells have the capacity to secrete an isotonic fluid through the active transcellular transport of Cl^-.[8–10] This process lubricates mucosal surfaces and facilitates the luminal extrusion of other secreted substances (e.g., secretory IgA and Paneth cell-derived cryptdins). Clinical diarrhea results when secretion exceeds colonic absorptive capacity. The cellular basis for epithelial Cl^- secretion involves Cl^- uptake across the basolateral membrane via a Na^+-K^+-$2Cl^-$ cotransporter followed by Cl^- extrusion across the apical membrane via Cl^- channels, including the cystic fibrosis transmembrane conductance regulator (CFTR) (Fig. 21.5).

Intestinal Immune Function

GENERAL CONSIDERATIONS

The mucosal immune system is critically important in defense against toxic and pathogenic threats from the luminal

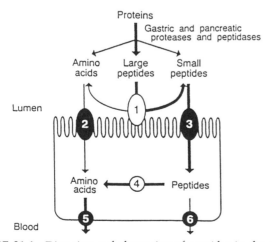

FIGURE 21.4. Digestion and absorption of peptides in the enterocyte by (1) brush border peptidases, (2) brush border amino acid transport systems, (3) brush border peptide transport systems, (4) cytoplasmic peptidases, (5) basolateral amino acid transport systems, and (6) basolateral peptide transport systems. (By permission from Johnson LR, ed. Physiology of the Digestive Tract, Philadelphia: Lippincott Williams & Wilkins, Third Ed. 1994.)

FIGURE 21.5. Model for active chloride secretion by crypt epithelial cells, the process underlying secretory diarrhea. Cl^- accumulates intracellularly by the combined action of a basolateral Na^+-K^+-$2Cl^-$ cotransporter, coupled to the Na^+-K^+ ATPase pump and K^+ channels. Cl^- exits the cell across the apical membrane by regulated Cl^- channels including the cystic fibrosis transmembrane conductance regulator (CFTR).

environment.[11,12] The lamina propria contains numerous immune cells including plasma cells, mast cells, and lymphocytes that produce not only immunoglobulins but also cytokine mediators.[13]

Secretory IgA and Epithelial Immune Function

Lamina propria plasma cells produce IgA in response to food antigens and microbes. IgA and IgM are secreted into the gut lumen by a mechanism that involves transcytosis through epithelial cells.[14] Secretory IgA prevents microbial pathogens from penetrating the epithelial layer. IgA–antigen interactions also occur within the intraepithelial and subepithelial compartments. In contrast to IgG, IgM, and IgE, antibodies of the IgA class evoke a much less proinflammatory (indeed, an antiinflammatory) response and thus contribute to the overall immunosuppressive tone of the mucosal immune system. In addition, intestinal epithelial cells themselves may also contribute to the immune function of the gut by transmitting important immunoregulatory signals to the underlying lymphocytic population.[15,16]

M Cells and Gut-Associated Lymphoid Tissue

Specialized cells known as M cells are found overlying Peyer's patches (Fig. 21.6) and serve as the major portal of entry for foreign material.[20] Specialized membrane invaginations in M cells create a pocket in which lymphocytes and macrophages gather. Luminal substances are immediately delivered to these professional antigen-processing cells, and this information is then directly conveyed to the underlying follicles. Antigen-specific lymphocyte proliferation occurs within Peyer's patches, and IgA-producing B cells migrate to regional lymph nodes and into the systemic circulation, from where they migrate back to diffusely populate the mucosa within the lamina propria. Within the lamina propria and submucosa, mature T cells, B cells, and macrophages carry out traditional cell-mediated immune responses including phagocytosis, cell killing, and secretion of cytokines.

Intestinal Neuroendocrine Function

General Considerations

The intestine is a rich source of regulatory peptides that control various aspects of gut function. These substances, released in response to luminal or neural stimuli, exert their biological actions either at distant sites (by entering the bloodstream in classical hormone fashion) or locally (as paracrine factors or neurotransmitters).

Secretin and Related Peptides

Secretin is a 27-amino-acid peptide released by enteroendocrine cells in the proximal small bowel in response to luminal acidification, bile salts, and fat. Its major function is to stimulate pancreatic ductal bicarbonate secretion. Secretin inhibits gastric release, gastric acid secretion, and gastrointestinal motility. Additionally, it stimulates bile flow by stimulating fluid secretion from cholangiocytes. Paradoxically, secretin stimulates rather than inhibits gastrin release in patients with gastrinoma, and this phenomenon forms the basis for the secretin infusion test in suspected Zollinger–Ellison syndrome. Other members of the secretin family that share substantial sequence homology and interact with similar G-protein-coupled receptors include vasoactive intestinal polypeptide (VIP), pituitary adenylate cyclase-activating polypeptide (PACAP), glucagon, gastric inhibitory polypeptide (GIP), and enteroglucagon.[17] Enteroglucagon and glucagon-like peptides (GLP) are secreted by neuroendocrine cells in the colon and small intestine and may be important in gut adaptation and glucose homeostasis.[18]

Cholecystokinin

Cholecystokinin (CCK) is released by specialized small-bowel enteroendocrine cells in response to luminal amino acids and medium- to long-chain fatty acids.[19] CCK release is inhibited by intraluminal trypsin and bile salts. Two major targets of CCK are the gallbladder and the sphincter of Oddi, where it causes coordinated contraction and relaxation, respectively,

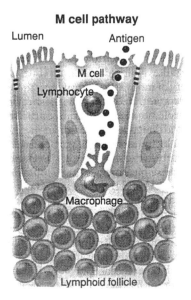

M cell pathway

Lumen — Antigen — M cell — Lymphocyte — Macrophage — Lymphoid follicle

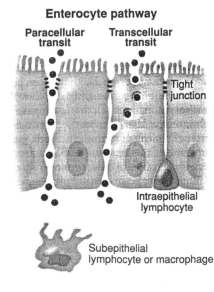

Enterocyte pathway

Paracellular transit — Transcellular transit — Tight junction — Intraepithelial lymphocyte — Subepithelial lymphocyte or macrophage

FIGURE 21.6. M cells and luminal pathways for antigen entry. Antigens can enter via M cells to deliver antigen directly to underlying immune cells. Alternatively, enterocytes may act as weak antigen-presenting cells. (From Madara,[120] with permission.)

to enhance luminal mixing of bile with ingested food.[20] Additionally, CCK stimulates pancreatic enzyme secretion. CCK stimulates cell growth in intestinal mucosa and pancreas, insulin release, and gut motility.

SOMATOSTATIN

Somatostatin is a 14-amino-acid peptide that exerts a wide variety of inhibitory functions in the gastrointestinal tract.[21] It is released from specialized enteroendocrine cells where it acts in paracrine fashion to inhibit intestinal, gastric, and pancreaticobiliary secretion as well as cell growth. Synthetic forms of somatostatin are used clinically in patients with enterocutaneous and pancreaticobiliary fistulae.[22]

OTHER PEPTIDES

Peptide YY is a 36-amino-acid peptide secreted by the distal small bowel. PYY appears to inhibit gastric acid secretion. It also decreases intestinal motility and inhibits pancreatic secretion and release of various intestinal hormones.[23–25] *Motilin* is secreted by the duodenum and proximal jejunum, where it acts to enhance contractility of smooth muscle and accelerate gastric emptying.[26] Erythromycin is a motilin receptor agonist, which may explain its utility for certain forms of delayed gastric emptying.[27] *Neurotensin* is produced in the ileum and enteric nerves. It appears to affect a variety of enteric functions including gastric acid secretion, gastric emptying, intestinal motility, and intestinal secretion, but its precise physiological role has not been defined. A number of gut peptides are released from enteric nerves and function as neurotransmitters, for example, VIP, calcitonin gene-related peptide (CGRP), galanin, bombesin, neuropeptide Y, gastrin-releasing peptides (GRP), and substance P.[28] The precise physiological roles of these substances have not been fully elucidated, but they are known to influence motility, local blood flow, and epithelial and exocrine secretion.

Motility of the Small Intestine

Intestinal motility consists of antegrade propulsion of luminal contents (peristalsis) combined with mixing action through segmentation. These functions are accomplished by the outer longitudinal and inner circular muscle layers of the intestinal wall, and, to a lesser extent, the *muscularis propria*, under the control of the myenteric and submucosal nerve plexi that interdigitate between these layers. The bowel is also innervated extrinsically by both vagal and sympathetic fibers. Cholinergic sympathetic input is excitatory while peptidergic input is probably inhibitory. Peristaltic waves are initiated by pacesetter potentials that originate in the duodenum. A nerve-related cell type known as the *interstitial cell of Cajal* appears to play a key role in the generation of pacemaker activity.[29]

The intestinal wall undergoes two distinct forms of contraction. Ring contractions are circumferential indentations that propagate caudally and grossly appear as classical peristaltic waves, whereas sleeve contractions consist of a subtler shortening of the intestinal wall. Small-intestinal motility varies with the fasted and fed state. During the interdigestive or fasting period between meals, a cyclical pattern of motor activity consisting of three phases is observed. This three-phase cycle, when viewed across the longitudinal axis of the small bowel, results in a pattern called the migrating motor complex.

Mechanical Obstruction of the Intestine

Clinical Presentation and Diagnosis

Obstruction of the intestine occurs when there is impairment in the normal flow of luminal contents caused by an extrinsic or intrinsic encroachment on the lumen. Intestinal pseudoobstruction, or adynamic ileus, can mimic mechanical obstruction, but differs in that the underlying problem is due to disordered motility. The key to management of small-intestinal obstruction is early diagnosis.

ETIOLOGY

Intestinal obstruction has a variety of causes, which differ as a function of age (Table 21.1).

CLINICAL PRESENTATION

In the setting of obstruction, the normal absorptive mechanisms of the small bowel are deranged such that excess fluid losses occur. Initially, there is vomitus, bowel wall edema, and transudative loss into the peritoneal cavity, but during the late stages of obstruction, venous pressure increases with resultant hemorrhage into the lumen, worsening hypovolemia. The normal relatively sterile environment of the proximal small intestine is altered under obstructed conditions such that bacterial overgrowth occurs, most notably involving the anaerobes such as *Bacteroides*. The feculant vomiting seen in cases of long-standing distal small-bowel obstruction is the result of this bacterial overgrowth and is virtually pathognomonic for a high-grade or complete distal mechanical small-bowel obstruction.

The diagnosis of intestinal obstruction is usually made on clinical grounds with the symptoms of crampy abdominal pain, decreased or absent flatus and stool, nausea, or vomiting. A prior history of small-bowel obstruction should be sought, because those patients with mechanical small-bowel obstruction caused by adhesions often experience recurrence. A history of other possible causes for small-bowel obstruction (e.g., Crohn's disease, radiation therapy) should be considered. The vomitus often contains occult blood and appears

TABLE 21.1. Common Causes of Mechanical Obstruction of the Small Intestine as a Function of Age.

Neonate	*Infant*	*Young adult*	*Adult*
Atresia	Groin hernia	Adhesions	Adhesions
Midgut volvulus	Intussusception	Groin hernia	Groin hernia
Meconium ileus	Meckel's diverticulum		

as "coffee grounds" in color, probably because of distension of the stomach with resultant mucosal hemorrhage. The level of the obstruction is often suggested on the basis of the pattern of the pain, with proximal obstructions usually causing more frequent cramps, perhaps every 3 to 5 min, whereas more distal obstructions cause less severe cramps with longer durations between episodes.

The obstructed patient often displays signs of dehydration with dry mouth and loss of skin turgor. The waves of abdominal pain, or colic, can actually be witnessed at the bedside and provide the strongest possible indication of a mechanically obstructed intestine. Occasionally, audible bowel sounds, or borborygmi, are present as a result of strong intestinal muscular contractions. Inspection of the abdomen usually reveals distension, although this may be absent in proximal obstruction. The presence of surgical scars should be noted, indicating the possibility of intraabdominal adhesions as the cause. An abdominal wall hernia might also be evident as the site of the obstruction. When hernia contents are soft and easily reducible in the obstructed patient, it is likely that an etiology other than the hernia exists. Although mild diffuse tenderness is a common feature in patients with distension from a mechanical obstruction, involuntary guarding or other signs of peritoneal irritation are unusual and suggest the possibility of ischemia or infarction of the bowel, perhaps even with perforation. Rectal examination is important to detect mass lesions and to check for the presence of stool, which is usually absent in cases of mechanical bowel obstruction, especially of long-standing nature.

DIAGNOSIS

Laboratory tests are not generally helpful in the diagnosis or management of patients with bowel obstruction. Routine blood counts reveal an elevated hematocrit indicative of intravascular volume depletion. Leukocytosis is sometimes present, but is often the result of hemoconcentration and an acute stress response rather than actual underlying infection. A markedly elevated white blood cell count should raise the suspicion for strangulation. The blood chemistry may reveal elevated blood urea nitrogen and creatinine, indicating hypovolemia with prerenal azotemia.

Plain X-rays of the abdomen are perhaps the most useful adjunctive test to confirm the diagnosis of bowel obstruction. Small-bowel obstruction leads to dilatation of the small bowel with air–fluid levels on an upright film. The presence of free air on a plain upright X-ray indicates perforation and the need for urgent operation. In small-bowel obstruction of long-standing nature, perhaps greater than 24 h, all the air and stool from the colon will have been evacuated, and this is evident on plain abdominal films. However, if the obstruction is in its early phase, or if it is only partial, then some air and

stool are present within the colon, making distinction between an early complete and a partial small-bowel obstruction very difficult.

Computed tomography (CT) is employed increasingly to evaluate patients with suspected bowel obstruction. The CT scan can often clearly identify dilated proximal and collapsed distal bowel, a feature that is aided by the administration of an oral contrast agent. The precise site and etiology of the obstruction may not be identified by CT, as in the case of adhesions, although in some instances an obstructing lesion can be seen. Based upon the high (up to 100%) sensitivity described in the literature, CT[30] has replaced the contrast small-bowel follow-through in many centers as the primary radiologic tool in suspected mechanical small-bowel obstruction.

Abdominal ultrasound has also been touted for patients with suspected small-bowel obstruction. Ultrasound can detect fluid-filled, dilated small bowel proximal to collapsed bowel and also the presence of peristaltic activity. Compared to plain radiographs, ultrasound has been shown in two studies[31,32] to be superior in detecting small-bowel obstruction. Ultrasonic evaluation is operator dependent, however, limiting its value to those who have expertise readily available.

Treatment of Small-Bowel Obstruction

GENERAL CONSIDERATIONS

Among the most important distinctions in the patient with a mechanical bowel obstruction is whether the site is within the small or large intestine. The differentiation between small- and large-bowel obstruction is critical in regard to both underlying cause (Table 21.2) and clinical management.

SIMPLE VERSUS STRANGULATING OBSTRUCTION

The most important issue to be addressed in patients with mechanical small-bowel obstruction is whether strangulation exists. Series that have compared mortality figures for simple versus strangulating obstruction have clearly demonstrated the importance of early recognition and treatment, as mortality for strangulated cases is generally 2- to 10-fold higher than that for simple obstruction.[33] Consequently, it has generally been accepted that only short periods of observation (<24 h) are appropriate in patients with apparent mechanical small-bowel obstruction, for fear of missing an unsuspected strangulation.

Because clinical criteria are imperfect in terms of differentiating simple from strangulating obstructions, a variety of radiologic tests have been employed. It is clear that plain abdominal radiographs can be helpful in diagnosing a bowel obstruction, but normal X-rays can be seen in as many as 20% of those patients with strangulation.[34,35] The presence of a

TABLE 21.2. Clinical Differences Between Small- and Large-Bowel Obstruction.

	Small-intestinal obstruction	*Large-intestinal obstruction*
Most common causes	Adhesions and groin hernias	Cancer and inflammatory diseases
Symptoms	Abdominal cramps and vomiting at regular/frequent intervals	Abdominal cramps and vomiting less prominent or frequent
Signs	Mild–moderate abdominal distension	Moderate–marked abdominal distension
Plain abdominal films	Dilated small intestinal loops with air/fluid levels; paucity of air and stool distally	Dilated air-filled colon with or without small-bowel distension and air/fluid levels

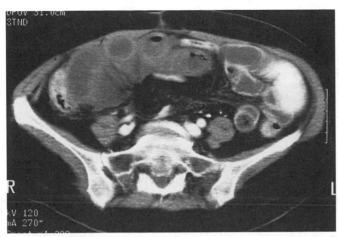

FIGURE 21.7. CT scan of a patient with a strangulating small-bowel obstruction. Dilated proximal small intestine is seen to be filled with the oral contrast agent. More distal loops are fluid filled but without luminal contrast because the "closed loop" is completely obstructing. In addition, the bowel wall appears thickened, and there is evidence of streaky inflammatory changes in the adjacent mesentery.

single loop of dilated small bowel in the setting of acute, severe abdominal pain should raise the suspicion of a strangulated closed-loop obstruction. Abdominal CT has been reported to be useful in identifying strangulation, usually on the basis of either bowel wall thickening, mesenteric edema, asymmetrical enhancement with contrast, pneumatosis, or portal venous gas. Figure 21.7 illustrates several features of strangulating obstruction detected by CT scan in a patient proven at operation to have a large segment of infarcted small intestine.

NONOPERATIVE TREATMENT

With improved surgical and anesthetic management, mortality from small-bowel obstruction has decreased during the past 50 to 60 years from approximately 25% to 5%.[33] Initial therapy is directed at correction of intravascular fluid and electrolyte abnormalities. The patient should be given nothing by mouth. Nasogastric tube suction can provide symptomatic improvement for patients with emesis. Resolution of the obstruction may occur after adequate hydration and decompression via a nasogastric tube, avoiding the need for surgical intervention. This nonoperative approach is often successful in those patients with either partial obstruction from adhesions or obstructions related to impaction of food particles at the sites of luminal narrowing, such as a Crohn's stricture. In addition to standard nasogastric tubes, a variety of long intestinal tubes have been used in an attempt at optimizing luminal decompression. However, no advantage in using these long tubes has been demonstrated.

Obstruction caused by incarcerated hernia can sometimes be relieved by reduction of the hernia, a procedure that should be performed cautiously and only by experienced clinicians. Excessive external pressure will lead to significant patient discomfort and, in rare circumstances, an inadvertent reduction "en masse" may occur, resulting in disappearance of the hernia bulge but with persistent bowel obstruction and possible strangulation within the constricting peritoneal sac.

OPERATIVE TREATMENT

Surgical intervention is indicated for those patients with a complete small-bowel obstruction who have any signs or symptoms indicative of strangulation or for those patients with simple obstruction that has not resolved within a reasonable period of nonoperative therapy, generally 24 to 48 h. Most clinicians would agree that constant or severe pain, especially associated with fever or signs of peritoneal irritation, are indications for urgent laparotomy.

The surgical approach to most patients with small-bowel obstruction is straightforward and includes laparotomy with adhesiolysis and resection of nonviable intestine. In most cases, all the adhesions should be lysed to ensure that the obstruction is relieved and perhaps to prevent future recurrences. When an obstructing lesion is identified, resection with primary anastomosis is performed.

Since the advent of minimally invasive surgical techniques in the 1980s, some surgeons have employed a laparoscopic approach to patients with small-bowel obstruction.[36] A single adhesive band may be lysed laparoscopically or a small laparotomy performed overlying the area of obstruction, thereby avoiding a long incision in the abdominal wall. Laparoscopy in the setting of a bowel obstruction can be performed safely, but the open technique is preferred to avoid the blind insertion of needles or trochars into the peritoneal cavity when distended loops of bowel are present.

Special Forms of Intestinal Obstruction

STRICTURE

Crohn's disease is among the most common etiologies for small intestinal stricture. Certain drugs[37,38] are known to cause mucosal ulceration and strictures, most notably enteric-coated potassium chloride preparations[39] and the nonsteroidal antiinflammatory agents.[40,41] Radiation therapy for intraperitoneal malignancy can lead to stricture formation, especially in the patient who has undergone previous surgery such that adhesions may "fix" the loops of intestine, allowing for greater exposure to isolated segments.[42] Because of problems with healing, obstructing segments of irradiated bowel either should be bypassed[43] or, if a resection is performed, at least one end of an anastomosis should include nonirradiated bowel.[44] Mesenteric ischemia can also lead to stricture formation, the distal ileum being at greatest risk because the ileocolic artery is the last branch of the superior mesenteric artery.[45] Various neoplasms, including carcinoma, carcinoid, and lymphoma, can also cause strictures within the small intestine.[46,47] In most cases of small-bowel stricture, the obstructive symptoms are chronic and progressive in nature, and the best surgical approach is resection whenever technically feasible.

INTERNAL HERNIAS

Internal herniation can be related to abnormalities created by prior operations, as from adhesions or in the paracolic or paraileal spaces adjacent to end stomas. In addition, congenital defects causing hernias have been described in the mesenteries of the ileum, transverse colon, sigmoid colon, and that of a Meckel's diverticulum, as well as in the left paracolic gutter and within the falciform ligament.[48] The presentation is generally indistinguishable from other causes of intestinal obstruction, so that an accurate preoperative diagnosis is rarely made. Surgical repair of the defect should be performed along with resection of any nonviable bowel.

GALLSTONE ILEUS

Gallstones account for approximately 1% to 2% of cases of intestinal obstruction, usually affecting patients older than 60 years.[49,50] To cause obstruction, the gallstone must be of large size (>2.5 cm) and therefore can enter the intestinal tract only by a process of ulceration and fistulization. The most common site of entry is a cholecystoduodenal fistula, although stones may also erode into the stomach, jejunum, ileum, colon, or through the distal common bile duct into the duodenum. The gallstone causes obstruction in the distal ileum or rarely at other areas of intestinal narrowing. The presentation is that of acute, perhaps recurrent, attacks of small-bowel obstruction, and is suggested by the concurrent radiologic features of intestinal obstruction along with air in the biliary tree. Surgical treatment mandates removal of the stone via enterotomy, or resection in cases where the stone has become severely impacted in the wall of the bowel. Whether to perform a cholecystectomy at the time of laparotomy remains controversial,[51] but so long as the gallbladder is emptied of all stones, the chances of recurrent intestinal obstruction are extremely low.[33]

EARLY POSTOPERATIVE SMALL-BOWEL OBSTRUCTION

In the early postoperative period (within 3–4 weeks) following laparotomy for any cause, small-bowel obstruction occurs in approximately 1% of patients. The differentiation between obstruction and adynamic ileus can usually be made on clinical grounds because an ileus rarely persists for more than 5 to 6 days. Clearly, many patients thought to have a "prolonged ileus" really have some degree of mechanical small-intestinal obstruction.[52] The diagnosis of early postoperative obstruction can be made in those patients who initially experience return of bowel function, only subsequently to develop nausea, vomiting, and abdominal distension. Plain radiographs may distinguish adynamic ileus from obstruction because a predominance of small-bowel gaseous distension would not be seen in most cases of ileus. CT scan has been reported to have 100% sensitivity and specificity in distinguishing mechanical small-bowel obstruction from paralytic ileus.[53]

It should be noted that the distinction between ileus and mechanical obstruction in the early postoperative period is rarely of clinical consequence because the treatment is usually nonoperative.[54] Many clinicians have suggested a relatively long trial of nonoperative therapy, perhaps 2 to 4 weeks, before considering surgical intervention. Clearly, there are some patients who have more severe forms of obstruction, for example, twisting of the mesentery, internal herniations, or bowel sutured in the abdominal closure, who will require prompt surgical correction, even in the early postoperative period.

PREVENTION

Adhesion formation can be reduced by avoiding excessive tissue ischemia, trauma, and manipulation. Because fibrin deposition is an initiating event in adhesion formation, anticoagulants (e.g., heparin and dextran) or thrombolytic agents (e.g., streptokinase and urokinase) have been used, but with minimal success. Several synthetic agents have been developed that may reduce the incidence of adhesions.

Crohn's Disease

Although the etiology of Crohn's disease remains a mystery, a number of factors, (environmental, genetic, and microbial) appear to play contributory roles.[55] The medical management of patients with Crohn's disease has focused primarily on the inflammatory process because activated T cells seem to be at the root of this disease. Indications for operation in Crohn's disease generally fall under the categories of either (1) intractibility, (2) luminal complications such as obstruction or hemorrhage, and (3) extraluminal complications such as perforation or fistula.

Intractibility

Elective operation in patients with Crohn's disease should be considered when nonoperative treatment has failed to control the symptoms. One must take into account side effects of medical therapy, notably steroid treatment that can lead to excessive bone loss, diabetes, and weight gain, among other problems. When the symptoms or drug side effects reach an intolerable point, then surgery should be considered. On the other hand, any discussion regarding elective surgery for Crohn's disease must include the issue of recurrent disease and the recognition that surgery rarely offers a permanent cure. Past experience shows that approximately 70% of patients with Crohn's disease ultimately come to operation at least once in their lifetime.[56]

Luminal Complications

Chronic inflammation with stricture formation can cause mechanical obstruction in some patients. The strictures may be either single or multiple with intervening "skip areas." Because luminal small-bowel obstruction related to Crohn's strictures does not lead to strangulation, initial nonoperative management is indicated and is usually successful. In Crohn's patients who have had prior surgery, however, the etiology for the obstruction could be an adhesive band, and in these cases a strangulating mechanism may exist. Therefore, a decision to operate for acute obstruction in Crohn's disease must include a careful consideration of the underlying mechanism with the important goal of avoiding bowel infarction and its adverse sequelae.

Although most patients with acute small-bowel obstruction caused by a Crohn's stricture will improve, recurrent bouts of obstruction can be an indication for operation. Depending upon the number, location, and length of the strictures, either resection or stricturoplasty should be performed. The benefit of stricturoplasty, where feasible, is that it avoids the need for resection and subsequent loss of bowel mucosal surface area, which may be important for preventing the short bowel syndrome that occurs in some patients with recurrent Crohn's disease.

If a Crohn's stricture is too long to perform a stricturoplasty, for example, greater than 8 to 10 cm, or if there are separate strictures that are too close to allow for individual stricturoplasties to be performed, resection is indicated. Recurrence rates are unaffected by the presence of microscopic disease at resection margins. As such, it appears that only grossly involved bowel needs to be resected.

The decision to operate for a Crohn's stricture should be based on clinical parameters and not on the radiologic picture. Many patients remain relatively asymptomatic despite the presence of a "string sign" that indicates severe luminal narrowing. Therefore, although it is important to document objective evidence of stricture formation in patients being considered for operation with Crohn's and obstructive symptoms, the radiologic appearance in and of itself should not be an indication for surgery.

Endoscopic dilatation has been used as an alternative to either resection or stricturoplasty in some patients with Crohn's strictures. This technique has generally been employed in patients with terminal ileal disease, a site that can be accessed at the time of colonoscopy. The results with endoscopic dilatation have been generally poor, however, with high failure rates and significant risks of complications such as perforation.[57]

There is an increase in the incidence of carcinoma in Crohn's disease. The presence of a neoplasm may be suggested in a patient with long-standing Crohn's who develops an unresolving obstruction. If carcinoma is suggested by the clinical or radiologic picture, then clearly surgical intervention is mandated. In most patients with small-intestinal carcinoma complicating Crohn's disease, however, the neoplasm is found incidentally.

Extraluminal Complications

Patients who present with acute abdominal pain and evidence of localized peritonitis often have an extraluminal complication of their disease. Small perforations or "microperforations" are usually manifested by signs of infection, including pain, fever, and leukocytosis. Occasionally, an inflammatory mass can be palpated, and radiologic evaluation by CT will show evidence of extraluminal inflammatory changes. A frank abscess may be amenable to radiologically guided catheter drainage, leading to a more rapid resolution of the infection. Most patients with microperforation respond to bowel rest, i.v. hydration, and i.v. antibiotics. The use of steroids in this setting is controversial because of concern that inhibition of the immune response could lead to rapid deterioration in regard to the underlying infection. Rarely, a gross perforation from Crohn's disease leads to diffuse peritonitis and to mandatory, urgent laparotomy with resection of the involved segment.

The extraluminal component of Crohn's inflammation can lead to the development of fistulae, whether enteroenteric, enterocutaneous, enterovesicle, or enterovaginal. The existence of a fistula is not in itself an indication for operation. Rather, initial therapy should be focused on ensuring the absence of undrained or ongoing sepsis. Once the infectious process is controlled, operative intervention to alleviate symptoms that may be related to the underlying fistula may be appropriate. Bypass procedures have been used in the past under such conditions, but with modern techniques resection of the involved bowel segment is safe and preferred because it avoids the potential for continued sepsis, as well as the development of sequelae such as carcinoma or bacterial overgrowth.

Recurrence

In patients operated on for small-bowel Crohn's disease, the most common site for recurrence is the neoterminal ileum, with the inflammatory changes typical ending abruptly at the anastomotic line. In contrast, in patients who initially present with ileocolitis, a majority (approximately 65%) of the recurrences also involve the colon. The reported clinical recurrence rates in Crohn's disease have varied widely but are generally in the range of 35% at 5 years, 55% at 10 years, and approximately 75% by 15 years. The presence of a symptomatic recurrence, however, does not always mandate surgery, and the need for reoperation is approximately 10 percentage points lower at each of the intervals.[58]

Perforative Versus Nonperforative Disease

Patients with Crohn's disease can be generally categorized into either "stricturing" or "fistulizing" groups. If a patient initially presents with fistulizing disease, that is, perforation or involvement of adjacent organs, then their recurrent disease following operation will generally manifest in a similar way. In contrast, those patients with stricturing disease who initially present with signs and symptoms of obstruction tend to have recurrent strictures following an initial operation. These data suggest that in the future we will be able to predict the course of one's future disease based upon its initial presentation, perhaps leading to improvements in treatment.

Laparoscopic Surgery for Crohn's Disease

A number of centers have reported early experiences with laparoscopic surgery for Crohn's disease. Unfortunately, the recurrent and inflammatory nature of Crohn's disease has limited the application of minimally invasive techniques. For example, those patients who have had multiple previous operations may have extensive adhesions throughout the peritoneal cavity, thereby precluding a laparoscopic approach. In addition, in some patients with marked thickening of the mesentery, including the presence of a mass or phlegmon, laparoscopic manipulation of the bowel can be difficult and even dangerous.

Laparoscopic Crohn's surgery generally involves an assisted technique in which the bowel is mobilized from its peritoneal attachments, and a small incision is then enlarged to deliver the intestine and perform an extracorporeal resection and anastomosis. The ideal candidate for such an approach would be a patient whose disease is limited to a segment of terminal ileum because mobilization of the distal small intestine and right colon can be easily accomplished using the laparoscopic approach.

The indications for a minimally invasive approach in Crohn's disease remain undefined. Clearly, if identical results in regard to the bowel disease can be attained through a smaller incision and with less morbidity, then such approaches should be pursued. Theoretically, the laparoscopic approach may be especially beneficial in Crohn's disease because the amount of adhesion formation may be minimized by this approach, thereby avoiding some of the morbidity associated with reoperative surgery in these patients.

Small-Bowel Fistula

A fistula is an abnormal communication between two epithelial-lined surfaces. The actual communication between the two surfaces can become completely epithelialized but in most cases is lined by simple granulation tissue. Internal fistulae can be surgically created (e.g., gastroenterostomy, cholodochojejunostomy), but internal fistulae can also occur as a complication of an underlying disease process and often require surgical correction. External fistulae, on the other hand, almost always require surgical intervention for physiological and/or psychosocial reasons.

Etiology

Almost all intestinal fistulae are acquired in the course of a disease process along with its associated operative interventions. To understand the principles of the management of patients with intestinal fistulae, it is important to recognize that most fistulae regardless of location or etiology will close spontaneously so long as the conditions are conducive to healing. If one or more of the following situations exist, however, then the fistula will not heal unless the underlying problem is addressed: distal obstruction, presence of a foreign body, malignancy, undrained associated abscess, radiation injury, or an underlying inflammatory process such as Crohn's disease. The management of any patient with a fistula must first address the issues of fluid, electrolytes, and nutrition. This step should be followed by an assessment of the underlying process and a determination as to whether or not the fistula is likely to heal spontaneously.

Nonoperative Management

Patients with intestinal fistulae often lose fluids and electrolytes in large amounts, especially when the site of involvement is the proximal gut. In these patients, adequate fluid and electrolyte replacement must be instituted and can ideally be accomplished via the enteral route, although parenteral supplementation may be required. In some cases, an attempt should be made to minimize fistula output, for example, bowel rest and treatment with the long-acting somatostatin analogue octreotide. Octreotide must be given parenterally and appears to be effective in reducing intestinal secretions. It is unclear, however, whether somatostatin treatment or the amount of fistula output actually affects the time to healing of the fistula. Thus, if the situation is such that fistula healing is expected, it is likely that allowing enteral nutrition and avoiding the potential side effects of octreotide outweigh the potential benefits of bowel rest and octreotide.

Skin breakdown at the site of an external (enterocutaneous) fistula must be prevented. Activated enzymes within the intestinal lumen can cause significant maceration of the skin, leading to irritation, cellulitis, and even frank tissue loss. Simple measures using stoma appliances or topical agents can usually prevent these problems.

Radiologic Evaluation

Depending on the clinical scenario, the site of the fistula can often be predicted. In some cases, however, contrast studies with either oral agents or via direct injection through an external fistula opening are required to precisely determine the site of the problem. Abdominal CT scanning can often be useful in identifying both the fistula site and possibly the underlying disease process.

Surgical Treatment

The surgical approach involves takedown of the fistula and resection of the underlying involved/diseased bowel. The margins of resection should be chosen based on the principles used in other surgery of the small intestine.

Small-Bowel Neoplasms

General Considerations

INCIDENCE

Although the small intestine represents 90% of the surface area of the gastrointestinal tract, tumors of this organ account for only 1% (0.6 to 1.4 per 100,000) of all gastrointestinal neoplasms and 0.3% of all tumors.[59,60]

CLINICAL PRESENTATION

The most common modes of presentation are intestinal obstruction and occult gastrointestinal hemorrhage. Obstruction is often intermittent or partial and may be associated with diarrhea. Obstruction may involve intussusception, particularly for benign neoplasms in adults. Malignant tumors may cause obstruction by circumferential growth, growth into adjacent structures causing fixation and adhesive obstruction, or kinking due to longitudinal growth along the bowel wall. Occasionally, the presentation involves the development of a palpable but otherwise asymptomatic abdominal mass. Perforation and gross bleeding are rare. The nonspecific nature of the symptoms makes diagnosis difficult.[61,62] A correct preoperative diagnosis is reached in only one-third of patients even in modern series.[61]

PATHOLOGY AND DIFFERENTIAL DIAGNOSIS

Benign lesions include adenoma, leiomyoma, fibroma, hamartoma, lipoma, hemangioma, lymphangioma, myxoma, and neurogenic tumors. The most common malignant tumors are adenocarcinoma, leiomyosarcoma, lymphoma, and carcinoid. The relative incidence varies from series to series due to the rarity of small-bowel tumors in general (Tables 21.3, 21.4). The differential diagnosis of neoplasms includes endometriosis, congenital pancreatic rest, splenosis, and duplication cysts.

DIAGNOSIS

Delay in the diagnosis of small-bowel tumors is frequently the result of failure to obtain appropriate imaging studies or misinterpretation of such studies.[63] A variety of diagnostic

TABLE 21.3. Relative Frequency of Benign Neoplasms of the Small Intestine.

Type	Relative frequency (%)
Leiomyoma	30–35
Adenoma	20–25
Lipoma	15
Hemangioma	10
Fibroma	5
Other	15

TABLE 21.4. Relative Frequency and Prognosis of Malignant Neoplasms of the Small Bowel.

Type	Frequency (%)	5-year Survival (%)
Adenocarcinoma	40	15–25
Carcinoid	25	50–60
Lymphoma	25	40–50
Sarcoma	10	35–50

tools are available in the setting of suspected small-bowel neoplasm (Table 21.5).

Benign Neoplasms

PRESENTATION AND MANAGEMENT

Many benign lesions cause no symptoms and are discovered only incidentally. Adenomas are the most common, but leiomyomas are the most common lesions that cause symptoms. The presentation is usually obstruction or occult hemorrhage. Surgical excision is almost always indicated because of the obstruction or hemorrhage, the potential risk of complications, and the inherent impossibility of definitively confirming benign disease in the absence of full microscopic evaluation. Occasionally, small lesions may be simply excised via enterotomy. More commonly, segmental resection and primary anastomosis is appropriate. The entire small bowel must be carefully inspected to exclude additional lesions.

PEUTZ–JEGHERS SYNDROME

Peutz–Jeghers syndrome is an inherited disorder consisting of mucocutaneous melanotic pigmentation and gastrointestinal polyps. The syndrome is autosomal dominant with a high degree of penetrance. The polyps are hamartomatous and occur primarily in the jejunum and ileum; however, more than half of patients also have polyps in the colon or rectum, and 25% have gastric polyps. The pigmented lesions are small, 1- to 2-mm brown or black spots that occur singly or multiply in the oral cavity or in perioral or perianal areas. Lesions may also be evident on the palms or fingers, forearms, or soles of feet. Polyposis may develop in the absence of pigmentation lesions. Because of the diffuse involvement of the intestinal tract, surgical therapy should be confined to limited segments of bowel clearly producing symptoms. Occasionally, prophylactic subtotal colectomy may be indicated if there is a substantial colonic polyp burden and if the hamartomas reveal adenomatous changes. The risk of gastrointestinal cancer in Peutz–Jeghers syndrome is estimated at 18 times greater than that expected in the general population.[64–66] The long-term natural history of the syndrome suggests emphatically that it is not a benign disease.[67] Therefore, screening upper endoscopy and colonoscopy are recommended starting at age 20, followed by annual flexible sigmoidoscopy, and by complete upper and lower examination every 3 years.

Malignant Neoplasms

PRESENTATION AND MANAGEMENT

Malignant neoplasms of the small intestine present much like benign lesions, typically with obstruction or occult bleeding. Delay in diagnosis is common, leading to advanced disease at presentation. Surgical resection is seldom curative for these advanced lesions.[62,68,69] Optimal treatment consists of wide resection including regional lymph nodes. For duodenal neoplasms, pancreaticoduodenectomy is recommended unless the lesion is locally advanced, in which case palliative gastrojejunostomy is indicated. For malignant tumors of the small bowel, resection should be performed even if cure is not pos-

TABLE 21.5. Comparison of Diagnostic Imaging Used in Evaluation of Suspected Small-Bowel Neoplasms.

	Advantage	Disadvantage
Plain abdominal film	May show obstruction	Nonspecific
UGI/SBFT	May show mass lesion, mucosal defect, or intussusception	No visualization outside lumen; not helpful in staging
Enteroclysis	More sensitive than conventional SBFT	Requires duodenal tube and additional technical skill
Computed tomography	Allows staging; may aid in diagnosis of tumor type	Lacks visualization of lumen or mucosal surface
Upper endoscopy	Direct visualization of mucosal surface of duodenum; allows for biopsy and/or polypectomy	Invasive; limited to duodenum and may miss submucosal lesions unless combined with endoscopic ultrasound
Push endoscopy	Extends visualization into proximal jejunum; allows for biopsy	Same as conventional endoscopy
Extended small-bowel endoscopy	Allows visualization of up to 70% of small bowel; more sensitive than enteroclysis	No biopsy capability; may take up to 8 h to pass scope; increased patient discomfort

UGI/SBFT, upper gastrointestinal series/small-bowel follow-through.

TABLE 21.6. Anatomical Distribution of Tumors (percent).

	Carcinoid	Adenocarcinoma	Lymphoma	Sarcoma
Duodenum	6	50	12	16
Jejunum	20	28	40	26
Ileum	74	22	48	58

Source: Disario et al. Am J Gastroenterol 1994;89:700.

sible, because possible complications of bleeding, obstruction, and perforation are prevented.

ADENOCARCINOMA

Adenocarcinoma represents about half of all small-bowel malignancies in hospital-based series. These lesions are twice as common in men than women. Adenocarcinoma typically presents with weight loss, bleeding, anemia, obstruction, or (when periampullary) jaundice. The adenoma-to-carcinoma sequence appears to apply for the small bowel,[70] and activating mutations in codon 12 of the oncogene K-*ras* are as common in proximal small-bowel cancers (~50% incidence) as in colorectal cancer.[71,72] Most lesions are located in the proximal bowel, except in the setting of Crohn's disease in which most are ileal (Table 21.6).[69,73] Carcinoma should be suspected in patients with longstanding Crohn's disease who develop a change in their clinical status.

Resection is the best treatment for small-bowel adenocarcinoma. At present, there is no convincing evidence that adjuvant chemotherapy or radiation treatments are effective.[69]

LEIOMYOSARCOMA AND MALIGNANT STROMAL TUMORS

Most small-bowel sarcomas are leiomyosarcomas, representing 10% to 20% of all malignant small-bowel tumors. These lesions may grow to considerable size before the development of symptoms. Leiomyosarcoma may spread by direct exten-

sion or may metastasize hematogenously to liver, lungs, or bone. As for other small-bowel neoplasms, wide en bloc resection with the associated mesentery is the treatment of choice. Extended lymphadenectomy is not indicated because lymphatic metastasis is rare. Palliative resections and bypass procedures are warranted because some of these tumors may be rather slow growing. There is no evidence that adjuvant chemotherapy or radiation therapy alone or in combination is effective.[69]

LYMPHOMA

Lymphomas represent 10% to 20% of malignant small-bowel tumors. The ileum is the most common site of involvement because of the presence of the greatest amount of gut-associated lymphoid tissue. Primary small-bowel lymphoma is the most common extranodal form of lymphoma.[74] Most are non-Hodgkin's lymphoma and predominantly B cell in origin,[75–77] although both Hodgkin's disease and plasma cell lymphoma have also been reported. Patients with small-bowel lymphoma commonly present with fatigue, weight loss, and abdominal pain.[78] A severe malabsorption syndrome is seen in about 10% of patients. Perforation, obstruction, bleeding, or intussusception are less common modes of presentation.[78] Individuals infected with HIV-1 have a markedly greater risk of developing non-Hodgkin's lymphoma, usually high grade.[79] The differences among the various intestinal lymphoma entities are summarized in Table 21.7.[74]

Intestinal lymphomas are staged according to a modification of the Ann Arbor system (Table 21.8). Treatment of primary small-bowel lymphoma (Western variety) is mainly surgical. Ideally, complete resection along with a wedge of mesentery is accomplished. However, for patients with positive margins, adjuvant therapy is recommended. Survival for completely resected intestinal lymphoma is about 50%.[80] Retrospective[81–87] and prospective[88] experiences suggest that the combination of surgery and adjuvant chemotherapy

TABLE 21.7. Primary Intestinal Lymphoma.

	Adult Western	Childhood	Immunoproliferative small-intestinal disease	Enteropathy-associated T-cell lymphoma
Population	Nonspecific	Children	Low socioeconomic class; parasitic infestation	Celiac disease, malabsorption
Geography	Worldwide	Worldwide	Common in Middle East, Mediterranean	Common in Middle East
Peak incidence (decade of life)	Sixth	First	Second, third	Fourth, fifth
Signs and symptoms	Pain, perforation, obstruction, hemorrhage	Tender abdominal mass, acute intussusception	Pain, fever, diarrhea, steatorrhea, vomiting, wasting disease, circulating IgA-α heavy chain	Deterioration in chronic condition, malnutrition, acute abdomen, rising IgA titers
Location	Small intestine	Ileum	Jejunum, duodenum	Distal small bowel, disseminates early
Pathology	Large tumors, B-cell in 75%, large-cell diffuse histology	Burkitt's type, small noncleaved B-cell	Nodularity of long segments of small intestine, IgA-producing B cells	Villous atrophy, crypt hyperplasia, large T-cell origin
Prognosis	By stage	Very good for stages I and II, tumor bulk important factor	May undergo spontaneous regression but overall poor prognosis	Poor due to early disseminated disease
Therapy	Surgery, adjuvant chemotherapy and radiation	Surgery for early stage, chemotherapy major role	Antibiotics, aggressive chemotherapy	Chemotherapy, surgery only for complications

Source: Modified after Turowski and Basson. Am J Surg 1995;169:435.

TABLE 21.8. Ann Arbor Classification of Primary Gastrointestinal Lymphoma.

Stage	Subgroups	Description
IE		Confined to single site
IIE		Confined below abdomen
	IIE1	Regional (mesenteric or perigastric) nodes
	IIE2	Distant (e.g., retroperitoneal) nodes
III		Involves organs on both sides of diaphragm
IV		Wide dissemination (liver, spleen)

Source: Modified after Musshoff K and Schmidt-Vollmer H. Prognostic sequence of primary site after radiotherapy in non-Hodgkins lymphoma. Lancet 1975 31(Suppl II):425–434.

(typically CHOP [cyclophosphamide-hydroxydaunomycin-vincristine-prednisone] or a variant thereof) improves outcome stage for stage. Primary gastric lymphoma tends to fare better than primary intestinal lymphoma.[88]

CARCINOID TUMORS

Carcinoid tumors of the gut represent about 20% to 40% of primary small-intestinal malignancies and are characterized by variable malignant potential and the secretion of multiple neurohormonal substances, notably serotonin and substance P. In population-based studies, carcinoid tumors are the most frequent of small-bowel neoplasms.[60] The highest incidence of occurrence is in the sixth decade, although carcinoids have been reported in patients aged 20 to over 80. Tumors are multicentric in 30%.[89] About 50% of intestinal carcinoids are located in the appendix. Of all nonappendiceal carcinoids, about half are present within the distal 2 feet of the ileum.

Carcinoid tumors often follow an indolent course, with median duration of symptoms up to 2 years before diagnosis. Symptoms tend to be nonspecific; like other small-bowel tumors, carcinoids may bleed, obstruct, or ulcerate. They may also present as segmental mesenteric ischemia associated with the mesenteric angiopathy that accompanies the intense desmoplasia surrounding the tumor.[90] Intestinal obstruction may occur not only because of the primary tumor but also due to kinking of the mesentery from bulky nodal metastases or mesenteric fibrosis.[91]

Radiologic findings may increase clinical suspicion of carcinoid tumors. Small-bowel follow-through examination typically reveals fixed loops of intestine, with angulation, luminal narrowing, or multiple filling defects. Mesenteric calcifications may be present. CT may show evidence of a fibrotic mesenteric reaction in the vicinity of a transition point between dilated proximal and distal collapsed small bowel. Hepatic metastatic lesions are characteristically hypervascular and thus brightly enhance with intravenous contrast administration. ^{131}I-Metaio-dobenzylguanidine (MIBG) scintigraphy may occasionally be useful to localize midgut carcinoid tumors, although the false-negative rate may be as high as 30%.[92]

Metastatic disease is already present in as many as 60% of cases at the time of diagnosis.[89,93] The malignant potential of carcinoid tumors is related to location, size, depth of penetration, and pattern of growth. Overall, 5-year survival is approximately 30% to 50%.[90,94] Treatment of carcinoid tumors of the small intestine is wide segmental resection.[94] For tumors of the distal ileum, the cecum and right colon should be resected en bloc,[90] and tumors involving the duodenum may require radical pancreaticoduodenectomy. Lesions without nodal metastases are almost always cured by resection. Palliative resections are probably worthwhile because most carcinoid tumors are slow growing.

Carcinoid tumors metastatic to the liver may produce the malignant carcinoid syndrome, which includes episodic diarrhea, flushing, abdominal cramps, and, later, right-sided valvular heart disease and asthma.[95] This syndrome is, in fact, quite uncommon. It is estimated that less than 10% of patients with metastatic carcinoid tumors will develop the carcinoid syndrome. Confirmation of malignant carcinoid syndrome is made by determination of urinary levels of 5-HIAA (5-hydroxyindoleacetic acid), the inactive breakdown product of 5-HT produced by metabolism in the lung and liver.

If possible, primary and metastatic lesions should be resected or at least debulked as this may produce substantial palliation of the symptoms of carcinoid syndrome. Ischemic therapy via hepatic artery embolization may be utilized in cases in which surgery is not possible and may produce dramatic, although frequently short-lived, relief of symptoms in about 90% of patients.[96,97] The long-acting somatostatin analogue octreotide also appears to be of some benefit, particularly in patients with carcinoid diarrhea.[98] Some response to the combination of 5-fluorouracil and streptozotocin has been reported, although in general chemotherapy appears to be of limited usefulness. Median survival of patients with carcinoid tumors metastatic to the liver is 3 years, compared to 5 years in patients with nonresectable abdominal disease in the absence of liver metastases.

OTHER TUMORS AND METASTATIC LESIONS

Gastrinoma, somatostatinoma, paraganglioma, and undifferentiated neuroendocrine carcinomas of the small intestine have been reported. These tumors may present as a hormone-specific hyperfunctional state or as nonfunctioning mass lesions. The small bowel is the most common site of melanoma metastatic to the gastrointestinal tract. Primaries from the breast, lung, and kidney metastatic to the small bowel, presumably via hematogenous spread, have also been described. Cervical, ovarian, and colonic tumors may involve the small bowel by direct extension. Treatment is, in general, palliative and consists of limited resection or bypass. In patients with small-bowel metastatic melanoma without a known primary, aggressive resection may improve the quality of life and disease-free survival.

Meckel's Diverticulum

Based on autopsy series, Meckel's diverticulum is present in 0.3% to 2.5% of the population. The size and shape of the diverticulum can vary greatly, although it is usually between 3 and 5 cm long and is found 10 to 150 cm from the ileocecal valve. Meckel's diverticula contain a mesentery with an independent blood supply from the ileal vessels. There is an association between Meckel's diverticulum and a number of other congenital malformations, including exomphalos, esophageal or anorectal atresia, and various central nervous system or cardiovascular malformations. Although usually lined by mucosa similar to that seen in the adjacent ileum, heterotopic mucosa has been described, including that of gastric, duodenal, colonic, or pancreatic nature.

Complications

Meckel's diverticula can be associated with various complications and often require surgical intervention. The presence of gastric mucosa with resultant acid production can lead to ulceration in the adjacent ileal mucosa, causing either hemorrhage or perforation. Perforation can also occur in the diverticulum itself, perhaps related to luminal obstruction from a foreign body. The resultant Meckel's diverticulitis presents with signs and symptoms that are generally indistinguishable from appendicitis. Meckel's diverticulum can also be associated with small-bowel obstruction, either from intussusception, volvulus, or an associated adhesive band. It has been estimated that the chances of a Meckel's diverticulum causing one of these complications to be 4.2% in children, dropping to 3% in adults and almost 0% in the elderly. As such, removal of a Meckel's diverticulum at the time of laparotomy for another reason is probably not indicated, especially in adults.

Diagnostic Studies

Meckel's diverticula are rarely demonstrated on routine barium studies. In the rare instance of an umbilical fistula, however, injection of contrast material directly into the external orifice demonstrates a communication with the underlying ileum, indicating a patent vitelline duct. Such a study will be able to differentiate the intestinal communication from a patent urachus that communicates with the urinary bladder. Tc 99m pertechnetate Meckel's scan detects the gastric mucosa within the Meckel's diverticulum and has been reported to be 90% accurate.[99] Meckel's diverticulum can also be detected angiographically.

Surgical Treatment

When a Meckel's diverticulum causes symptoms or complications, resection is indicated. Either excision of the diverticulum alone or resection of the adjacent segment of ileum containing the diverticulum is acceptable.

Short Bowel Syndrome

Maintenance of adequate nutrition is dependent on the normal digestive and absorptive function of the small intestinal mucosa. A normal, healthy adult possesses an excess of gut mucosa such that limited resection or loss of bowel surface area through other means is usually well tolerated. However, depending on the amount of bowel removed and the specific level of resection, symptoms can ensue following surgery, in some cases leading to a condition known as the "short bowel syndrome." Because of the important functional capacities of the duodenum in regard to iron and calcium, and of the distal ileum in regard to vitamin B_{12} and bile salts, resections of these specific regions tend to be poorly tolerated. In contrast, up to 40% of the mid-small bowel can be removed with only moderate clinical sequelae. As a general rule, resection of 50% of the small intestine produces significant malabsorption, and

if 70% or more of the intestine is resected, survival is threatened.

The minimal amount of small intestine required to sustain life is variable. Prolonged survival has been recorded in isolated patients with as little as 1 foot of jejunum along with an intact duodenum, but in general survival is threatened in patients with less than 2 feet (60 cm) of intestine beyond the duodenum. An intact ileocecal valve is thought to be important in regard to improving function of the remaining small intestine, and clearly the colon is vitally important for preventing water loss. Patients with short bowel syndrome have impairment in the absorption of water and electrolytes as well as that of all nutrients, that is, fat, protein, carbohydrates, and vitamins. Fluid losses can be greater than 5 to 10 l/day. As a result, patients with short bowel syndrome suffer weight loss, fatigue, calorie deprivation, electrolyte abnormalities, and vitamin deficiencies.

Treatment

Initial therapy involves maintenance of fluid and electrolyte balance. Total parenteral nutrition (TPN) is often indicated and, depending on the extent of resection, may be required throughout the lifetime of the patient. It is likely that even small amounts of enteral nutrition are beneficial, however, because the luminal nutrients appear to enhance the adaptive response of the remaining gut. Various antidiarrheal and stool-bulking agents have also been used with some benefit. Gastric hypersecretion should be treated with either H_2-blockers or proton pump inhibitors. Cholestyramine may be beneficial in patients with limited ileal resections, but if the bile salt pool has been depleted, then cholestyramine is contraindicated.[100]

Because of the increased risk of cholelithiasis in patients with short gut syndrome, prophylactic cholecystectomy should be considered if long-term survival is anticipated.

Surgical Approach

The surgical treatment of patients with short bowel syndrome has been disappointing. In small numbers of patients, various procedures including intestinal lengthening, reversal of short segments, and plication of excessively dilated bowel have been used.[101,102] Although some improvement has been seen in isolated cases, such operations have not become universally adopted. The results of small-intestinal transplantation have been disappointing, primarily because of a high incidence of rejection.[103]

Malabsorption Syndromes

Clinical Aspects

Malabsorption results from the pathological disturbance of the normal sequence of digestion, absorption, and nutrient transport.[104] A wide range of clinical features result from malabsorption syndromes and may yield clues as to the specific etiology. Classically, malabsorption produces both intestinal and extraintestinal symptoms. Chronic diarrhea, consisting of watery, bulky, frequent stools, is common. Patients with steatorrhea may note pale, foul-smelling, greasy, floating stool. Anorexia, hyperphagia, nausea, vomiting, abdominal distention, gassiness, excessive flatus, or borborygmus are common symptoms. Pain is unusual. Several malabsorption syndromes are particularly relevant to surgical disease.[105] Celiac disease, tropical sprue, and lactase deficiency are not considered further here.

Bile Acid Malabsorption

Bile salts are necessary for proper absorption of dietary fats and fat-soluble substances. Normally, more than 90% of excreted bile is reabsorbed in the small intestine as part of the enterohepatic circulation system. In the terminal 100 cm of ileum, bile salt absorption is mediated by a Na^+-coupled bile salt transporter.[6,7] Primary or idiopathic bile salt malabsorption is unusual. More commonly, bile salt malabsorption is the result of resection of the terminal ileum, such as in Crohn's disease.[106,107] Some patients develop bile salt malabsorption after cholecystectomy or after vagotomy.[108] Bile salt malabsorption is manifest as diarrhea and is the consequence of excessive concentrations of bile salts (>3 mM) reaching the colon. Cholestyramine is effective in more than 90% of cases of bile salt diarrhea.[108]

Vitamin B$_{12}$ Malabsorption

Inadequate absorption of vitamin B$_{12}$ and folic acid leads to macrocytic anemia. Vitamin B$_{12}$ undergoes a complex process of absorption involving the salivary glands (protein R), the stomach (intrinsic factor), a pancreatic protease, and active absorption in the terminal ileum. Treatment is by periodic parenteral administration of vitamin B$_{12}$ and, where relevant, the addition of specific therapy to reverse the underlying disorder.

Bacterial Overgrowth Syndrome

A variety of conditions predispose to bacterial overgrowth in the small bowel. Bacterial overgrowth in poorly emptying or stagnant small-intestinal segments leads to a syndrome of diarrhea and steatorrhea accompanied by abdominal pain, weight loss, anemia (usually macrocytic), fat-soluble vitamin deficiencies, and, in late stages, neurological deficits.[109,110] This situation is sometimes referred to as the blind loop syndrome but can occur in a variety of conditions not involving the presence of a self-filling, nonemptying intestinal segment. The pathophysiology of the syndrome involves excessive bacterial metabolism of vitamin B$_{12}$, leading to its insufficient availability for intestinal absorption. Furthermore, bile salt deconjugation by luminal bacteria leads to inadequate micellization of dietary fat and, consequently, steatorrhea. Deconjugated bile salts are toxic to enterocytes and may directly elicit diarrhea and cellular damage that leads to further malabsorption of other nutrients. Medical treatment consists of intermittent oral antibiotic therapy. If feasible, the underlying anatomical arrangement favoring bacterial overgrowth should be surgically corrected.

Evaluation of Malabsorptive Conditions

The etiology of a malabsorptive condition is often suggested by a thorough history followed by inspection of the stool and an estimation of its volume.[111] Specific testing may confirm the diagnosis, although in general specificity and sensitivity are suboptimal and many specialized examinations are not routinely performed in many centers.[105] Fat malabsorption is usually detectable by quantitative measurements of fecal fat content in a 24-h collection or by Sudan stain of feces. Breath tests utilizing ^{14}C-labeled carbohydrates are used to detect lactose intolerance or other syndromes of carbohydrate malabsorption.[112–114] D-Xylose absorption and detection in either plasma or urine can be used as a general test of intestinal absorptive function.[115] There are currently no accurate tests to confirm or exclude bile salt malabsorption; the response to an empiric trial of bile salt-binding agents such as cholestyramine may be useful. Vitamin B$_{12}$ malabsorption is detected with 94% accuracy by dual-label Schilling test.[116]

Pancreatic insufficiency leading to malabsorption and steatorrhea is usually suspected on clinical or radiologic grounds. A symptomatic response to pancreatic enzyme replacement therapy is useful supporting evidence, but occasionally detailed testing of pancreatic exocrine function is necessary. Bacterial overgrowth can be confirmed by quantitative culture of endoscopically aspirated small-bowel luminal contents or by ^{14}C-xylose breath testing.[117,118] However, the empiric response to antibiotic therapy using agents such as tetracycline or metronidazole is usually more helpful in establishing the presumptive diagnosis. A Schilling test that reverts to normal after a 3- to 5-day course of tetracycline but not after addition of exogenous intrinsic factor confirms the diagnosis and is 86% accurate.[116]

Miscellaneous Conditions

Pneumatosis Intestinalis

Pneumatosis intestinalis refers to the presence of gas or air within the wall of the intestine, as seen either at the time of surgery or by a radiographic study. So-called benign pneumatosis is generally an incidental finding and does not imply an underlying intestinal pathology, such that the clinical course is not characterized by intestinal perforation or sepsis. In contrast, when pneumatosis intestinalis occurs as a result of primary intestinal pathology, urgent surgery is usually required.

Small-Bowel Ulceration

Ulcerative lesions of the small bowel are most commonly the result of ingested medications such as enteric-coated potassium chloride, nonsteroidal antiinflammatory drugs, and corticosteroids. Less often, small-bowel ulcers are caused by segmental arterial or venous occlusion or vasculitis.[119] Heterotopic gastric mucosa within a Meckel's diverticulum may lead to peptic ulceration of the small-bowel mucosa. Rarely, gastrinoma may be associated with small-bowel ulceration. Ulceration may develop in association with Crohn's disease and with small-bowel lymphoma. Finally, a number of infectious causes of small-bowel ulceration are recognized, including tuberculosis, syphilis, and typhoid fever. In a distinct minority of patients, no definable etiology of the small bowel ulceration will be found. In this situation, the ulceration is usually single and located in the terminal ileum.

About two-thirds of cases present as intermittent small-bowel obstruction. Preoperative localization in this setting can be difficult, and even when a site of partial obstruction can be identified during radiographic evaluation (e.g., by enteroclysis), the precise cause for the obstruction may not be determined even at the time of surgical exploration. The treatment of a symptomatic small-bowel ulcer is surgical resection. Suture repair of perforated small-bowel ulceration is not recommended due to an unacceptably high rate of complications. Recurrence after resection is extremely unusual, particularly if the offending medication is stopped.

Foreign-Body Ingestion

Emergency department evaluation for the accidental or intentional ingestion of sharp or pointed foreign bodies including fish bones, pins, toothpicks, and broken razor blades is not rare. Although there is a small potential for intestinal perforation, the vast majority of ingested foreign objects pass through the gastrointestinal tract without incident. Radiopaque objects may be followed by serial plain films of the abdomen. The development of abdominal pain associated with tenderness and leukocytosis strongly suggests that a contained local perforation has occurred. Surgical resection is indicated, because nonoperative antibiotic therapy is associated with the occasional development of chronic infection or stricture formation. Perforation after passage into the colon is rare, because by that time the object generally has become safely embedded within solid fecal matter. Occasionally, larger objects such as whistles or coins may lead to intestinal obstruction if they become lodged, typically near the ileocecal valve.

References

1. Hermiston ML, Gordon JI. Organization of the crypt-villus axis and evolution of its stem cell hierarchy during intestinal development. Am J Physiol 1995;268:G813–G822.
2. Simon TC, Gordon JI. Intestinal epithelial cell differentiation: new insights from mice, flies and nematodes. Curr Opin Genet Dev 1995;5:577–586.
3. Potten C. Epithelial cell growth and differentiation. II. Intestinal apoptosis. Am J Physiol 1997;273:G253–G257.
4. Mitic LL, Anderson JM. Molecular architecture of tight junctions. Annu Rev Physiol 1998;60:121–142.
5. Anderson JM, Van Itallie CM. Tight junctions and the molecular basis for regulation of paracellular permeability. Am J Physiol 1995;269:G467–G475.
6. Schneider BL, Dawson PA, Christie DM, Hardikar W, Wong MH, Suchy FJ. Cloning and molecular characterization of the ontogeny of a rat ileal sodium-dependent bile acid transporter. J Clin Invest 1995;95:745–754.
7. Dawson PA, Oelkers P. Bile acid transporters [see comments]. Curr Opin Lipidol 1995;6:109–114.
8. Hansen MB, Skadhauge E. New aspects of the pathophysiology and treatment of secretory diarrhoea. Physiol Res 1995;44:61–78.
9. Ooms L, Degryse A. Pathogenesis and pharmacology of diarrhea. Vet Res Commun 1986;10:355–397.
10. Bridges RJ, Rummel W. Mechanistic basis of alterations in mucosal water and electrolyte transport. Clin Gastroenterol 1986; 15:491–506.
11. Mowat AM, Viney JL. The anatomical basis of intestinal immunity. Immunol Rev 1997;156:145–166.
12. Neutra MR. Current concepts in mucosal immunity. V. Role of M cells in transepithelial transport of antigens and pathogens to the mucosal immune system. Am J Physiol 1998;274:G785–G791.
13. Perdue MH, McKay DM. Integrative immunophysiology in the intestinal mucosa. Am J Physiol 1994;267:G151–G165.
14. Lamm M. Current concepts in mucosal immunity: how epithelial transport of IgA antibodies relates to host defense. Am J Physiol 1998;274:G614–G617.
15. Mayer L. Current concepts in mucosal immunity: I. Antigen presentation in the intestine: new rules and regulations. Am J Physiol 1998;274:G7–G9.
16. Kraehenbuhl JP, Pringault E, Neutra MR. Review article: Intestinal epithelia and barrier functions. Aliment Pharmacol Ther 1997;11(suppl 3):3–8; discussion 8–9.
17. Ulrich C II, Holtmann M, Miller L. Secretin and vasoactive intestinal peptide receptors: members of a unique family of G protein-coupled receptors. Gastroenterology 1998;114:382–397.
18. Drucker DJ. Glucagon-like peptides. Diabetes 1998;47:159–169.
19. Liddle RA. Regulation of cholecystokinin secretion by intraluminal releasing factors. Am J Physiol 1995;269:G319–G327.
20. Raybould HE, Lloyd KC. Integration of postprandial function in the proximal gastrointestinal tract. Role of CCK and sensory pathways. Ann N Y Acad Sci 1994;713:143–156.
21. Reichlin S. Somatostatin. N Engl J Med 1983;309:1495–1501.
22. Farthing MJ. Octreotide in the treatment of refractory diarrhoea and intestinal fistulae. Gut 1994;35:S5–S10.
23. Sheikh SP. Neuropeptide Y and peptide YY: major modulators of gastrointestinal blood flow and function. Am J Physiol 1991;261:G701–G715.
24. Hill FL, Zhang T, Gomez G, Greeley GH Jr. Peptide YY, a new gut hormone (a mini-review). Steroids 1991;56:77–82.
25. Gehlert DR. Multiple receptors for the pancreatic polypeptide (PP-fold) family: physiological implications. Proc Soc Exp Biol Med 1998;218:7–22.
26. Geoghegan J, Pappas TN. Clinical uses of gut peptides. Ann Surg 1997;225:145–154.
27. Tonini M. Recent advances in the pharmacology of gastrointestinal prokinetics. Pharmacol Res 1996;33:217–226.
28. Holzer P, Holzer-Petsche U. Tachykinins in the gut. Part II. Roles in neural excitation, secretion and inflammation. Pharmacol Ther 1997;73:219–263.
29. Der-Silaphet T, Malaysz J, Hagel S, Arsenault A, Huizinga J. Interstitial cells of Cajal direct normal propulsive contractile activity in mouse small intestine. Gastroenterology 1998;114: 724–736.
30. Balthazar E. CT of small bowel obstruction. AJR 1994;162:225–261.
31. Ko Y, Lim J, Lee D, Lee H, Lim J. Small bowel obstruction: sonographic evaluation. Radiology 1993;188:649–653.
32. Ogata M, Mateer J, Condon R. Prospective evaluation of abdominal sonography for the diagnosis of bowel obstruction. Am Surg 223;1996:223:237–241.
33. Maignot R. Maignot's abdominal operation. In: Seymour Shwartz, Harold Ellis, Husser WC, eds. 1989. East Norwalk CT: Appleton and Lange.
34. Silen W, Hein M, et al. Strangulation obstruction of the small intestine. Arch Surg 1962;85:12.
35. Becker W. Intestinal obstruction: an analysis of 1007 cases. South Med J 1955;48:41.
36. Reissman P, Wexner S. Laparoscopic surgery for intestinal obstruction. Surg Endosc 1995;9(8):365–868.
37. Lee F. Drug-related pathological lesions of the intestinal tract. Histopathology 1994;25:303–308.
38. George C. Drugs causing intestinal obstruction: a review. J R Soc Med 1994;73:200.
39. Abbruzzese A, Gooding C. Reversal of small bowel obstruction: withdrawal of hydrochlorothiazide potassium chloride therapy. JAMA 1965;192:781.
40. Speed C, Bramble M, Corbett W, Haslock I. Non-steroidal anti-inflammatory induced diaphragm disease of the small intestine: complexities of diagnosis and management. Br J Rheumatol 1994;33:778–780.

41. Levi S, De Lacey G, Price A, Grumpel M, Levi A, Bjarnson I. Diaphragm-like strictures of the small bowel in patients with nonsteroidal anti-inflammatory drugs. Br J Radiol 1990;63:186–189.

42. Jackson B. Bowel damage from irradiation. Proc R Soc Med 1976;69:683.

43. Mann W. Surgical management of radiation enteropathy. Surg Clin North Am 1991;71:977–990.

44. Galland R, Spencer J. Surgical management of radiation enteritis. Surgery (St. Louis) 1986;99:133–139.

45. Thaker P, Weingarten L, Friedman I. Stenosis of the small intestine due to nonconclusive ischemic disease. 1977;112:1216–1217.

46. Zollinger RJ. Primary neoplasms of the small intestine. Am J Surg 1986;151:654–658.

47. Martin R. Malignant tumors of the small intestine. Surg Clin North Am 1986;66:779–785.

48. Janin Y, Stone A, Wise L. Mesenteric hernia. Surg Gynecol Obstet 1980;150:747–754.

49. Mclaughlin C, Raines M. Obstruction of the alimentary tract from gall stones. Am J Surg 1951;81:424.

50. Stitt R, Heslin D, Currie DJ. Gallstone ileus. Br J Surg 1967;54:673.

51. Buetow G, Glaubitz J, et al. Recurrent gallstone ileus. Surgery (St. Louis) 1963;54:716.

52. Silen W. Cope's Early Diagnosis of the Acute Abdomen. Oxford: Oxford University Press, 1996.

53. Frager D, Baer J, Rothpearl A, Bossart P. Distinction between postoperative ileus and mechanical small-bowel obstruction: value of CT compared with clinical and other radiographic findings. AJR 1995;164:891–894.

54. Ludwig K, Condon R. Surgical Consultations. St. Louis: Mosby Year-Book, 1993.

55. Fiocchi C. Inflammatory bowel disease: etiology and pathogenisis. Gastroenterology 1998;115:182–205.

56. Clotzer D. Surgical therapy for Crohn's disease. Gastroenterol Clin North Am 1995;24:577–596.

57. Couckuyt H, Gevers A, Coremans G, Hiele M, Rutgeerts P. Efficacy and safety of hydrostatic balloon dilation of ileocolonic Crohn's strictures: a prospective long term analysis. 1995;36:577–580.

58. Felder J, Adler D, Korelitz B. The safety of corticosteroid therapy in Crohn's disease with an abdominal mass. Am J Gastroenterol 1991;86:1450–1455.

59. Barclay TH, Schapira DV. Malignant tumors of the small intestine. Cancer (Phila) 1983;51:878–881.

60. DiSario JA, Burt RW, Vargas H, McWhorter WP. Small bowel cancer: epidemiological and clinical characteristics from a population-based registry. Am J Gastroenterol 1994;89:699–701.

61. Ciccarelli O, Welch JP, Kent GG. Primary malignant tumors of the small bowel. The Hartford Hospital experience, 1969–1983. Am J Surg 1987;153:350–354.

62. Ashley SW, Wells SA Jr. Tumors of the small intestine. Semin Oncol 1988;15:116–128.

63. Maglinte DD, O'Connor K, Bessette J, Chernish SM, Kelvin FM. The role of the physician in the late diagnosis of primary malignant tumors of the small intestine. Am J Gastroenterol 1991;86:304–308.

64. Giardiello FM, Welsh SB, Hamilton SR, et al. Increased risk of cancer in the Peutz-Jeghers syndrome. N Engl J Med 1987;316:1511–1514.

65. Boardman LA, Thibodeau SN, Schaid DJ, et al. Increased risk for cancer in patients with the Peutz-Jeghers syndrome. Ann Intern Med 1998;128:896–899.

66. Hizawa K, Iida M, Matsumoto T, Kohrogi N, Yao T, Fujishima M. Neoplastic transformation arising in Peutz-Jeghers polyposis. Dis Colon Rectum 1993;36:953–957.

67. Foley TR, McGarrity TJ, Abt AB. Peutz-Jeghers syndrome: a clinicopathologic survey of the "Harrisburg family" with a 49-year follow-up. Gastroenterology 1988;95:1535–1540.

68. Norberg KA, Emas S. Primary tumors of the small intestine. Am J Surg 1981;142:569–573.

69. Cunningham JD, Aleali R, Aleali M, Brower ST, Aufses AH. Malignant small bowel neoplasms: histopathologic determinants of recurrence and survival. Ann Surg 1997;225:300–306.

70. Perzin KH, Bridge MF. Adenomas of the small intestine: a clinicopathologic review of 51 cases and a study of their relationship to carcinoma. Cancer (Phila) 1981;48:799–819.

71. Younes N, Fulton N, Tanaka R, Wayne J, Straus FH II, Kaplan EL. The presence of K-12 ras mutations in duodenal adenocarcinomas and the absence of ras mutations in other small bowel adenocarcinomas and carcinoid tumors. Cancer (Phila) 1997;79:1804–1808.

72. Sutter T, Arber N, Moss SF, et al. Frequent K-ras mutations in small bowel adenocarcinomas. Dig Dis Sci 1996;41:115–118.

73. Ouriel K, Adams JT. Adenocarcinoma of the small intestine. Am J Surg 1984;147:66–71.

74. Turowski GA, Basson MD. Primary malignant lymphoma of the intestine. Am J Surg 1995;169:433–441.

75. Radaszkiewicz T, Dragosics B, Bauer P. Gastrointestinal malignant lymphomas of the mucosa-associated lymphoid tissue: factors relevant to prognosis. Gastroenterology 1992;102:1628–1638.

76. Hansen PB, Vogt KC, Skov RL, Pedersen-Bjergaard U, Jacobsen M, Ralfkiaer E. Primary gastrointestinal non-Hodgkin's lymphoma in adults: a population-based clinical and histopathologic study. J Intern Med 1998;244:71–78.

77. Gisbertz IA, Schouten HC, Bot FJ, Arends JW. Cell turnover parameters in small and large cell varieties of primary intestinal non-Hodgkin's lymphoma. Cancer (Phila) 1998;83:158–165.

78. Contreary K, Nance FC, Becker WF. Primary lymphoma of the gastrointestinal tract. Ann Surg 1980;191:593–598.

79. Beck P, Gill J, Sutherland L. HIV-associated non-Hodgkin's lymphoma of the gastrointestinal tract. Am J Gastroenterol 1996;91:2377–2381.

80. Taggart DP, McLatchie GR, Imrie CW. Survival of surgical patients with carcinoma, lymphoma and carcinoid tumours of the small bowel. Br J Surg 1986;73:826–828.

81. ReMine SG. Abdominal lymphoma. Role of surgery. Surg Clin North Am 1985;65:301–313.

82. ReMine SG, Braasch JW. Gastric and small bowel lymphoma. Surg Clin North Am 1986;66:713–722.

83. Amer MH, el-Akkad S. Gastrointestinal lymphoma in adults: clinical features and management of 300 cases. Gastroenterology 1994;106:846–858.

84. Lin KM, Penney DG, Mahmoud A, Chae W, Kolachalam RB, Young SC. Advantage of surgery and adjuvant chemotherapy in the treatment of primary gastrointestinal lymphoma. J Surg Oncol 1997;64:237–241.

85. Auger MJ, Allan NC. Primary ileocecal lymphoma. A study of 22 patients. Cancer (Phila) 1990;65:358–361.

86. Fleming ID, Turk PS, Murphy SB, Crist WM, Santana VM, Rao BN. Surgical implications of primary gastrointestinal lymphoma of childhood. Arch Surg 1990;125:252–256.

87. Sanchez-Bueno F, Garcia-Marcilla JA, Alonso JD, et al. Prognostic factors in primary gastrointestinal non-Hodgkin's lymphoma: a multivariate analysis of 76 cases. Eur J Surg 1998;164:385–392.

88. Ruskone-Fourmestraux A, Aegerter P, Delmer A, Brousse N, Galian A, Rambaud JC. Primary digestive tract lymphoma: a prospective multicentric study of 91 patients. Groupe d'Etude des Lymphomes Digestifs. Gastroenterology 1993;105:1662–1671.

89. Burke AP, Thomas RM, Elsayed AM, Sobin LH. Carcinoids of the jejunum and ileum: an immunohistochemical and clinicopathologic study of 167 cases. Cancer (Phila) 1997;79:1086–1093.

90. Peck JJ, Shields AB, Boyden AM, Dworkin LA, Nadal JW. Carcinoid tumors of the ileum. Am J Surg 1983;146:124–132.

91. Dawes L, Schulte WJ, Condon RE. Carcinoid tumors. Arch Surg 1984;119:375–378.

92. Hanson MW, Feldman JM, Blinder RA, Moore JO, Coleman RE.

Carcinoid tumors: iodine-131 MIBG scintigraphy. Radiology 1989;172:699–703.

93. Stinner B, Kisker O, Zielke A, Rothmund M. Surgical management for carcinoid tumors of small bowel, appendix, colon, and rectum. World J Surg 1996;20:183–188.

94. Strodel WE, Talpos G, Eckhauser F, Thompson N. Surgical therapy for small-bowel carcinoid tumors. Arch Surg 1983;118:391–397.

95. Wareing TH, Sawyers JL. Carcinoids and the carcinoid syndrome. Am J Surg 1983;145:769–772.

96. Persson BG, Nobin A, Ahren B, Jeppsson B, Mansson B, Bengmark S. Repeated hepatic ischemia as a treatment for carcinoid liver metastases. World J Surg 1989;13:307–311; discussion 311–312.

97. Carrasco CH, Charnsangavej C, Ajani J, Samaan NA, Richli W, Wallace S. The carcinoid syndrome: palliation by hepatic artery embolization. AJR (Am J Roentgenol) 1986;147:149–154.

98. Saslow SB, O'Brien MD, Camilleri M, et al. Octreotide inhibition of flushing and colonic motor dysfunction in carcinoid syndrome. Am J Gastroenterol 1997;92:2250–2256.

99. Cooney D, Duszynski D, et al. The abdominal technetium scan (a decade of experience). J Pediatr Surg 1982;17:611.

100. Thompson J. Management of the short bowel syndrome. Gastroenterol Clin North Am 1994;23:403–420.

101. Thompson J, Edgar J. Poth Memorial Lecture. Surgical aspects of the short-bowel syndrome. Am J Surg 1995;170:532–536.

102. Thompson J, Langnas A, Pinch L, Kaufman S, Quigley E, Vanderhoff J. Surgical approach to short-bowel syndrome. Experience in population of 160 patients. Ann Surg 1995;222:600–605.

103. Abu-Elmagd K, Reyes J, Todo S, et al. Clinical intestinal transplantation: new perspectives and immunologic considerations. J Am Coll Surg 1998;186:512–525.

104. Hermann-Zaidins MG. Malabsorption in adults: etiology, evaluation, and management. J Am Diet Assoc 1986;86:1171–1178,1181.

105. Brasitus TA, Sitrin MD. Intestinal malabsorption syndromes. Annu Rev Med 1990;41:339–347.

106. Fromm H, Malavolti M. Bile acid-induced diarrhoea. Clin Gastroenterol 1986;15:567–582.

107. Aldini R, Roda A, Festi D, et al. Bile acid malabsorption and bile acid diarrhea in intestinal resection. Dig Dis Sci 1982;27:495–502.

108. Sciarretta G, Furno A, Mazzoni M, Malaguti P. Post-cholecystectomy diarrhea: evidence of bile acid malabsorption assessed by SeHCAT test. Am J Gastroenterol 1992;87:1852–1854.

109. Mathias JR, Clench MH. Review: pathophysiology of diarrhea caused by bacterial overgrowth of the small intestine. Am J Med Sci 1985;289:243–248.

110. Brin MF, Fetell MR, Green PH, et al. Blind loop syndrome, vitamin E malabsorption, and spinocerebellar degeneration. Neurology 1985;35:338–342.

111. Romano TJ, Dobbins JW. Evaluation of the patient with suspected malabsorption. Gastroenterol Clin North Am 1989;18:467–483.

112. Kotler DP, Holt PR, Rosensweig NS. Modification of the breath hydrogen test: increased sensitivity for the detection of carbohydrate malabsorption. J Lab Clin Med 1982;100:798–805.

113. DiPalma JA, Narvaez RM. Prediction of lactose malabsorption in referral patients. Dig Dis Sci 1988;33:303–307.

114. King CE, Toskes PP. The use of breath tests in the study of malabsorption. Clin Gastroenterol 1983;12:591–610.

115. Casellas F, Chicharro L, Malagelada JR. Potential usefulness of hydrogen breath test with D-xylose in clinical management of intestinal malabsorption. Dig Dis Sci 1993;38:321–327.

116. Domstad PA, Choy YC, Kim EE, DeLand FH. Reliability of the dual-isotope Schilling test for the diagnosis of pernicious anemia or malabsorption syndrome. Am J Clin Pathol 1981;75:723–726.

117. King CE, Toskes PP, Guilarte TR, Lorenz E, Welkos SL. Comparison of the one-gram d-[^{14}C]xylose breath test to the [^{14}C]bile acid breath test in patients with small-intestine bacterial overgrowth. Dig Dis Sci 1980;25:53–58.

118. King CE, Toskes PP. Comparison of the 1-gram [^{14}C]xylose, 10-gram lactulose-H$_2$, and 80-gram glucose-H$_2$ breath tests in patients with small intestine bacterial overgrowth. Gastroenterology 1986;91:1447–1451.

119. Perlemuter G, Chaussade S, Soubrane O, et al. Multifocal stenosing ulcerations of the small intestine revealing vasculitis associated with C$_2$ deficiency. Gastroenterology 1996;110:1628–1632.

120. Madara JL. The chameleon within: improving antigen delivery [comment]. Science 1997;277:910–911.

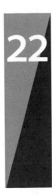

Appendix

David I. Soybel

Anatomy and Physiology

In the adult,[1] the average length of the appendix is 9 cm. Its outside diameter varies between 3 and 8 mm and the luminal diameter is between 1 and 3 mm. The tip of the appendix can be located anywhere in the right lower quadrant of the abdomen or pelvis. The base of the appendix can be located by following the longitudinally oriented *tenia coli* to their confluence at the cecum.

The appendix receives its arterial supply from the appendicular branch of the ileocolic artery. This artery originates posterior to the terminal ileum, entering the mesoappendix close to the base of the appendix. A small arterial branch arises at this point that runs to the cecal artery. The arterial supply to the appendix is illustrated schematically in Figure 22.1. The lymphatic drainage of the appendix flows into lymph nodes that lie along the ileocolic artery. Innervation of the appendix is derived from sympathetic elements contributed by the superior mesenteric plexus (T10–L1), afferents from parasympathetic elements brought in via the vagus nerve.[12]

The histological features of the appendix include the following: first, the muscularis layers are not well defined and may be deficient in some locations.[1] Second, in the submucosa and mucosa, lymphoid aggregates occur with or without the typical structure of a germinal center. Lymph vessels are prominent in regions underlying these lymphoid aggregates. Third, the mucosa is like that of the large intestine, except for the density of the lymphoid follicles. The crypts are irregularly sized and shaped, in contrast to the more uniform appearance of the crypts in the colon. Neuroendocrine complexes composed of ganglion cells, Schwann cells, neural fibers, and neurosecretory cells are positioned just below the crypts. Serotonin is a prominent secretory product and has been implicated in mediating pain arising from the noninflamed appendix.[3,4] These complexes may be the source of carcinoid tumors, for which the appendix is known to be the most common site of origin.[1,4,5]

With regard to function, the widely held notion that the appendix is a vestigial organ is not consistent with the facts. Curiously, the appendix seems more highly developed in the higher primates, and it is possible that the appendix may play a role in immune surveillance.[6,7] In addition, although the unique function of the appendix remains unclear, the mucosa of the appendix, like any mucosal layer, is capable of secreting fluid, mucin, and proteolytic enzymes.[1]

Diseases of the Vermiform Appendix

Acute Appendicitis

ETIOLOGY AND PATHOGENESIS

ROLE OF ENVIRONMENT: DIET AND HYGIENE
Given the relatively lower frequency of appendicitis and other bowel disorders among peoples with high fiber diets, it has been proposed that low-fiber diets contribute to changes in motility, flora, or luminal conditions that predispose to development of fecaliths. Striking, however, is the observation that most patients with acute appendicitis do not have obvious fecalith or stone in either population group.

ROLE OF OBSTRUCTION
Early descriptions conceptualized acute appendicitis as a closed-loop obstruction with the obstruction usually being caused by a fecalith. More recently, it has become dogma that, in the absence of a fecalith, many cases of obstruction are caused by hyperplasia of lymphoid tissue in the mucosa and submucosa. In a very small percentage of cases, perhaps 2%, obstruction is caused by neoplasm (carcinoma or carcinoid tumor) or, very rarely, a foreign body.[8–10]

In the evolution of acute appendicitis, the following sequence of events is envisioned: first, luminal obstruction leads to secretion of mucus and fluid, with a consequent rise

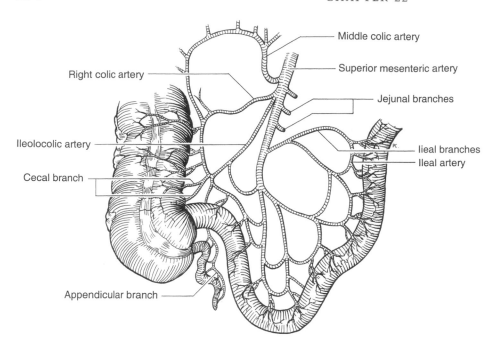

Right colic artery

Ileocolic artery

Cecal branch

Appendicular branch

Middle colic artery

Superior mesenteric artery

Jejunal branches

Ileal branches
Ileal artery

FIGURE 22.1. Details of the arterial blood supply to the terminal ileum, cecum, and appendix showing the normal divisions of the ileocolic artery. (After Keighley MRB, Williams NS. Surgery of the Anus, Rectum and Colon. London: Saunders, 1993.)

in luminal pressure; second, when the rise in luminal pressure exceeds pressure within the submucosal venules and lymphatics, outflow of blood and lymph is obstructed, leading to increases in pressure within the appendiceal wall; and third, when capillary pressure is exceeded, mucosal ischemia, inflammation, and ulceration are the result. Eventually, bacterial overgrowth within the lumen and bacterial invasion into the mucosa and submucosa lead to transmural inflammation, edema, vascular stasis, and necrosis of the muscularis. Perforation ensues.

Accompanying the local changes within the appendix is a regional inflammatory response mediated by the mesothelium and blood vessels in the parietal peritoneum and serosa of nearby visceral structures. This leads to formation of a walled-off, periappendiceal abscess. Alternatively, if surrounding structures fail to wall off the evolving phlegmon, perforation of the appendix would cause spillage into the peritoneal cavity, leading to spreading peritonitis, massive third-spacing of fluid, shock, prostration, and then death.

Although it is widely accepted that obstruction is the inciting event in most cases of acute appendicitis, it is worth pointing out some observations that are not consistent with this hypothesis. The first observation is that impacted fecaliths have been observed with no accompanying local inflammation or syndrome of appendicitis.[11] In addition, fecalith impaction or functional evidence of obstruction cannot be demonstrated in a substantial number, up to half, of cases.[10,12–14] Thus obstruction may be just one of many factors involved in the etiology and pathogenesis of acute appendicitis.

ROLE OF NORMAL COLONIC FLORA

The flora of the inflamed appendix differs from that of the normal appendix. About 60% of aspirates of inflamed appendices have anaerobes, compared to 25% of aspirates from normal appendices.[15–17] Presumably, the lumen is the source of organisms that invade the mucosa when mucosal integrity is

compromised by increased luminal pressure or intramural ischemia. Tissue specimens from the inflamed appendix wall (not luminal aspirates) virtually all culture out *E. coli* and *Bacteroides* species.[16,17] In fact, studies indicate that invasion of tissue by *Bacteroides* elicits specific humoral responses. Moreover, as is discussed next, in many cases in which acute appendicitis is highly likely, antibiotic therapy alone can reverse the evolving clinical syndrome and permit individuals to get well without an operation. Thus, the normal colonic flora play a key role in the evolution of acute appendicitis to gangrene and perforation.

NATURAL HISTORY AND COMPLICATIONS

As classically conceptualized, acute appendicitis progresses inexorably, from obstruction to mucosal and then transmural inflammation, necrosis, and then gangrene with local inflammatory responses from the visceral and parietal peritoneum, to perforation with local abscess formation or spreading peritonitis. One time-honored observation has been that perforation is not common if symptoms have been present for less than 24 h. In one recent study,[18] 95 consecutive adult patients with symptoms and signs of acute appendicitis were monitored prospectively. Fifteen patients ultimately were shown to have a perforation. Of these, 3 (20%) developed perforation earlier than 24 h after onset of symptoms; in 1 patient, perforation occurred as early as 10 h after the onset of symptoms. Average time from onset of symptoms to perforation was 64 h.

Once necrotic or perforated, other complications can result. These rarer complications are listed in Table 22.1. What should be emphasized about such complications is that they are observed generally in the very young and the very old. In other words, these complications occur in patients who cannot speak for themselves or infirm patients who do not experience the acute lower abdominal symptoms that would ordinarily motivate the patient to see a physician more quickly.

TABLE 22.1. Complications of Acute Appendicitis.

Complication	Management
Spreading peritonitis	Antibiotics, appendectomy
Abscess	Antibiotics, appendectomy
Abdominal	Percutaneous drainage reserved
Retroperitoneal	for poor surgical risk patients; interval appendectomy in 6 weeks recommended
Intestinal obstruction	Antibiotics, appendectomy
Bacteremia/systemic sepsis	Antibiotics, appendectomy, or percutaneous drainage of appendiceal abscess until acute episode resolves
Fistula	
Abdominal wall	Antibiotics until acute episode resolved, then bladder interval appendectomy and closure of fistula
Liver abscess	Broad-spectrum antibiotics; percutaneous drainage of liver and appendiceal abscess; interval appendectomy
Pyelophlebitis	Broad-spectrum antibiotics; systemic anticoagulation; percutaneous drainage of liver and appendiceal abscesses; interval appendectomy

CLINICAL PRESENTATION

SYMPTOMS

At the onset of the episode, the patient typically reports crampy (colicky) abdominal pain. This quality of the pain is attributable to the initial response of the muscularis of the appendix (or any hollow-lumen organ) to obstruction. The pain is described as diffuse or perhaps centered about the umbilicus; this is because the appendix arises from the midgut, an embryonic midline structure that derives its innervation from autonomic afferents related to the spinal cord centered around T10. Typically, this pain does not radiate, nor do the patients describe it as being exacerbated by changes in body position, meals, urination, or defecation. As the response to luminal obstruction evolves to include luminal distension, intramural edema, and ischemia, the pain becomes constant. Vomiting is often reported by younger patients but is not a prominent symptom in mature adult and aged patients. In general, patients with appendicitis report nausea and loss of appetite; a patient reporting a normal appetite is very uncommon.

SIGNS

The invasion of bacteria with ensuing inflammatory response within the appendiceal wall and the surrounding visceral structures leads to appearance of pain and tenderness localized to the area of parietal peritoneum overlying the inflamed tissue ("phlegmon"). Fever above 100°F or 38.2°C rarely occurs early in the appendicitis syndrome and usually appears after the time when localizing tenderness appears. In many cases, the localized pain and tenderness are accompanied by peritoneal findings that are localized to the right lower quadrant of the abdomen. These symptoms include rebound tenderness, referred tenderness, and involuntary guarding in the area overlying the phlegmon. Although its predictive power is disputed,[19–21] McBurney's point is supposed to be the place where the appendix lies and therefore the place of maximum tenderness.[20,22]

The visceral pain of distension and ischemia that is centered about the umbilicus does not necessarily go away, and it is not accurate to describe the pain as having "migrated."

When the inflamed portion of the appendix (usually the tip) is not located near the parietal peritoneum, the place of maximal tenderness is not necessarily in the right lower quadrant. In fact, there may be no localizing area of tenderness[38] when the appendix is located in a retroperitoneal or retroileal position or in the true pelvis. Theoretically, an acutely inflamed appendix in the true pelvis can be suspected by means of rectal examination when the examiner elicits localized tenderness or palpates a mass.

Classic texts also recognize three diagnostic maneuvers: *Rovsing's sign* is positive when pressure applied in the left lower quadrant of the abdomen elicits pain on the right side, reflecting peritoneal irritation. The *psoas sign* is elicited by positioning the patient on the left side and extending the right hip. Pain produced with this maneuver reflects irritation of the right psoas muscle and indicates retrocecal and retroperitoneal irritation from a phlegmon or an abscess. The *obturator sign* is produced by positioning the patient supine and then rotating the flexed right thigh internally, from lateral to medial. Pain produced with this maneuver indicates inflammation near the obturator muscle in the true pelvis. It should be recognized that each of these "signs" is sought as a way of establishing the location of the inflamed or perforated appendix. It is only in the context of a characteristic history and examination that the diagnosis of appendicitis itself is made. These considerations emphasize that no one symptom or finding, observed at any single point in time, reliably establishes or excludes the diagnosis of acute appendicitis: It is the overall clinical picture that counts.

LABORATORY FINDINGS

Routine laboratory studies are helpful in diagnosing acute appendicitis, largely through exclusion of other conditions. Perhaps the only truly routine study is the leukocyte count. It is well recognized that the white blood cell (WBC) count is usually elevated in bona fide cases of appendicitis. However, a substantial number of patients have the diagnosis and a normal WBC count. Depending on the clinical circumstances, three other types of studies should be performed routinely. First, urine analysis with microscopic examination should be performed in all patients with suspected appendicitis.[23,24] The goal of performing the test is to exclude ureteral stones (hematuria) and to evaluate the possibility of urinary tract infection (pyuria, bacteruria) as a cause of lower abdominal pain, particularly in elderly diabetic patients. Lower urinary tract infection (UTI) is not infrequent among patients with acute appendicitis, especially women. The presence of UTI thus does not exclude acute appendicitis, but does need to be identified. The newer "dipsticks" that contain indicators for bacterial infection can be used to supplant the microscopic examination.

Second, measurement of serum liver enzymes and amylase levels can be very helpful in diagnosing liver, gallbladder, or pancreatic inflammation if the pain is described as being more in the midabdomen or even right upper quandrant. Serum amylase levels are reported elevated in 3% to 10% of patients with acute appendicitis or acute lower abdominal pain not attributable to pancreatitis.[25,26] If pancreatitis is the cause, the pattern of amylase elevation is usually higher and is accompanied by elevations of serum lipase. Measurements of serum amylase are not recommended for all patients with abdominal pain, but should be considered in patients with atypical clinical features.

Third, serum β-HCG (human chorionic gonadotropin) levels should be measured in women of childbearing years if there is any possibility of pregnancy.

IMAGING STUDIES

Four types of imaging studies may assist in the diagnosis of acute appendicitis (Table 22.2). Plain abdominal films have been used regularly in evaluation of patients with acute abdominal pain. The finding most commonly associated with acute appendicitis is the fecalith. However, although fecaliths are found in 10%–40% of patients with appendicitis, it is difficult to formulate estimates of the sensitivity and specificity of the finding of a fecalith. It would appear, however, that in the setting of acute abdominal pain, the presence of fecalith is likely to be associated with acute appendicitis about 90% of the time. It may thus be regarded as a sensitive sign of acute appendicitis and predictive of a high likelihood of progression to perforation.

In older patients, where perforated viscus is a major part of the differential diagnosis, it is difficult to argue against the plain film as the initial imaging study. In younger patients, the low likelihood of finding a fecalith suggests that obtaining plain films is not cost-effective. If such films are done, it is best to obtain a complete series of plain films, including flat and upright views. A follow-up barium enema can be helpful but is not more helpful than other modalites.

Ultrasound examination of the abdomen has become increasingly popular in recent years. Key findings of this study include (1) thickening of the wall and loss of the normal layers ("target" sign); (2) loss of wall compressibility; (3) increased echogenicity of the surrounding fat; and (4) loculated pericecal fluid (Fig. 22.2). Although this test has a relatively low sensitivity level (80%), it has a relatively high specificity (90%). This imaging modality is very helpful in excluding other causes of abdominal pain in women, particularly those in their childbearing years. When gynecological causes of pain are difficult to exclude, vaginal ultrasound may be a useful adjunct in these patients.

Computerized tomography (CT) may be considered the gold standard for noninvasive imaging of acute appendicitis. The CT scan can detect and localize inflammatory mass and abscess (Fig. 22.3); if orally administered contrast fills the appendiceal lumen and no inflammatory changes are present, the diagnosis is essentially excluded. In addition, other abdominal pathology can be detected, including lesions in the

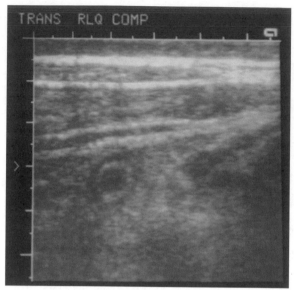

FIGURE 22.2. Sonographic detection of an acutely inflamed, unruptured appendix. A "target" sign is demonstrated just below the abdominal wall musculature. Edema (water density) in the wall separates the more dense mucosa and submucosa of the appendix from surrounding structures. (Courtest of Fay Lang, MD, Dept. of Radiology, Brigham and Women's Hospital, Boston, MA.)

pelvis. Although technological innovation has produced high-resolution images with standard or helical imaging protocols, a technique for focused helical CT of the appendix has recently been introduced as a means of saving time and cost without reducing accuracy. However, it is not clear that such cost savings can be realized in institutions that do not have access to this technology.

EVALUATION AND MANAGEMENT OF THE PATIENT WITH SUSPECTED APPENDICITIS

STRUCTURED AND HISTORY EXAMINATION

A structured approach to the patient with acute abdominal pain improves diagnostic accuracy and accelerates the initiation of the correct management plan.[27] Table 22.3 provides an example of a structured history, physical, and basic laboratory examination. Three points deserve repeat emphasis: first, the evolution of symptoms and signs is the key to correct diagnosis and one examination alone is not usually sufficient to render a diagnosis; second, the examination is incomplete unless digital rectal and (in women) speculum/bimanual examinations of the pelvis are performed; third, urine analysis and pregnancy test should be performed to

TABLE 22.2. Imaging Modalities in the Diagnosis of Acute Appendicitis.

Modality	Key findings	Sensitivity (%)	Specificity (%)
Plain abdominal film	Fecalith Loss of fat stripe Sentinel loop/ileus	30	50–80
Barium enema	Nonfilling of appendix; cecal wall irregularity/mass effect	85	95
Ultrasound	"Target" sign abscess; loss of motility	80	90
CT scan	Phlegmon abscess	95	90

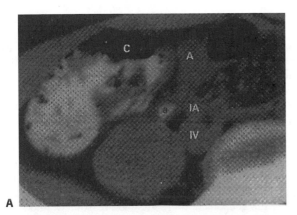

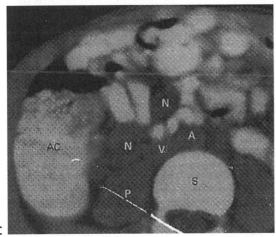

FIGURE 22.3. Computerized tomography of three patients with lower abdominal pain, suspected of having acute appendicitis. **A**. In a 17-year-old male, an unopacified appendix (*A*) and the appendicolith itself (*a*) are seen. Also visualized are the cecum (*C*), iliac artery (*IA*), and iliac vein (*IV*). **B**. In a 21-year-old woman, the opacified appendix (*A*) is normal. **C**. In a 8-year-old girl, enlarged lymph nodes (*N*) are seen at the level of the ascending colon (*AC*), consistent with a diagnosis of mesenteric adenitis. Also shown are the aorta (*A*), vena cava (*V*), and psoas muscle (*P*). (From Rao et al. N Engl J Med 1998;338:141–146, with permission.)

avoid missing a diagnosis of urinary tract processes and pregnancy, as well as to prevent unknowing exposure of an unborn fetus to X-ray radiation.

DIFFERENTIAL DIAGNOSIS

Causes of lower abdominal pain other than appendicitis are listed in Table 22.4, based on location. In young men, given the appropriate clinical setting, acute appendicitis is the like-

TABLE 22.3. Structured Format for Diagnosis of Acute Appendicitis.

Patient identification

History
    Previous laparotomy
    Previous RLQ pain
    Other relevant medical problems
    1st degree relative with acute appendicitis
    Ob/gyn history and last menses (date)
Clinical assessment
    Initial exam date/time/examiner/duration of illness
    Repeat exam date/time/examiner/duration of illness

Symptoms/signs	*1st exam*	*2nd exam*
Classic history of pain (onset, quality, location, radiation, associated symptoms)		
Pain shift to RLQ		
Pain with cough/movement		
Facial flush		
Tenderness at McBurney's point		
Guarding at McBurney's point		
Rectal exam: increased pain on right		
Pelvic exam: absence of discharge/ adnexal tenderness		
Temperature		
Urinalysis Sugar WBCs RBCs β-HCG		
Blood test Hematocrit/hemoglobin WBC count Left shift?		

Indication for surgery
    Clear indications
    Uncertain indications

Operation
    Date/time/surgeon
    Postoperative diagnosis
    Findings
    Operation performed
Lessons learned:

liest cause of acute right lower quadrant pain. Inflammation of a Meckel's diverticulum is extremely uncommon, but is not that different in pathogenesis or natural history from appendicitis.[28] Gastroenteritis may be suspected when GI disturbances (vomiting, diarrhea) are prominent in the symptom complex; it should be suspected particularly when such symptoms precede the development of abdominal pain and when fever or leukocytosis occur very early in the course of the illness. Crohn's disease should also be considered with a chronic or relapsing history of pain, diarrhea, fever, or weight loss.

In middle-aged and older men, consideration must be given to inflammatory conditions such as perforating peptic ulcer with fluid tracking along the right colonic gutter, acute cholecystitis, and acute pancreatitis. These conditions are not commonly confused with acute appendicitis. More difficult to distinguish are episodes of acute diverticulitis, especially if the diverticulum is located in the cecum or ascending colon.[29]

TABLE 22.4. Differential Diagnosis of Acute Appendicitis.

A. When the appendix is located above the cecum:
 Cholecystitis
 Inflamed or perforated duodenal ulcer (fluid tracking down
  the right gutter)
 Perinephric abscess
 Hydronephrosis (acute or subacute)
 Kidney/upper ureteral stone
 Omental torsion
 Pneumonia with pleurisy
 Hepatitis
 Pancreatitis

B. When appendix is in the iliac position:
 Inflamed or perforated duodenal ulcer (fluid tracking down
  the right gutter)
 Crohn's disease
 Cecal carcinoma
 Lymphoma
 Ureteral stone
 Yersinia, CMV, tuberculous infection
 Inflamed Meckel's diverticulum
 Psoas abscess (tuberculosis or other cause)
 Rupture or hematoma of the rectus abdominis muscle
 Cecal ulcer
 Typhoid fever (*Salmonella typhi* or *Salmonella paratyphi*)

C. When the appendix is in the pelvic position:
 Intestinal obstruction
 Diverticulitis of the colon
 Perforation of a typhoid ulcer
 Gastroenteritis

D. In women:
 Ectopic pregnancy
 Ovarian cyst ruptured or twisted on its pedicle
 Pelvic inflammatory disease (including rupture of pyosalpinx)
 Ruptured ovarian follicle
 Ruptured corpus luteum cyst

Malignancies must also be considered. Perforating carcinomas of the cecum or ascending colon may present with acute pain and peritoneal findings, or abscess.[30] Rarely, a cecal carcinoma itself obstructs the lumen of the appendix, leading secondarily to an episode of acute appendicitis.[31] Lymphomas of the terminal ileum can also present with acute obstruction or perforation, mimicking an episode of complicated appendicitis. Most such abdominal malignancies, however, are usually accompanied by findings of guaiac-positive stool, anemia, history of weight loss, or chronic changes in bowel habits.

In young women, common causes of right lower quadrant pain include those mentioned for young men and the following problems: rupture of an ovarian follicle or cyst, torsion of an ovary, ectopic pregnancy, and acute salpingitis with or without tuboovarian abscess. In older but premenopausal women, endometriosis is a cause of chronic lower abdominal pain that, in very acute episodes, can sometimes be mistaken for appendicitis.[32] With regard to all these gynecological conditions, differentiation from acute appendicitis can usually be made based on gynecological history and association of the episode with the phases of the menstrual cycle.

INITIAL MANAGEMENT

It is a truism, but a necessity, to point out that patients with acute abdominal pain can be separated into those who are clearly sick and getting worse, those who are clearly not very sick and getting better, and those in whom the evolution of symptoms and signs is not certain. Those patients who are clearly sick require a management plan that includes the placement of intravenous access, initiation of intravenous fluid infusion to replace calculated losses and to anticipate future losses, and the inability to take fluids orally. In general, pain medication and antibiotic therapy should not be administered if the diagnosis is undecided. Although this point of management remains controversial, it should be emphasized that therapy can be initiated intelligently only when the diagnosis is known or when the failure to treat could result in unacceptable morbidity or mortality. When the diagnosis is not certain, it is this author's view that early use of pain medication and antibiotics can obscure and delay the diagnosis and initiation of appropriate therapy. On the other hand, if the diagnosis of appendicitis is decided, there are good reasons to make the patient comfortable and to initiate antibiotic therapy while awaiting definitive management. Such patients should be admitted to the care of the surgeon, who must then decide whether further diagnostic imaging is needed or whether the situation requires immediate operative exploration.

Patients who seem to be not very ill and getting better should be evaluated with the following question in mind: Is it possible that the apparent improvement of symptoms is only temporary? It is well recognized that perforation of a gangrenous appendix can temporarily be accompanied by relief of some aspects of the patient's discomfort. In this situation, however, such patients never quite lose their apprehensiveness and the abdominal wall rigidity persists. In other circumstances, the perforation may be accompanied by formation of a walled-off abscess, which is associated with improvement in pain and tenderness and even a recovery in appetite. Such patients may return several days later with a mass that was not suspected at the initial evaluation. However, most such patients can be recognized by a rather slow progression of improvement. Most patients who present with acute abdominal pain that subsides within a few hours and is not accompanied by local tenderness, leukocytosis, anorexia, or signs of systemic illness can safely be assumed not to have appendicitis and can be discharged. All such patients should receive warnings to return for evaluation if their symptoms return.

The patient who is not clearly progressing in either direction requires a high level of vigilance. Intravenous access and fluids should be initiated. Pain medication and antibiotic therapy should not be started. It is a safe principle of management to admit all such patients to the hospital ward or to an observation ward in the emergency department. The progression of symptoms and signs, and perhaps the white blood cell (WBC) count, should be evaluated over 6 to 24 h, preferably by the same examiner. In such cases, the progression of symptoms clarifies the diagnosis and the interval of observation poses little real risk in terms of outcome.[33] In other cases, it may be preferable and cost-effective to obtain imaging studies early on.

IMAGING

There is not a published consensus regarding the use of the different imaging modalities to evaluate patients with suspected appendicitis. In older patients, the decreased incidence of appendicitis relative to other diagnoses, particularly malignancy, makes it reasonable to consider the use of abdominal and pelvic CT to confirm the diagnosis and to exclude other processes.

In younger patients, particularly women in the childbearing years, ultrasound can be useful in excluding gynecological processes and in evaluating the appendix. Used in conjunction with a carefully obtained history and examination, it reduces the need for laparotomy and laparoscopy simply to establish a diagnosis. As it is generally an inexpensive test, it is our preferred modality in pediatric and young adult patients in whom the diagnosis is in doubt.

Although plain abdominal films have been included in the traditional evaluation of such patients,[34] it is difficult to justify their routine use unless there is concern for the possibility of a perforated viscus (e.g., duodenal ulcer or diverticulitis). Except in unusual circumstances, barium enema would not be used to evaluate a patient in whom acute appendicitis is strongly suspected.

INDICATIONS FOR OPERATION

When the diagnosis of appendicitis has been made with a reasonable degree of certainty, operation is indicated except in unusual circumstances. One such circumstance involves the patient in whom the acute illness has passed but is now complicated by formation of a well-circumscribed abscess. CT is excellent at delineating such lesions. In some cases, antibiotic therapy alone can be used to help the mass resolve; in others, the use of CT directs a percutaneous approach to drainage.[35,36] In this situation, the base of the cecum and appendix are not recognizable in the inflammatory mass. A secure operative closure is not feasible and operative intervention is not likely to accomplish much more than percutaneous drainage of the abscess. CT-directed drainage avoids laparotomy until definitive (so-called interval) appendectomy is performed some weeks later. This approach is particularly suited to the elderly, infirm patient who is at risk for more morbidity in the acutely ill and debilitated state. It should be emphasized that a nonoperative approach is employed most successfully when the acute illness is passed or when the abscess is circumscribed. Most patients are better served by early operation once the diagnosis is made.[37]

It should be pointed out that a number of clinicians have also evaluated the possibility of treating acute appendicitis, in its early phases, using intravenous antibiotics alone. However, limited data suggest that it would be difficult to argue that this nonoperative approach is a cost-effective approach in most clinical situations.

PREOPERATIVE PREPARATION

Once the diagnosis is made and operative management is chosen, the patient should be made comfortable with pain medication. Fluid status should be monitored closely, using clinical indicators (pulse, blood pressure, urine output). Electrolyte balance is not usually a problem, unless the illness has been prolonged and other complications (i.e., bowel obstruction) have supervened. If such imbalances are detected in the admitting serum chemistry evaluation, they should also be addressed.

When the decision to operate has been made, antibiotic therapy is started, usually consisting of a second-generation cephalosporin alone or a combination regimen that includes broad-spectrum coverage of gram-negative aerobes (principally *E. coli*) and anaerobes (*Bacteroides* spp.).[38] *It should be emphasized that ordinarily, the goal of antibiotic therapy is not to treat the appendicitis itself.* In uncomplicated cases antibiotics are used to reduce the incidence of wound and deep peritoneal infections that may occur after the operation and to protect against the consequences of bacteremia. In cases complicated by abscess formation or bacteremia, antibiotics are used to treat the complications. The literature regarding antibiotic prophylaxis is complicated, but there does seem to be consensus about the following: (1) in uncomplicated cases, a second-generation cephalosporin is as effective in reducing wound complications as multiple drug regimens; (2) antibiotics are most effective when given just before or at the time of surgery, to obtain good tissue levels as the incision is being made; and (3) in uncomplicated cases, one dose is enough and additional doses after the operation do not further reduce infection rates.

OPERATIVE DECISIONS

The first decision to be made is whether the procedure will be performed through a traditional "open" approach or with the assistance of laparoscopy (see Table 22.5). Numerous trials comparing open and laparoscopically assisted approaches have been performed since the technique was popularized in the early 1990s. A number of outcome–cost and meta-analyses have been published in the last few years as well.[39–42] Based on the most recent information available, it seems clear that, in uncomplicated cases where the diagnosis is secure, the laparoscopic approaches may offer a small reduction in pain scores, a mild reduction in hospital stay, and possibly a reduction in wound infection rates. Return to work may also occur earlier. In these cases, however, the operating time and overall hospital costs of the laparoscopic approach are higher. Thus, in a cost analysis, the benefit of laparoscopically assisted appendectomy can only be realized if the patients routinely return to work and productive activity sooner than pa-

TABLE 22.5.

Advantages of Laparotomy versus Laparoscopy Approaches to Appendectomy.

Laparotomy	Laparoscopy
Shorter time in operating room	Diagnosis of other conditions
Lesser cost of operation	Decreased wound infection
Overall lesser cost of hospital stay	Minimal decrease in hospital stay
Possibly less risk of intraabdominal abscess in perforated cases	Possible decrease in time for convalescence and return to work or normal activity

Source: Based on meta-analysis and reviews of prior prospective controlled randomized trials (Level I Evidence), including Br J Surg 1997;84:1045–1050, Dis Colon Rectum 1998;41:398–403, J Am Coll Surg 1998;186:545–553.

tients undergoing open procedures. This advantage has not yet been shown. Patients with complications of appendicitis have not yet been included in large enough numbers to reach conclusions about the relative advantages of either approach. In the meantime, the optimal choice for operative approach should be based on likelihood of diagnosis, complexity of the appendicitis, and severity of illness.

The one circumstance in which laparoscopic approach may offer a definite advantage is when the diagnosis is in doubt. The diagnosis is particularly difficult to make in young women. In this group, as many as 25% to 50% of patients explored for the diagnosis of acute appendicitis will actually have another disorder.[43,44] Although the rate of "negative exploration" is expected to decrease with increasing use of imaging modalities such as ultrasound and appendix-directed CT, it seems likely that this group of patients will continue to pose a challenge. Thus, it will probably turn out that patients in this subgroup will benefit from a laparoscopic approach.

At the time of the operation, the appendix is removed if it appears inflamed. A key point in the operation includes dissection of appendix to its true base at the confluence of the tenia on the cecal wall. Failure to fully dissect the appendix may lead to retention of an appendiceal stump that is sufficiently large to harbor recurring appendicitis. A number of such cases have been reported, occurring even many years later. Such cases should serve as a warning to the wary clinician: even when a patient reports a prior appendectomy and has a scar to prove it, there may yet be a recurrent appendicitis.

Once identified, the appendix is amputated close to the base. When the operation is performed open, it is customary to invert the appendiceal stump into the cecal lumen. However, there is no evidence that this reduces postoperative leak or fistula formation, either being exceedingly rare events in uncomplicated cases. When surgery is performed laparoscopically, the appendix is usually amputated at its base using a stapling device, and no inversion is performed. When the base of the appendix cannot be identified because inflammation or abscess formation precludes safe dissection, a closed suction drain may be placed into the cavity. If the lumen of the appendix has not been obliterated, the drain allows fecal contents to drain to the outside, thereby preventing accumulation of pus and fecal material inside the peritoneal cavity.

If the exploration or laparoscopy fails to reveal acute appendicitis, a search for the cause of the acute abdominal pain must be undertaken. If no other source of pain can be identified, it is reasonable to remove the appendix. There are three reasons for removing the appendix, even if it appears grossly normal: first, the presence of a scar and history of exploration for the diagnosis may lead future care providers to assume the appendix has been removed; second, if the pain recurs, removal of the appendix eliminates this diagnosis from the differential (with the caveat just noted); and third, even in grossly normal appendices, early intramural or serosal inflammatory changes (so-called periappendicitis) have been noted with regularity (25%–50%) in microscopic evaluation or with special stains for inflammatory cytokines.[45,46]

The last intraoperative decision is whether the wounds should be left open, with the risk of wound infection, or whether they can be closed primarily. Although most authors recommend leaving the incisions open when there is gross contamination by pus and fecal material, there is increasing evidence that this may be no more unsafe and less cost-effective than closing all wounds (where it is feasible) and later treating any wound infections that result.[47] This decision should be individualized to each patient.

POSTOPERATIVE CARE

In uncomplicated cases, patients may take liquids and then solid food as soon as they feel able, and discharge should be anticipated within 24 to 48 h. Postoperative antibiotics and nasogastric decompression are not indicated routinely in such patients. Patients with perforation, abscess, or other complications have a variable course. With established peritonitis or abscess formation, a longer course of antibiotics may be needed, from 5 to 7 days after surgery.

SPECIAL CONSIDERATIONS

ADVANCED AGE

It is widely recognized that elderly patients with appendicitis present with less acute symptoms, less impressive clinical signs, and leukocytosis.[48–50] Up to 30% of elderly patients present more than 48 h into the illness, and between 50% and 70% have a perforation at the time of surgery. In addition, the elderly are susceptible to malignancy and other processes that are in the differential diagnosis, making correct preoperative diagnosis of acute appendicitis more difficult. Perioperative complications and mortality of delayed intervention increase with age as well. However, timely intervention can result in very acceptable complication rates, even in the most elderly patients. Therefore, in this age group, it is reasonable to be diagnostically aggressive (i.e., use CT scan) to establish the diagnosis or to identify other pathology and to move as quickly as possible to the appropriate intervention.

PREGNANCY

The diagnosis of acute appendicitis during pregnancy is one of the most challenging of all clinical problems. Pregnancy itself, especially in the early stages, is associated with nausea, vomiting, and pain. In the first and early second trimester, the evolution of symptoms and signs is not different from that in nonpregnant women. After the fifth month, the cecum and appendix are shifted upward by the expanding uterus. In the last trimester, localized tenderness from the appendix may be found in the upper flank and right upper quadrant of the abdomen. Ultrasound is very helpful in this setting, as it may provide images of the appendix, gallbladder, uterus, and other pelvic organs.[51] X-rays should be avoided if at all possible.

When the diagnosis of appendicitis is considerred likely, the patient should be explored. The following considerations should be borne in mind if the diagnosis is not certain[52–54]: (1) appendicitis is not more common in any of the three trimesters; (2) progression to perforation seems to be more common in the last trimester, presumably because of delays in seeking treatment and delays in recognition of the need for surgery; (3) fetal mortality is probably less than 5% if the appendix is removed before rupture and as high as 20% if the appendix is removed after rupture; and (4) maternal mortality is small (less than 1%) but has been reported almost exclusively in patients who had a ruptured appendix. On the other hand, patients and relatives need to be counseled about the risks of negative laparotomy to the fetus. Overall, however, it would seem that, while the risk of preterm labor in increased, the actual harm to the fetus is not associated with increased perinatal mortality.[55] These considerations strongly argue for a proactive approach to exploration in doubtful cases and probably justify the higher negative laparotomy rates of 25% to 40% that have been reported.

One additional consideration is whether it is safe and appropriate to submit the pregnant patient to laparoscopic exploration and appendectomy. In the last trimester of pregnancy, it is technically too difficult for laparoscopic instruments to reach the appendix, which lies above or behind the uterus, and the procedure is most expeditiously performed using an open incision. In the first and early second trimester, however, it is feasible to perform laparoscopy and, if needed, appendectomy with laparoscopic assistance. The safety of laparoscopic surgery in pregnancy remains a controversial subject, with some groups reporting no adverse events and some groups reporting higher than expected incidents of adverse fetal outcomes.[56,57] When the diagnosis of appendicitis seems likely, an open procedure is probably the most expeditious approach.

IMMUNOCOMPROMISE

Immunocompromise alters responses of patients to localized infection and systemic stress, as well as hindering normal processes of wound healing. Because appendicitis strikes patients in all age groups and walks of life, it must be considered in the differential diagnosis of acute abdominal pain of patients who have undergone organ transplantation, patients who have received chemotherapy for malignancy, patients with hematological malignancy or bone marrow failure, and patients who are infected with HIV or HTLV. A comprehensive discussion of abdominal pain in the immunocompromised state is beyond the scope of this chapter. However, it is worth pointing out that the differential diagnosis is broad, including pancreatitis from medication or viral [cytomegalovirus (CMV)] infection, viral hepatitis, acalculous cholecystitis (viral, *Campylobacter*, ischemia), intraabdominal infection due to opportunistic organisms, secondary malignancies such as lymphoma, graft-versus-host disease, or neutropenic enterocolitis.

The patient with known HIV infection and AIDS may pose a particularly difficult diagnostic dilemma and therapeutic challenge. The pain syndrome is frequently atypical, and delays in recognition and treatment are not uncommon. Expeditious use of CT is recommended, both to verify the diagnosis and to exclude other pathological processes. Morbidity and mortality rates from acute appendicitis were thought to be almost prohibitive; even now, it is clear that patients with AIDS may well have higher than expected complication and death rates after emergency laparotomy. However, early diagnosis and treatment are associated with excellent short-term survival and discharge. The presence of AIDS should not be viewed as a contraindication for aggressive diagnosis and operative intervention.[58–61]

CAMPYLOBACTER JEJUNI AND YERSINIA ENTEROCOLITICA

These two bacteria are responsible for a small percentage of cases of acute appendicitis.[62] Antibiotics are recommended only in cases that do not resolve quickly or if fever and symptoms are intense.

CHRONIC APPENDICITIS

Chronic right lower quadrant pain is sometimes attributed to chronic appendicitis. In careful reviews of individual cases, it has generally been possible to recognize an initial, acute episode that might have been recognized as acute appendicitis.[63,64] However, cases of chronic or recurrent acute appendicitis are now well documented. In addition, there are cases in which it is reasonable to explore or perform laparoscopy for selected patients with recurring pain and removing the appendix if no other lesion or source can be identified.[65]

INCIDENTAL APPENDECTOMY

This term refers to the removal of the appendix when the laparotomy or laparoscopy is being performed to address an unrelated clinical problem. The stated goal of this practice is to prevent an episode of acute appendicitis later on. It may be reasonable to perform incidental appendectomy in children and young adults, but it is difficult to justify the practice in patients over the age of 30 years. Incidental appendectomy should not be performed if, in the surgeon's judgment, there is a possibility that it would incur any additional morbidity.

Neoplasms of the Appendix

Neoplasms are found in about 0.5% of appendices.[66,67] The major categories are primary adenocarcinoma, cystic neoplasms, carcinoid tumor, and metastatic tumors. Stromal tumors (leiomyoma, leiomyosarcoma, lipoma) have been reported also, but are extremely rare. Lymphoma has also been increasingly recognized, arising in patients with AIDS and causing significant complications.

PRIMARY ADENOCARCINOMA

The diagnosis of primary appendiceal adenocarcinoma is almost never suspected before surgery. The most common presentation is that of acute appendicitis or of carcinoma of the right colon. The staging system for these lesions is similar to that for colon carcinoma. In a series reported by the Mayo Clinic,[66] Dukes stages A, B, C, and D were associated with 5-year survival rates of 100%, 67%, 50%, and 6%, respectively. The optimal treatment is right hemicolectomy. When the lesion has been diagnosed by the pathologist in a simple appendectomy specimen, it is recommended that the patient undergo reexploration and formal hemicolectomy.[66,68]

CYSTIC NEOPLASMS AND PSEUDOMYXOMA PERITONEI

On occasion, the appendix may be transformed into a cystic structure, called a mucocele.[69–71] Neoplastic lesions (cystadenoma, cystadenocarcinoma) are found in approximately 75% to 85% of mucoceles, although most of these lesions are benign cystadenoma. These lesions generally present as incidental findings on CT or painless masses. When the mucocele has ruptured, appendectomy is curative if the lesion is benign. If the lesion is malignant, however, cancer cells are spilled into the peritoneum and carcinomatosis may ensue. Pseudomyxoma peritonei is caused by spillage of implantation of mucin-secreting cells into the peritoneal cavity. Wide resection of the primary disease, if at all possible, is recommended.

CARCINOID TUMORS

Carcinoids represent the great majority of tumors found in the appendix, and the appendix is the most common site in the alimentary tract where carcinoids are found.[67,69] About 50% of the time these tumors are found incidently at surgery and about 50% of the time they present with acute appendicitis. About 75% of the time, the lesions are less than 1 cm in size; about 10% of the time they are more than 2 cm. Most lesions are found at the tip or in the distal third of the appendix. Lymph node and distant metastases have been reported almost exclusively when lesions are greater than 2 cm in size, although regional and distant spread have been reported in small tumors. It is very rare for the carcinoid syndrome to accompany an appendiceal carcinoid.

These lesions are best managed according to size. When less than 2 cm, simple appendectomy is sufficient because the likelihood of lymph node metastasis is low. When larger than 2 cm, right hemicolectomy is recommended to obviate the possibility of leaving diseased regional nodes undiagnosed. Patients with distant metastasis are treated by combination chemotherapy protocols used for carcinoid tumors in other regions. The metastases of these lesions grow slowly, so that 5-year survival rates are greater than 50% even when distant disease is present.

References

1. Williams RA, Myers P. Pathology of the Appendix. London: Chapman & Hall, 1994:1–7.
2. Myers S, Miller TA. Acute abdominal pain: physiology of the acute abdomen. In: Miller TA, ed. St. Louis: Quality Medical, 1998:641–667.
3. Dhillon AP, Rode J. Serotinin and its possible role in the painful non-inflamed appendix. Diagn Histopathol 1983;6:239–246.
4. Dhillon AP, Williams RA, Rode J. Age, site, and distribution of subepithelial neurosecretory cells in the appendix. Pathology 1992;24:56–59.
5. Rode J, Dhillon AP, Papadaki L, Griffiths D. Neurosecretory cells of the lamina propria of the appendix, and their possible relationship to carcinoids. Histopathology 1982;6:69–73.
6. Bockman DE, Cooper MD. Early lymphoepithelial relationships in human appendix. Gastroenterology 1975;68:1160–1168.
7. Spencer J, Finn T, Isaacson PG. Gut-associated lymphoid tissue: a morphological and immunocytochemical study of the human appendix. Gut 1985;26:672–679.
8. Peck JJ. Management of carcinoma discovered unexpectedly at operation for acute appendicitis. Am J Surg 1988;155:683–685.
9. Armstrong CP, Ahsan Z, Hinchley G, Prothero DL, Brodribb AJ. Appendicectomy and carcinoma of the cecum. Br J Surg 1989;76:1049–1053.
10. Klingler PJ, Smith SL, Abendstein BJ, Brenner E, Hinder RA. Management of ingested foreign bodies within the appendix: a case report with review of the literature. Am J Gastroenterol 1997;92:2295–2298.
11. Jones BA, Demetriades D, Segal I, Burkitt DP. The prevalence of appendiceal fecaliths in patients with and without appendicitis. A comparative study from Canada and South Africa. Ann Surg 1985;202:80–82.
12. Pieper R, Kager L, Tidefeldt. Obstruction of appendix vermiformis causing acute appendicitis. Acta Chir Scand 1982;148:63–72.
13. Sisson RG, Ahlvin RC, Hartlow MC. Superficial mucosal ulcerationand the pathogenesis of acute appendicitis in childhood. Am J Surg 1971;122:378–380.
14. Nitecki S, Karmeli R, Sarr MG. Appendiceal calculi and fecaliths as indications for appendectomy. Surg Gynecol Obstet 1990;171:185–188.
15. Thadepalli H, Mandal AK, Chuah SK, Lou MA. Bacteriology of the appendix and the ileum in health and in appendicitis. Am Surg 1991;57:317–322.
16. Pieper R, Kager L, Weintraub A, Lindberg AA, Nord CE. The role of Bacteroides fragilis in acute appendicitis. Acta Chir Scand 1982;148:39–44.
17. Bennion RS, Baron EJ, Thompson JE Jr, et al. The bacteriology of gangrenous and perforated appendicitis—revisited. Ann Surg 1990;211:165–171.
18. Temple CL, Huchcroft SA, Temple WJ. The natural history of appendicitis in adults: a prospective study. Ann Surg 1995;221:278–281.
19. Ramsden WH, Mannion RA, Simpkins KC, DeDombal FT. Is the appendix where you think it is—and if not does it matter? Clin Radiol 1993;47:100–103. (See also published erratum: Clin Radiol 1993;48:148.)
20. Karim OM, Boothroyd AE, Wyllie JH. McBurney's point—fact or fiction. Ann R Coll Surg 1990;72:304–308.
21. Guidry SP, Poole GV. The anatomy of appendicitis. Am Surg 1994;60:68–71.
22. McBurney CM. Experience with early operative interference in cases of disease of the vermiform appendix. NY Med J 1889;50:676–684.
23. Scott JH, Amin M, Harty JI. Abnormal urinalysis in appendicitis. J Urol 1983;129:1015–1018.
24. Puskar D, Bedalov G, Fridrih S, Vickovic I, Banek T, Pasini J. Urinalysis ultrasound analysis, and renal dynamic scintigraphy in acute appendicitis. Urology 1995;45:108–112.
25. Swensson EE, Maull KI. Clinical significance of elevated serum and urine amylase levels in patients with appendicitis. Am J Surg 1981;142:667–670.
26. Gumaste W, Roditis N, Mehta D, Dave PB. Serum lipase levels in non-pancreatic abdominal pain. Am J Gastroenterol 1993;88:2051–2055.
27. Korner H, Sondenaa K, Soreide JA, Anderson E, Nysted A, Lende TH. Structured data collection improves the diagnosis of appendicitis. Br J Surg 1998;85:341–344.
28. Cullen JJ, Kelly KA, Moir CR, Hodge DO, Zinsmeister AR, Melton LJ. Surgical management of Meckel's diverticulum: an epidemiologic, population-based study. Ann Surg 1994;220:564–568.
29. Harada RN, Whelan TJ. Surgical management of cecal diverticulitis. Am J Surg 1993;166:666–669.
30. Soybel DI, Bliss DP, Wells SA. Colorectal carcinoma. Curr Probl Cancer 1987;11:259–356.
31. Bizer LS. Acute appendicitis is rarely the presentation of cecal cancer in the elderly patients. J Surg Oncol 1993;54:45–46.
32. Singh KK, Lessells AM, Adam J, et al. Presentation of endometriosis to general surgeons: a ten year experience. Br J Surg 1995;82:1349–1351.
33. Graff L, Radford MJ, Werne C. Probability of appendicitis before and after observation. Ann Emerg Med 1991;20:503–507.
34. Campbell JP, Gunn AA. Plain abdominal radiographs and acute abdominal pain. Br J Surg 1988;75:554–556.
35. Hurme T, Nylamo E. Conservative vs. operative treatment of appendicular abscess. Experience of 147 consecutive patients. Ann Chir Gynaecol 1995;84:33–36.
36. Jeffrey RB Jr, Federle MP, Tolentino CS. Periappendiceal inflammatory masses: CT-directed management and clinical outcome in 70 patients. Radiology 1988;167:13–16.
37. Wilcox RT, Traverso LW. Have the evaluation and treatment of acute appendicitis changed with new technology? Surg Clin North Am 1997;77:1355–1370.

38. Nichols RL. Surgical antibiotic prophylaxis. Surg Clin North Am 1995;79:509–522.

39. McCahill LE, Pellegrini CA, Wiggins T, Helton WS. A clinical outcome and cost-analysis of laparoscopic versus open appendectomy. Am J Surg 1996;171:533–537.

40. Minne L, Varner D, Burnell A, Ratzer E, Clark J, Haun W. Laparoscopic vs. open appendectomy. Prospective randomized study of outcomes. Arch Surg 1997;132:708–711.

41. McCall JL, Sharples K, Jadallah F. Systematic review of randomized controlled trials comparing laparoscopic with open appendectomy. Br. J Surg 1997;84:1045–1050.

42. Golub R, Siddiqui F, Pohl D. Laparoscopic versus open appendectomy: a metaanalysis. J Am Coll Surg 1998;186:545–553.

43. Cox MR, McCall JL, Padbury RT, Wilson TG, Wattchaw DA, Toouli J. Laparoscopic surgery in women with a clinical diagnosis of appendicitis. Med J Aust 1995;162:130–132.

44. Laine S, Rentala A, Gullichsen R, Ovaska J. Laparoscopic appendectomy—is it worthwhile? A prospective randomized study in young women. Surg Endosc 1997;11:95–97.

45. Fink AS, Kosakowski CA, Hiatt JR, Cochran AJ. Peri-appendicitis is a significant clinical finding. Am J Surg 1990;159:564–568.

46. Wang Y, Reen DJ, Puri P. Is a histologically normal appendix following emergency appendicectomy always normal? Lancet 1996;347:1076–1079.

47. Brasel KJ, Borgstorm DC, Weigelt JA. Cost-utility analysis of contaminated appendectomy wounds. J Am Coll Surg 1997;184:23–30.

48. Watters JM, Blakslee JM, March RJ, Redmond ML. The influence of age on the severity of peritonitis. Can J Surg 1996;39:142–146.

49. Braveman P, Schaaf VM, Egerter S, Bennett T, Schecter W. Insurance-related differences in the risk of ruptured appendix. New Engl J Med 1994;330:444–449.

50. Paajanen H, Kettunen J, Kostiainen S. Emergency appendectomy in patients over 80 years. Am Surg 1994;60:950–953.

51. Lim HK, Bae SH, Seo GS. Diagnosis of acute appendicitis in pregnant women: value of ultrasound. AJR 1992;159:539–542.

52. Tamir IL, Bongard FS, Klein SR. Acute appendicitis in the pregnant patients. Am J Surg 1990;160:571–575.

53. To WW, Ngai CS, Ma HK. Pregnancies complicated by acute appendicitis. Aust N Z J Surg 1995;65:799–803.

54. Mahmoodian, S. Appendicitis complicating pregnancy. South Med J 1992;85:19–24.

55. Kort B, Katz VL, Watson WJ. The effect of non-obstetric operation during pregnancy. Gynecol Obstet 1993;177:371–376.

56. Amos JD, Schorr SJ, Norman PF, et al. Laparoscopic surgery during pregnancy. Am J Surg 1996;171:435–437.

57. Gurbuz AT, Peetz ME. The acute abdomen in the pregnant patient. Is there a role for laparoscopy? Surg Endosc 1997;11:98–102.

58. Whitney TM, Macho JR, Russell TR, Bossart KJ, Heer FW, Schecter WP. Appendicitis in the acquired immunodeficiency syndrome. Am J Surg 1992;164:467–470.

59. Lowy AM, Barie PS. Laparotomy in patients infected with human immunodeficiency virus: indications and outcome. Br J Surg 1994;81:942–945.

60. Savioz D, Lironi A, Zurbuchen P, Leissing C, Kaiser L, Morel P. Acute right iliac fossa pain in acquired immunodeficiency. Br J Surg 1996;83:644–646.

61. Flum DR, Steinberg SD, Sarkis AY, Wallack MK. Appendicitis in patients with acquired immunodeficiency syndrome. Am Coll Surg 1997;184:481–486.

62. Van Noyen R, Selderslaghs R, Bekaert J, Wauters G, Vandepitte J. Causative role of *Yersinia* and other enteric pathogens in the appendicular syndrome. Eur J Clin Microbiol Infect Dis 1991;10: 735–741.

63. Mattei P, Sola JE, Yeo CJ. Chronic and recurrent appendicitis are uncommon entities often misdiagnosed. J Am Coll Surg 1994;178:385–389.

64. Barber MD, McLaren J, Rainey JB. Recurrent appendicitis. Br J Surg 1997;84:110–112.

65. Klingensmith ME, Soybel DI, Brooks DC. Laparoscopy for abdominal pain. Surg Endosc 1996;10:1085–1087.

66. Nitecki SS, Wolff BG, Schlinkert R, Sarr MG. The natural history of surgically treated primary adenocarcinoma of the appendix. Ann Surg 1994;219:51–57.

67. Deans GT, Spence RA. Neoplastic lesions of the appendix. Br J Surg 1995;82:299–306.

68. Cortina R, McCormick J, Kolm P, Perry RR. Management and prognosis of adenocarcinoma of the appendix. Dis Colon Rectum 1995;38:848–852.

69. Carr NJ, McCarthy WF, Sobin LH. Epithelial noncarcinoid tumors and tumor-like lesions of the appendix. Cancer (Phila) 1995;75:757–768.

70. Madwed D, Mindelzun R, Jeffrey RB. Mucocele of the appendix. AJR 1993;159:69–72.

71. Qizilbash AH. Mucoceles of the appendix: their relationship to hyperplastic polyps, mucinous cystadenomas, and cystadenocarcinomas. Arch Pathol 1995;99:548–555.

23

Colon, Rectum, and Anus

Mark L. Welton, Madhulika G. Varma, and Andreas Amerhauser

Anatomy and Physiology

Anatomy

COLONIC ANATOMY

The colon is one structural unit with two embryological origins. The cecum and right and midtransverse colons are of midgut origin and as such are supplied by the superior mesenteric artery. The distal transverse, splenic flexure, and descending and sigmoid colon are of hindgut origin and receive blood from the inferior mesenteric artery. The entire colon starts as a midline structure that rotates during development and attaches laterally to the right and left posterior peritoneum. The right and left colonic mesenteries are obliterated, fusing to the posterior peritoneum in these regions, leaving these portions of the colon covered by peritoneum on the lateral, anterior, and medial surfaces. The transverse and sigmoid colons, in contrast, are completely covered with peritoneum and are attached by long mesenteries, allowing for great variation in the location of these structures.

COLONIC HISTOLOGY

Three layers form the mucosa of the colon: epithelium, lamina propria, and muscularis mucosa. The epithelium is columnar with crypts made of straight nonbranching tubules (glands of Lieberkuhn). The cells around the crypts are simple columnar cells with occasional goblet cells. The crypts are mostly lined with goblet cells, except at the bases, where undifferentiated cells, amine precursor uptake and decarboxylation cells (APUD), and enterochromaffin cells predominate. The lamina propria is connective tissue surrounding a network of capillaries. The muscularis mucosa is a thin sheet of muscle fibers containing a network of lymphatics. The submucosa is a layer of connective tissue containing vessels, lymphatics, and Meissner's plexus. The muscularis propria is composed of circular and longitudinal muscle. The inner circular muscle completely encompasses the entire colon and rectum, ending in the anus as the internal sphincter muscle. The myen-

teric plexus of Auerbach lies on the circular muscle. The longitudinal muscle is grouped into three dominant cables of muscle called taeniea coli that originate in the cecum and fuse together to form a circumferential coat at the junction of the sigmoid and rectum. The colon is covered with serosa on the intraperitoneal surfaces, but not where it is attached to the retroperitoneum on the posterior aspects of the ascending and descending colon.

COLONIC ARTERIAL SUPPLY

The blood supply to the colon is quite variable, but general patterns exist (Fig. 23.1). The ileocolic artery, a constant structure, is the terminal branch of the superior mesenteric artery. It commonly gives rise to cecal, appendiceal, ileal, and ascending branches, some of which anastomose with ileal and right colic vessels. The right colic artery may originate from the superior mesenteric, middle colic, or ileocolic vessels and is present in 10% to 98% of cases.[1,2] The middle colic artery arises from the superior mesenteric artery, branches early into the right and left branches, and anastomoses with the ascending branches of both the right and left colic arteries. The artery is present in 95% to 98% of cases.[2,3] The inferior mesenteric artery originates from the aorta 3 to 4 cm above the bifurcation.[4] It gives rise to the left colic artery, to the sigmoid vessels, and ends in the superior rectal artery. The left colic artery divides into ascending and descending branches. The ascending branch anastomoses with branches off the middle colic and the descending branch anastomoses with the sigmoid vessels. Collateral circulation between the vessels of superior mesenteric and inferior mesenteric arteries is through two named arteries: the marginal artery of Drummond and the "Arc of Riolan" or "meandering mesenteric."

COLONIC VENOUS DRAINAGE

The venous drainage of the colon is through veins that bear the same name as the arteries with which they run except for the inferior mesenteric vein that runs alone in the mesentery of the left colon to join the splenic vein.

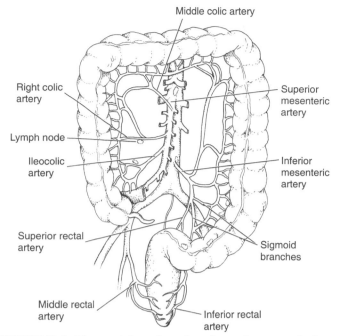

FIGURE 23.1. The arterial supply to the colon and rectum. The lymphatic drainage parallels the arterial supply.

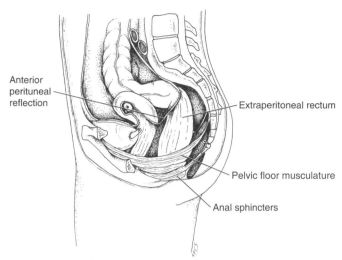

FIGURE 23.2. The rectum transitions from completely intraperitoneal to extraperitoneal as it passes into the pelvis. The point at which it becomes completely extraperitoneal is the anterior peritoneal reflection. The muscles of the pelvic floor create a broad sheet suspending the rectum.

COLONIC LYMPHATIC DRAINAGE

The lymphatic drainage of the colon starts as a network of vessels within the muscularis mucosa, which drain into the extramural system. The extramural lymphatic vessels and nodes follow along the arteries to their origins at the superior and inferior mesenteric vessels.

COLONIC INNERVATION

The colon is innervated via the sympathetic and parasympathetic nervous systems. Sympathetic stimulation inhibits peristalsis whereas it is promoted by the parasympathetic system.

ANORECTAL ANATOMY

The rectum is approximately 12 to 15 cm long. It extends from the rectosigmoid junction, marked by the fusion of the tenia, to the anal canal, marked by the passage of the bowel into the pelvic floor musculature. The rectum lies in the sacrum and forms three distinct curves, creating folds that when visualized endoscopically are known as the valves of Houston. The rectum gradually transitions from intraperitoneal to extraperitoneal, beginning posteriorly at 12 to 15 cm from the anus and becoming completely extraperitoneal at the anterior peritoneal reflection, 6 to 8 cm from the anus (Fig. 23.2). The rectum is "fixed" posteriorly, laterally, and anteriorly by the presacral or Waldeyer's fascia, the lateral ligaments, and Denonvilliers fascia, respectively.[5–7]

The anatomical anal canal starts at the dentate line and ends at the anal verge. However, a practical definition is the surgical anal canal, which extends from the termination of the muscular diaphragm of the pelvic floor to the anal verge.[8] The internal sphincter is a specialized continuation of the circular muscle of the rectum. It is an involuntary muscle that is normally contracted at rest. The external sphincter is com-

posed of voluntary striated muscle. The conjoined longitudinal muscle separates the internal and external sphincter. This intersphincteric plane is created by the continuation of the longitudinal muscle of the rectum, joined by fibers from the levator ani and puborectalis forming the conjoined muscle.[9]

Hemorrhoids are found in the subepithelial tissue above and below the dentate line. These are cushions composed of vascular and connective tissues and supportive muscle fibers. Internal hemorrhoids originate above the dentate line and are lined with insensate rectal columnar and transitional mucosa. External hemorrhoids are similar vascular complexes except that they are underlying the richly innervated anoderm rather than insensate rectal mucosa.

ANORECTAL HISTOLOGY

The rectum is composed of an innermost layer of mucosa that lies over the submucosa, two continuous sheaths of muscle, the circular and longitudinal muscles, and in the upper rectum, serosa. The mucosa is subdivided into three layers: (1) epithelial cells, (2) lamina propria, and (3) muscularis mucosa. The muscularis mucosa is a fine sheet of muscle containing a network of lymphatics. Lymphatics are not present above this level, making the muscularis mucosa critical in defining metastatic potential of malignancies.[10]

ANORECTAL ARTERIAL SUPPLY

The arterial supply of the anorectum is via the superior, middle, and inferior rectal arteries.[11] The superior rectal artery is the terminal branch of the inferior mesenteric artery and descends in the mesorectum. It supplies the upper and middle rectum. The middle rectal arteries generally arise from the internal pudendal artery, but may come off the inferior gluteal or internal iliac arteries. They enter the rectum anterolaterally in the distal third of the rectum at the level of the pelvic floor musculature.[6,11] They supply the lower two-thirds of the rectum. The inferior rectal arteries, branches of the internal pudendal arteries, enter posterolaterally, do not anastomose extramurally with the blood supply to the rectum, and provide blood supply to the anal sphincters and epithelium.

ANORECTAL VENOUS DRAINAGE

The venous drainage of the anorectum is via the superior, middle, and inferior rectal veins draining into the portal and systemic systems. The superior rectal vein drains the upper and middle third of the rectum. It empties into the portal system via the inferior mesenteric vein. The middle rectal veins drain the lower rectum and upper anal canal into the systemic system via the internal iliac veins. The inferior rectal veins drain the lower anal canal, communicating with the pudendal veins and draining into the internal iliac veins. There is communication between the venous systems, which allows low rectal cancers to spread via the portal and systemic systems.

ANORECTAL LYMPHATIC DRAINAGE

Lymphatic drainage of the upper and middle rectum is into the inferior mesenteric nodes. Lymph from the lower rectum may also drain into the inferior mesenteric system but may drain to the systems along the middle and inferior rectal arteries, posteriorly along the middle sacral artery, and anteriorly through channels in the retrovesical or rectovaginal septum. These drain to the iliac nodes and ultimately to the periaortic nodes. Lymphatics from the anal canal above the dentate line drain via the superior rectal lymphatics to the inferior mesenteric lymph nodes and laterally to the internal iliac nodes. Below the dentate line drainage occurs primarily to the inguinal nodes but can occur to the inferior or superior rectal lymph nodes.

ANORECTAL INNERVATION

The innervation of the rectum is via the sympathetic and parasympathetic nervous systems. The sympathetic nerves originate from the lumber segments L1–L3, form the inferior mesenteric plexus, travel through the superior hypogastric plexus, and descend as the hypogastric nerves to the pelvic plexus.[12]

The parasympathetic nerves arise from sacral roots S2–S4 and join the hypogastric nerves anterior and lateral to the rectum to form the pelvic plexus. Sympathetic and parasympathetic fibers pass to the rectum and internal anal sphincter as well as the prostate, bladder, and penis. Injury to these nerves or plexi can lead to impotence, bladder dysfunction, and loss of normal defecatory mechanisms.[13–15]

The internal anal sphincter is innervated by the autonomic nervous system. It receives excitatory sympathetic innervation via the hypogastric nerves (L5) and inhibitory parasympathetic innervation by the pelvic splanchnic nerves S2–S4. The inferior rectal branch of the pudendal nerve S2–S4 innervates the external anal sphincter.

Sensations of noxious stimuli above the dentate line are conducted through afferent fibers of these parasympathetic nerves and experienced as an ill-defined dull sensation. Below the dentate line, the epithelium is exquisitely sensitive and richly innervated by somatic nerves.[16] Cutaneous sensations of heat, cold, pain, and touch are conveyed through the inferior rectal and perineal branches of the pudendal nerve.

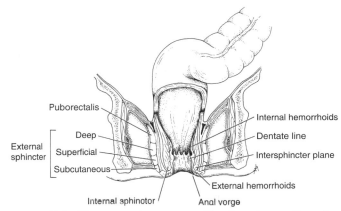

FIGURE 23.3. The rectum is compressed by the puborectalis and external sphincter complex as it transitions into the surgical anal canal.

PELVIC FLOOR ANATOMY

The pelvic floor is a consortium of funnel-shaped muscles that separate the pelvis and the perineum. It is composed of the levator ani and puborectalis muscles. The puborectalis serves as a bridge between the broad sheetlike component of the funnel created by the levators and the narrow spout of the funnel created by the external anal sphincter (Fig. 23.3). The puborectalis in the contracted state is responsible for the normal acute anorectal angle between the levators and the external sphincters. It is also responsible for the shelf that is normally palpable on digital exam as one passes from the distal narrow lumen of the "anus" to the more proximal capacious lumen of the "rectum."[17–19] Innervation of the pelvic floor is from branches of ventral nerve roots of S2–S4.

Physiology

COLONIC PHYSIOLOGY

The major functions of the colon are absorption, storage, propulsion, and digestion of the output of the proximal intestinal tract.

Absorption of the salts and water of the ileal output is critical in the maintenance of normal fluid and electrolyte balance. In normal individuals, the ileum expels approximately 1500 ml of fluid per day, of which 1350 ml is absorbed by the colon. The right colon is more active in this process than the left. Water absorption is driven by active sodium absorption against concentration and electrical gradients.[20,21] An Na^+/K^+-ATPase pump at the basolateral membrane is responsible for the net absorption of Na^+. Chloride is actively absorbed in exchange for bicarbonate.[22] Urea is secreted into the lumen of the colon, metabolized by bacteria into ammonia, and absorbed passively in the nonionized form.[20] The colon also actively secretes mucus that is high in K^+.

The propulsive and storage functions of the colon are difficult to study. Radiographic studies have revealed three types of contractions: segmental nonpropulsive,[23] retrograde,[24,25] and antegrade propulsive mass movements.[26] Segmental contractions occur primarily in the right colon and move contents over short distances distally or proximally. Retrograde contractions also mix the contents and slow transit, forcing the fluid into more proximal bowel and increasing absorption times.[27,28] Mass movements move intraluminal contents rapidly over long distances.

Digestion is an underrecognized activity of the colon. Primarily anaerobic bacteria that ferment proteins, dietary fiber, and carbohydrates accomplish digestion. Carbohydrate fermentation produces short-chain fatty acids that are important mucosal fuels.[29] Their absorption is associated with sodium and water absorption and bicarbonate secretion.[30] The bacteria produce substances that the colon could not otherwise absorb, such as ammonia and vitamin K,[31] and detoxify carcinogens.[32]

ANORECTAL PHYSIOLOGY

The levator ani create a broad funnel cone suspending the rectum in a muscular sling that ends where the puborectalis pulls the rectum forward at the anorectal junction, creating an acute anorectal angle "at rest." The levators may contain sensory fibers that report pelvic fullness and therefore may be important in the sensation of the urge to defecate. The acuity of the angle created by the puborectalis is critical for maintaining continence.

The internal sphincter, composed of smooth muscle, generates 85% of the resting tone. It is innervated with sympathetic and parasympathetic fibers. Both are inhibitory and keep the sphincter in a constant state of contraction.[33] The external sphincters are skeletal muscles innervated by the pudendal nerve with fibers that originate from S2–S4. The muscles provide 15% of the resting tone and 100% of the voluntary squeeze pressures. Voluntary contraction of the external sphincter should double the resting pressure but cannot be sustained longer than 3 min.[34,35]

Hemorrhoids are important participants in maintaining continence and minimizing trauma during defecation. They function as protective pillows that engorge with blood during the act of defecation, protecting the anal canal from direct trauma due to passage of stool.[36] They also seal the anal canal and prevent leakage of gas and stool. The internal and external sphincters alone cannot close the anal canal but when combined with interdigitating internal hemorrhoidal cushions, continence is achieved.[37–39] Hemorrhoidal tissues engorge when intraabdominal pressure is increased, as occurs with obesity, pregnancy, lifting, and defecation.

Colon and Rectum: Benign Diseases

Inflammatory Bowel Disease: Crohn's Disease

Crohn's disease was originally described as an inflammation of the terminal ileum that led to stricture and fistula formation. Since then, this nonspecific, transmural, inflammatory bowel disease has been found throughout the gastrointestinal tract, from the oropharynx to the anus.[40] It also manifests itself in many extraintestinal symptoms of the eyes, skin, and joints. Crohn's colitis is distinguished from ulcerative colitis on the basis of gross and microscopic pathology (Table 23.1). Approximately 10% to 15% of patients will be diagnosed with indeterminate colitis[6] and have features of both diseases.

The incidence of Crohn's disease ranges from 0.30 to 10 per 100,000 population; the prevalence is approximately 10 to 90 cases per 100,000 population. There is a bimodal age distribution, with the first peak at age 15 to 30 years and the second at 55 to 80 years. Some studies have shown that women, Jewish people, cigarette smokers, urban dwellers, and oral contraceptive users are at increased risk.[41–44] Although Crohn's disease has been noted in families, no genetic transmission has been found. The etiology of Crohn's disease remains elusive, as does the etiology of ulcerative colitis with which it shares many similarities.

The presentation of Crohn's disease can be difficult to appreciate. Patients have a variety of symptoms that are directly related to the extent, character, and location of the inflammation. The classic symptoms are abdominal pain, diarrhea, which can be bloody, and weight loss. Other signs and symptoms include fever, nausea, vomiting, anorexia, palpable abdominal mass, aphthous ulcerations of the mouth, cholelithiasis, and renal calculi.

The nature of Crohn's disease can be divided into three categories: inflammatory, stricturing, and fistulizing. Patients with stricturing Crohn's disease may only have symptoms of obstruction, whereas those with a fistula or abscess may have a more septic presentation.

The disease occurs most commonly in the ileocolic region (30%–45%), followed by isolated small bowel (20%–40%) and colonic (16%–40%) disease.[45–48] Five percent of patients will present with perianal disease and no evidence of other disease. For those with Crohn's disease limited to the colon, two of three will have total colonic involvement.[6]

The evaluation for Crohn's disease verifies the diagnosis and assesses the severity and extent of the disease. Upper and lower endoscopy with directed and random biopsies and radiographic imaging will help to elucidate the diagnosis. Stool cultures may find evidence of infectious enterocolitis that may mimic Crohn's disease. Colonoscopy is the most sensitive test for identifying a patchy distribution of inflammation, terminal ileal involvement, and rectal sparing that are highly suggestive of Crohn's. Endoscopic findings include mucosal edema and erythema, aphthous or linear ulcerations, and fibrotic strictures. Biopsy is diagnostic when a sarcoid-type giant cell granuloma is found.

It is important to distinguish Crohn's colitis from ulcerative colitis. Therefore, thorough evaluation of the rest of the GI tract is critical. Many patients with colonic disease also have small-bowel findings, which distinguishes Crohn's from ulcerative colitis. To evaluate the extent of the disease an upper GI with small-bowel follow-through is imperative to find lesions of the stomach, duodenum, or small intestine such as strictures or fistulas.

The most common symptoms found outside the gastrointestinal tract involve the skin, eyes, and joints. Erythema nodosum and pyoderma gangrenosum are dermatological diseases that occur with both ulcerative colitis and Crohn's disease. Multiple subcutaneous nodules that are tender, red, raised, and microscopically composed of lymphocytes and histiocytes characterize erythema nodosum. Pyoderma gangrenosum develops from an erythematous lesion into a tender necrotizing ulcer.

Ocular manifestations include uveitis, iritis, episcleritis, vasculitis, and conjunctivitis. These findings are more commonly associated with colonic disease and infrequently precede any intestinal symptoms.

Arthritis, synovitis, ankylosing spondylitis, and sacroiliitis are all joint complications of ulcerative colitis and

Crohn's disease. Although arthritis and synovitis may improve with treatment of intestinal disease, the latter two can only be abated.

The incidence of carcinoma is increased in the setting of Crohn's disease and should be suspected in patients with a severe or chronic stricture.

Surgical specimens have certain classic characteristics. The intestinal wall is generally thickened and hyperemic with a corkscrewing of the vessels. The mesentery is thickened and tends to wrap around the bowel wall as "creeping fat." Mesenteric lymph nodes can be quite enlarged. The segment of intestine removed may contain an abscess cavity or direct fistulous communication to another loop of intestine or adjacent organ. The mucosal appearance is similar to that seen on endoscopy with inflammatory pseudopolyps and cobblestoning. The microscopic characteristics include submucosal inflammation with edema, lymphocyte and plasma cell infiltrates, and fibrosis. The granulomas specific for the disease are found in only 50% to 60% of resected specimens.

MEDICAL THERAPY

The primary treatment of Crohn's disease is medical. Surgery is indicated for complications of the disease process.

AMINOSALICYLATES

Sulfasalazine and mesalamine are the two aminosalicylates used for Crohn's disease. Sulfasalazine works after the azo bond is cleaved in the colon, making the 5-ASA active component available. Thus, the drug is useful for patients with Crohn's colitis or ileocolitis.[49,50] Unbound mesalamine (5-ASA) is absorbed in the proximal small bowel and is therefore useful in proximal and mid small bowel Crohn's disease. However, mesalamine may be coated with an inert substance that slows absorption making it useful in the treatment of ileocolic and colonic Crohn's disease. Mesalamine (5-ASA) delivered rectally in enema or suppository form allows direct topical therapy for rectal and descending colonic disease.

CORTICOSTEROIDS

For patients with exacerbations leading to moderate or severe Crohn's disease, steroids are the primary therapy. However, they do not help to maintain remission and are detrimental when used for long-term treatment (more than 6–9 consecutive months). They inhibit the release of arachidonic acid, IL-1, and IL-2, thus exerting an immunosuppressive effect. They can be administered orally, rectally, and for severe cases parenterally.[51]

ANTIBIOTICS

Although antibiotics are not used to treat specific bacterial organisms, they have been found to be effective in the treatment of Crohn's disease, especially for the perianal area. Metronidazole is the most common agent employed, although ciprofloxacin has also been used. By decreasing the amount of bacterial flora in the intestinal lumen, they act to prevent the infectious complications of Crohn's disease such as abscesses and fistulas. Clinical trials have shown their efficacy in inducing remission.[52–54]

IMMUNOMODULATORS

As increasing evidence points to an immunological etiology of inflammatory bowel disease, efforts have been made to utilize various immunotherapies. The drugs most commonly used are azathioprine and its metabolite, 6-mercaptopurine (6-MP), antimetabolites that inhibit DNA synthesis. The mechanism of these drugs stems from their inhibition of T-cell clones. A meta-analysis of nine trials found that azathioprine and 6-MP are effective in patients with active disease but the adverse side effects approached 10%.[55] The most important criteria for the success of azathioprine and 6-MP are adequate dosing, initial treatment with corticosteroids, and adequate duration of treatment. Withdrawal of drug has shown a 70% relapse rate.[55]

Methotrexate is a folate analogue that inhibits purine and pyrimidine synthesis and has been shown in a number of trials to be effective in treating Crohn's disease.[56] However, this drug has significant side effects including hepatotoxicity and bone marrow suppression and thus is reserved for patients with severe Crohn's that is refractory to other therapies. Other drugs shown to be effective include cyclosporine, tacrolimus, mycophenolate mofetil, and infliximab.

SURGICAL THERAPY

As previously stated, the primary treatment of Crohn's disease is medical and surgery is considered for patients with specific complications of the disease. Crohn's disease cannot be cured by an operation, but it can help ameliorate certain situations (Table 23.2). The goal in the surgical management of Crohn's disease is to minimize the amount of healthy small bowel and colon resected and the amount of healthy perianal tissue divided while treating the complication that led to surgery. This goal can be achieved through sufficient preoperative assessment of disease and nutritional status, bowel rest, TPN (total parenteral nutrition), percutaneous drainage of abscesses, and maximal medical therapy to minimize the amount of inflammation in surrounding uninvolved normal tissue.

The three classic indications for surgery are stricture, bleeding, and perforation. Patients with symptoms of obstruction not responsive to medical treatment with radiographic evidence of a stricture, and without a predominant component of inflammation, require operative intervention for the stenotic diseases. Medical therapy may be adequate for fistulizing diseases of the perineum or between two loops of bowel, but if the fistulas result in undrained abscesses, either intraabdominal or perineal, or if they result in free perforation of the intestine, urgent surgical consultation is indicated. Finally, patients who are on maximal medical therapy but are continuing to have severe symptoms of bleeding, pain, or malabsorption may benefit from resection of the diseased segment.

Small intestinal or ileocolic stenotic disease is treated by resection with primary anastomosis. Only grossly involved intestine should be resected because wide resection or microscopically negative margins of resection have no impact on the recurrence rate of disease.[57] Stricturoplasty should be considered for strictures widely separated by normal bowel and when multiple previous bowel resections have been performed.

Patients who present with fistulizing disease with either established fistulas or undrained sepsis require the greatest amount of judgment and caution. The surgical inclination is to operate urgently. However, percutaneous drainage, TPN, and bowel rest control sepsis and allows the inflammation of the uninvolved bowel and surrounding structures to resolve.

For isolated Crohn's colitis, a total proctocolectomy with ileostomy or total abdominal colectomy with ileorectal anastomosis or ileostomy and rectal stump are the primary

TABLE 23.1. Comparison of Ulcerative Colitis and Crohn's Colitis

Manifestation	Ulcerative colitis	Crohn's colitis
Clinical Features		
Bleeding per rectum	3+	1+
Diarrhea	3+	3+
Abdominal pain	1+	3+ Especially with involvement of ileum
Vomiting	R	3+
Fever	R	2+
Palpable abdominal mass	R	2+
Weight loss	+	3+
Clubbing	R	1+
Rectal involvement	4+	1+
Small bowel involvement	0	4+
Anal and perianal involvement	R	4+
Risk of carcinoma	1+	1+
Clinical course	Relapses/remission	Slowly progressive
Radiologic		
Thumb printing sign on barium enema	R	1+
Endoscopic		
Distribution	Symmetric	Asymmetric
Continuous involvement	4+	1+
Rectal	4+	1+
Vascular architecture	Absent	1+
Friability	4+	1+
Erythema	3+	1+
Spontaneous petechiae	2+	R
Profuse bleeding	1+	R
Aphthous ulcer	0	4+
Serpiginous ulcer	R	4+
Deep longitudinal ulcer	0	4+
Cobblestoning	0	4+
Mucosa surrounding ulcer	Abnormal	±Normal
Pseudopolyps	2+	2+
Bridging	R	1+
Gross Appearance		
Thickened bowel wall	0	4+
Shortening of bowel	2+	R
Fat creeping onto serosa	0	4+
Segmental involvement	0	4+
Aphthous ulcer	R	4+
Linear ulcer	0	4+
Microscopic Picture		
Depth of involvement	Mucosa and submucosa	Full thickness
Lymphoid aggregation	0	4+
Sarcoid-type granuloma	0	4+
Fissuring	0	2+
Goblet cell mucin depletion	4+	1+
Intramural sinuses	0	1+
Operative Treatment		
Total proctocolectomy	Excellent option in selected patients	Indicated in total large bowel involvement
Segmental resection	R	Frequent
Ileal pouch procedure	"Gold standard"	Contraindicated

(continued)

TABLE 23.1. (continued)

Manifestation	Ulcerative colitis	Crohn's colitis
Prognosis		
Recurrence after total proctocolectomy	0	3+
Complications		
Internal fistula	R	4+
Intestinal obstruction (stricture or infection)	0	4+
Hemorrhage	1+	1+
Sclerosing cholangitis	1+	R
Cholelithiasis	0	2+
Nephrolithiasis	0	2+

R, rare; 0, not found; 1+, may be present; 2+, common; 3+, usual finding; 4+, characteristic (not necessarily common).

Source: From Nivatvongs S. The colon, rectum, and anal canal. In: James EC, Corry RJ, Perry JF Jr, eds. Basic Surgical Practice. Philadelphia: Hanley & Belfus, 1987:325; Ogorek CP, Fisher RS. Differentiation between Crohn's disease and ulcerative colitis. Med Clin North Am 1994;78;1249–1258.

therapies. The choice of operations is dependent on the extent of disease in the rectum and anus and the overall health of the patient. Segmental colon resections for Crohn's disease are usually not recommended.

Perianal complications of Crohn's disease are common, and surgical management controversial. Liberal placement of drainage catheters and noncutting Setons, advancement flap closure of perineal fistulas, and selective construction of diverting stomas have good results when combined with opti-

TABLE 23.2. Indications for Surgical Treatment of Crohn's Disease.

- Failure of medical treatment
  - ➤ Persistence of symptoms despite corticosteroid therapy for longer than six months
  - ➤ Recurrence of symptoms when high-dose corticosteroids tapered
  - ➤ Worsening symptoms or new onset of complications with maximal medical therapy
  - ➤ Occurrence of steroid-induced complications (Cushingoid features, cataracts, glaucoma, systemic hypertension, aseptic necrosis of the head of the femur, myopathy, or vertebral body fractures
- Obstruction
  - ➤ Intestinal obstruction (partial or complete)
- Septic complications
  - ➤ Inflammatory mass or abscess (intraabdominal, pelvic, perineal)
  - ➤ Fistula if
    - — Drainage causes personal embarrassment (e.g. enterocutaneous, enterovaginal fistula, fistula-in-ano)
    - — Fistula communicates with the genito-urinary system (e.g. entero- or colo-vesical fistula)
    - — Fistula produces functional or anatomic bypass of a major segment of intestine with consequent malabsorption and/or profuse diarrhea (e.g., duodenocolic or enterorectosigmoid fistula)
    - — Free perforation
- Hemorrhage
- Carcinoma
- Growth retardation
- Fulminant colitis with or without toxic megacolon

Source: Reprinted with permission from Operative Strategies in Inflammatory Bowel Disease, Michelassi and Milsom, Editors. ©1999 Springer-Verlag, New York, Inc.

mal medical therapy to induce remission of inflammation. Protectomy, which is infrequently required, can often be postponed for several years when complementary surgical and medical treatments are provided. As with Crohn's disease proximally, palliation of symptoms and preservation of functional bowel are the priorities guiding surgical intervention. Likewise, the aim of therapy is the treatment of complications of disease rather than the disease itself. Two mandates clarify these principles with respect to perianal disease: (1) the management of a septic focus is an indication for surgery, and (2) the sphincter should be preserved so long as the patient is coping well.

When treating perirectal or perianal abscesses in the Crohn's patient, we prefer catheter drainage to standard open incision and drainage, as this avoids the large incision and prolonged healing that are often required. Fistulotomy, which is the standard treatment for fistulas associated with cryptoglandular abscesses, is also the first-line treatment for superficial Crohn's fistula-in-ano.[58,59] The cutting Seton is associated with an unacceptable incontinence rate and should be avoided. The purpose of a noncutting Seton is to maintain a patent external opening to the fistulous tract and thereby control local sepsis in the patient who has recurrent abscesses. With free drainage of the tract, no abscess forms. The internal opening of the fistula persists because of Crohn's disease activity, and it will not close until medical therapy induces remission. The Seton can be safely removed or exchanged at that time.

The rectal mucosal advancement flap is the optimal operation for management of rectovaginal and anterior perineal fistulas as well as perineal fistulas refractory to other therapy.[58] In the male patient, an anourethral or rectourethral fistula can similarly be closed with an advancement flap after diagnostic urethroscopy and proctoscopy have been performed.

The creation of a diverting ileostomy or colostomy is typically unsuccessful when used alone to address perineal Crohn's disease. However, temporary diversion combined with (1) control of perineal sepsis, (2) advancement flap repair of fistulas, and (3) maximal medical therapy may allow sphincter preservation for 10 to 15 years.[60] In those patients who fail to have control of perianal disease with combination therapy, diverting ileostomy or colostomy can be regarded as a staging procedure; patients have the opportunity to live with a stoma and prepare psychologically for protectomy.

Skin tags in Crohn's perineal disease have been described as "pseudo-skin tags" because they are usually inflamed skin between fissures and ulcers rather than redundant skin, which constitutes skin tags. Biopsy of these pseudo-skin tags can show the presence of granulomas and can, therefore, be helpful in securing the diagnosis of Crohn's disease. In general, local skin care and control of diarrhea are the cornerstones of treatment. Excision invites complications such as delayed healing or chronic ulceration.[61]

Fissures that are off midline or are multiple may indicate the presence of Crohn's disease. However, because the majority of Crohn's-related fissures are on the midline, this diagnosis should be considered whenever a midline fissure fails to respond to conventional therapy.[60] Although lateral sphincterotomy is the standard operative treatment of routine anal fissures, it is to be avoided in the setting of Crohn's disease.

The anorectum that is stenosed as a result of inflammation but is still somewhat supple may be amenable to digital dilation with one finger. More commonly, the stricture that results from chronic inflammation is rigid and unyielding. Such strictures are unresponsive to dilation and are an indication for protectomy when symptomatic.

When hemorrhoids are coincident with Crohn's disease, operative interventions are associated with a high rate of complications. Every effort should be made to avoid surgery.

Although the risk of developing squamous cell carcinoma of the anus is not increased in the Crohn's perineum, diagnosis may be delayed because of the presence of chronic inflammation. Failure of fissures to heal or persistence of painful ulcers should prompt consideration for biopsy of the lesion.[62]

Inflammatory Bowel Disease: Ulcerative Colitis

Ulcerative colitis (UC) is a mucosal inflammatory condition of the gastrointestinal tract confined to the colon and rectum. Like Crohn's, it is considered a manifestation of inflammatory bowel disease (IBD). Although the medical therapy is similar for Crohn's disease and ulcerative colitis, the surgical therapies for each differ greatly, and it is imperative that a clear diagnosis is made whenever possible. The anatomical location and microscopic pathology of the two diseases helps to differentiate them. However, in about 15% of patients with inflammatory bowel disease, a definitive diagnosis cannot be made. These patients are diagnosed with indeterminate colitis with features more consistent with ulcerative colitis or Crohn's but with elements suggestive of both diseases present on pathological evaluation. The treatment of these patients is complicated and individualized in consultation with a gastroenterologist, the patient, and the patient's support system.

The incidence of ulcerative colitis ranges from 2 to 15 per 100,000 population and has remained relatively constant for the past 20 years. Previously, the higher incidence appeared to correlate with northern countries and more developed nations, but the incidence in Asia has been increasing. The prevalence of UC is 50 to 70 cases per 100,000 population per year. There is a bimodal age distribution, with the peak incidence occurring between 20 to 29 years of age and the second peak at 60 to 70 years.[63] No environmental or genetic factors have been found that are directly implicated in this disease, although smokers have a decreased incidence of UC and a familial aggregation has been noted. Also, 20% to 30% of patients with ulcerative colitis have another family member with the disease.[64,65] The etiology of inflammatory bowel disease is unknown.

The clinical manifestations of ulcerative colitis vary with the severity of the disease. Patients may have active disease with intervening periods of quiescence. The most common symptom of ulcerative colitis is bloody diarrhea. Patients with mild disease may have occasional blood and mucus and a moderate number of stools. Frequent, explosive diarrhea with significant bleeding or discharge of mucus and pus manifests more severe disease. Massive hemorrhage from ulcerative colitis is rare. Severe disease may also be associated with fever, abdominal pain, tenesmus, malaise, anemia, or weight loss. Some may have fecal incontinence with severe disease activity. Most patients present with mild to moderate disease involving the rectum and a contiguous segment of the distal colon. About 20% of patients present with pancolitis. The so-called toxic "megacolon" is a presentation of fulminant colitis with fever, abdominal pain, and leukocytosis that may or may not be associated with radiographic evidence of colonic dilatation. Patients may require emergent operation for perforation or resistance to medical therapy.

Physical examination findings are dependent on the severity of the disease. In mild cases, the examination may be normal. In more severe cases, patients may have abdominal distension and tenderness or localized peritoneal signs. Digital rectal examination may reveal tenderness, and blood, mucus, or pus in the rectal vault.

The diagnosis of ulcerative colitis is made endoscopically. A sigmoidoscopy may be diagnostic and colonoscopy hazardous (perforation) when active disease is present. There may be loss of the submucosal vascular pattern and edema with mild disease, a granular, hyperemic, and friable mucosa with moderate disease, and a deep-red, velvety appearance with more active disease. A mucopurulent exudate may obscure ulcerations. Pseudopolyps may also be seen. Assessment of severity is important in choosing therapy and assessing endpoints.

Once the disease has become more quiescent, a colonoscopy should be performed to determine the extent of the disease. Barium enema (BE) is useful to establish the extent of bowel involved and, in long-standing disease, to reveal strictures and foreshortening of the colon. There is a loss of haustrations, and a rigid pipe appearance develops as the colon narrows and shortens. This test should not be performed in the setting of acute disease because of the risk of perforation. Strictures seen on BE should be considered malignant until proven otherwise.

Surveillance by colonoscopy in ulcerative colitis is important because of the increased risk of colorectal dysplasia and carcinoma. Patients at higher risk are those with colitis proximal to the splenic flexure and those with long-standing disease, at least 8 to 10 years.[66–70] Patients with ulcerative proctitis are not at increased risk for developing cancer. Other factors correlated with the risk of cancer are a positive family history of colorectal cancer and the presence of primary sclerosing cholangitis.[71,72] The incidence of colorectal cancer in ulcerative colitis[73,74] is estimated to be approximately 0.5% to 1.0% per year after 8 to 10 years of disease.[75,76] For surveillance of these patients, dysplasia is used as a premalignant marker for carcinoma. As a result, the current recommendations are for patients with pan-colitis to undergo colonoscopy every 1 to 2 years after the eighth year of disease and yearly after the fifteenth year. Biopsies should be taken at 10-cm intervals, resulting in a total of at least 30 biopsies. Pathological studies have confirmed that up to 33 biopsies may be required to have a 90% chance of detecting dysplasia.[77] In patients with left-sided colitis, yearly colonoscopy should be performed after the fifteenth year. Similar biopsies should be obtained as for pan-colitis.

The extraintestinal manifestations of ulcerative colitis (UC) are similar to those of Crohn's disease with the exception of hepatobiliary complications, which are more common and can be quite severe. Primary sclerosing cholangitis (PSC) is uncommon with Crohn's disease and occurs in 7.5% of patients with UC. Most patients are men under 40. Hepatobiliary symptoms may precede intestinal manifestations by as much as 7 years.[78] Treatment of the colonic disease with total proctocolectomy does not affect the clinical course of PSC but may reverse the fatty infiltration and liver function abnormalities seen with UC.[79]

Other manifestations of ulcerative colitis include involvement of the skin, eyes, and joints. Patients with ulcerative colitis have also been noted to have a higher risk of thromboembolic disease and vasculitis. The most significant extracolonic manifestation that can be reversed with surgical therapy is malnutrition and, in younger patients, growth retardation.

Ulcerative colitis is a disease of the mucosa and submucosa. It starts in the rectum and extends proximally to include a variable amount of colon. The pathological characteristics vary depending on disease state (acute or chronic), severity, and presence of complications. Generally, the outer wall of the colon will look completely normal or the serosa may have dilated blood vessels. However, in chronic cases, the bowel may be foreshortened secondary to a thickening and contraction of the muscularis mucosae. The mesentery remains normal, unlike the thickened mesocolon of Crohn's disease. The mucosa may be erythematous, thickened, friable, or granular and can have ulcerations, superficial fissures, or pseudopolyps. A mucopurulent exudate may be present on the mucosa. The mucosal inflammation always starts in the rectum and is continuous. If "skip lesions" with intervening normal mucosa are seen, Crohn's disease should be suspected. In about 10% of patients with pancolitis, the distal ileum may appear inflamed and ulcerated. This finding is secondary to reflux of colonic contents through the ileocecal valve and is termed backwash ileitis. It should not be confused with Crohn's disease, as this inflammation generally is contiguous with the rest of the inflammation of the colon.

Microscopic characteristics include the presence of polymorphonuclear leukocytes (PMN) in the epithelium of the crypts of Lieberkuhn forming crypt abscesses. Progression of the disease leads to coalescence of these crypts into broad-based ulcers eroding the mucosa. The residual normal mucosa that remains at the borders of these crypt abscesses is what projects into the lumen as a "pseudopolyp."

MEDICAL THERAPY

The medical therapy for ulcerative colitis overlaps significantly with those therapies used for Crohn's disease.

Sulfasalazine (Azulfidine) was the first drug developed for the treatment of ulcerative colitis. Sulfasalazine is a sulfapyridine linked to 5-aminosalicylic acid (5-ASA) by an azo bond. Sulfasalazine is cleaved in the colon making the active 5-ASA component available to act on the large intestine. A dosage of 4 g/day can reduce the relapse rate at 1 year from 70% to 9%.[80] Mesalamine (unbound 5-ASA) is absorbed in the small intestine and is not effective in ulcerative colitis. Preparations to delay the release of 5-ASA in the intestinal tract with resin, Asacol, or slow-release microspheres regulated by pH, Pentasa, are available. Other sulfa-free aminosalicylates, Olsalazine, two 5-ASA linked by an azo bond, and Balsalazide, 5-ASA linked to an inert carrier molecule, have been developed. Both drugs have shown benefit in maintaining remission of ulcerative colitis.[81,82] Rowasa is a topical enema preparation of 5-ASA useful in the treatment of ulcerative proctitis. Topical preparations, used in conjunction with oral therapy, have been found to be more effective in maintaining remission than oral agents alone.[83]

For patients with moderate or severe exacerbations of ulcerative colitis, steroids exert an antiinflammatory effect. However, they do not help to maintain remission and are detrimental when used long term.

As increasing evidence points to an immunological etiology of inflammatory bowel disease, efforts have been made to utilize various immunotherapies. The most commonly used drugs are azathioprine and its metabolite, 6-mercaptopurine, antimetabolites that inhibit DNA synthesis. Other effective drugs include cyclosporine and tacrolimus.

SURGICAL THERAPY

According to longitudinal studies, approximately 30% of all patients with ulcerative colitis ultimately have surgery. Within the first year of diagnosis, 10% require operative intervention, and the colectomy rate then is about 3% per year for the next 4 years and 1% per year thereafter.[84] The surgical treatment of ulcerative colitis involves removing the colon and, in most cases, the rectum. Segmental colectomies have a limited role in ulcerative colitis as the entire colon is at risk for subsequent problems. The indications for surgery depend on the severity and duration of the patient's disease. For patients with active disease, emergency operation may be indicated for fulminant colitis unresponsive to medical therapy with bleeding, perforation, or toxic colitis. In these situations, the safest procedure is a total abdominal colectomy with end ileostomy, leaving the rectum in place. This allows an extremely ill patient to undergo a shorter, less complicated procedure that does not prevent a subsequent restorative procedure. It is the preferred operation for those who require emergent surgery, or are debilitated, malnourished, or receiving excessive doses of steroids or immunosuppressive agents.

For patients with chronic active or quiescent disease, the indications for surgery include an inability to wean from steroids, extracolonic manifestations that may respond to colectomy, and the presence of dysplasia or carcinoma on colonoscopy for screening. Children with UC may require surgery to treat delayed growth and maturation secondary to medical therapy or malnutrition. For these patients, a number of surgical options may be entertained; these include total proctocolectomy with end ileostomy, continent ileostomy or ileal pouch–anal anastomosis, and total abdominal colectomy with ileorectal anastomosis. In a majority of situations, a total proctocolectomy is performed because the disease in the rectum is severe enough to warrant excision.

Total proctocolectomy with end ileostomy was the gold standard procedure with the lowest morbidity and mortality. Unfortunately, it relegates patients to a permanent ileostomy and has largely been replaced by ileal pouch procedures. The advantage of a standard proctocolectomy is that all the disease is removed. The disadvantage, however, is that the patient is left with an "incontinent" end ileostomy that passes stool and flatus in an uncontrolled fashion. To remedy this, various continence-restoring procedures have been performed.

The continent ileostomy allowed patients with ileostomies to control elimination from the pouch by fashioning a "nipple" that maintained continence. The patient empties the pouch with a catheter and is not required to wear an appliance. Unfortunately, this procedure has a high rate of early and late complications and has been supplanted by the ileal pouch–anal procedure.

The ileal pouch–anal anastomosis has become the standard operation for ulcerative colitis. The advantage of the procedure is that it allows the patient to void per anus, thus avoiding a stoma. The disadvantage is that the procedure is associated with significant morbidity and the risk of cancer is not completely eliminated, as it is when a standard proctocolectomy is performed. Contraindications to this procedure are preoperative fecal incontinence, possibility of Crohn's disease, previous significant small-bowel resection, and distal rectal cancer.

The issue of mucosectomy has been raised in relation to the subsequent risk of carcinoma or disease in the retained rectal mucosa. Studies have shown evidence of active disease or even dysplasia in specimens of stripped anorectal mucosa,[85,86] leading some authors to argue that a mucosectomy must always be performed. Others believe that the remnant mucosa is transitional mucosa (cuboidal epithelium) and does not represent true rectal mucosa at risk for malignancy or inflammation. Our preference is to perform a stapled anastomosis within 1 to 1.5 cm of the dentate without a mucosectomy and to recommend yearly surveillance with anoscopy and digital exam of the residual mucosa.

The mortality from this surgery is extremely low, less than 1%, and is especially low when performed in an elective setting. In contrast, the morbidity is significant, even in an experienced surgeon's hands.[87] Pelvic abscess and pouch anastomotic leaks occur about 4% and 10% of the time. Urinary retention and sexual dysfunction are related to injury or disruption of the presacral nerves during rectal dissection. These sequelae occur about 1% to 3% of the time.[88,89] Late complications include pouchitis, anal strictures, pouch fistulas, bleeding, and excessive stools with dehydration or incontinence. A small number of patients may require pouch excision or permanent ileostomy to treat these complications.

Diverticular Disease

Diverticular disease of the left colon is an acquired disease effecting primarily Western cultures.[90] The incidence increases with age, with estimates of the incidence ranging from 5% in the fifth decade to 75% in the ninth decade of life.[91,92] Neither sex is more clearly affected.[91–95] The etiology is not clearly understood but the most accepted hypothesis is that diverticulosis occurs as a result of a highly refined, low-residue diet.[96]

Although diverticulosis is common, complications requiring surgery occur in only approximately 1% of patients with the disease,[97] 30% of symptomatic patients,[91,98] and 15% to 30% of those who require hospital admission.[90,99] Hospital admission and recurrent attacks increase the likelihood of significant complications and need for surgery.

Colonoscopy is preferred over barium enema in the initial workup of suspected diverticular disease because of its superior sensitivity and specificity.[100] However, colonoscopy is less rewarding and more dangerous in the evaluation of acute complications of perforated diverticular disease. In these instances, CT scan of the abdomen and pelvis with intravenous, oral, and rectal contrast is the preferred test.

Fiber is the mainstay of the medical management of uncomplicated diverticulosis or mild diverticulitis. A high-fiber diet is believed to reduce intracolonic pressures, presumably eliminating the "cause" of diverticular disease. The fiber increases stool bulk and water content, generating a softer formed stool that requires the colon to generate less pressure to pass the stool in a shorter time.[101,102] Despite popular beliefs that dietary seeds may occlude a diverticulum, there is no evidence to suggest that patients with diverticulosis should avoid seeds.

Complications of colonic diverticula that may require surgical consultation or intervention are hemorrhage and the complications of perforation of a diverticulum, which include chronic left lower quadrant pain, phlegmon, abscess, peritonitis, fistula, and stricture. Hemorrhage occurs in up to 20% of patients with diverticulosis. In 5%, the hemorrhage is massive.[103] The source of the bleeding is generally right sided even though diverticula are predominately present on the left.[104,105] The majority of patients (70%–82%) stop bleeding, but 12% to 30% continue to bleed and require intervention.[103,105,106] The cause of the hemorrhage appears to be an erosion into the vasa recta that courses along the diverticulum.[107]

Patients with gastrointestinal hemorrhage need to be worked up and treated in a similar fashion no matter the cause. Once resuscitation is under way, attention is directed toward localization of the source. If the nasogastric tube and proctosigmoidoscopic evaluation suggests a distal source, a nuclear medicine test is the preferred first step. Bleeding at a rate as low as 0.1 ml/min can be detected.[108] Success in localization is operator dependent and varies widely between institutions, but sensitivities as high as 97% and specificities of 85% are reported from multiple centers.[109–111] Most centers require this before angiography because of the higher sensitivity of the nuclear medicine test compared to angiography, 0.1 ml/min versus 0.5 to 1.0 ml/min.

Angiographic localization is attempted in those with a positive nuclear medicine scan. This technique allows for confirmation of location and therapeutic intervention[105] with either microembolization of a terminal arcade or pitressin infusion via the catheter positioned in a distal branch.[112] Both techniques have a greater than 90% success rate.

Urgent colonoscopy after rapid bowel cleansing has been successfully performed in select institutions with dedicated teams as both a diagnostic and therapeutic technique, but this has not gained wide acceptance despite excellent results.[108,113,114] The indications for surgery and the choice of operation remain controversial and require a good deal of clinical judgment. Efforts to localize the bleeding source are maximized to allow therapeutic intervention as mentioned and to direct the segmental resection if a colectomy is necessary. Urgent segmental colectomy is indicated after localization (1) if the bleeding cannot be controlled with the aforementioned nonoperative measures or (2) if blood products are limited or unavailable while awaiting spontaneous cessation (Jehovah's Witness, or antibodies on cross match). "Blind" segmental colectomy is not recommended because of the high recurrence rates and the difficulty in managing patients with postoperative hemorrhage. "Blind" total colectomy may be necessary when there is massive hemorrhage and the lesion cannot be localized preoperatively or with intraoperative techniques (enteroscopy/colonoscopy). An algorithm for treatment of lower gastrointestinal hemorrhage is presented in Fig. 23.4.

Diverticulitis develops when a diverticulum ruptures. In most cases the perforation is microscopic, causing localized inflammation in the colonic wall or paracolic tissues. In more severe cases an abscess may form, or the diverticulum may freely rupture into the peritoneal cavity, causing generalized peritonitis. The average age at presentation is the early sixties; more than 90% of cases occur after 50 years of age. Fifty percent to 90% of cases in the United States occur in the left colon, particularly the sigmoid. However, among the Asian population, up to 75% right-sided disease has been reported.[115–117] Fifty percent of patients have been symptomatic for less than 1 month before presentation; the duration of symptoms is inversely correlated with the severity of disease.

Patients with acute diverticulitis typically present with the gradual onset of left lower quadrant pain and low-grade fever. The pain is constant and does not radiate. The localized inflammatory process may lead to irritation of the contiguous small bowel, colon, and bladder, which may cause anorexia, nausea, vomiting, diarrhea, constipation, dysuria, frequency, or urgency. On physical examination, tenderness to palpation is usually present in the left lower quadrant or suprapubic region. A mass suggestive of a peridiverticular abscess or phlegmon may also be palpable. Rectal examination may reveal a boggy mass anteriorly if a pelvic abscess is present. Unlike diverticulosis, acute diverticulitis is usually not associated with hemorrhage, but 30% to 40% of cases have guaiac-positive stool. Pneumaturia or fecaluria suggest the presence of a colovesical fistula.

The clinical presentation is often sufficient to establish the diagnosis. Laboratory studies are nonspecific and frequently unrevealing. Leukocytosis may be absent in up to half of cases. Urinalysis may be abnormal with microscopic pyuria or hematuria. In elderly or immunocompromised patients, the presentation may be subtle, and immunocompromised patients are more likely to have complications of diverticulitis. The differential diagnosis is listed in Table 23.3.

Plain film abdominal series including an upright chest X-ray should be obtained to rule out free intraperitoneal air or lower lobe pneumonia. These studies may be normal or may demonstrate a distal large-bowel obstruction, localized ileus, or extracolonic air. Computed tomography with i.v., oral, and rectal contrast is the study of choice.[118] It is superior to bar-

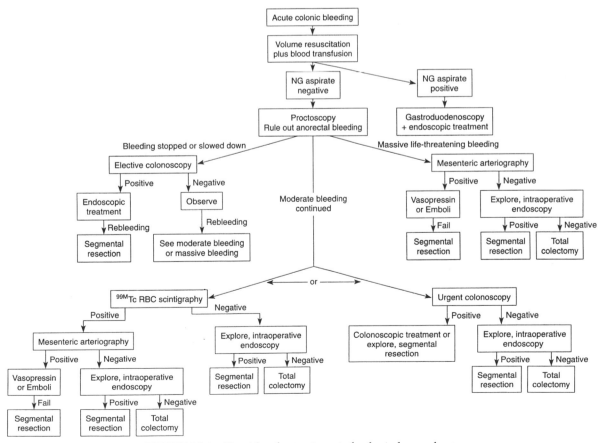

FIGURE 23.4. Algorithm for treatment of colonic hemorrhage.

TABLE 23.3. Differential Diagnosis of Acute Diverticulitis.

Appendicitis
Carcinoma
Colonic spasm
Gastroenteritis
Infectious colitis
Ischemia
Irritable bowel
Inflammatory bowel disease
Pelvic inflammatory disease
Perforated peptic ulcer
Foreign body perforation
Volvulus
Urosepsis
Pneumonia

ium enema in that it can directly demonstrate extraluminal complications of the disease such as abscess, phlegmon, free intraperitoneal air, or colovesical fistula and allows for therapeutic intervention with percutaneous drainage.

Interval contrast enema studies may be helpful in establishing the diagnosis in patients with mild disease and in ruling out adenocarcinoma of the proximal bowel when colonoscopy is incomplete. Barium should be avoided in the acute setting because of the risk of extravasation into the peritoneum, peritonitis, and vascular collapse. If an urgent contrast study must be done, water-soluble agents may be used.

Endoscopy is generally contraindicated in the setting of acute diverticulitis. It is hazardous and may aggravate a free perforation or convert a controlled perforation to a free perforation. Further, it is often difficult to visualize the involved segment as inflammation renders the bowel impassable and the patient experiences pain as the lesion is approached.

Mild cases of acute diverticulitis in immunocompetent patients can be managed on an outpatient basis with clear liquids and oral antibiotics.[115,119] Ideal patients for outpatient management are those who are able to tolerate a diet, have no systemic symptoms or peritoneal signs, and are reliable with a reliable family. Immunocompromise, steroid therapy, and advanced age are contraindications to outpatient therapy.

If outpatient therapy is elected, patients need to watch for systemic signs or progression of symptoms, and should be instructed to return if these develop. Follow-up with the treating physician must occur within 48 to 72 h after presentation. Patients in whom any of the foregoing criteria are not met should be admitted to the hospital for total bowel rest, intravenous antibiotics for gram-negative organisms and anaerobes, serial exams, and further evaluation as indicated.

CT should be ordered liberally in patients with moderate or severe disease, in the immunocompromised patient, and in patients in whom the diagnosis is unclear. If the patient worsens under observation or does not improve over 48 h, as occurs in 10% to 25% of patients, then reassessment is needed. Imaging with triple-contrast CT, if not already performed, to detect an unsuspected abscess is acceptable. Otherwise, immediate surgical exploration is indicated. Of the patients having emergency surgery, 70% have no antecedent history of diverticulitis.

Abscess or phlegmon is the most common complication

of acute diverticulitis, and may occur in the mesocolon, abdomen, pelvis, retroperitoneum, buttocks, or scrotum. The location and size of the abscess dictate the clinical presentation and management. Small intramesenteric abscesses may resolve with conservative therapy, whereas large intraabdominal abscesses may mandate surgical intervention or percutaneous drainage by interventional radiology.[115,120]

Purulent or fecal peritonitis may develop secondary to rupture of a contained abscess or free perforation of a diverticulum. Most present with an acute abdomen and some degree of septic shock. Aggressive intravenous resuscitation, antibiotics, and surgery are recommended for patients who present in this fashion. They are explored urgently, and a resection with descending colostomy and oversewing of the rectal stump is performed in all but the sickest patients.[115,121] The reported mortality rates for purulent and fecal peritonitis are 6% and 35%, respectively.[115]

Fistulas develop in only 2% of patients with diverticulitis, but fistula is the indication for surgery in 20% of those undergoing surgery for diverticulitis and its associated complications. Eight percent have multiple fistulas.[115] The incidence is greater in men than in women presumably because the uterus separates the colon from the bladder, and the uterus, being a thick muscular structure, is resistant to fistula formation. Most women who develop fistulas have had a prior hysterectomy, but colouterine and colosalpingo fistulas have been reported. Colocutaneous fistulas generally develop in the postoperative setting as an anastomotic complication.[115]

A thorough preoperative evaluation including abdominal–pelvic CT and colonoscopy to rule out colonic malignancy at the site of the fistula or in the proximal colon is suggested. Patients may be prepared for a completely elective procedure after an interval suitable to allow the acute inflammation to resolve. A colectomy with primary anastomosis should be anticipated.

Diverticulitis is the cause of approximately 10% of all large-bowel obstruction.[115] The obstruction is usually partial, with complete obstruction occurring rarely. The obstruction is secondary to edema, spasm, and chronic inflammatory changes.

The indications for surgery for diverticulitis are recurrent attacks, a severe attack, and age less than 50 years, the immunocompromised state, a severe complication of perforation such as significant phlegmon/abscess, peritonitis, fistula, or stricture. The goals of surgical therapy are to minimize morbidity and mortality, remove the septic focus and diseased colon, avoid or at least minimize the risks of a second operation, and convert an emergent situation to an urgent or elective operation. These goals should guide the surgeon both pre- and intraoperatively.

Patients are best managed by resection of the diseased bowel with or without primary anastamosis. In the rare circumstance when the disease obliterates the pelvic space or the patient or operating team are unable to proceed, drainage and diversion are acceptable despite the high morbidity and mortality associated with this procedure.[122,123]

Infectious Colitides

Infections of the large bowel usually cause diarrhea and can produce fever or abdominal pain. Infectious colitis must be differentiated from other etiologies of colitis. It is critical to elicit a complete history from the patient including recent travel, unusual ingestions suspect for food poisoning, similar illnesses among family members, recent hospitalizations, and treatment with antibiotics, sexual history, immunosuppression, and evidence of systemic disease. The pertinent positives of the history will help tailor the diagnostic workup. Patients often have physical signs of dehydration such as decreased skin turgor, dry mucous membranes, tachycardia, or hypotension. Additionally, the abdominal exam may reveal tenderness or local peritoneal signs. A rectal is done to check for blood and tenderness.

The diagnostic workup includes testing for fecal leukocytes, *Clostridium difficile* toxin, and stool cultures for bacteria, ova, and parasites. Endoscopic evaluation may be useful in patients who require biopsy for diagnosis.[124] Occasionally, radiographic imaging is necessary to assess the degree of colonic involvement and to look for evidence of necrosis or perforation. Once the source of colitis is found, the treatment depends on the severity of the patient's illness and the need for supportive care and antibiotics. Certain infections can result in fulminant colitis that is refractory to medical treatment and requires surgery.

CLOSTRIDIUM DIFFICILE

Diarrhea that develops during antibiotic administration may be related to a change in the bacterial flora of the colon. This resolves spontaneously after cessation of therapy. However, a minority of patients on antibiotics will have a proliferation[125] of the toxin-producing strains of *C. difficile*, a gram-positive, anaerobic organism. The toxins produce mucosal damage and inflammation. Although clindamycin was considered to be the primary culprit in producing this disease,[126] it is now known that any antibiotic can produce this colitis. Humans can transmit the organism in hospitals and nursing homes via an oral–fecal route.

Patients present with watery diarrhea, fever, and leukocytosis. Abdominal pain and tenderness are also common. Some patients develop toxic megacolon. Symptoms can occur both during antibiotic administration or weeks to months after cessation of treatment. The diagnosis is made by rapid immunoassays that test for antigens or toxins in the stool.[127] On endoscopic exam the mucosa can look inflamed or develop plaque-like membranes, which is why it has been called "pseudomembranous" colitis (Fig. 23.5). Fecal leukocytes, although not specific for *C. difficile* colitis, are present about 50% of the time.

The mainstay of therapy involves cessation of the antibiotics previously administered if the patient is still under treatment. Additionally, oral vancomycin and metronidazole are very effective against *C. difficile*. For those patients unable to tolerate an oral dose because of abdominal surgery or ileus, intravenous metronidazole is effective, with bactericidal levels of the drug in the stool. Vancomycin is only effective if delivered orally.[128]

Antidiarrheal agents should be avoided. Cholestyramine and colestipol are anion-exchange binding resins that can bind toxin but will also bind antibiotic. Therefore, they are generally effective for patients with mild colitis only. Patients who develop toxic megacolon may require emergent surgical therapy. The mortality rate with emergent surgery is reported to be about 24% to 43%.[129]

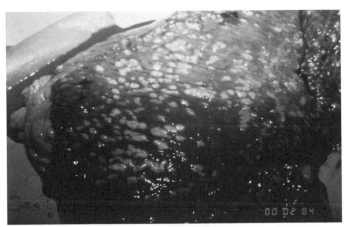

FIGURE 23.5. Colonic specimen with the yellow-white "plaque-like" membranes that led to the name pseudomembranous colitis.

BACTERIAL COLITIS

Patients with bacterial colitis develop these infections from a fecal–oral route. Most patients have self-limiting infections and require only supportive care and rehydration. However, a minority of these patients develop toxic megacolon, bleeding, or perforation that requires surgery with an associated high morbidity and mortality. The most common causative organisms are *Shigella*, *Campylobacter*, *Salmonella*, and *Escheria* (*E. coli*).

PROTOZOAL COLITIDES

ENTAMOEBA HISTOLYTICA

E. histolytica is a water-borne organism that is transmitted by contaminated food or water. Many patients are asymptomatic but the classic presentation includes chronic intermittent diarrhea, abdominal pain, weight loss, and flatulence. Examination of the stool and identification of cysts or trophozoites confirms the diagnosis. Metronidazole is the treatment of choice.

GIARDIA

This organism comes from contaminated drinking water and is very common in the western United States and eastern Europe. Patients present with frequent diarrhea, mucus, steatorrhea, bloating, weight loss, and fatigue. Checking the stool for ova and parasites provides the diagnosis. As the diagnosis is sometimes difficult to make, patients are treated with metronidazole empirically when the disease is suspected.

CRYPTOSPORIDIUM PARVUM

Cryptosporidiosis is a common cause of diarrhea in immunosuppressed patients and health care workers. Patients present with fever, abdominal pain, and watery diarrhea. Colonic biopsy or acid-fast staining of the stool will reveal oocysts. The disease is self-limiting, lasting about 2 weeks. The treatment is supportive with rehydration. No medication is known to be effective.

VIRAL COLITIDES

CYTOMEGALOVIRUS

Immunocompromised patients frequently develop cytomegalovirus infections. Patients present with fever, abdominal pain, and weight loss. The stools are usually watery, but they can also be bloody. Diagnosis is made by tissue biopsy showing intranuclear viral inclusions. Treatment includes supportive care and the use of antiviral agents such as ganciclovir (DHPG) or foscarnet.

HERPES SIMPLEX VIRUS

HSV causes similar symptoms as CMV in this population. Patients are treated with acyclovir and require the same supportive care.

Ischemic Colitis

Ischemic colitis is the most common form of intestinal ischemia. It is thought to affect "watershed" areas of the colon where two blood supplies may incompletely overlap; that is, the splenic flexure supplied by the left branch of the middle colic (SMA origin) and the ascending left colic (IMA origin). It may result from vascular occlusion or a low flow state. The severity of injury appears to be related to multiple factors including duration of ischemia, vessel caliber, acuity of ischemia onset, collateral circulation, and virulence of intestinal bacteria.[130]

Patients are often elderly, debilitated patients in the intensive care unit with multiple medical problems in which an inciting event is difficult to determine. The onset may be insidious, not recognized, or attributed to the medical comorbidities. The outcome depends as much on the reversibility of these comorbidities as it does on factors such as severity of disease and rapidity of disease onset. Onset of acute colonic ischemia is heralded by the sudden onset of cramping abdominal pain. This may be associated with bloody diarrhea, fever, abdominal distension, anorexia, nausea, or vomiting. Physical exam may reveal abdominal distension and tenderness, particularly over the involved segment. In the gangrenous form, an abdominal catastrophe may be apparent with septic shock.[131]

Ischemic colitis is classified by the degree of colonic injury.[132] The three stages include transient ischemia, ischemic stricture, and gangrenous colitis. The majority of cases are transient and reversible, with fewer than 5% with infarction.[133] In the transient form, the injury is localized primarily to the mucosa and submucosa. Superficial sloughing of the mucosa, submucosal hemorrhage, and edema generally resolve within 1 to 2 weeks without permanent sequelae. An ischemic stricture may develop if the injury extends beyond the submucosa into the muscular layers and healing with fibrosis results in compromise of the lumen. Gangrenous ischemic colitis is full thickness and represents a surgical emergency. On initial presentation these three subgroups cannot be distinguished unless the patient presents in extremis where gangrene would be clearly suspected.

The workup of patients with suspected ischemic colitis should be focused on resuscitation and correction of the underlying medical conditions. Plain films of the abdomen may reveal the classic findings of "thumbprinting" of the bowel wall caused by the submucosal hemorrhages. Free air, pneumatosis, or portal venous gases all suggest gangrenous bowel and mandate emergent exploration. CT scans may reveal nonspecific findings such as thickened loops of bowel but may also demonstrate associated occlusion of the IMA and unsuspected vascular disease. Most abnormal laboratory values are nonspecific and occur late after the patient has declared clinically. Colonoscopy is the preferred diagnostic test.

The differential diagnosis includes vascular catastrophes involving the remainder of the gastrointestinal tract, bowel obstruction or perforation, peptic ulcer disease, volvulus, infectious colitis, pseudomembranous colitis, diverticulitis, and inflammatory bowel disease.[134]

The initial management of ischemic colitis is bowel rest, intravenous hydration, and intravenous antibiotics. Underlying medical conditions must be optimized and confounding medications discontinued when possible. Serial exams are mandatory. As noted above, most ischemic colitis resolves without long-term sequelae. Patients resume a diet when their pain, abdominal tenderness, and ileus resolve.

If the patient presents with an acute abdomen, worsens or fails to improve on maximal medical therapy, or develops refractory hemorrhage, surgery is indicated. At surgery, wide resection of all nonviable bowel should be carried out. An anastomosis is created or a stoma and mucous fistula or oversewing of the distal stump is performed. A second-look operation at 24 to 48 h may be indicated if there is concern for ongoing ischemia. Late stricture formation, if symptomatic, is an indication for segmental colectomy.

The prognosis for ischemic colitis is dependent on the medical comorbidities.[133,135] Overall, roughly 90% of the patients recover and less than 5% progress to bowel infarction.[133] However, with disease that mandates surgery, mortality is significantly increased and ranges from 29% to 88%.[133,135–138]

Volvulus

Intestinal volvulus is a closed-loop obstruction of the bowel resulting from an axial twist of the intestine upon its mesentery of at least 180°; this results in luminal obstruction and progressive strangulation of the blood supply. Early diagnosis and treatment of volvulus is important to avoid intestinal ischemia or gangrene that can lead to a high morbidity and mortality.

The incidence of colonic volvulus varies based on geographic and epidemiological factors. In some parts of the world, sigmoid volvulus causes up to 50% to 85% of all bowel obstructions. In the United States, however, it is responsible for only 5% of all intestinal obstructions and 10% of colonic obstructions.[139] Sigmoid volvulus is the most common site (61%), followed by cecum/right colon (34%) and transverse colon (4%).[139]

Intestinal volvulus has been found to be associated with conditions that may result in a chronically dilated or elongated colon. Previous abdominal surgery, coarse high-fiber diets, chronic constipation, Parkinson's disease, neurological disorders, Hirschsprung's disease, diabetes, infectious and ischemic colitis, and pregnancy have all been implicated.[140–148]

Patients with sigmoid volvulus usually present with the triad of abdominal pain, distension, and obstipation. Upon questioning one will often elicit a history of previous attacks. On exam, the abdomen will be dramatically distended, with high-pitched bowel sounds and tympany to percussion. Minimal tenderness may be elicited in spite of this presentation. Patients with gangrene may present with a more fulminant picture of systemic illness and an acute abdomen. Interestingly, no correlation has been found with the length of history and the presence of gangrene or mortality.[149–151]

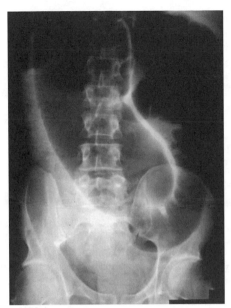

FIGURE 23.6. Classic sigmoid volvulus. Note that pelvis of kidney bean–shaped volvulus points to origin of volvulus.

The diagnosis can be confirmed with a radiograph of the abdomen, which will show an extremely dilated sigmoid colon shaped as a "bent inner tube" with the apex extending up to the right upper quadrant (Fig. 23.6). The ends of the loop sit in the pelvis or left lower quadrant. There can be an air–fluid level in the two sides of the loop at different levels ("pair of scales"). Gastrografin enema will show a "birds beak" or "ace of spades" at the point of the twist (Fig. 23.7). When the plain films or enema are nondiagnostic (30%–40%), CT scan can also be used; this will show a dilated sigmoid loop around a "whirl sign," mesenteric fat with engorged vessels converging toward the center.

The goals of treatment are to untwist and decompress the bowel before strangulation and to prevent recurrences. Those

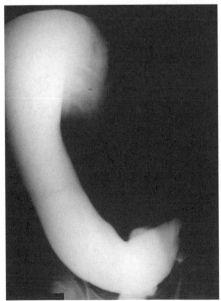

FIGURE 23.7. Barium enema with "bird's beak" deformity at site of volvulus.

patients admitted with signs of sepsis indicative of gangrenous bowel must be aggressively resuscitated and taken emergently to the operating room. These patients will require resection of the gangrenous colonic segment with a primary anastomosis or colostomy and Hartman's pouch. The mortality in patients with gangrenous bowel ranges from 40% to 80%.[152]

When patients do not show signs of intestinal strangulation, the initial treatment of choice of sigmoid volvulus is endoscopic decompression; this allows the volvulus to reduce so that surgical treatment can be performed electively, after a full mechanical bowel preparation, with lower morbidity and mortality. Rigid sigmoidoscopy can reduce and decompress the bowel, evaluate the rectal and colonic mucosa, and allow for the passage of a rectal tube to keep the bowel decompressed. The rectal tube should then be left in place for at least 48 h. Endoscopic decompression is successful about 85% of the time.[153–159] If the patient cannot be reduced endoscopically, strangulation should be suspected and emergent laparotomy performed.

Although the mortality from this mode of therapy is low (5%–8%), the recurrence rate is high (40%–70%).[155,158,160,161] Therefore, once the patient is decompressed and can undergo a bowel prep, the most effective treatment is sigmoid resection; this results in a recurrence rate of less than 1% and a mortality of only 3%.[155] Colopexy, mesosigmoidoplasty, and sigmoidostomy tube placement have higher recurrence rates.[140]

Cecal volvulus is the second most common type of volvulus, although it is the cause of only 1% of all intestinal obstructions. Most patients are younger and there is a predominance of women. Most patients present with symptoms of a small-bowel obstruction: nausea, vomiting, cramping abdominal pain, and distension. Abdominal plain films will show a markedly dilated cecum (coffee bean); it can be anywhere in the abdomen but the "pelvis of the bean" will point to the colon segment of origin. Thus, for a cecal volvulus, a large air-filled "coffee bean" will occupy the abdomen and the "pelvis of the bean" will be facing the right lower quadrant. Gastrografin study can reveal a birds beak and CT may show a whirl sign.

These patients cannot be reduced endoscopically and require operation for definitive treatment. If the bowel is gangrenous, right hemicolectomy with ileostomy is the standard treatment. The mortality of this procedure ranges from 22% to 40%.[162,163] However, if no perforation is present and the patient is hemodynamically stable, then an ileocolectomy and primary anastomosis may be safely performed.[162–164] Reduction of the volvulus alone results in a high recurrence rate, 20%.[165]

Volvulus of the transverse colon and splenic flexure do occur, although rarely. Generally the fixation of the transverse colon by the hepatic and splenic flexure and the relatively short mesocolon keep it in place. Anatomical and acquired conditions can predispose patients to this problem. Patients present with symptoms similar to a small-bowel obstruction. These cases are generally treated by endoscopic decompression, followed by resection or colopexy.[166–169]

Colonic Inertia

Colonic inertia and obstructed defecation (discussed later) may lead to complaints of constipation. Constipation is a very common condition, and most patients with complaints of infrequent or difficult bowel movements do not require extensive workup after colorectal malignancy has been ruled out with either colonoscopy or barium enema and sigmoidoscopy. A thorough history often uncovers a change in diet, medication, or physical activity that is easily corrected. It will also establish the patient's definition of constipation. Patients and physicians alike often confuse constipation with straining at stool or firm bowel movements.[170] Constipation is defined as two bowel movements per week, or fewer than three per week in women or five per week in men while on a high-fiber diet (30 g dietary fiber/day).[171,172] The nature of the complaint (infrequent bowel movements, firm bowel movements, or straining at stool) determines the tests required to establish the diagnosis. Prolonged or repeated straining at stool without result or sense of incomplete evacuation or digital anal–perianal maneuvers suggests a defecation disorder (discussed later under pelvic floor dysfunction).

There are many causes of constipation including dietary factors, daily routine, structural and functional disorders, iatrogenic causes, extracolonic neurological diseases, psychiatric disorders, and endocrine diseases. These disorders are listed in Table 23.4.

The initial management of the patient with constipation is directed toward ruling out structural (colorectal malignancy, stricture, volvulus) and systemic (hypothyroidism, diffuse dysmotility disorders, scleroderma, diabetes) diseases. Once these issues have been addressed, a trial of increased dietary fiber and water is instituted with resolution of symptoms in most patients. Should symptoms persist, evaluation of colonic transit times and pelvic floor function are indicated. Pelvic floor function is assessed with defecography and anorectal manometry. If the patient has isolated colonic inertia without evidence of pelvic floor dysfunction or proximal dysmotility, then a total abdominal colectomy with ileorectal anastomosis may be considered in selected patients. Rare (disabled or institutionalized) patients with colonic inertia and either uncertain pelvic floor function or pelvic floor dysfunction may benefit from creation of an end ileostomy after total abdominal colectomy or total abdominal proctocolectomy.

Malignant Diseases: Colorectal Polyps and Cancer

INCIDENCE

Colorectal cancer is the second leading cause of death by cancer in the United States (estimated at 15% of all malignancies). It is the third leading cause of death from carcinoma in men and women when analyzed by sex (lung and prostate, and lung and breast, are first and second, respectively, in men and women). Approximately 55,000 deaths and 134,000 new cases are predicted for each year.

EPIDEMIOLOGY

The epidemiology of colorectal cancer shows a dramatic variation in disease incidence and mortality rates by country. In general, countries of the Western world have the highest incidence of colorectal cancer. There is an increased risk in urban populations when compared to rural populations.

AGE

Carcinoma of the large intestine is predominantly a disease of older patients, with the peak incidence being in the sev-

---

TABLE 23.4. Common Causes of Constipation.

Faulty Diets and Habits	**Neurologic Abnormalities (Outside Colon)**
Inadequate bulk (fiber)	Central nervous system (cerebral neoplasm, Parkinson's disease)
Excessive ingestion of foods that harden stools (e.g., cheese)	Trauma
Lack of exercise	Spinal cord (neoplasm, multiple sclerosis)
Ignoring call to stool	Defective innervation (resection of nervi erigentes)
Laxative abuse	
Environmental changes (e.g., hospitalization, vacation)	**Psychiatric Disorders**
	Depression
Structural or Functional Disorders	Psychoses
Colonic obstruction	Anorexia nervosa
Neoplasm, volvulus, inflammation (diverticulitis),	
ameboma, tuberculosis, syphilis, lymphogranuloma	**Iatrogenic Causes**
venereum, ischemic colitis, anastomotic stricture,	Medication (codeine, antidepressants, iron,
endometriosis, intussusception	anticholinergics)
Diverticular disease	Immobilization
Anorectal outlet obstruction	
Anal obstruction (stenosis, fissure)	**Endocrine and Metabolic Causes**
Rectocele	Hypothyroidism
Rectal procidentia	Hypercalcemia
Spastic pelvic floor syndrome (anismus)	Pregnancy
Descending perineum syndrome	Diabetes mellitus
Visceral neuropathy or myopathy	Dehydration
Congenital aganglionosis (Hirschsprung's disease)	Hypokalemia
Acquired aganglionosis (Chagas' disease)	Uremia
Slow-transit constipation (colonic inertia)	Pheochromocytoma
Megarectum (sometimes with megacolon)	Hypopituitarism
Chronic intestinal pseudo-obstruction (Ogilvie's	Lead poisoning
syndrome)	Porphyria
Irritable bowel syndrome (visceral hypersensitivity)	Mucoviscidosis

Source: From Gordon and Nivatvongs,[134] with permission.

enth decade. It has been estimated that only 5% of colorectal carcinomas occur in patients younger than 40 years of age.

SITE

In the past 50 years there has been a shift in the location of carcinomas from the rectum to the right colon. Reasons for the shift are not entirely clear. As a consequence, screening of large bowel should be directed at the entire colon rather than being limited to the distal 25 cm of the large intestine. As reported, 30% are located in the rectum, 28% in the sigmoid, 9% in the descending colon, 11% in the transverse colon, 9% in the ascending colon, and 13% in the cecum.[173]

FAMILY HISTORY

There is a twofold to fourfold increased incidence of colorectal carcinomas in first-order relatives of patients who have suffered from the disease.[174]

DIET

Diets low in animal fat and protein and high in cruciferous fiber (whole grains, fruits, and vegetables) are protective.[175,176]

CHEMOPREVENTION

Numerous epidemiological studies point to a chemopreventive effect of either aspirin or NSAIDs on the incidence of sporadic colorectal cancer.[177,178] Nevertheless there is no double-blind prospective study to prove these data. However, a recent prospective randomized study[179] showed the protective effect of calcium supplementation in the development of recurrent colorectal adenomas.

INFLAMMATORY BOWEL DISEASE

There is an increased risk to develop colorectal cancer with long-standing ulcerative colitis and Crohn's disease. There is an increased risk for cancer development with long-standing ulcerative colitis of 3%, 5%, and 13% after 15, 20, and 25 years, respectively.[180] The incidence for colorectal cancer in Crohn's patients is 4 to 20 times greater than in the general population.[181]

GENETICS

Three major categories of genes have been implicated in the development of colorectal cancer, namely oncogenes such as K-*ras*, tumor suppressor genes such as APC, DCC, p53, and MCC, and the mismatch repair genes hMSH2, hMLH1, hPMS, and hPMS2 (Table 23.5).

SCREENING AND SURVEILLANCE

Cancer screening refers to the testing of a population of apparently asymptomatic individuals to determine the risk of developing colorectal cancer. Surveillance refers to the ongoing monitoring of individuals who have an increased risk for the development of a disease. Various screening and surveillance modalities are available to detect colorectal cancers and adenomatous polyps (Tables 23.6 and Table 23.7).

FECAL OCCULT BLOOD TESTING (FOBT)

Testing the stool for fecal occult blood was one of the first tests used in colorectal cancer screening. The advantage of fecal occult testing includes availability, convenience, good patient compliance, and low cost. Limitations include low sensitivity and low specificity.[182–184] However, we believe the test is effective in reducing the mortality of colorectal malignancy and is cost-effective when compared to the cost of treating an undetected malignancy.[185] Further level I evidence suggests that when the test is repeated annually after the age of 50, as it should be, the sensitivity is improved and the malignancy is detected at an earlier stage than if no screening is performed (Table 23.7).

FLEXIBLE SIGMOIDOSCOPY

The benefit of proctosigmoidoscopy in screening programs has been suggested by several studies using the rigid sigmoidoscope.[186,187] The advantage of the flexible sigmoidoscope over the rigid is that the 60-cm flexible sigmoidoscope allows the clinician to reach the descending colon or even the splenic flexure, suggesting more polyps and carcinomas would be identified with the flexible scope and the screening benefit enhanced.[188,189] Both rigid and flexible sigmoidoscopies are inexpensive, require no conscious sedation, are relatively safe, and afford direct visualization and biopsy of polyps and can-

TABLE 23.5. Genes Commonly Altered in Colorectal Cancer.

Gene	Chromosome	Gene class	Function	Comment
APC	5q	Tumor suppressor	Adhesion and intercellular communication	Mutated in FAP, Gardner's, and Turcot's syndrome
DCC	18q	Oncogene	Cell-cell adhesion and interactions	Tumor growth, invasion, and metastasis
P53	17p	Tumor suppresor	Transcription factor for genes that inhibit tumor growth	>50% colon cancers have p53 mutation
K-ras	12p	Oncogene	Signal transduction	50% of colon cancers have K-*ras* activity
hMSH2, hMLH1, hPMS1, hPMS2	2p	Mismatch repair	Corrects DNA replication errors	HNPCC

TABLE 23.6. Patients Who Should Be Screened or in Surveillance Programs.

	Screen		Surveillance	
Average risk & symptoms:	*Average risk & age >50*	*Average risk & request screen*	*Increased risk:*	*Personal history*
Change in bowel habits, per anal bleeding, unclear abdominal pain, unclear anemia			Family history of CRC, adenomas in 1st degree relatives <60 years old, genetic family syndrome (HNPCC, FAP)	IBD, previous adenomas, previous CRC, genetic syndromes

cers. The disadvantage is the entire colon is not visualized with either procedure and lesions may be missed in the proximal bowel. Three case-controlled studies suggest rigid sigmoidoscopy can effectively reduce the risk of death from sigmoid and rectal cancer (Table 23.8).[190–192] We believe flexible sigmoidoscopy is a safe (fewer than 1–2 perforations per 10,000) screening tool that may be repeated every 5 years. If adenomatous disease is found, full colonoscopy is recommended.

BARIUM ENEMA

Barium enema combined with sigmoidoscopy allows for visualization of the entire colon and rectum. Single-contrast barium enema is significantly less sensitive and specific than double-contrast barium enema (DCBE) and should not be used as a screening tool for colorectal malignancy. Double-contrast barium enema has a sensitivity of 50% to 80% for polyps less than 1 cm, 70% to 90% for polyps greater than 1 cm, and 55% to 85% for Dukes' A and B carcinomas, suggesting most clinically important lesions are detected with DCBE.[193–195]

COLONOSCOPY

Examination of the entire colon by colonoscopy is currently recommended for patients with any benign neoplasm found at the time of flexible sigmoidoscopy. When performed by trained endoscopists, colonoscopy with polypectomy is a safe procedure with a perforation incidence of 0.1%, a hemorrhage incidence of 0.3%, a mortality of 0.01% to 0.03%, and the

cecum is visualized in up to 98.6% of patients.[196–201] A DCBE is required when the cecum is not reached. Table 23.9 summarizes the risks and benefits of screening tests for colorectal malignancy.

SIGNS AND SYMPTOMS

The presentation of large-bowel malignancy generally falls into three categories; the most common presentation is that of an insidious onset of chronic symptoms (77%–92%), followed by obstruction (6%–16%) and perforation with local or diffuse peritonitis (2%–7%).[202–204]

Bleeding is the most common symptom of colorectal malignancy.[205] Unfortunately, patient and physician alike often attribute the bleeding to hemorrhoids. Bleeding may be occult or it may be seen as stool that is black, maroon, dark purple, or bright red depending on the location of the malignancy. Occult bleeding may present with iron-deficiency anemia and associated fatigue.

Change in bowel habits is the second most common complaint, with patients noting either diarrhea or constipation.[205] Constipation is more often associated with left-sided lesions because the diameter of the colon is smaller and the stool is more formed than on the right side. Patients may report a gradual change in the caliber of the stool or may have diarrhea if the narrowing has progressed sufficiently to cause obstruction. Carcinomas of the right side of the colon do not typically present with changes in bowel habits, but large

TABLE 23.7.

Impact of FOBT on Mortality from Colorectal Malignancy.

Author	*Level of evidence*	*n*	*Design*	*Result*
Mandel[347]	I	46,551	Annual FOBT vs biennial FOBT vs usual care	Annual FOBT → 33% ↓ mortality, biennial no Δ
Hardcastle[348]	I	152,850	Biennial FOBT vs usual care	Biennial FOBT → 15% ↓ mortality
Kronborg[349]	I	61,933	Biennial FOBT vs usual care	Biennial FOBT → 18% ↓ mortality
Winawer[350]	I	21,756	Annual FOBT plus rigid sigmoidoscopy vs annual rigid sigmoidoscopy alone	Annual FOBT → 43% ↓ mortality over rigid sigmoidoscopy alone
Kewenter[351]	I	21,347 initial and 19,991 @ follow-up	FOBT initial evaluation and @ 16–24 months	Mortality Δ pending but earlier stage tumors

TABLE 23.8.

Impact of Sigmoidoscopy on Mortality from Colorectal Malignancy.

Author	Level of evidence	n	Design	Result	Comments
Selby[190]	III	1129	Case control study of rigid sigmoidoscopy (261 case subjects)	59% ↓ in mortality	↓ in mortality only for portion of bowel visualized
Newcomb[191]	III	262	Case control study of rigid sigmoidoscopy (66 case subjects)	80% ↓ in mortality	
Muller[192]	III	—	Case control study of diagnostic procedures of the large bowel	59% ↓ in mortality	Greatest benefit with "tissue removal"

amounts of mucus generated by a tumor may cause diarrhea, and large right-sided lesions or lesions involving the ileocecal valve may cause obstruction.

Abdominal pain is as common a presentation as change in bowel habits.[206] Left-sided obstructing lesions may present with cramping abdominal pain, associated with nausea and vomiting, and relieved with bowel movements. Right-sided malignancies may result in vague pain that is difficult to localize. Rectal lesions may present with tenesmus, but pelvic pain is generally associated with advanced disease after the tumor has involved the sacral or sciatic nerves. Less common symptoms include weight loss, malaise, fever, abdominal mass, and symptoms of urinary tract involvement (frequency, pneumaturia, and fecaluria). Bacteremia with *Streptococcus bovis* is highly suggestive of colorectal malignancy.[207,208]

Acute onset of intestinal obstruction was the presenting feature of 15% of about 23,500 patients reported in 26 series.[209] Physical exam is often unrevealing because the abdomen is distended and masses, primary or metastatic, are not palpable. Colorectal malignancy should always be considered when patients present with large-bowel obstruction. The history, physical exam, and plain films of the abdomen may suggest the diagnosis. It may be confirmed with contrast enema, rigid or flexible endoscopy, or CT scans of the abdomen and pelvis.

Perforation may result in localized peritonitis or generalized peritonitis or, if walled off, it may present with obstruction or fistula to an adjacent structure such as the bladder. When the perforation occurs proximal to the obstructing lesion, as with perforation of a dilated cecum proximal to an obstructing sigmoid carcinoma, the patients present with diffuse peritonitis and sepsis. Emergent surgical intervention after adequate fluid resuscitation is clearly indicated. However, in the case of perforation at the tumor, possibly secondary to tumor necrosis, the more indolent course may lead to confusion of the perforated tumor with inflammation associated with appendicitis, diverticulitis, or Crohn's disease.

STAGING

Staging systems are important for predicting outcomes, selecting patients for various therapies, and comparing therapies for like patients across institutions. For a tumor to be considered as an invasive cancer and staged, it must penetrate through the muscularis mucosa. Malignant cells superficial to this layer are thought to lack metastatic potential because of a paucity of lymphatics and are considered carcinoma in situ. In 1932, Dukes proposed a classification based on the extent of direct extension along with the presence or absence of regional lymphatic metastases for the staging of rectal cancer. Dukes' A lesions are those in which the depth of penetration of the primary tumor is confined to the bowel wall. Dukes' B tumors have primary tumor penetration through the full thickness of the bowel to include serosa or fat. Dukes' C lesions have local (C_1) or regional (C_2) nodal involvement. Although not initially described, it became accepted by common practice to add a fourth category for distant spread (D) outside the resected specimen. The Astler-Coller Modification divided the Dukes' B and C cases depending on the depth

TABLE 23.9. Summary of the Characteristics of Screening Tests for Colorectal Malignancy.

Screening test	Overall performance	Complexity	Potential effectiveness	Evidence of effectiveness	Screening test risk
FOBT	Intermediate for carcinomas, low for polyps	Lowest	Lowest	Strongest	Lowest
Flexible sigmoidoscopy	High for up to half of the colon	Intermediate	Intermediate	Intermediate	Intermediate
FOBT plus flexible sigmoidoscopy	Same as flexible sigmoidoscopy and FOBT	Intermediate	Intermediate	Intermediate	Intermediate
DCBE	High	High	High	Weakest	Intermediate
Colonoscopy	Highest	Highest	Highest	Weakest	Highest

FOBT, fecal occult blood test; DCBE, double-contrast barium enema.

Source: From Winawer SJ, Fletcher H, Miller L, et al. Colorectal cancer screening: clinical guidelines and rationale. Gastroenterology 1997;112:594–642.

TABLE 23.10. AJCC Definition of TNM for Colon and Rectum Cancers Staging System.

Primary Tumor (T)

TX	Primary tumor cannot be assessed
T0	No evidence of primary tumor
Tis	Carcinoma *in situ*: intraepithelial or invasion of lamina propria*
T1	Tumor invades submucosa
T2	Tumor invades muscularis propria
T3	Tumor invades through the muscularis propria into the subserosa, or into non-peritonealized pericolic or perirectal tissues
T4	Tumor directly invades other organs or structures, and/or perforates visceral peritoneum**,***

*Note: Tis includes cancer cells confined within the glandular basement membrane (intraepithelial) or lamina propria (intramucosal) with no extension through the muscularis mucosae into the submucosa.

**Note: Direct invasion in T4 includes invasion of other segments of the colorectum by way of the serosa; for example, invasion of the sigmoid colon by a carcinoma of the cecum.

***Tumor that is adherent to other organs or structures, macroscopically, is classified T4. However, if no tumor is present in the adhesion, microscopically, the classification should be pT3. The V and L substaging should be used to identify the presence or absence of vascular or lymphatic invasion.

Regional Lymph Nodes (N)

NX	Regional lymph nodes cannot be assessed*
N0	No regional lymph node metastasis
N1	Metastasis in 1 to 3 regional lymph nodes
N2	Metastasis in 4 or more regional lymph nodes

*Note: A tumor nodule in the pericolorectal adipose tissue of a primary carcinoma without histologic evidence of residual lymph node in the nodule is classified in the pN category as a regional lymph node metastasis if the nodule has the form and smooth contour of a lymph node. If the nodule has an irregular contour, it should be classified in the T category and also coded as V1 (microscopic venous invasion) or as V2 (if it was grossly evident), because there is a strong likelihood that it represents venous invasion.

Distant Metastasis (M)

MX	Distant metastasis cannot be assessed
M0	No distant metastasis
M1	Distant metastasis

Source: Used with permission of the American Joint Committee on Cancer (AJCC), Chicago, IL. The original source for this material is the AJCC Cancer Staging Manual, Sixth Edition (2002) published by Springer-Verlag New York, www.springer-ny.com

TABLE 23.11. Comparison of AJCC Definition of TNM System to Duke's Classification.

Stage	T	N	M	Dukes*
0	Tis	N0	M0	—
I	T1	N0	M0	A
	T2	N0	M0	A
IIA	T3	N0	M0	B
IIB	T4	N0	M0	B
IIIA	T1-T2	N1	M0	C
IIIB	T3-T4	N1	M0	C
IIIC	Any T	N2	M0	C
IV	Any T	Any N	M1	—

Source: *Dukes B is a composite of better (T3 N0 M0) and worse (T4 N0 M0) prognostic groups, as is Dukes C (Any TN1 M0 and Any T N2 M0). Used with permission of the American Joint Committee on Cancer (AJCC), Chicago, IL. The original source for this material is the AJCC Cancer Staging Manual, Sixth Ed. (2002) published by Springer-Verlag New York, www.springer-ny.com

PREOPERATIVE STAGING FOR COLORECTAL CANCER

The general physical examination remains a cornerstone in assessing a patient preoperatively to determine the extent of local disease, disclosing distant metastases, and appraising the general operative risk. Special interest should be paid to weight loss, pallor as a sign of anemia, and signs of portal hypertension. In addition, a complete workup should include the investigations listed in Table 23.12.

POLYPS: COLONIC

NATURAL HISTORY

In healthy colonic epithelium, there is a normal, constant renewal of the surface epithelium approximately every 6 days by cellular proliferation and differentiation of crypt cells. As cells move up the crypt, differentiation and maturation occur, and the cells lose their capacity to divide again. Eventually cells die and are shed into the colonic lumen. In the adenoma, this is markedly altered. There is continued mitosis and lack of differentiation of cells so that the proliferative compartment may envelop the entire crypt. The persistent replication of cells near the crypt surface, coupled with retarded cell maturation and extrusion, results in an increased number of replicating surface cells.

A colorectal polyp is defined as a mass that protrudes into the lumen of the colon. These masses may either be sessile or pedunculated. The clinical significance of polyps is defined by their histological classification. The main distinction is between neoplastic and nonneoplastic polyps. Adenomas are benign neoplasms with dysplasia. Nonneoplastic polyps are without dysplastic features and include mucosal, hyperplastic, inflammatory, and hamartomatous (including juvenile) polyps. Approximately 70% of colonoscopically removed polyps are adenomas. Their growth patterns as tubular, villous, or tubulovillous further classifies adenomas.

In autopsy series, the prevalence of sporadic colorectal adenomas is: 30% at 50 years of age, 40% to 50% at 60 years, and 50% to 65% at 70 years of age. Endoscopic studies reveal lower rates, between 10% and 20%, in individuals, even

of primary spread, with Dukes' B_1 including tumors with penetration confined to the bowel wall and B_2 lesions including tumors that penetrate the bowel wall. If nodal disease is present, the tumor depth of penetration determines whether the lesion is C_1 [B_1 with (+) nodes] or C_2 [B_2 with (+) nodes].

The TNM (tumor/node/metastasis) classification was proposed by the American College of Surgeons' Commission on Cancer to incorporate findings at laparotomy. The stages of the TNM system roughly correlate to the stages with Dukes' classification: stage 1 equivalent to Dukes' A; stage 2 equivalent to Dukes' B; stage 3 equivalent to Dukes' C; and stage 4 equivalent to Dukes' D (Tables 23.10, 23.11).

Classification of histological grade, cell type, lymphatic, venous or perineural invasion, tumor ploidy, carcinoembryonic antigen (CEA) level, bowel perforation, and distal and tangential margins allow for further subclassification of the tumors and improved prognostication.

TABLE 23.12. Preoperative Evaluation for Colorectal Malignancy.

Routine blood work	CBC, LFT, CEA
Colonoscopy	Tissue diagnosis, synchronous disease
Radiographs	CXR, seleced CT abdomen/pelvis
Ultrasound	Transrectal ultrasound

though these studies are performed in populations with a high prevalence of adenomas.

The overall risk of an adenoma progressing to cancer is between 2.5% and 8% over a 10-year period and increases with the size of the polyp.[210,211] After 20 years the relative risk increases to 24%, and having multiple adenomas increases the risk for developing subsequent adenomas and adenocarcinomas. Polyp type also impacts the rate at which cancer is found in the polyp.[212]

MALIGNANT POLYPS

A malignant polyp is an adenoma in which carcinoma has invaded across the muscularis mucosa. Endoscopic polypectomy is curative in 99.7% of cases of pedunculated and 98.5% of cases of sessile malignant polyps. In the case of incomplete resection, poor differentiation, lymphatic or vascular invasion, cure rates following endoscopic polypectomy decrease to 91% and segmental colectomy may be indicated.

COLORECTAL DISTRIBUTION

The distribution of adenomas changes with age. In patients older than 55 years the incidence of proximal polyps increases.[213]

ENDOSCOPIC MANAGEMENT OF BENIGN ADENOMAS

Colonscopy has revolutionized the management of large-bowel polyps. Most polyps throughout the colon can be removed through the colonoscope using the snare polypectomy technique. When performed by trained endoscopists, colonoscopy with polypectomy is a safe procedure, with a perforation incidence of 0.3% to 1% and a hemorrhage incidence of 0.7% to 2.5%.[214,215]

INDICATIONS FOR SURGERY

The majority of colorectal polyps found at endoscopy are suitable for snare excision via colonoscope. However, because of location and size, some are deemed unsafe to treat in this manner and therefore require colectomy. Surgical options include segmental bowel resection via laparotomy and colotomy with open polypectomy. Laparoscopic segmental colon resection, as well as laparoscopic-assisted endoscopic polypectomy, are also available in selected cases.[216]

Special problems arise with better understanding of the molecular changes in the development of colorectal cancer. The term aggressive adenoma was created because the adenoma–carcinoma sequence seems to be accelerated in patients with HNPCC. It has therefore been recommended that subtotal colectomy be offered to HNPCC patients with polyps. A less radical approach is hemicolectomy in the case of multiple polyps confined to an anatomical region.

POLYPS: RECTAL

About 8% of colorectal polyps are located in the rectum.[212] They represent a unique situation as they can be palpated with the finger or visualized through a sigmoidoscope. If invasive cancer is considered, rectal ultrasound can be performed. It is well recognized that larger polyps carry a higher risk for dysplasia and carcinoma.

SURGICAL OPTIONS

Most rectal polyps are removed during colonoscopy or proctoscopy using different snaring devices. Most polyps up to 2 cm can be removed with a single snare. Larger polyps may be snared in pieces or removed per anus if within the distal 10 cm of the rectum. Piece-by-piece snaring may be performed in multiple sessions at 4- to 6-week intervals.

Large villous or tubulovillous adenomas are removed by transanal excision. If the tumor is not indurated or ulcerated, the chance that it is benign is 90%.[217] Preoperative biopsies are unreliable as they have a false-negative rate up to 30%.[218] The entire tumor is removed in one piece whenever possible to ensure adequate histological evaluation.

Cancer of the Colon

NATURAL HISTORY

Surgery remains the cornerstone of treatment for colorectal cancer but has inherent limitations imposed by the biology and stage of the tumor as well as its location. Ultimately, 50% of patients who undergo curative resection develop local, regional, or widespread recurrence; this presumably occurs as a result of progression of micrometastases present at the time of initial operation. Colorectal tumors are relatively slow-growing neoplasms, and metastases occur relatively late. Five-year survival rates are presented in Table 23.13.

BOWEL PREPARATION

Mechanical cleansing may be accomplished by the use of vigorous laxatives along with repeated enemas until clearing. Commonly used products include GoLYTELY, Phospho-Soda, and Fleet enemas.

ANTIBIOTIC ADMINISTRATION

Although there is no question that preoperative antibiotic administration is beneficial in elective and emergency colorectal surgery, the route of administration and antibiotic combination remains a matter of debate. Most surgeons start antibiotic prophylaxis at the day of operation using a combination to cover gram-positive and gram-negative, aerobic and anaerobic bacteria. Whether the antibiotic is given orally or intravenously does not appear to matter so long as the antibiotic is administered before skin incision. There is no evidence that antibiotic administration after the first initial postoperative day is beneficial.

SURGICAL STAPLERS IN COLORECTAL SURGERY

Surgical staplers have gained increased popularity in recent years and can be acceptably used as long as the general principles of anastomoses are maintained: adequate blood supply, absence of tension, and accurate apposition of healthy tissue.

CANCER OF THE CECUM, ASCENDING COLON, OR HEPATIC FLEXURE

For lesions located in the cecum or ascending colon, a right hemicolectomy to encompass the bowel served by the ileo-

TABLE 23.13. The Stage-Dependent Relative 5-Year Survival Rate.

Location	Stage 1 (% survival)	Stage 2 (% survival)	Stage 3 (% survival)	Stage 4 (% survival)
Colon	70	60	44	7
Rectum	72	54	39	7

Source: Beart et al. (1995)[206]; Jessup et al. (1996).[352]

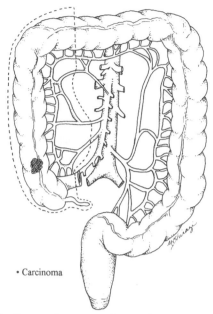

FIGURE 23.8. Extent of resection for cecal, ascending colon, or hepatic flexure carcinoma. (Adapted from Gordon and Nivatvongs.[134])

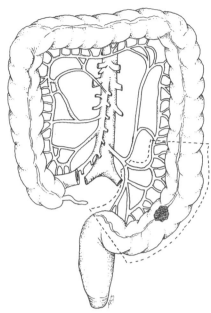

FIGURE 23.10. Extent of resection for sigmoid colon carcinoma. (Adapted from Gordon and Nivatvongs.[134])

colic, right colic, and right branch of the middle colic vessels is recommended (Fig. 23.8).

For lesions involving the hepatic flexure, a more extended resection is indicated including the right colon and proximal and midtransverse colon including both branches of the middle colic artery. This is often referred to as "an extended right hemicolectomy." The method of bowel division depends on the preferred method of anastomoses.

Cancer of the Transverse Colon

Depending on the exact location of the tumor, the transverse colon is often resected including either the hepatic or splenic

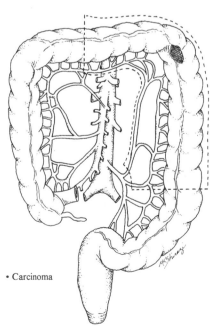

FIGURE 23.9. Extent of resection for a splenic flexure colon carcinoma. (Adapted from Gordon and Nivatvongs.[134])

flexure. As the resection needs to fulfill oncological principles, the appropriate lymphatic drainage must be included. The lymphatic drainage may occur through the middle colic and or the right or left colic branches. For technical reasons it is usually easier to include the ascending colon in the resection rather than mobilizing both flexures.

Cancer of the Splenic Flexure

Splenic flexure lesions require removal of the distal half of the transverse colon and the descending colon (Fig. 23.9). After resection, a tension-free anastomosis is performed between the distal transverse colon and the proximal sigmoid colon.

Cancer of the Sigmoid Colon

Sigmoid lesions are treated by removal of the sigmoid colon. The exact boundaries of resection depends on the level of the tumor (Fig. 23.10). Resections of higher sigmoid lesions include the descending–sigmoid junction, whereas resections for lower lesions include the recto–sigmoid junction. More radical procedures such as high ligation of the inferior mesenteric artery at its root have not been shown to increase survival and are associated with increased complications.[219]

Total Abdominal Colectomy

The incidence of synchronous lesions (more than one carcinoma at different sites) is reported to be between 1.5% and 7.6%.[220,221] The 5-year survival rate by stage was 87% for stage 1, 69% for stage 2, 50% for stage 3, and 14% for stage 4.[222] Subtotal colectomy is the treatment of choice for patients with synchronous lesions at different sites. If synchronous lesions are located in the same anatomical region, a conventional resection may be performed.[222] The rectum is not removed unless it has pathological lesions as well. When the rectum is removed, an ileoanal pouch procedure may be performed if intestinal continuity is to be restored. However, creation of the pouch after adequate pathological staging and treat-

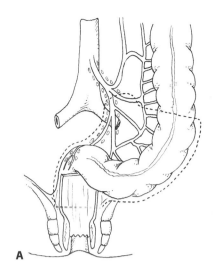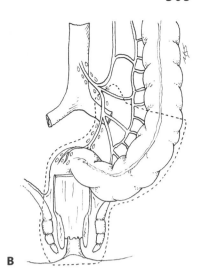

FIGURE 23.11. Extent of resection with either (**A**) low anterior resection of the rectum or (**B**) abdominal perineal resection for rectal adenocarcinoma. (Adapted from Gordon and Nivatvongs.[134])

ment of a rectal cancer would seem advisable as the small bowel does not tolerate radiation well.

Cancer of the Rectum

NATURAL HISTORY

About 30% of all colorectal cancers are rectal. In 1995, the American Cancer Society estimated 40,000 new cases in the United States.

SELECTION OF OPERATION AND ASSESSMENT OF RESECTABILITY

Rectal cancer has traditionally been treated with abdominoperineal resection, which removes the whole rectum and anus. More recently, the low anterior resection and local excision with and without radiation have gained popularity. Both preserve continence and can result in equal 5-year survival rates in properly selected patients. Thus, preoperative staging is critical to the selection of the appropriate operation.

Depending on the depth of invasion, location, distal and proximal margins, involvement of lymph nodes, and status of distant disease, the surgeon chooses between local transanal and transabdominal techniques with mesenteric resection. Local excision is performed in small tumors for cure and in advanced disease for palliation where excision of the mesentery does not improve survival. In the case of mid- to distal rectal

cancers, a low anterior resection (LAR) is attempted, with a goal of transecting the rectum at least 2 cm inferior to the lower end of the carcinoma. If this is technically not achievable, an abdominoperineal resection (APR) is performed (Fig. 23.11). In an APR, a very low anterior resection is done in combination with a complete perineal excision of the anus and rectum, and an endcolostomy is brought out on the anterior abdominal wall.

LOCAL PER ANAL EXCISION OR DESTRUCTION

Generally, lesions within 8 cm of the anal verge that are less than 4 cm, well or moderately well differentiated, mobile, not ulcerated, and without evidence of nodal involvement are considered for transanal excision. Nodal involvement may be as high as 18% in T1 lesions and up to 38% in T2 lesions,[223,224] leaving about 5% of rectal cancers as suitable for attempt at cure with local excision alone[225] (Table 23.14). However, if one plans local excision followed by chemoradiation or radiation, excellent local control has been achieved for T1 and T2 lesions[226] (Table 23.15).

Transanal destruction with electrocautery or radiation therapy may also be used to control the tumor within the pelvis. The radiation therapy may be delivered as the sole treatment or may be combined with excisional therapy.

TRANSANAL ENDOSCOPIC MICROSURGERY (TEM)

Transanal endoscopic microsurgery has been used for the local treatment of benign and malignant rectal tumors.[227] The

TABLE 23.14.

Results for Selected Series of Local Excision of Rectal Cancer Alone With Intent to Cure.

Author	No. patients	Margins	Stage	Local recurrence (%)	Salvage surgery[a] (%)	Cancer-specific survival (%)	Follow-up (months)
Morson[353]	91	Negative	T1, T2	3	66	100	
Hager[354]	36	Negative	T1	8	NS	90	33
	18	Negative	T2	17	NS	78	40
Heimann[355]	14	Negative	T1, T2	21	100	93	48
Obrand[356]	19	Negative	T1, T2 (one T3)	26	60	82	58
Garcia-Aguilar[357]	57	Negative	T1	15	70	97	48
	28	Negative	T2	39	87	84	55

Source: Reprinted with permission from Ambulatory Anorectal Surgery, edited by Bailey and Synder, ©2000, Springer-Verlag New York.

TABLE 23.15.

Results for Selected Series of Local Excision of Rectal Cancer and Postoperative Radiation or Chemoradiotherapy.

Author	No. patients	Negative margins (%)	Stage	Radiation (cGy)	Chemo-therapy	Local recurrence (%)	Salvage surgery[a] (%)	Survival (%)	Follow-up (months)
Rosenthal[358]	16	100	2 T1 9 T2 5 T3	2700–5700	No	12.50	100	94 (3 years)	33
Bailey[359]	53	100	35 T1 18 T2	4500–5000[b]	No	8	50	90	44
Minsky[360]	22	95	4 T1 12 T2 6 T3	4500–7380	Variable	18	75	79 (4 years)	37
Fortunato[361]	21	66	2 T1 15 T2 4 T3	2700–6300	10%	19	75	58	56
Ota[362]	46	100	16 T1 15 T2 15 T3	5300	Variable	8	NS	NS	35
Bleday[363]	21	100	21 T2	5400	Yes	0	—	100	43

Source: Reprinted with permission from Ambulatory Anorectal Surgery, edited by Bailey and Synder, ©2000, Springer-Verlag, New York.

system uses a special rectoscope, which allows continuous carbon dioxide insufflation to keep the rectum open for exposure. The surgeon operates with instruments similar to those used in laparoscopic surgery. Vision is provided through a magnifying optical system, which is hooked up to a TV screen. The procedure is used for lesions in the upper, middle, and low rectum. The excision is done with electrocautery and the defect is closed with a running suture. Complication rates are low as reported, but include bleeding, breakdown of suture line, and rectovaginal fistula.[228–230]

Obstructing Colon Cancer

Colon cancer is the most common cause of large-bowel obstruction. This complication occurs as a presenting manifestation in up to 15% to 20% of patients with colorectal cancer.[231] Obstructing colon cancers are generally caused by larger tumors and have a poorer prognosis. The incidence of obstruction correlates with advancing patient age and is most commonly seen with left-sided colon cancer.

The treatment is dependent on the location of the obstruction. Primary resection and anastomosis generally treat right-sided and transverse tumors. A diverting colostomy or ileostomy is rarely needed. The anastomosis can be performed using either hand suturing or stapling techniques. The leak rate should not exceed 3% with either technique.[232]

The treatment of descending and more distal tumors is more complex and controversial. Historically, there are three procedures: the three-stage procedure, the Hartmann's procedure, and the subtotal colectomy with primary anastomosis. The three-stage operation with a transverse colostomy, as an initial procedure, followed by a resection and anastomosis and finally by closure of the colostomy, is generally of historical interest only. However, if the patient is too sick to tolerate a definitive procedure, this is certainly an option.

The second option, and that most commonly utilized, is to resect the colon and tumor, fashion a colostomy from the proximal bowel, and oversew the distal bowel. This is commonly referred to as a Hartmann's procedure, which is incorrect because that procedure is for rectal cancer in particular. Alternatively, if the distal bowel is of adequate length, if may

be brought up to the abdominal wall, opened, and sutured to the skin as a mucous fistula. Overall operative mortality is about 10%.[233] Colostomy closure rates are approximately 60%.

Subtotal colectomy with primary anastomosis has become increasingly popular recently. The procedure is a one-stage operation. Although this operation seems more extensive, good results can be achieved with a single shorter hospitalization, no stoma problems, and removal of possible synchronous proximal lesions. Mortality rates are as low as 3% in experienced hands, and morbidity ranges between 6% and 31%,[234] competitive with the more accepted resection and colostomy procedure. These data suggest that a subtotal colectomy and primary anastomosis is the preferred approach in the patient with an obstructing colon cancer on the left side.

Perforated Colon Cancer

Perforation of colorectal cancer is associated with a poor prognosis and a high recurrence rate. About 3% to 9% of patients with colorectal carcinoma present with a perforation as their initial manifestation. In about 66%, localized perforation with abscess occurs, while in about 33% free perforation with peritonitis occurs.[203] The tumor itself may be perforated or there may be a right-sided perforation with a left-sided tumor. Whenever possible, the perforated bowel segment should be resected at the initial operation. Reanastomosis is feasible in many patients and should be accompanied by a protective proximal stoma in most cases. If the patient has generalized peritonitis, colectomy, colostomy formation, and oversewing of the distal bowel or mucous fistula creation should be considered. In the case of a perforation remote from the diseased segment, a subtotal colectomy should be considered as the therapy of choice.

Cancer Arising in a Colon Polyp

There is now a general consensus that most colon cancers arise from preexisting polyps. The lifetime risk of an adenoma transforming into a malignancy is estimated to be 5% to 10%, and the time for transforming is estimated to be 5 to 15 years.[235] Colonoscopy and complete polypectomy are curative in 99% of the patients with carcinoma in situ, as these lesions appear to have no potential for metastases. On the other hand, lymph node metastases can be demonstrated in approximately 12% of patients, with carcinoma invading into the submucosa.[236] In otherwise healthy patients with submucosal invasive carcinoma arising in a polyp, formal colon resection is recommended to remove any residual cancer. Discovery of lymph node metastases justifies adjuvant chemotherapy.

Therapy for Metastatic Colorectal Cancer

Of 100 patients with colorectal cancer, 50 will be cured by surgery, 15 will develop local recurrence, and 35 will develop blood-borne distant metastases. The organs most frequently involved are the liver in 75%, the lung in 15%, and the bone and the brain in 5%.[237] In patients who develop colorectal liver metastases, the main cause of death is liver failure. Patients with untreated diffuse liver metastases have a median survival of 7 to 10 months.[238] By comparison, patients with multiple metastases limited to one lobe have a mean survival of 15 months, and those with only one lesion have a median survival of 21 months without resection.

The mode of treatment of liver metastases from colorectal carcinoma is still a matter of debate. Chemotherapeutic regimens including systemic, intraarterial, and intraportal administration have only had moderate benefit. Systemic chemotherapy has resulted in response rates of 18% to 28%, but with the cost of considerable toxicity and anxiety.[239] Thus, the lack of effective therapeutic alternatives has made hepatic resection or cryoablation a primary treatment consideration.

Pulmonary metastases alone are more common in patients with rectal primaries. Only 1% to 4% of all patients develop pulmonary metastases that are amenable for surgery. Ideally, in determining resectability, the metastasis should be solitary, the primary should be controlled, there should be no evidence of other metastases, and the patient should be a good surgical candidate. A chest CT scan is essential to characterize the extent and locations of pulmonary lesions. The median survival after pulmonary resection of colorectal metastases is approximately 24 months. Operative mortality rates are 0% to 5%.[240–242]

Therapy for Local Recurrent Colorectal Cancer

Of all colorectal recurrences, 70% occur within 2 years of operation.[243] Local recurrences vary between 1% and 20% for colon cancer and between 3% and 32% for rectal cancer.[244–247]

OPERATIVE TREATMENT

In selected circumstances, when technically possible the best chance for cure is resection of the recurrent lesion. Radical surgery may need to be considered in selected patients, and the type of operation varies on the location. Debulking operations play only a minor role except for palliation of symptoms such as bleeding, bowel obstruction, and severe pain.

ENDOSCOPIC LASER THERAPY

For the recurrent unresectable tumor, relief of obstruction and control of bleeding may be obtained by the user of a laser. This procedure offers no relief of pain nor does it prolong survival.[248] It can be performed as an outpatient procedure, and only very little sedation is needed.

TUMOR STENTING

Relief of obstruction may also be obtained by the use of a bowel stent. This procedure offers no relief of pain nor does

it prolong survival, but in select patients it may relieve obstruction, allowing for subsequent radiation therapy, and even bowel preparation and attempted resection.

RADIOTHERAPY

External beam radiotherapy is the therapy most frequently used to control local recurrences of rectal cancer. The average survival rate after palliative radiation therapy is about 20 months.[249] External beam radiotherapy has proven of no benefit for recurrent colon cancer, mainly because of the effects of radiation on the remaining abdominal viscera. Intraoperative radiotherapy or brachytherapy have shown promise in the treatment of recurrent colon and rectal adenocarcinoma.

CHEMOTHERAPY

Systemic chemotherapy has not demonstrated dramatic or long-term effects. Some palliation has been reported with the use of intraarterial 5-FU and mitomycin.[250]

Adjuvant Therapy: Colon Cancer

CHEMOTHERAPY

The use of adjuvant chemotherapy is recommended by the National Institutes of Health (NIH) as "standard" for patients with stage 3 disease (any T, $N_{1,2}$). The recommendation was based on two studies that showed that the combination of 5-FU and levamisole had a reduced risk of carcinoma recurrences of 43% in stage 3 patients and that the overall death rate was reduced by 33%.[251,252] A similar benefit was seen with 5-FU and leucovorin with a 30% and 32% reduction in recurrences and mortality, respectively.[253] The benefit of chemotherapy in the treatment of stage 2 disease remains unclear, and it is administered on an individualized basis because of contradictory evidence.[254,255]

RADIOTHERAPY

There is only a limited role for radiotherapy in the treatment of colon cancer, although it plays a major role in the treatment of rectal cancer. If the margins are grossly or microscopically positive, improved palliation and survival have been reported with radiation therapy.[256–261]

IMMUNOTHERAPY

There is no conclusive evidence that immunotherapy improves either survival or recurrence rates.

ADJUVANT THERAPY: RECTAL CANCER

Radiation therapy may be delivered, with or without chemotherapy, preoperatively, intraoperatively, or postoperatively, in the treatment of rectal cancer. The potential benefits of preoperative radiation therapy (with or without chemotherapy) are (1) large tumors may shrink, increasing resectability of the tumor; (2) tumors cells within the lymphatics may be sterilized, decreasing seeding of viable tumor cells at the time of surgery; (3) radiation therapy works better in well-oxygenated tissues and the postoperative tissue may be relatively hypoxic; (4) surgical complications may lead to a long delay in therapy; and (5) preoperative radiation minimizes the risk of radiating the same loop of small bowel that may be fixed in the pelvis after surgery. The reputed disadvantages are possible overtreatment of stage 1 and 2 lesions assumed to be stage 3 lesions on pre-

TABLE 23.16.

Results of Randomized Trials of Preoperative Radiotherapy (Level I Evidence).

Trial (author(s))	No. of patients	Dose (Gy/Fractions)	Dukes' stage C (%)	Local recurrence (%)	Distant metastases (%)	Overall 5-year survival (%)
MRC 1[364] (1984)	824	Control	46	No difference	No difference	38
		5/1	45			41
		20/10	36*			40
VASOG 2[365] (Higgins, Humphrey, and Dweight, 1986)	361	Control	41			42
		31.5/18	35			43
EORTC[366] (Gerard et al., 1988)	466	Control	59	30	39	59
		34.5/15	55	15*	39	69
Sao Paulo[367] (Reis Neto, Guilic, and Reis Neto, 1989)	68	Control	47	47	32	34
		40/20	26*	15*	15*	80*
Norway[368] (Dahl et al., 1990)	309	Control	28	21	21	58
		31.5/18	18*	15	23	57
ICRF[369] (Goldberg et al., 1994)	468	Control	No difference	24		40
		15/3		17*		39
Northwest Region[370] (Marsh, James, and Schofield, 1994)	284	Control		37	36	70
		20/4		13*	43	70
Stockholm I[371] (Cedermark et al., 1995)	849	Control	28	28	37	36
		25/5-7	28	14*	30	36
Stockholm II[372] (Cedermark et al., 1996)	557	Control		21	26	56
		25/5		10*	19*	70*
SRCT[373] (1997)	1168	Control		27		48
		25/5		11		58*

MRC = Medical Research Council; VASOG = Veterans' Administration Surgical Oncology Group Trial II; EORTC = European Organization for Research and Treatment of Cancer; ICRF = Imperial Cancer Research Foundation; SRCT = Swedish Rectal Cancer Trial.

*Statistically significant.

Source: From Gordon and Nivatvongs,[134] with permission.

operative evaluation, loss of accurate pathological staging at the time of resection because of "downstaging," delay in "definitive resection," and risk of increased operative complications secondary to radiation injury. The results for randomized trials suggest that regardless of whether it is delivered preoperatively or postoperatively, radiation therapy appears to have a significant impact on local recurrence but does not appear to improve survival. (Tables 23.16 and 23.17)

The addition of chemotherapy to radiation may improve

TABLE 23.17.

Results of Randomized Trials of Postoperative Radiotherapy (Level I Evidence).

Trial (author(s))	No. of patients	Dose (Gy/Fractions)	Dukes' stage	Local recurrence (%)	Distant metastases (%)	Overall 5-year survival (%)
GITSG[262] (1985)	227	Operation alone	B$_2$ and C	24	34	43
		CT		27	27	57
		40–48 Gy/22–27		20	30	50
		CT + 40-44 Gy/22–24		11	26	59
Denmark[374] (Balsev et al., 1986)	494	Operation alone	B/C	18	14	Similar
		50 Gy/25		16	19	
NSABP[375] (Fisher et al., 1988)	555	Operation alone	B and C	25	27	43
		CT		21	24	53*
		46–47 Gy/26–27		16	31	50
Netherlands[376] (Treurniet-Donker et al., 1991)	172	Operation alone	B$_2$/C	33	26	57
		50 Gy/25		20	36	45
MRC3[377] (Gates et al., 1995)	469	Operation alone	B/C	34	35	38
		40 Gy/20		21*	31	41

CT = Chemotherapy; GITSIG = Gastrointestinal Tumor Study Group; MRC = Medical Research Council; NSABP = National Surgical Adjuvant Breast and Bowel Project.

*Statistically significant.

Source: From Gordon and Nivatvongs,[134] with permission.

local control and survival. A four-arm study compared surgery alone, postoperative chemotherapy, postoperative radiation, and postoperative radiation plus chemotherapy. The best results were achieved with the combination of postoperative chemoradiation, with a local recurrence rate of 11%, a distant metastases rate of 26%, and a 5-year overall survival of 59%. In comparison, the local recurrence rate for surgery alone was 24%, the distant metastases rate was 34%, and the 5-year survival rate was 43%.[262] In a study of 660 patients treated with postoperative radiation therapy with either bolus or continuous intravenous chemotherapy, local recurrence rates of 8% (bolus) to 11% (continuous) with an overall survival rate of 60% (bolus) to 70% (continuous) were reported. The distant metastases rate varied between 40% (bolus) and 31% (continuous).[263] Results of randomized trials of combined chemoradiation are presented in Table 23.18.

Intraoperative radiation is used in selected cases such as primary carcinomas and local recurrences considered unresectable for cure. A local control rate of 80% to 82% versus 24% to 67% without intraoperative radiation[264] and improved survival rates of 20% compared to the expected 5% are reported[134] when there is no evidence of tumor outside the pelvis.

Our preference is to deliver preoperative chemoradiation to large bulky lesions, to those tumors with obvious nodal or full-thickness disease where postoperative therapy seems certain. This decision is made after lengthy and frank discussions with the patient and family members about the risks and benefits of the various protocols. Intraoperative radiation is recommended for carefully selected patients with primary or recurrent disease that appears close to but not invading unresectable structures in the pelvis (nerves and bone).

POLYPOSIS COLI SYNDROMES

FAMILIAL ADENOMATOUS POLYPOSIS

Familial adenomatous polyposis (FAP) is an inherited, non-sex-linked, dominant disease characterized by the progressive development of hundreds of polyps. The mutated gene is found on the long arm of chromosome 5 and is called the APC gene. Polyps occur at a mean age of 16 years and almost all affected persons exhibit adenomas by age 35 years. Seven percent of untreated individuals have cancer by age 21, 50% by age 39, and 90% by the age of 45 years. Large-bowel cancer is virtually inevitable if the colon is not removed.

Upper gastrointestinal manifestations of FAP include gastric polyps in 50% to 100% of affected persons and duodenal polyps in 90% to 100%. Duodenal polyps are adenomatous polyps that also bear some malignant risk because a 10% to 12% lifetime occurrence of periampullary duodenal cancer has been reported.

Extraintestinal manifestations of FAP include osteomas, soft tissue tumors of the skin, supernumerary teeth, desmoid tumors, and congenital hypertrophy of the retinal pigment epithelium.

All first-degree relatives of an individual with newly diagnosed FAP should undergo colonoscopy to screen for the disease. In a family already known to have FAP, sigmoidoscopy screening in younger at-risk patients should begin between ages 10 to 12 years and be repeated every 1 to 2 years.

For a colon without polyps, it takes about 5 years to develop an adenoma and about another 5 years to develop invasive cancer.[265] Thus, removal of polyps is prophylactic against colon cancer. Timing of operation depends on the number of polyps found in the colon and rectum. Most centers recommend total colectomy with ileorectal anastamo-

TABLE 23.18.

Results of Randomized Trials of Combined Chemoradiation (Level I Evidence).

Trial (author(s))	No. of patients	Dose (Gy/Fraction)	Local recurrence (%)	Distant metastases (%)	Overall 5-year survival (%)
EORTC[378] (Boulis-Wassif et al., 1984)	247	Preop 34.5 Gy/15.0 Preop 34.5 Gy/15.0 + 5-FU	15 15	30 30	59 46
GITSG[262] (1985)	227	Operation alone CT Postop 40-48 Gy/22–27 CT + 40-44 Gy/22–21	24 27 20 11	34 27 30 26	43 57 50 59
NCCTG[379] (Krook et al.,1991)	209	Postop 45 Gy/25 + 5.4 Gy boost Postop 45 Gy/25 + 5-FU	23 14*	46 29*	38 53*
GITSG[380] (1992)	210	Postop 44.4 Gy/23 + 5-FU Postop 41.4 Gy/23 + 5-FU + Semustine	15 11	25 33	44 46
Intergroup[263] (O'Connell et al., 1994)	660	50.4/28 Gy + CT bolus 54 Gy/30 + CT continuous	11 8	40 31	60 70*
NSABP[381] (Hyams et al., 1996)	741	MOF 5-FU-leucovorin 5-FU + postop 46 Gy (26.5) 5-FU-leucovorin + postop 46 Gy	14 9*		66 68

CT = Chemotherapy; EORTC = European Organization for Research and Treatment of Cancer; GITSG = Gastrointestinal Tumor Study Group; MOF = methyl CCNU, vincristine sulfate (Oncovin), 5-FU; NCCTG = North Central Cancer Treatment Group; NSABP = National Surgical Adjuvant Breast and Bowel Project.

*Statistically significant.

Source: From Gordon and Nivatvongs,[134] with permission.

sis or restorative proctocolectomy with ileoanal pouch by the age of 25 years.

FAP families that exhibit frequent and prominent benign extraintestinal lesions, particularly osteomas and soft tissue tumors, are said to have Gardner's syndrome.

When central nervous system malignancies occur together with colonic polyposis, it is called Turcot's syndrome.

Hundreds or even thousands of polyps may be distributed throughout the entire colon and rectum, and the disease, called juvenile polyposis, may also involve the stomach and small bowel. This type of polyp is a hamartoma, however, and is not premalignant.

HEREDITARY NONPOLYPOSIS COLI SYNDROMES (HNPCC)

HNPCC is an autosomal dominant inherited disease with a high risk of colon cancer. The average age of colon cancer diagnosis is 45 years, and the lifetime risk of colon cancer is 80% in gene carriers. Despite its name, polyps are features of HNPCC as well in 8% to 17% of first-degree relatives.[266]

HNPCC has four major subtypes: Lynch 1, Lynch 2, Muir-Torr syndrome, and a variant of Turcot's syndrome. The Amsterdam criteria are clinical criteria developed to confirm the diagnosis of HNPCC: (1) at least three relatives with histologically verified colorectal carcinoma, one of whom should be first degree relative of the other two; (2) at least two successive generations should be affected; (3) in one of the relatives, colorectal carcinoma should have been diagnosed when the patient was younger than 50 years of age.

All patients with HNPCC need to be entered in a surveillance program by the age of 20 to 25 years. Screening should not only be directed to the colon but also to the pancreas, breast, cervix, and bladder.[463] Colonoscopic surveillance should be performed every other year until 30 years of age and annually thereafter. Some experts recommend prophylactic subtotal colectomy if no colorectal cancer is present at age 25, but others cite an extracolonic carcinoma incidence of 30% as reason for performing a standard hemicolectomy for malignancy should it develop.[267]

Anus: Benign Diseases and Neoplasms

Benign Diseases

ANORECTAL ABSCESS AND FISTULA

Perirectal abscess fistulous disease not associated with a specific systemic disease is most commonly cryptoglandular in origin.[237,268–270] The anal canal has 6 to 14 glands that lie in or near the intersphincteric plane between the internal and external sphincters. Projections from the glands pass through the internal sphincters and drain into the crypts at the dentate line. Glands may become infected when a crypt is occluded, trapping stool and bacteria within the gland. If the crypt does not decompress into the anal canal, an abscess may develop in the intersphincteric plane. Abscesses are classified by the space they invade (Fig. 23.12). Regardless of abscess location, the extent of disease is often difficult to determine without examination under anesthesia.

Antibiotics given while allowing the abscess to "mature" are not helpful. Early surgical consultation and operative

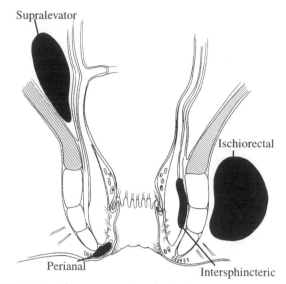

FIGURE 23.12. Abscesses are classified by location. (Reprinted with permission from Vasilevsky CA. Fistula-in-ano and abscess. In: Beck DE, Wexner SD (eds.), Fundamentals of Anorectal Surgery, ©1992, McGraw-Hill.)

drainage are the best measures to avoid the disastrous complications associated with undrained perineal sepsis. When drained, either surgically or spontaneously, 50% will have persistent communication with the crypt, creating a fistula from the anus to the perianal skin or fistula in ano. A fistula in ano is not a surgical emergency because the septic focus has drained.

An abscess typically causes severe continuous throbbing anal pain that may worsen with ambulation and straining.[271] Swelling and discharge are noted less frequently. A patient with fistula in ano may report a history of severe pain, bloody purulent drainage associated with resolution of the pain, and subsequent chronic mucopurulent discharge.

Physical examination of the patient with an abscess reveals a tender perianal or perirectal mass. A fistula is present when an internal and external opening are identified. A firm connecting tract is often palpable.

No imaging studies are necessary in uncomplicated abscess fistulous disease, but imaging studies such as sinograms, transrectal ultrasound, CT, and MRI may be useful in the evaluation of complex or recurrent disease.

Abscess fistula disease of cryptoglandular origin must be differentiated from complications of Crohn's disease, pilonidal disease, hidradenitis suppurativa, tuberculosis, actinomycosis, trauma, fissures, carcinoma, radiation, chlamydia, local dermal processes, retrorectal tumors, diverticulitis, and uretheral injuries.

The complications of an undrained anorectal abscess may be severe. If the abscess is not drained surgically or spontaneously, the infection may spread rapidly, which may result in extensive tissue loss, sphincter injury, and even death. In contrast, a fistula in ano, which may develop when the abscess is drained, is not a surgical emergency. A chronic fistula may be associated with recurring perianal abscesses and, rarely, with cancer of the fistulous tract.

Abscesses should be drained surgically. Patients often require drainage in the operating room where anesthesia allows for adequate evaluation of the extent of the disease. Intersphincteric abscesses are treated by internal sphincterotomy,

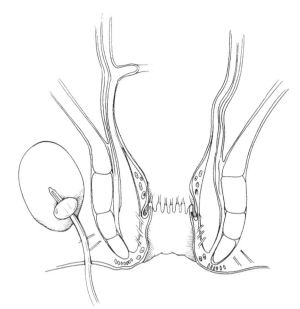

FIGURE 23.13. Catheter drainage of an ischiorectal abscess. The catheter is sewn to the skin with a 2-0 nylon that is cut after 1 week, and the "mushroom" anchors the tube in place. (Reprinted with permission from *Ambulatory Anorectal Surgery*, edited by Bailey and Synder, ©2000, Springer-Verlag, New York.)

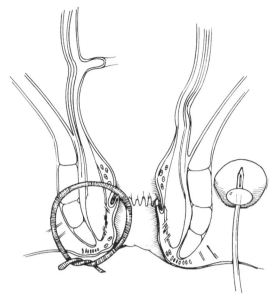

FIGURE 23.14. Control of perianal sepsis with a Seton and mushroom catheter for complex abscess fistulous disease or Crohn's disease. (Reprinted with permission from *Ambulatory Anorectal Surgery*, edited by Bailey and Synder, ©2000, Springer-Verlag, New York.)

which drains the abscess and destroys the crypt. Perirectal and ischiorectal abscesses should be drained by a catheter or with adequate excision of skin to prevent premature closure and reaccumulation of the abscess (Fig. 23.13).

Patients with a chronic or recurring abscess after apparent adequate surgical drainage often have an undrained deep postanal space abscess that communicates with the ischiorectal fossa via a "horseshoe fistula." Treatment involves opening the deep postanal space and counterdraining the tract through the ischiorectal external opening. Once the postanal space heals, the counterdrain may be removed.

Immunocompromised patients are a particular challenge. In the moderately compromised host, such as the diabetic patient, urgent drainage in the operating room is required because these patients are more prone to necrotizing anorectal infections. In the severely compromised host, patients receiving chemotherapy, an infection may be present without an "abscess" due to neutropenia. In these patients, it is important to attempt to localize the process, establish "drainage," localize the internal opening, and biopsy the tissue for pathology and culture (to rule out leukemia and select antibiotics).

The treatment of fistulas is dictated by the course of the fistula. If the tract passes superficially and does not involve sphincter muscle, then a simple incision of the tract with ablation of the gland and "saucerization" of the skin at the external opening is all that is necessary. A fistula that involves a small amount of sphincter (except anterior midline in women) may be treated similarly. A tract that passes deep, or that involves an undetermined amount of muscle, is best treated with a mucosal advancement flap. Immediate or delayed muscle division with a cutting Seton is associated with a high rate of incontinence, but a noncutting Seton may be used to control sepsis while preparing for definitive therapy of a complex fistula (Fig. 23.14). Anterior midline fistulas in women are best treated with advancement flap repair because

the external sphincter is a particularly thin band of muscle in this location and the risk of sphincter injury resulting in significant incontinence is increased.

Goodsall's rule is of particular assistance in identifying the direction of the tract (Fig. 23.15) in fistulas with posterior external openings,[272] but reliability is decreased anteriorly and in particular as distance from the verge is increased.[273]

The prognosis for cryptoglandular abscess fistula disease is excellent once the source of infection is identified. Fistulas persist when the source has not been identified or adequately drained, when the diagnosis is incorrect, or when postoperative care is insufficient.

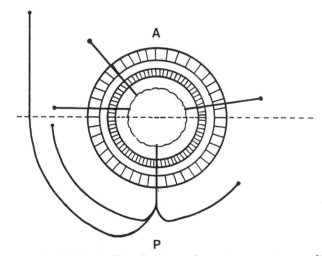

FIGURE 23.15. Goodsall's rule: External openings anterior to a line drawn between 3 and 9 o'clock will communicate with an internal opening along a straight line drawn toward the dentate line. Posterior external openings will communicate with the posterior midline in a nonlinear fashion. The exception may be an anterior opening that is greater than 3 cm from the dentate line. (Reprinted with permission from *Surgical Management of Anorectal and Colonic Diseases*, 2nd Ed., edited by Marti and Givel, ©1999, Springer-Verlag, Heidelberg.)

FISSURES

An anal fissure is a split in the anoderm. An ulcer is a chronic fissure. When mature, an ulcer is associated with a skin tag (sentinel pile), and a hypertrophied anal papilla. Fissures occur in the midline just distal to the dentate line, and the majority are in the posterior position.

Fissures result from forceful dilation of the anal canal, most commonly during defecation. The anoderm is disrupted, exposing the underlying internal sphincter muscle. This results in muscle spasm that fails to relax with the next dilatation.[274–280] This leads to further tearing, deepening of the fissure, and increased muscle irritation and spasm.[278] The persistent muscle spasm leads to relative ischemia of the overlying anoderm and inhibits healing.[38,281,282]

Classically, the initial insult is believed to be a firm bowel movement. The pain associated with the initial bowel movement is great, and the patient therefore ignores the urge to defecate for fear of experiencing the pain again. This delay allows a harder stool to form, which tears the anoderm more as it passes because of its size and the poor relaxation of the sphincter. A self-perpetuating cycle of pain, poor relaxation, and reinjury results.

Fissures cause pain and bleeding with defecation. The pain is often tearing or burning, worst during defecation, and subsides over a few hours. Blood is noted on tissue and on the stool but is not mixed in the stool or toilet water.

Physical examination by simple gentle traction on the buttocks will evert the anus sufficiently to reveal a disruption of the anoderm in the midline at the mucocutaneous junction. In the acute fissure, this may be all that is present. In the chronic fissure, a sentinel pile may be visualized at the inferior margin of the ulcer. Gentle, limited, digital examination will confirm internal sphincter spasm. Anoscopy and proctosigmoidoscopy should be deferred until healing occurs or the procedure can be performed under anesthesia. Under anesthesia, the classic triad of a proximal hypertrophied anal papilla above a fissure with the sentinel pile at the anal verge may be identified. If a midline fissure fails to heal, it must be biopsied to exclude Crohn's disease or malignancy.

Stool softeners, bulk agents, and sitz baths are successful in healing 90% of anal fissures. A second episode has a 60% to 80% chance of healing with this regimen. Sitz baths after painful bowel movements soothe the muscle spasm. Stool softeners and bulk agents make the stool more malleable, decreasing the trauma of each successive bowel movement. Chronic (1-month history) or chronic recurrent ulcers should be considered for surgery, botulinum toxin (Botox) injection to paralyze the internal sphincter spasm, or nitroglycerin ointment to relax the internal sphincter and improve blood flow. If a patient requires surgery, lateral internal anal sphincterotomy is the procedure of choice.[283] Fewer than 10% of patients so treated are incontinent to mucous and gas. Recurrence is less than 10%.

HEMORRHOIDS

Hemorrhoidal tissues are part of the normal anatomy of the distal rectum and anal canal.

The disease state of "hemorrhoids" exists when the internal complex becomes chronically engorged or the tissue prolapses into the anal canal as the result of laxity of the surrounding connective tissue and dilatation of the veins.[36] External hemorrhoids may thrombose, leading to acute onset of severe perianal pain. When the thrombosis resolves, the overlying skin may remain enlarged, creating a skin tag.

Internal hemorrhoids are traditionally classified by the following scheme: first-degree hemorrhoids bleed; second-degree hemorrhoids bleed and prolapse, but reduce spontaneously; third-degree hemorrhoids bleed, prolapse, and require manual reduction; and fourth-degree hemorrhoids bleed, and cannot be reduced.

Internal hemorrhoids typically do NOT cause pain but rather bright-red bleeding per rectum, mucous discharge, and a sense of rectal fullness or discomfort. Infrequently, internal hemorrhoids will prolapse into the anal canal, incarcerate, thrombose, and necrose. In this instance, patients may complain of pain. Anoscopy may reveal tissue with evidence of chronic venous dilatation, friability, mobility, and squamous metaplasia. Rigid sigmoidoscopy should be performed to rule out other disease of the distal colon and rectum.

External hemorrhoids may develop an acute intravascular thrombus, which is associated with acute onset of extreme perianal pain. No precipitating causes have been identified. The thrombus occasionally may cause ischemia and necrosis of the overlying anoderm, resulting in bleeding. The pain usually peaks within 48 h. The acutely thrombosed external hemorrhoid is seen as a purplish, edematous, tense subcutaneous perianal mass that is quite tender.

Chronic bleeding from internal hemorrhoids may cause anemia. However, until all other sources of blood loss have been ruled out, anemia must not be attributed to hemorrhoids regardless of the patient's age. Barium enema or colonoscopy are necessary to rule out malignancy and inflammatory bowel disease. Defecography is helpful when obstructed defecation or rectal prolapse are suspected.

The complications of internal or external hemorrhoids are the indications for medical or surgical intervention: these are bleeding, pain, necrosis, mucous discharge, moisture, and, rarely, perianal sepsis. Initial medical management for all but the most advanced cases is recommended. Dietary alterations, including elimination of constipating foods (e.g., cheeses), addition of bulking agents, stool softeners, and increased intake of liquids are advised. Changing daily routines by adding exercise and decreasing time spent on the commode is often beneficial.

First- and second-degree hemorrhoids generally respond to medical management.[284,285] Hemorrhoids that fail to respond to medical management may be treated with elastic band ligation, sclerosis, photocoagulation, cryosurgery, excisional hemorrhoidectomy, and many other local techniques that induce scarring and fixation of the hemorrhoids to the underlying tissues.

The acutely thrombosed external hemorrhoid may be treated with excision of the hemorrhoid or clot evacuation if the patient presents within 48 h of onset of symptoms. Excision removes the clot and hemorrhoidal tissues, thereby decreasing the incidence of recurrence. However, many surgeons simply evacuate the thrombus, relieving the pressure and pain. If the patient presents more than 48 h after onset of symptoms, conservative management with warm sitz baths, high-fiber diet, stool softeners, and reassurance is advised. The thrombus has begun to organize, evacuation will not be successful, and excision will not reduce the amount or duration of anal pain.

The prognosis for recurrence of hemorrhoidal disease is

related most to success in changing the patient's bowel habits. Increasing dietary fiber, decreasing constipating foods, introducing exercise, and decreasing time spent on the toilet all decrease the amount of time spent straining in the squatting position. These behavioral modifications are the most important steps in preventing recurrence.

PILONIDAL DISEASE

The incidence of pilonidal disease is highest in Caucasian males (3:1 male/female ratio) between ages 15 and 40 with a peak incidence between 16 and 20 years of age.[286]

Patients with pilonidal disease may present with small midline pits or an abscess(es) off the midline near the coccyx or sacrum. The patients are generally heavy, hirsute males. The workup is limited to a physical exam unless one suspects Crohn's disease, where a more extensive evaluation may be necessary. The differential diagnosis includes abscess/fistulous disease of the anus, hidradenitis suppurativa, furuncle, and actinomycosis.

Pilonidal abscesses may be drained under local anesthesia. A probe may be inserted into the primary opening and the abscess unroofed. Granulation tissue and inspissated hair are curetted out, but definitive therapy is not required at the first procedure. Cure rates of 60% to 80% have been reported after primary unroofing.[287] For those who fail to heal after 3 months or develop a chronic draining sinus, definitive therapy is recommended. Nonoperative therapy with meticulous skin care (shaving of the natal cleft, perineal hygiene) and drainage of abscesses may significantly reduce the need for surgery.[288]

Conservative excision of midline pits with removal of hair from lateral tracts and postoperative weekly shaving has an 89% success rate.[289] Excision with open packing, marsupialization, or primary closure with or without flaps have all been advocated.[286] Open packing and marsupialization both leave the patient with painful wounds that are slow to heal, and marsupialization has a reported recurrence rate of 6% to 10%.[290] Our preference is to excise the pilonidal disease and primarily close the defect with rotational flaps over closed suction drainage. Simple primary closure has an unacceptably high dehiscence rate.

PELVIC FLOOR DYSFUNCTION

INCONTINENCE

Continence is maintained through a complex integrated pathway that involves rectal compliance, anorectal sensation, anorectal reflexes, and anal sphincter function.[34] The incidence of fecal incontinence is difficult to assess because of underreporting and lack of standardization of what represents incontinence. Incontinence in one patient may be acceptable normal staining in another.

Obstetrical trauma during delivery is the major cause of mechanical injury to the external sphincter and potentially a cause of neurological injury.[291,292] There is an increased incidence of incontinence after third-degree perineal tears, multiple vaginal deliveries, and infection of an episiotomy repair.[134] The injury after prolonged labor may be twofold, with mechanical disruption of the sphincter and stretch of the pudendal nerve.[293]

Incontinence may result from the treatment of cryptogenic abscess/fistula disease, or perianal Crohn's disease, where the external sphincter may be divided during a fistu-

lotomy. If it is surgically disrupted, or destroyed by chronic inflammation, continence is lost.

Neurogenic causes of incontinence include pudendal nerve stretch secondary to prolonged labor or multiple births, or chronic history of straining to defecate.[292,294,295] Vaginal deliveries are associated with reversible pudendal nerve injury in 80% of primagravida births.[296]

Other causes of incontinence include iatrogenic muscle disruption (anal dilatation, internal sphincterotomy, hemorrhoidectomy), systemic diseases effecting either the muscular or neurological systems (i.e., scleroderma, multiple sclerosis, dermatomyositis diabetes), and causes unrelated to the function of the sphincter itself (severe diarrhea, fecal impaction with overflow incontinence, radiation proctitis with fibrosis, tumors of the distal colon and rectum, low pelvic colorectal anastomoses).

Complete incontinence is lack of control of gas, liquid, and solid stool. Inability to control liquid and gas or gas alone is partial incontinence. Elicitation of these symptoms is important in localizing the deficit. Patients who complain of soiling with urgency may have poor rectal compliance and normal sphincters, whereas those patients complaining of inability to sense stool until it has passed may have a neurological injury. The physical signs of incontinence may include a patulous anus, focal loss of corrugation of the anal verge, flattening and maceration of the perineum, exaggerated descent of the perineum with straining, decreased sphincter tone, diminished voluntary squeeze pressures, and loss of anal sensation.

Evaluation with anorectal manometry, transanal ultrasound, pudendal nerve latency studies, EMG, and defecography may all be part of the evaluation of the incontinent patient. No particular study is diagnostic in all patients, and appropriate tests must be chosen based on history and physical examination.

The decision tree for the diagnosis and treatment of incontinence is summarized in Fig. 23.16. If a muscular defect is limited and there is no neurological injury, surgical correction with an overlapping sphincter reconstruction restores continence by reestablishing a complete ring of muscle. However, if there is extensive loss of sphincter muscle or severe neurological injury, simple overlapping repair is not as successful and consideration must be given to muscle flap procedures or encirclement procedures. Incontinence from muscular weakness or decreased sensation secondary to incomplete neurologic injury may respond to retraining with biofeedback.[297]

OBSTRUCTED DEFECATION

Obstructed defecation may result from anal stenosis, pelvic floor dysfunction, or abnormal rectal fixation. The most common cause of anal stenosis is scarring after anal surgery. Other causes include anal tumors, Crohn's disease, radiation injury, recurrent anal ulcers, infection, and trauma.

Patients with anal stenosis present with increasing difficulty and straining at defecation, thin and sometimes painful bowel movements, and bloating. Examination may reveal postsurgical changes and a stenotic anal canal. Digital exam may be quite painful or impossible.

Causes of anal pain that must be distinguished from anal stenosis include fissure, external hemorrhoids, perirectal abscess, malignancy, foreign body, and proctalgia fugax. Proctalgia fugax (levator syndrome), a diagnosis of exclusion, is

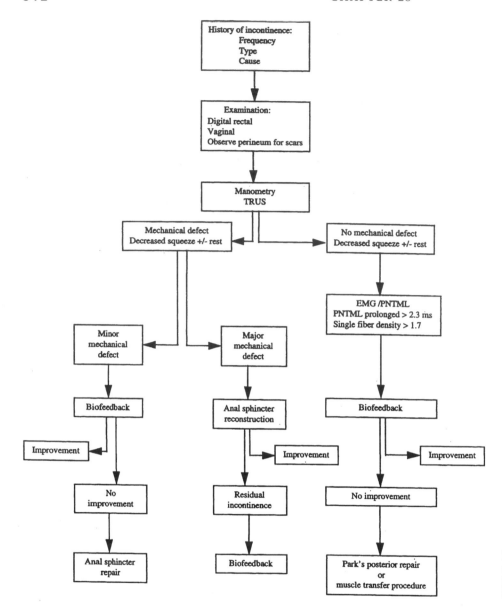

FIGURE 23.16. Algorithm for the workup and treatment of fecal incontinence. (From Shelton AA, Weltop ML. The pelvic floor. W J Med 1997;167(2):90–98.)

suggested when a patient complains of pain that awakens them from sleep. The pain is generally left sided, short lived, and relieved by heat, dilatation, or muscle relaxants. The patient often has a history of migraines and may report the occurrence of pain in relation to stressful events.

Mild anal stenosis may be treated successfully with gentle dilatation and bulk agents. Severe anal stenosis is treated surgically if there is no evidence of active disease (i.e., Crohn's disease) and healthy tissue is available to perform the anoplasty. The prognosis for anal stenosis is excellent if there is no evidence of active disease.

Pelvic floor dysfunction alternatively referred to as nonrelaxing puborectalis syndrome, anismus, or paradoxical pelvic floor contraction, is a functional disorder in that the muscle is normal but control is dysfunctional. In health, the puborectalis is contracted "at rest," maintaining the anorectal angle. During defecation, the muscle relaxes and evacuation occurs. In nonrelaxing puborectalis syndrome the muscle does not relax and maintains or increases the anorectal

angle. The patient therefore performs a Valsalva maneuver against an obstructed outlet, and elimination either does not occur or is significantly diminished. Patients may complain of straining and anal or pelvic pain, constipation, incomplete evacuation, or a need to perform digital maneuvers to evacuate rectal contents. Those who have developed internal intussusception complain of such but may also note mucous discharge, rectal bleeding, or tenesmus.

Digital examination of the patient with nonrelaxing puborectalis syndrome may reveal a tender pelvic muscular diaphragm but it is otherwise unremarkable. Sigmoidoscopic examination may reveal a solitary rectal ulcer if intussusception has occurred chronically. The ulcer develops 4 to 12 cm from the anal verge, is anterior, and is the ischemic traumatized lead point of the internal intussusception.

Nonrelaxing puborectalis syndrome is best treated with biofeedback. The puborectalis is retrained to relax during the act of defecation, allowing the act to proceed without obstruction. Biofeedback results are excellent,[297] but patients may require occasional retraining before education is complete.

Mild to moderate intusssception is treated with bulk agents, modification of bowel habits, and reassurance. Severe intussusception with impending pudendal nerve damage is treated surgically.

Patients with rectal procidentia complain of mucous discharge, progressive incontinence, pain, and bleeding; on direct questioning, they may report their rectum "falls out." Physical examination of the patient who presents with an acute episode of rectal prolapse is not difficult. A large mass of prolapsed tissue with concentric mucosal rings will be apparent (Fig. 23.17). This finding is in contrast to the patient with prolapsed hemorrhoids where physical exam reveals prolapsing tissue with deep radial grooves between areas of edematous tissue.

Patients with rectal prolapse may need anorectal manometry, electromyography, pudendal nerve latency studies, defecography, and barium enema or colonoscopy. Defecography may document the prolapse if not clinically apparent. Evaluation of the entire colon with either barium enema or colonoscopy is necessary to rule out a malignancy. The surgical approach may be chosen based on the pudendal nerve latency studies and EMG.

There are two classes of operations for rectal prolapse, abdominal and perineal. The abdominal procedures have a lower recurrence rate and preserve the reservoir capacity of the rectum but submit the patients to a higher-risk intraabdominal procedure. The perineal procedures do not require an abdominal incision and do not have an intraabdominal anastomosis, but do remove the rectum, eliminating the rectal reservoir. Thus, the abdominal procedures may be preferred over the perineal procedures in low-risk active patients less than 50 years of age and in patients who otherwise require an abdominal procedure.

The abdominal procedures for patients with severe intussusception or rectal prolapse with normal sphincter function are sigmoid resection, with or without rectopexy, and rectopexy alone. The perineal approaches to rectal prolapse include anal encirclement and the transanal Delorme procedure and Altemeier procedures. For those patients with prolapse who either have prohibitively high operative risk or who are elderly with limited life expectancy, an anal encirclement procedure may be performed, where an outlet obstruction is created and laxatives or enemas are required for rectal evacuation. The encirclement procedures are complicated by erosion of the foreign material into the rectum and infection. The Delorme procedure is essentially a mucosal proctectomy with imbrication of the prolapsing rectal wall, resulting in functional success 74–93% of the time. The Altemeier procedure is a complete proctectomy and often partial sigmoidectomy, with resection of the redundant bowel and primary reanastamosis. Recurvence rates for the Altemeier procedure range from 3–11% at a mean follow-up of up to 2 years.

SEXUALLY TRANSMITTED DISEASES

Sexually transmitted diseases of the anorectum are found frequently in urban men who have sex with men,[298–300] but these diseases are not limited to this population. The anorectum appears more susceptible to certain infections and it is therefore important to inquire into sexual practices, regardless of sex or sexual preference. The external genitalia, oral cavity, and anorectum should be examined for evidence of infection. It should be remembered that the infections are often multiple and the exact location, whether anus, perineum, or rectum, is helpful in making the pathological diagnosis. Herpes simplex virus type 2, *Treponema pallidum*, *Neisseria gonorrhoeae*, and *Chlamydia trachomatis* often cause proctitis. Anusitis or perineal infections suggest syphilis, chancroid, herpes, or lymphogranuloma verereum (LGV). Once a diagnosis is made, the patient should be counseled on safe sex practices, and the partner or partners evaluated. Suggested treatments are listed in Table 23.19.

CONDYLOMATA ACUMINATA

Human papilloma virus (HPV) is the cause of condylomata acuminatum. Multiple types have been identified. Types HPV-6 and HPV-11 are associated with the common "benign" genital wart,[301–303] whereas HPV-16 and HPV-18 are associated with the development of high-grade dysplasia and anal cancer.[304] In the United States, condylomata acuminatum is the most common sexually transmitted viral disease, with 1 million new cases reported each year.[305] It is the most common anorectal infection within homosexual men[306] and is particularly prominent in HIV(+) patients.[307] However, the disease is not limited to men or women who practice anoreceptive intercourse. In women, the virus may pull and track down from the vagina, and in men, it may pool and tract from the base of the scrotum. Immunosuppression, either with drugs after kidney transplant or from HIV, significantly impact the incidence of condylomatous disease, with rates up to 4% and 86%, respectively.[307,308]

The most frequent complaint is that of a perianal growth. Pruritus, discharge, bleeding odor, and anal pain are present to a lesser degree. Physical exam reveals the classic cauliflower-like lesion that may be isolated, clustered, or coalescent. The warts tend to run in radial rows out from the anus. The lesions may be surprisingly large at the time of presentation.

Anoscopy and proctosigmoidoscopy are essential because the disease extends internally in more than three-fourths of

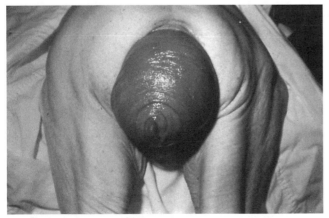

FIGURE 23.17. Rectal prolapse with concentric rings of mucosa, not masses of tissue with deep radial grooves as is seen with prolapsed internal hemorrhoids.

TABLE 23.19. Sexually Transmitted Diseases of the Anorectum and Their Treatments.

Organism	Suggested treatment for STDs Treatment
Neisseria gonorrhoeae	Ceftriaxone, 250 mg, IM once plus doxycycline, 100 mg, PO bid for 7 days
Chlamydia trachomatis	Doxycycline, 100 mg, bid for 21 days, or azithromycin, 1 g, PO as a single dose
Campylobacter sp.	Erythromycin, 500 mg, qid for 7 days, or ciprofloxacin, 500 mg, q 12 h for 7 days
Shigella sp.	Trimethoprim-sulfamethoxazole double strength PO bid for 5 days
Haemophilus ducreyi	Azithromycin, 1 g, PO as a single dose, or ceftriaxone, 250 mg, IM one time
Donovania sp.	Tetracycline, 500 mg, qid for 10 days
Treponema pallidum	Benzathine penicillin G, 2.4 million U, IM, or tetracycline, 500 mg, qid for 30 days
Herpes virus	Acyclovir, 200 mg, 5 times a day for 5 days
Hepatitis virus	Symptomatic
Entamoeba histolytica	Metronidazole, 750 mg, tid for 10 days, plus diloxanide furoate, 500 mg, tid for 10 days
Giardia lamblia	Metronidazole, 250 mg, PO tid for 7 days

Source: From Gordon and Nivatvongs,[134] with permission.

patients, and 94% of homosexual men have intraanal disease.[306,309] Cultures and serologies for other venereal diseases may be taken from the penis, anus, mouth, and vagina.

These lesions must be distinguished from condylomata lata and anal squamous cell carcinoma. Condylomata lata are the lesions of secondary syphilis. They are flatter, paler, and smoother than condylomata acuminata. Anal squamous cell carcinoma is generally painful and may be tender and ulcerated, whereas condylomata are not tender or ulcerated.

The extent of the disease or the risk of malignancy (dysplasia treatment is discussed later) determines the treatment. Minimal disease is treated in the office with topical agents such as bichloracetic acid[310] or 25% podophyllin in tincture of benzoin.[311] Patients should be seen again at regular intervals until the treatment is complete. More extensive disease may require initial treatment under anesthesia in which random lesions may be excised for pathological evaluation to rule out dysplasia and the remainder coagulated. Refractory disease may respond to excision or destruction followed by intralesional interferon or autogenous vaccine created from excisional biopsies of the lesions.[312–317] Recurrence rates of only 4.6% have been reported for destruction and vaccination combined, but the preparation of the vaccine is tedious and therefore this technique has not gained wide acceptance.[314,317]

Other sexually transmitted diseases of the anorectum and their treatments are listed in Table 23.19.

Anal Neoplasms

Prediction of the biology and planning for treatment of tumors of the perianal region is dependent on precise localization of the tumor with respect to anal landmarks such as the dentate line, the anal verge, and the anal sphincters. These landmarks define two classes of perianal neoplasms: tumors of the anal margin and tumors of the anal canal. Historically, the anal canal has been defined as the region above the anal verge and the anal margin as the area below the anal verge.[318–321] Squamous cell tumors of the anal margin are

TABLE 23.20. AJCC Definition of TNM and Stage Groupings for Anal Cancer.

Primary Tumor (T)

TX	Primary tumor cannot be assessed
T0	No evidence of primary tumor
Tis	Carcinoma *in situ*
T1	Tumor 2 cm or less in greatest dimension
T2	Tumor more than 2 cm but not more than 5 cm in greatest dimension
T3	Tumor more than 5 cm in greatest dimension
T4	Tumor of any size invades adjacent organ(s), e.g., vagina, urethra, bladder*

*Note: Direct invasion of the rectal wall, perirectal skin, subcutaneous tissue, or the sphincter muscle(s) is not classified as T4.

Regional Lymph Nodes (N)

NX	Regional lymph nodes cannot be assessed
N0	No regional lymph node metastasis
N1	Metastasis in perirectal lymph node(s)
N2	Metastasis in unilateral internal iliac and/or inguinal lymph node(s)
N3	Metastasis in perirectal and inguinal lymph nodes and/or bilateral internal iliac and/or inguinal lymph nodes

Distant Metastasis (M)

MX	Distant metastasis cannot be assessed
M0	No distant metastasis
M1	Distant metastasis

Stage Grouping

Stage	T	N	M
Stage 0	Tis	N0	M0
Stage I	T1	N0	M0
Stage II	T2	N0	M0
	T3	N0	M0
Stage IIIA	T1	N1	M0
	T2	N1	M0
	T3	N1	M0
	T4	N0	M0
Stage IIIB	T4	N1	M0
	Any T	N2	M0
	Any T	N3	M0
Stage IV	Any T	Any N	M1

Source: Used with permission of the American Joint Committee on Cancer (AJCC), Chicago, IL. The original source for this material is the AJCC Cancer Staging Manual, Sixth Ed. (2002) published by Springer-Verlag New York, www.springer-ny.com

well-differentiated, keratinizing tumors that behave similarly to squamous cell tumors of the skin elsewhere. Tumors of the anal canal are aggressive high-grade tumors with significant risk for metastasis. The staging system for anal tumors is shown in Table 23.20.

Overall, anal cancers occur in 7 of 1,000,000 men and 9 of 1,000,000 women. In the immunocompromised patient (transplant, HIV+) the rate is increased. At particular risk are men who have sex with men where the estimated rates are 35 of 100,000 and 70 of 100,000 for HIV− and HIV+ men, respectively. There is a high incidence of anal dysplasias, 15%, in the HIV(+) patients, and the rate of anal cancers may increase as lives are prolonged with highly active retroviral therapies.[324] Screening analagous to Pap smears in this hig-risk population may help to identify areas of dysplasia that may then be excised or destroyed prior to development of malignant lesions.

Tumors of the Anal Margin

SQUAMOUS CELL CARCINOMA

Patients frequently complain of a lump, bleeding, itching, pain, or tenesmus (complaints common to most lesions of this region). Typically the lesions are large, centrally ulcerated with rolled everted edges, and have been present for more than 2 years before detection.[325–327]

All chronic or nonhealing ulcers of the perineum should be biopsied to rule out squamous cell carcinoma. Small well-differentiated lesions of 4 cm or less are treated by wide local excision.[328] Deep lesions that involve the sphincters require an abdominoperineal resection of the rectum. Chemoradiation is used for less favorable lesions.[329,330] Spread is to the inguinal lymph nodes, which are generally included in the radiation fields. T stage determines survival with reports of 5- and 10-year survival of 100% for T1 lesions compared to 60% and 40% for T2 lesions at 5 and 10 years, respectively.[330]

BASAL CELL CARCINOMA

Bleeding, itching, and pain are presenting symptoms. The lesions appear with raised edges and central ulceration. They are more frequent in men.

As with squamous cell carcinoma of the margin, treatment is wide local excision when possible. Deeply invasive lesions may require abdominal perineal resection. Metastasis is rare, but local recurrence rates are 29%.[331] Local recurrences are treated with reexcision.

BOWEN'S DISEASE

As with the previous lesions, patients often complain of perianal burning, itching, or pain. Lesions are often found on routine histological evaluation of specimen acquired at unrelated procedures.[332] When grossly apparent, the lesions appear scaly, discrete, erythematous, and sometimes pigmented. Wide local excision with four quadrant biopsies to establish that no residual disease persists has been the treatment of choice.[332] Less than 10% of the patients with Bowen's develop invasive squamous cell carcinoma of the anus.[333,334]

PAGET'S DISEASE

In contrast to the three diseases just discussed, this disease occurs predominantly in women. Patients are usually in the seventh or eighth decade. Severe intractable pruritus is characteristic. On physical examination, an erythematous, eczematoid rash is apparent. As before, biopsy of any nonhealing lesion should be taken to rule out this diagnosis. If Paget's disease is diagnosed, a thorough workup for an occult malignancy is indicated because 50% of patients have a coexistent carcinoma.[332]

Wide local excision with multiple perianal biopsies is the treatment of choice. An abdominal perineal resection may be indicated for advanced disease. Lymph node dissection should only be for palpable adenopathy. The role for chemoradiotherapy is less clear.[335,336] The prognosis is good unless there is metastatic disease or an underlying neoplasm, in which case patients do poorly.

Tumors of the Anal Canal

EPIDERMOID (SQUAMOUS, BASALOID, MUCOEPIDERMOID) CARCINOMA

Generally there is a long history of minor perianal complaints such as bleeding, itching, or perianal discomfort.[337,338] A mass may or may not be associated with these symptoms. These cancers are more common in women, which may reflect an HPV effect. Digital rectal and anoscopy are useful in determining depth of invasion, size, presence of pararectal nodes, and proximal extent of disease. The mass is biopsied under anesthesia to confirm the diagnosis. Both groins should be palpated for gross disease. Abdominal CT and chest radiographs evaluate the liver and chest for distant disease. Endorectal ultrasound can determine the depth of invasion and may identify pararectal nodes.

Early lesions that are small, mobile, confined to the submucosa, and well differentiated may be treated with local excision. Overall reported recurrence rates with local excision alone are high, with survival of 45% to 85% at 5 years.[339,340] Radiation therapy or chemoradiotherapy are the preferred treatment options for larger lesions of the anal canal.[341–343]

There are reports of excellent 5- and 10-year survivals for T1–T3 node-negative disease of 88% and T1–T3 non-positive disease of 52%.[344] Metastatic disease is more likely with increasing depth of invasion, size, and worsening histological grade.[336,345,346] Distant disease is uncommon at the time of diagnosis but most commonly involves the liver when present. Subsequent metastasis out of the pelvis is not uncommon, and 40% of patients die of disease outside the pelvis.[336] The presence of lymph nodes at the time of presentation is a bad prognostic sign.[337]

References

1. Michels NA, Siddharth P, Kornblith PL, Parke WW. The variant blood supply to the small and large intestines: its import in regional resections. J Int Coll Surg 1963;39:127–170.
2. Garcia-Ruiz A, Milsom JW, Ludwig KA, Marchesa P. Right colonic arterial anatomy. Implications for laparoscopic surgery. Dis Colon Rectum 1996;39(3):906–911.
3. Steward JA, Rankin FW. Blood supply of the large intestine. Arch Surg 1933;26:843–891.

4. Griffith JD. Surgical anatomy of the blood supply of the distal colon. Ann R Coll Surg Engl 1956;19:241–256.

5. Crapp AR, Cuthbertson AM. William Waldeyer and the rectosacral fascia. Surg Gynecol Obstet 1974;138(2):252–256.

6. Sato K, Sato T. The vascular and neuronal composition of the lateral ligament of the rectum and the rectosacral fascia. Surg Radiol Anat 1991;13(1):17–22.

7. Walsh PC. Radical retropubic prostatectomy. In: Walsh PC, Gittes RF, Perlmutter AD, Stamey TA, eds. Campbell's Urology, Vol. 3. Philadelphia: Saunders, 1986:2754–2755.

8. Milligan ETC, Morgan CN. Surgical anatomy of the anal canal. Lancet 1933;2:1150–1156.

9. Shafik A. New concept of the anatomy of the anal sphincter mechanism and the physiology of defecation. II. Anatomy of the levator ani muscle with special reference to puborectalis. Invest Urol 1975;13(3):175–182.

10. Fenoglio CM, Kaye GI, Lane N. Distribution of human colonic lymphatics in normal, hyperplastic, and adenomatous tissue. Its relationship to metastasis from small carcinomas in pedunculated adenomas, with two case reports. Gastroenterology 1973;64(1):51–66.

11. Ayoub SF. Arterial supply to the human rectum. Acta Anat (Basel) 1978;100(3):317–327.

12. Havenga K, DeRuiter MC, Enker WE, Welvaart K. Anatomical basis of autonomic nerve-preserving total mesorectal excision for rectal cancer [see comments]. Br J Surg 1996;83(3):384–388.

13. Pearl RK, Monsen H, Abcarian H. Surgical anatomy of the pelvic autonomic nerves. A practical approach. Am Surg 1986;52(5):236–237.

14. Lepor H, Gregerman M, Crosby R, Mostofi FK, Walsh PC. Precise localization of the autonomic nerves from the pelvic plexus to the corpora cavernosa: a detailed anatomical study of the adult male pelvis. J Urol 1985;133(2):207–212.

15. Babb RR, Kieraldo JH. Sexual dysfunction after abdominoperineal resection. Am J Dig Dis 1977;22(12):1127–1129.

16. Duthie HL, Gairns FW. Sensory nerve-endings and sensation in the anal region of man. Br J Surg 1960;47:585–594.

17. Dickson VA. Maintenance of anal continence: a review of pelvic floor physiology (progress report). Gut 1978;19:1163–1174.

18. Duthie HL. Progress report. Anal continence. Gut 1971;12(10):844–852.

19. Cherry DA, Rothenberger DA. Pelvic floor physiology. Surg Clin North Am 1988;68(6):1217–1230.

20. Duthie HL, Wormsley KG. Absorption from the human colon. In: Shields R, ed. Scientific Basis of Gastroenterology. Edinburgh: Churchill Livingstone, 1979.

21. Devroede GJ, Phillips SF. Conservation of sodium, chloride, and water by the human colon. Gastroenterology 1969;56(1):101–109.

22. Powell DW. Transport in the large intestine. In: Giebisch G, Tosteson DC, Ussing HH, eds. Membrane Transport in Biology. New York: Raven Press, 1978:1389–1418.

23. Ritchie JA. Movement of segmental constrictions in the human colon. Gut 1971;12(5):350–355.

24. Cannon WB. The movements of the intestines studied by the means of the roentgen rays. Am J Physiol 1902;6:251–277.

25. Elliott TR, Baarclay-Smith E. Antiperistalsis and other muscular activities of the colon. J Physiol (Lond) 1904;31:272–304.

26. Herz AF. The passage of food along the human alimentary canal. Guy's Hosp Rep 1907;61:389–427.

27. Ritchie JA, Truelove SC, Ardan GM, Tuckey MS. Propulsion and retropulsion of normal colonic contents. Am J Dig Dis 1971;16(8):697–704.

28. Cohen S, Snape WJ. Movement of the small and large intestine. In: Fordtran J, Sleisenger M, eds. Gastrointestinal Disease, 3rd Ed. New York: McGraw-Hill, 1983:859–873.

29. Latella G, Caprilli R. Metabolism of large bowel mucosa in health and disease. Int J Colorectal Dis 1991;6:127–132.

30. Gaginella TS. Absorption and secretion in the colon. Curr Opin Gastroenterol 1995;11:2–8.

31. Simon GL, Gorbach SL. Intestinal flora and gastrointestinal function. In: Johnson JR, ed. Physiology of the Gastrointestinal Tract, 2nd Ed. New York: Raven Press, 1987:1729–1747.

32. Bokkenheuser V. The friendly anerobes. Clin Infect Dis 1993;15(suppl 4):S427–S434.

33. Henry MM, Thompson JP. The anal sphincters. Scand J Gastroventerol 1984;19:53–58.

34. Madoff RD, Williams JG, Caushaj PF. Fecal incontinence. N Engl J Med 1992;326(15):1002–1007.

35. Parks AG, Porter NH, Melzack J. Experimental study of the reflex mechanisms controlling muscles of the pelvic floor. Dis Colon Rectum 1962;5:407–410.

36. Thomson WH. The nature of haemorrhoids. Br J Surg 1975;62(7):542–552.

37. Loder PB, Kamm MA, Nicholls RJ, Phillips RK. Haemorrhoids: pathology, pathophysiology and aetiology. Br J Surg 1994;81(7):946–954.

38. Gibbons CP, Trowbridge EA, Bannister JJ, Read NW. Role of anal cushions in maintaining continence. Lancet 1986;1(8486):886–888.

39. Lestar B, Penninckx F, Rigauts H, Kerremans R. The internal anal sphincter can not close the anal canal completely. Int J Colorectal Dis 1992;7(3):159–161.

40. Janowitz HD. Crohn's disease—50 years later [editorial]. N Engl J Med 1981;304(26):1600–1602.

41. Odes HS, Locker C, Neumann L, et al. Epidemiology of Crohn's disease in southern Israel. Am J Gastroenterol 1994;89(10):1859–1862.

42. Anseline PF. Crohn's disease in the Hunter Valley region of Australia. Aust N Z J Surg 1995;65(8):564–569.

43. Katchinski B, Fingerle D, Scherbaum B, et al. Oral contraceptive use and cigarette smoking in Crohn's disease. Dig Dis Sci 1993;38:1596–1600.

44. Cottone M, Rosselli M, Orlando A, et al. Smoking habits and recurrence in Crohn's disease. Gastroenterology 1994;106(3):643–648.

45. Farmer RG, Hawk WA, Turnbull RB Jr. Clinical patterns in Crohn's disease: a statistical study of 615 cases. Gastroenterology 1975;68(4 pt 1):627–635.

46. Greenstein AJ. The surgery of Crohn's disease. Surg Clin North Am 1987;67(3):573–596.

47. Ritchie JK. The results of surgery for large bowel Crohn's disease. Ann R Coll Surg Engl 1990;72(3):155–157.

48. Platell C, Mackay J, Collopy B, Fink R, Ryan P, Woods R. Anal pathology in patients with Crohn's disease. Aust N Z J Surg 1996;66(1):5–9.

49. Malchow H, Ewe K, Brandes JW, et al. European Cooperative Crohn's Disease Study (ECCDS): results of drug treatment. Gastroenterology 1984;86(2):249–266.

50. Summers RW, Switz DM, Sessions JT Jr, et al. National Cooperative Crohn's Disease Study: results of drug treatment. Gastroenterology 1979;77(4 pt 2):847–869.

51. Hanauer SB. Drug therapy: inflammatory bowel disease. New Engl J Med 1996;334:841–848.

52. Sutherland L, Singleton J, Sessions J, et al. Double blind, placebo controlled trial of metronidazole in Crohn's disease. Gut 1991;32(9):1071–1075.

53. Brandt LJ, Bernstein LH, Boley SJ, Frank MS. Metronidazole therapy for perineal Crohn's disease: a follow-up study. Gastroenterology 1982;83(2):383–387.

54. Turunen U, Farkkila V, Valtonen V. Long-term outcome of ciprofloxacin treatment in severe perianal or fistulous Crohn's disease. Gastroenterology 1993;104:A793.

55. Pearson DC, May GR, Fick GH, Sutherland LR. Azathioprine and 6-mercaptopurine in Crohn disease. A meta-analysis. Ann Intern Med 1995;123(2):132–142.

56. Feagan BG, Rochon J, Fedorak RN, et al. Methotrexate for the treatment of Crohn's disease. The North American Crohn's Study Group Investigators [see comments]. N Engl J Med 1995; 332(5):292–297.

57. Fazio VW, Marchetti F, Church M, et al. Effect of resection margins on the recurrence of Crohn's disease in the small bowel. A randomized controlled trial. Ann Surg 1996;224(4):563–571; discussion 571–573.

58. Williams JG, Rothenberger DA, Nemer FD, Goldberg SM. Fistula-in-ano in Crohn's disease. Results of aggressive surgical treatment [see comments]. Dis Colon Rectum 1991;34(5):378–384.

59. Sangwan YP, Schoetz DJ Jr, Murray JJ, Roberts PL, Coller JA. Perianal Crohn's disease. Results of local surgical treatment. Dis Colon Rectum 1996;39(5):529–535.

60. Levein DH, Gross EL, Auriemma WS. Anal Crohn's disease. In: Mazier WP, Levein DH, et al., eds. Surgery of the Colon, Rectum, and Anus. Philadelphia: Saunders, 1995.

61. Cohen Z, McLeod RS. Perianal Crohn's disease. Gastroenterol Clin North Am 1987;16(1):175–189.

62. Buchman AL, Ament ME, Doty J. Development of squamous cell carcinoma in chronic perineal sinus and wounds in Crohn's disease. Am J Gastroenterol 1991;86(12):1829–1832.

63. Stewenius J, Adnerhill I, Ekelund G, et al. Ulcerative colitis and indeterminate colitis in the city of Malmo, Sweden. A 25-year incidence study. Scand J Gastroenterol 1995;30(1):38–43.

64. Farmer RG, Michener WM, Mortimer EA. Studies of family history among patients with inflammatory bowel disease. Clin Gastroenterol 1980;9(2):271–277.

65. Lashner BA, Evans AA, Kirsner JB, Hanauer SB. Prevalence and incidence of inflammatory bowel disease in family members. Gastroenterology 1986;91(6):1396–1400.

66. Willenbucher RF. Inflammatory bowel disease. Semin Gastrointest Dis 1996;7(2):94–104.

67. Greenstein AJ, Sachar DB, Smith H, Janowitz HD, Anfses AH Jr. A comparison of cancer risk in Crohn's disease and ulcerative colitis. Cancer 1981;48:2742–2745.

68. Gyde SN, Prior P, Allan RN, et al. Colorectal cancer in ulcerative colitis: a cohort study of primary referrals from three centres. Gut 1988;29(2):206–217.

69. Sugita A, Sachar DB, Bodian C, Ribeiro MB, Aufses AH Jr, Greenstein AJ. Colorectal cancer in ulcerative colitis. Influence of anatomical extent and age at onset on colitis-cancer interval. Gut 1991;32(2):167–169.

70. Choi PM, Kim WH. Colon cancer surveillance. Gastroenterol Clin North Am 1995;24(3):671–687.

71. Ekbom A, Helmick C, Zack M, Adami HO. Ulcerative colitis and colorectal cancer. A population-based study. N Engl J Med 1990;323(18):1228–1233.

72. Broome U, Lindberg G, Lofberg R. Primary sclerosing cholangitis in ulcerative colitis—a risk factor for the development of dysplasia and DNA aneuploidy? [see comments]. Gastroenterology 1992;102(6):1877–1880.

73. Devroede G. Risk of cancer in inflammatory bowel disease. In: Winawer SJ, Shottenfeld D, Sherlock P, eds. Colorectal Cancer: Prevention, Epidemiology, and Screening. New York: Raven Press, 1980.

74. Devroede GJ, Taylor WF, Sauer WG, Jackman RJ, Stickler GB. Cancer risk and life expectancy of children with ulcerative colitis. N Engl J Med 1971;285(1):17–21.

75. Ransohoff DF, Riddell RH, Levin B. Ulcerative colitis and colonic cancer. Problems in assessing the diagnostic usefulness of mucosal dysplasia. Dis Colon Rectum 1985;28(6):383–388.

76. Sachar DB, Greenstein AJ. Cancer in ulcerative colitis: good news and bad news. Ann Intern Med 1981;95(5):642–644.

77. Rubin CE, Haggitt RC, Burmer GC, et al. DNA aneuploidy in colonic biopsies predicts future development of dysplasia in ulcerative colitis. Gastroenterology 1992;103(5):1611–1620.

78. Broome U, Lofberg R, Lundqvist K, Veress B. Subclinical time span of inflammatory bowel disease in patients with primary sclerosing cholangitis. Dis Colon Rectum 1995;38(12):1301–1305.

79. Cangemi JR, Wiesner RH, Beaver SJ, et al. Effect of proctocolectomy for chronic ulcerative colitis on the natural history of primary sclerosing cholangitis. Gastroenterology 1989;96:790–794.

80. Sutherland LR, May GR, Shaffer EA. Sulfasalazine revisited: a meta-analysis of 5-aminosalicylic acid in the treatment of ulcerative colitis. Ann Int Med 1993;118:540–549.

81. Travis SP, Tysk C, de Silva HJ, Sandberg-Gertzen H, Jewell DP, Jarnerot G. Optimum dose of olsalazine for maintaining remission in ulcerative colitis. Gut 1994;35(9):1282–1286.

82. Green JR, Swan CH, Rowlinson A, et al. Short report: comparison of two doses of balsalazide in maintaining ulcerative colitis in remission over 12 months. Aliment Pharmacol Ther 1992;6:647–652.

83. d'Albasio G, Pacini F, Camarri E, et al. Combined therapy with 5-aminosalicylic acid tablets and enemas for maintaining remission in ulcerative colitis: a randomized double-blind study. Am J Gastroenterol 1997;92(7):1143–1147.

84. Langholz E, Munkholm P, Davidsen M, Binder V. Course of ulcerative colitis: analysis of changes in disease activity over years [see comments]. Gastroenterology 1994;107(1):3–11.

85. Curran FT, Sutton TD, Jass JR, Hill GL. Ulcerative colitis in the anal canal of patients undergoing restorative proctocolectomy (abstract). Br J Surg 1990;77:1420.

86. Tsunoda A, Talbot IC, Nicholls RJ. Incidence of dysplasia in the anorectal mucosa in patients having restorative proctocolectomy. Br J Surg 1990;77(5):506–508.

87. Amerhauser A, Welton ML. Complications of ileal pouche-anal anastomosis. In: Becker J, ed. Problems in General Surgery, Vol. 16. Philadelphia: Lippincott Williams & Wilkins, 1999:132–138.

88. Dozois RR, Kelly KA, Welling DR, et al. Ileal pouch-anal anastomosis: comparison of results in familial adenomatous polyposis and chronic ulcerative colitis [see comments]. Ann Surg 1989;210(3):268–271; discussion 272–273.

89. Oresland T, Fasth S, Nordgren S, Hulten L. The clinical and functional outcome after restorative proctocolectomy. A prospective study in 100 patients. Int J Colorectal Dis 1989;4(1):50–56.

90. Almy TP, Howell DA. Diverticula of the colon. N Eng J Med 1980;302:324–331.

91. Parks TG. Natural history of diverticular disease of the colon. Clin Gastroenterol 1975;4(1):53–69.

92. Rodkey GV, Welch CE. Changing patterns in the surgical treatment of diverticular disease. Ann Surg 1984;200(4):466–478.

93. Hughes LE. Postmortem survey of diverticular disease of the colon. I. Diverticulosis and diverticulitis. Gut 1969;10(5):336–344.

94. Eide TJ, Stalsberg H. Diverticular disease of the large intestine in Northern Norway. Gut 1979;20(7):609–615.

95. Morson BC. Pathology of diverticular disease of the colon. Clin Gastroenterol 1975;4(1):37–52.

96. Painter NS. Diverticular disease of the colon. The first of the Western diseases shown to be due to a deficiency of dietary fibre. S Afr Med J 1982;61(26):1016–1020.

97. Roberto PL, Veidenheimer MC. Current management of diverticulitis. Adv Surg 1994;27:189–208.

98. Ulin AW, Pearce AE, Weinstein SF. Diverticular disease of the colon: surgical perspectives in the past decade. Dis Colon Rectum 1981;24(4):276–281.

99. Ryan P. Two kinds of diverticular disease [see comments]. Ann R Coll Surg Engl 1991;73(2):73–79.

100. Boulos PB, Karamanolis DG, Salmon PR, Clark CG. Is colonoscopy necessary in diverticular disease? Lancet 1984;1(8368): 95–96.

101. Taylor I, Duthie HL. Bran tablets and diverticular disease. Br Med J 1976;1(6016):988–990.

102. Thompson WG, Patel DG. Clinical picture of diverticular disease of the colon. Clin Gastroenterol 1986;15:903–916.

103. McGuire HH Jr, Haynes BW Jr. Massive hemorrhage for diverticulosis of the colon: guidelines for therapy based on bleeding patterns observed in fifty cases. Ann Surg 1972;175(6):847–855.

104. Casarella WJ, Galloway SJ, Taxin RN, Follett DA, Pollock EJ, Seaman WB. "Lower" gastrointestinal tract hemorrhage: new concepts based on arteriography. Am J Roentgenol 1974;121:357–368.

105. McGuire HH Jr. Bleeding colonic diverticula. A reappraisal of natural history and management. Ann Surg 1994;220(5):653–656.

106. Bokhari M, Vernava AM, Ure T, Longo WE. Diverticular hemorrhage in the elderly—is it well tolerated? Dis Colon Rectum 1996;39(2):191–195.

107. Baer JW. Pathogenesis of bleeding colonic diverticulosis: new concepts. Crit Rev Diagn Imaging 1978;11:1–20.

108. Rossini FP, Ferrari A, Spandre M, et al. Emergency colonoscopy. World J Surg 1989;13(2):190–192.

109. Nicholson ML, Neoptolemos JP, Sharp JF, Watkin EM, Fossard DP. Localization of lower gastrointestinal bleeding using in vivo technetium-99m-labelled red blood cell scintigraphy. Br J Surg 1989;76(4):358–361.

110. Emslie JT, Zarnegar K, Siegel ME, Beart RW Jr. Technetium-99m-labeled red blood cell scans in the investigation of gastrointestinal bleeding. Dis Colon Rectum 1996;39(7):750–754.

111. Suzman MS, Talmor M, Jennis R, Binkert B, Barie PS. Accurate localization and surgical management of active lower gastrointestinal hemorrhage with technetium-labeled erythrocyte scintigraphy [see comments]. Ann Surg 1996;224(1):29–36.

112. Athanasoulis CA. Angiography in the management of patients with gastrointestinal bleeding. Adv Surg 1983;16(2 pt 1):1–23.

113. Jensen DM, Machicado GA. Diagnosis and treatment of severe hematochezia. The role of urgent colonoscopy after purge. Gastroenterology 1988;95(6):1569–1574.

114. Gostout CJ, Wang KK, Ahlquist DA, et al. Acute gastrointestinal bleeding. Experience of a specialized management team. J Clin Gastroenterol 1992;14(3):260–267.

115. Rothenberger DA, Wiltz O. Surgery for complicated diverticulitis. Surg Clin North Am 1993;73(5):975–992.

116. Roberts P, Abel M, Rosen L, et al. Practice parameters for sigmoid diverticulitis. The Standards Task Force, American Society of Colon and Rectal Surgeons. Dis Colon Rectum 1995;38:125–132.

117. Schoetz DJ Jr. Uncomplicated diverticulitis. Indications for surgery and surgical management. Surg Clinics North Am 1993;73:965–974.

118. Hachigian MP, Honickman S, Eisenstat TE, Rubin RJ, Salvati EP. Computed tomography in the initial management of acute left-sided diverticulitis [published erratum appears in Dis Colon Rectum 1993;36(2):193] [see comments]. Dis Colon Rectum 1992;35(12):1123–1129.

119. Montgomery RA, Venbrux AC, Bulkley GB. Mesenteric vascular insufficiency. Curr Prob Surg 1997;34(12):941–1025.

120. Detry R, Jamez J, Kartheuser A, et al. Acute localized diverticulitis: optimum management requires accurate staging. Int J Colorectal Dis 1992;7(1):38–42.

121. Belmonte C, Klas JV, Perez JJ, et al. The Hartmann procedure. First choice or last resort in diverticular disease? Arch Surg 1996;131(6):612–615; discussion 616–617.

122. Smirniotis V, Tsoutsos D, Fotopoulos A, Pissiotis AC. Perforated diverticulitis: a surgical dilemma. Int Surg 1992;77(1):44–47.

123. Kronborg O. Treatment of perforated sigmoid diverticulitis: a prospective randomized trial. Br J Surg 1993;80(4):505–507.

124. Schmitt SL, Wexner SD. Bacterial, fungal, parasitic, and viral colitis. Surg Clin North Am 1993;73(5):1055–1062.

125. Bartlett JG, Chang TW, Gurwith M, Gorbach SL, Onderdonk AB. Antibiotic-associated pseudomembranous colitis due to toxin-producing clostridia. N Engl J Med 1978;298(10):531–534.

126. Tedesco FJ, Barton RW, Alpers DH. Clindamycin-associated colitis. A prospective study. Ann Intern Med 1974;81(4):429–433.

127. Kelly CP, Pothoulakis C, LaMont JT. *Clostridium difficile* colitis [see comments]. N Engl J Med 1994;330(4):257–262.

128. Kleinfeld DI, Sharpe RJ, Donta ST. Parenteral therapy for antibiotic-associated pseudomembranous colitis [letter] [see comments]. J Infect Dis 1988;157(2):389.

129. Jobe BA, Grasley A, Deveney KE, Deveney CW, Sheppard BC. *Clostridium difficile* colitis: an increasing hospital-acquired illness. Am J Surg 1995;169(5):480–483.

130. Kaleya RN, Boley SJ. Colonic ischemia. Perspect Colon Rectal Surg 1990;3:62–81.

131. Gandhi SK, Hanson MM, Vernava AM, Kaminski DL, Longo WE. Ischemic colitis. Dis Colon Rectum 1996;39(1):88–100.

132. Marston A, Pheils MT, Thomas ML, Morson BC. Ischaemic colitis. Gut 1966;7(1):1–15.

133. Longo WE, Ballantyne GH, Gusberg RJ. Ischemic colitis: patterns and prognosis. Dis Colon Rectum 1992;35(8):726–730.

134. Gordon PH, Nivatvongs S, eds. Principles and Practice of Surgery for the Colon, Rectum, and Anus, 2nd Ed. St. Louis: Quality Medical, 1999.

135. Guttormson NL, Bubrick MP. Mortality from ischemic colitis. Dis Colon Rectum 1989;32(6):469–472.

136. Reeders JWAJ, Tytgat GNJ, Rosenbusch G. Ischemic Colitis. Dordrecht, The Netherlands: Martinus Nijhoff, 1984.

137. Abel ME, Russell TR. Ischemic colitis. Comparison of surgical and nonoperative management. Dis Colon Rectum 1983;26(2):113–115.

138. Parish KL, Chapman WC, Williams LF Jr. Ischemic colitis. An ever-changing spectrum: Am Surg 1991;57(2):118–121.

139. Ballantyne GH. Review of sigmoid volvulus. Clinical patterns and pathogenesis. Dis Colon Rectum 1982;25(8):823–830.

140. Gibney EJ. Volvulus of the sigmoid colon. Surg Gynecol Obstet 1991;173(3):243–255.

141. Bruusgaard C. Volvulus of the sigmoid colon and its treatment. Surgery (St. Louis) 1947;22:466–478.

142. String ST, DeCosse JJ. Sigmoid volvulus. An examination of the mortality. Am J Surg 1971;121(3):293–297.

143. Shepherd JJ. The epidemiology and clinical presentation of sigmoid vovulus. Br J Surg 1969;56(5):353–359.

144. Berenyl MR, Schwartz GS. Megasigmoid syndrome in diabetes and neurologic disease; review of 13 cases. Am J Gastroenterol 1967;47:310–320.

145. Habr-Gama A, Haddad J, Simonsen O, et al. Volvulus of the sigmoid colon in Brazil: a report of 230 cases. Dis Colon Rectum 1976;19:314–320.

146. Glazer IM, Aldersberg D. Volvulus of the colon: a complication of sprue. Gastroenterology 1953;24:159–172.

147. Meyers MA, Ghahremani GG, Govoni AF. Ischemic colitis associated with sigmoid volvulus: new observations. AJR Am J Roentgenol 1977;128(4):591–595.

148. Lord SA, Boswell WC, Hungerpiller JC. Sigmoid volvulus in pregnancy. Am J Surg 1995;62:380–382.

149. Hall-Craggs ECB. Sigmoid volvulus in an African population. Br Med J 1960;1:1015–1017.

150. Mishra SB, Sahoo KP. Primary resection and anastomosis for volvulus of sigmoid colon. J Indian Med Assoc 1986;84(9):265–268.

151. Griffin WD, Barton CR, Meyer KA. Volvulus of the sigmoid colon. Report of 25 cases. Surg Gynecol Obstet 1945;81:287–294.

152. Reilly PM, Jones B, Bulkley GB. Volvulus of the colon. In: Cameron JL, ed. Current Surgical Therapy, 4th Ed. St. Louis: Decker, 1992:170–175.

153. Wuepper KD, Otteman MG, Stahlgren LH. An appraisal of the operative and nonoperative treatment of sigmoid volvulus. Surg Gynecol Obstet 1966;122(1):84–88.

154. Drapanas T, Stewart JD. Acute sigmoid volvulus: concepts in surgical treatment. Am J Surg 1961;101:70–77.

155. Shepherd JJ. Treatment of volvulus of sigmoid colon: a review of 425 cases. Br Med J 1968;1:280–283.

156. Biery DL, Hoffman SM. Colonoscopic reduction of sigmoid volvulus. J Am Osteopath Assoc 1978;77(7):543–545.

157. Orchard JL, Mehta R, Khan AH. The use of colonoscopy in the treatment of colonic volvulus: three cases and review of the literature. Am J Gastroenterol 1984;79(11):864–867.

158. Wertkin MG, Aufses AH Jr. Management of volvulus of the colon. Dis Colon Rectum 1978;21(1):40–45.

159. Priuiti FW, Holt RW. Detorsion of sigmoid volvulus by flexible fiberoptic sigmoidoscopy. J Med Soc NJ 1984;78:289–290.

160. Brothers TF, Strodel WE, Ekhauser FE. Endoscopy in colonic volvulus. Ann Surg 1977;206:1–4.

161. Mangiante EC, Croce MA, Fabian TC, Moore OF, Britt LG. Sigmoid volvulus. A four-decade experience. Am Surg 1989;55(1):41–44.

162. Todd GJ, Forde KA. Volvulus of the cecum: choice of operation. Am J Surg 1979;138(5):632–634.

163. Rabinovich R, Simansky DA, Kaplan O, Mavor E, Manny J. Cecal volvulus. Dis Colon Rectum 1990;33:765–769.

164. Burke JB, Ballantyne GH. Cecal volvulus. Low mortality at a city hospital. Dis Colon Rectum 1984;27(11):737–740.

165. Haskin PH, Teplick SK, Teplick JG, Haskin ME. Volvulus of the cecum and right colon. JAMA 1981;245(23):2433–2435.

166. Gumbs MA, Kashan F, Shumofsky E, Yerubandi SR. Volvulus of the transverse colon. Reports of cases and review of the literature. Dis Colon Rectum 1983;26(12):825–828.

167. Kerry RL, Ransom HK. Volvulus of the colon. Arch Surg 1969;99(2):215–222.

168. Fishman EK, Goldman SM, Patt PG, Berlanstein B, Bohlman ME. Transverse colon volvulus: diagnosis and treatment. South Med J 1983;76(2):185–189.

169. Zinkin LD, Katz LD, Rosin JD. Volvulus of the transverse colon: report of case and review of the literature. Dis Colon Rectum 1979;22(7):492–496.

170. Moore-Gillon V. Constipation: what does the patient mean? J R Soc Med 1984;77(2):108–110.

171. Drossman DA, Sandler RS, McKee DC, Lovitz AJ. Bowel patterns among subjects not seeking health care. Use of a questionnaire to identify a population with bowel dysfunction. Gastroenterology 1982;83(3):529–534.

172. Devroede G. Constipation: mechanisms and management. In: Sleisenger MH, Fordtran JS, eds. Gastrointestinal Disease, 3rd Ed. Philadelphia: Saunders, 1983.

173. Allen JI. Molecular biology of colo rectal cancer: A clinician's view. Perspect Colon Rectal Surg 1995(8):181–202.

174. Lovett E. Family studies in cancer of the colon and rectum. Br J Surg 1976;63(1):13–18.

175. Nigro ND, Bull AW. Prospects for the prevention of colorectal cancer. Dis Colon Rectum 1987;30(10):751–754.

176. Galloway DJ, Indran M, Carr K, Jarrett F, George WD. Dietary manipulation during experimental colorectal carcinogenesis: a morphological study in the rat. Int J Colorectal Dis 1987;2(4):193–200.

177. Thun MJ, Namboodiri MM, Heath CW Jr. Aspirin use and reduced risk of fatal colon cancer [see comments]. N Engl J Med 1991;325(23):1593–1596.

178. Rosenberg L, Palmer JR, Zauber AG, Warshauer ME, Stolley PD, Shapiro S. A hypothesis: nonsteroidal anti-inflammatory drugs reduce the incidence of large-bowel cancer [see comments]. J Natl Cancer Inst 1991;83(5):355–358.

179. Baron JA, Beach M, Mandel JS, et al. Calcium supplements for the prevention of colorectal adenomas. Calcium Polyp Prevention Study Group. N Engl J Med 1999;340(2):101–107.

180. Lennard-Jones JE, Morson BC, Ritchie JK, Williams CB. Cancer surveillance in ulcerative colitis. Experience over 15 years. Lancet 1983;2(8342):149–152.

181. Greenstein AJ, Sachar DB, Smith H, Janowitz HD, Aufses AH Jr. A comparison of cancer risk in Crohn's disease and ulcerative colitis. Cancer (Phila) 1981;48(12):2742–2745.

182. Toribara NW, Sleisenger MH. Screening for colorectal cancer [see comments]. N Engl J Med 1995;332(13):861–867.

183. Lang CA, Ransohoff DF. Fecal occult blood screening for colorectal cancer. JAMA 1994;271:1011–1013.

184. Ahlquist DA, Wieand HS, Moertel CG, et al. Accuracy of fecal occult blood screening for colorectal neoplasia. A prospective study using Hemoccult and HemoQuant tests [see comments]. JAMA 1993;269(10):1262–1267.

185. Bond JH. Screening for colorectal cancer: confuting the refuters [editorial]. Gastrointest Endosc 1997;45(1):105–109.

186. Gilbertson VA. Proctosigmoidoscopy and polypectomy in reducing the incidence of rectal cancer. Cancer (Phila) 1974;34(3):suppl:936–939.

187. Neugut AI, Pita S. Role of sigmoidoscopy in screening for colorectal cancer: a critical review. Gastroenterology 1988;95(2):492–499.

188. Bohlman TW, Katon RM, Lipshutz GR, McCool MF, Smith FW, Melnyk CS. Fiberoptic pansigmoidoscopy. An evaluation and comparison with rigid sigmoidoscopy. Gastroenterology 1977;72(4 pt 1):644–649.

189. Zucker GM, Madura MJ, Chmiel JS, Olinger EJ. The advantages of the 30-cm flexible sigmoidoscope over the 60-cm flexible sigmoidoscope. Gastrointest Endosc 1984;30(2):59–64.

190. Selby JV, Friedman GD, Quesenberry CP Jr., Weiss NS. A case-control study of screening sigmoidoscopy and mortality from colorectal cancer [see comments] N Engl J Med 1992;326:653–657.

191. Newcomb PA, Norfleet RG, Storer BE, Surawicz TS, Marcus PM. Screening sigmoidoscopy and colorectal cancer mortality [see comments] J Natl Cancer Inst 1992;84:1572–1575.

192. Müller AD, Sonnenberg A. Protection by endoscopy against death from colorectal cancer. A case-control study among veterans [see comments] Arch Int Med 1995;155:1741–1748.

193. Fork FT. Double contrast enema and colonoscopy in polyp detection. Gut 1981;22(11):971–977.

194. Steine S, Stordahl A, Lunde OC, Loken K, Laerum E. Double contrast barium enema versus colonoscopy in the diagnosis of neoplastic disorders: aspects of decision making in general practice. Fam Pract 1993;10:288–291.

195. Hixson LJ, Fennerty MB, Sampliner RE, Garewal HS. Prospective blinded trial of the colonoscopic miss-rate of large colorectal polyps. Gastrointest Endosc 1991;37(2):125–127.

196. Rex DK, Lehman GA, Hawes RH, Ulbright TM, Smith JJ. Screening colonoscopy in asymptomatic average-risk persons with negative fecal occult blood tests [see comments]. Gsatroenterology 1991;100(1):64–67.

197. Godreau CJ. Office-based colonoscopy in a family practice. Fam Pract Res J 1992;12(3):313–320.

198. Jorgensen OD, Kronborg O, Fenger C. The Funen Adenoma Follow-up Study. Incidence and death from colorectal carcinoma in an adenoma surveillance program. Scand J Gastroenterol 1993;28(10):869–874.

199. Waye JD, Lewis BS, Yssayan S. Colonoscopy: a prospective report of complications. J Clin Gastroenterol 1992;15(4):347–351.

200. McAfee JH, Katon RM. Tiny snares prove safe and effective for removal of diminutive colorectal polyps. Gastrointest Endosc 1994;40(3):301–303.

201. Jentschura D, Raute M, Winter J, Henkel T, Kraus M, Manegold BC. Complications in endoscopy of the lower gastrointestinal tract. Therapy and prognosis. Surg Endosc 1994;8:672–676.

202. Aldridge MC, Phillips RK, Hittinger R, Fry JS, Fielding LP. Influence of tumour site on presentation, management and subsequent outcome in large bowel cancer. Br J Surg 1986;73(8):663–670.

203. Mandava N, Kumar S, Pizzi WF, Aprile J. Perforated colorectal carcinomas. Am J Surg 1996;172:236–238.

204. Runkel NS, Schlag P, Schwarz V, Herfarth C. Outcome after emergency surgery for cancer of the large intestine. Br J Surg 1991;78(2):183–188.

205. Beart RW, Melton LJd, Maruta M, Dockerty MB, Frydenberg HB,

O'Fallon WM. Trends in right and left-sided colon cancer. Dis Colon Rectum 1983;26(6):393–398.

206. Beart RW, Steele GD Jr, Menck HR, Chmiel JS, Ocwieja KE, Winchester DP. Management and survival of patients with adenocarcinoma of the colon and rectum: a national survey of the Commission on Cancer. J Am Coll Surg 1995;181(3):225–236.

207. Belinkie SA, Narayanan NC, Russell JC, Becker DR. Splenic abscess associated with *Streptococcus bovis* septicemia and neoplastic lesions of the colon. Dis Colon Rectum 1983;26(12):823–824.

208. Silver SC. *Streptococcus bovis* endocarditis and its association with colonic carcinoma. Dis Colon Rectum 1984;27(9):613–614.

209. Ohman U. Prognosis in patients with obstructing colorectal carcinoma. Am J Surg 1982;143(6):742–747.

210. Stryker SJ, Wolff BG, Culp CE, Libbe SD, Ilstrup DM, MacCarty RL. Natural history of untreated colonic polyps. Gastroenterology 1987;93(5):1009–1013.

211. Hoff G, Foerster A, Vatn MH, Sauar J, Larsen S. Epidemiology of polyps in the rectum and colon. Recovery and evaluation of unresected polyps 2 years after detection. Scand J Gastroenterol 1986;21(7):853–862.

212. O'Brien MJ, Winawer SJ, Zauber AG, et al. The National Polyp Study. Patient and polyp characteristics associated with high-grade dysplasia in colorectal adenomas. Gastroenterology 1990;98(2):371–379.

213. Ponz de Leon M, Antonioli A, Ascari A, Zanghieri G, Sacchetti C. Incidence and familial occurrence of colorectal cancer and polyps in a health-care district of northern Italy. Cancer (Phila) 1987;60(11):2848–2859.

214. Shahmir M, Schuman BM. Complications of fiberoptic endoscopy. Gastrointest Endosc 1980;26(3):86–91.

215. Smith LE. Fiberoptic colonoscopy: complications of colonoscopy and polypectomy. Dis Colon Rectum 1976;19(5):407–412.

216. Hensman C, Luck AJ, Hewett PJ. Laparoscopic-assisted colonoscopic polypectomy. Technique and preliminary experience. Surg Endosc 1999;13(3):231–232.

217. Nivatvongs S, Nicholson JD, Rothenberger DA, et al. Villous adenomas of the rectum: the accuracy of clinical assessment. Surgery (St. Louis) 1980;87(5):549–551.

218. Taylor EW, Thompson H, Oates GD, Dorricott NJ, Alexander-Williams J, Keighley MR. Limitations of biopsy in preoperative assessment of villous papilloma. Dis Colon Rectum 1981;24(4):259–262.

219. Dwight RW, Higgins GA, Keehn RJ. Factors influencing survival after resection in cancer of the colon and rectum. Am J Surg 1969;117(4):512–522.

220. Chu DZ, Giacco G, Martin RG, Guinee VF. The significance of synchronous carcinoma and polyps in the colon and rectum. Cancer (Phila) 1986;57(3):445–450.

221. Bussey HJ, Wallace MH, Morson BC. Metachronous carcinoma of the large intestine and intestinal polyps. Proc R Soc Med 1967;60(3):208–210.

222. Passman MA, Pommier RF, Vetto JT. Synchronous colon primaries have the same prognosis as solitary colon cancers. Dis Colon Rectum 1996;39(3):329–334.

223. Billingham RP. Conservative treatment of rectal cancer. Extending the indications. Cancer (Phila) 1992;70(5 suppl):1355–1363.

224. Hojo K, Koyama Y, Moriya Y. Lymphatic spread and its prognostic value in patients with rectal cancer. Am J Surg 1982;144(3):350–354.

225. Killingback MJ. Indications for local excision of rectal cancer. Br J Surg 1985;72(suppl):S54–S56.

226. Varma MG, Rogers SJ, Schrock TR, Welton ML. Local excision of rectal carcinoma. Arch Surg 1999;134(8):863–867; discussion 867–868.

227. Buess G, Kipfmuller K, Hack D, Grussner R, Heintz A, Junginger T. Technique of transanal endoscopic microsurgery. Surg Endosc 1988;2(2):71–75.

228. Buess G, Mentges B, Manncke K, Starlinger M, Becker HD. Technique and results of transanal endoscopic microsurgery in early rectal cancer. Am J Surg 1992;163(1):63–69; discussion 69–70.

229. Mayer J, Mortensen NJ. Transanal endoscopic microsurgery: a forgotten minimally invasive operation. Br J Surg 1995;82(4):435–437.

230. Smith LE, Ko ST, Saclarides T, Caushaj P, Orkin BA, Khanduja KS. Transanal endoscopic microsurgery. Initial registry results. Dis Colon Rectum 1996;39(10 suppl):S79–S84.

231. McGregor JR, O'Dwyer PJ. The surgical management of obstruction and perforation of the left colon. Surg Gynecol Obstet 1993;177(2):203–208.

232. Stephenson BM, Shandall AA, Farouk R, Griffith G. Malignant left-sided large bowel obstruction managed by subtotal/total colectomy. Br J Surg 1990;77(10):1098–1102.

233. Deans GT, Krukowski ZH, Irwin ST. Malignant obstruction of the left colon. Br J Surg 1994;81(9):1270–1276.

234. Lau PW, Lo CY, Law WL. The role of one-stage surgery in acute left-sided colonic obstruction. Am J Surg 1995;169(4):406–409.

235. Muto T, Bussey HJ, Morson BC. The evolution of cancer of the colon and rectum. Cancer (Phila) 1975;36(6):2251–2270.

236. Tanaka S, Haruma K, Teixeira CR, et al. Endoscopic treatment of submucosal invasive colorectal carcinoma with special reference to risk factors for lymph node metastasis. J Gastroenterol 1995;30(6):710–717.

237. Morson BC, Dawson IMP. Gastrointestinal Pathology. London: Blackwell, 1972.

238. Scheele J, Stangl R, Altendorf-Hofmann A. Hepatic metastases from colorectal carcinoma: impact of surgical resection on the natural history. Br J Surg 1990;77(11):1241–1246.

239. Ramming KP, O'Toole K. The use of the implantable chemoinfusion pump in the treatment of hepatic metastases of colorectal cancer. Arch Surg 1986;121(12):1440–1444.

240. Shirouzu K, Isomoto H, Hayashi A, Nagamatsu Y, Kakegawa T. Surgical treatment for patients with pulmonary metastases after resection of primary colorectal carcinoma. Cancer (Phila) 1995;76(3):393–398.

241. Sauter ER, Bolton JS, Willis GW, Farr GH, Sardi A. Improved survival after pulmonary resection of metastatic colorectal carcinoma. J Surg Oncol 1990;43(3):135–138.

242. van Halteren HK, van Geel AN, Hart AA, Zoetmulder FA. Pulmonary resection for metastases of colorectal origin [see comments]. Chest 1995;107(6):1526–1531.

243. Russell AH, Tong D, Dawson LE, Wisbeck W. Adenocarcinoma of the proximal colon. Sites of initial dissemination and patterns of recurrence following surgery alone. Cancer (Phila) 1984;53(2):360–367.

244. Sagar PM, Pemberton JH. Surgical management of locally recurrent rectal cancer. Br J Surg 1996;83(3):293–304.

245. Olson RM, Perencevich NP, Malcolm AW, Chaffey JT, Wilson RE. Patterns of recurrence following curative resection of adenocarcinoma of the colon and rectum. Cancer (Phila) 1980;45(12):2969–2974.

246. Obrand DI, Gordon PH. Incidence and patterns of recurrence following curative resection for colorectal carcinoma. Dis Colon Rectum 1997;40(1):15–24.

247. Gunderson LL, Sosin H, Levitt S. Extrapelvic colon—areas of failure in a reoperation series: implications for adjuvant therapy. Int J Radiat Oncol Biol Phys 1985;11(4):731–741.

248. Wodnicki H, Goldberg R, Kaplan S, Yahr WZ, Kreiger B, Russin D. The laser: an alternative for palliative treatment of obstructing intraluminal lesions. Am Surg 1988;54(4):227–230.

249. Dobrowsky W, Schmid AP. Radiotherapy of presacral recurrence following radical surgery for rectal carcinoma. Dis Colon Rectum 1985;28(12):917–919.

250. Patt YZ, Peters RE, Chuang VP, Wallace S, Claghorn L, Mavligit G. Palliation of pelvic recurrence of colorectal cancer with intra-arterial 5-fluorouracil and mitomycin. Cancer (Phila) 1985;56(9):2175–2180.

251. Moertel CG, Fleming TR, Macdonald JS, et al. Levamisole and fluorouracil for adjuvant therapy of resected colon carcinoma [see comments]. N Engl J Med 1990;322(6):352–358.

252. Laurie JA, Moertel CG, Fleming TR, et al. Surgical adjuvant therapy of large-bowel carcinoma: an evaluation of levamisole and the combination of levamisole and fluorouracil. The North Central Cancer Treatment Group and the Mayo Clinic [see comments]. J Clin Oncol 1989;7(10):1447–1456.

253. Wolmark N, Rockette H, Fisher B, et al. The benefit of leucovorin-modulated fluorouracil as postoperative adjuvant therapy for primary colon cancer: results from National Surgical Adjuvant Breast and Bowel Project protocol C-03. J Clin Oncol 1993;11(10):1879–1887.

254. Mamounas EP, Rockette H, Jones J, et al. Comparative efficacy of adjuvant chemotherapy in paients with Dukes B vs. Dukes C colon cancer: results from four NSABP adjuvant studies (C-01, C-02, C-03, C-04) [abstract 461]. Proc Am Soc Clin Oncol 1996;15:205.

255. Investigators IMPAoCCTI. Efficacy of adjuvant fluorouracil and folinic acid in colon cancer. Lancet 1995;345:939–944.

256. Duttenhaver JR, Hoskins RB, Gunderson LL, Tepper JE. Adjuvant postoperative radiation therapy in the management of adenocarcinoma of the colon. Cancer (Phila) 1986;57(5):955–963.

257. Ghossein NA, Samala EC, Alpert S, et al. Elective postoperative radiotherapy after incomplete resection of colorectal cancer. Dis Colon Rectum 1981;24(4):252–256.

258. Wong CS, Harwood AR, Cummings BJ, Keane TJ, Thomas GM, Rider WD. Postoperative local abdominal irradiation for cancer of the colon above the peritoneal reflection. Int J Radiat Oncol Biol Phys 1985;11(12):2067–2071.

259. Kopelson G. Adjuvant postoperative radiation therapy for colorectal carcinoma above the peritoneal reflection. I. Sigmoid colon. Cancer (Phila) 1983;51(9):1593–1598.

260. Kopelson G. Adjuvant postoperative radiation therapy for colorectal carcinoma above the peritoneal reflection. II. Antimesenteric wall ascending and descending colon and cecum. Cancer (Phila) 1983;52(4):633–636.

261. Minsky BD. Adjuvant radiation therapy for colon cancer. Cancer Treat Rev 1995;21(5):407–414.

262. GITSG. Prolongation of the disease-free interval in surgically treated rectal carcinoma. Gastrointestinal Tumor Study Group. N Engl J Med 1985;312(23):1465–1472.

263. O'Connell MJ, Martenson JA, Wieand HS, et al. Improving adjuvant therapy for rectal cancer by combining protracted-infusion fluorouracil with radiation therapy after curative surgery. N Engl J Med 1994;331(8):502–507.

264. Valentini V, De Santis M, Morganti AG, Trodella L, Cellini N, Dobelbower RR. Intraoperative radiation therapy (IORT) in rectal cancer: methodology and indications. Rays (Rome) 1995; 20(1):73–89.

265. Morson BC. The polyp-cancer sequence in the large bowel. Proc R Soc Med 1974;67:451–457.

266. Lynch HT, Smyrk T. Hereditary nonpolyposis colorectal cancer (Lynch syndrome). An updated review. Cancer (Phila) 1996;78(6): 1149–1167.

267. Mecklin JP, Järvinen HJ. Tumor spectrum in cancer family syndrome (hereditary nonpolyposis colorectal cancer). Cancer (Phila) 1991;68(5):1109–1112.

268. Parks AG. Pathogenesis and treatment of fistula-in-ano. Br Med J 1961;1:463–469.

269. Eisenhammer S. The internal anal sphincter and the anorectal abscess. Surg Gynecol Obstet 1956;103:501–506.

270. Eisenhammer S. A new approach to the anorectal fistulous abscess on the high intramuscular lesion. Surg Gynecol Obstet 1958;106:595–599.

271. Vasilevsky C-A. Results of treatment of fistula-in-ano. Dis Colon Rectum 1984;28:225–231.

272. Cirocco WC, Reilly JC. Challenging the predictive accuracy of Goodsall's rule for anal fistulas. Dis Colon Rectum 1992;35(6): 537–542.

273. Marks CG, Ritchie JK. Anal fistulas at St. Mark's Hospital. Br J Surg 1977;64:84–91.

274. Chowcat NL, Araujo JG, Boulos PB. Internal sphincterotomy for chronic anal fissure: long term effects on anal pressure. Br J Surg 1986;73(11):915–916.

275. Xynos E, Tzortzinis A, Chrysos E, Tzovaras G, Vassilakis JS. Anal manometry in patients with fissure-in-ano before and after internal sphincterotomy. Int J Colorectal Dis 1993;8(3):125–128.

276. McNamara MJ, Percy JP, Fielding IR. A manometric study of anal fissure treated by subcutaneous lateral internal sphincterotomy. Ann Surg 1990;211(2):235–238.

277. Farouk R, Duthie GS, MacGregor AB, Bartolo DC. Sustained internal sphincter hypertonia in patients with chronic anal fissure. Dis Colon Rectum 1994;37(5):424–429.

278. Keck JO, Staniunas RJ, Coller JA, Barrett RC, Oster ME. Computer-generated profiles of the anal canal in patients with anal fissure. Dis Colon Rectum 1995;38(1):72–79.

279. Williams N, Scott NA, Irving MH. Effect of lateral sphincterotomy on internal anal sphincter function. A computerized vector manometry study. Dis Colon Rectum 1995;38(7):700–704.

280. Prohm P, Bonner C. Is manometry essential for surgery of chronic fissure-in-ano? Dis Colon Rectum 1995;38(7):735–738.

281. Kuypers HC. Is there really sphincter spasm in anal fissure? Dis Colon Rectum 1983;26(8):493–494.

282. Schouten WR, Briel JW, Auwerda JJ, De Graaf EJ. Ischaemic nature of anal fissure. Br J Surg 1996;83(1):63–65.

283. Cirocco WC. Lateral internal sphincterotomy remains the treatment of choice for anal fissures that fail conservative therapy [letter; comment]. Gastrointest Endosc 1998;47(2):212–214.

284. Moesgaard F, Nielsen ML, Hansen JB, Knudsen JT. High-fiber diet reduces bleeding and pain in patients with hemorrhoids: a double-blind trial of Vi-Siblin. Dis Colon Rectum 1982;25(5): 454–456.

285. Senapati A, Nicholls RJ. A randomised trial to compare the results of injection sclerotherapy with a bulk laxative alone in the treatment of bleeding haemorrhoids. Int J Colorectal Dis 1988;3(2):124–126.

286. Nivatvongs S. Pilonidal disease. In: Gordon PH, Nivatvongs S, eds. Principles and Practice of Surgery for the Colon, Rectum, and Anus. St. Louis: Quality Medical, 1992:269–299.

287. Jensen SL, Harling H. Prognosis after simple incision and drainage for a first-episode acute pilonidal abscess. Br J Surg 1988; 75(1):60–61.

288. Armstrong JH, Barcia PJ. Pilonidal sinus disease. The conservative approach. Arch Surg 1994;129(9):914–917; discussion 917–919.

289. Edwards MH. Pilonidal sinus: a 5-year appraisal of the Millar-Lord treatment. Br J Surg 1977;64(12):867–868.

290. Allen-Mersh TG. Pilonidal sinus: finding the right track for treatment. Br J Surg 1990;77(2):123–132.

291. Ctercteko GC, Fazio VW, Jagelman DG, Lavery IC, Weakley FL, Melia M. Anal sphincter repair: a report of 60 cases and review of the literature. Aust N Z J Surg 1988;58(9):703–710.

292. Ryhammer AM, Laurberg S, Hermann AP. Long-term effect of vaginal deliveries on anorectal function in normal perimenopausal women. Dis Colon Rectum 1996;39(8):852–859.

293. Laurberg S, Swash M, Henry MM. Delayed external sphincter repair for obstetric tear. Br J Surg 1988;75(8):786–788.

294. Kiff ES. Swash M. Slowed conduction in the pudendal nerves in idiopathic (neurogenic) faecal incontinence. Br J Surg 1984;71(8): 614–616.

295. Womack NR, Morrison JF, Williams NS. The role of pelvic floor denervation in the aetiology of idiopathic faecal incontinence. Br J Surg 1986;73(5):404–407.

296. Snooks SJ, Henry MM, Swash M. Fecal incontinence due to external anal sphincter division in childbirth with damage of the

innervation of the pelvic floor musculature: a double pathology. Br J Obstet Gynecol 1985;92:824–828.

297. Ko CY, Tong J, Lehman RE. Shelton AA, Schrock TR, Welton ML. Biofeedback is effective therapy for fecal incontinence and constipation. Arch Surg 1997;132(8):829–833; discussion 833–834.

298. Wilcox RR. Epidemiology of anorectal disease. J R Soc Med 1980;73:508–509.

299. Augenbraun MH, McCormack WM. Sexually transmitted diseases in HIV-infected persons. Infect Dis Clin North Am 1994; 8(2):439–448.

300. Modesto VL, Gottesman L. Sexually transmitted diseases and anal manifestations of AIDS. Surg Clin North Am 1994;74(6): 1433–1464.

301. Gissmann L, Schwarz E. Persistence and expression of human papillomavirus DNA in genital cancer. Ciba Found Symp 1986; 120(5437):190–207.

302. Parker BJ, Cossart YE, Thompson CH, Rose BR, Henderson BR. The clinical management and laboratory assessment of anal warts. Med J Aust 1987;147(2):59–63.

303. Labropoulou V, Balamotis A, Tosca A, Rotola A, Mavromara-Nazos P. Typing of human papillomaviruses in condylomata acuminata from Greece. J Med Virol 1994;42(3):259–263.

304. Palmer JG, Scholefield JH, Coates PJ, et al. Anal cancer and human papillomaviruses. Dis Colon Rectum 1989;32(12):1016–1022.

305. Rockley PF, Tyring SK. Interferons alpha, beta and gamma therapy of anogenital human papillomavirus infections. Pharmacol Ther 1995;65(2):265–287.

306. Sohn N, Robilotti JG Jr. The gay bowel syndrome. A review of colonic and rectal conditions in 200 male homosexuals. Am J Gastroenterol 1977;67(5):478–484.

307. Breese PL, Judson FN, Penley KA, Douglas JM Jr. Anal human papillomavirus infection among homosexual and bisexual men: prevalence of type-specific infection and association with human immunodeficiency virus. Sex Transm Dis 1995;22(1):7–14.

308. Landsberg K, Bear RA. Severe condylomata acuminata in a renal transplant recipient. Am J Nephrol 1986;6(4):325–326.

309. Schlappner OL, Shaffer EA. Anorectal condylomata acuminata: a missed part of the condyloma spectrum. Can Med Assoc J 1978;118(2):172–173.

310. Swerdlow DB, Salvati EP. Condyloma acuminatum. Dis Colon Rectum 1971;14(3):226–231.

311. Culp OS, Kaplan IW. Condylomata acuminata: two hundred cases treated with podophyllin. Ann Surg 1944;120:251–256.

312. Abcarian H, Sharon N. Long-term effectiveness of the immunotherapy of anal condyloma acuminatum. Dis Colon Rectum 1982;25(7):648–651.

313. Eftaiha MS, Amshel AL, Shonberg IL, Batshon B. Giant and recurrent condyloma acuminatum: appraisal of immunotherapy. Dis Colon Rectum 1982;25(2):136–138.

314. Wiltz OH, Torregrosa M, Wiltz O. Autogenous vaccine: the best therapy for perianal condyloma acuminata? Dis Colon Rectum 1995;38(8):838–841.

315. Schonfeld A, Nitke S, Schattner A, et al. Intramuscular human interferon-beta injections in treatment of condylomata acuminata. Lancet 1984;1(8385):1038–1042.

316. Fleshner PR, Freilich MI. Adjuvant interferon for anal condyloma. A prospective, randomized trial. Dis Colon Rectum 1994; 37(12):1255–1259.

317. Mayeaux EJ Jr, Harper MB, Barksdale W, Pope JB. Noncervical human papillomavirus genital infections [see comments]. Am Fam Phys 1995;52(4):1137–1146, 1149–1150.

318. Brown DK, Oglesby AB, Scott DH, Dayton MT. Squamous cell carcinoma of the anus: a twenty-five year retrospective. Am Surg 1988;54(6):337–342.

319. Greenall MJ, Quan SH, Urmacher C, DeCosse JJ. Treatment of epidermoid carcinoma of the anal canal. Surg Gynecol Obstet 1985;161(6):509–517.

320. Pintor MP, Northover JM, Nicholls RJ. Squamous cell carcinoma

of the anus at one hospital from 1948 to 1984. Br J Surg 1989; 76(8):806–810.

321. Nigro ND. Multidisciplinary management of cancer of the anus. World J Surg 1987;11(4):446–451.

322. Deans GT, McAleer JJ, Spence RA. Malignant anal tumours. Br J Surg 1994;81(4):500–508.

323. Penn I. Cancers of the anogenital region in renal transplant recipients. Analysis of 65 cases. Cancer (Phila) 1986;58(3):611–616.

324. Melbye M, Cote TR, Kessler L, Gail M, Biggar RJ. High incidence of anal cancer among AIDS patients. The AIDS/Cancer Working Group. Lancet 1994;343(8898):636–639.

325. Beahrs OH, Wilson SM. Carcinoma of the anus. Ann Surg 1976; 184(4):422–428.

326. Papillon J, Chassard JL. Respective roles of radiotherapy and surgery in the management of epidermoid carcinoma of the anal margin. Series of 57 patients. Dis Colon Rectum 1992;35(5): 422–429.

327. Möller C, Saksela E. Cancer of the anus and anal canal. Acta Chir Scand 1970;136(4):340–348.

328. Cummings BJ. Editorial. Oncology 1996;10(12):1853–1854.

329. Fuchshuber PR, Rodriguez-Bigas M. Anal canal and perianal epidermoid cancers. J Am Coll Surg 1997;185:494–505.

330. Touboul E, Schlienger M, Buffat L, et al. Epidermoid carcinoma of the anal margin: 17 cases treated with curative-intent radiation therapy. Radiother Oncol 1995;34(3):195–202.

331. Nielsen OV, Jensen SL. Basal cell carcinoma of the anus—a clinical study of 34 cases. Br J Surg 1981;68(12):856–857.

332. Beck DE. Paget's disease and Bowen's disease of the anus. Semin Colon Rectal Surg 1995;6(3):143–149.

333. Graham JH, Helwig EB. Bowen's disease and its relationship to systemic cancer. Arch Dermatol 1961;83:738–758.

334. Marfing TE, Abel ME, Gallagher DM. Perianal Bowen's disease and associated malignancies. Dis Colon Rectum 1987;30(10): 782–785.

335. Berardi RS, Lee S, Chen HP. Perianal extramammary Paget's disease. Surg Gynecol Obstet 1988;167(4):359–366.

336. Goldman S, Ilhre T, Lagerstedt U, Svensson C. Perianal Paget's disease: report of five cases. Int J Colorect Dis 1992;7:167–169.

337. Stearns MW Jr, Quan SH. Epidermoid carcinoma of the anorectum. Surg Gynecol Obstet 1970;131(5):953–957.

338. Welch JP, Malt RA. Appraisal of the treatment of carcinoma of the anus and anal canal. Surg Gynecol Obstet 1977;145(6):837–841.

339. Gordon PH. Current status—perianal and anal canal neoplasms. Dis Colon Rectum 1990;33(9):799–808.

340. Jensen SL, Hagen K, Harling H, Shokouh-Amiri MH, Nielsen OV. Long-term prognosis after radical treatment for squamous-cell carcinoma of the anal canal and anal margin. Dis Colon Rectum 1988;31(4):273–278.

341. Papillon J, Montbarron JF. Epidermoid carcinoma of the anal canal. Dis Colon Rectum 1987;30(5):324–333.

342. Cummings BJ, Keane TJ, O'Sullivan B, Wong CS, Catton CN. Epidermoid anal cancer: treatment by radiation alone or by radiation and 5-fluorouracil with and without mitomycin C [see comments]. Int J Radiat Oncol Biol Phys 1991;21(5):1115–1125.

343. Allal A, Kurtz JM, Pipard G, et al. Chemoradiotherapy versus radiotherapy alone for anal cancer: a retrospective comparison. Int J Radiat Oncol Biol Phys 1993;27(1):59–66.

344. Myerson RJ, Shapiro SJ, Lacey D, et al. Carcinoma of the anal canal. Am J Clin Oncol 1995;18(1):32–39.

345. Boman BM, Moertel CG, O'Connell MJ, et al. Carcinoma of the anal canal. Cancer (Phila) 1984;54(1):114–125.

346. Cummings BJ. Treatment of primary epidermoid carcinoma of the anal canal. Int J Colorectal Dis 1987;2(2):107–112.

347. Mandel JS, Bond JH, Church TR, et al. Reducing mortality from colorectal cancer by screening for fecal occult blood. Minnesota Colon Cancer Control Study [published erratum appears in N Engl J Med 1993;329(9):672] [see comments]. N Engl J Med 1993;329(19):1365–1371.

348. Hardcastle JD, Chamberlain JO, Robinson MH, et al. Randomised

controlled trial of faecal-occult-blood screening for colorectal cancer [see comments]. Lancet 1996;348(9040):1472–1477.

349. Kronborg O, Fenger C, Olsen J, Jorgensen OD, Sondergaard O. Randomised study of screening for colorectal cancer with faecal-occult-blood test [see comments]. Lancet 1996;348(9040): 1467–1471.

350. Winawer SJ, Flehinger BJ, Schottenfeld D, Miller DG. Screening for colorectal cancer with fecal occult blood testing and sigmoidoscopy [see comments]. J Natl Cancer Inst 1993;85(16): 1311–1318.

351. Kewenter J, Brevinge H, Engaras B, Haglind E, Ahren C. Results of screening, rescreening, and follow-up in a prospective randomized study for detection of colorectal cancer by fecal occult blood testing. Results for 68,308 subjects. Scand J Gastroenterol 1994;29(5):468–473.

352. Jessup JM, McGinnis LS, Steele GD Jr, Menck HR, Winchester DP. The National Cancer Data Base. Report on colon cancer. Cancer (Phila) 1996;78(4):918–926.

353. Morson BC, Bussey HJ, Samoorian S. Policy of local excision for early cancer of the colorectum. Gut 1977;18:1045–1050.

354. Hager TH GF, Hermanek P. Local excision of cancer of the rectum. Dis Colon Rectum 1983;26:149–151.

355. Heimann TM, Oh C, Steinhagen RM, Greenstein AJ, Perez C, Aufses AH Jr. Surgical treatment of tumors of the distal rectum with sphincter preservation. Ann Surg 1992;216:432–436; discussion 436–437.

356. Obrand DI, Gordon PH. Results of local excision for rectal carcinoma. Can J Surg 1996;39:463–468.

357. Garcia-Aguilar J MA, Sivatvongs P, et al. Local excision of early rectal cancer: the Minnesota experience. Ann Surg 1998 Submitted.

358. Rosenthal SA, Yeung RS, Weese JL, et al. Conservative management of extensive low-lying rectal carcinomas with transanal local excision and combined preoperative and postoperative radiation therapy. A report of a phase I-II trial. Cancer 1992;69: 335–341.

359. Bailey HR, Huval WV, Max E, Smith KW, Butts DR, Zamora LF. Local excision of carcinoma of the rectum for cure. Surgery 1992;111:555–561.

360. Minsky BD, Cohen AM, Enker WE, Mies C. Sphincter preservation in rectal cancer by local excision and postoperative radiation therapy. Cancer 1991;67:908–914.

361 Fortunato L, Ahmad NR, Yeung RS, et al. Long-term follow-up of local excision and radiation therapy for invasive rectal cancer. Dis Colon Rectum 1995;38:1193–1199.

362. Ota DM SJ, Rich TA. MD Anderson Cancer Center experience with local excision and multimodality therapy for rectal cancer. Surg Clin North Am 1992;1:147–152.

363. Bleday R BE, Jessup JM, et al. Prospective evaluation of local excision for small rectal cancers. Dis Colon Rectum 1997;40:388–392.

364. The evaluation of low dose pre-operative X-ray therapy in the management of operable rectal cancer; results of a randomly controlled trial. Br J Surg 1984;71:21–25.

365. Higgins GA, Humphrey EW, Dwight RW, Roswit B, Lee LE, Jr., Keehn RJ. Preoperative radiation and surgery for cancer of the rectum. Veterans Administration Surgical Oncology Group Trial II. Cancer 1986;58:352–359.

366. Gérard A, Buyse M, Nordlinger B, et al. Preoperative radiotherapy as adjuvant treatment in rectal cancer. Final results of a randomized study of the European Organization for Research and Treatment of Cancer (EORTC). Ann Surg 1988;208:606–614.

367. Reis Neto JA, Quilici FA, Reis JA, Jr. A comparison of nonoperative vs. preoperative radiotherapy in rectal carcinoma. A 10-year randomized trial. Dis Colon Rectum 1989;32:702–710.

368. Dahl O, Horn A, Morild I, et al. Low-dose preoperative radiation postpones recurrences in operable rectal cancer. Results of a randomized multicenter trial in western Norway. Cancer 1990;66:2286–2294.

369. Goldberg PA, Nicholls RJ, Porter NH, Love S, Grimsey JE. Long-term results of a randomized trial of short-course low-dose adjuvant pre-operative radiotherapy for rectal cancer: reduction in local treatment failure [see comments]. Eur J Cancer 1994;30A: 1602–1606.

370. Marsh PJ, James RD, Schofield PF. Adjuvant preoperative radiotherapy for locally advanced rectal carcinoma. Results of a prospective, randomized trial. Dis Colon Rectum 1994;37:1205–1214.

371. Cedermark B, Johansson H, Rutqvist LE, Wilking N. The Stockholm I trial of preoperative short term radiotherapy in operable rectal carcinoma. A prospective randomized trial. Stockholm Colorectal Cancer Study Group. Cancer 1995;75:2269–2275.

372. Cedermark B. Randomized study on preoperative radiation therapy in rectal carcinoma. Ann Surg Oncol 1996;3:423–430.

373. Improved survival with preoperative radiotherapy in resectable rectal cancer. Swedish Rectal Cancer Trial [see comments] [published erratum appears in N Engl J Med 1997 May 22;336:1539]. New Engl J Med 1997;336:980–987.

374. Balslev I, Pedersen M, Teglbjaerg PS, et al. Postoperative radiotherapy in Dukes' B and C carcinoma of the rectum and rectosigmoid. A randomized multicenter study. Cancer 1986;58: 22–28.

375. Fisher B, Wolmark N, Rockette H, et al. Postoperative adjuvant chemotherapy or radiation therapy for rectal cancer: results from NSABP protocol R-01. J Natl Cancer Inst 1988;80:21–29.

376. Gates G obotMRCWP. Results of the MRC trial of postoperative radiotherapy for operable rectal cancer. UKCCR Meeting on Colorectal Cancer. Oxford, UK 1995, March 20.

377. Treurniet-Donker AD, van Putten WL, Wereldsma JC, et al. Postoperative radiation therapy for rectal cancer. An interim analysis of a prospective, randomized multicenter trial in The Netherlands [see comments]. Cancer 1991;67:2042–2048.

378. Boulis-Wassif S, Gerard A, Loygue J, Camelot D, Buyse M, Duez N. Final results of a randomized trial on the treatment of rectal cancer with preoperative radiotherapy alone or in combination with 5-fluorouracil, followed by radical surgery. Trial of the European Organization on Research and Treatment of Cancer Gastrointestinal Tract Cancer Cooperative Group. Cancer 1984;53: 1811–1818.

379. Krook JE, Moertel CG, Gunderson LL, et al. Effective surgical adjuvant therapy for high-risk rectal carcinoma [see comments]. N Engl J Med 1991;324:709–715.

380. Radiation therapy and fluorouracil with or without semustine for the treatment of patients with surgical adjuvant adenocarcinoma of the rectum. Gastrointestinal Tumor Study Group. J Clin Oncol 1992;10:549–557.

381. Hymans D ME, Wolmark N, et al. The effects of postoperative radiation therapy used with adjuvant chemotherapy in Dukes' B and C rectal cancer. Results from NSABP R-02 [Abstract 2] Proc Am Soc Surg Oncol 1996.

24

Spleen

Alan T. Lefor and Edward H. Phillips

Embryology and Anatomy

The splenic primordium becomes evident during the fifth week of gestation as an outgrowth of the dorsal mesogastrium, which migrates to the left upper quadrant. The gross appearance of the spleen is the result of its development from multiple anlage, resulting in an organ with multiple clefts. The normal spleen weighs 150 to 250 g and is located in the left upper quadrant, beneath the ninth, tenth, and eleventh ribs. This location offers some protection to this fragile organ, but also explains why the spleen is the organ most commonly injured in blunt abdominal trauma. The parietal surface of the spleen is related to the diaphragm and the visceral surface is related to the left colon, left kidney, tail of the pancreas, and stomach.[1] The capsule of the spleen is thin and consists of mesothelial cells.

The spleen receives its arterial supply from the splenic artery, which originates in the celiac axis. It is easy to identify on angiographic studies by its characteristic tortuous appearance. After its origin, the splenic artery courses along the superior edge of the pancreas, with multiple branches into the pancreatic parenchyma. The artery then gives off several branches into the spleen, the first being the superior polar artery. There are other arterial vessels to the spleen from the left gastroepiploic artery and the short gastric artery. The splenic veins follow the arterial distribution closely, and the main splenic vein emerges from the spleen following a course to join the superior mesenteric vein, forming the portal vein.

The spleen is held in place by a number of peritoneal attachments, which are commonly referred to as "ligaments":

Splenogastric ligament: also called the gastrosplenic omentum, contains the short gastric vessels

Splenocolic ligament: a fold of peritoneum from the splenic flexure of the colon to the lower pole of the spleen

Splenorenal ligament: posterior peritoneum that splits anterior to the underlying kidney to envelop the hilar vessels and tail of the pancreas

Splenophrenic ligament: usually very attenuated, from the superior pole of the spleen to the diaphragm

Splenoomental ligament: a constant fold of peritoneum connecting the lower pole of the spleen to the omentum near the splenic flexure of the colon. Intraoperative traction on this structure is most commonly responsible for iatrogenic injuries to the lower pole.

There are occasionally other folds of peritoneum attached to the spleen, but those listed remain the most constant, and are those with which the surgeon must be familiar at the time of splenic surgery.

Functions and Pathological Conditions of the Spleen

Circulation through the spleen is about 150 to 200 ml/min, or about 5% of the cardiac output.[2] The spleen has traditionally been ascribed four functions: (1) filtration, (2) immunological, (3) reservoir, and (4) hematopoietic.[3] The filtration function is the most dominant splenic function in humans and refers to the removal of abnormal or senescent red blood cells from the circulation. Other particles removed include particulate antigens such as microorganisms or antigen–antibody complexes. The immunological functions of the spleen include trapping of antigens, homing of lymphocytes, antibody and lymphokine production, and macrophage activation. The spleen is the main site for immunoglobulin and antibody synthesis in the body, and affects the capability of cellular populations in other lymphoid organs through largely unknown mechanisms.[2] The reservoir function refers to the fact that the spleen harbors about one-third of the total platelet mass and a large number of granulocytes. The hematopoietic functions are minimal in humans and much more prominent in other species. It is clear that a majority of pathological processes in the spleen are related to the filtration and immunological functions of the spleen.

TABLE 24.1. Disorders Associated with Hypersplenism.

1. Disorders associated with sequestration of abnormal blood cells in an intrinsically normal spleen.
   A. Congenital disorders of erythrocytes
      1. Hereditary spherocytosis
      2. Hereditary elliptocytosis
      3. Hemoglobinopathies
   B. Acquired disorders of erythrocytes
      1. Autoimmune hemolytic anemia
      2. Parasitic diseases (e.g., malaria, babesiosis)
   C. Autoimmune thrombocytopenia
   D. Autoimmune neutropenia
2. Disorders of the spleen resulting in sequestration of normal blood cells
   A. Disorders of cordal macrophages: Banti's syndrome, storage diseases, parasitic diseases (e.g., kala-azar), Langerhan's cell histiocytosis, malignant histiocytosis
   B. Infiltrative disorders: leukemias, lymphomas, plasma cell dyscrasias, myeloid metaplasia, metastatic carcinoma
   C. Vascular abnormalities
   D. Splenic cysts
   E. Hamartomas
3. Miscellaneous conditions
   A. Hyperthyroidism
   B. Hypogammaglobulinemia
   C. Progressive multifocal leukoencephalopathy

Source: Reiman (1997).[3]

Conditions associated with defective or absent splenic function are grouped together as being conditions of *hyposplenism*. These conditions are characterized by the presence of Howell–Jolly bodies in the peripheral circulation. Conditions associated with *hypersplenism* remain the most frequent indication for elective splenectomy; these can be divided into those conditions in which the spleen is normal but increased destruction of abnormal blood elements causes hypersplenism, and those in which there is a primary disorder of the spleen that results in increased destruction of normal blood cells (Table 24.1).[3]

SPLENIC RUPTURE

The spleen can rupture from three underlying causes: trauma, spontaneous rupture, and pathological rupture. Traumatic rupture of the spleen remains the most frequent indication for splenectomy. Pathological causes of splenic rupture include infiltration of the spleen by reactive lymphoid cells or by neoplastic cells. Most cases attributed to spontaneous rupture of the spleen are actually due to an undiagnosed pathological process.[3]

Benign Lesions of the Spleen

HEMANGIOMA

This is the most common benign primary neoplasm of the spleen, and is frequently an incidental finding after splenectomy for other causes. Lesions can be solitary or multiple, and are usually blue-red, well-circumscribed nodules. Microscopically, they usually appear as endothelium-lined spaces, and are known as cavernous hemangiomas. The process can affect the entire spleen as a diffuse hemangiomatosis that can present with splenomegaly. Treatment of these lesions is usually splenectomy, although partial splenectomy may be indicated for isolated lesions.

LYMPHANGIOMA

These lesions are less common than hemangiomas, and are usually subcapsular, appearing as soft, compressible, multicystic lesions on the splenic surface. When located within the parenchyma, they may be solitary or multiple. When large, they present with splenomegaly as an indication for resection. There are case reports of patients presenting with hypersplenic syndromes, consumptive coagulopathy, and even portal hypertension with these lesions.[4]

PELIOSIS

These rare lesions bear a superficial resemblance to vascular neoplasms of the spleen. They consist of blood-filled cysts distributed in patches or diffusely, and can result in splenomegaly.[4] Intraperitoneal hemorrhage can result from the rupture of these lesions.[5]

HEMANGIOENDOTHELIOMA

This rare lesion is thought to be intermediate between hemangioma and angiosarcoma. They usually contain cellular atypia, differentiating them from hemangiomas. These lesions may present with splenomegaly or rupture, and should suggest the possibility of a malignant vascular neoplasm.[4]

HAMARTOMAS

These are focal developmental abnormalities within the normal spleen, rather than being true neoplasms. They consist of normal cellular elements in disarray, and are usually found incidentally.

OTHER BENIGN LESIONS

There are a number of other benign neoplasms, including hemangipericytoma, bacillary angiomatosis, inflammatory pseudotumors, and mycobacterial spindle cell pseudotumors. These are all extremely rare lesions and are rarely found except as incidental findings when the spleen is removed for other reasons.

NONPARASITIC CYSTS

Nonparasitic cysts have been reported in patients of all ages, and are probably the result of a development anomaly. Patients with these benign lesions usually present with left upper quadrant pain. Evaluation of these patients usually reveals splenomegaly. These lesions are round and well circumscribed on imaging studies. In general, cysts that are less than 4 cm in size and asymptomatic can be observed; those that are greater than 4 cm or are symptomatic should be resected.[4] Partial splenectomy is the preferred method of resection when possible.[6]

PARASITIC CYSTS

The only parasitic cyst of importance is the echinococcal cyst. This condition is endemic in the Near East, New Zealand, Australia, and the western United States. The complement fixation test is used for diagnosis. The treatment of this condition is splenectomy.[4]

Malignant Lesions of the Spleen

There are many malignancies that affect the spleen. A list of these conditions is given in Table 24.2.[7]

NON-HODGKIN'S LYMPHOMA

Non-Hodgkin's lymphoma is a diverse group of diseases with a wide range of biological behaviors. They may be very aggressive and rapidly fatal, or may behave as one of the most indolent and well-tolerated malignancies afflicting man.[8] The therapy for these patients is still evolving, and surgical staging is generally reserved for the very small minority of patients who will receive radiation therapy alone if the disease is localized.

The role of the surgeon in the care of patients with non-Hodgkin's lymphoma is, therefore, usually limited to the biopsy of a single peripheral lymph node to establish a tissue diagnosis. Abdominal surgery is rarely required except in the absence of peripheral lymphadenopathy, when laparotomy or laparoscopy may be necessary to obtain adequate tissue for diagnosis of intraabdominal disease. In non-Hodgkin's lymphoma, the precise definition of disease location, unlike Hodgkin's lymphoma, has less impact on therapeutic decision making.[9] In general, non-Hodgkin's lymphomas are systemic diseases at the time of diagnosis, and require the use of systemic therapy (e.g., chemotherapy) rather than regional therapy (e.g., radiation) for treatment. This fact coupled with increasingly more sensitive and specific diagnostic tests has limited the number of operative staging procedures needed to assist in treatment planning.

HODGKIN'S DISEASE

Hodgkin's lymphoma usually originates in a single nodal group and predictably proceeds in a stepwise progression from one contiguous node group to the next.[10] The disease originates above the diaphragm in 80% to 90% of patients[11] and is limited to the lymph nodes in 85% of cases.[12] Below the diaphragm, the spleen becomes involved by Hodgkin's lymphoma before proceeding along the periaortic lymph nodes to the iliac and inguinal nodal basins.[11] Rarely, the disease originates below the diaphragm and proceeds cephalad in reverse sequence.[11] The need for surgical staging is, therefore, more clearly defined for Hodgkin's than non-Hodgkin's lymphoma. The rationale is that the staging will more reliably predict disseminated disease in Hodgkin's because an orderly progression is the norm and abdominal involvement will alter the type of therapy.

It is critical to understand the role of stage of disease in determining therapy as staging operations are only performed when the outcomes from the procedures will directly impact the plan of treatment. Clearly, if chemotherapy is to be used no matter what result the staging procedure yields, then it is doubtful that the procedure should be performed at all. The staging of Hodgkin's lymphoma takes into account the lymph node involvement above and below the diaphragm as well as the presence or absence of constitutional symptoms with the designations "A" or "B."

Patients with pathological stage I and IIA disease are usually successfully treated with radiation therapy alone.[13,14] Exceptions to this paradigm are the subgroup of patients who present with bulky mediastinal disease [greater than one-third the greatest transverse diameter of the chest on posteroanterior (PA) chest X-ray]. This group will receive chemotherapy as either primary or adjuvant therapy. Surgical staging, therefore, will only benefit this group of patients if it has a significant likelihood of upstaging the groups who are intended to receive radiation therapy alone. Should the disease relapse after radiation therapy, patients can be salvaged with chemotherapy without jeopardizing their long-term survival.[15]

Patients with stage IIB disease can be approached in two different ways. In institutions that would primarily treat this group with chemotherapy, surgical staging is unnecessary and clinical staging suffices. If radiation is to be the sole mode of treatment, then these patients need to be staged surgically, then treated with subtotal lymph node radiotherapy. Should the disease recur they then can be salvaged with chemotherapy. Clearly, the type of staging used for this group is dependent on the treatment philosophy of the individual oncologists caring for a specific patient.

In the early 1980s, staging laparotomy was recommended for all patients with clinical stage III disease. By the addition of surgical staging to the evaluation, many patients could be "downstaged" and therefore needed less chemotherapy. Nonetheless, many patients with pathological stage III disease were still treated with radiation therapy alone to avoid the side effects of chemotherapy.[16] Currently, there is enough evidence that radiotherapy can only be used in a small subset of stage III patients designated as stage III$_1$ (upper abdominal lymph nodes involvement) while those with pathological stage III$_2$ (lower abdominal lymph nodes involvement) require chemotherapy.[13] Patients with pathological stage IIIB and stage IV disease require a combination of radiotherapy and chemotherapy, negating the need for surgical staging.

Staging laparotomy is now performed in only 30% of patients.[18] With refinement of noninvasive imaging techniques, as well as changes in the medical management of the disease, the value of surgical staging of lymphoma has been reevaluated. This has resulted in significant decreases in the proportion of splenectomies performed for staging lymphoma. The role of splenectomy, however, is still in evolution. There is growing evidence that combined chemo–radiation therapy for Hodgkin's lymphoma may be associated with a signifi-

---

TABLE 24.2. Malignant Lesions of the Spleen.

I. Lymphoproliferative disorders
  a. Non-Hodgkin's lymphoma
  b. Hodgkin's disease
  c. Chronic lymphocytic leukemia
  d. Hairy cell leukemia
  e. Plasmacytoma
  f. Waldenström's macroglobulinemia

II. Myeloproliferative disorders
  a. Chronic myelogenous leukemia
  b. Polycythemia vera
  c. Myelofibrosis (agnogenic myeloid metaplasia)
  d. Essential thrombocythemia

III. Vascular tumors
  a. Hemangiosarcoma
  b. Lymphangiosarcoma

IV. Metastatic tumors: breast, lung, melanoma, etc.

V. Other lesions
  a. Sarcoma: fibrosarcoma, leiomyosarcoma, Kaposi's sarcoma

Source: Adapted from Giles and Lim (1997).[7]

cantly increased risk of developing a second malignant disease.[12] If this risk proves to hold true, it follows that surgical staging may again provide significant benefits for patients with Hodgkin's lymphoma by reducing their need for combination therapy. Further study is obviously needed.

Thus, at the present time, the role of the surgeon in patients with Hodgkin's lymphoma includes lymph node biopsy to establish a diagnosis, and staging laparotomy in a very select group of patients, usually limited to those patients with stage IIB disease after imaging evaluation. Patients with obvious stage III or stage IV disease should rarely be subjected to staging laparotomy because they will be treated with chemotherapy, and patients with stage I disease are usually treated with radiation alone, obviating the need for staging laparotomy. When indicated, laparoscopic approaches have been successfully employed.

CHRONIC LYMPHOCYTIC LEUKEMIA (CLL)

This is the most common of the chronic leukemias, usually found in patients over 60 years of age. It is usually of B-cell lineage and is characterized by an accumulation of incompetent lymphocytes.[17] CLL is incurable, but it is managed with a variety of chemotherapeutic agents and sometimes splenectomy. Splenectomy is indicated in those patients who progress despite chemotherapy, often with massive splenomegaly.

HAIRY CELL LEUKEMIA

This is a rare lymphoproliferative disorder that affects middle-aged men; it presents with pancytopenia and splenomegaly and is characterized by the identification of "hairy cells" in the peripheral circulation. Splenectomy has long been the therapy of choice for this disease. However, more recently, systemic chemotherapy employing 2-chloro-deoxyadenosine has been shown to induce remission in 80% to 90% of patients.[18] Splenectomy is thus reserved for patients who fail to respond to systemic chemotherapy or who have massive symptomatic splenomegaly.

MYELOPROLIFERATIVE DISORDERS

These diseases include chronic myelogenous leukemia (CML), myelofibrosis (also called agnogenic myeloid metaplasia), polycythemia vera, and essential thrombocythemia. These diseases are often considered as being along a spectrum with considerable overlap in clinical and laboratory findings. Early splenectomy has not been shown to delay the onset of blast transformation or prolong survival, and so the role of splenectomy remains controversial.

PRIMARY LYMPHOMA OF THE SPLEEN

This is a subset of non-Hodgkin's lymphoma (NHL) in which the disease begins in the spleen, and the bulk of disease is concentrated in the spleen with additional involvement of hilar lymph nodes.[19] Splenomegaly is a prominent feature of this disease, but peripheral adenopathy is absent. In a single institutional series, data suggest that patients with localized splenic and splenic hilar disease have the same prognosis as other patients with stage I NHL and that those patients with other sites of involvement have a similar prognosis to patients with similarly staged forms of NHL.[19]

HEMANGIOSARCOMA

This is a rare primary tumor of the spleen in humans. Treatment is surgical, and no effective adjuvant therapies have been identified.

Indications for Splenectomy

There are two surgical procedures performed in reference to the spleen: partial splenectomy and splenectomy. A splenectomy can be conducted by conventional open technique (OS) or by laparoscopic means (LS). The indications for splenectomy are unrelated to the technique that will be used to remove the spleen.

Splenectomy for Trauma

The spleen is the organ most commonly injured in blunt abdominal trauma, and thus the majority of splenectomies in the United States are performed for trauma. At this time, it appears prudent that splenic surgery for trauma is conducted by OS techniques, although it is conceivable that there may be rare instances in which LS is a reasonable alternative.

Splenic injury is often suspected in the injured patient on the basis of mechanism of injury and the presence of associated injuries such as left lower rib fractures. Some patients undergo CT scan of the abdomen and reveal injuries such as those seen in Figure 24.1. Once splenic injury is identified, there are three options: nonoperative management, splenic salvage (repair of the injury or partial splenectomy), or splenectomy. There is no role for splenic salvage in the critically injured trauma patient with multiple intraabdominal injuries. In these patients, splenectomy is the only procedure to be considered.

Splenic autotransplantation is easy to carry out, but its efficacy is not really known. The concept is to preserve splenic function by transplanting fragments of the excised spleen elsewhere in the abdomen, usually within an omental pouch. There is no consensus about the number, mass, or size of implants used. The only proven immunological result of replantation is the normal IgM levels. It is unclear whether lymphocyte function is normal.

The specific management of a patient with a splenic injury is guided by the overall stability of the injured patient,

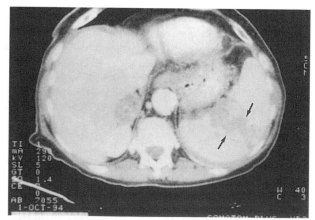

FIGURE 24.1. Splenic fracture (*arrows*). There is a small amount of fluid adjacent to the spleen posteriorly.

TABLE 24.3. Grading of Traumatic Splenic Injuries.

I	Hematoma	Subcapsular, nonexpanding, <10% surface
	Laceration	Capsular tear, nonbleeding, <1 cm parenchymal depth
II	Hematoma	Subcapsular, nonexpanding, 10%–50% surface area
	Laceration	Capsular tear, active bleeding, 1–3 cm, not involving a trabecular vessel
III	Hematoma	Subcapsular, >50% surface area or expanding, ruptured subcapsular hematoma with active bleeding, intraparenchymal hematoma, <2 cm or expanding
	Laceration	>3 cm parenchymal depth or involving trabecular vessels
IV	Hematoma	Ruptured intraparenchymal hematoma with active bleeding
	Laceration	Laceration involving segmental or hilar vessel with major devascularization (>25%)
V	Laceration	Completely shattered spleen
	Vascular	Hilar vascular injury with devascularized spleen

Source: Adapted from Lipshy et al. (1996).[20]

mechanism of injury, age, interval from time of injury, associated injuries, and preexisting medical conditions. Splenic injuries are graded by severity (Table 24.3). In a recent series of adults with splenic injuries, 18% were treated nonoperatively, 22% underwent splenorrhaphy, and 60% underwent splenectomy.[20]

MANAGEMENT OF SPLENIC INJURIES IN CHILDREN

The nonoperative management of splenic injury has been applied primarily (and most uniformly) in children. Hemodynamic stability and transfusion requirement less than 50% of the blood volume is essential to manage these injuries without surgery. Obviously, nonoperative management assumes no other intraabdominal injuries requiring exploration. Three factors form the basis for this approach: bleeding from splenic lacerations often ceases by the time of laparotomy; the spleen is immunologically important; and CT scanning permits accurate localization of intraabdominal solid organ injury. Delayed splenic rupture remains a possibility in patients managed nonoperatively.

Guidelines for the nonoperative management of splenic injuries in children include documentation of splenic injury by imaging studies, admission to the ICU with close observation, hemodynamic stability, serial hematocrit determination, absence of other intraabdominal injuries, transfusion requirements less than 50% of total blood volume, and absence of neurotrauma permitting patient cooperation with serial history and physical examination.

MANAGEMENT OF SPLENIC INJURIES IN ADULTS

The nonoperative management of splenic injuries in adults is less established as a standard than in children. It is an evolving practice with success rates reported from 27% to 100%. Patients are considered candidates for nonoperative management by meeting criteria such as hemodynamic stability, minimum transfusion requirement, absence of associated intraabdominal injury, and an ability to perform reliable serial abdominal examinations.[21] A stable defect on repeat imaging also supports this approach. Patients treated without exploration should be carefully observed and undergo repeat CT scan at 3 weeks to assess stability of the defect.

The decision to embark on splenorrhaphy in the adult with a splenic injury is based on hemodynamic stability, pres-

ence of other injuries, and extent of splenic injury.[22] Adequate mobilization is essential. Grade I and II injuries (capsular avulsions and superficial parenchymal fractures) are managed by topical hemostatic agents. The argon beam coagulator may be helpful in the management of these lesions. Mattress sutures over Teflon pledgets may be useful to close deeper wounds. Grade III and IV splenic injury requires complete mobilization of the spleen to expose the hilum. Division of the short gastric vessels is required. Partial splenectomy may be indicated. Most authors report low incidence of reoperation (0%–2%) following splenic preservation. Not surprisingly, the laparoscopic control of splenic injury with splenic preservation has also been reported.[23]

Splenectomy for Hematological Disorders

Common indications for elective splenectomy are listed in Table 24.4.

HEREDITARY SPHEROCYTOSIS

This clinically heterogeneous condition is characterized by a deficiency in spectrin, resulting in a defective erythrocyte membrane that causes the cell to be less deformable and thus more susceptible to trapping within the spleen.[24] It is a congenital condition, transmitted in an autosomal dominant fashion, and is the most common hemolytic anemia for which splenectomy

TABLE 24.4. Indications for Elective Splenectomy.

ITP (idiopathic thrombocytopenia purpura)
Hereditary spherocytosis
Autoimmune hemolytic anemia
Staging for Hodgkin's disease
Lymphoma
Thrombocytopenic thrombotic purpura
AIDS-related thrombocytopenia
Leukemia
Splenic abscess
Gaucher's disease
Myelofibrosis
Splenic infarct

is performed. Patients with this condition present with anemia, splenomegaly, and jaundice. The diagnosis is established by examination of the peripheral blood smear. Therapy of this disease is splenectomy, with a nearly 100% response rate.

THALASSEMIA

This is a disease of hemoglobin synthesis, transmitted in a dominant fashion, and common in people of Mediterranean descent. The diagnosis is established by examining the peripheral blood smear, which demonstrates target cells. Splenectomy is reserved for patients with symptomatic splenomegaly or pain from splenic infarcts.

SICKLE CELL ANEMIA

This hereditary condition is predominantly seen in African-Americans. The peripheral blood smear demonstrates sickle-shaped erythrocytes, caused by abnormal Hb-S, which has replaced the normal Hb-A. Splenectomy may benefit some patients in whom acute splenic sequestration of red blood cells is demonstrated.[25]

IDIOPATHIC AUTOIMMUNE HEMOLYTIC ANEMIA

This disease is characterized by hemolysis of normal erythrocytes after exposure to circulating antibodies. It is believed that the spleen serves as a source of antibody in this process. The initial therapy is steroid administration, reserving splenectomy for patients in whom steroids are ineffective or contraindicated.

IDIOPATHIC THROMBOCYTOPENIA PURPURA (ITP)

The most common indication for elective splenectomy in most series, this is an acquired disorder caused by the destruction of platelets exposed to IgG antiplatelet factors.[25] These factors are produced in the spleen, and the spleen also serves as the location for platelet sequestration and destruction. Imaging studies demonstrate that these patients have normal-sized spleens. Laboratory studies usually demonstrate a platelet count under 50,000/mm^3 or even lower.

Therapy of this disease is usually begun with steroid administration. This protocol is often supplemented with intravenous immunoglobulin (IVIG), and these measures result in cure in about 15% to 20% of patients.[26] Failure of nonoperative therapy is usually followed by splenectomy, which results in a cure in about 85% of patients. Patients who do not respond with normalization of platelet counts usually have no recurrences of petechiae and ecchymoses. Patients who do not respond to splenectomy or who relapse at a later date may have accessory splenic tissue that was not identified at the time of surgery.

THROMBOTIC THROMBOCYTOPENIA PURPURA (TTP)

TTP is characterized by a pentad of clinical findings: microangiopathic hemolytic anemia, consumptive thrombocytopenia, CNS abnormalities, renal failure, and fever. Damage to the endothelium resulting in platelet aggregation and microvascular occlusion is central to the pathophysiology.[27] Therapy for this illness includes plasmapheresis, steroids, splenectomy, dextran, antiplatelet agents, and vinca alkaloids.[28] Splenectomy is reserved for patients who relapse after

plasmapheresis and plasma exchange. Splenectomy has a clear role in the treatment of this complex illness, but first-line therapy remains medical.

FELTY'S SYNDROME

This syndrome consists of rheumatoid arthritis, splenomegaly, and neutropenia. Patients are usually treated with steroids, but failure to respond to steroids may be an indication for splenectomy.

OTHER CONDITIONS

Splenectomy may be indicated for some patients with a variety of diseases that result in hypersplenism or splenomegaly, including sarcoidosis, Gaucher's disease, porphyria erythropoietica, and systemic mast cell disease.

Operative Approach to the Spleen

Patient Preparation

In preparation for splenectomy, patients should be immunized against *Pneumococcus*, *Haemophilus influenza* B, and *Meningococcus* at least 2 weeks before operation, if possible. Preoperative splenic artery embolization, used only in selected patients with splenomegaly or AIDS or in obese patients, should be performed on the day of surgery because patients may experience considerable pain after infarction of the spleen. Platelets are not administered in the preoperative period for patients with ITP, regardless of the level of thrombocytopenia.[25] Platelet transfusions are withheld for patients with significant intraoperative bleeding after removal of the spleen. Patients must be given a thorough discussion of overwhelming postsplenectomy infection before the procedure.

Open Splenectomy

The technique of open splenectomy has remained largely unchanged for many years. The patient is placed on the operating table in the supine position. The incision used is dependent on the preference of the operating surgeon, as splenectomy can be performed with facility through a midline incision or a left subcostal incision.

The splenic artery can be managed in several ways. Some have suggested ligation of the artery in the lesser sac at the beginning of the procedure for patients with massive splenomegaly.[29] Others have suggested that patients should undergo preoperative splenic artery occlusion using radiologic techniques.[30] However, even in cases of splenomegaly, not all surgeons believe that it is necessary to approach the splenic artery before a routine splenectomy.

After removal of the spleen, drains are not usually required, but when desired, closed suction drains are employed. In those patients for whom splenectomy is performed for hematological diseases, a search for accessory splenic tissue is conducted.

Laparoscopic Splenectomy

The technique of laparoscopic splenectomy was first described in 1992[31,32] and has become a well-accepted procedure. Initially, there was concern that the procedure would result in excessive blood loss, splenosis, and inaccurate pathological examination of the specimen. For the most part, these fears have been proven unwarranted. While splenomegaly remains a technical challenge, LS has become the preferred surgical technique for ITP and other diseases with normal spleen size.

To begin, the patient is placed in supine, lithotomy, lateral, or semilateral position. The supine position is preferred for initiating pneumoperitoneum, inserting trocars, exploring for accessory spleens, and ligating the splenic artery in the lesser sac, while the lateral position offers excellent exposure of the hilum to facilitate dissection and vessel ligation.[33] At present, preoperative embolization is used infrequently by most surgeons, and the methods of hilar dissection and vessel ligation vary according to the surgeon's preference.

Increasing operative experience and technical refinements have produced good results relative to open splenectomy (OS) in terms of outcome, patient discomfort, length of hospitalization, and costs. It is anticipated that the procedure may have greatest benefit in patients at greatest risk of complications of laparotomy, including those with hypersplenism who are treated with steroids and other immunosuppressive regimens. Wound problems, infections, and pulmonary complications, which are particularly troublesome with conventional splenectomy techniques, may be avoided with LS.

COLLECTED EXPERIENCE

Approximately 900 laparoscopic splenectomies have been reported. There are no prospective randomized trials recorded in the literature because for the most part the results are strongly in support of the laparoscopic approach. Overall success rates for the procedures are better than 90%, with bleeding by far the most common reason for conversion. Comparing LS with OS, most authors have reported significantly shorter postoperative hospital stay, no difference in blood loss, earlier recovery of bowel function, but significantly greater operative times for laparoscopic splenectomy.

It is inaccurate, however, to compare the results of LS to OS in a heterogenous population. Most LS series contain patients with ITP primarily, while OS series include patients with trauma, splenectomy performed in conjunction with other procedures, and a greater number of patients with diseases other than ITP. It is therefore important to keep indication in mind when evaluating technique. Still, in the few series where OS and LS are compared according to similar indication, LS appears to be the more favorable approach.

Partial Splenectomy

The principal indication for partial splenectomy is trauma, where one desires to maintain the splenic immune function to decrease the incidence of postoperative infectious complications. It is clear that this procedure is much more technically demanding than splenectomy. It is a particularly useful technique in children, for whom the risk of OPSI is greatest. Laparoscopic partial splenectomy has been described and is obviously technically feasible.[34]

Accessory Splenic Tissue

Accessory splenic tissue is identified in 10% to 20% of patients undergoing splenectomy and remains an important issue in the operative management of these patients. The search for accessory splenic tissue remains an integral part of the procedure when performed for certain hematological conditions such as ITP because residual splenic tissue can hypertrophy and cause relapse of the disease, sometimes years after splenectomy.[35] Knowledge of the location of this tissue is important. Most commonly, accessory splenic tissue is located at or near the splenic hilum, but it has been reported along the left gutter and even into the left scrotum.

A patient who presents with relapse of ITP should be assumed to have retained accessory splenic tissue until proven otherwise. The initial diagnostic test should be a technetium-99–sulfur colloid liver–spleen scan. If a focus of uptake is identified, then CT scan may be useful to locate the residual tissue. Long-term remission after excision of the accessory splenic tissue has been reported.[35] Both open and laparoscopic techniques have been used.

Incidental Splenectomy

The spleen is easily injured during procedures in the upper abdomen involving the stomach, esophageal hiatus, vagus nerves, pancreas, left colon, and left kidney. Most commonly this involves capsular tears, resulting in continuous bleeding. When the splenic capsule is injured during the conduct of other procedures, attempts should be made at splenic salvage to minimize the necessity for incidental splenectomy.

Complications of Splenectomy

Published series of OS[36–40] report morbidity rates that range from 15% to as high as 61%. Series of LS[33,41–45] report morbidity rates of 0% to 14%. The mortality rates reported for OS range from 6% to 13% and those for LS from 0% to 5%. However, most series of OS include splenectomies performed for trauma or iatrogenic operative injury, for which morbidity and mortality rates may be higher (36% and 16%, respectively).[38] Factors predisposing to complications include the underlying indication for the splenectomy, the patient's age, and associated diseases.

Operative Complications

CARDIOVASCULAR EFFECTS OF PNEUMOPERITONEUM

Cardiovascular effects of pneumoperitoneum are minimal and rarely result in hypotension or arrhythmia.[46] Hemodynamic problems, usually during insufflation, occur in approximately 0.2% of patients and are associated with vasovagal reflex or decreased venous return. Most often, the problems are minor and can be corrected with administration of fluids or atropine.

BOWEL INJURY

Injury to the bowel is rare and usually occurs during creation of the pneumoperitoneum. Reported frequency, in the gynecology literature, is 0.16% to 0.27%.[47] Patients who have had prior abdominal surgery are at increased risk of accidental enterotomy, regardless of the technique used. Prior abdominal surgery is a relative contraindication to LS.

VASCULAR INJURY

Injury to blood vessels may occur during Veress needle or trocar insertion. Use of the open technique eliminates the risk of injury to major intraabdominal vessels as a blunt-tipped trocar is inserted. Major vascular injuries requiring further intervention occur in 0.64% of laparoscopic procedures.[47] Minor bleeding that causes abdominal wall hematomas may occasionally occur from trocar injuries to abdominal wall vessels. These areas should be identified by careful inspection of the trocar sites before the conclusion of the operation; simple ligation of the vessels usually contains the hemorrhage.

HEMORRHAGE

The most common intraoperative complication of splenectomy is hemorrhage, which occurs in roughly 5% of cases. In our series of LS, it occurred in 6%. Hemorrhage was responsible for 75% of conversions to an open procedure. Defects of clotting factors and platelets cause bleeding from raw surfaces of the splenic bed, diaphragm, retroperitoneum, and less frequently from the pancreatic surface. Meticulous hemostasis and accurate dissection can avoid this problem.

INJURY TO ADJACENT ORGANS

Injuries to structures adjacent to the spleen (pancreas, stomach, diaphragm), reported in 1% to 3% of OS, have been rare during LS. The magnification of the laparoscopic technique seems to afford a better view of the organs and will probably decrease iatrogenic injuries.

Postoperative Complications

RESPIRATORY

Respiratory complications affect 10% to 48% of patients after OS (atelectasis, 15%; pleural effusion, 11%; pneumonia, 7%–13%).[38] To avoid diaphragmatic irritation from blood and irrigant, the subphrenic space should be aspirated dry at the conclusion of the operation.

SUBPHRENIC ABSCESS

Subphrenic abscesses are reported to occur in 4% to 8% of OS[39,40] but to date have not been reported in the laparoscopic literature. No laparoscopic cases were performed for trauma, where associated bowel injuries increase the risk of subphrenic infection.

WOUND PROBLEMS

Wound complications such as hematoma, seroma, and infection occur because of impaired wound healing, coagulation abnormalities, steroid use, and immune defects. Wound infections occur in 3% of OS performed for diagnostic indications and 6% performed for therapeutic indications, and in 11% of patients who require perioperative steroids.[36,48]

ILEUS AND SMALL-BOWEL OBSTRUCTION

Postoperative ileus and small-bowel obstruction have been reported in 1% to 10% of OS for Hodgkin's disease, with a reoperation rate of 2% to 7%.[48] In the laparoscopic series, there is only one report of a prolonged postoperative ileus.[49]

FEVER

Postoperative fever unrelated to any of the common postoperative causes has been reported in the open splenectomy literature. It is believed to be secondary to circulating leukoagglutinizing antibodies and is self-limited.[38] This complication has not been reported in the laparoscopic literature.

THROMBOEMBOLISM

Thromboembolism complicates 2% to 11% of OS[38,40] and is more common in patients who have hypersplenism or myeloproliferative disorders. The presumed causes include eradication of splenic sequestration, removal of regulatory humoral factors produced by the spleen, altered platelet function, thrombocytosis, and thrombus extending from the splenic vein remnant secondary to intimal injury and stasis. Treatment with antiplatelet medication may be of some use if platelets exceed 500,000/mm^3, but no prospective studies have been performed. In addition, thrombolytic agents and anticoagulants may prove to be lifesaving.

SPLENOSIS

Splenosis is defined as the autotransplantation of splenic tissue in an ectopic position and is usually seen following traumatic splenic rupture in children; the reported incidence is 48% to 66%.[50] This is worrisome to the laparoscopic surgeon, because the ideal grasper for the spleen has not been developed, and fracture of the spleen may occur. Nevertheless, there have been no reports of splenosis following LS.

OVERWHELMING POSTSPLENECTOMY INFECTION

Overwhelming postsplenectomy infection (OPSI) follows 4% of splenectomies, with a mortality rate of 1.7%. It is important to apprise patients of their risks related to OPSI before surgery when possible. Splenectomy reduces phagocytosis and the clearance of microorganisms, the elaboration of specific immune responses, and the production of splenic opsonins.[51] More than 66% of these cases and 80% of deaths occur within the first 2 years of splenectomy. The incidence of this complication following LS should be the same as after OS.

Most importantly, patients who are to undergo elective splenectomy must be given appropriate vaccines as noted above (see "Patient Preparation"). OPSI is a condition that occurs most commonly in young children. Other preventive measures include the use of prophylactic penicillin for all children less than 2 years of age after splenectomy, and providing adults with a prescription for penicillin to be filled at the first onset of symptoms. The role of prophylactic antibiotics appears somewhat controversial, especially in light of low documented compliance rates. Patients who undergo splenectomy after trauma should undergo vaccination immediately after surgery. Some physicians advise patients to wear a "Medic-Alert" bracelet.

References

1. Morgenstern L. A history of splenectomy. In: Hiatt JR, Phillips EH, Morgenstern L, eds. Surgical Diseases of the Spleen. New York: Springer, 1997.
2. Llende M, Santiago-Delpin EA, Lavergne J. Immunobiological

consequences of splenectomy: a review. J Surg Res 1986;40:85–94.

3. Reiman RS. Pathology of the spleen. In: Hiatt JR, Phillips EH, Morgenstern L, eds. Surgical Diseases of the Spleen. New York: Springer, 1997.

4. Morgenstern L. Benign neoplasms of the spleen. In: Hiatt JR, Phillips EH, Morgenstern L, eds. Surgical Diseases of the Spleen. New York: Springer, 1997.

5. Kohr RM, Haendiges M, Taube RR. Peliosis of the spleen: a rare cause of spontaneous splenic rupture with surgical implications. Am Surg 1993;59:197–199.

6. Ehrlich P, Jamieson CG. Nonparasitic splenic cysts: a case report and review. Can J Surg 1990;33:306–308.

7. Giles FJ, Lim SW. Malignant splenic lesions. In: Hiatt JR. Phillips EH, Mogenstern L, eds. Surgical Diseases of the Spleen. New York: Springer, 1997.

8. Rosenberg SA. Non-Hodgkin's lymphoma—selection of treatment on the basis of histologic type. N Engl J Med 1979;301:924–928.

9. Longo DL, Devita VT, Jaffe ES, et al. Lymphocytic lymphomas. In: Devita VT, Hellman S, Rosenberg SA, eds. Cancer: Principles and Practice of Oncology, 4th Ed. Philadelphia: Lippincott, 1993:1859–1937.

10. Rosenberg SA, Kaplan HS. Evidence for an orderly progression in the spread of Hodgkin's disease. Cancer Res 1966;26:1225–1231.

11. Moormeier JA, Williams SF, Golomb HM. The staging of Hodgkin's disease. Hematol Oncol Clin North Am 1989;3:237–251.

12. Williams SF, Golomb HM. Perspective on staging approaches in the malignant lymphomas. Surg Gynecol Obstet 1986;163:193–201.

13. Urba WJ, Longo DL. Hodgkin's disease. N Engl J Med 1992;326:678–687.

14. Mai DHW, Peschel RE, Portlock C, et al. Stage I and II subdiaphragmatic Hodgkin's disease. Cancer (Phila) 1991;68:1476–1481.

15. Lefor AT. Laparoscopic staging of abdominal lymphomas. In: Greene F, Rosin RD, eds. Minimal Access Surgical Oncology. New York: Radcliffe, 1995.

16. Grieco MB, Cady B. Staging laparotomy in Hodgkin's disease. Surg Clin North Am 1980;60:369–379.

17. Thiruvengadam R, O'Brien S, Kantarjian H, et al. Splenectomy in advanced chronic lymphocytic leukemia. Leukemia 1990;4:758–760.

18. Tallman MS, Hakimian D, Variakojis D, et al. A single cycle of 2-chlorodeoxy-adenosine results in complete remission in the majority of patients with hairy cell leukemia. Blood 1992;2203–2209.

19. Kehoe J, Straus DJ. Primary lymphoma of the spleen. Cancer (Phila) 1988;62:1433–1438.

20. Lipshy KA, Shaffer DJ, Denning DA. An institutional review of the management of splenic trauma. Contemp Surg 1996;48:330.

21. Godley CD, Warren RL, Sheridan RL, McCabe CJ. Nonoperative management of blunt splenic injury in adults: age over 55 years as a powerful indicator for failure. J Am Coll Surg 1996;183:133.

22. Pickhardt B, Moore EE, Moore FA, McCroskey BL, Moore GE. Operative splenic salvage in adults: a decade perspective. J Trauma 1989;29:1386–1393.

23. Rizk N, Chapault G, Boutelier P. Laparoscopic splenic salvage in blunt abdominal trauma. Acta Chir Belg 1995;95:202.

24. Croom RD, McMillan CW, Sheldon GW, Orringer EP. Hereditary spherocytosis. Ann Surg 1986;203:34–39.

25. Schwartz SI. Splenectomy for hematologic disorders. In Hiatt JR, Phillips EH, Morgenstern L, eds. Surgical Diseases of the Spleen. New York: Springer, 1997.

26. Schwartz SI. Role of splenectomy in hematologic disorders. World J Surg 1996;20:1156–1159.

27. Winslow GA, Nelson EW. Thrombotic thrombocytopenic purpura: indications for and results of splenectomy. Am J Surg 1995;170:558–563.

28. Schneider PA, Rayner AA, Linker CA, et al. The role of splenectomy in multimodality treatment of thrombotic thrombocytopenia purpura. Ann Surg 1985;202:318–322.

29. Hiatt JR, Allins A, Kong LR. Open splenectomy. In: Hiatt JR, Phillips EH, Morgenstern L, eds. Surgical Diseases of the Spleen. New York: Springer, 1997.

30. Fujitani RM, Johs SM, Cobb SR, et al. Preoperative splenic artery occlusion as an adjunct for high risk splenectomy. Am Surg 1988;54:602–608.

31. Carroll BJ, Phillips EH, Semel CJ, et al. Laparoscopic splenectomy. Surg Endosc 1992;6:183–185.

32. Delaitre B, Maignien B. Laparoscopic splenectomy: technical aspects. Surg Endosc 1992;6:305–308.

33. Phillips EH, Carroll BJ, Fallas MJ. Laparoscopic splenectomy. Surg Endosc 1994;8:931–933.

34. Poulin EC, Thibault C, DesCoteaux JG, Cote G. Partial laparoscopic splenectomy for trauma: technique and case report. Surg Laparosc Endosc 1995;5:306–310.

35. Walters DN, Roberts JL, Votaw M. Accessory splenectomy in the management of recurrent immune thrombocytopenic purpura. Am Surg 1998;64:1077–1078.

36. Musser G, Lazar G, Hocking W, Busuttil RW. Splenectomy for hematologic disease: the UCLA experience with 306 patients. Ann Surg 1984;200(1):40–45.

37. Aksnes J, Abdelnoor M, Mathisen O. Risk factors associated with mortality and morbidity after elective splenectomy. Eur J Surg 1995;161:253–258.

38. Ellison EC, Fabri PJ. Complications of splenectomy: etiology, prevention and management. Surg Clin N Am 1983;63(6):1313–1330.

39. Horowitz J, Smith JL, Weber TK, Rodriguez-Bigas MA, Petrelli NJ. Postoperative complications after splenectomy for hematologic malignancies. Ann Surg 1996;223:290–296.

40. MacRae HM, Yakimets WW, Reynolds T. Perioperative complications of splenectomy for hematologic disease. Can J Surg 1992;35:432–436.

41. Friedman RL, Fallas MJ, Carroll BJ, et al. Laparoscopic splenectomy for ITP. The gold standard. Surg Endosc 1996;10:991–995.

42. Gigot JF, Jamar F, Ferrant A, et al. Inadequate detection of accessory spleens and splenosis with laparoscopic splenectomy. Surg Endosc 1998;12:101–106.

43. Lefor AT, Melvin WS, Bailey RW, Flowers JL. Laparoscopic splenectomy in the management of immune thrombocytopenia purpura. Surgery (St. Louis) 1993;114:613–618.

44. Rhodes M, Rudd M, O'Rourke N, Nathanson L, Fielding G. Laparoscopic splenectomy and lymph node biopsy for hematologic disorders. Ann Surg 1995;222:43–46.

45. Yee LF, Carvajal SH, Lorimier A, Mulvihill SJ. Laparoscopic splenectomy: an initial experience at University of California, San Francsico. Arch Surg 1995;130:874–878.

46. Hanley ES. Anesthesia for laparoscopic surgery. Surg Clin North Am 1992;72:1013–1019.

47. Phillips JM. Laparoscopy. Baltimore: Williams & Wilkins, 1977:220–246.

48. Jockovich M, Mendenhall NP, Sombeck MD, Talbert JL, Copeland EM III, Bland KI. Long-term complications of laparotomy in Hodgkin's disease. Ann Surg 1994;219:615–624.

49. Poulin EC, Thibault C, Mamazza J. Laparoscopic splenectomy. Surg Endosc 1995;9:172–177.

50. Mintz SJ, Petersen SR, Cheson B, Cordell LJ, Richards RC. Splenectomy for immune thrombocytopenic purpura. Arch Surg 1981;116:645–650.

51. Shaw JHF, Print CG. Postsplenectomy sepsis. Br J Surg 1989;76:1074–1081.

Hernias and Abdominal Wall Defects

Daniel J. Scott and Daniel B. Jones

Groin Hernias

Definitions

A hernia is a protrusion of visceral contents through the abdominal wall. There are two key components of a hernia. The first is the defect itself, namely the size and location of the fascial opening, and the second component is the hernia sac, which is a protrusion of peritoneum through the defect. The hernia sac may contain abdominal contents such as small intestine, colon, or bladder, or the sac may be empty. A *sliding hernia* exists when a retroperitoneal organ, usually the sigmoid colon, cecum, bladder, or ureter, forms part of the wall of the sac; these organs may be injured during hernia repair. A *Richter's hernia* exists when the antimesenteric portion of intestine (not the complete circumference of bowel) protrudes into the hernia sac. A *Littre's hernia* exists when the sac contains a Meckel's diverticulum. If the sac and its contents can be returned to the abdominal cavity, a hernia is termed reducible. If it cannot be returned to the abdominal cavity, as is sometimes the case with a small fascial defect and a large hernia, the hernia is termed irreducible or incarcerated. If an irreducible hernia contains intestine or other viscera whose blood supply is compromised, the hernia is *strangulated*. This condition can lead to a life-threatening situation in which the hernia sac contains gangrenous bowel and requires emergent exploration.

Anatomy

Successful repair of a groin hernia requires a thorough knowledge of the anatomy of the abdominal wall, inguinal canal, and femoral canal. The layers of the abdominal wall, from superficial to deep, include skin, Camper's fascia, Scarpa's fascia, the external oblique aponeurosis and muscle, the internal oblique aponeurosis and muscle, the transversus abdominis aponeurosis and muscle, the transversalis fascia, the preperitoneal fat, and the peritoneum. These layers continue in the region of the groin as they form their insertions in the inguinal canal.

INGUINAL CANAL

Several structures course within the inguinal canal (Fig. 25.1) and require familiarity to avoid iatrogenic injury during herniorraphy. The canal contains the spermatic cord in males and the round ligament of the uterus in females. The canal lies obliquely between the internal or deep inguinal ring, derived from transversalis fascia, and the external or superficial inguinal ring, derived from external oblique aponeurosis.

The spermatic cord courses from the internal ring through the inguinal canal and exits through the external ring to join the testicle within the scrotum. The spermatic cord contains multiple structures including the superficial spermatic fascia, derived from Camper's and Scarpa's fascia; the external spermatic fascia, derived from external oblique muscle; a circumferential layer of cremaster muscle, derived from internal oblique muscle; the cremasteric or external spermatic artery; the internal spermatic fascia, derived from transversalis fascia; the vas deferens and arteries to the vas deferens; the testicular or internal spermatic artery, which arises from the aorta just inferior to the renal arteries; the pampiniform venous plexus, which coalesces into the testicular veins and drains into the inferior vena cava on the right and the renal vein on the left; the ilioinguinal nerve; the genital branch of the genitofemoral nerve; and sympathetic fibers from the hypogastric plexus.

The inguinal canal can be defined by its borders. The inguinal canal is bound anteriorly by the external oblique aponeurosis, superiorly by internal oblique and transversus abdominis muscles and aponeuroses, and inferiorly by the inguinal and lacunar ligaments. The posterior wall or floor is formed by transversalis fascia. A defect in this layer may allow peritoneum and the contents of the abdominal cavity to herniate. *Hesselbach's triangle* is formed by the inguinal ligament laterally, the rectus sheath medially, and the inferior epigastric vessels superiorly (Fig. 25.2). A *direct hernia*

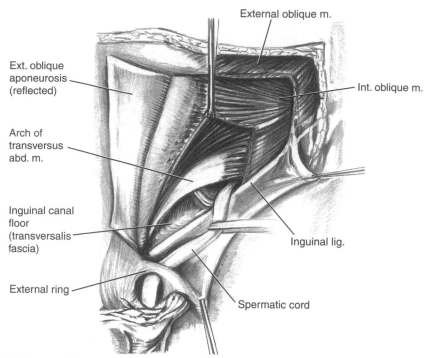

FIGURE 25.1. The left inguinal canal with the external oblique aponeurosis incised and reflected.

protrudes through the floor of the inguinal canal within this triangle (medial to the inferior epigastric vessels). Thus, a direct hernia is a protrusion of peritoneum through the transversalis fascia; it lies adjacent to (not within) the spermatic cord. The hernia sac exits the canal with the cord through the external ring into the scrotum. An *indirect hernia* forms lateral to the inferior epigastric vessels. An indirect hernia lies within the spermatic cord and with the cord it passes through the internal ring. The hernia sac courses through the inguinal canal and can exit with the cord through the external ring into the scrotum. The sac of an indirect hernia is usually found on the anteromedial aspect of the cord. Hernias with both a direct and an indirect component are called pantaloon hernias because the two components drape over the inferior epigastric vessels like the legs of a pair of trousers.

FEMORAL CANAL

A femoral hernia is a visceral protrusion through the femoral ring, which is bounded laterally by the femoral vein, anteriorly by the inguinal ligament, medially by the lacunar ligament, and posteriorly by Cooper's ligament. The femoral canal (see Fig. 25.2) represents an extension of the femoral ring for approximately 2 cm inferiorly into the thigh. The femoral sheath is derived from transversalis fascia and contains the femoral artery, vein, and canal. The femoral triangle is bounded by the inguinal ligament, the sartorius muscle, and the adductor longus muscle and contains, from lateral to medial, the femoral nerve, artery, vein, "empty" space (femoral canal), and lymphatics (hence the pneumonic *NAVEL*).

NERVES

The nerves of the ilioinguinal region arise from the lumbar plexus, innervate the abdominal musculature, and provide sensation for the skin and parietal peritoneum. Entrapment

usually causes severe pain, whereas transection results in numbness. Careful technique and anatomical knowledge are necessary to avoid nerve injury during herniorraphy. The iliohypogastric nerve (T12,L1) emerges from the lateral edge of

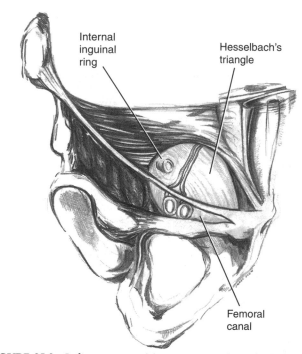

FIGURE 25.2. Indirect inguinal hernias occur through the internal ring. Direct inguinal hernias occur in Hesselbach's triangle, which lies between the inguinal ligament, the rectus sheath, and the inferior epigastric vessels. Femoral hernias occur through the femoral canal, which lies between the inguinal ligament, the lacunar ligament, Cooper's ligament, and the femoral vein. Fruchaud's myopectineal orifice refers to the entire musculoaponeurotic area through which inguinal and femoral hernias can occur.

the psoas muscle and courses within the layers of the abdominal wall. It penetrates the external oblique muscle within 1 to 2 cm of the superomedial aspect of the external ring where it supplies the skin in the suprapubic region with sensory fibers.

The ilioinguinal nerve (L1) courses with the iliohypogastric nerve and then joins the spermatic cord or round ligament through the internal and external inguinal rings to innervate the skin of the base of the penis or mons pubis, the scrotum or labia majora, and the medial aspect of the thigh.

The genitofemoral nerve (L1, L2) runs along the anterior aspect of the psoas muscle and divides before reaching the internal inguinal ring. The genital branch penetrates the iliopubic tract lateral to the internal inguinal ring and then enters the ring to join the cord. It supplies the anterior scrotum with sensory fibers, the cremaster muscle with motor fibers, and is the efferent limb for the cremasteric reflex. The femoral branch courses beneath the inguinal ligament to provide sensation to the anteromedial thigh and is the afferent limb for the cremasteric reflex.

The lateral femoral cutaneous nerve (L2, L3) emerges at the lateral edge of the psoas muscle, courses along the iliac fossa, lateral to the iliac vessels, and beneath the iliopubic tract and inguinal ligament to provide sensation to the lateral thigh. Injury of this nerve may be common with inexperienced surgeons performing laparoscopic hernia repair.

The femoral nerve (L2–L4) emerges from the lateral aspect of the psoas muscle and courses beneath the inguinal ligament lateral to the femoral vessels and outside of the femoral sheath to provide motor and sensory innervation for the thigh. Care must be taken to avoid femoral nerve injury during femoral hernia repair.

BLOOD VESSELS

The external iliac artery and vein lie on the medial aspect of the psoas muscle and course deep to the iliopubic tract to form the femoral artery and vein.

The inferior epigastric artery and vein cross over the iliopubic tract at the medial aspect of the internal ring and ascend along the posterior surface of the rectus muscles, invested in a fold of peritoneum called the lateral umbilical ligament. Near its takeoff the inferior epigastric artery gives off two branches, the cremasteric and the pubic. The cremasteric branch penetrates the transversalis fascia and joins the spermatic cord. The pubic branch courses in a vertical fashion inferiorly, crossing Cooper's ligament, and anastomoses with the obturator artery.

The testicular vessels follow the ureter into the pelvis on its lateral border, and then course along the lateral edge of the external iliac artery, cross the iliopubic tract, and join the spermatic cord at the lateral aspect of the internal ring. The testicular veins drain into the inferior vena cava on the right and the renal vein on the left.

The deferential artery arises from the inferior vesicle artery, forming a microvascular network with the adventitia of the vas deferens. The deferential vein drains into the pampiniform plexus and the vesical plexus.

INGUINAL LIGAMENT

The inguinal ligament or Poupart's ligament forms from the thickened lateral inferior edge of the external oblique aponeurosis (see Fig. 25.1). The ligament courses between the anterior superior iliac spine and the pubic tubercle.

ILIOPUBIC TRACT

The iliopubic tract is a thickened lateral extension of the transversalis fascia, which runs from the superior pubic ramus to the iliopectineal arch. It is anterior to Cooper's ligament and posterior to the inguinal ligament. Although intimately associated with the inguinal ligament, the iliopubic tract is a separate structure.

LACUNAR LIGAMENT

The lacunar ligament or Gimbernat's ligament is the most inferior and posterior portion of the inguinal ligament. The ligament is triangular, and its fibers curve to meet Cooper's ligament as it inserts onto the pubic symphysis, forming the medial aspect of the femoral canal.

COOPER'S LIGAMENT

Cooper's ligament or the pectineal ligament is a condensation of transversalis fascia and periosteum of the superior pubic ramus lateral to the pubic tubercle. It is several millimeters thick, densely adherent to the pubic ramus, and joins the iliopubic tract and lacunar ligaments at their medial insertions.

CONJOINED TENDON

The existence of this structure is debated or at least variable, but it is thought to be a fusion of the lower fibers of the internal oblique muscle and the aponeurosis of the transversus abdominis muscle at their insertions onto the pubic tubercle.

PREPERITONEAL SPACE

In both open and laparoscopic preperitoneal approaches to hernia repair, a sound understanding of the anatomical structures in the groin from a seemingly reversed perspective are necessary. The preperitoneal space (Fig. 25.3) is bounded internally by the peritoneum and externally by the transversalis fascia and contains fat, blood vessels, lymphatics, nerves, and the vas deferens. The testicular vessels and the vas deferens at the internal ring form the apex of a theoretical triangle called the triangle of doom. Within this triangle lie the external iliac artery and vein, as well as the genital and femoral branches of the genitofemoral nerve, which are hidden under peritoneum and transversalis fascia, thus placing them at high risk of injury. The *triangle of pain* lies lateral to this, and its apex is formed inferomedially by the testicular vessels and superolaterally by the iliopubic tract. Within this triangle lie the femoral branch of the genitofemoral nerve, the femoral nerve, and the lateral cutaneous femoral nerve. Stapling of these structures during a laparoscopic hernia repair results in painful neuralgias and should be avoided.

Etiology

Inguinal hernias may be caused by congenital factors, as in indirect hernias occurring through a patent processus vaginalis, or in a variety of connective tissue abnormalities, such as Ehler–Danlos syndrome and Marfan syndrom. In addition, increased intraabdominal pressure has also been associated with hernia formation; this is especially true with peritoneal

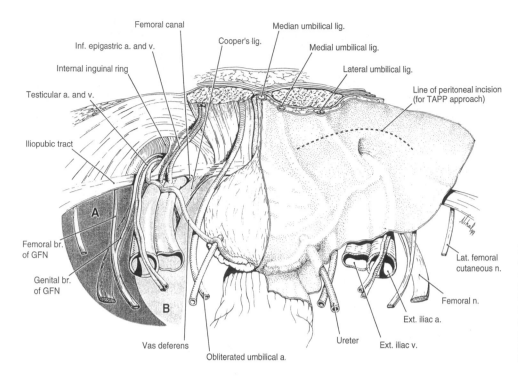

FIGURE 25.3. The preperitoneal space as viewed from within the abdomen. *Shaded area A* designates the triangle of pain; *shaded area B* designates the triangle of doom. These areas contain nerves and blood vessels that are at risk of injury during hernia repair. *GFN,* genitofemoral nerve; *TAPP,* transabdominal preperitoneal laparoscopic repair.

dialysis and ascites.[1] Obesity and advanced age are also risk factors. Chronic cough in patients with chronic obstructive pulmonary disease (COPD), straining in patients with benign prostatic hyperplasia (BPH) or chronic constipation, or strenuous labor may increase the wear-and-tear effect on the abdominal wall and increase the risk of hernia formation.[2]

Diagnosis

The gold standard for hernia diagnosis is a history and physical exam. Patients usually complain of a persistent or intermittent bulge in the groin associated with some degree of discomfort, aggravated by physical exertion. If the hernia is reducible, the pain may wax and wane. A more persistent pain is typical of an incarcerated hernia. If fever, tachycardia, exquisite tenderness on palpation, erythema of the overlying skin, leukocytosis, and obstructive symptoms are present, an irreducible hernia is likely strangulated and warrants immediate operative intervention.

To examine a patient for a groin hernia, the physician is seated and the disrobed patient stands and faces the examiner. First, the groin is visually inspected for evidence of a bulge, and palpated with the patient straining either by coughing or by performing a valsalva maneuver. In males, the examiner's gloved finger is inserted into the redundant scrotal skin reaching onto the abdominal wall and into the external inguinal ring, just lateral to the pubic tubercle. During the straining exercise, an inguinal hernia will be evident as a bulge or mass pushing downward onto the examiner's fingertip. In females, the same examination is performed by inserting the finger into the labia majus to gain access to the external ring.

A femoral hernia will appear as a mass below the inguinal ligament in the area medial to the femoral pulse and can be elicited by similar straining techniques. Femoral hernias may be difficult to diagnose, especially in obese patients, and a second opinion is frequently reassuring.

After examining the patient for both an inguinal and femoral hernia with the patient standing, the patient should be reexamined in a similar fashion in the supine position. It is important to note that both groins should be examined to exclude bilateral hernias. Masses other than hernias must be ruled out, and this can usually be done by physical exam (Table 25.1).

Epidemiology and Classification

Approximately 680,000 inguinal hernia repairs are performed annually in the United States.[3] More than 90% are performed on males. Female patients undergo three times as many femoral repairs as males, although females undergo three times as many inguinal repairs as femoral repairs. Indirect inguinal hernias are more common on the right side, possibly related to the later descent of the right gonad and delayed closure of the processus vaginalis.

Multiple classification schemes have been developed; the most widely accepted is the Nyhus classification (Table 25.2).[4]

Management

Traditionally, hernias are electively repaired because the natural history of hernias dictates that they only become larger,

TABLE 25.1. Differential Diagnosis of Groin Masses.

Inguinal hernia	Hydrocele
Femoral hernia	Testicular mass
Lipoma	Testicular torsion
Lymphadenitis	Epididymitis
Lymphadenopathy	Ectopic testicle
Abscess	Femoral aneurysm or pseudoaneurysm
Hematoma	Cyst
Varicocele	Seroma

TABLE 25.2. Nyhus Classification of Groin Hernias.

Type 1. Indirect inguinal hernia—normal internal inguinal ring

Type 2. Indirect inguinal hernia—enlarged internal inguinal ring but intact inguinal canal floor

Type 3. Posterior wall defect
    A. Direct inguinal hernia
    B. Indirect inguinal hernia—enlarged internal inguinal ring with destruction of adjacent inguinal canal floor, e.g., massive scrotal, sliding, or pantaloon hernias
    C. Femoral hernias

Type 4. Recurrent hernia
    A. Direct
    B. Indirect
    C. Femoral
    D. Combined

do not resolve spontaneously, and can lead to intestinal obstruction or strangulation. The only exception to this dictum is in patients too debilitated to undergo repair or in patients whose operative risks are excessively high.

Generally, it is safe to attempt reduction of an incarcerated hernia in the absence of evidence of strangulation. Analgesics may be required, and Trendelenberg positioning may be helpful. Any hernia that cannot be successfully reduced requires prompt operative intervention.

Repairs

ANTERIOR APPROACHES

The goal of all repairs is to close the myofascial defect through which the hernia protrudes. This closure can be done from a number of approaches with or without placement of a prosthetic mesh. The classic tissue repairs use permanent suture to reinforce the internal inguinal ring and the floor of the inguinal canal and do not employ the use of a prosthesis. These techniques include the Marcy, Bassini, Shouldice, and McVay repairs. The Lichtenstein repair uses prosthetic mesh, as does the plug technique. Common to all these methods is the anterior dissection of the inguinal canal and hernia sac, followed by a myofascial repair, and closure of the canal. The basic technique of inguinal canal and sac dissection is the same for all anterior approaches, whereas the repair of the myofascial defect differs.

After incising and dividing the layers of the anterior abdominal wall to expose the inguinal canal, the spermatic cord is isolated at the level of the pubic tubercle, and mobilized to the level of the internal ring. The cord is then dissected by dividing cremasteric muscle fibers to identify an indirect sac, if present. The sac is usually found on the anteromedial side of the cord. The sac is opened and its contents reduced back into the abdominal cavity. The sac is ligated at its base with a pursestring suture and amputated. If an indirect sac extends inferiorly beyond the pubic tubercle, the distal sac should simply be divided and left open.

If a direct hernia sac is identified, it generally should not be operated but should be reduced bluntly back into the abdominal cavity and imbricated with one or more sutures placed superficially in the transversalis fascia. This maneuver effectively avoids injury to any organs such as the colon or bladder, which may form a sliding component in a direct hernia.

MARCY REPAIR

The Marcy repair refers to a high ligation of the sac and closure of the internal inguinal ring along its medial aspect, displacing the cord laterally. This technique can be used only to repair indirect inguinal hernias, and its main utility is in pediatric patients or in adults (especially women) with a small indirect hernia and minimal damage to the internal ring. Patients with a direct inguinal hernia require the addition of another type of repair.

BASSINI REPAIR

After a complete and deliberate dissection of the inguinal canal, the floor is reconstructed by approximating the internal oblique muscle, the transversus abdominis muscle, and the transversalis fascia (the Bassini triple layer) with the iliopubic tract and shelving edge of the inguinal ligament using interrupted sutures (Fig. 25.4). This repair may be used for both indirect and direct inguinal hernias.

SHOULDICE REPAIR

This technique is remarkably similar to the Bassini operation in that the layers approximated to reconstruct the inguinal canal floor are the same for both. However, the Shouldice technique uses a series of running sutures to imbricate the reconstruction into several layers (Fig. 25.5). As in the Bassini operation, the cord is mobilized, the cremaster muscle is divided, a high ligation of the sac is performed, and the transversalis fascia forming the floor of the inguinal canal is incised. The floor is reconstructed by placing a series of running sutures to approximate the lateral edge of the rectus abdominis muscle near the pubic tubercle, the internal oblique muscle, the transversus abdominis muscle, and the transversalis fascia to the iliopubic tract and the shelving edge of the inguinal ligament.

McVAY (COOPER'S LIGAMENT) REPAIR

The McVay repair approximates the transversus abdominis arch to Cooper's ligament, the iliopubic tract, and the inguinal

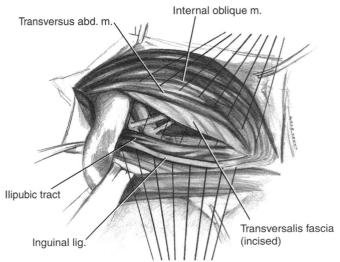

FIGURE 25.4. The Bassini repair reconstructs the canal floor using interrupted sutures to approximate the internal oblique muscle, the transversus abdominis muscle, and transversalis fascia (Bassini's triple layer) with the iliopubic tract and inguinal ligament.

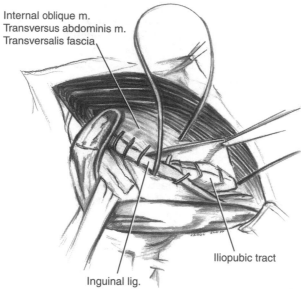

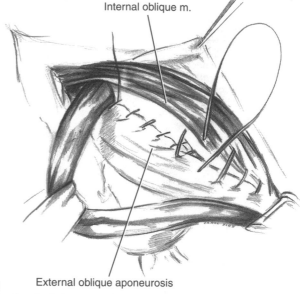

FIGURE 25.5. The Shouldice repair reconstructs the canal floor using a series of running sutures. **A.** The first suture is started at the pubis and run laterally to approximate the internal oblique muscle, transversus abdominis muscle, and transversalis fascia with the iliopubic tract and inguinal ligament. The same suture is reversed at the level of the internal inguinal ring and run back to the pubis. **B.** A second suture is started at the internal inguinal ring and run medially to approximate the internal oblique muscle with the external oblique aponeurosis. The same suture is reversed at the pubis and run back to the internal inguinal ring.

ligament (Fig. 25.6). The McVay repair may be used for inguinal and femoral hernias.

LICHTENSTEIN REPAIR

The Lichtenstein approach is a tension-free method that uses prosthetic mesh to reinforce the transversalis fascia forming the canal floor without attempting to use any attenuated native tissues in the repair (Fig. 25.7). Polypropylene mesh is trimmed to extend 4 cm lateral to the internal ring and 2 cm medial to the public tubercle, and is then secured to the inguinal ligament laterally and the lateral edge of the rectus sheath and internal oblique muscle and aponeurosis medially using permanent monofilament suture. Local anesthesia may be used, and several studies have shown that this repair enables a quicker return to work, is associated with less postoperative pain, and has fewer recurrences than tissue repairs.[5] The Lichtenstein repair may be used for direct and indirect inguinal hernias but does not address femoral hernias.

Given the results of several studies which have compared the tension-free to classical tissue repair techniques, the Lichtenstein repair has reshaped the way surgeons perform

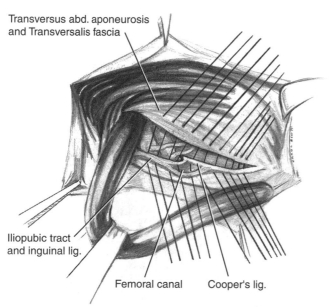

FIGURE 25.6. The McVay repair reconstructs the canal floor using interrupted sutures to approximate transversus abdominis aponeurosis and transversalis fascia with Cooper's ligament, the iliopubic tract, and the inguinal ligament. Transition sutures in Cooper's ligament and the anterior femoral fascia close the femoral canal.

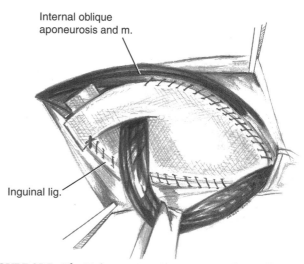

FIGURE 25.7. The Lichtenstein repair uses a mesh prosthesis to reinforce the canal floor. Tails are fashioned around the spermatic cord to reconstruct the internal inguinal ring.

open herniorrhaphy. It has reduced patient discomfort and hernia recurrence rates dramatically. It has also reversed the notion that bilateral hernias should not be repaired simultaneously. The short- and long-term recurrence rates seem better than the results previously achieved with tissue repairs. The procedure is readily reproducible by those who do not specialize in hernia repair, with comparable excellent results.[6]

MESH PLUG REPAIR

A variety of techniques have been developed that use a polypropylene mesh plug to fill the hernia defect and effect a repair. These techniques are championed as tension free and arc becoming quite popular in combination with a mesh patch repair. There may be particular utility in using this approach for recurrent hernias, as remobilization of the cord may be avoided, which may decrease the risk of ischemic orchitis.

OPEN PREPERITONEAL APPROACH

Nyhus introduced the open preperitoneal repair in 1960.[7] He has championed this method for the repair of all recurrent and complicated groin hernias, namely those involving incarcerated or strangulated intestine, as well as for femoral hernias. For the recurrent hernia, densely scarred tissue in the inguinal canal is avoided, possibly reducing the risk of nerve injury and cord damage.[8,9] In strangulated hernias, proximal unaffected intestine can be controlled and necrotic intestine may be isolated before its reduction. The peritoneal cavity can be opened to perform an intestinal resection and anastamosis. Sliding hernias can also be readily reduced. For femoral hernias, ample access is afforded to reduce and repair the hernia without disturbing the floor of the inguinal canal, which is necessitated by anterior approaches. Preperitoneal repairs can be performed both with and without mesh. Although the use of mcsh provides lower recurrence rates, contamination may preclude its use if bowel resection is necessary.

GIANT PROSTHETIC REINFORCEMENT OF THE VISCERAL SAC (GPRVS OR STOPPA) REPAIR

Placing a giant prosthetic reinforcement of the visceral sac in the preperitoneal space using a large sheet of unsutured polyester mesh, is commonly referred to as the Stoppa repair (Fig. 25.8).[10] In contrast to other approaches, no attempt is made at repairing the musculofascial defect creating the hernia.[11] Instead, the transversalis fascia is functionally replaced by the insertion of a large chevron-shaped piece of mesh into the preperitoneal space after all hernias have been reduced. The transverse dimension of the mesh is equal to the distance between both anterior superior iliac spines minus 2 cm. The height is the distance between the umbilicus and the pubis with an average mesh size of 24 × 16 cm. By adhering to the visceral sac, the mesh renders the peritoneum indistensible so that it cannot protrude through any abdominal wall defects. The Stoppa repair can be very useful in complex hernias including recurrent and bilateral hernias, and hernias at high risk for recurrence such as in patients with connective tissue disorders, ascites, obesity, or advanced age. The Stoppa repair is contraindicated if contamination is present because the risk of prosthetic infection is high.

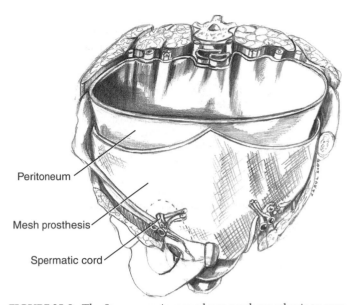

FIGURE 25.8. The Stoppa repair uses a large mesh prosthesis to completely encompass the visceral sac and prevent inguinal or femoral hernia formation.

LAPAROSCOPIC APPROACHES

Since its introduction, three techniques of laparoscopic repair have proved more effective and emerged as the most popular. These techniques are the transabdominal preperitoneal (TAPP), the intraperitoneal onlay mesh (IPOM), and the totally extraperitoneal (TEP). These repairs approach the myopectineal orifice posteriorly, similar in anatomical perspective to the open preperitoneal approaches. A clear understanding of the anatomy from this perspective (see Fig. 25.3) is crucial to avoid a number of complications, mainly vascular and nerve injuries. Laparoscopy provides a clear view of the entire myopectineal orifice, and repairs of both inguinal and femoral hernias can be performed.

In the TAPP procedure, three trocars are placed through the abdominal wall into the peritoneal cavity after a pneumoperitoneum has been created. The peritoneum cephalad to the groin is then transversely incised from the median umbilical fold to several centimeters lateral to the internal ring, taking care not to injure the underlying inferior epigastric vessels. The hernia is reduced using blunt dissection and gentle traction. The vas deferens and testicular vessels are parietalized by carefully freeing them from their proximal and lateral peritoneal attachments. The inferior epigastric vessels are defined but not completely skeletonized, which can lead to bleeding. A large piece of polypropylene mesh (at least 10 × 15 cm) is then placed over the entire myopectineal orifice with generous overlap of its borders, and secured in place with helical fasteners or staples. The fasteners are applied medially into the rectus muscle, superiorly to the transversus abdominis arch, inferiorly to Cooper's ligament up to the medial aspect of the external iliac vein, and laterally to the iliopubic tract. The peritoneum is reapproximated using staples or sutures. Care must be taken to completely close the peritoneum without leaving gaps that can allow small-bowel entrapment or adherence to the mesh.

The IPOM repair uses an intraabdominal approach and places a large piece of mesh against the peritoneum after hernia contents have been reduced. The mesh is secured with staples placed into the same anatomical structures as in the TAPP repair but is placed in an intraperitoneal position instead of a preperitoneal position.

The TEP technique gains access to the groin via a completely extraperitoneal approach. A small infraumbilical incision is made and carried down through the anterior rectus sheath. The rectus muscle is retracted away from the midline and the anterior surface of the posterior rectus sheath is clearly visualized. A balloon dissector is placed along this surface, advanced inferiorly to the pubic bone, and inflated with air or saline, creating a working space between the peritoneum and the abdominal wall. After the preperitoneal working space has been developed, a cannula is inserted and the preperitoneal space is insufflated. Two additional trocars are placed in the midline under direct visualization without violation of the peritoneum. The hernia is reduced using blunt dissection and gentle traction. The remainder of the operation, including the dissection of the myopectineal orifice, parietalization of the cord and testicular vessels, and mesh placement, is identical to the TAPP procedure.

The results of several randomized trials comparing laparoscopic and open repairs are summarized in Table 25.3.[2,12–22] Many of the data support laparoscopic repairs as being effective and safe. Although many of the earlier trials had short follow-up, several of the more recent trials provide encouraging results, showing recurrence rates of 0% to 6% at follow-up as long as 28 months (mean).[2,13–15]

The incidence of complications associated with laparoscopic repairs is comparable to or better than that of open repairs, especially after the learning curve has been overcome.[15,21,23–25] Almost all the trials show that laparoscopic repairs are associated with less postoperative pain and a decreased time for return to work, but take longer to perform and cost more than conventional open repairs. A large, prospective, randomized VA trial is currently under way to further compare TEP, TAPP, and Lichtenstein repairs.

Several studies have compared the various types of laparoscopic repairs, as summarized in Table 25.4.[27–29] They all indicate that TAPP, IPOM, and TEP are effective and have low recurrence rates.

Complications

Complication rates following open inguinal hernia repairs average 7% to 12%.[23] Reports on laparoscopic approaches are widely variable, but the rates of complications for both conventional and laparoscopic repairs is now thought to be comparable.[18,21,23–25] It is still important to inform patients that the long-term durability of laparoscopic repairs may not yet be known.

RECURRENCE

Ten percent is reported as the average recurrence rate for groin hernias, although most surgeons boast their rates are well below the average.[3] Recurrence rates following conventional repairs vary from 1% to 7% for indirect inguinal hernias, from 4% to 10% for direct inguinal hernias, from 1% to 7% for femoral hernias, and from 5% to 35% for recurrent hernia repair.[3,30] Failure to diagnose multiple hernias at the time of initial operation, failure to close an enlarged internal ring, and breakdown of the repair under tension have all been implicated in the causes of recurrences.[31,32]

For laparoscopic repairs, the reasons for recurrence are surgeon inexperience, inadequate dissection, insufficient prosthesis size, insufficient prosthesis overlap of hernia defects, inadequate fixation, prosthesis folding or twisting, missed hernias or lipomas, and mesh dislodgment secondary to hematoma formation.[2,26,33–35] Recurrence is directly related to surgeon experience, with failures occurring much more frequently early in the surgeon's learning curve.[2,26,36]

NERVE ENTRAPMENT

Injury results in numbness, pain, and parasthesias in the distribution of the nerve, which can be mild or incapacitating.[37] Complete nerve transection is likely to cause only numbness and little long-term morbidity, whereas partial transection or entrapment with a staple, suture, or subsequent encroachment by scar tissue is likely to cause neuroma formation and chronic pain.[9,38] Symptoms usually appear immediately postoperatively and intensify during the first 2 weeks; most kresolve within 8 weeks.[39] Treatment consists of rest and injections with local anesthetic and corticosteroids until symptoms resolve.[39] In a minority of patients, symptoms persist, necessitating exploration and entrapment release or neurectomy.[40] The incidence of nerve injuries following conventional open repairs is less than 2%.[39–41]

Entrapment of the lateral femoral cutaneous nerve is the most common nerve injury encountered in laparoscopic repairs. It results in pain and numbness in the upper lateral thigh and is called meralgia paraesthetica.[42] To avoid nerve entrapment, dissection and stapling should be above the iliopubic tract. Entrapment of the ilioinguinal, iliohypogastric, and genital branch of the genitofemoral nerve can be entrapped during laparoscopic repairs if excessive pressure is applied externally during mesh fixation, compressing the muscles enough to allow the staples to reach the nerves.[39]

ISCHEMIC ORCHITIS/TESTICULAR ATROPHY/VAS DEFERENS INJURY

Ischemic orchitis is a potentially devastating but rare complication of hernia repair, caused by surgical trauma to the veins of the spermatic cord. Anterior approaches are more apt to cause testicular atrophy than posterior approaches because they require more dissection and handling of the cord. This complication is more likely to occur in recurrent hernias that involve scar tissue and a difficult dissection or when the distal sac is dissected. The result is a swollen and hard cord, testicle, and epididymis. Fever and leukocytosis may occur, but infection is not part of the natural history of this phenomenon. The symptoms become apparent 2 to 5 days postoperatively. The pain usually lasts several weeks, but the swelling and induration may last 4 to 5 months. Ischemic orchitis may resolve without sequelae, or may cause the testicle to shrink, resulting in a completely atrophic testicle. There is no known treatment of ischemic orchitis that prevents progression to testicular atrophy. Only rarely does the testicle become necrotic or require removal. An atrophic testicle is painless, not prone to malignant degeneration, and does not diminish serum testosterone or fertility.[9]

The incidence of ischemic orchitis following laparoscopic repair is not well documented, but is thought to be sufficiently low because a minimum of cord handling and dissection is required, similar to the open preperitoneal approach.[41]

Direct injury to the vas deferens itself can result in infertility if the contralateral side is abnormal. Injury usually manifests as a painful spermatic granuloma, formed by highly antigenic spermatozoa once they have escaped the vas. Excision of the granuloma and microsurgical repair of the vas is the treatment of choice.[24]

BOWEL OBSTRUCTION AND INTRAABDOMINAL ADHESIVE COMPLICATIONS

Unique to the laparoscopic approach is the potential for intraabdominal adhesions and intestinal obstruction. There have been multiple case reports of such occurrences, most of which followed TAPP repairs, but the overall incidence remains small, of the order of less than 1%.[22,43–48]

Incisional hernias at trocar sites can occur after laparoscopic repairs and cause intestinal obstruction and strangulation.[49] They are more common after TAPP repairs, occurring in up to 1% of patients, necessitating fascial closure of all ports larger than 5 mm.[26,43] Preexisting umbilical hernias can substantially increase the risk of postoperative umbilical hernias, despite routine closure, and require additional attention.[50]

VASCULAR INJURIES

In laparoscopic repairs, the inferior epigastric, external iliac, femoral, and testicular vessels are at risk. Injuries may result in intraoperative hemorrhage or may present as postoperative hematomas. The reported incidence of postoperative hematoma formation is 1% to 8%.[24]

In open repairs, bleeding is not a common intraoperative problem, but the incidence of hematoma formation may be as high as 31%.[18] Meticulous efforts to achieve complete hemostasis should be made. Hematomas may be self limited or may necessitate evacuation.

VISCERAL INJURIES

At risk are the small intestine, colon, and bladder, and although rare, injuries to these structures can be the source of considerable morbidity, especially if their diagnosis and treatment are delayed.[25] Many of these injuries can occur if an attempt is made to open the sac of a direct sliding hernia. If direct sacs are not opened but are simply reduced and inverted, the risk of injury may be minimized.

In laparoscopic repairs, risk of injury may be minimized by bladder decompression with a Foley catheter, use of an open Hasson cannula technique, insertion of trocars under direct visualization, and thorough anatomical knowledge with cautious dissection.[51] Confining dissection to the area lateral to the medial umbilical ligament is helpful in avoiding bladder injury.[24] Entering the peritoneal cavity with the TAPP and IPOM techniques increases the potential for visceral injury.

WOUND INFECTIONS

Hernia repair is regarded as a clean operation and as such should have an infection rate of less than 2%.[52] Antibiotic prophylaxis has been the area of controversy. For clean cases, prophylaxis is normally not indicated. However, implantation of a mesh prosthesis has been used as an indication, and

some surgeons routinely give prophylactic antibiotics to all hernia repairs.

Special Considerations

FEMORAL REPAIRS

Femoral hernias are much less common than inguinal hernias, but are more often associated with complicated presentations, with a 20% incidence of incarceration.[23] Some authors have suggested that the ideal way to repair femoral hernias is via a preperitoneal approach, either open or laparoscopic.[53] This method facilitates control of hernia contents, avoids the disruption of the inguinal floor mandated by an anterior approach, and avoids the difficulty associated with approaching a femoral hernia through a thigh incision. The McVay repair has been used, however, with successful results.[54] Strangulated femoral hernias require proximal control, resection, and anastamosis of intestine and may best be approached through a preperitoneal incision or a midline laparotomy.

COMPLICATED GROIN HERNIAS

Approximately 10% of inguinal hernias and 20% of femoral hernias present incarcerated.[23] Incarcerated hernias can cause intestinal obstruction or strangulation and infarction, resulting in a high incidence of infection, hernia recurrence, and operative mortality, especially in elderly patients. The possibility of such complications has prompted the recommendation that all hernias be repaired electively and promptly as soon as the diagnosis is made.[55]

PEDIATRIC HERNIAS

The incidence of inguinal hernias in children is between 10 and 20 per 1000 live births, with a 4:1 male-to-female ratio. The overall incidence, incidence of bilaterality, male predominance, and incidence of incarceration are higher in premature infants. The incidence of bilaterality is at least 10% in full-term infants and as high as 55% in premature infants. The incidence of inguinal hernia in cryptorchid infants approaches 65%. Approximately 55% to 70% of inguinal hernias in children are on the right side, and 1% have a direct component.[56] The higher incidence of right-sided hernias is thought to be caused by the later descent of the right gonad and delayed closure of the processus vaginalis. Incarceration occurs in 9% to 20% of cases, is more frequent in children less than 6 months of age, and, in the absence of signs of strangulation, can usually be managed by manual reduction followed by prompt elective repair. Elective repair is associated with a much lower incidence of complications compared to emergent operations, especially in low birth weight infants. Elective repair should be performed as soon as possible to avoid reincarceration, which occurs in as many as 16% of cases.[57]

The most widely accepted repair of pediatric inguinal hernias is a high ligation of the sac. This technique alone is usually sufficient because most pediatric hernias are indirect with no laxity of the internal ring. If ring laxity exists, a few sutures can be placed in the transversalis fascia to approximate the tissues. Recurrence rates of less than 1% are reported.[56]

Considerable debate exists concerning routine contralateral groin exploration. Historically, this has been advocated, given the high incidence of bilaterality. Selective contralat-

TABLE 25.3.

Prospective Randomized Trials Comparing Laparoscopic and Open Repairs (Level I Evidence).

Reference	Study design	Average follow-up (months)	No. of repairs	Complications (not including recurrences)	Recurrences
Paganini et al. 1998, Italy[13]	TAPP vs. Lichtenstein	28	TAPP: 52	14 (26.9%) total complications 4 (7.6%) hematoma 1 (1.9%) hydrocele 5 (9.6%) parasthesia 4 (7.6%) seroma*	2 (3.8%)
			Licht.: 56	15 (26.7%) total complications 8 (14.2%) hematoma 2 (3.5%) hydrocele 5 (8.9%) parasthesia 0 seroma*	0
Zieren et al. 1998, Germany[14]	TAPP vs. Plug & Patch vs. Shouldice	25	TAPP: 80	2 (3%) intraop bleeding* 15 (19%) postop complications	0
			Plug: 80	12 (15%) postop complications	0
			Shouldice: 80	13 (16%) postop complications	0
Liem et al. 1997, Netherlands[2]	TEPP vs. open (Marcy, Lichtenstein, Bassini, Shouldice, McVay)	20.2	TEP: 487	24 (5%) Conversion to TAPP or open 54 (11%) total postop complications 0 deep wound infection* 10 (2%) chronic pain* 7 (1%) seroma* 3 (1%) pneumoscrotum >1 day	17 (3%)*
			Open: 507	99 (19.5%) total postop complications 6 (1%) deep wound infection* 70 (14%) chronic pain* 0 seroma*	31 (6%)*
Champault et al. 1997, France[15]	TEP vs. Stopps	20.2	TEP: 51	4% total complications* 3 (6%) conversions to open	3 (6%)
			Stoppa: 49	20% total complications*	1 (2%)
Kald et al. 1997, Sweden[16]	TAPP vs. Shouldice	12	TAPP: 122	8 (6.6%) total complications	0*
			Shouldice: 89	9 (10.1%) total complications	3 (3.4%)*
Bessell et al. 1966, Australia[17]	TEP vs. Shouldice	7.3	TEP: 39	6 conversion to open 3 conversion to TAPP 4 (10%) postop complications	2 (5.1%)
			Shouldice: 74	7 (9.5%) postop complications	0
Wright et al. 1996, Scotland[18]	TEP vs. open (Lichtenstein or preperitoneal)	—	TEP: 67	6 (9%) conversion to open 15 (22%) postop complications 1 (2%) hematoma* 0 seroma*	—
			Open: 64	46 (72%) postop complications 20 (31%) hematoma* 7 (11%) seroma*	—

Operative time (min)	Cost	Postoperative pain	Return to work (days)	Conclusions/details
66.6 Unilateral Primary* 71.1 Unilateral Recurrent 85.7 Bilateral	$1,249	↓ pain score @ 48 h*	15	95% of Lichtenstein repairs performed under local anesthesia. TAPP had less postop pain. TAPP should not be adopted routinely unless its cost can be reduced.
48.2 Unilateral Primary* 41.2 Unilateral Recurrent 75.9 Bilateral	$306	↑ discomfort @ 7 d, 3 mon	14	
61*	$1,211		16	Plug & Patch and TAPP cause less pain and have faster return to work than Shouldice; Plug & Patch cost less than TAPP and can be performed faster and under local anesthesia.
36	$124		18	
47	$69	↑ pain score *	26*	
45*	—	↓ pain score *	14*	TEPP has more rapid recovery and fewer recurrences than open repairs, but takes slightly longer to perform.
40*	—		21*	
"Significantly longer"*	—	↓ pain score * ↓ meds *	17*	45% bilateral, 43% recurrent. Mesh for TEP was not fixed in place; mesh size increased from 6 × 11 cm to 12 × 15 cm due to early recurrences. Single piece of mesh for bilateral hernias believed to reduce recurrence rates. TEP has the same long-term recurrence rate as the Stoppa procedure, but confers a real advantage in the early postop period.
	—		35*	
72*	+ $483 direct cost	—	10*	TAPP had faster recovery and return to work with comparable complication rates. TAPP more cost effective if indirect cost compared, which included income lost by a delay in return to work.
62*	+ $1,364 indirect cost	—	23*	
87.5*	—	↓ pain score * ↓ meds	30.5	Study biased because of large crossover to open group. Substantial conversion rate to open and TAPP repairs. TEPP has significant decrease in pain, equivalent return to work, but longer operative time. TEPP alleviates the inherent dangers associated with TAPP, but further studies needed.
50*	—		32	
58*	—	↓ pain score * ↓ meds	—	Acute study focusing on early outcome. No data for length of follow-up or recurrences. Significant decrease in pain but increased OR time for TEPP. Significant conversion rate. Very high complication rates for both groups. Also looked at pulmonary and metabolic measures; no differences found.
45*	—		—	

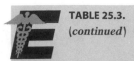

TABLE 25.3.
(continued)

Reference	Study design	Average follow-up (months)	No. of repairs	Complications (not including recurrences)	Recurrences
Tschudi et al. 1996, Switzerland[19]	TAPP vs. Shouldice	6.7	TAPP: 52	6 (12%) total complications	1 (1.9%)
			Shouldice: 56	9 (16%) total complications	2 (3.5%)
Barkun et al. 1995, Canada[20]	TAPP or IPOM vs. open (Bassini, Mcvay, Shouldice, Lichtenstein, Plug & Patch)	14	TAPP: 33 IPOM: 10	10 (22.5%) total complications	0
			Open: 49	6 (11.9%) total complications	1 (2%)
Vogt et al. 1994, US[12]	IPOM (with meshed PTFE) vs. open (Bassini, McVay)	8	IPOM: 30	5 (17%) total complications 1 (3.3%) bladder perforation	1 (3.3%)
			Open: 31	5 (16%) total complications	2 (6.4%)
Stoker et al. 1994, UK[21]	TAPP vs. open (nylon darn plication)	7	TAPP: 83	6 (8%) total complications* 1 deep wound infection 3 persistent pain 1 hematoma	0
			Open: 84	16 (21%) total complications* 5 deep wound infection 6 persistent pain 3 hematoma	0
Payne et al. 1994, US[22]	TAPP vs. Lichtenstein	10	TAPP: 48	6 (12%) total complications 0 groin pain >1 mon. 2 (4%) conversions to open 1 (2%) incarcerated omentum in peritoneal flap	0
			Licht: 52	9 (18%) total complications 4 (8%) groin pain >1 mon.	0

TAPP, transabdominal preperitoneal approach; IPOM, intraperitoneal onlay mesh repair; TEP, totally extraperitoneal approach; PTFE, polytetrafluoroethylene.
*, Statistically significant.

Operative time (min)	Cost	Postoperative pain	Return to work (days)	Conclusions/details
87 unilateral* 124 bilateral	—	↓ pain score * ↓ meds *	25	Study biased because patients undergoing open repairs told not to resume activity for 4–6 weeks. Significantly less pain with TAPP., but longer OR time. Long-term follow-up needed for analysis of recurrences.
59 unilateral* 79 bilateral	—		48	
43	$1,718	↓ meds *	9.6	Improved quality of life and decreased pain with laparoscopic repairs, but at increased cost. Laparoscopic repairs are feasible and comparable to open repairs.
49	$1,224		10.9	
62.5	—	↓ med	7.5	Less pain and faster return to work with IPOM, with comparable efficacy and morbidity. Longer follow-up needed.
80.9	—		18.5	Two patients had IPOM under local anesthesia.
50 unilateral* 92 bilateral	+£168	↓ pain score * ↓ meds *	14*	TAPP has less pain, faster return to work, and fewer complications, but increased operative time. Substantial economic savings in lost work days.
35 unilateral* 60 bilateral			28*	
68 unilateral 87 bilateral 67 recurrent	$3,093 *	—	9 unilat.* 7.5 bilat. 11.4 recurr.	TAPP can be performed with similar operative times and short-term recurrence rates, with faster return to work, but an increased cost. 90% of Lichtenstein's used local anesthesia. Biggest impact on faster return to work and increased ability to perform straight leg raises seen in manual labor population.*
56 unilateral 93 bilateral 73 recurrent	$2,494 *	—	17 unilat.* 25 bilat. 26 recurr.	

TABLE 25.4.
Trials Comparing Different Types of Laparoscopic Repairs.

Reference	Study design	Average follow-up (months)	No. of repairs	Complications (not including recurrences)	Recurrences	Operative time (min)	Return to work (days)	Conclusions/details
Kald et al. 1997, Sweden[26]	Prospective Nonrandomized TAPP vs. TEP (level II evidence)	TAPP: 23 TEP: 7	TAPP: 393 TEP: 98	0 conversions to open 31 (7.8%) total complications 2 bowel obstructions (at 12 & 19 weeks postop) 3 trocar hernias 8 conversions to TAPP 1 conversion to open 7 (8.0%) total complications 0 bowel obstructions 0 trocar hernias	7 (1.8%) 0	80 80	12* 8*	High-quality hernia repairs can be performed with both TAPP and TEP. TEP is technically more difficult but results in fewer major complications and a faster return to work. TEP avoids the potential dangers of a trans-abdominal approach and may be the procedure of choice.
Ramshaw et al. 1996 US[27]	Retrospective TAPP vs. TEP (level III evidence)		TAPP: 300 TEP: 300	2 conversions to open 32 (10.6%) total complications 1 enterotomy 1 cystotomy 1 trocar hernia 6 parasthesia 2 conversions to open 7 conversions to TAPP 10 (3.3%) total complications 2 enterotomies 1 cystotomy 0 trocar hernia 1 parasthesia	6 (2.0%) 1 (0.3%)			TAPP and TEP have acceptable complication and recurrence rates, but TEP has fewer. TEP has the advantage of avoiding entering the abdominal cavity and using epidural anesthesia (47 patients), and is the preferred technique. Previous lower abdominal surgery is a relative contraindication to TEP (all recurrences and visceral injuries occurred in these patients). TEP is more technically difficult.

Study	Evidence/Design	No.	Procedures	Complications	Complication rate	Recurrence (%)	Time to activity	Comments
Fitzgibbons et al. 1995, US[28]	Prospective Nonrandomized (level II evidence)	23	TAPP vs. IPOM (with polypropylene mesh) vs. TEP					Laparoscopic hernia repair is effective with acceptable early recurrence rates.
			TAPP: 562	Total complications 2 bowel adhesions/obstructions 5% neuralgias	28 (5%)	—		TAPP, IPOM, and TEP appear to be equally effective, although TEP more difficult technically. IPOM and TEP may be better suited for small indirect inguinal hernias, whereas TAPP may be better for complicated recurrent hernias.
			IPOM: 217	12% neuralgias 1 prosthetic infection (appendicitis vs. cecal erosion)	11 (5.1%)	—		Other procedures can be safely performed at the same time as hernia repair (61 additional procedures performed with 1 associated complication). The incidence of neuralgias decreases with increased surgeon experience.
			TEP: 87	0% neuralgias	0	—		This series represents a very well done multicenter trial, but the total complication rate is high
			All three groups analyzed together	2 conversions to open 29.2% total complications 5 (0.7%) trocar hernias 1 (0.1%) cystotomy 1 (0.1%) enterotomy 24 (3.5%) bleeding (2 requiring transfusion) 6 (0.87%) 2nd abdominal procedure required (for bleeding, infection, adhesion, enterotomy, neuralgia)	4.5%	70 unilateral 90.6 bilateral		The authors stress the need for prospective randomized trials to further evaluate laparoscopic repairs.
Felix et al. 1995, US[29]	Retrospective (level III evidence)	TAPP: 24 TEP: 9	TAPP vs. TEP				7 days for "normal activity" for TAPP and TEP	Time to return to work was the same in TAPP and TEP, but was 8 days for noncompensated patients vs. 16 days for compensated.
			TAPP: 733	9 (1.2%) intraabdominal complications 1 bowel obstruction 2 enterotomies 6 trocar hernias 10% seroma 7 hydroceles	2 (0.3%)	—		TEP is less invasive, minimizes the risk of intraabdominal complications, and is the procedure of choice, except for incarcerated hernias and large scrotal hernias, which are more easily handled by TAPP.
			TEP: 382	7 (1.8%) conversions to TAPP 1 (1.2%) intraabdominal complications 0 bowel obstruction 0 enterotomies 1 trocar hernias (in TAPP conversion) 10% seroma 2 hydroceles	1 (0.3%)	—		Slit in mesh associated with transient scrotal hyperesthesia. Parietalization of the cord more easily achieved in TEP, alleviating the need for a slit in the mesh. 50% of all repairs done with double buttress technique; there were no recurrences but all hydroceles occurred in this group

TAPP, transabdominal preperitoneal approach; IPOM, intraperitoneal onlay mesh repair; TEP, totally extraperitoneal approach.
*, Statistically significant.

eral exploration on the basis of a laparoscopic evaluation for a patent processus vaginalis performed through the opened hernia sac decreases the number of negative explorations and may be the best option.[58]

Abdominal Wall Defects

Ventral Hernias

Approximately 90,000 ventral hernias are repaired in the United States each year.[59] Important to remember is the anatomical structure of the anterior abdominal wall, which above the semilunar line of Douglas consists of skin, subcutaneous fat, anterior rectus sheath, rectus muscle, posterior rectus sheath, and peritoneum. Below the semilunar line, the layers are the same except that there is no posterior rectus sheath. Laterally, the layers are skin, subcutaneous fat, external oblique aponeurosis and muscle, internal oblique aponeurosis and muscle, traversus abdominis aponeurosis and muscle, transversalis fascia, and peritoneum. A ventral hernia is a defect in the abdominal wall. Ventral hernias present as a protrusion or bulge and may contain preperitoneal fat or intestinal contents. The size may range from very small to massive. Patients may or may not be symptomatic. The fascial edge along the circumference of the defect is usually palpable on exam. In obese patients, a CT scan or ultrasound examination may help confirm the diagnosis. As with groin hernias, ventral hernias may present with incarceration, strangulation, or bowel obstruction; elective repair is preferred to emergent repair.

Umbilical hernias are caused by an error in the embryological development of the abdominal wall. Umbilical hernias occur in 10% to 30% of live births, but frequently close during the first few years of life. If larger than 2 cm, the likelihood of the defect spontaneously closing is much less, and repair is not delayed. Otherwise, repair is usually postponed until the child reaches 4 years of age to allow time for spontaneous closure. Most infants are asymptomatic, and incarceration or strangulation is extremely rare.[56] Repair consists of simple fascial closure. Defects may persist, become evident in adulthood, and should be repaired.

Epigastric hernias arise in the upper abdomen along the linea alba, and usually appears in adulthood, often in association with obesity or pregnancy. Epigastric hernias frequently present as small defects with incarcerated preperitoneal fat or omentum, causing pain and warranting repair. Diastasis recti is a condition in which the medial borders of the rectus muscles slowly spread apart with thinning and stretching of the rectus sheath, resulting in a diffuse bulge in the upper midline abdomen. In contrast to epigastric hernias, diastasis recti is not a fascial defect or hernia per se, and consequently presents no threat of complication; diastasis recti is merely a cosmetic deformity. Excision of the thinned fascia and placement of a mesh prosthesis alleviate the deformity.

Incisional hernias occur in at least 2% to 11% of abdominal wound closures.[60–62] Many risk factors for developing an incisional hernia have been cited, including obesity, wound infection, advanced age, postoperative pulmonary complications, jaundice, abdominal distension, emergency operation, reuse of a previous incision, pregnancy, postoperative chemotherapy, steroids, malnutrition, ascites, and peritoneal dialysis. Most of these risk factors are associated with excessive strain on the incision or poor wound healing. Wound infection is the most important risk factor, with hernias four times more likely to occur after a wound infection.[63] Obesity has also been clearly established as a risk factor.[62,64] Reuse of an incision has been shown to double the incidence of subsequent incisional hernias.[65] Suture technique has been extensively studied, with no difference in hernia incidence shown between continuous and interrupted suture techniques, or layered versus mass wound closure.[60,66]

REPAIR TECHNIQUES

A variety of repair methods exists and a prosthetic mesh may or may not be used. In open repairs, the hernia is approached through a skin incision placed directly over the fascial defect, usually incorporating the scar from the previous incision. The sac is dissected free from subcutaneous tissues and the fascial edges. The sac may be opened to facilitate lysis of adhesions and inspection and reduction of sac contents. If possible, the sac is not completely excised, so that there is a sufficient amount of sac to close over the intestinal contents. This method provides protection against adhesive complications if mesh is to be used in the repair. The superficial and deep surfaces of the fascia are exposed several centimeters back from the hernia defect. Attenuated fascia is excised. A thorough search for concomitant hernias is performed. Depending on the type of repair, fascia may then be closed with or without placing a mesh buttress. Fascia should only be closed when it can be done so without tension. Closed suction drains may be placed in the dead space superficial to the fascia to minimize seroma formation.

PRIMARY REPAIR

Ventral hernias may be repaired by primary closure so long as the repair can be performed in a tension-free fashion. The direction of closure is not important. Primary closure is the preferred technique for umbilical hernias in children and some small epigastric or umbilical hernias in adults. Permanent suture is used and the fascial edges are approximated. Unfortunately, the results of primary repair in all but the smallest of incisional hernias are poor,[67,68] with failure rates as high as 49% to 58%[69,70]; this is likely because patients with incisional hernias have fascia that is weakened and that does not have sufficient tensile strength to hold sutures when placed under mechanical stress.

MESH ONLAY REPAIR

Significantly better results have been reliably achieved with mesh repairs, with rates of complications comparable to that of primary repairs.[71] Recurrence rates average 6% for mesh repairs. In the mesh onlay technique, a mesh prosthesis is placed superficial to the anterior rectus sheath. The mesh is then held in place by full-thickness horizontal mattress sutures. Ideally, this method allows for a barrier between the abdominal contents and the mesh to prevent adhesions and fistula formation.

MESH INLAY AND PATCH REPAIRS

The inlay method of repair places a prosthetic mesh deep to the posterior rectus fascia. The mesh is placed in either an intraperitoneal or a preperitoneal position. Mattress sutures are placed from the deep aspect of the mesh through the abdominal wall. Once all sutures have been placed, they are tied on the anterior fascial surface. The patch method simply sutures the prosthesis to the fascial edge circumferentially. With either the inlay or patch technique, if the prosthesis is placed in an intraperitoneal position or, if no tissue can be interposed between bowel and the prosthesis, the potential for adhesions and fistulization is created.

STOPPA REPAIR

Stoppa[72] and Wantz[73] have both described the use of a giant Mersilene mesh prosthesis in the repair of large (>10 cm) incisional hernias. This approach is similar to the inlay method but overlaps the defect by 8 to 10 cm and avoids raising extensive subcutaneous flaps by passing sutures through separate stab incisions. The hernia is reduced, and adhesiolysis is performed to widely expose the deep surface of the abdominal wall. Peritoneum is dissected free from the posterior rectus sheath, and the mesh is inserted in the preperitoneal space. Alternatively, the mesh may be inserted between the posterior rectus sheath and the rectus muscle. Before mesh insertion, the peritoneum, hernia sac, or posterior rectus sheath is closed to prevent contact between abdominal contents and mesh, to minimize potential adhesive complications.

LAPAROSCOPIC REPAIR

Laparoscopy has recently gained momentum in the area of ventral hernias. Most reports describe a transabdominal approach, placing several trocars in an intraperitoneal position, reducing the hernia through sharp adhesiolysis and blunt manipulation, leaving the hernia sac in situ, and using a mesh prosthesis to close the defect. Mesh is sized externally to provide at least 2 cm of overlap on all sides of the defect. A suture is placed through each corner and tied, with tails left long. The skin is marked at the sites where the four corner sutures will exit, and small stab incisions are made. Mesh is then rolled and passed intraabdominally through a port, unfolded, and positioned over the defect. A fascial closure device is passed through the skin stab incision and used to individually retrieve the tails of each corner suture. The tails are tied superficial to fascia in a subcutaneous position. Hernia staples or helical fasteners are used to secure the mesh to peritoneum and fascia, preventing herniation of bowel or omentum between the mesh and the abdominal wall.

Although randomized controlled trials are lacking, preliminary reports suggest that this approach is safe and effective, and may offer a shortened postoperative course and faster resumption of normal activities, compared to the conventional open approaches.[59,74,75]

Emergency Abdominal Wall Defects

Abdominal wall closure can be difficult and morbid in the emergency setting. Emergency closures are often required in the face of vigorous resuscitation with massive tissue edema or in the case of tissue loss secondary to trauma, surgical debridement for necrotizing infections, or resection of tumors. Such wounds may be heavily contaminated, and postoperative wound sepsis is common. Primary fascial approximation may create a closure under tension and result in abdominal compartment syndrome, dehiscence, evisceration, or fistula formation.[76,77] A prosthetic repair provides tension-free closure and is effective in alleviating evisceration and restoring abdominal wall continuity in the acute phase.[78] Prosthetic repairs, however, can be fraught with long-term complications, such as mesh extrusion or enteric fistulas.

The use of absorbable mesh provides a lower incidence of fistulization and wound complications but universally leads to ventral hernias, which must be cared for at a later date. The proponents of absorbable mesh note that it is effective in closing acute abdominal wall defects that are contaminated. Unlike permanent mesh, absorbable mesh does not chronically harbor infection; this allows complete clearance of infection before definitive ventral hernia repair, providing a better chance of a successful repair. It also provides no residual foreign body to complicate wound management should a fistula form.

The ideal method of preventing acute evisceration and long-term ventral hernia formation in acute full-thickness abdominal wall defects in the face of contamination has yet to be determined. Much of the evidence supports the use of absorbable mesh with planned definitive ventral hernia repair at a later date. A protocol using permanent or absorbable mesh with early mesh removal, wound coverage, and planned ventral hernia repair yields good results as well but requires an additional operation for mesh removal.

Other Abdominal Hernias

SPIGELIAN

The Spigelian or semilunar line marks the transition from muscle to aponeurosis of the transversus abdominis muscle. The Spigelian fascia lies between this line and the lateral border of the rectus sheath. A defect in this fascia results in a Spigelian hernia. As many as 90% are located 0 to 6 cm cranial to the interspinal plane (the horizontal plane through both anterior iliac spines).[79] The defect originates in the transversus abdominis muscle and may or may not involve the more superficial layers; hernia sac and contents often lie in an intramural location between the abdominal wall layers and may not be palpable. Consequently, patients often present with vague complaints of pain and nonspecific tenderness on exam. Computed tomography or ultrasound scanning may aid in the diagnosis. Ultimate diagnosis may not be made until the time of surgical exploration.

Exploration may be undertaken via an incision directly over the defect if palpable. If it is nonpalpable, exploration via a preperitoneal approach through a midline or paramedian incision avoids an extensive subcutaneous dissection. The defect is usually small and can be repaired primarily. Recently, success has been reported using laparoscopic approaches.[80,81]

LUMBAR

Lumbar hernias occur either spontaneously, posttraumatically, or as incisional hernias (such as following nephrectomy). These hernias represent defects through the transversalis fascia and transversus abdominis muscle aponeurosis. Retroperitoneal fat or a peritoneum-lined sac may herniate through the defect. Patients present with a symptomatic posterior bulge but rarely with a strangulated hernia. There are two lumbar triangles. The inferior or Petit's triangle is bordered by the latissimus dorsi muscle, the external oblique muscle, and the iliac crest; it is covered only by superficial fascia. The superior or Grynfeltt's triangle is bordered by the twelfth rib, internal oblique muscle, and sacrospinalis muscle; it is covered by the lattissimus dorsi muscle.

Repair can be performed primarily if the defect is small, but a myofascial flap, such as a gluteus maximus fascial flap for inferior triangle hernias, or mesh repairs are necessary for larger defects. An oblique incision from the twelfth rib medially to the iliac crest laterally provides adequate exposure. Recent reports document success with laparoscopic repairs using mesh.[82]

PELVIC FLOOR HERNIAS

Pelvic floor hernias include (in decreasing frequency) obturator, perineal, and sciatic hernias. Obturator hernias occur when abdominal contents herniate through the obturator canal along the course of the obturator neurovascular bundle. The obturator membrane, which covers the obturator foramen and forms the canal, is indistensible, and herniated bowel often becomes incarcerated and strangulated. These hernias are most often seen in emaciated females in their eighth decade, almost always occurring on the right side. A preoperative diagnosis is difficult and infrequently made. Patients usually present with partial or complete acute small bowel obstruction without a palpable hernia. Rarely a mass may be palpable on the anteromedial aspect of the thigh or on pelvic and rectal examinations. Computed tomography or abdominopelvic ultrasound scanning can confirm the diagnosis. Exploration may be carried out via a number of incisions, but a lower midline provides the best exposure for resecting compromised bowel and adequate repair of the hernia defect.[83] The defect may be closed primarily, with mesh, or by advancing adductor longus muscle flap. Recently success has also been reported using laparoscopic approaches.[84] Even with appropriate operative treatment, mortality rates may be as high as 75% because of the advanced age and debilitated states of most patients and delays in diagnosis. Therefore, prompt treatment should be rendered.[85]

Perineal hernias may occur spontaneously or as incisional hernias after procedures such as abdominoperineal resections or pelvic exenterations. These hernias occur anteriorly in women, involving the urogenital diaphragm and passing into the labia majora. Posterior perineal hernias are defects in the levator ani muscles that occur in the ischiorectal fossa between the bladder and the rectum. Patients present with soft reducible masses. A primary repair or a repair with mesh may be performed through either a perineal or an abdominal approach.[86]

Sciatic hernias, the rarest of all hernias, occur in the greater or lesser sciatic foramen through a defect in the piriformis muscle. Patients may be symptomatic with sciatic nerve palsy and a palpable mass, or may simply present with intestinal obstruction. Repair can be performed via a gluteal approach or a transabdominal approach.[87]

PARASTOMAL

Parastomal hernias occur through defects adjacent to ostomy sites. The incidence of paracolostomy hernias is 12% to 32%, and for paraileostomy hernias is less than 10%.[88] Construction of the ostomy through an appropriately small fascial defect in the rectus sheath and not maturing the ostomy through the laparotomy incision decrease the risk of subsequent hernia formation. The majority of patients are asymptomatic. Patients may, however, present with obstruction, incarceration, a poorly fitting appliance, or local pain, warranting repair. Options include primary fascial repair, prosthetic fascial repair, or stomal relocation. Local procedures pose an infectious risk if a prosthetic is used, but avoid a laparotomy and potentially extensive adhesiolysis. On the other hand, formal laparotomy alleviates ostomy contamination of prosthetic material and provides access for repair or relocation. No prospective randomized trials have been performed to date. Because parastomal hernias are generally well tolerated and all types of repair are associated with significant morbidity and high recurrence rates, repair should be avoided if possible.

INTERNAL HERNIAS

Internal hernias occur when intraperitoneal contents prolapse through a normal or abnormal orifice. Normally existing orifices include the foramen of Winslow (known as the hernia of Blandin). Abnormally existing orifices are congenital peritoneal fossae and include left and right paraduodenal, pericecal, intersigmoid, paravascular, supravesicular, and hernias inside the broad ligament of the uterus. These hernias account for up to 2% of all abdominal hernias.[89] Patients present with a closed-loop intestinal obstruction, and diagnosis is usually made at the time of operation. The operation involves reduction of incarcerated bowel, resection of nonviable segments, and primary closure of the hernia orifice.

Internal hernias may also be iatrogenic, occurring after a previous operation in which a defect in mesentery or omentum was not adequately closed. If such a hernia occurs, reduction and closure are necessary at laparotomy.

CONGENITAL ABDOMINAL WALL DEFECTS

Gastroschisis refers to herniation of the abdominal viscera without a sac and in the presence of an intact umbilical cord. It is now thought to be a separate entity from omphalocele. It is twice as common as omphalocele but associated with half as many anomalies. The most common associated anomaly is intestinal atresia, which is present in 10% of cases. The eviscerated intestine is edematous, matted with fibrinous adhesions, and shortened, resulting in intestinal absorptive and motility dysfunction.[90] Repair can be performed by primary fascial closure or a staged procedure with closure of skin followed by subsequent fascial closure. Gentle stretching of the abdominal wall can enlarge the abdominal cavity and help facilitate repair. If visceroabdominal disproportion is severe, the eviscerated intestine is enclosed within a prosthetic silo attached at its base to the abdominal wall. As the edema diminishes, sequential compression of the top of the silo returns the herniated contents into the abdomen and allows fascial closure. Mortality is less than 10%.

Omphalocele refers to herniation of the abdominal viscera into the umbilical cord, resulting in a sac lined internally by peritoneum and externally by amnion. Structural and chromosomal anomalies are present in up to 50% of cases. Repair of the abdominal defect can be performed similar to the methods used for gastroschisis. The severity of associated anomalies largely determines long-term survival.

CONGENITAL DIAPHRAGMATIC HERNIAS

Congenital diaphragmatic hernias occur in 1 of every 2100 pregnancies (including spontaneously aborted pregnancies) and 1 of every 4800 live births.[91] They can be characterized by their location. Bochdalek's hernias are located posterolaterally and Morgagni hernias are located anteriorly.

Bochdalek's hernias occur between the costal and spinal diaphragmatic attachments and account for the majority of congenital diaphragmatic hernias. Nonrotation of the intestine is usually associated with the defect. Hernia contents are enclosed within a sac in only 10% to 20% of cases. Because abdominal contents occupy the thoracic cavity during fetal development, pulmonary hypoplasia can be severe. Mortality rates are as high as 80% in the first month of life. Repair is via an abdominal approach and consists of reduction of hernia contents, sac excision, primary or prosthetic (usually PTFE) diaphragm repair, and a Ladd procedure. Occasionally, Bochdalek's hernias may be diagnosed in older children exhibiting only mild symptoms. Elective repair is indicated to avoid potential complications.

Morgagni hernias occur between the sternal and costal diaphragmatic attachments in a retrosternal or parasternal position. Associated cardiac anomalies are frequent. Contents are usually enclosed within a sac, and 90% of hernias are right-sided. In infants, respiratory distress is usually present. When discovered in adults, symptoms are often mild or absent. Repair is indicated in all cases to prevent incarceration. The repair can be performed via an abdominal or thoracic approach, similar to the repair of Bochdalek's hernias. Recently, success in adult patients has been reported using laparoscopic approaches.[92]

References

1. Hurst RD, Butler BN, Soybel DI, et al. Management of groin hernias in patients with ascites. Ann Surg 1992;216:696–700.
2. Liem MSL, Van Der Graff Y, Van Steensel CJ, et al. Comparison of conventional anterior surgery and laparoscopic surgery for inguinal hernia repair. N Engl J Med 1997;336:1541–1547.
3. Rutkow IM, Robbins AW. Demographic, classificatory, and socioeconomic aspects of hernia repair in the United States. Surg Clin North Am 1993;73:413–426.
4. Nyhus LM. Individualization of hernia repair: a new era. Surgery (St. Louis) 1993;114:1–2.
5. Kark AE, Kurzer MN, Belsham PA. 3175 primary inguinal hernia repairs: advantages of ambulatory open mesh repair using local anesthesia. J Am Coll Surg 1998;186:447–456.
6. Beecherl EE, Jones DB, Carrico CJ. McVay to Lichtenstein: evolution of inguinal herniorrhaphy at a teaching institution. Presented at North Texas Chapter of American College of Surgeons, Dallas, TX, Feb. 27, 1998.
7. Nyhus LM, Condon RE, Harkins HN. Clinical experiences with the preperitoneal hernia repair for all types of hernia of the groin: with particular reference to the importance of transversalis fascia analogues. Am J Surg 1960;100:234–244.
8. Reid I, Devlin HB. Testicular atrophy as a consequence of inguinal hernia repair. Br J Surg 1994;81:91–93.
9. Wantz GE. Testicular atrophy and chronic residual neuralgia as risks of inguinal hernioplasty. Surg Clin North Am 1993;73:571–582.
10. Stoppa RE, Quintyn M. Les deficiences de la paroi abdominale chez le suget age: colloque avec le praticien. Semin Hop (Paris) 1969;45:2182–2184.
11. Stoppa RE, Rives JL, Warlaumont CR, et al. The use of Dacron in the repair of hernias of the groin. Surg Clin North Am 1984;64:269–285.
12. Vogt DM, Curet MJ, Pitcher DE, et al. Preliminary results of a prospective randomized trial of laparoscopic onlay versus conventional inguinal herniorrhaphy. Am J Surg 1995;169:84–90.
13. Paganini AM, Lezoche E, Carle F, et al. A randomized, controlled, clinical study of laparoscopic vs open tension-free inguinal hernia repair. Surg Endosc 1998;12:979–986.
14. Zieren J, Zieren H, Jacobe CA, et al. Prospective randomized study comparing laparoscopic and open tension-free inguinal hernia repair with Shouldice's operation. Am J Surg 1998;175:330–333.
15. Champault G, Rizk N, Catheline JM, et al. Inguinal hernia repair: totally pre-peritoneal laparoscopic approach versus Stoppa operation, randomized trial: 100 cases. Hernia 1997;1:31–36.
16. Kald A, Anderberg B, Carlsson P, Park PO, et al. Surgical outcome and cost-minimization analyses of laparoscopic and open hernia repair: a randomized prospective trial with one year follow-up. Eur J Surg 1997;163:505–510.
17. Bessell JR, Baxter P, Riddell P, Watkin S, et al. A randomized controlled trial of laparoscopic extraperitoneal hernia repair as a day surgical procedure. Surg Endosc 1996;10:495–500.
18. Wright DM, Kennedy A, Baxter JN, et al. Early outcome after open versus extraperitoneal endoscopic tension-free hernioplasty: a randomized clinical trial. Surgery (St. Louis) 1996;119:552–557.
19. Tschudi J, Wagner M, Klaiber C, Brugger JJ, et al. Controlled multicenter trial of laparoscopic transabdominal preperitoneal hernioplasty vs Shouldice herniorrhaphy. Surg Endosc 1996;10:845–847.
20. Barkun JS, Wexler MJ, Hinchey EJ, Thibeault D, et al. Laparoscopic versus open inguinal herniorrhaphy: preliminary results of a randomized controlled trial. Surgery (St. Louis) 1995;118:703–710.
21. Stoker DL, Spiegelhalter DJ, Singh R, Wellwood JM. Laparoscopic versus open inguinal hernia repair: randomized prospective trial. Lancet 1994;343:1243–1245.
22. Payne JH, Grininger LM, Izawa MT, et al. Laparoscopic or open inguinal herniorrhaphy? A randomized prospective trial. Arch Surg 1994;129:973–981.
23. MacFadyen BV, Mathis CR. Inguinal herniorraphy: complications and recurrences. Semin Laparosc Surg 1994;1:128–140.
24. Payne JH Jr. Complications of laparoscopic inguinal herniorrhaphy. Semin Laparosc Surg 1997;4:166–181.
25. Sayad P, Hallak A, Ferzli G. Laparoscopic herniorrhaphy: review of complications and recurrence. J Laparoendosc Surg 1998;8:3–10.
26. Kald A, Anderberg B, Smedh K, Karlsson M. Transperitoneal or totally extraperitoneal approach in laparoscopic hernia repair: results of 491 consecutive herniorrhaphies. Surg Laparosc Endosc 1997;7:86–89.
27. Ramshaw BJ, Tucker JG, Conner T, Mason EM, et al. A comparison of the approaches to laparoscopic herniorrhaphy. Surg Endosc 1996;10:29–32.
28. Fitzgibbons RJ, Camps J, Cornet D, Nguyen NX, et al. Laparoscopic inguinal herniorrhaphy: results of a multicenter trial. Ann Surg 1995;221:3–13.
29. Felix EL, Michas CA, Gonzalez MH. Laparoscopic hernioplasty: TAPP vs TEP. Surg Endosc 1995;9:984–989.
30. Condon RE, Nyhus LM. Complications of groin hernias. In: Nyhus LM, Condon RE, eds. Hernia. Philadelphia: Lippincott, 1995.
31. Lichtenstein IL, Shulman AG. Ambulatory outpatient hernia surgery, including a new concept, introducing tension-free repair. Int Surg 1986;71:1–4.
32. LeBlanc KA, Booth WV. Avoiding complications with laparoscopic herniorrhaphy. Surg Laparosc Endosc 1993;3:420–424.
33. Lowham AS, Filipi CJ, Fitzgibbons, et al. Mechanisms of hernia recurrence after preperitoneal mesh repair: traditional and laparoscopic. Ann Surg 1997;225:422–431.
34. Deans GT, Wilson MS, Royston CMS, et al. Recurrent inguinal hernia after laparoscopic repair: possible cause and prevention. Br J Surg 1995;82:539–541.
35. Phillips EP, Rosenthal R, Fallas MJ, et al. Reasons of early recurrences following laparoscopic hernioplasty. Surg Endosc 1995;9:140–145.
36. Liem MSL, Van Steensel CJ, Boelhouwer RU, et al. The learning curve for totally extraperitoneal laparoscopic inguinal hernia repair. Am J Surg 1996;171:281–285.

37. Cunningham J, Temple WJ, Mitchell P, et al. Cooperative hernia study: pain in the postrepair patient. Ann Surg 1996;224:598–602.

38. Sampath P, Yeo C, Campbell JN. Nerve injury associated with laparoscopic inguinal herniorrhaphy. Surgery (St. Louis) 1995; 118:829–833.

39. Seid AS, Amos E. Entrapment neuropathy in laparoscopic herniorrhaphy. Surg Endosc 1994;8:1050–1053.

40. Choi PD, Nath R, Mackinnon SE. Iatrogenic injury to the ilioinguinal and iliohypogastric nerves in the groin: a case report, diagnosis, and management. Ann Plast Surg 1996;37:60–65.

41. Skandalakis JE, Skandalakis LJ, Colborn GL. Testicular atrophy and neuropathy in herniorrhaphy. Am Surg 1996;62:775–782.

42. Eubanks SE, Newman L, Goehring L, et al. Meralgia paraesthetica: a complication of laparoscopic herniorrhaphy. Surg Laparosc Endosc 1993;3:381–385.

43. Felix EL, Michas CA, Gonzalez MH. Laparoscopic hernioplasty: TAPP vs TEP. Surg Endosc 1995;9:984–989.

44. Hendrickse CW, Ewans DS. Intestinal obstruction following laparoscopic inguinal hernia repair. Br J Surg 1993;80:1432.

45. Neugebauer E, Troidl H, Kum CK, et al. The EAES consensus development conferences on laparoscopic cholecystectomy, appendectomy, and hernia repair. Surg Endosc 1995;9:550–563.

46. Milkins R, Wedgwood K. Intestinal obstruction following laparoscopic inguinal hernia repair. Br J Surg 1994;81:471.

47. Spier LN, Lazzaro RS, Procaccino A, et al. Entrapment of small bowel after laparoscopic herniorrhaphy. Surg Endosc 1993;7: 535–536.

48. Petersen TI, Qvist N, Wara P. Intestinal obstruction—a procedure-related complication of laparoscopic inguinal hernia repair. Surg Laparosc Endosc 1995;5:214–216.

49. Jones DB, Callery MP, Soper NJ. Strangulated incisional hernia at trocar site. Surg Laparosc Endosc 1996;6:152–154.

50. Azurin DJ, Schuricht AL, Stoldt HS, et al. Small bowel obstruction following endoscopic extraperitoneal-preperitoneal herniorrhaphy. J Laparoendosc Surg 1995;5:263–266.

51. Carter SI, Jones DB. Complications of laparoscopic surgery. In: Jones DB, Wu JS, Soper NJ, eds. Laparoscopic surgery: principles and procedures. St. Louis: Quality Medical, 1997;89–96.

52. Cruse PJE, Foord R. The epidemiology of wound infection. Surg Clin North Am 1980;60:27–40.

53. Condon RE. Surgical treatment of inguinal hernia, 1997 [editorial]. J Gastrointest Surg 1997;1:299–300.

54. Rutledge RH. A 25 year experience with a single technique for all groin hernias in adults. Surgery (St. Louis) 1988;103:1–10.

55. Oishi SN, Page CP, Schwesinger WH. Complicated presentation of groin hernias. Am J Surg 1991;162:568–571.

56. Skinner MA, Grosfeld JL. Inguinal and umbilical hernia repair in infants and children. Surg Clin North Am 1993;73:439–449.

57. Gahukamble DB, Khamage AS. Early versus delayed repair of reduced incarcerated inguinal hernias in the pediatric population. J Pediatr Surg 1996;31:1218–1220.

58. Wulkan ML, Wiener ES, VanBalen N, et al. Laparoscopy through the open ipsilateral sac to evaluate presence of contralateral hernia. J Pediatr Surg 1996;31:1174–1177.

59. Toy FK, Bailey RW, Carey S, et al. Prospective, multicenter study of laparoscopic ventral hernioplasty: preliminary results. Surg Endosc 1998;12:955–959.

60. Santora TA, Roslyn JJ. Incisional hernia. Surg Clin North Am 1993;73:557–570.

61. Carlson MA, Ludqig KA, Condon RE. Ventral hernia and other complications of 1,000 midline incisions. South Med J 1995;88: 450–453.

62. Israelsson LA, Jonsson T, Knutsson A. Suture technique and wound healing in midline laparotomy incisions. Eur J Surg 1996;162:605–609.

63. Gislason H, Gronbech JE, Soreide O. Burst abdomen and incisional hernia after major gastrointestinal operations—comparison of three closure techniques. Eur J Surg 1995;161:349–354.

64. Sugerman HJ, Kellum JM, Reines D, et al. Greater risk of incisional hernia with morbidly obese than steroid-dependent patients and low recurrence with prefascial polypropylene mesh. Am J Surg 1996;171:80–84.

65. Lamont PM, Ellis H. Incisional hernia in re-opened abdominal incisions: an overlooked risk factor. Br J Surg 1988;75:374–376.

66. Trimbos JB, Smit IB, Holm JP, et al. A randomized clinical trial comparing two methods of fascia closure following midline laparotomy. Arch Surg 1992;127:1232–1234.

67. Mudge M, Hughes LE. Incisional hernia: a 10 year prospective study of incidence and attitudes. Br J Surg 1985;72:70–71.

68. Read RC, Yonder G. Recent trends in the management of incisional herniation. Arch Surg 1989;124:485–488.

69. Van Der Linden FTPM, Van Vroonhoven THJMV. Long-term results after correction of incisional hernia. Neth J Surg 1988; 40:127–129.

70. Koller R, Miholic J, Jakl RJ. Repair of incisional hernias with expanded polytetrafluoroethylene. Eur J Surg 1997;163:261–266.

71. George CD, Ellis H. The results of incisional hernia repair: a twelve year review. Ann R Coll Surg 1986;68:185–187.

72. Stoppa RE. The treatment of complicated groin and incisional hernias. World J Surg 1989;13:545–554.

73. Wantz GE. Incisional hernioplasty with Mersiline. Surg Gynecol Obstet 1991;172:129–137.

74. Holzman MD, Purut CM, Reintgen K, et al. Laparoscopic ventral and incisional hernioplasty. Surg Endosc 1997;11:32–35.

75. Park A, Gagner M, Pomp A. Laparoscopic repair of large incisional hernias. Surg Laparosc Endosc 1996;6:123–128.

76. Fabian TC, Croce MA, Pritchard FE, et al. Planned ventral hernia: staged management for acute abdominal wall defects. Ann Surg 1994;219:643–653.

77. Stone HH, Fabian TC, Turkleson ML, et al. Management of acute full-thickness losses of the abdominal wall. Ann Surg 1981;193:612–618.

78. Voyles CR, Richardson JD, Bland KI, et al. Emergency abdominal wall reconstruction with polypropylene mesh: short-term benefits versus long-term complications. Ann Surg 1981;194: 219–223.

79. Spangen L. Spigelian hernia. Surg Clin N Am 1984;64:351–366.

80. Felix EL, Michas C. Laparoscopic repair of spigelian hernias. Surg Laparosc Endosc 1994;4:308–310.

81. Amendolara M. Videolaparoscopic treatment of spigelian hernias. Surg Laparosc Endosc 1998;8:136–139.

82. Heniford BT, Iannitti DA, Gagner M. Laparoscopic inferior and superior lumbar hernia repair. Arch Surg 1997;132:1141–1144.

83. Marchal F, Parent S, Tortuyaux JM, et al. Obturator hernias—report of seven cases. Hernia 1997;1:23–26.

84. Bryant TL, Umstot RK. Laparoscopic repair of an incarcerated obturator hernia. Surg Endosc 1996;10:437–438.

85. Ziegler D, Rhoads JE. Obturator hernia needs a laparotomy, not a diagnosis. Am J Surg 1995;170:67–68.

86. So JB, Palmer MT, Shellito PC. Postoperative perineal hernia. Dis Colon Rectum 1997;40:954–957.

87. Cali RL, Pitsch RM, Blatchford GJ, et al. Rare pelvic floor hernias: report of a case and review of the literature. Dis Colon Rectum 1992;35:604–612.

88. Martin L, Foster G. Parastomal hernia. Ann R Coll Surg Engl 1996;78:81–84.

89. Armstrong O, Letessier E, Genier F, et al. Internal hernia: report of nine cases. Hernia 1997;1:143–145.

90. Langer JC. Gastroschisis and ophalocele. Semin Pediatr Surg 1996;5:124–128.

91. Heiss KF. Congenital diaphragmatic hernia in 1994: a hard look at the need for 'emergency surgery.' Semin Thorac Cardiovasc Surg 1994;6:221–227.

92. Orita M, Okino M, Yamashita K, et al. Laparoscopic repair of a diaphragmatic hernia through the foramen of Morgagni. Surg Endosc 1997;11:668–670.

26

Abdominal Trauma

Robert C. Mackersie

Traumatic injury remains the great killer of young adults, accounting for a greater percentage of productive years of life lost than heart disease and cancer combined. Of all the injury-related deaths in the United States, approximately 39% involve blunt impact injury, principally vehicular accidents, falls, and pedestrians struck by motor vehicles. Interpersonal assault and violence, principally stab wounds and gunshot wounds, account for the bulk of penetrating trauma deaths, representing approximately 25%. The remainder of injury-related deaths are caused by burns, drowning, strangulation, or poisoning.[1] Abdominal injuries have been reported to occur in approximately 25% of major trauma victims, and often involve multiple organ injuries (Table 26.1A).[2] Multiple system injuries involving head and/or thoracic injuries are common, and may complicate the management of abdominal injuries (Table 26.1B).

The principal causes of morbidity and mortality in abdominal trauma are associated with delays in diagnosis or treatment. They have been identified as (1) hemorrhage, as might occur with hepatic, splenic, or mesenteric injuries, and (2) secondary inflammatory injury, sepsis, and multiple organ failure (MOF) syndromes as may occur with bowel, pancreas, or biliary tract injuries.[3]

Initial Management

The initial management of abdominal injuries begins with the rapid restoration of cardiopulmonary function and the prioritized management of airway, breathing, and circulation. Rapid identification and control of major hemorrhage and the identification and treatment of traumatic brain injury (TBI) are typically the two most important diagnostic and therapeutic goals. Resuscitation from compensated and decompensated shock, neurological injury, and airway management are discussed in detail in other chapters.

The initial clinical presentation may include signs of compensated ("normal" blood pressure) or decompensated (hy-potension) hemorrhagic shock. Decompensated shock is more clinically overt but may be overlooked in the presence of ongoing fluid resuscitation. Persistent or recurrent hypotension (systolic BP <90–100) or relative hypotension (more than a 40-mmHg blood pressure drop from expected) usually represent clear evidence of decompensated shock. In many cases, during the course of fluid resuscitation, blood pressure responds (increases) and then decreases, producing a classical "saw-toothed" pattern reflecting ongoing hemorrhage. Under most circumstances, decompensated hemorrhagic shock of this type should be regarded as potential impending death. In the absence of other suspected sources of major hemorrhage (e.g., chest, pelvis), immediate resuscitation with blood and blood products and direct transport to the operative room for exploratory laparatomy offer the best opportunity for survival. Compensated shock, occurring in the absence of significant decreases in systolic blood pressure, may be manifested by more subtle clinical findings such as narrowed pulse pressure, tachycardia, decreased capillary refill, cool extremities, or abnormally high arterial base deficit.

In addition to hemorrhagic shock from a suspected abdominal source, relative indications for immediate operative exploration include (1) signs of peritonitis, (2) evisceration, (3) chest radiographic evidence of diaphragmatic rupture, (3) abdominal impalement, and (4) ALL gunshot wounds to the abdomen unless substantial suspicion exists that the wounds are tangential and extraabdominal. Under these circumstances, patients should be transported immediately to the operating room following initial airway management, establishment of large-bore resuscitative intravenous catheters, and immediate institution of fluid and blood therapy.

Initial Diagnostic Evaluation

Unlike the head, chest, and, to a lesser extent, the pelvis, the abdomen is a frequent location of occult injury that may not be manifested initially by physical findings, lab

TABLE 26.1A. Representative Incidence of Intraabdominal Injuries Requiring Exploratory Laparotomy for Blunt and Penetrating Injuries.

	Blunt (%)	Penetrating (%)
Spleen	47	7
Liver/biliary	51	28
Pancreas or duodenum	10	11
Colon	5	23
Stomach or small bowel	9	42

TABLE 26.1B. Approximate Incidence of Combined Regional Injuries with Blunt Abdominal Trauma (SFGH 1994–1998).

Head injuries	23%
Thoracic injuries	11%
Axial spine/spinal cord injuries	8%
Pelvic fractures	21%
Major long bone fractures	31%

studies, or routine radiographic evaluation. Thus, it is perhaps not surprising that one of the most common errors made during the resuscitative phase of trauma evaluation is a failure to adequately evaluate the abdomen.[4] As the morbidity and mortality of intraabdominal traumatic injuries are often associated with delayed or misdiagnosis, the guiding philosophy in the evaluation of abdominal trauma is the avoidance of missed injuries or delayed diagnoses through the liberal use of objective diagnostic evaluation. Objective diagnostic studies are those that rely on well-defined radiographic or laboratory findings or discrete observations: diagnostic peritoneal lavage (DPL), computed tomography (CT scan), ultrasonography, diagnostic laparoscopy, and local wound exploration for penetrating trauma patients.

Laboratory studies in the setting of acute abdominal trauma may be of limited value. Serial measurement of hemoglobin/hematocrit is a useful monitor of hemorrhage over a period of time, but rapid hemorrhage or crystalloid hemodilution in the absence of major hemorrhage may produce misleading false-negative and false-positive results, respectively. Arterial base deficit provides an accessible index of metabolic acidosis (lactate accumulation) in the setting of major hemorrhage and is an important indicator of major hemorrhage. Coagulation studies may be important for the early detection of injury-induced coagulopathy, particularly from organ injuries associated with high tissue thromboplastin (brain, liver, long bones).

In addition to standardized "trauma blood studies," all major trauma patients, and particularly those with evidence of significant blood loss or serious injury, should have appropriate blood and blood products available, requiring a blood specimen to be obtained early during resuscitation. Routine type and cross-matching for major trauma patients, however, is relatively contraindicated by time constraints. The principal determining factor dictating the blood bank process for releasing allogenic blood should be the time needed to transfusion. Immediate transfusion mandates uncrossed-matched type O. Emergent transfusion needs may be met by using (ABO) type-specific uncross-matched blood, and urgent needs may allow for typing and major antigen screening.

Diagnostic Peritoneal Lavage

DPL, originally introduced in 1965 by Root et al.,[5] is performed by the insertion of a small flexible catheter into the peritoneal cavity, the installation of 1000 ml saline solution, and the passive (siphon) return of the lavasate with quantatative analysis of the constituents. The incidence of complications is typically less than 1% with a high degree of sensitivity (Table 26.2).[5–18] DPL has the advantage of being a very rapid test, usually performed in less than 10 min. It has been strongly advocated for use in patients with shock or with other serious organ injury.[19]

Cell count thresholds for blunt abdominal trauma vary somewhat, with the threshold for a positive lavage generally set at 100,000 cells/mm³ on lavasate return. This has resulted in high sensitivity, and a low incidence of false-negative exams, with an acceptable incidence of nontherapeutic laparotomy (see Table 26.2). Diagnostic peritoneal lavage thresholds for penetrating trauma are somewhat more controversial, varying in reported series from 1,000 to as high as 50,000 cells/mm³. High thresholds result in higher incidence of delayed diagnoses and potential missed injuries but a very low incidence of nontherapeutic laparotomy, whereas low cell count thresholds miss very few injuries but result in a relatively higher incidence of nontherapeutic laparotomies. Establishment of diagnostic threshold for penetrating abdominal trauma, therefore, is to a large degree a function of philosophy and institutional experience.

Computed Tomography

The principal advantages of CT for blunt abdominal trauma relate to its high degree of sensitivity and specificity in staging solid organ injuries (liver, spleen, kidney), thereby permitting expectant (nonoperative) management of injuries selected, in part, based on the CT scan (Table 26.2). Injuries to the retroperitoneal structures (kidney, pancreas, pelvic fractures) are usually well defined by the CT scan as compared to DPL. The principal pitfalls of CT scanning for blunt abdominal trauma are its ability to miss small amounts of free intraperitoneal fluid associated with blunt intestinal injury,[20,21] the requirement that the patient be transported to a relatively unmonitored portion of the hospital and the time required for completion of this study. This makes the use of CT relatively contraindicated, at most centers, for patients in decompensated shock.

Ultrasonography (US)

Use of ultrasonography in blunt injury, principally for the detection of hemoperitoneum, has been associated with good sensitivity as experience has accumulated (see Table 26.2). The focused abdominal ultrasound for trauma (FAST) has been developed as a protocol-driven US exam for the primary purpose of detecting hemoperitoneum and hemopericardium. In this exam, the hepatic and splenic gutters, pelvis, and pericardium are examined for fluid (blood) (Fig. 26.1). The advantages of US are its speed and convenience (given

TABLE 26.2.
Comparison of Diagnostic Methods for Evaluating Blunt and Penetrating Abdominal Trauma.

Test	Time required (min)	Pros	Cons	Sensitivity [specificity] @ injury type	Reference	Utility: blunt vs. penetrating
Diagnostic peritoneal lavage (DPL)	5–15	Fast. Very sensitive. Minimal equipment required. Specialized training not required. May be performed in a variety of locations. Results are quantitative, objective, and operator-independent.	Invasive. Not recommended if prior laparotomy. Not injury specific. May miss retroperitoneal and diaphragm injuries.	97% [99%] blunt 85–93% [67–99] pen 99% [43%] penetr 99% [86%] penetr 100% [84%] blunt	Alyonc[6] Alyonc[6] Oreskcvich[7] Merlotti[8] Liu[9]	Good sensitivity for both blunt and penetrating trauma. Nonspecific for both. Sensitivity and specificity highly dependent on cell count criteria used.
Abdominal CT	30–50	Very specific with good sensitivity. Good for evaluating posterior (back & flank, retroperitoneal) injuries. Allows staging of blunt organ injuries for nonoperative management. Most major injuries operator (reader) independent.	Not useful for most anterior penetrating injuries. Requires time and patient transport. Some operator (reader) dependence. May miss blunt intestinal injuries and, initially, some pancreatic injuries. Limited finding-specific or quantitative criteria mandating operation exist.	85% [100] blunt 99% [100] blunt 97% [95] blunt	Fabian[10] Peitzman[11] Liu[9]	Good sensitivity and specificity for blunt injuries and most posterior penetrating injuries. Insensitive for anterior penetrating injuries.
Abdominal ultrasonography (FAST)	5–10	Fast. Sensitive for hemoperitoneum in experienced hands. Noninvasive & no contrast required. May be performed in a variety of locations if equipment is available.	Not useful for penetrating injuries. Requires immediately accessible equipment & specialized training & experience. Nonquantitative and substantially operator dependent.	92% [95] 83% [100] 95% [95] 97% [97] 82% [99]	Liu[9] McKenney[12] Yoshii[13] Singh[14] Rozycki[15]	Good sensitivity for clinically significant blunt injuries. Poor sensitivity for penetrating injuries.
Diagnostic laparoscopy (DL)	20–60++	Excellent for diagnosis of diaphragmatic injuries. Good for nonquantitative dx. of hemoperitoneum. Good for determining peritoneal penetration for SW/GSW. High degree of injury specificity when visualized.	Invasive. Poor sensitivity for some injuries. Requires specialized training, experience, and equipment. Nonquantitative and substantially operator dependent. Typically requires more conscious sedation than other methods. General anesthesia may be needed in some circumstances.	88% liver/spleen 83% diaphragm 50% panc/kidney 25% hollow viscous 100% periton penetr 18% GI injuries	Ortega[16] Ortega[16] Ortega[16] Ortega[16] Sosa[17] Ivatury[18]	Good sensitivity for peritoneal penetration, hemoperitoneum, & diaphragmatic injuries. Poor sensitivity for GI and retroperitoneal injuries.

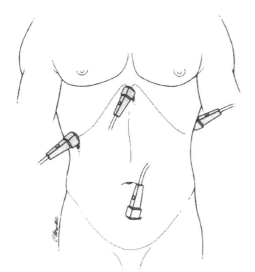

FIGURE 26.1. Focused abdominal sonography for trauma (FAST) exam showing four areas of examination.

equipment availability), but it requires specialized training and proctored experience.

Laparoscopy for Abdominal Trauma

As technical improvements have expanded the use of laparoscopy in recent years, efforts have been made to apply these minimally invasive techniques to the diagnosis and, in some cases, the treatment of abdominal injuries. Although the specificity is good, the diagnostic sensitivity for hollow viscous or retroperitoneal injuries has been unacceptably low, making it ill advised as a definitive diagnostic test for penetrating abdominal trauma.

The use of diagnostic laparoscopy (DL) in blunt abdominal trauma has not been associated with higher sensitivity or specificity than that obtained with CT scan, but does offer the potential for therapeutic intervention for solid organ injuries and possibly selected diaphragm injuries.[24,25]

Until better techniques utilizing DL are developed, its principal advantage appears to be for the evaluation of tangential gunshot wounds to the abdomen that might otherwise require laparotomy and for the assessment of potential diaphragmatic injuries which may be missed by both CT scans and DPL.

Protocol for the Evaluation of Blunt Abdominal Trauma

The specific diagnostic processes and methods used for abdominal trauma vary from institution to institution depending on expertise, equipment availability, patient population, historical experience, and, to a certain degree, physician preference. One such process algorithm for the initial evaluation of blunt abdominal trauma is shown in Fig. 26.2.

Protocol for the Evaluation of Penetrating Abdominal Trauma

With respect to penetrating injuries, the "abdomen" should more appropriately be considered the torso, with anterior boundaries extending from the nipple line to the inguinal lig-

ament and posterior boundaries extending from the inferior tip of the scapula to the inferior gluteal fold. Most penetrating injuries consist of firearm injuries (gunshot wounds) or piercing-type injuries (stab wounds). With a 95+% incidence of associated serious intraabdominal injuries, all gunshot wounds to the abdomen should undergo exploratory laparotomy with the exception of those strongly suspected to be tangential in nature. Although blast injury to hollow viscous structures may occur occasionally, most of these patients may be treated nonoperatively. The use of diagnostic laparoscopy has been used successfully to evaluate the potential for blast injury and the presence of peritoneal penetration in wounds more difficult to assess.

Stab wounds to the abdomen may be stratified into those involving the anterior abdomen (anterior to the midaxillary line) and those involving the back and flank (posterior to the midaxillary line). Stab wound patients with clear clinical signs of shock, evisceration, or peritonitis should go directly to the operating room. Wounds penetrating the anterior fascia should prompt further diagnostic evaluation. It is recommended that patients without previous major abdominal incisions, and with positive local wound explorations, in the absence of other operative indications should undergo routine diagnostic peritoneal lavage to exclude significant intraperitoneal injuries from anterior abdominal stab wounds (Fig. 26.3).

Posterior stab wounds to the back and flank are more problematic due to the relative low incidence of significant injury (typically <15%) associated with stab wounds to this area.[26] The optimal method of evaluating these injuries remains unclear. Diagnostic peritoneal lavage and computed tomography have both been used successfully. CT scanning has the advantage of providing better imaging of retroperitoneal structures, including the kidneys. While it is the preferred method at many centers, the low incidence of major injury and cost have restricted its more widespread use.[27-29]

Intraoperative Management of Specific Injuries

Although the majority of abdominal operations for trauma may be conducted under routine, carefully controlled circumstances, this may not always be possible in patients with life-threatening hemorrhage or severe multiple system injuries. Special consideration should be given to the effects of general anesthesia and positive pressure ventilation in these patients, as well as the potential need for access to the chest for specific abdominal injuries (Table 26.3).

The principal technical objective for abdominal exploration for penetrating trauma is to carefully examine the path or potential path of the stab or gunshot wound until (1) the tract is completely defined and all injuries treated, or (2) the wound tract is found to pass beyond any vital structures, or (3) all structures possibly subject to injury are completely evaluated. This "trace-the-track" approach coupled with a systematic evaluation of all intraperitoneal and retroperitoneal structures is critical to avoid missed intraabdominal injuries.

Damage Control

Experience in recent years has suggested that prolongation of operative procedures in the setting of major intraabdominal

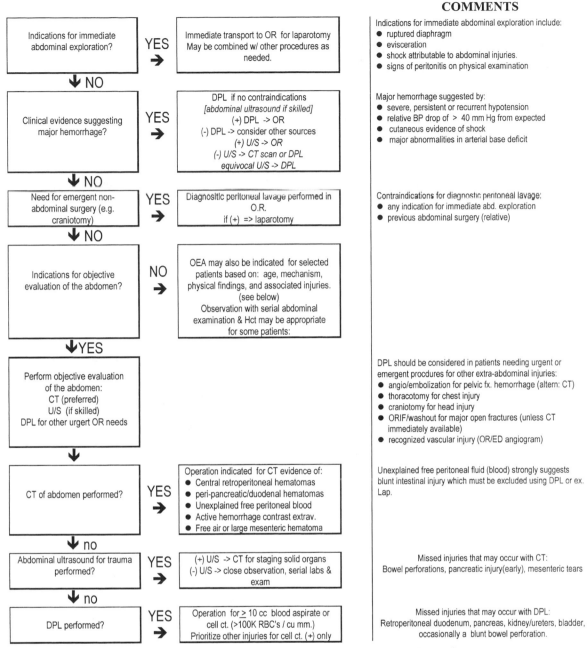

COMMENTS

Indications for immediate abdominal exploration include:
- ruptured diaphragm
- evisceration
- shock attributable to abdominal injuries.
- signs of peritonitis on physical examination

Major hemorrhage suggested by:
- severe, persistent or recurrent hypotension
- relative BP drop of > 40 mm Hg from expected
- cutaneous evidence of shock
- major abnormalities in arterial base deficit

Contraindications for diagnostic peritoneal lavage:
- any indication for immediate abd. exploration
- previous abdominal surgery (relative)

DPL should be considered in patients needing urgent or emergent procdures for other extra-abdominal injuries:
- angio/embolization for pelvic fx. hemorrhage (altern: CT)
- thoracotomy for chest injury
- craniotomy for head injury
- ORIF/washout for major open fractures (unless CT immediately available)
- recognized vascular injury (OR/ED angiogram)

Unexplained free peritoneal fluid (blood) strongly suggests blunt intestinal injury which must be excluded using DPL or ex. Lap.

Missed injuries that may occur with CT:
Bowel perforations, pancreatic injury(early), mesenteric tears

Missed injuries that may occur with DPL:
Retroperitoneal duodenum, pancreas, kidney/ureters, bladder, occasionally a blunt bowel perforation.

FIGURE 26.2. Suggested algorithm for the evaluation of blunt abdominal trauma.

vascular or hepatic injuries and massive transfusion have been associated with worsening metabolic acidosis, coagulapathy, hypothermia, and early mortality. In "damage control" mode, definitive control and repair of all injuries are deferred and the operative procedure concluded. A variety of techniques have been utilized, including hepatic packing (discussed later in this chapter), preemptory splenectomy, stapled control of GI laceration (often deferring reanastomosis), ligation of (carefully selected) vascular injuries, and tamponade packing of other areas of dissection or injury. Preliminary data suggest that this strategic approach to severe, multiple abdominal injuries may improve outcome.[30,31] Timing for planned return to the operating room is generally based on the correction of coagulopathy and metabolic derangements and the specific injuries left incompletely treated.[32]

Hepatic Injuries

Along with vascular injuries, hepatic injuries are a leading cause of attributable death from intraabdominal injuries in patients surviving to hospital arrival. The potential lethality of these injuries stems from inherent difficulties in gaining rapid hepatic vascular control, operative accessibility, and the high frequency of multiple bleeding sites and associated injuries. The key elements in the management of hepatic injuries are outlined in Table 26.4. Hepatic injuries may be graded (grades 1–6) according to size, location, and involvement of vascular structures.[33]

Perhaps the most important development in the management of hepatic injuries over the past decade has been an increased trend toward nonoperative management in carefully se-

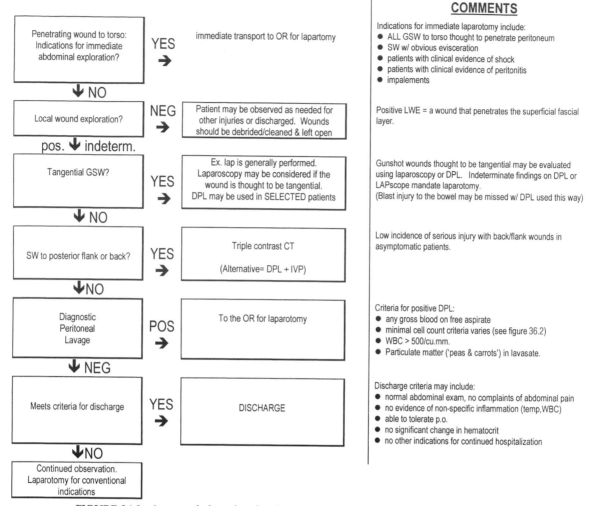

FIGURE 26.3. Suggested algorithm for the evaluation of penetrating abdominal trauma.

lected patients.[34] This trend has resulted from a number of factors, including the increasing use of CT scanning in blunt abdominal trauma and the ability to better define the extent of injury and degree of associated hemorrhage. Hepatic injury patients without clinical signs of shock (compensated or decompensated), ongoing hemorrhage (continued transfusion requirements or active extravasation of intravascular contrast seen on CT scan), massive hemoperitoneum, or other findings mandating operative exploration (e.g., peritonitis, free air), may be managed nonoperatively with close physiological monitoring.

TABLE 26.3. Initial Considerations in the Operative Management of Major Abdominal Trauma.

Positioning & preparation	"Chin to knees": for combined or severe abdominal injuries. Consider 30° lateral rotation for combined thoracoabdominal injuries.
Induction of GA	Positive pressure ventilation increases mean intrathoracic pressure, decreases venous return, and may worsen hypotension or even precipitate hypotensive arrest in severe cases. Surgical team should be scrubbed and in attendance.
Control of profound hypotension	Proximal aortic control may be needed. Options include thoracotomy vs. abdominal approach.
Incision	Midline for virtually all injuries.
Initial maneuvers	• Pack control of hemorrhage (all 4 quadrants) • Immediate solid organ assessment (blunt) • Immediate assessment of proximal mesentery & retroperitoneum for major vascular injury (penetrating)
Exploratory maneuvers (used as needed)	• Mobilization of right & left colon & organ block, to midline as needed (Catel/Mattox) (colon, vascular injuries) • Mobilization of spleen & pancreatic tail (spleen, pancreatic injuries) • "Kocherization" of duodenum & pancreatic head • Lesser sac exploration (body of pancreas) • Mobilization of right & left triangular (hepatic) ligaments + falciform. • Proximal control of renal a. & v. followed by mobilization of kidney (renal injuries)

TABLE 26.4. Key Elements in the Intraoperative Management of Specific Abdominal Injuries.

Hepatic injuries
  Principal therapeutic goals — Control of hemorrhage, control/containment of biliary drainage.
  Diagnosis/staging — CT staging preferred if possible for blunt injury. Selection for nonoperative management based on clinical behavior & CT findings. DPL or U/S(blunt) if unstable. DPL for SW.
  Intraoperative maneuvers (options) for control & access — Packing. Inflow occlusion (Pringle). Hepatic mobilization. Sternotomy extension for exposure. Hepatic isolation (including aortic clamp) or atrial-caval shunt.
  Therapeutic options (singly or in combination) — Simple hepatorraphy. Packing w/planned return to OR. "Hepatotomy or wound tractotomy" w/oversew of bleeding. R. hepatic artery ligation for selected injuries. Resectional debridement if necessary.

Splenic injuries
  Principal therapeutic goals — Control of hemorrhage. Preservation of splenic function if possible.
  Diagnosis/staging — Same as for hepatic injuries. Lower threshold for operative intervention based on CT.
  Intraoperative maneuvers (options) for control & access — Complete mobilization of spleen. Proximal hilar control. Necessary for splenectomy or splenorrhaphy.
  Therapeutic options — Splenectomy. Splenorrhaphy: suture, pledgets, wrapping, partial splenectomy.

Pancreatic injuries
  Principal therapeutic goals — Control of associated hemorrhage. Control of exocrine secretions.
  Diagnosis/staging — CT for diagnosis. (Injuries may be missed by DPL.) Threshold for operative exploration should be low. DPL or U/S if unstable. DPL for SW.
  Intraoperative maneuvers (options) for control & access — Complete exposure of area of suspected injury. Thorough assessment of major pancreatic duct (MPD) injury (inspection, pancreatogram, ERCP).
  Therapeutic options — Drainage only (contusions, minor lacerations). Distal resection (MPD injuries) of body/tail. Drainage w/sphincterotomy vs. resection (Whipple) for major injuries to pancreatic head.

Duodenal injuries
  Principal therapeutic goals — Control of associated hemorrhage. Control of GI secretions with reestablishment of duodenal continuity. Maximizing suture line durability.
  Diagnosis/staging — Same as for pancreas. Isolated intramural hematomas may be treated expectantly. Low threshold for operative exploration. DPL or U/S if unstable. DPL for SW.
  Intraoperative maneuvers (options) for control & access — Complete mobilization of duodenum: Kocher + ligament of Treitz takedown as needed.
  Therapeutic options — Simple repair. Repair w/tube duodenostomy. "Jordan" modified diversion (see text). Roux-en-Y jejunoduodenostomy for augmentation. Resection for combined pancreatic head injuries only.

Colorectal injuries
  Principal therapeutic goals — Reestablishment of GI continuity. Prevention of colon-related septic complications.
  Diagnosis/staging — CT poor for diagnosis of hollow-viscous injuries. DPL for SW.
  Intraoperative maneuvers (options) for control & access — Complete mobilization of involved region of colon. Flexible sigmoidoscopy for rectal evaluation.
  Therapeutic options — Primary repair for most penetrating colon & selected rectal injuries. Diversion + repair/resection reserved for more severe combined injuries (colon) & most rectal injuries.

Retroperitoneal hematoma
  Principal therapeutic goals — Control of hemorrhage, avoidance of missed injuries.
  Diagnosis/staging — CT preop. DPL insensitive and nonspecific. Hematomas graded according to location: central, pelvic, perinephric.
  Intraoperative maneuvers (options) for control & access — Retroperitoneal exploration indicated for all central hematomas. Exploration indicated for all large, expanding, or pulsatile perinephric hematomas. Pelvic fracture hematomas may be packed if necessary, but should be explored only for suspected major vascular injuries.
  Therapeutic options — Repair of associated vascular, pancreatic, or renal injuries. Pelvic fracture hemorrhage controlled by angiography + embolization ± pelvic external fixation.

Splenic Injuries

Splenic injuries are among the more common, are potentially life threatening when encountered following major abdominal trauma, and are an important cause of potentially preventable morbidity and mortality in nontrauma systems. Injuries may be relatively occult without symptoms of abdominal pain or early signs of hemorrhage. Splenic injuries are typically described by grade (1–5),[33] which is a function of size, and by location. CT scanning offers the best means of diagnosis and grading of splenic injuries, with DPL reserved for penetrating injuries or those blunt trauma patients presenting with clinical signs of shock potentially attributable to intraabdominal injury. Splenectomy remains the definitive treatment for major splenic injuries, and may be rapidly and easily accomplished by mobilization of the spleen with ligation or division of the hilar and short gastric vessels and avoidance of iatrogenic injury to the pancreatic tail.

Splenic repair (splenorrhaphy) is generally performed for controlled splenic hemorrhage and may be accomplished through a variety of technical means, including simple suture, pledgeted suture, or absorbable mesh wrap, or through the use of topical hemostatic agents (fibrin glue, topical collagen, foam-adsorbed thrombin, etc.) The technical results with splenorrhaphy have been good, with a low incidence of reoperation and an estimated 70% to 90% intraoperative success rate.

Although more time consuming, the rationale for splenorrhaphy is related to the observations that splenectomy for trauma acts to compromise immune function and has been associated with a higher incidence of posttraumatic infectious complications[35] including overwhelming postsplenectomy sepsis (OPSS).

The nonoperative management of blunt splenic injuries, a practice once confined almost exclusively to children, has been extended to adults in more recent years. Patients to be considered reasonable candidates for nonoperative splenic management should generally meet the following conditions: (1) no evidence of hypovolemic shock, persistent or recurrent splenic hemorrhage, massive hemoperitoneum, or grade V injury; (2) no anticipated need for transfusion requirements as the result of splenic injury; (3) no evidence of active extravasation or splenic vascular injury seen on abdominal CT scan; (4) no other indications for exploratory laparotomy; (5) age less than 50 to 55 years; and (6) no exacerbating factors such as coagulopathy or portal hypertension.

Pancreatic Injuries

Because of the protected anatomical location of the pancreas and duodenum, the incidence of significant injuries to these structures is relatively low, typically between 5% and 7%. These injuries often occur in conjunction with hepatic, splenic, gastric, vascular, renal, or thoracic injuries. The unique therapeutic goal with respect to the pancreas is the need to control pancreatic exocrine secretions in the setting of ductal or glandular disruption and the prevention of secondary hemorrhage or septic complications (see Table 26.4).

CT scanning remains the diagnostic method of choice for blunt pancreatic and duodenal injuries because of its sensitivity in detecting retroperitoneal fluid or free air and in visualizing the pancreas. CT is not, however, completely reliable in detecting all pancreatic injuries, particularly when utilized early in the postinjury course. Scans should be performed using both oral and i.v. contrast. Serum enzymes (lipase, amylase) as indicators of major pancreatic injury do not have the sensitivity to be used as a means of exclusion for blunt trauma. The diagnosis of pancreatic and duodenal penetrating injuries is usually made at the time of exploratory laparotomy based on a positive DPL or shock state.

The key to intraoperative diagnosis of pancreatic injury is thorough exploration of the potentially injured portion of the gland. The technical maneuvers for this exploration include separate exposure of the duodenum and pancreatic head, pancreatic body, and pancreatic tail. The specific treatment of pancreatic injuries depends primarily on two factors: (1) the presence or absence of main pancreatic duct (MPD) injury and (2) the anatomical location of the injury.[36] Most pancreatic injuries consist of simple contusions or minor superficial lacerations. Almost without exception, these can be managed satisfactorily with the use of simple closed suction drainage placed adjacent to the laceration or contusion.

Duodenal Injuries and Combined Pancreaticoduodenal Injuries

The diagnosis, initial management, and exploration of duodenal injuries are similar to those for pancreatic injuries (see Table 26.4). The main therapeutic goals are reestablishment of duodenal (GI) continuity and creation of a durable duodenal suture line. Most duodenal injuries are simple lacerations (blunt and penetrating) and may be managed safely using conventional two-layered anastomotic techniques. These injuries do not generally require any adjunctive measures such as duodenal decompression or localized drainage. In some instances, more extensive lacerations involving the fourth portion of the duodenum, which anatomically behaves more like the small bowel, may be resected with primary jejunoduodenal anastomosis depending on the extent of destruction.

For combined duodenal and pancreatic injuries, several authors have advocated the use of duodenal "exclusion," involving diversion of the gastric stream via a gastrojejunostomy with staple or suture (temporary) closure of the pylorus, and primary repair plus drainage of the duodenal and pancreatic injuries.[37] This technique theoretically protects the duodenal suture line by diverting the GI stream. Results with this approach have been satisfactory, and the oversewn or stapled pylorus typically reopens after 6 to 10 weeks.[38]

Stomach and Small Bowel

Gastric injuries and most small-bowel injuries occur primarily as the result of penetrating abdominal trauma.[39] Initial presentation may involve hematemesis or presence of gross blood on nasogastric tube aspiration or early signs of peritonitis. During exploration, particularly for penetrating wounds, it is critical that the small bowel be meticulously inspected and that even small adjacent hematomas be carefully evaluated, looking for tiny transmural lacerations. Mesenteric hematomas from penetrating injuries may rebleed if not also carefully examined for potential lacerations to small mesenteric vessels.

The majority of gastric and small-bowel lacerations are simple lateral or tangential injuries amenable to primary repair. More severe small-bowel injuries involving near transections or involving the small bowel mesentery are generally best managed by resection and primary reanastomosis. Multiple repairs or primary anastomoses may be performed in the small bowel without any additional morbidity if extensive resections are avoided.

Contusions or traction injuries to the small bowel may occur in the setting of blunt abdominal trauma, causing full-thickness tears or "blow-out" perforations, devascularizing mesenteric injuries, or full-thickness bowel wall ischemic injury. Although these blunt intestinal injuries (BII) are often associated with solid organ injuries requiring immediate exploration, they may also occur in isolation. They can be difficult to detect during the initial evaluation and represent an important cause of potentially preventable morbidity in the blunt trauma patient. The sensitivity of diagnostic peritoneal lavage in BII has been reported as approximately 90% to 93%.[40,41] Computed tomography, more commonly used for blunt abdominal trauma, has reported sensitivities for BII between 40% and 92%.[42–44]

Colon and Rectal Injuries

Most colon and rectal injuries are the result of stab or gunshot wounds and are discovered at laparotomy performed on the basis of clinical exam findings or a positive DPL. Occasionally, extraperitoneal wounds in proximity to the rectum are diagnosed preoperatively using sigmoidoscopy. The intraoperative diagnosis of rectal injuries suspected on the basis of a pelvic hematoma or missile trajectory may be made difficult by the limited exposure. For this reason, all patients with the potential for rectal injuries should be positioned in a modified lithotomy (e.g., Lloyd–Davies) position to allow access to the perineum and rectum for "on-table" sigmoidoscopy, preferably using a flexible scope.

One of the primary goals in the management of colorectal injuries is the prevention of associated postoperative septic complications (see Table 26.4). Previously held concepts predicting a high incidence of septic complications and leaks when repairs or anastomoses were performed in the setting of significant fecal contamination, other associated abdominal injuries, significant hemorrhage, or destructive colon injuries have not necessarily been borne out. The extensive experience with penetrating colon injuries has led recently to the development of clinical management guidelines[45] that support the practice of routine repair of nondestructive colon lesions in the absence of established peritoneal infection (early treatment). These data also suggest that even resection and anastomosis of colon injuries, typically performed for more destructive wounds, may also be safe in the absence of persistent shock, other major associated intraabdominal injuries, or established peritonitis.[45]

Diaphragmatic Injuries

Injuries to the diaphragm occur in approximately 3% of blunt and 1% of penetrating abdominal injuries. They may vary from clinically insignificant lacerations involving the right side to complete "blowout" involving large tears of the diaphragm, including the pericardial portion, with herniation of the heart.[46] Clinical diagnosis of diaphragm lacerations or rupture, particularly in the absence of other significant abdominal trauma, may be challenging. DPL allows diagnosis in many cases, but may be falsely negative because bleeding from the diaphragm either may be minimal or may be obscured by its suction evacuation via an associated tube thoracostomy.

Blunt diaphragmatic rupture may be suspected by a variety of chest radiographic findings including an indistinct or elevated diaphragm, but radiographs may be completely normal in as many as 50% of cases. A definitive diagnosis is made when CXR shows a gastric bubble in the left chest or a nasogastric tube positioned above the left diaphragm. Computed tomography may be useful in some cases, but reports of its diagnostic efficacy are mixed.[47–49] Laparoscopy, as discussed earlier, has been found to be very sensitive in evaluating potential diaphragmatic injuries, and may be particularly useful for assessing smaller, left-sided, asymptomatic injuries, particularly in the setting of proximal penetrating trauma.[50] Continued suspicion of a diaphragmatic rupture or laceration based on inconclusive radiographs, CT scans, or even DPL should prompt laparoscopic inspection in patients without other indications for exploratory laparotomy.

The approach to an acute diaphragmatic injury should almost always be through the abdomen due to the frequency of associated injuries. Control of associated intraabdominal

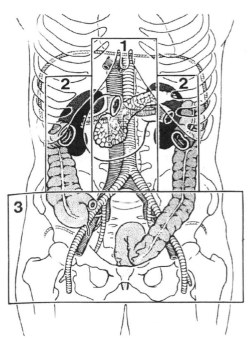

FIGURE 26.4. Classification of retroperitoneal hematomas. (Reprinted from Selivanov et al. 1986,[134] with permission.)

hemorrhage, often from splenic injury, remains the first priority. In injuries involving the GI tract with intrathoracic contamination, it is important to thoroughly cleanse the chest of any debris and establish good pleural drainage because the pleural space is relatively intolerant of GI contamination. Most diaphragmatic injuries are simple tears or lacerations amenable to repair using interrupted sutures of nonabsorbable material.

Retroperitoneal Hematomas and Pelvic Fracture Hemorrhage

Retroperitoneal hematomas, while not strictly intraabdominal injuries, can be associated with major hemorrhage, with and without surgically repairable lesions. Retroperitoneal hematomas caused by blunt injury may be classified into three zones[51] (Fig. 26.4): pelvic hematomas (zone 3), perinephric hematomas (zone 2), and central retroperitoneal hematomas (zone 1). The decision to explore a blunt injury retroperitoneal hematoma is based principally on location (see Table 26.4) and the clinical behavior of the hematoma (e.g., expanding or pulsatile).

Priorities in the Management of Multisystem Injuries

Major abdominal injuries may be associated with continued, uncontrolled hemorrhage, often making their treatment the highest priority in multisystem trauma. In some cases of less acute abdominal injuries, however, other organ systems may take priority. Although no general set of guidelines can apply to every case, injuries can be loosely prioritized on the basis of treatment goals. (see Table 26.5)

Table 26.5. Priorities in the Management of Multisystem Injuries.

Priority	Treatment goals
1st	1. Identification and control of primary site of life-threatening hemorrhage: abdomen, chest, pelvis. 2. Diagnosis and treatment of major traumatic brain injury (TBI).
2nd	1. Diagnosis and treatment of blunt aortic injury. 2. Control of secondary source of hemorrhage: pelvis, chest, abdomen, fracture site.
3rd	Containment of contamination; infection risk reduction. Control of tertiary sites of hemorrhage: pelvis, fracture sites, etc. Confirmation and treatment of suspected spinal cord injury. Treatment of critical orthopedic injuries.
4th	Diagnosis and treatment of major but noncritical orthopedic, maxillofacial injuries, repair of nonbleeding lacerations.
5th	Repeat of head to toe exam, review/reordering of radiology studies, labs. Diagnosis of potential noncritical occult injuries, "rule-out" injuries, etc.

Interdisciplinary collaboration and clear communication are important in managing these more complex injuries, and the general or trauma surgeon's role in guiding overall therapy ("captain of the ship") is critical.

Postoperative and Postinjury Complications

The spectrum of adverse sequelae following the treatment of intraabdominal injuries is not dissimilar to that which occurs in a variety of other abdominal surgical conditions. Recurrent hemorrhage, wound and intraabdominal infection, fistulas, and posttraumatic systemic inflammatory response syndromes (SIRS, ARDS, MODS) occur following major traumatic injury and are discussed elsewhere in this book.

Missed Injuries

Missed injuries and delayed diagnosis are some of the more troublesome complications following intraabdominal injury. As previously discussed, one of the most common etiologies for these diagnostic errors is failure to adequately evaluate the abdomen. This particular error constituted approximately 19% of all identifiable errors made in a trauma system.[4]

Intraabdominal Compartment Syndrome

The observed association between severe intraabdominal injuries, massive fluid resuscitation, high abdominal wall tension, and a variety of adverse physiological sequelae, including decreased urine output, high peak airway pressures, and compromised organ perfusion, has led to the description of what is now called the intraabdominal compartment syndrome (IACS).[52] Although not completely unique to trauma, the characterization and management of IACS has been described mainly following severe abdominal injuries. IACS is produced by excessive intraabdominal pressures as the result of massive bowel edema, 'third space' fluid, intraperitoneal hemorrhage, or retroperitoneal hematomas. This increased pressure may cause decreases in splanchnic, renal, and abdominal wall perfusion and may produce venous capacitance pooling in the pelvis and lower extremities from a tourniquet-like effect on the midtorso.[53–57]

Several techniques have been used for monitoring intraabdominal pressure. Among the simplest and most effective is the measurement of intravesicular (bladder) pressure, performed by instilling 50 to 100 ml fluid in the bladder and measuring pressure via Foley catheter using either manometry or a pressure transducer. Pressure readings that are greater than 30 cm H_2O are consistent with IACS. This measurement correlates well with experimentally placed intraabdominal pressure catheters and provides a quick, simple bedside means of estimating intraabdominal pressures.[58]

The treatment of IACS has generally involved decompression of the abdominal compartment and the placement of a temporary abdominal wall prosthesis. In many instances, resolution of abdominal compartment edema allows either single or staged closure of the abdominal wall.

References

1. National Center for Injury Prevention and Control: *http://www.cdc.gov/ncipc/*.
2. Fabian TC, Croce MA. Abdominal trauma, including indication for celiotomy. In: Mattox KL, Moore EE, Feliciano DV, eds. Trauma, 3rd Ed. Stamford: Appleton & Lange, 1996.
3. Shackford SR, Mackersie RC, Holbrook TL, et al. The epidemiology of traumatic death: a population-based analysis. Arch Surg 1993;128:571–575.
4. Davis JW, Hoyt DB, McArdle MS, et al. An analysis of errors causing morbidity and mortality in a trauma system: a guide for quality improvement. J Trauma 1992;32:660–666.
5. Root HD, Hauser CW, McKinley CR, et al. Diagnostic peritoneal lavage. Surgery (St. Louis) 1965;57:633–637.
6. Alyono D, Morrow CE, Perry JF. Reappraisal of diagnostic peritoneal lavage criteria for operation in penetrating and blunt trauma. Surgery (St. Louis) 1982;92:751–757.
7. Oreskovich MR, Carrico CJ. Stab wounds of the anterior abdomen: analysis of a management plan using local wound exploration and quantitative peritoneal lavage. Ann Surg 1983;198:411–418.
8. Merlotti GJ, Marcet E, Sheaff CM, et al. Use of peritoneal lavage to evaluate abdominal penetration. J Trauma 1985;25:228–231.
9. Liu M, Lee CH, P'eng FK. Prospective comparison of diagnostic peritoneal lavage, computed tomographic scanning, and ultrasonography for the diagnosis of blunt abdominal trauma. J Trauma 1993;35(2):267–270.
10. Fabian TC, Mangiante EC, White TJ, et al. A prospective study of 91 patients undergoing both computed tomography and peritoneal lavage following blunt abdominal trauma. J Trauma 1986;26:602.
11. Peitzman AB, Makaroun MS, Slasky BS, Ritter P. Prospective study of computed tomography in initial management of blunt abdominal trauma. J Trauma 1986;26:585–592.
12. McKenney M, Lentz K, Nunez D, et al. Can ultrasound replace diagnostic peritoneal lavage in the assessment of blunt trauma? [see comments]. J Trauma 1994;37(3):439–441.
13. Yoshii H, Sato M, Yamamoto S, et al. Usefulness and limitations of ultrasonography in the initial evaluation of blunt abdominal trauma. J Trauma 1998;45(1):45–50.
14. Singh G, Arya N, Safaya R, et al. Role of ultrasonography in blunt abdominal trauma. Injury 1997;28(9-10):667–670.
15. Rozycki GS, Ochsner MG, Schmidt JA, et al. A prospective study of surgeon-performed ultrasound as the primary adjuvant modality for injured patient assessment. J Trauma 1995;39(3):492–498.
16. Ortega AE, Tang E, Froes ET, Asensio JA, Katkhouda N, Demetriades D. Laparoscopic evaluation of penetrating thoracoabdominal traumatic injuries. Surg Endosc 1996;10(1):19–22.
17. Sosa JL, Arrillaga A, Puente I, Sleeman D, Ginzburg E, Martin

L. Laparoscopy in 121 consecutive patients with abdominal gunshot wounds. J Trauma 1995;39(3):501–504, discussion 504–506.

18. Ivatury RR, Simon RJ, Stahl WM. A critical evaluation of laparoscopy in penetrating abdominal trauma. J Trauma 1993; 34(6):822–827, discussion 827–828.

19. Blow O, Bassam D, Butler K, et al. Speed and efficiency in the resuscitation of blunt trauma patients with multiple injuries: the advantage of diagnostic peritoneal lavage over abdominal computerized tomography. J Trauma 1998;44(2):287–290.

20. Sherck J, Shatney C, Sensaki K, Selivanov V. The accuracy of computed tomography in the diagnosis of blunt small-bowel perforation. Am J Surg 1994;168(6):670–675.

21. Udekwu PO, Gurkin B, Oller DW. The use of computed tomography in blunt abdominal injuries. Am Surg 1996;62(1):56–59.

22. Han DC, Rozycki GS, Schmidt JA, Feliciano DV. Ultrasound training during ATLS: an early start for surgical interns. J Trauma 1996;41(2):208–213.

23. Rozycki GS, Ochsner MG, Feliciano DV, et al. Early detection of hemoperitoneum by ultrasound examination of the right upper quadrant: a multicenter study. J Trauma 1998;45(5):878–883.

24. Chen RJ, Fang JF, Lin BC, et al. Selective application of laparoscopy and fibrin glue in the failure of nonoperative management of blunt hepatic trauma. J Trauma 1998;44(4):691–695.

25. Slim K, Bousquet J, Chipponi J. Laparoscopic repair of missed blunt diaphragmatic rupture using a prosthesis. Surg Endosc 1998;12(11):1358–1360.

26. Peck JJ, Berne TV. Posterior abdominal stab wounds. J Trauma 1981;21(4):298–306.

27. Kirton OC, Wint D, Thrasher B, et al. Stab wounds to the back and flank in the hemodynamically stable patient: a decision algorithm based on contrast-enhanced computed tomography with colonic opacification. Am J Surg 1997;173(3):189–193.

28. Meyer DM, Thal ER, Weigelt JA, Redman HC. The role of abdominal CT in the evaluation of stab wounds to the back [see comments]. J Trauma 1989;29(9):1226–1228.

29. McAllister E, Perez M, Albrink MH, et al. Is triple contrast computed tomographic scanning useful in the selective management of stab wounds to the back? J Trauma 1994;37(3):401–403.

30. Rotondo MF, Schwab CW, McGonigal MD, et al. 'Damage control': an approach for improved survival in exsanguinating penetrating abdominal injury. J Trauma 1993;35(3):375–382.

31. Carrillo EH, Spain DA, Wilson MA, Miller FB, et al. Alternatives in the management of penetrating injuries to the iliac vessels. J Trauma 1998;44(6):1024–1029.

32. Morris JA Jr, Eddy VA, Blinman TA, et al. The staged celiotomy for trauma. Issues in unpacking and reconstruction. Ann Surg 1993;217(5):576–584; discussion, 584–586.

33. Moore EE, Cogbill TH, Jurkovich GJ, et al. Organ injury scaling: spleen and liver (1994 revision). J Trauma 1995;38(3):323–324.

34. Brasel KJ, DeLisle CM, Olson CJ, Borgstrom DC. Trends in the management of hepatic injury. Am J Surg 1997;174(6):674–677.

35. Hebbler RF, Ward RE, Miller PW, et al. The management of splenic injury. J Trauma 1982;22:492.

36. Bradley EL III, Young PR Jr, Chang MC, et al. Diagnosis and initial management of blunt pancreatic trauma: guidelines from a multiinstitutional review. Ann Surg 1998;227(6):861–869.

37. Vaughan GD III, Frazier OH, Graham DY, et al. The use of pyloric exclusion in the management of severe duodenal injuries. Am J Surg 1977;134(6):785–790.

38. Martin TD, Feliciano DV, Mattox KL, Jordan GL Jr. Severe duodenal injuries. Treatment with pyloric exclusion and gastrojejunostomy. Arch Surg 1983;118(5):631–635.

39. Durham RM, Olson S, Weigelt JA. Penetrating injuries to the stomach. Surg Gynecol Obstet 1991;172(4):298–302.

40. Wisner DH, Chun Y, Blaisdell FW. Blunt intestinal injury. Keys to diagnosis and management. Arch Surg 1990;125(10):1319–1322; discussion 1322–1333.

41. Munns J, Richardson M, Hewett P. A review of intestinal injury from blunt abdominal trauma. Aust N Z J Surg 1995;65(12):857–860.

42. Udekwu PO, Gurkin B, Oller DW. The use of computed tomography in blunt abdominal injuries. Am Surg 1996;62(1):56–59.

43. Hagiwara A, Yukioka T, Satou M, et al. Early diagnosis of small intestine rupture from blunt abdominal trauma using computed tomography: significance of the streaky density within the mesentery. J Trauma 1995;38(4):630–633.

44. Sherck J, Shatney C, Sensaki K, Selivanov V. The accuracy of computed tomography in the diagnosis of blunt small-bowel perforation. Am J Surg 1994;168(6):670–675.

45. Internet website: Eastern Association for the Surgery of Trauma (EAST). *http://www.east.org*.

46. VanLoenhout RM, Schiphorst TM, Wittens CA, et al. Traumatic intrapericardial diaphragmatic hernia. J Trauma 1986;26:271.

47. Murray JG, Caoili E, Gruden JF, Evans SJ, Halvorsen RA, Mackersie RC. Acute rupture of the diaphragm due to blunt trauma: diagnostic sensitivity and specificity of CT. Am J Roentgenol 1996;166(5):1035–1039.

48. Flancbaum L, Dauber M, Demas C, et al. Early diagnosis and treatment of blunt diaphragmatic injury. Am Surg 1988;54:195.

49. Morgan AS, Flancbaum L, Esposito T, Cox EF. Blunt injury to the diaphragm: an analysis of 44 patients. J Trauma 1986;26(6):565–568.

50. Murray JA, Demetriades D, Asensio JA, et al. Occult injuries to the diaphragm: prospective evaluation of laparoscopy in penetrating injuries to the left lower chest. J Am Coll Surg 1998;187(6):626–630.

51. Selivanov V, Chi HS, Alverdy JC, et al. Mortality in retroperitoneal hematoma. J Trauma 1984;24(12):1022–1027.

52. Burch JM, Moore EE, Moore FA, Franciose R. The abdominal compartment syndrome. Surg Clin North Am 1996;76(4):833–842.

53. Saggi BH, Sugerman HJ, Ivatury RR, Bloomfield GL. Abdominal compartment syndrome. J Trauma 1998;45(3):597–609.

54. Bloomfield GL, Ridings PC, Blocher CR, et al. A proposed relationship between increased intra-abdominal, intrathoracic, and intracranial pressure. Crit Care Med 1997;25(3):496–503.

55. Rosenthal RJ, Friedman RL, Kahn AM, et al. Reasons for intracranial hypertension and hemodynamic instability during acute elevations of intra-abdominal pressure: observations in a large animal model. J Gastrointest Surg 1998;2(5):415–425.

56. Diebel LN, Dulchavsky SA, Wilson RF. Effect of increased intra-abdominal pressure on mesenteric arterial and intestinal mucosal blood flow. J Trauma 1992;33(1):45–48.

57. Diebel L, Saxe L, Dulchavsky S. Effect of intra-abdominal pressure on abdominal wall blood flow. Am Surg 1992;58(9):573–575.

58. Iberti TJ, Lieber CE, Benjamin E. Determination of intra-abdominal pressure using a transurethral bladder catheter: clinical validation of the technique. Anesthesiology 1989;70(1):47–50.

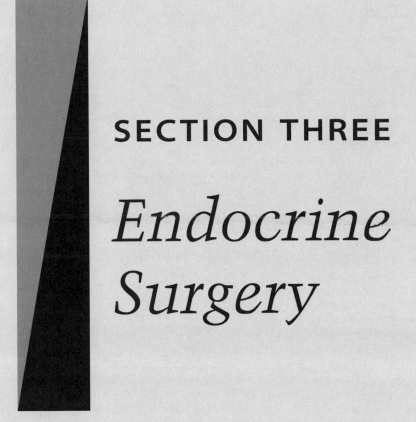

SECTION THREE

Endocrine Surgery

27

Parathyroid

Hop N. Le and Jeffrey A. Norton

Calcium Physiology

Accurate diagnoses, proper selection of patients for surgical treatment, and management of hyperparathyroidism require a detailed understanding of the homeostatic mechanisms of calcium. An average daily dietary intake of calcium is between 500 and 1000 mg.[1] The duodenum and upper jejunum are the principal sites of active calcium absorption, involving vitamin D metabolites. The diurnal variation in the level of serum calcium is 5% or less. This homeostasis is achieved by the balance between gastrointestinal absorption, bone deposition and release, and urinary excretion of calcium.

Serum calcium is regulated by a closely integrated interplay of three hormones: parathyroid hormone (PTH), vitamin D_3 (1,25-dihydroxycholecalciferol), and calcitonin (Fig. 27.1). The key target organs include the parathyroids, skeletal system, kidneys, and intestine. PTH is synthesized in the parathyroid glands as a larger molecule, pre-pro-PTH, which is cleaved into its inactive form, pre-PTH.[2] Pre-PTH is further cleaved into PTH, which is released into the circulation and broken down further into amino- and carboxyl-terminal fragments by the liver and kidney. Only the whole intact PTH molecule and the amino-terminal fragment are physiologically active. The double-antibody immunoradiometric assay (IRMA) is the current method of intact PTH detection.[3] PTH exerts its effect by activating membrane-bound adenylate cyclases generating cyclic adenosine monophosphate. PTH regulates serum calcium level by directly and indirectly affecting calcium exchange at the intestine, bone, and kidney. PTH directly increases serum calcium by inhibiting the synthetic function of osteoblast and stimulating renal tubular calcium reabsorption. PTH indirectly contributes to calcium regulation by stimulating osteoclast maturation and inducing renal phosphate clearance and synthesis of calcitriol, which in turn promotes gastrointestinal absorption of calcium.

Vitamin D is another key regulator of bone mineral metabolism. Calcitriol is the major active form of vitamin D. It stimulates calcium-binding protein in the gut and enhances absorption of calcium and phosphorus.

Calcitonin is produced by the parafollicular C cells of the thyroid. Calcitonin decreases bone resorption by antagonizing the effects of PTH. Its physiological role has been implicated in minimizing calcium loss during development, pregnancy, and nursing.[4] Although calcitonin receptors are found in the kidneys, brain, and throughout the body, the complete absence or supernormal levels of calcitonin do not seem to have any significant clinical manifestations.

Embryology, Anatomy, and Pathophysiology

Despite the wide deviation in gland distribution, the location of parathyroid glands is predictable from knowledge of embryology. The parathyroid glands develop at about the fifth week of gestation. The upper parathyroid glands arise from the dorsal part of the fourth branchial pouches along with the lateral lobes of the thyroid. The upper glands only descend slightly and stay in close association with the upper portion of the lateral thyroid lobes.[5,6] This position remains fairly constant into adult life. On the other hand, the lower parathyroids develop from the dorsal part of the third branchial pouches along with the thymus. The lower glands descend a great distance with the thymus, thus accounting for a wide range of distribution in adulthood. The range of location includes just beneath the mandible at the level of the hyoid, anteromedial to the carotid bifurcation to the pericardium, and anteromedial to the recurrent laryngeal nerve (Fig. 27.2).

Facility in the identification of normal and abnormal parathyroid glands is essential. Parathyroid glands vary in color from a light yellow to a reddish brown, and the consistency is usually soft and pliable.[5] Typically, there are four parathyroid glands, and the average weight of a normal gland is 35 to 50 mg. Normal glands tend to be flat and ovoid; with enlargement, they become globular. The normal measure-

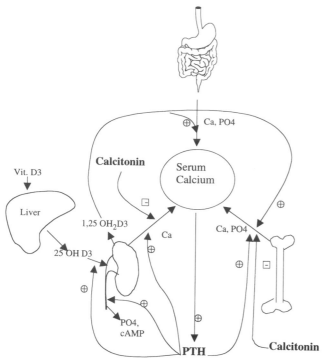

FIGURE 27.1. The interplay of parathyroid hormone (PTH), vitamin D, and calcitonin on calcium and phosphorus regulation at specific target organs. A decrease in serum calcium stimulates PTH secretion by the parathyroid glands. PTH directly and indirectly affects calcium exchange at the intestine, bone, and kidney to elevate the serum level of calcium. Calcitriol [1,25(OH)$_2$D], the major active form of vitamin D, enhances calcium and phosphorus absorption in the intestine while inhibiting PTH. There is a negative feedback loop between serum calcium and calcitonin levels. An increase in serum calcium results in calcitonin secretion, which regulates bone and kidney to decrease serum calcium.

ments are 5 to 7 mm × 3 to 4 mm × 0.5 to 2 mm. The combined weight of all parathyroid glands is 90 to 130 mg, and the superior glands are usually smaller than the inferior glands.[7] Most parathyroid glands are suspended by a small vascular pedicle and enveloped by a pad of fatty tissue.[8]

Approximately 5% of humans have supernumerary (more than four) parathyroid glands.[9] Supernumerary glands and fragments of parathyroid glands are most commonly found within the thymus.

Clinical Features

Primary hyperparathyroidism (PHPT) is characterized by an inappropriately elevated secretion of PTH relative to the level of serum calcium. PHPT accounts for 50% to 60% of hypercalcemia in the ambulatory setting, whereas malignancy accounts for 65% of hypercalcemia in the inpatient setting[10] (Table 27.1). Certain factors such as a family history of PHPT or multiple endocrine neoplasia (MEN), childhood radiation to the head and neck, postmenospausal state, renal calculi, peptic ulcer, hypertension, or thiazide-induced hypercalcemia are more consistent with PHPT. Clinical presentations of primary hyperparathyroidism may be in one of three forms: (1) asymptomatic hypercalcemia; (2) nephrolithiasis; or (3) bone disease with more marked hypercalcemia, fatigue, gen-

eral debility, bone pain, weight loss, sometimes pathological fractures, and even parathyroid crisis. The most common presentation is asymptomatic hypercalcemia. The diagnosis of primary hyperparathyroidism is based on concomitant measurements of elevated serum levels of total calcium[11,12] or ionized calcium[13] and intact parathyroid hormone (PTH).[14–17] Measurement of 24-h urinary calcium excretion, which is elevated in patients with PHPT, helps confirm the diagnosis.

Prognostic Indicators of Parathyroid Pathology

Primary hyperparathyroidism is caused by parathyroid adenoma or a single abnormal gland (85%), parathyroid hyperplasia or multiple abnormal glands (10%–12%), double adenoma (1%–2%), or carcinoma (1%). It is up to the operating surgeon to correctly diagnose the precise etiology of PHPT. Certain symptoms and signs may suggest specific types of parathyroid pathology. Parathyroid adenoma is rarely ever palpable, but parathyroid carcinoma is palpable in a high percentage of cases.[18,19] Exceptionally high concentrations of serum PTH or calcium (>13 mg/dl) also may suggest parathyroid cancer.[19] Parathyroid hyperplasia is often inherited in familial syndromes such as MEN I or MEN IIA.[20,21] There are no physical signs characteristic of MEN I or MEN II. Recent studies have identified the genetic defect in patients with MEN I as the MENIN mutation on chromosome 11q13[22] and

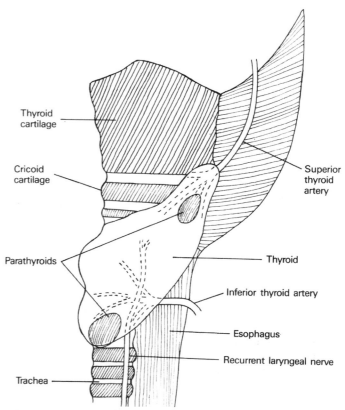

FIGURE 27.2. A lateral view of the anatomical relationship of the parathyroids to their arterial blood supply and the recurrent laryngeal nerve. The superior parathyroid glands are usually located in the upper portion of the lateral thyroid lobes and are supplied by either the superior or inferior thyroid artery. The location of the inferior parathyroid glands is more variable but can usually be found in the lower pole of the thyroid. The inferior parathyroids are supplied by the inferior thyroid artery, which runs just lateral to the recurrent laryngeal nerve.

TABLE 27.1. Differential Diagnosis of Hypercalcemia.

Endocrine
    Primary hyperparathyroidism
    Thyrotoxicosis
    Pheochromocytoma
    Addison's disease
    VIPomas
Malignancy
    Solid tumors
    Lytic bone metastasis
    Parathyroid hormone-related protein
    Lymphoma and leukemia
Granulomatous diseases
    Sarcoidosis
    Tuberculosis
    Histoplasmosis
    Coccidioidomycosis
    Leprosy
Medication
    Calcium
    Vitamin A or D intoxication
    Thiazides
    Lithium
    Estrogens and antiestrogens
Others
    Milk alkali syndrome
    Familial hypocalciuric hypercalcemia
    Immobilization
    Paget's disease
    Renal insufficiency

Malignancy is the most common cause of hypercalcemia in the inpatient setting; primary hyperparathyroidism is the most common cause in the outpatient setting.

in patients with MEN II as the RET proto-oncogene mutation on chromosome 10q11.2.[23] MEN IIb patients do not have primary hyperparathyroidism. Familial hypocalciuric hypercalcemia (FHH) is an autosomal dominant trait presenting usually as asymptomatic mild hypercalcemia and relative hypocalciuria.[24,25] Mutations in the calcium-sensing receptor gene on chromosome 3 have been identified in its heterozygous form in benign FHH.[19] In patients with FHH, the hypercalcemia is PTH dependent and associated with mild parathyroid hyperplasia; however, subtotal parathyroidectomy is rarely successful in correcting hypercalcemia and is contraindicated.

Hypercalcemic Crisis

Hypercalcemic crisis is an unusual state of progressive, marked primary hyperparathyroidism producing accelerated bone resorption and excessive elevation in serum and urinary levels of calcium. Clinical manifestations include anorexia, vomiting, constipation, dehydration, acute pancreatitis, shortened QT interval, increased sensitivity to digitalis, polyuria, polydipsia, nephrocalcinosis, apathy, drowsiness, coma, and, if untreated, death.[26–29] Serum levels of calcium should not be the only defining criteria for a hypercalcemic crisis because there have been reports of asymptomatic patients with serum calcium levels of 20 mg/dl and of patients in hypercalcemic crisis with serum calcium less than 14 mg/dl.[30]

Management of the severe hypercalcemia in patients with parathyroid crisis centers on achieving four basic goals: (1) correct dehydration, (2) enhance renal excretion of calcium, (3) inhibit accelerated bone resorption, and (4) treat the underlying disorder. Initial treatment is administration of large volumes of saline to correct dehydration. Once fluid status is corrected, intravenous administration of saline followed by a loop diuretic (i.e., furosemide) is usually effective in reducing the hypercalcemia by inhibiting calcium reabsorption in the ascending limb of the loop of Henle. Thiazide diuretics are contraindicated because they enhance distal tubular reabsorption of calcium. In patients with low serum concentration of phosphate, normal renal function, and moderate hypercalcemia, oral phosphate may also be used. If hydration and treatment with furosemide intravenously are not effective in reducing the hypercalcemia, treatment with diphosphonates, mithramycin, calcitonin, or gallium should be started as necessary to normalize serum levels of calcium.[29]

Localization Techniques

Localization Before Initial Parathyroidectomy

Because radiographic parathyroid localization adds to the costs and does not improve the efficacy of most parathyroid surgeons, localization studies are usually not recommended for previously unoperated cases. However, recent studies indicate that ultrasound and sestamibi scintigraphy may be useful (see below).

Localization Before Reoperative Parathyroidectomy

In patients with failed initial procedures for PHPT or in individuals who subsequently develop recurrent hypercalcemia, the probability of successful repeat surgery is reduced[31,32] and the incidence of complications is greater.[33] Therefore, a maximum effort at preoperative gland localization should be made, commencing with the noninvasive procedures (US, CT, MRI, sestamibi) and proceeding (if necessary) to the more invasive studies. Review of the recent literature indicates that localization studies were helpful in the majority of reoperative parathyroidectomies (Table 27.2). Currently, noninvasive techniques can localize an abnormal gland in about 75% to 80% of patients requiring repeat surgery.[34–36] Invasive localizing studies usually provide some useful information in the remainder.[37] An important principle in reviewing the results of any radiographic imaging technique is that identification of one abnormal parathyroid gland does not exclude the presence of another additional pathological gland or glands in other locations. Approximately 30% of patients undergoing reoperations have more than one abnormal gland.[32,38]

Ultrasound

US is the least expensive and least invasive technique to image abnormal parathyroid glands. It is particularly effective for localizing enlarged glands in the neck and correctly identifies approximately 60% of the abnormal glands in patients requiring reoperation.[31,36,39,40]

Sestamibi Scintigraphy

Sestamibi–technetium 99m scanning has a superior resolution and sensitivity of 70% to 90% for solitary parathyroid tumors.[41] Both the thyroid and parathyroid take up sestamibi, but its uptake is stronger and the signal persists longer in abnormal parathyroid glands. Overall, sestamibi is the single

TABLE 27.2.
Imaging Modalities in Reoperative Parathyroidectomies: Overall Results.

References	Level of evidence[a]	n	Imaging modalities: true-positive/false-positive (%)						
			Sestamibi	Tech-thal	Ultrasound	CT	MRI	Angiography	Venous sampling
Mariette 1998[94]	III	38	69/—	—	—	16/—	—	—	63/—
Peeler 1997[95]	III	25	74/—	—	45/—	68/—	—	—	—
Jaskowiak 1996[42]	II	227	67/0	42/8	48/21	52/16	48/14	59/9	76/4
Shen 1996[32]	III	102	77/—	68/—	57/—	42/—	77/—	—	77/—
MacFarlane 1994[86]	III	42	42/15	—	67/9	56/10	36/8	68/14	69/8
Rodriguez 1994[43]	III	152	70/0	60/16	53/16	42/12	69/12	—	69/15
Doherty 1992[96]	III	27/—	—	4/23	0/20	35/13	19/13	84/7	—

[a]I, randomized prospective study; II, prospective study; III, retrospective study, review or anecdotal.
[b]Values represent sensitivities.

best imaging study for abnormal parathyroid glands. It has achieved sensitivities as high as 86% with specificities varying from 77% to 100%.[42,43]

Computed Tomography

CT is particularly effective for abnormal parathyroid glands in the anterior mediastinum and the tracheoesophageal groove.[44] It correctly identifies the adenoma in about 70% of initial cases.[45–49] Ectopic mediastinal glands usually lie within the fat-replaced thymus, and even small adenomas are readily visualized. Further, the tracheoesophageal groove in the posterosuperior mediastinum is the most common location of missed parathyroid adenomas.[50–51] CT localizes parathyroid pathology in 50% to 60% of the reoperative patient group.[35,44,50] CT is poor at detecting intrathyroid or juxtathyroidal tumors.

Magnetic Resonance Imaging

MRI with surface coils provides exquisite anatomy of the neck and enhanced resolution.[52] Results indicate that approximately 57% to 90% of abnormal parathyroid glands can be correctly imaged in patients undergoing reoperations.[53] With gadolinium MRI, and T_1- and T_2-weighted images, MRI can now provide a higher sensitivity at identifying ectopic parathyroid tumors than CT scan. In addition, MRI does not require intravenous contrast, and surgical clips do not cause artifacts. However, MRI is more expensive than CT.

Fine-Needle Aspiration

To unequivocally confirm that the mass is parathyroid, a lesion may be aspirated with a very thin needle under CT or US guidance and the concentration of parathyroid hormone in the aspirate measured.[33] CT-guided fine-needle aspiration (FNA) for PTH has a sensitivity of 70% and a specificity of 100%.[54]

Angiography

Intravenous digital angiography for parathyroid localization has been successful in less than 30% of cases.[54] Patient mo-

tion degrades subtraction images, and motion artifacts produce a high incidence of false-positive examinations. On the other hand, the intraarterial digital technique requires no highly selective catheter positioning, so it can be accomplished expeditiously at nearly every hospital. However, improved results with noninvasive imaging studies have dramatically reduced the need for angiography.

Selective Venous Sampling

Selective venous sampling requires the greatest experience and is the most poorly performed study in nonreferral centers. It is indicated in only a small proportion of reoperative patients who have significant primary hyperparathyroidism and no apparent localizing information after completing all noninvasive studies and angiography.

Summary of Radiographic Modalities

An algorithm for use of the various radiographic modalities is given in Figure 27.3.

Intraoperative Determination of Parathyroid Hormone

Generally, after successful removal of a single parathyroid adenoma or adequate resection of hyperplastic glands, serum levels of intact PTH fall immediately and reach normal range within 30 to 90 min after removal of the tissue involved.[56] Most studies suggest that a 50% decline from the baseline level predicts a successful outcome. Serum levels of intact PTH are measured during surgery by rapid RIA. Studies demonstrate that serum levels of intact PTH decline rapidly, and a significant drop (>50% from baseline) will be detectable only 15 min following resection of a parathyroid adenoma.[56,57] Furthermore, the rate of decline is less in patients with hyperplasia and may provide an additional clue to its diagnosis.[57] Currently, however, these determinations are not the standard of care and should be used as adjuncts to surgery. To determine the exact role of intraoperative PTH assay, if any, requires additional prospective studies.

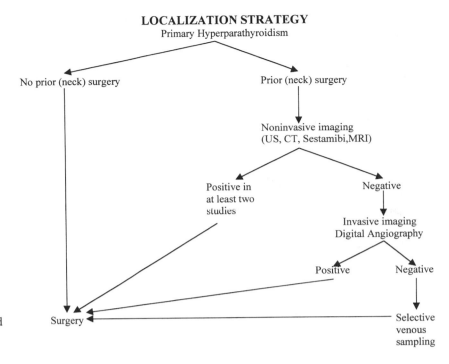

LOCALIZATION STRATEGY
Primary Hyperparathyroidism

No prior (neck) surgery   Prior (neck) surgery

Noninvasive imaging
(US, CT, Sestamibi,MRI)

Positive in   Negative
at least two
studies

Invasive imaging
Digital Angiography

Positive   Negative

Surgery   Selective
venous
sampling

FIGURE 27.3. Algorithm for a suggested approach toward imaging studies for localization of parathyroid adenomas in initial and reoperative parathyroidectomies.

Indications for Surgery

In general, we suggest surgical exploration for all patients with clear biochemical evidence of primary hyperparathyroidism and documented signs or symptoms of the disease[58,59] (Table 27.3).

The best treatment for totally asymptomatic patients is controversial.[58] Younger patients with apparently asymptomatic primary hyperparathyroidism may require earlier surgery given a low operative risk and long temporal exposure

to the disease. In apparently asymptomatic, older patients with primary hyperparathyroidism, we recommend careful observation and follow-up, with surgery reserved for patients who develop evidence of progression or symptoms. Progression is documented by a decrease in bone density on serial studies, kidney stones, serum calcium level greater than 12 mg/dl, or elevated serum levels of bone alkaline phosphatase.

Indications agreed upon by the Proceedings of the NIH Consensus Development Conference on Diagnosis and Mangement of Asymptomatic PHPT include (1) serum calcium greater than 11.5 to 12 mg/dl, (2) creatinine clearance reduced more than 30% for age in absence of another cause, (3) 24-h urinary Ca^{2+} greater than 400 mg/dl, (4) bone mass reduced more than 2 SD compared with age, gender, and race-matched controls, (5) patients who request surgery or in whom long-term surveillance is unsuitable, and (6) young patients (<50 years old).[58] There is certainly no urgent need for surgery in this group, but regular follow-up once or twice a year is indicated to guard against progression of disease. Studies suggest that approximately 20% of patients with asymptomatic primary hyperparathyroidism develop symptoms with long-term follow-up.[59,60]

Surgical Management of Primary Hyperparathyroidism

Surgery is the only curative treatment for patients with primary hyperparathyroidism. In general, abnormal gland or glands can be correctly identified at exploration in approximately 95% of patients.[30,61–65] Complication rates are low. Recurrent laryngeal nerve injury occurs in less than 1% of initial operations and approximately 5% of repeat operations for primary hyperparathyroidism.[33,66] Fortunately, symptoms in many of these nerve injuries are temporary, and full recovery may be seen at 3- to 6-month follow-up. Hypoparathyroidism is a complication that usually does not occur following initial explorations[66] but may occur in 2.7% to 16% of individ-

TABLE 27.3. Manifestations of Primary Hyperparathyroidism That Warrants Surgery.

System	Signs and symptoms
Serum	Calcium level >12 mg/dl
Skeletal	Decreased bone density
	Pain
	Pathological fracture
	Bone cysts
	Brown tumors
	Osteitis fibrosa cystica
	Gout and pseudogout
	Nonspecific arthralgias
Renal	Urinary calcium >350 mg/24 h
	Renal colic
	Nephrocalcinosis
	Decreased creatinine clearance
Gastrointestinal	Peptic ulcer disease
	Pancreatitis
Neurological	Emotional lability
	Slow mentation
	Poor memory
	Depression
	Easy fatigability
Neuromuscular	Proximal muscular weakness
	Muscular atrophy
Other	Anemia

uals following reoperations.[38,51,67–68] Another undesired outcome is unsuccessful surgery. Initial procedures are successful in approximately 85% to 95% of cases[61–65,69] and repeat procedures in 78% to 90%.[38,51,67,70,71]

General Technique of Exploration

We recommend identification and biopsy of all four parathyroid glands. Abnormal glands are completely removed. However, others recommend identification of all glands and excision of any abnormal glands and biopsy of only one normal parathyroid gland. A minority of endocrine surgical centers practice unilateral neck exploration for primary hyperparathyroidism.

Dissection of the neck requires meticulous hemostatic technique. Blood-stained tissue alters the color, making identification of parathyroid glands more difficult. The upper glands are usually posterior and lateral to the recurrent laryngeal nerve, and the lower glands are usually anteromedial to it. Because the upper glands are most constant in location, they should be identified first. If the upper glands are biopsied and found to be normal but the lower glands cannot be located, then the thyrothymic ligament should be carefully explored because 44% of inferior glands are within this ligament. If the ligament does not contain parathyroid tissue, then both superior horns of the thymus in the lower neck should be dissected and removed; 17% of inferior glands are found within the thymus. If the inferior gland is not within the thymus, then the thyroid lobe on the side of the missing gland may be removed; 3% of inferior parathyroid glands are found within the thyroid lobe.[72] Some recommend that intraoperative ultrasound be used during the operation before thyroid lobectomy to determine whether a suspicious sonolucent mass lesion (parathyroid adenoma) is present within the thyroid.[44,73]

Failure of the initial exploration, even with diligent search of the areas just noted, calls for stopping the procedure. Reevaluation of the diagnosis and then localization procedures should be performed before initiating a median sternotomy. Median sternotomy is indicated in only 1% to 2% of patients undergoing initial explorations.[74]

Special Issues in Surgery

Adenoma

Regarding operative strategy for presumed adenoma, review of the recent literature shows that the surgical results of either a bilateral or unilateral approach can achieve similar overall success rates, and the complication rates of a unilateral approach do not appear to be any lower than that of a bilateral approach. Key is the assured removal of the affected gland(s). In either method, the most important indicators of normal or abnormal tissue are appearance of the gland and histopathologic confirmation of the biopsied tissue.

Hyperplasia

The surgical management of parathyroid hyperplasia is more difficult and the results less satisfactory. There are two possible surgical procedures designed for this diagnosis: subtotal (3.5-gland) parathyroidectomy or four-gland parathyroidectomy with immediate autograft.

Our approach to nonfamilial parathyroid hyperplasia is subtotal (3.5-gland) parathyroidectomy, leaving approximately 50 mg of the most normal-appearing parathyroid tissue marked with a surgical clip in the neck. The incidence of either persistent disease or hypoparathyroidism has been low, and we expect our incidence of recurrent disease to be between 10% and 20% based on long-term follow-up data from others.[64] For familial hyperplasia, we use total parathyroidectomy and immediate parathyroid autograft to the forearm because the incidence of recurrent disease is high (38%–64%).[20,75–77] If recurrent hypercalcemia develops in these patients, a portion of the transplanted tissue can be removed under local anesthesia. In patients with recurrent disease after subtotal parathyroidectomy, total parathyroidectomy with cryopreservation of resected tissue is required.[78]

Secondary and Tertiary Hyperparathyroidism

Almost all patients with advanced renal failure on chronic dialysis have evidence of bone disease secondary to hyperparathyroidism and elevated serum levels of PTH. Secondary hyperparathyroidism should be suppressed in these individuals by measures that normalize serum levels of calcium and phosphorus. Failure of these measures occurs in a minority of individuals, and parathyroidectomy is then used to decrease the mass of hyperplastic parathyroid tissue.

Potential indications for parathyroidectomy in patients with chronic renal failure and autonomous hyperplastic parathyroid glands (tertiary hyperparathyroidism) include (1) hypercalcemia in prospective renal transplant patients; (2) pathological fractures secondary to renal osteodystrophy; (3) symptoms secondary to hyperparathyroidism including pruritus, bone pain, and extensive soft tissue calcification and calciphylaxis; (4) hypercalcemia in patients with renal transplants that are functioning well; and (5) a calcium times phosphate product greater than 70.[79,80] Improvements in medical management have reduced these complications in many patients so that surgery is less often needed.

Controversy exists about whether to perform a subtotal parathyroidectomy,[81] a total parathyroidectomy without autograft,[82] or a total parathyroidectomy with immediate autograft.[76] No overwhelming evidence suggests one procedure over the other in this patient population.

Reoperations for Primary Hyperparathyroidism

Patients with hypercalcemia following initial operations for primary hyperparathyroidism can be classified as having persistent or recurrent disease. In persistent disease there is hypercalcemia in the immediate postoperative period or within 6 months of the initial neck exploration. In recurrent disease, there is either an initial period of hypocalcemia or normalization of the serum levels of calcium for at least 6 months after neck exploration and then the reappearance of hypercalcemia. The complexity of repeat neck surgery for primary hyperparathyroidism makes it imperative to confirm again the diagnosis and the presence of significant symptoms and to attempt precise preoperative localization, as outlined here, before embarking on a second exploration.[32,38]

The surgeon should use the first operation report, pathology results, and the localization data to plan the reexploration. For example, if two abnormal parathyroid glands were removed and the family history is positive for parathyroid disease, the surgeon must use a working diagnosis of hyperplasia and remove two additional abnormal glands. A biopsy-proven normal gland found at the initial procedure and radiologic localization studies suggesting a mediastinal adenoma would prompt a direct approach to the identified abnormal parathyroid gland by either transcervical approach or median sternotomy.[82] For cervical glands, we use an alternate route in the neck along the medial border of the sternocleidomastoid muscle instead of between the strap muscles.[32,38,83] This route requires a separate approach on each side of the neck. Intraoperative ultrasound (IOUS) using a 10-MHz transducer is performed after the right or left side of the neck is opened. In our experience,[84,85] IOUS can image most abnormal glands during reoperations.[45] It is especially helpful for intrathyroidal, intrathymic, and paraesophageal parathyroid adenomas.[74]

Another strategy for reoperative parathyroid surgery is minimally invasive radioguided parathyroidectomy (MIRP). This strategy includes a preoperative dual-phase sestamibi scan and injection of Tc-99m–sestamibi approximately 0.75–2.5 h before surgery. A unilateral neck exploration is guided by a handheld gamma probe. The advantage of this technique includes smaller incisions, shorter operative time, decreased risk of nerve injury complications, outpatient surgery with use of local anesthetics, and no frozen section analysis requirement. The disadvantage includes the possibility of missing a second lesion on the contralateral side of the neck.

It should be remembered that even at reoperations for primary hyperparathyroidism the majority of abnormal glands can be removed through a cervical incision.[86] Slow, meticulous exploration in a bloodless field is generally necessary to find these "ectopic" glands. Cryopreservation of removed parathyroid tissue during reoperations is indicated because the existence of remaining normal parathyroid tissue in these cases is unpredictable.

With careful attention to confirmation of diagnosis, prior operative records, judicious use of preoperative localization, and postoperative autografting, successful outcome may be achieved in more than 90% of reoperations[38,87,88] (Table 27.4).

Parathyroid Carcinoma

Parathyroid carcinoma should be suspected in patients with primary hyperparathyroidism who have a very high serum level of calcium, evidence of recurrence of the abnormal gland at the same site in which an abnormal gland was previously removed,[19,89] or a palpable neck mass that is firm and nonmobile.[19,90]

Parathyroid cancer usually invades along the tracheoesophageal groove, and the patient may present with hoarseness secondary to a recurrent laryngeal nerve injury. At neck exploration, the cancerous tissue appears gray with a thick, hard capsule. We recommend, based on suspicion (e.g., mass, local recurrence, high serum level of calcium), wide excision including thyroid lobectomy in continuity with the tumor.[91] Recurrent laryngeal nerve injury, either from the tumor itself or from the surgeon attempting to completely resect the tumor mass with the ipsilateral thyroid lobe, is probable and occurs in 75% of patients.[19] Locally recurrent benign parathyroid adenomas may occur and be confused with parathyroid carcinomas. Recurrent adenomas generally present with a longer disease-free interval, a lower serum level of calcium, and a history of either incomplete resection or spillage of tumor at the time of initial surgery.[19] Nevertheless, both locally recurrent parathyroid adenoma and cancer appear to respond favorably to aggressive local resection, and most patients can be rendered either hypocalcemic or normocalcemic for a reasonable period of time.[19,92] In patients with distant metastases, surgery appears to have a lesser role in treatment and chemotherapy has been shown to be of little benefit.[93] Therapy for these patients has been directed primarily at controlling the severe hypercalcemia.[29]

Postoperative Management

Successful parathyroidectomy leads to dramatic changes in calcium metabolism. Levels of serum calcium usually reach a nadir below normal on the second or third postoperative day but may take even longer to drop in patients with renal disease. Most patients who have undergone successful surgery

TABLE 27.4.
Surgical Outcome for Reoperative Surgery.

References	n	Level of evidence[a]	Success (%)	RLN paresis	RLN paralysis	Permanent hypocalcemia	Transient hypocalcemia	Wound infection	Mortality (%)
Mariette 1998[94]	38	III	92	—	3	2	—	—	—
Jaskowiak 1996[42]	222	II	97	6	3	12	49	0	0
Shen 1996[32]	102	III	95	1	1	1	6	—	—
Rodriquez 1994[43]	152	III	93	1	0	1	6	—	—
Weber 1994[97]	51	III	92	1	0	1	11	1	2
Carty 1991[31]	206	III	95	12	1	17	—	—	0.5
Jarhult 1993[98]	93	III	82	—	9	15	—	—	—
Rothmund 1990[99]	70	III	96	—	4	19	—	—	—
Cheung 1989[100]	83	III	86	2	1	8	10	1	1.2
Grant 1986[67]	157	III	89	13	6	20	27	—	0

[a]I, randomized prospective study; II, prospective study; III, retrospective study, review or anecdotal.

for primary hyperparathyroidism have some symptoms of hypocalcemia and may even develop a positive Chvostek sign. Treatment is guided primarily by the serum level of calcium, which should be maintained above 8.0 mg/dl.

If the symptoms of hypocalcemia are severe and the patient appears to be on the verge of tetany (occurring most frequently in patients with "hungry bone syndrome"), the clinician may need to treat with i.v. calcium. These symptoms can usually be rapidly corrected by the infusion of 2 mg/kg of elemental calcium over 15 min.

When hypocalcemia persists despite maximal oral replacement doses and hyperphosphatemia develops, we recommend the use of $1,25(OH)_2D_3$ (calcitriol), which is the major biologically active metabolite of vitamin D. The usual initial dose is calcitriol 0.25 to 1.0 μg/day given on a twice-daily schedule. Serum levels of calcium should be monitored weekly following discharge to further adjust oral calcium and calcitriol doses.

References

1. Mallette LE. Regulation of blood calcium in humans. Endocrinol Metabol Clin North Am 1989;18(3):601–610.
2. Pocotte SL, Ehrenstein G, Fitzpatrick LA. Regulation of parathyroid hormone secretion. Endocr Rev 1991;12(3):291–301.
3. Kao P, van Heerden JA, Grant CS, Klee GG, Khosla S. Clinical performance of parathyroid hormone immunometric assays. May Clin Proc 1992;67:637–645.
4. McDermott MT, Perloff JJ, Kidd GS. Effects of mild asymptomatic primary hyperparathyroidism on bone mass in women with and without estrogen replacement therapy. J Bone Miner Res 1994;9(4):509–514.
5. Akerstrom G, Malmaeus J, Bergstrom R. Surgical anatomy of human parathyroid glands. Surgery (St. Louis) 1984;95:14.
6. Thompson NW, Vinik AI. The technique of initial parathyroid exploration and reoperative parathyroidectomy. In: Thompson NW, Vinik AI, eds. Endocrine Surgery Update. New York: Grune & Stratton, 1983:368.
7. Wells SA, Leight GF, Ross A. Primary hyperparathyroidism. Curr Probl Surg 1980;17:398.
8. Wang CA. The anatomic basis of parathyroid surgery. Ann Surg 1975;183:271.
9. Wang CA, Mahaffey JE, Axelrod L, et al. Hyperfunctioning supernumerary parathyroid glands. Surg Gynecol Obstet 1979;148:711.
10. Lafferty FW. Differential diagnosis of hypercalcemia. J Bone Miner Res Suppl 1991;2:s51–s59.
11. Christensson T, Hellstrom K, Wengle B, et al. Prevalence of hypercalcemia in a health screening in Stockholm. Acta Med Scand 1976;200:131–137.
12. Christensson T, Hellstrom K, Wengle B. Hypercalcemia and primary hyperparathyroidism: prevalence in patients receiving thiazides as detected in a health screen. Arch Intern Med 1977; 137:1138–1142.
13. Landenson JH, Lewis JH, McDonald JM, et al. Relationship of free and total calcium in hypercalcemia conditions. J Clin Endocrinol Metab 1978;48:393–397.
14. Papapoulos SE, Manning RM, Hendy GN, et al. Studies of circulating parathyroid hormone in man using a homologous amino-terminal specific immunoradiometric assay. Clin Endocrinol 1980;13:57–67.
15. Mallette LE, Tuma SN, Berger RE, et al. Radioimmunoassay for the middle region of human parathyroid hormone using a homologous antiserum with carboxy-terminal fragment of bovine parathyroid hormone as radioligand. J Clin Endocrinol Metab 1982;54:1017–1024.
16. Hitzler W, Schmidt-Gayk H, Spiropoulos P, et al. Homologous

17. Lindall AW, Elting J, Ells J, et al. Estimation of biologically active intact parathyroid hormone in normal and hyperparathyroid sera by sequential N-terminal immunoextraction and mid-region radioimmunoassay. J Clin Endocrinol Metab 1983;57: 1007–1014.
18. Shane E, Bilezikian JP. Parathyroid carcinoma: a review of 62 patients. Endocr Rev 1982;3:218.
19. Fraker DL, Travis WD, Merendino JJ Jr, et al. Locally recurrent parathyroid neoplasms as a cause for recurrent and persistent primary hyperparathyroidism. Ann Surg 1991;213:58–65.
20. Rizzoli R, Green J III, Marx SJ. Primary hyperparathyroidism in familial multiple endocrine neoplasia type I: long-term follow-up of serum calcium levels after parathyroidectomy. Am J Med 1985;78:467–474.
21. Keiser HR, Beaven MA, Doppman J, et al. Sipple's syndrome: medullary thyroid carcinoma, pheochromocytoma and parathyroid disease. Ann Intern Med 1973;78:561–579.
22. The European Consortium on MEN 1. Identification of the multiple endocrine neoplasia type 1 (MEN1) gene. Hum Mol Genet 1997;6:7.
23. Lairmore TC, Howe JR, Korte JA, et al. Familial medullary thyroid carcinoma and multiple endocrine neoplasia type 2B map to the same region of chromosome 10 as multiple endocrine neoplasia type 2A. Genomics 1991;9:181–192.
24. Marx SJ, Spiegel AM, Levine MA, et al. Primary hyperparathyroidism in familial multiple endocrine neoplasia type I: long-term follow-up of serum calcium after parathyroidectomy . Am J Med 1982;307:416–426.
25. Levin KE, Clark OH. The reasons for failure in parathyroid operations. Arch Surg 1989;124:911–915.
26. Maselly MJ, Lawrence AM, Brooks M, et al. Hyperparathyroid crisis. Surgery (St. Louis) 1981;90:741–746.
27. MacLeod WAJ, Holloway C. Hyperparathyroid crisis: a collective review. Ann Surg 1967;166:1012.
28. Fitzpatrick LA, Bilezikian JP. Acute primary hyperparathyroidism: a review of 48 patients. Am J Med 1987;82:272–282.
29. Bilezikian JP. Management of acute hypercalcemia. N Engl J Med 1992;326:1196–1203.
30. Brasier AR, Nussbaum SR. Hungry bone syndrome: clinical and biochemical predictors of its occurrence after parathyroid surgery. Am J Med 1988;84:654–660.
31. Carty SE, Norton JA. Management of patients with persistent or recurrent primary hyperparathyroidism. World J Surg 1991;15: 716–723.
32. Shen W, Duren M, Morita E, et al. Reoperation for persistent or recurrent primary hyperparathyroidism. Arch Surg 1996;131: 861–869.
33. Patow CA, Norton JA, Brennan MF. Vocal cord paralysis and reoperative parathyroidectomy. Ann Surg 1986;203:282–285.
34. Doppman JL, Krudy AG, Marx SJ, et al. Aspiration of enlarged parathyroid glands for parathyroid hormone assay. Radiology 1983;148:31–35.
35. Bergenfelz A, Forsberg L, Hederström E, et al. Preoperative localization of enlarged parathryoid glands with ultrasonically guided fine needle aspiration for parathyroid hormone assay. Acta Radiol 1991;32:403–405.
36. Miller DL, Doppman JL, Shawker TH, et al. Localization of parathyroid adenomas in patients who have undergone surgery. Part I. Noninvasive imaging methods. Radiology 1987;162:133–137.
37. Miller DL. Preoperative localization and interventional treatment of parathyroid tumors: when and how? World J Surg 1991; 15:706–715.
38. Lange JR, Norton JA. Surgery for persistent or recurrent primary hyperparathyroidism. Curr Pract Surg 1992;4:56–62.
39. Krudy AG, Shawker TH, Doppman JL, et al. Ultrasonic parathy-

16. (continued) radioimmunoassay for human parathyrin (residues 53–84). Clin Chem 1982;28:1749–1753.

roid localization in previously operated patients. Clin Radiol 1984;35:113–118.

40. Reading CC, Charboneau JW, James EM, et al. Postoperative parathyroid high-frequency sonography: evaluation of persistent or recurrent hyperparathyroidism. AJR 1985;144:399–400.

41. Wei JP, Burke GJ, Mansberger AR. Preoperative imaging of abnormal parathyroid glands in patients with hyperparathyroid disease using combination Tc-99m-pertechnetate and Tc-99m-sestamibi radionuclide scans. Ann Surg 1994;219:5.

42. Jaskowiak N, Norton JA, Alexander HR, et al. A prospective trial evaluating a standard approach to reoperation for missed parathyroid adenoma. Ann Surg 1996;224:308–322.

43. Rodriquez JM, Tezelman S, Siperstein AE, et al. Localization procedures in patients with persistent or recurrent hyperparathyroidism. Arch Surg 1994;129.211–216.

44. Doppman JL, Brennan MF, Kohler JO, et al. CT scanning for parathyroid localization. J Comput Assist Tomogr 1977;1:30–36.

45. Sommer B, Welter HF, Spelsberg F, et al. Computed tomography for localiziing enlarged parathyroid glands in primary hyperparathyroidism. J Comput Assist Tomogr 1982;6:521–526.

46. Stark DD, Gooding JW, Moss AA, et al. Parathyroid scanning by computer tomography. Radiology 1983;148:297.

47. Stark DD, Gooding JW, Moss AA, et al. Parathyroid imaging: comparison of high resolution CT and high resolution sonography. AJR 1983;141:633–638.

48. Krubsack AJ, Wilson SD, Lawson TL, et al. Prospective comparison of radionuclide, computed tomographic, and sonographic localization of parathyroid tumors. World J Surg 1986;10:579–585.

49. Carmalt HL, Gillett DJ, Chu J, et al. Prospective comparison of radionuclide, ultrasound, and computed tomography in the preoperative localization of parathyroid glands. World J Surg 1988;12:830–834.

50. Doppman JL, Krudy AG, Brennan MR, et al. CT appearance of enlarged parathyroid glands in the posterior-superior mediastinum. J Comput Assist Tomogr 1982;6:1099–1102.

51. Wang C. Parathyroid re-exploration: a clinical and pathological study of 112 cases. Ann Surg 1977;186:140–145.

52. Auffermann W, Guis M, Tavares NJ, et al. MR signal intensity of parathyroid adenomas: correlation with histopathology. AJR 1989;153:873–876.

53. Higgins CB, Auffermann W. MR imaging of thyroid and parathyroid glands: a review of current status. AJR 1988;151:1095–1106.

54. Auffermann W, Gooding GAW, Okerlund MD, et al. Diagnosis of recurrent hyperparathyroidism: comparison of MR imaging and other imaging techniques. AJR 1988;150:1027–1033.

55. Krudy AG, Doppman HL, Miller DL, et al. Abnormal parathyroid glands: comparison of nonselective arterial digital arteriography, selective parathyroid arteriography and venous digital arteriography as methods of detection. Radiology 1983;148:23–29.

56. Patel PC, Pellitteri PK, Patel NM, Fleetwood MK. Use of rapid intraoperative parathyroid hormone assay in the surgical management of parathyroid disease. Arch Otolaryngol Head Neck Surg 1998;123:559–562.

57. Bergenfelz A, Isaksson A, Lindblom P, Westerdahl J, Tibblin S. Measurement of parathyroid hormone in patients with primary hyperparathyroidism undergoing first and reoperative surgery. 1998;85:1129–1132.

58. Consensus Development Conference Panel. Diagnosis and management of asymptomatic primary hyperparathyroidism: consensus development conference statement. Ann Intern Med 1991;114:593–597.

59. Norton JA. Controversies and advances in primary hyperparathyroidism. Ann Surg 1992;215:1–3.

60. Scholz DA, Purnell DC. Asymptomatic primary hyperparathyroidism: 10 year prospective study. Mayo Clin Proc 1981;56:473–478.

61. Tibblin S, Bondeson A-G, Bondeson L, et al. Surgical strategy in hyperparathyroidism due to solitary adenoma. Ann Surg 1984;200:776–784.

62. Piemonte M, Miani P, Bacchi G. Parathyroid surgery in primary hyperparathyroidism: an update. Arch Otorhinolaryngol 1989;246:324–327.

63. Poole GV Jr, Albertson DA, Myers RT. Causes of the failed cervical exploration for primary hyperparathyroidism. Am Surg 1988;54:553–557.

64. Rudberg C, Akerström G, Palmer M, et al. Late results of operation for primary hyperparathyroidism in 441 patients. Surgery (St. Louis) 1986;99:643–651.

65. Lavelle MA. Parathyroid adenoma stained with methylene blue. J R Soc Med 1980;73:462.

66. Cowie AGA. Morbidity in adult parathyroid surgery. J R Soc Med 1982;75:942–945.

67. Grant CS, van Heerden JA, Charboneau JW, et al. Clinical management of persistent and/or recurrent primary hyperparathyroidism. World J Surg 1986;10:555–565.

68. Brennan MF, Norton JA. Reoperation for persistent and recurrent hyperparathyroidism. Ann Surg 1985;201:40–44.

69. van Heerden JA, James EM, Caselle PR, et al. Small part ultrasonography in primary hyperparathyroidism. Ann Surg 1982;195:774–780.

70. Brennan MF, Marx SJ, Doppman J, et al. Results of reoperation for persistent and recurrent hyperparathyroidism. Ann Surg 1981;194:671.

71. Prinz RA, Gamvros OI, Allison DJ, et al. Reoperations for hyperparathyroidism. Surg Gynecol Obstet 1981;152:760–764.

72. Thompson NW, Eckhauser F, Harness J. Anatomy of primary hyperparathyroidism. Surgery (St. Louis) 1982;92:814.

73. Paloyan E, Lawrence AM, Oslapas R. Subtotal parathyroidectomy for primary hyperparathyroidism: long-term results in 292 patients. Arch Surg 1983;118:425.

74. Nathanials EK, Nathaniels AM, Wang C. Mediastinal parathyroid tumors: a clinical and pathological study of 84 cases. Ann Surg 1970;171:165.

75. Lamers CBHW, Froeling PGAM. Clinical significance of hyperparathyroidism in familial multiple endocrine adenomatosis type I (MEA I). Am J Med 1979;66:422.

76. Romanus ME, Farndon JR, Wells SA Jr. Transplantation of the parathyroid glands. In: Johnston IDA, Thompson NW, eds. Endocrine Surgery. Stoneham: Butterworth, 1983:25–40.

77. Wells SA Jr, Farndon JR, Dale JK, et al. Long-term evaluation of patients with primary parathyroid hyperplasia managed by total parathyroidectomy and heterotopic autotransplantation. Ann Surg 1980;192:451.

78. Worsey MJ, Carty SE, Watson CG. Success of unilateral neck exploration for sporadic PHPT. Surgery (St. Louis) 1993;114(6):1024–1030.

79. Andress DL, Ott SM, Maloney NA, et al. Effect of parathyroidectomy on bone aluminum accumulation in chronic renal failure. N Engl J Med 1985;312:468–473.

80. Clark OH. Secondary hyperparathyroidism. In: Clark OH, ed. Endocrine Surgery of the Thyroid and Parathyroid Glands. St. Louis: Mosby, 1985:241.

81. Johnson WJ, McCarthy JT, van Heerden JA, et al. Results of subtotal parathyroidectomy in hemodialysis patients. Am J Med 1988;84:23–32.

82. Wang C, Gaz RD, Moncure AC. Mediastinal parathyroid exploration: a clinical and pathologic study of 47 cases. World J Surg 1986;10:687–695.

83. Satava RM Jr, Beahrs OH, Scholz DA. Success rate of cervical exploration for hyperparathyroidsim. Arch Surg 1975;110:625–628.

84. Norton JA, Shawker TH, Jones BL, et al. Intraoperative ultrasound and reoperative parathyroid surgery: an initial evaluation. World J Surg 1986;10:631–639.

85. Kern KA, Shawker TH, Doppman JL, et al. The use of high-resolution ultrasound to locate parathyroid tumors during reop-

erations for primary hyperparathyroidism. World J Surg 1987;11: 579–585.

86. McFarland MP, Fraker DL, Shawker TH, et al. Use of preoperative fine-needle aspiration in patients undergoing reoperation for primary hyperparathyroidism. Surgery (St. Louis) 1994;116:959–964.

87. Norman J, Chheda H. Minimally invasive parathyroidectomy facilitated by intraoperative nuclear mapping. Surgery (St. Louis) 1997;122:998–1004.

88. Fraker DL, Doppman JL, Shawker TH, et al. Undescended parathyroid adenoma: an important etiology for failed operations for primary hyperparathyroidism. World J Surg 1990;14:342–348.

89. Wang C, Gaz RD. Natural history of parathyroid carcinoma: diagnosis, treatment, and results. Am J Surg 1985;149:522–527.

90. Schantz A, Castleman B. Parathyroid carcinoma? a study of 70 cases. Cancer (Phila) 1973;31:600.

91. van Heerden JA, Weiland LH, Re Mine WH, et al. Cancer of the parathyroid glands. Arch Surg 1979;114:475.

92. Haff RC, Ballinger WF. Causes of recurrent hypercalcemia after parathyroidectomy for primary hyperparathyroidism. Ann Surg 1971;173:884.

93. Flye MW, Brennan MF. Surgical resection of metastatic parathyroid carcinoma. Ann Surg 1981;193:425.

94. Mariette C, Pellissier L, Combemale F, Quievreuz JL, Carnaille B, Proye C. Reoperation for persistent or recurrent primary hyperparathyroidism. Langenbecks Arch Surg 1998;383(2):174–179.

95. Peeler BB, Martin WH, Sandler MP, Goldstein RE. Sestamibi parathyroid scanning and preoperative localization studies for patients with recurrent/hyperparathyroidism or significant comorbid conditions: development of an optimal localization. Am Surg 1997;63(1):37–46.

96. Doherty GM, Doppman JL, Miller DL, et al. Results of a multidisciplinary strategy for management madiastinal parathyroid adenoma as a cause of persistent hyperparathyroidism. Ann Surg 1992;215(2):101–106.

97. Weber CJ, Sewell CW, McGarity WC. Persistent and recurrent sporadic primary hyperparathyroidism: histopathology, complications, and results of operation. Surgery (St. Louis) 1994;116: 991–998.

98. Jarhult J, Nordenstrom J, Perbeck L. Reoperation for suspected primary hyperparathyroidism. Br J Surg 1993;80:453–456.

99. Rothmund M, Wagner PK, Seesko H, Zielke A. Lessons from reoperations in 55 patients with primary hyperparathyroidism. Dtsch Med Wochenschr 1990;115(42):1579–1585.

100. Cheung PSY, Borgstrom A, Thompson NW. Strategy in reoperative surgery for hyperparathyroidism. Arch Surg 1989;124:676–680.

Thyroid

Ronald J. Weigel

Anatomy and Physiology

The common indications for thyroidectomy include a suspicion of cancer, local symptoms of a large neck mass (e.g., difficulty breathing or swallowing), and abnormal thyroid function (e.g., hyperthyroidism). Surgical management of thyroid problems requires a thorough understanding of the anatomy and pathophysiology of the thyroid gland.

Surgical Approach

The normal thyroid weighs approximately 20 g and is situated anterior and slightly inferior to the thyroid cartilage. Figure 28.1 depicts the relevant anatomy and surgical approach to the thyroid. The thyroid is highly vascular and derives its blood supply from paired superior and inferior thyroid arteries. The superior thyroid artery is a branch of the external carotid artery, and the inferior thyroid artery is derived from the thyrocervical trunk. Thyroid ima vessels are branches directly from the aorta and enter the gland inferiorly. The recurrent laryngeal nerve ascends from the superior mediastinum and runs in the tracheoesophageal groove. The nerve courses directly posterior to the thyroid lobe and passes through the cricopharyngeus to innervate the intrinsic muscles of the larynx. The location of the parathyroid glands is variable but the glands are usually found lateral and posterior to the thyroid. The identification of these structures is critical during neck exploration.

Thyroid Function Tests and Thyroid Imaging

The thyroid synthesizes thyroid hormone, which is necessary for normal metabolism. The secretion of thyroid hormone is precisely regulated. The hypothalamus secretes thyrotropin-releasing hormone (TRH), which induces the anterior pituitary to secrete thyroid-stimulating hormone (TSH). TSH stimulates growth and function of the follicle cells of the thyroid. In response to TSH, the thyroid concentrates iodine and synthesizes the thyroid hormones thyroxine (T4) and the more metabolically active form of thyroxine, T3. Free thyroxine is the active form of the hormone and exerts a negative feedback on the pituitary and probably the hypothalamus. The plasma concentrations of these hormones provides the clinician with a reliable means of assessing thyroid physiological function. The half-lives of T4 and T3 are approximately 7 and 3 days, respectively. For this reason, thyroid tests are commonly examined 4 to 6 weeks after altering dosages of thyroid medications.

The commonly employed thyroid function tests are listed in Table 28.1. TSH is the single best test for diagnosis of hyper- and hypothyroidism. In hyperthyroid states, TSH is suppressed. In mild cases of hyperthyroidism, the TSH may be suppressed although thyroid hormone levels remain in the normal range. However, in most cases all three parameters of thyroxine measurement [free T4 (FT4), total T4, and total T3] are increased simultaneously. Additionally, there are cases of hyperthyroidism in which only T3 is measurably increased (T3 thyrotoxicosis). In hypothyroid states, TSH is elevated and the thyroxine parameters are below normal. In instances of mild hypothyroidism, TSH is elevated with normal thyroxine parameters. Under certain physiological conditions, such as pregnancy, patients on thyroid hormone replacement require increased thyroid hormone dosage, as can be evidenced by a measured increase in TSH.

Thyroid scan using ^{123}I is a useful test to help diagnose diseases of the thyroid involving abnormal thyroid function. The thyroid scan has limited usefulness in the setting of a suspicion of thyroid malignancy. The common findings of thyroid scans include cold nodules, hot nodules (solitary or multiple), and Graves' disease.

Hyperthyroidism

Hyperthyroidism is caused by thyroid hormone excess. The usual pathological states causing hyperthyroidism are toxic nodule, toxic multinodular goiter, Graves' disease, and the

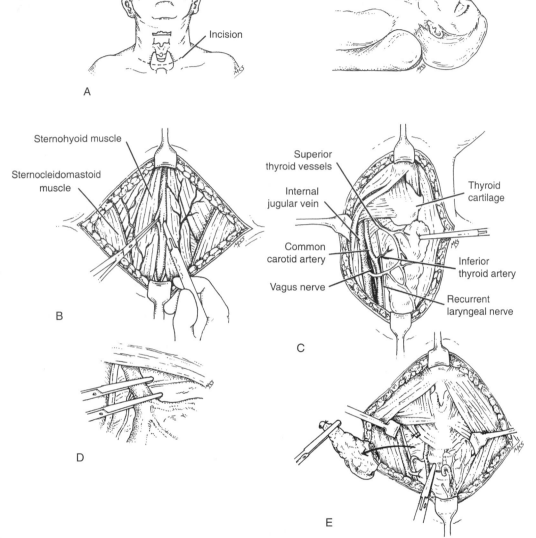

A

Sternohyoid muscle

Sternocleidomastoid muscle

B

Superior thyroid vessels

Internal jugular vein

Common carotid artery

Vagus nerve

Thyroid cartilage

Inferior thyroid artery

Recurrent laryngeal nerve

C

D

E

FIGURE 28.1. Thyroidectomy. **A.** The patient is placed with the neck in extension. The thyroid is approached through a Kocher collar incision, which is commonly made approximately 2.0 cm superior to the sternal notch. **B.** The strap muscles are divided in the midline to expose the thyroid gland. **C.** The strap muscles are retracted laterally and the thyroid is retracted medially, exposing the structures of the mid-neck. The recurrent laryngeal nerve can be seen lying within the tracheoesophageal groove. **D.** The superior pole vessels are individually clamped and ligated as they enter the thyroid gland. Inferior thyroid vessels, as well as the vessels of the thyroid (ima), are individually suture-ligated. **E.** The dissection is completed by dissection of the thyroid gland off the trachea. The isthmus is then transected and can be oversewn with a suture for hemostasis. (Redrawn, with permission, from Macdonald J. Haller D. Weigel R: Endocrine System. Abeloff MD (ed): Clinical Oncology. Churchill Livingstone, 1995, p. 1051.)

early stage of subacute thyroiditis. Iatrogenic thyrotoxicosis can be caused by inappropriate dosage of thyroid hormone replacement. Symptoms associated with hyperthyroidism include heat intolerance, sweating, weight loss, tremulousness, palpitations, restlessness, emotional instability, and insom-

nia. Atrial fibrillation is a common finding in older patients. A severe form of hyperthyroidism called thyroid storm can be precipitated by surgery, sepsis, or trauma in patients with untreated or incompletely treated Graves' disease.[1,2] Storm can have mortality rates of 20% to 30% and is characterized by fever, hypotension, congestive heart failure (CHF), and circulatory collapse. Treatment involves initial resuscitation with i.v. fluids and cooling blankets. Potassium iodine is given to suppress thyroid synthesis, and steroids are given to treat associated adrenal insufficiency. Administration of β-blockade, usually propranolol, is helpful in managing the cardiac manifestations. Propylthiouracil (PTU) is used to suppress thyroid hormone synthesis and also blocks the peripheral conversion of T4 to the more active metabolite T3.

Graves' Disease

Graves' disease is characterized by hyperthyroidism, goiter, and exophthalmos. These features may occur singly or in any

TABLE 28.1. Laboratory Evaluation of the Thyroid Patient.

Test	Normal values
Free T$_4$	0.73–2.01 ng/dl
TSH	0.4–4.0 μIU/ml
T$_3$, total	100–190 ng/dl
T$_4$, total	6.2–11.8 μg/dl
Thyroglobulin	With thyroid gland: <20 ng/ml
	Athyreotic on T$_4$: <2 ng/ml
	Athyreotic off T$_4$: <5 ng/ml
Antithyroid microsomal	Negative: <0.3 U/ml
24 hr ^{131}I uptake	5%–30%

TSH, thyroid-stimulating hormone.

combination; approximately one-third of patients have manifestations of thyrotoxicosis and eye findings with initial presentation. The pathophysiology of Graves' disease is attributable to thyroid autoantibodies that recognize and stimulate the TSH receptor.[3] These antibodies stimulate growth of the thyroid and increase synthesis of hormone.

The thyroid in Graves' disease is diffusely enlarged although the enlargement can be asymmetrical. Distinct nodules are unusual and should raise the suspicion of malignancy. Thyroid carcinoma has been reported to occur in 5% to 7% of patients undergoing surgery for Graves' disease.[4,5] Thyroid function tests should be used to confirm the diagnosis of hyperthyroidism. Normally patients present with a suppressed TSH and elevated FT4. Thyroid uptake is increased, with 50% to 90% of administered iodine dose localized to the thyroid. The thyroid scan in patients with Graves' disease demonstrates diffuse uptake, lacking nodularity. The presence of a cold nodule noted on radioiodine scan should raise the suspicion of malignancy and is an indication for thyroidectomy.[6]

The initial treatment of Graves' disease is aimed at establishing a euthyroid state. In the United States, the two commonly used antithyroid medications are PTU and methimazole (Tapazole). These drugs inhibit thyroid hormone synthesis by interfering with organification of iodine in the thyroid. Additionally, PTU inhibits peripheral conversion of T4 to T3. Following medical treatment, most patients achieve a euthyroid state in approximately 6 weeks. For patients with cardiac manifestations associated with thyrotoxicosis, a β-blocker such as propranolol may be added until a euthyroid state is achieved.

Although some clinicians treat patients with long-term medical therapy, definitive treatment of Graves' disease is accomplished with either radioactive iodine (RAI) or surgery. In the United States, RAI treatment has become the preferred treatment option.[7] The thyroid gland in Graves' disease is extremely sensitive to RAI. Using this approach, thyrotoxicosis can be cured in 80% to 90% of patients. In some instances, retreatment or surgery is required. Contraindications to the use of RAI include pregnancy and a suspicion of thyroid malignancy.

Thyroidectomy is an alternative treatment option for Graves' disease. There are two basic approaches to surgical treatment. Some surgeons perform a lobectomy on one side and a subtotal thyroidectomy on the contralateral lobe leaving approximately 4 g of tissue. The intent of this approach is to render the patients euthyroid without the need for medication. An alternative approach is to perform a total or near-total thyroidectomy and treat patients with thyroxine replacement postoperatively. There is a reported incidence of recurrent hyperthyroidism of 4% to 15% in patients treated by subtotal thyroidectomy.[8,9] Total thyroidectomy has a lower recurrence rate and has been shown to result in lower antithyroid antibodies compared to subtotal thyroidectomy.[8]

Toxic Multinodular Goiter

The thyroid in patients with toxic multinodular goiter (MNG) usually contains several palpable nodules. Local symptoms of difficulty in breathing or swallowing are more common than in Graves' disease. Thyroid function tests indicate hyperthyroidism with a suppressed TSH although a normal FT4 and T3 is a common finding. Thyroid scan demonstrates several nodules that usually have varying degrees of uptake. Cold areas noted on scan are also commonly seen. For patients with overt thyrotoxicosis, medical treatment with antithyroid medications is the initial treatment.

Definitive treatment for toxic MNG can be accomplished with RAI or surgery. Compared to RAI, thyroidectomy has been shown to render patients euthyroid sooner.[10] Total thyroidectomy is the preferred surgical procedure for toxic MNG because it is more likely to cure hyperthyroidism compared to subtotal thyroidectomy or thyroid lobectomy.[10]

Toxic Nodule

A solitary hot nodule is usually caused by a follicular adenoma, although in children hot nodules may be malignant. Nodules larger than 3 cm often cause overt thyrotoxicosis. Thyroid scan demonstrates a hot nodule with partial or complete suppression of the remaining thyroid. After the patient is rendered euthyroid, definitive treatment can be accomplished with RAI or surgery (most often lobectomy). The rates of persistent hyperthyroidism and posttreatment hypothyroidism after RAI are both approximately 10%.[11]

Hypothyroidism

Hypothyroidism is the result of a deficiency of thyroid hormone and is characterized by cold intolerance, weight gain, constipation, dry skin, brittle hair, hoarse voice, difficulty concentrating, and fatigue. Hypothyroidism is usually the result of thyroiditis or the result of surgery or RAI ablation. Thyroid function tests demonstrate an increased TSH and a low FT4 and T3. Hypothyroidism is treated with thyroxine replacement starting with a low dose and increasing the dose to achieve a euthyroid state.

Hashimoto's Thyroiditis

Hashimoto's thyroiditis, also known as chronic lymphocytic thyroiditis, is the most common form of thyroiditis. The disease occurs almost exclusively in women, usually in middle age. Nodules may be present, and some patients develop local symptoms of compression. Usually, however, patients have no local symptoms and lack thyroid tenderness that is characteristic of subacute thyroiditis. Antithyroid antibodies can be detected in the serum of patients with Hashimoto's thyroiditis. Antimicrosomal and antithyroglobulin antibodies are usually measured. Treatment involves supplementation with thyroxine. Surgery is rarely indicated and is reserved for patients with local compression or in cases in which malignancy is suspected.

Subacute Thyroiditis

Subacute thyroiditis is characterized by a tender swelling of the thyroid that usually lasts for 2 to 4 months. The initial presentation may be associated with hyperthyroidism. Treatment during this stage of the disease relies on nonsteroidal antiinflammatory drugs to treat local symptoms. Steroids have been used but may be associated with a protracted course. Several months following initial presentation, patients may develop hypothyroidism. The disease is characterized by recurrence but is usually self-limited. Surgery is rarely indicated, and patients are treated with thyroid replacement.

Goiter

Goiter is a term commonly used to refer to a benign enlargement of the thyroid gland. Goiters can be diffuse or multinodular. Iodine deficiency has been shown to cause goiters. These patients also demonstrate an elevated TSH that is likely to be the etiology of thyroid enlargement in this condition. In most cases, thyroid function is normal and there is little to be gained from treatment with thyroxine.

Goiters often cause symptoms from local compression. These large glands concentrate iodine poorly as compared to their size. Therefore, RAI is not effective in treating goiters that occur in the euthyroid setting. Surgical resection is indicated in most cases because of local compression. Postoperatively, patients should be treated with thyroid hormone replacement.

Evaluation of the Thyroid Nodule

Figure 28.2 outlines one approach to the evaluation of thyroid nodules. Determining the clinical setting is the first step of evaluation. The treatment of asymptomatic nodules is largely dependent upon the results of FNA.[12,13] The use of ra-

dioiodine scan has limited value in the evaluation of thyroid nodules.[12-14] Nodules that are symptomatic, causing difficulty swallowing or breathing, usually require surgery. The occurrences of large nodules (usually >5 cm), recurrent cysts, or nodules with a clear history of growth are also indications for surgical treatment. However, FNA can help guide the choice of surgical procedure. The finding of lymphoma or anaplastic cancer in this setting also significantly alters the treatment plan.

Fine-Needle Aspiration

Most thyroid nodules are benign, and the use of FNA has reduced the number of patients requiring surgical excision. Results from FNA can be characterized into one of four categories.[12,13]

PAPILLARY CANCER OR SUSPICIOUS FOR PAPILLARY CANCER

A number of cytological criteria are present in papillary thyroid cancer (PTC). When the majority of these features are present, the diagnosis of papillary cancer is made and is confirmed in 98% of cases on permanent sections.[15]

INDETERMINATE

The finding of indeterminate FNA refers to follicular neoplasms that are either follicular adenoma (FA), follicular thyroid carcinoma (FTC), or Hürthle cell neoplasms. Approximately 20% of indeterminate FNAs are found to be malignant on permanent section.[16]

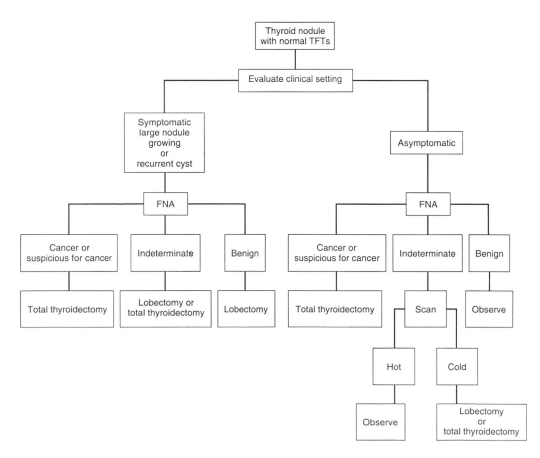

FIGURE 28.2. Flow diagram for evaluation of thyroid nodule in patients with normal thyroid function tests (TFTs).

BENIGN

The chance that a thyroid cancer will yield a benign result on FNA is approximately 4%.[15,16]

INADEQUATE

The category designated inadequate indicates a poor aspirate and should be repeated.

Frozen Section Evaluation of Thyroid Nodules

There is some debate as to the role of frozen section evaluation at the time of surgery to aid in determining the extent of operation. At this time, it cannot unequivocally be recommended for use in determining extent of resection.

Thyroid Cancer

There are approximately 17,000 new cases of thyroid cancer annually in the United States.[17] However, the annual mortality from thyroid malignancies is only 1,200, indicating that most patients with thyroid cancer have an excellent prognosis. The male to female ratio of thyroid cancer incidence is 1:2.7, but the ratio of cancer-associated mortality is 1:2, indicating that the tumors may be slightly more aggressive in men. Table 28.2 summarizes the common histological types of thyroid malignancies. The majority of thyroid cancers are well-differentiated tumors that are derived from thyroid follicular epithelium. Anaplastic cancer is also derived from follicular epithelial cells and may represent a more malignant transformation of well-differentiated tumors. Medullary thyroid cancer (MTC) is derived from the calcitonin-secreting C-cells or parafollicular cells of the thyroid. Thyroid lymphomas and metastases to the thyroid account for 5% to 6% of thyroid malignancies.

Radiation-Associated Thyroid Cancer

Ionizing radiation exposure increases the incidence of benign and malignant thyroid nodules. Most of the radiation-induced thyroid malignancies are PTC.

Molecular Genetics of Thyroid Cancer

One of the earliest observations indicating a genetic basis for thyroid cancer was the recognition of the association between familial adenomatous polyposis (FAP) and the development of

TABLE 28.2. Types of Thyroid Cancers.

Tumor histology	Incidence (%)
Well-differentiated	85
Papillary (80%–90%)	
(papillary and follicular variant)	
Follicular (10%–20%)	
(micro- and macroinvasion, Hürthle)	
Medullary	6–8
Anaplastic	2–4
Lymphoma	4–5
Metastatic	<1

PTC.[18] Inheritance of a mutation of the adenomatous polyposis coli (APC) gene results in predisposition to FAP. The increased incidence of PTC in FAP patients implies a role for APC mutations in thyroid oncogenesis.

There is a familial form of PTC that occurs independent of FAP. As with other familial cancers, these tumors demonstrate vertical transmission in consecutive generations.[19] Although the cancers do not appear to occur at an earlier age, they are more often multifocal and bilateral. The gene responsible for familial PTC has not been identified.

The *ret* proto-oncogene is a receptor tyrosine kinase that has been identified as the gene responsible for inheritance of MEN2A, MEN2B, and familial MTC.[20–22] Ret mutations have also been examined in PTC.[23] Three chromosomal rearrangements have been reported between *ret* and one of three loci designated PTC1, PTC2, and PTC3.[24–27] These rearrangements result in overexpression of ret chimeric proteins.

N-*ras* activation has been examined in thyroid cancer.[28,29] and was also shown to be an independent prognostic factor for increased mortality. Other data, however, have suggested a role for *ras* activation in early thyroid tumorigenesis.[30]

Clinical studies have demonstrated that p53 overexpression is an independent prognostic factor for survival of patients with thyroid cancer.[31] These studies support the hypothesis that p53 mutation in thyroid cancer plays a role in progression to a more aggressive phenotype.

Well-Differentiated Thyroid Cancer

Papillary thyroid cancer (PTC) accounts for 80% to 90% of well-differentiated thyroid cancers. Within the last decade, it has become recognized that there is a follicular variant of papillary cancer that lacks the normal papillary architecture. The follicular variant is recognized by cytological features shared with other PTC, and the clinical course of this tumor is consistent with the papillary phenotype.[32] Occult papillary carcinoma (OPC) of the thyroid has been reported in a significant percentage of the population. OPC has histological features that are indistinguishable from clinically evident PTC; however, OPC is less than 10 mm and is generally considered to be a benign entity because it is found incidentally in thyroid specimens or at autopsy in approximately 20% of the general population.[33]

EXTENT OF SURGERY

There has been long-standing controversy concerning the appropriate extent of surgical resection for well-differentiated thyroid cancer.[34,35] Studies examining the outcome of thyroidectomy for patients with thyroid cancer are all retrospective.

PROPONENTS OF LESS THAN TOTAL THYROIDECTOMY

The basis for this position is that there is insignificant improvement of recurrence or mortality to justify the potential risk of recurrent laryngeal nerve injury or permanent hypoparathyroidism for performing more than a lobectomy in most cases. The reported incidence of recurrent nerve injury (0%–7%) and permanent hypoparathyroidism (0%–8%) varies with the extent of operation, the history of previous neck surgery, and the experience and training of the surgeon.[34,36–40] The majority of studies advocating lobectomy have focused on the low-risk group [based upon AMES (age, metastasis, extent, size) criteria].[41] For low-risk patients, lobectomy appears to be adequate.[42–45]

PROPONENTS OF TOTAL THYROIDECTOMY

A number of considerations argue in favor of treating thyroid cancer patients with a total thyroidectomy. First, patients with thyroid cancer are usually treated with thyroid hormone replacement to suppress TSH so there is no functional reason to preserve a thyroid lobe. Second, thyroid cancer is multifocal in 10% to 30% of cases, and resecting the contralateral lobe removes foci of cancer that might otherwise metastasize. Third, total thyroidectomy facilitates treatment with radioactive iodine (RAI) because it removes normal thyroid tissue that would take up iodine and also allows treatment under a hypothyroid protocol. Fourth, patients treated with total thyroidectomy and RAI often have undetectable or very low thyroglobulin (Tg) levels, thus facilitating the use of this test as a screen for recurrence. Fifth, there is evidence that total thyroidectomy results in fewer recurrences and less mortality compared to lesser procedures. Given the low complication rate for thyroidectomy among most endocrine surgeons, total thyroidectomy seems to be evolving into the treatment of choice for well-differentiated thyroid cancer.[46]

RADIOACTIVE IODINE

RAI has been successfully used for many years to ablate normal thyroid remnants and residual carcinoma following surgical resection. The usual protocol after thyroidectomy withholds thyroid hormone replacement for 4 to 6 weeks to induce a hypothyroid state. The elevation in TSH stimulates iodine uptake in residual thyroid tissue and thyroid carcinoma. In the face of elevated TSH, an increase in Tg levels is also usually evident.

The rates of complications from RAI treatment, which include radiation thyroiditis, chronic sialoadenitis, odynophagia, and facial edema, are low. Complication rates and the need for repeated treatments are higher with less extensive surgery.[47,48] RAI does not appear to have adverse effects on female fertility[49] but at least one study indicated an association with transient impairment of testicular function.[50]

PROGNOSIS OF WELL-DIFFERENTIATED THYROID CANCER

A number of variables that have been shown to influence prognosis for well-differentiated thyroid cancer are listed in Table 28.3. Fixed characteristics are based on clinical parameters that are present at the time of diagnosis. Variable characteristics can be influenced by treatment and may give clinicians an opportunity to improve outcome in patients.

TABLE 28.3. Prognosis.

Fixed factors affecting prognosis	Variable factors affecting prognosis
Age of patient	Extent of thyroidectomy
Clinical stage of primary	Use of RAI
Size	Time from diagnosis to treatment
Extension	
Lymph node metastasis	
Distant metastasis	
Histology	
Gender	

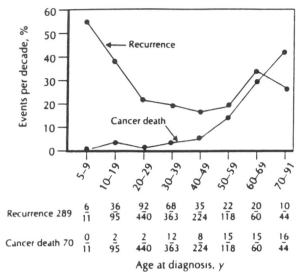

FIGURE 28.3. Recurrence rate and cancer death for well-differentiated thyroid cancer as a function of patient's age at diagnosis. (From Mazzaferri and Jhiang,[51] with permission.)

AGE

Some series have demonstrated that age is the single most significant variable affecting mortality.[41,45] Interestingly, recurrence has a bimodal distribution with age (Fig. 28.3). Although recurrence rates are higher in younger patients, mortality remains relatively low.[51,52] By contrast, recurrence in patients over the age of 45 is a poor prognostic indicator, and overall mortality rates increase linearly with age of patients at presentation.

SIZE

There is a nearly linear increase in mortality with the diameter of the primary tumor at presentation.[51] Tumors less than 1 to 1.5 cm have negligible cancer-related mortality and a 30-year recurrence rate of 11%.[51] Tumors more than 3 to 4 cm in diameter have a 30-year disease-specific mortality of 20% to 30%.[51,53]

EXTENT OF TUMOR INVASION

Extrathyroidal tumor invasion carries a worse prognosis than tumors that are intrathyroidal or have minor capsular invasion. Tumors that invade adjacent structures such as strap muscles or trachea are associated with high recurrence and mortality.[41,51,53,54] As may be expected, inability to completely resect tumor is associated with a worse outcome,[53,55] and completely resecting disease can improve outcome even in the presence of local invasion.[55]

METASTASIS

Patients over age 45 with distant metastatic disease at presentation have 15-year and 30-year mortality rates of 50% to 65% and 65% to 70%, respectively.[51,53] Papillary cancer frequently metastasizes to lung, and this is exclusively the site of metastasis in children. Bone metastasis is also common in older patients and in patients with follicular cancer. Other less common sites of metastasis include brain and liver.[56]

Lymph node metastasis is common in well-differentiated thyroid cancer. However, lymph node involvement has a modest effect on prognosis. In patients with T1–T3 primary tumors, the 30-year mortality rates for patients with nodal involvement is 4% to 6% compared to 0% to 1% without nodal metastasis.[51,57] Nodal metastasis has been found to influence prognosis except in cases of T4 tumors (extrathyroidal invasion), supporting the role of lymphadenectomy as part of the initial surgical treatment.[57]

HISTOLOGY

Many studies have demonstrated prognostic differences between papillary and follicular cancers,[58–60] but results are inconsistent.

GENDER

Women with well-differentiated thyroid cancer tend to demonstrate an improved prognosis compared to men.[51,61]

TREATMENT VARIABLES

A number of retrospective studies have reported that treatment modalities can influence the prognosis of thyroid cancer. As noted earlier, extent of surgery and use of RAI have been reported to improve recurrence and mortality from thyroid cancer. Time from first recorded tumor manifestation to initial treatment has been reported to have a significant effect on outcome. In a study of 1,355 patients, those who died of cancer had a mean delay of 18 months compared to 4 months for those who survived ($p < 0.001$).[51]

TUMOR STAGING

Based upon the variables determined to affect prognosis, several staging systems have been devised for thyroid cancer. The AMES (Age, Metastasis, Extent, Size)[41] and AGES (Age, Grade, Extent, Size)[62] systems use similar categories and have been shown to be predictive of high- and low-risk patients. Clinical class has been applied with good success and is based on tumor spread: class I, intrathyroidal disease; class II, lymph node metastases; class III, extrathyroidal invasion; class IV, distant metastases.[53] The TNM system[63] has been developed

TABLE 28.4. TNM Classification of Malignant Tumors of the Thyroid Gland.

Primary tumor (T stage)
  Tx Tumor cannot be assessed
  T0 No clinical evidence of tumor
  T1 Tumor ≤1 cm
  T2 Tumor >1 cm and <4 cm
  T3 Tumor ≥4 cm
  T4 Tumor extending beyond thyroid capsule

Regional lymph nodes (N stage)
  N0 No palpable nodes
  N1 Regional nodal metastases
      N1a Ipsilateral nodes
      N1b Contralateral, bilateral, or mediastinal nodes
Distant metastases (M stage)
  Mx Metastases cannot be assessed
  M0 No evidence of distant metastases
  M1 Distant metastases present

TABLE 28.5. Clinical Staging of Thyroid Cancer.

Medullary

Stage I	T1	N0	M0
Stage II	T2	N0	M0
Stage III	Any$_T$	N1	M0
Stage IV	Any$_T$	Any$_N$	M1

Undifferentiated: all cases stage IV
Papillary or follicular

	Cases <45 yr of age			Cases >45 yr of age		
Stage I	Any$_T$	Any$_N$	M0	T1	N0	M0
Stage II	Any$_T$	Any$_N$	M1	T2	N0	M0
Stage III				T3,T4	N0	M0
Stage IV				Any$_T$	Any$_N$	M1

and can be used to assess tumor stage as shown in Tables 28.4 and 28.5. The approximate 30-year mortality rates for stages I, II, III, and IV are 0% to 1%, 6%, 10% to 15%, and 65% to 80%, respectively.[51,53,64]

FOLLOW-UP FOR PATIENTS WITH THYROID CANCER

After initial treatment for thyroid cancer, patients are followed for tumor recurrence at 6-month intervals for the first 3 years and yearly thereafter.[13] The plan for following patients is influenced by the suspicion of possible recurrence based on prognostic factors. Patients are usually treated with suppressive doses of thyroxine. The goal of thyroid suppression is to have TSH levels at the lower limit of normal or slightly below normal without signs or symptoms of hyperthyroidism. Thyroglobulin (Tg) levels are a useful means to detect tumor recurrence.[13,65,66] In the setting of a rising Tg level, patients should have thyroid replacement withheld and a thyroid scan performed. As a general guideline, recurrences detected by scan alone can be treated with RAI. Recurrences that can be detected clinically by either physical exam or imaging (ultrasound, CT, or MRI) should undergo surgical resection followed by RAI.[67] It is important to obtain cytological confirmation of thyroid cancer before subjecting a patient to exploration. Ultrasound-guided biopsy is a particularly useful technique to confirm the presence of local recurrence.[68] Recent imaging modalities with real-time MRI using a split magnet have also been successful for biopsy of potential recurrence not accessible with ultrasound.

Medullary Thyroid Cancer

Medullary thyroid cancer (MTC) is derived from the calcitonin-secreting C-cells or parafollicular cells of the thyroid. Because MTC can occur in association with familial cancer syndromes (MEN2A, MEN2B, and familial MTC), family members should be screened for the presence of *ret* mutations.[69] Surgical treatment at a young age, before the development of carcinoma, can be performed safely and will likely cure patients of an otherwise incurable disease.[70] Patients with MTC should also be screened for pheochromocytoma because this tumor occurs in approximately 40% of MEN2 patients.[71]

Primary surgical treatment for MTC is a total thyroidectomy and central node dissection.[69,72] Patients with pheochromocytoma should undergo adrenalectomy first, although combination procedures have been described with excellent results. The cancer-specific mortality for MTC at 5 and 10 years is approximately 30% and 40%, respectively. Calcitonin and carcinoembryonic antigen (CEA) levels may be followed for evidence of recurrence.[73,74]

Anaplastic Thyroid Cancer

Patients with anaplastic thyroid cancer (ATC) usually present with a rapidly enlarging neck mass, often associated with dysphagia or airway obstruction. ATC has the worst prognosis of all thyroid malignancies, with 5-year survival rates of approximately 10%.[75] The goal of surgical treatment is to maintain a patent airway and, if possible, clear the neck of disease. Surgery has a limited role in the primary treatment. Once the diagnosis is established, patients should be treated with hyperfractionated radiotherapy and doxorubicin-based chemotherapy.[76]

References

1. Tietgens ST, Leinung MC. Thyroid storm. Med Clin North Am 1995;79:169–184.
2. Yoshida D. Thyroid storm precipitated by trauma. J Emerg Med 1996;14:697–701.
3. Brown RS. Editorial: Immunoglobulins affecting thyroid growth: a continuing controversy. J Clin Endocrinol Metab 1996;80:1506–1508.
4. Razack MS, Lore JM, Lippes HA, Schaefer DP, Rassael H. Total thyroidectomy for Graves' disease. Head Neck 1997;19:378–383.
5. Linos DA, Karakitsos D, Pappademetriou J. Should the primary treatment of hyperthyroidism be surgical? Eur J Surg 1997;163:651–657.
6. Joseph UA, Jhingran SG. Graves' disease and concurrent thyroid carcinoma: the importance of thyroid scintigraphy in Graves' disease. Clin Nucl Med 1995;20:416–418.
7. Levy EG. Treatment of Graves' disease: the American way. Bailliere's Clin Endocrinol Metab 1997;11:585–595.
8. Miccoli P, Vitti P, Rago T, et al. Surgical treatment of Graves' disease: subtotal or total thyroidectomy? Surgery (St. Louis) 1996;11:1020–1025.
9. Sugino K, Mimura T, Ozaki O, et al. Management of recurrent hyperthyroidism in patients with Graves' disease treated by subtotal thyroidectomy. J Endocrinol Invest 1995;18:415–419.
10. Erickson D, Gharib H, Li H, vanHeerden JA. Treatment of patients with toxic multinodular goiter. Thyroid 1998;8:277–282.
11. Siegel RD, Lee SL. Toxic nodular goiter. Endocrinol Metab Clin North Am 1998;27:151–168.
12. Mazzaferri EL. Management of a solitary thyroid nodule. N Engl J Med 1993;328:553–559.
13. Singer PA, Cooper DS, Daniels GH, et al. Treatment guidelines for patients with thyroid nodules and well-differentiated thyroid cancer. Arch Intern Med 1996;156:2165–2172.
14. Sabel MS, Staren ED, Gianakakis LM, Dwarakanathan S, Prinz RA. Effectiveness of the thyroid scan in evaluation of the solitary thyroid nodule. Am Surg 1997;63:660–664.
15. Agrawal S. Diagnostic accuracy and role of fine needle aspiration cytology in management of thyroid nodules. J Surg Oncol 1995;58:168–172.
16. Woeber KA. Cost-effective evaluation of the patient with a thyroid nodule. Endocr Surg 1995;75:357–363.
17. Landis SH, Murray T, Bolden S, Wingo PA. Cancer statistics, 1998. CA—Cancer J Clin 1998;48:6–30.
18. Smith WG, Kern BB. The nature of the mutation in familial multiple polyposis: papillary carcinoma of the thyroid, brain tumors, and familial multiple polyposis. Dis Colon Rectum 1973;16:264–271.
19. Grossman RF, Tu S-H, Duh Q-Y, Siperstein AE, Novosolov F, Clark OH. Familial nonmedullary thyroid cancer. Arch Surg 1995;130:892–897.
20. Mulligan LM, Kwok JBJ, Healey CS, et al. Germ-line mutations of the *RET* proto-oncogene in multiple endocrine neoplasia type 2A. Nature (Lond) 1993;363:458–460.
21. Donis-Keller H, Dou S, Chi D, et al. Mutations in the RET proto-oncogene are associated with MEN 2A and FMTC. Hum Mol Genet 1993;2:851–856.
22. Eng C, Smith DP, Mulligan LM, et al. Point mutation within the tyrosine kinase domain of the *RET* proto-oncogene in multiple endocrine neoplasia type 2B and related sporadic tumours. Hum Mol Genet 1994;3:237–241.
23. Santoro M, Carlomagno F, Hay ID, et al. Ret oncogene activation in human thyroid neoplasms is restricted to the papillary cancer subtype. J Clin Invest 1992;89:1517–1522.
24. Pierotti MA, Santoro M, Jenkins RB, et al. Characterization of an inversion on the long arm of chromosome 10 juxtaposing *D10S170* and *RET* and creating the oncogenic sequence *RET/PET*. Med Sci 1992;89:1616–1620.
25. Tong Q, Li Y, Smanik PA, Fithian LJ, Xing S, Mazzaferri EL, Jhiang SM. Characterization of the promoter region and oligomerization domain of H4 (D10S170), a gene frequently rearranged with the *ret* proto-oncogene. Oncogene 1995;10:1781–1787.
26. Sozzi G, Bongarzone I, Miozzo M, et al. A t(10;17) translocation creates the *RET/PTC2* chimeric transforming sequence in papillary thyroid carcinoma. Genes Chromosomes Cancer 1994;9:244–250.
27. Bongarzone I, Butti MG, Coronelli S, et al. Frequent activation of *ret* protooncogene by fusion with a new activating gene in papillary thyroid carcinomas. Cancer Res 1994;54:2979–2985.
28. Farid NR, Shi Y, Zou M. Molecular basis of thyroid cancer. Endocr Rev 1994;15:202–232.
29. Hara H, Fulton N, Yashiro T, Ito K, DeGroot LJ, Kaplan EL. N-Ras mutation: an independent prognostic factor for aggressiveness of papillary thyroid carcinoma. Surgery (St. Louis) 1994;116:1010–1016.
30. Namba H, Rubin SA, Fagin JA. Point mutations of *ras* oncogenes are an early event in thyroid tumorigenesis. Mol Endocrinol 1990;4:1474–1479.
31. Nishida T, Nakao K, Hamaji M, Nakahara M-A, Tsujimoto M. Overexpression of p53 protein and DNA content are important biologic prognostic factors for thyroid cancer. Surgery (St. Louis) 1996;119:568–575.
32. Grebe SKG, Hay ID. Follicular thyroid cancer. Endocrinol Metab Clin North Am 1995;24:761–801.
33. Martinez-Tello FJ, Martinez-Cabruja R, Fernandez-Martin J, Lasso-Oria C, Ballestin-Carcavilla C. Occult carcinoma of the thyroid. Cancer (Phila) 1993;71:4022–4029.
34. Patwardhan N, Cataldo T, Braverman LE. Surgical management of the patient with papillary cancer. Surg Clin North Am 1995;75:449–464.
35. Soh EY, Clark OH. Surgical considerations and approach to thyroid cancer. Endocrinol Metab Clin North Am 1996;25:115–139.
36. Stephenson BM, Wheeler MH, Clark OH. The role of total thyroidectomy in the management of differentiated thyroid cancer. Curr Opin Gen Surg 1994;53–59.
37. Harness JK, Thompson NW, McLeod MK, Pasieka JL, Fukuuchi A. Differentiated thyroid carcinoma in children and adolescents. World J Surg 1992;16:547–554.
38. Hoelting T, Buhr HJ, Herfarth C. Intraoperative tumour classification in papillary thyroid cancer—a diagnostic dilemma. Eur J Surg Oncol 1995;21:353–356.
39. Liu Q, Djuricin G, Prinz RA. Total thyroidectomy for benign thyroid disease. Surgery (St Louis) 1998;123:2–7.
40. Burge MR, Zeise T-M, Johnsen MW, Conway MJ, Qualls CR. Risks of complication following thyroidectomy. J Gen Intern Med 1998;13:24–31.
41. Cady B, Rossi R. An expanded view of risk-group definition in

differentiated thyroid carcinoma. Surgery (St. Louis) 1988;104: 947–953.

42. Nguyen KV, Dilawari RA. Predictive value of AMES scoring system in selection of extent of surgery in well differentiated carcinoma of thyroid. Am Surg 1995;61:151–155.

43. Shaha AR, Shah JP, Loree TR. Low-risk differentiated thyroid cancer: the need for selective treatment. Ann Surg Oncol 1997; 4:328–333.

44. Sanders LE, Cady B. Differentiated thyroid cancer: reexamination of risk groups and outcome of treatment. Arch Surg 1988; 133:419–425.

45. Wanebo H, Coburn M, Teates D, Cole B. Total thyroidectomy does not enhance disease control or survival even in high-risk patients with differentiated thyroid cancer. Ann Surg 1998;227: 912–921.

46. Weigel RJ. Advances in the diagnosis and management of well-differentiated thyroid cancers. Curr Opin Oncol 1996;8: 37–43.

47. Lin J-D, Kao P-F, Chao T-C. The effects of radioactive iodine in thyroid remnant ablation and treatment of well differentiated thyroid carcinoma. Br J Radiol 1998;71:307–313.

48. DiRusso G, Kern KA. Comparative analysis of complications from I-131 radioablation for well-differentiated thyroid cancer. Surgery (St. Louis) 1994;116:1024–1030.

49. Dottorini ME, Lomuscio G, Mazzucchelli L, Vignati A, Colombo L. Assessment of female fertility and carcinogenesis after iodine-131 therapy for differentiated thyroid carcinoma. J Nucl Med 1995;36:21–27.

50. Pacini F, Gasperi M, Fugazzola L, et al. Testicular function in patients with differentiated thyroid carcinoma treated with radioiodine. J Nucl Med 1994;35:1418–1422.

51. Mazzaferri EL, Jhiang SM. Long-term impact of initial surgical and medical therapy on papillary and follicular thyroid cancer. Am J Med 1994;97:418–428.

52. Newman KD, Black T, Heller G, et al. Differentiated thyroid cancer: determinants of disease progression in patients <21 years of age at diagnosis. Ann Surg 1998;227:533–541.

53. DeGroot LJ, Kaplan EL, McCormick M, Straus FH. Natural history, treatment and course of papillary thyroid carcinoma. J Clin Endocrinol Metab 1990;71:414–424.

54. Loh K-C, Greenspan FS, Gee L, Miller TR, Yeo PPB. Pathological tumor-node-metastasis (pTNM) staging for papillary and follicular thyroid carcinomas: a retrospective analysis of 700 patients. J Clin Endocrinol Metab 1997;82:3553–3562.

55. Andersen PE, Kinsella J, Loree TR, Shaha AR, Shah JP. Differentiated carcinoma of the thyroid with extrathyroidal extension. Am J Surg 1995;170:467–470.

56. Samaan NA, Schultz PN, Hickey RC, et al. The results of various modalities of treatment of well differentiated thyroid carcinoma: a retrospective review of 1599 patients. J Clin Endocrinol Metab 1992;75:714–720.

57. Scheumann GFW, Gimm O, Wegener G, Hundeshagen H, Dralle H. Prognostic significance and surgical management of locoregional lymph node metastases in papillary thyroid cancer. World J Surg 1994;18:559–568.

58. DeGroot LJ, Kaplan EL, Shukla MS, Salti G, Straus FH. Mor-

bidity and mortality in follicular thyroid cancer. J Clin Endocrinol Metab 1995;80:2946–2953.

59. Schlumberger MJ. Papillary and follicular thyroid carcinoma. N Engl J Med 1998;338:297–305.

60. Brennan MD, Bergstralh EJ, van Heerden JA, McConahey WM. Follicular thyroid cancer treated at the Mayo Clinic, 1946 through 1970: initial manifestations, pathologic findings, therapy, and outcome. Mayo Clin Proc 1991;66:11–22.

61. Ruiz de Almodovar JM, Ruiz-Garcia J, Olea N, Villalobos M, Pedraza V. Analysis of risk of death from differentiated thyroid cancer. Radiother Oncol 1994;31:207–212.

62. Hay ID, Grant CS, Taylor WF, McConahey WM. Ipsilateral lobectomy versus bilateral lobar resection in papillary thyroid carcinoma: a retrospective analysis of surgical outcome using a novel prognostic scoring system. Surgery (St. Louis) 1987;102:1088–1095.

63. Shah JP, et al. Part II: Head and Neck. In: Greene FL, Page DL, Fleming ID, et al. editors. AJCC Cancer Staging Manual 6th Ed. New York: Springer-Verlag, 2002.

64. Noguchi S, Murakami N, Kawamoto H. Classification of papillary cancer of the thyroid based on prognosis. World J Surg 1994;18:552–558.

65. Ladenson PW. Optimal laboratory testing for diagnosis and monitoring of thyroid nodules, goiter, and thyroid cancer. Clin Chem 1996;42:183–187.

66. Ozata M, Suzuki S, Takahide M, et al. Serum thyroglobulin in the follow-up of patients with treated differentiated thyroid cancer. J Clin Endocrinol Metab 1994;79:98–105.

67. Coburn M, Teates D, Wanebo H. Recurrent thyroid cancer. Ann Surg 1994;291:587–595.

68. Carmeci C, Jeffrey RB, McDougall IR, Nowels KW, Weigel RJ. Ultrasound-guided fine-needle aspiration biopsy of thyroid masses. Thyroid 1998;8:283–289.

69. Moley JF. Medullary thyroid cancer. Surg Clin North Am 1995;75:405–420.

70. Wells SA, Chi DD, Toshima K, et al. Predictive DNA testing and prophylactic thyroidectomy in patients at risk for multiple endocrine neoplasia type 2A. Ann Surg 1994;220:237–250.

71. Howe JR, Norton JA, Wells SA. Prevalence of pheochromocytoma and hyperparathyroidism in multiple endocrine neoplasia type 2A: results of long-term follow-up. Surgery (St. Louis) 1993; 114:1070–1077.

72. Kallinowski F, Buhr HJ, Meybier H, Eberhardt M, Herfarth C. Medullary carcinoma of the thyroid—therapeutic strategy derived from fifteen years of experience. Surgery (St. Louis) 1993; 114:491–496.

73. Dottorini ME, Assi A, Sironi M, Sangalli G, Spreafico G, Colombo L. Multivarate analysis of patients with medullary thyroid carcinoma. Cancer (Phila) 1996;77:1556–1565.

74. Hoie J, Jorgensen OG, Stenwig AE, Langmark F. Medullary thyroid cancer in Norway. Acta Chir Scand 1988;154:339–343.

75. Tan RK, Robert K, Finley I, et al. Anaplastic carcinoma of the thyroid: a 24-year experience. Head Neck 1995;17:41–48.

76. Tennvall J, Lundell G, Hallquist A, Wahlberg P, Wallin G, Tibblin S. Combined doxorubicin, hyperfractionated radiotherapy, and surgery in anaplastic thyroid carcinoma. Cancer (Phila) 1994;74:1348–1354.

29

Adrenal

Robert Udelsman

Anatomy

The adrenal glands are paired retroperitoneal organs located in close contact to the superior surface of either kidney. They are surrounded by a loose layer of areolar connective tissue and have multiple fibrous bands and vascular attachments through which they are associated with the superior poles of the kidneys. They are recognizable by their firm texture and chromate yellow color, which is distinctly darker than the pale retroperitoneal fat. The normal adrenal gland is slightly nodular and generally weighs between 4 and 5 g in the adult.[1] The presence of adrenal nodules is not uncommon, and their frequency increases with age.[2]

The anatomical relationships of the adrenal glands are important and have significant surgical ramifications. The CT findings of the normal adrenal glands (Fig. 29.1) are easily visualized on most CT scans, and the width of each adrenal gland limb is similar to that of the nearby diaphragm. Their anatomical relationships have been summarized by Mihai and Farndon[1] (Table 29.1). The location of the adrenal gland deep in the retroperitoneum has in the past made them relatively inaccessible. However, laparoscopic adrenalectomy has dramatically changed the surgical management of adrenal tumors.

Each adrenal gland is supplied by small arterial branches that originate from three distinct sources. The major supplying vessels are the inferior phrenic artery, the aorta, and the ipsilateral renal artery. Occasional additional sources include the intercostal and ovarian vessels. The arterial branches ramify over the capsule of the gland and form a subcapsular plexus.[1,3] The major source of adrenal medullary blood appears to be via the adrenal cortex from which blood rich in glucocorticoids flows from the cortical layers into the medulla.[3] This intraadrenal "portal venous" circulation has significant physiological ramifications. The final pathway for the catecholamine epinephrine requires the enzyme phenylethanolamine N-methyltransferase (PNMT), and glucocorticoids are required for this final step.[4] Thus, there is significant functional interaction between the adrenal medulla and cortex.

The venous drainage of the adrenal gland is more constant than the arterial supply. The right adrenal gland usually drains by one short vein, which empties directly into the vena cava. Accessory adrenal veins are not infrequently present. The left major adrenal vein is often joined by the inferior phrenic vein, which drains into the left renal vein. There may be associated small additional veins. Lymphatic drainage from the adrenal glands drains directly into adjacent, periaortic and paracaval nodes. These structures are important when operating for malignant adrenal lesions.[3]

Physiology

The adrenal gland is composed of two distinct organs, the adrenal cortex and the adrenal medulla. The cortex is divided into three functional zones: the outer glomerulosa, the intermediate fasciculata, and the inner reticularis. These three zones are associated with the production of mineralocorticoids, glucocorticoids, and sex steroids, respectively. Of these three hormone classes, the only one absolutely required for life is glucocorticoids.

Glucocorticoids exert a myriad of effects on essentially every tissue in the body. A partial list of the effects of glucocorticoids is presented in Table 29.2. Cortisol is the major glucocorticoid in humans. The rate-limiting step in adrenal steroid synthesis, which is controlled by adrenocorticotropic hormone (ACTH), is the cleavage of the cholesterol side chain to yield pregnenolone.[5,6] Glucocorticoids are secreted directly into the circulation immediately upon their synthesis. Cortisol circulates in both the bound form (95%) and in a free unbound state (5%). The free form passes into target cells by diffusion and binds to cytosolic receptors. All physiological actions of glucocorticoids are mediated through binding to steroid receptors, which are present in virtually every nucleated cell.[7] The actions of glucocorticoids are both "permissive," allowing other hormones to function in the basal state, as well as "regulatory," which are observed under stress-induced conditions.[8]

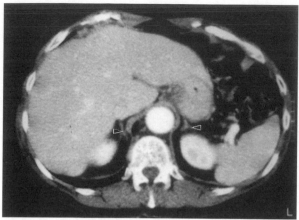

FIGURE 29.1. CT scan demonstrating normal adrenal glands (*arrowheads*). (From Sosa JA, Udelsman R. Imaging of the adrenal gland. In: Kurtzman S, ed. Surgical Oncology Clinics of North America. Philadelphia: Saunders, 1998;109–127, with permission.)

The autonomic nervous system develops in parallel to the hypothalamic–pituitary–adrenal (HPA) axis. The adrenal medulla is embryologically analogous to a peripheral sympathetic ganglia. The medullary chromaffin cells have rudimentary nerve fibers and the ability to synthesize, store, and secrete catecholamines.[9] The primary secretory product of the adrenal medulla is epinephrine. The proximity of the adrenal

medulla and the adrenal cortex results in a unique site of catecholamine–glucocorticoid interactions.[10,11]

The biosynthetic pathway for catecholamines is demonstrated in Figure 29.2.[12] Epinephrine constitutes approximately 80% of adrenal medullary secretion.[13]

Adrenal Imaging

The adrenal glands are relatively inaccessible retroperitoneal organs that are surrounded by perinephric fat. Plain abdominal films have a very limited role in adrenal imaging. However, they can detect calcifications, especially in children who have had neonatal hemorrhage or have neuroblastoma. In adults, calcifications of the adrenal glands are highly suggestive of granulomatous disease including tuberculosis, histoplasmosis, and sarcoidosis. Ultrasonography can detect adrenal lesions and is a relatively inexpensive method to serially follow small adrenal adenomas. Adrenal ultrasound has a limited role for diagnostic purposes and is largely supplemented by computed tomography (CT) or magnetic resonance imaging (MRI) scans. Intraoperative ultrasound performed during laparoscopic adrenalectomy has proven to be a useful modality. It can identify the location of small adrenal glands and delineate their vasculature.[14]

CT Scans

Computed tomography scanning of the adrenal gland has proven to be the diagnostic procedure of choice for most patients. Simple cysts and myelolipomas can be diagnosed with virtual certainty based on their CT characteristics. Intravenous contrast is generally not required, and a low attenuation value on an unenhanced CT scan can help differentiate benign (low density) from malignant lesions as well as metastases, which generally have a higher density.[15–17] Lesions with low Hounsfield units (HU) are most likely benign, whereas lesions that have a HU density greater than 20 are more likely to be malignant.[18] Accordingly, it has been suggested that a cutoff point of 30 HU should be accepted for discriminating malignant and benign lesions.[19]

MRI Scan

Magnetic resonance imaging (MRI) has a significant role in the evaluation of adrenal tumors. Nonfunctioning adenomas appear on T_2-weighted images like normal adrenal tissue. Functional adenomas tend to demonstrate a slightly increased signal intensity, whereas adrenal metastases or primary adrenal cortical carcinomas tend to be relatively bright. Enhancement on T_2-weighted images is particularly useful for pheochromocytomas and therefore MRI appears to be the imaging study of choice in patients with suspected pheochromocytomas.

Radioisotope Scan

Iodocholesterol-labeled agents including ^{131}I-6-β-iodomethyl-19-norcholesterol (NP59) are incorporated into steroidogenesis pathways in the form of intracellular cholesterol and therefore have the ability to visualize functional adrenal cortical lesions.[20] However, NP59 is not readily available at most in-

TABLE 29.1. Anatomical Relations of the Adrenal Glands.

Surface	Area	Description
Right Adrenal		
Anterior	Medial area	Not covered by peritoneum; posterior to the inferior vena cava
	Lateral area	Upper part in contact with the inferomedial angle of bare area of liver; lower part may be covered by peritoneum, reflected onto it from the inferior layer of the coronary ligament
Posterior	Upper area	Rests against the diaphragm
	Lower area	In contact with the superior pole and the adjacent anterior surface of right kidney
Medial border		Right celiac ganglion
		Right inferior phrenic artery
Left Adrenal		
Anterior	Superior area	Covered with peritoneum of the omental bursa, which separates it from the cardia
	Inferior area	Not covered by peritoneum; in direct contact with the tail of pancreas and splenic artery
Posterior	Medial part	In contact with left crus of diaphragm
	Lateral part	Close to the kidney
Medial border		Left celiac ganglion
		Left inferior phrenic artery
		Left gastric arteries

Source: Reprinted with permission from Mihai R, Farndon JR. Surgical embryology and anatomy of the adrenal glands. In: Clark OH, Duh QY, eds. Textbook of Endocrine Surgery. Philadelphia: Saunders, 1997:452.

TABLE 29.2. Glucocorticoid Actions.

Area	Increase	Decrease
Liver	Gluconeogenesis, glycogenesis, protein synthesis	Glycogenolysis
Muscle	Lactate release	Protein synthesis
Peripheral tissues		Glucose uptake and use (increased insulin levels)
Adipose tissue	Lipolysis, redistribution of body fat	
Bone	Osteoporosis, osteoclast activity, PTH	Intestinal absorption of calcium, renal reabsorption of calcium
Cardiovascular	Vascular tone, binding to mineralocorticoid receptor, catecholamine synthesis	
Immunological	Immunosuppression	Production and activity of prostaglandins, kinins, and histamine
	Leukocyte distribution	Leukocyte movement, antigen processing
Wound healing		Collagen formation, glycosaminoglycan, and fibroblast function
CNS	Behavior and mood effects	

CNS, central nervous system; PTH, parathyroid hormone.

Source: Udelsman R, Holbrook NJ. Endocrine and molecular responses to surgical stress. Curr Prob Surg 1994;8:653–728, with permission.

stitutions and dexamethasone pretreatment is required.[21] These two factors limit its clinical utility.

Meta-iodobenzylguanidine (MIBG) is frequently used for the evaluation of pheochromocytoma as well as neuroblastoma. ^{131}I-MIBG and ^{123}I-MIBG are concentrated in catecholamine storage vesicles and therefore are useful in suspected cases of pheochromocytoma.[22,23] In cases of extraadrenal disease, which has a lower propensity for MIBG uptake, positron emission tomography (PET) utilizing 2-fluorine-18-fluoro-2-deoxy-D-glucose (FDG) may be useful.[24]

Angiography

Angiography and venography were at one time more commonly employed for the evaluation of adrenal tumors. These procedures have been largely replaced by noninvasive imaging.

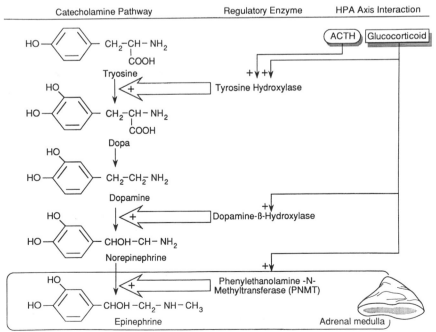

FIGURE 29.2. Biosynthetic pathway for catecholamines, their regulatory enzymes, and interactions with the hypothalamic–pituitary–adrenal (*HPA*) axis. ACTH, adrenocorticotropic hormone. (From Udelsman R, Holbrook NJ. Endocrine and molecular responses to surgical stress. Curr Probl Surg 1994;31:653–728, with permission.)

Pertucaneous Biopsy

Percutaneous biopsy of the adrenal gland can be performed under either CT or ultrasound guidance. However, there are very few appropriate indications for this procedure. A percutaneous biopsy cannot reliably distinguish between an adrenal adenoma and an adrenal carcinoma.[25] The most common indication is in the setting of suspected metastatic disease to the adrenal gland. In such a case, when a fine-needle aspiration demonstrates nonadrenal malignant tissue the diagnosis of metastasis is confirmed. This procedure should never be performed in a patient until a biochemical workup has been completed to rule out a pheochromocytoma because sudden death has been reported following biopsy of unsuspected pheochromocytoma.

Incidentaloma

Adrenal "incidentalomas" are adrenal tumors discovered on an imaging study that has been obtained for indications exclusive of adrenal-related conditions. The frequent use of CT scans, which can detect adrenal lesions greater than 1 cm, has resulted in their detection in 0.35% to 5% of studies.[2] The evaluation and decision paradigm for an incidentaloma hinges on three issues: (1) Is it functional? (2) Is it likely to be a malignant adrenal tumor? (3) Is it metastatic? The evaluation is focused on answering each of the foregoing questions.

Hormone Evaluation

All evaluations begin with a detailed history and physical examination. If symptoms or signs suggesting a functional adrenal neoplasm are detected, then, in addition to a routine screening evaluation, specific hormone studies are indicated. However, most patients are asymptomatic. The CT findings of a specific subset of adrenal masses including simple adrenal cysts and myelolipomas can be pathognomonic. In these instances, hormonal screening studies are not required.[26,27]

Screening studies are directed at three specific syndromes: pheochromocytoma, aldosteronoma, and Cushing's syndrome. Pheochromocytomas are rare. However, because the risk of complications associated with an occult pheochromocytoma is significant, virtually all investigators agree that all incidentaloma patients should be screened for catecholamine hypersecretion.[27–29] Most commonly, urinary collections over 24 h are obtained in bottles containing acid. These collections are analyzed for metanephrines, vanillylmandelic acid (VMA), or fractionated catecholamines.

The screen for aldosteronoma in the setting of an incidentaloma is often limited. If the patient is normotensive and not receiving hypertension or diuretic therapy and has a normal serum potassium (>3.5 mEq/l), then an aldosteronoma is very unlikely. If the patient does not satisfy these criteria, then an aldosteronoma evaluation is performed as delineated later in this chapter.

Cushing's syndrome is important to consider in all patients with adrenal tumors. Patients with advanced Cushing's syndrome present with classic symptoms and signs of glucocorticoid excess and are therefore not difficult to diagnose. However, patients not uncommonly present with subtle stigmata of Cushing's syndrome or with occult or "subclinical" disease. In this situation the patient has an adrenal adenoma that has attained functional autonomy in its ability to secrete

glucocorticoids but has not yet manifest findings of Cushing's syndrome.[30] This silent but subtle hypercortisolism occurs in approximately 15% of patients with incidentalomas.[30] It is important to rule out subclinical Cushing's syndrome for two reasons: (1) if one elects not to perform an adrenalectomy, then the endocrinopathy will continue and deleterious effects will occur, and (2) if one does perform an adrenalectomy, the contralateral adrenal will be suppressed, and if perioperative glucocorticoids are not administered the patient will be at risk for Addisonian crisis.

It is important to recognize that an incidentaloma may represent a metastatic lesion in the adrenal gland. The majority of patients with metastatic disease to one or both adrenal glands have both a history of malignant disease and metastases to multiple additional sites. In the setting of widespread metastatic disease, the adrenal disease is not treated directly as it represents only a small focus of total tumor burden. Patients with bilateral adrenal metastases are at some risk for adrenal insufficiency.

An important and unresolved issue in the management of incidentalomas is the determination of what size of adrenal tumor is in itself an indication for extirpation. In the absence of scientific trials an empiric approach has been employed. Virtually all experts agree that any lesion greater than 5 cm on initial presentation should be excised because of the risk of malignancy. Lesions less than 3 cm are generally followed with serial imaging studies. Several experienced investigators have recommended excision of all adrenal tumors greater than 4 cm.[31,32] If one elects not to excise an incidentaloma, then a follow-up imaging study should be obtained at a relatively short interval (approximately 3 months) to determine if serial growth has occurred. Lesions that grow should be excised.

An algorithm for the evaluation of incidentally discovered adrenal masses is depicted in Figure 29.3. It is based upon a

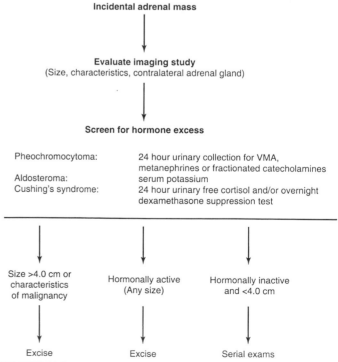

FIGURE 29.3. Recommended evaluation for incidentally discovered adrenal mass.

systematic literature review and the acceptance of 4.0 cm as a size that is in itself an indication for adrenalectomy.

Hyperaldosteronism

Excessive secretion of aldosterone results in hypertension and hypokalemia. It may be caused by primary aldosteronism, an intrinsic abnormality of one or both adrenal glands. It can also be caused by excessive renin secretion, which results from a low effective arterial blood volume, in which case it is termed secondary aldosteronism.[33] Primary aldosteronism is rare, with a prevalence among hypertensive patients estimated to range between 0.05% and 2%.[34] Aldosteronomas occur in approximately 65% of patients with primary aldosteronism. They are almost always unilateral and are often less than 2 cm in size.

It is extremely important to distinguish a unilateral aldosteronoma from idiopathic hyperaldosteronism (IHA), which occurs in 25% of patients with primary aldosteronism and is caused by bilateral adrenal hyperplasia. In this case both adrenal glands contain multiple macro- and microscopic nodules. Importantly, unilateral adrenalectomy in the setting of IHA is not curative. Unfortunately, the distinction between aldosterone-producing adenoma (APA) and IHA can be difficult.

Additional, but less common, surgically correctable causes of primary aldosteronism include primary adrenal hyperplasia and renin-response aldosterone-producing adenoma. Primary adrenal hyperplasia may be unilateral or bilateral, and the glands appear histologically like those seen in patients with IHA. The biochemical profile, however, is similar to that seen in an APA and unilateral adrenalectomy appears to be beneficial in patients with unilateral lesions.[35,36] Renin-responsive aldostrone-producing adenomas appear biochemically like IHA, and they also respond to surgical resection.[35,37] Adrenal cortical aldosterone-producing carcinoma is extremely rare and represents another surgically treatable form of primary aldosteronism.[38]

Clinical Presentation

The signs and symptoms of primary aldosteronism are nonspecific and include hypertension and hypokalemia. The mean age at presentation ranges from 30 to 50 years, and it is twice as common in women.[39,40] The hypertension is generally indistinguishable from that seen in the population with essential hypertension.

Screening for Primary Aldosteronism

The presence of spontaneous hypokalemia in a hypertensive individual strongly suggests the diagnosis. Unfortunately, the common use of diuretics, as well as antihypertensive agents including angiotension-converting enzyme inhibitors and spironolactone, interfere with the ability to establish the diagnosis.[41,42] Most endocrinologists recommend discontinuation of all diuretic and antihypertensive therapy for at least 4 weeks before a diagnostic evaluation. If the patient's blood pressure requires control during this interval, prazosin can be used as it will not interfere with the workup.[41] A wide variety of biochemical tests have been recommended, but there is no clear consensus as to which tests are the most appro-

priate. Hypokalemia, although highly suggestive of the diagnosis, should not be considered as a necessary criterion.[43]

PLASMA ALDOSTERONE/RENIN RATIO

Excess autonomous secretion of aldosterone results in salt retention, hypertension, and suppression of plasma renin activity. However, single isolated measurements of either plasma renin or aldosterone are of limited diagnostic value.[43–45] Because primary aldosteronism results in elevated aldosterone and suppressed plasma renin levels, simultaneous determination appears more useful and is less affected by physiological or pharmacological variables.[46,47]

SALINE INFUSION TEST

The saline infusion test is used to demonstrate autonomous aldosterone secretion that does not decrease appropriately following sodium loading.[47–49] Failure to suppress plasma aldosterone below 8.5 mg/dl after 2 l of intravenous normal saline is considered diagnostic of primary aldosteronism.[49]

DISTINCTION BETWEEN APA AND IHA

The majority of cases of primary aldosteronism are caused by either an APA (65%) or IHA (25%). It is important to discriminate between these as an APA is treated by unilateral adrenalectomy, whereas IHA is generally treated with spironolactone.[50] A variety of biochemical and imaging studies are available to make this distinction (Table 29.3).

Localization

Once the biochemical criteria for an APA have been satisfied, the next step is tumor localization. High-quality CT scans have simplified this workup for the majority of patients. If a unilateral adrenal mass is detected and the contralateral adrenal gland is normal, then proceeding directly to unilateral adrenalectomy appears reasonable.[35,42,51]

Treatment

There is an ever-expanding body of literature to suggest that laparoscopic adrenalectomy is the procedure of choice for al-

TABLE 29.3. Aldosteronoma Screening Studies.

Test	Results
Aldosterone-producing adenoma (APA)	
Plasma aldosterone after postural stimulation	Decrease or <30% increase
18-Hydroxycorticosterone	>100 ng/dl
Computed tomography scan	Unilateral mass
Iodocholesterol scan	Localization
Adrenal venous sampling	Localization
Idiopathic aldosteronism	
Plasma aldosterone after postural stimulation	>30% increase
18-Hydroxycorticosterone	<100 ng/dl
Computed tomography scan	? Bilateral masses
Iodocholesterol scan	Bilateral uptake
Adrenal venous sampling	No localization

Source: Udelsman R. Tumors of the adrenal cortex. In: Cameron JL, ed. Current Surgical Therapy, 6th Ed. St. Louis: Mosby, 1998:577–580, with permission.

dosteronomas.[52–54] This technique results in improvement in length of stay, morbidity, and costs. In addition the patient is able to return to normal activity in a much shorter interval.[14,55] The traditional surgical treatment has required a unilateral total adrenalectomy. Recently, aldosteroma enucleation or subtotal adrenalectomy has been suggested as an equally effective technique.[56,57]

Results

The surgical treatment of APA results in correction of hypokalemia in almost all cases.[58] Hypertension is usually improved, but may persist, particularly if the patient has long-standing hypertension at the time of surgery.[58] The incidence of persistent hypertension is approximately 30%.[59] Risk factors associated with persistent hypertension include age greater than 50 at the time of surgery, male sex, and the presence of "multiple adenomas" or inappropriately diagnosed IHA.[39]

Cushing's Syndrome

Harvey Cushing described eight patients in 1932 with moon facies, truncal obesity, hypertension, polyphagia, polydipsia, polycythemia, and pulmonary infections. Pituitary basophil adenomas were noted in autopsy in four of these patients, and he correctly associated this syndrome with pituitary adenomas.[60] The most common cause of Cushing syndrome is iatrogenic administration of glucocorticoids. Endogenous Cushing syndrome is, for the most part, either ACTH dependent or ACTH independent (Table 29.4). The most common cause of endogenous Cushing's syndrome, accounting for nearly 85% of all cases, is Cushing's disease, glucocorticoid excess caused by a pituitary adenoma. The majority of ACTH-independent causes of Cushing's syndrome are adrenal in origin, consisting of adrenal adenoma and rare adrenal carcinomas. The management of ACTH-dependent Cushing's syndrome requires accurate tumor identification and extirpation whenever possible. In some circumstances, pituitary surgery is unsuccessful or the source of the ectopic ACTH secretion cannot be identified. In this situation bilateral adrenalectomy may be required to alleviate the sequela of life-threatening glucocorticoid excess.

The treatment of choice of ACTH-independent Cushing's syndrome is surgical resection. Patients with endogenous Cushing's syndrome caused by a unilateral adrenal tumor will have an elevated 24-h urinary free cortisol and 17-hydroxy-corticosteroid levels. Because these tumors produce glucocorticoids in the absence of ACTH stimulation, the normal

TABLE 29.4. Endogenous Causes of Cushing's Syndrome.

ACTH-dependent
  Cushing's disease (pituitary adenoma)
  Ectopic ACTH syndrome
ACTH-independent
  Adrenal adenoma
  Adrenal carcinoma
  Primary pigmented nodular adrenal dysplasia (PPNAD)
ACTH-variable
  Macronodular adrenal hyperplasia

pituitary secretion of ACTH is suppressed. Therefore, an elevated plasma ACTH level in this setting is inconsistent with the diagnosis. The dexamethasone suppression test can be extremely useful in discriminating between ACTH-dependent and ACTH-independent causes of Cushing's syndrome. It is also crucial to carefully evaluate the imaging studies. In the setting of an adrenal adenoma one anticipates unilateral adrenal enlargement and a contralateral normal or slightly suppressed adrenal gland. In the setting of adrenocortical carcinoma, the ipsilateral adrenal gland should be significantly enlarged and may be associated with local tumor invasion. The contralateral adrenal gland should be normal in size. In addition, in the setting of an adrenal carcinoma one is likely to find elevated levels of adrenal androgens.[61]

Surgical treatment of adrenal causes of Cushing syndrome has undergone significant changes.[62] Adrenal surgery can be performed safely with low morbidity and operative mortality in the 2% to 3% range. The recent advent of laparoscopic adrenalectomy has dramatically changed the management of these patients.[14,53] Unilateral adrenalectomy is the treatment of choice for most patients with a tumor causing ACTH-independent endogenous Cushing's syndrome.

Bilateral Adrenalectomy

Bilateral adrenalectomy will continue to play a small but significant role in the management of selected patients with Cushing's disease.[63] These include patients who have not been cured following pituitary resection, patients with primary pigmented nodular adrenal dysplasia, and patients with macronodular adrenal hyperplasia refractory to medical management with receptor blockers.

Bilateral adrenalectomy is associated with significant long-term morbidity. These patients require lifelong replacement with both mineralocorticoids and glucocorticoids. Occult adrenal insufficiency may occur and can be life threatening.[64]

Pheochromocytoma

Pheochromocytomas are rare tumors that arise from the neuroectodermally derived chromaffin cells. The majority of pathologists believe that all pheochromocytomas are of adrenal origin, and they refer to extraadrenal chromaffin tumors as paragangliomas, which may or may not be functional. However, most clinicians designate catecholamine-secreting tumors as either adrenal or extraadrenal pheochromocytomas.[65]

The majority of pheochromocytomas (90%) in adults are located in the adrenal gland. However, in children the incidence of extraadrenal pheochromocytomas is much higher (35%).[65] Most pheochromocytomas (90%) are unilateral. However, the incidence of synchronous or metachronous pheochromocytomas are more common in patients with familial forms of pheochromocytomas. These syndromes and their associated findings are listed in Table 29.5. The majority of pheochromocytomas (90%) are thought to be benign. However, because the criteria for malignancy requires the demonstration of distant metastasis or direct invasion into surrounding organs, it is possible that surgical extirpation of a subset of presumptively benign pheochromocytomas results

TABLE 29.5. Genetic Syndromes Associated with Pheochromocytoma.

Syndrome	Findings
MEN2A (Sipple's syndrome)	Medullary carcinoma of the thyroid Pheochromocytoma Hyperparathyroidism
MEN 2B	Medullary carcinoma of the thyroid Pheochromocytoma Mucosal neuroma Marfanoid habitus Ganglioneuromas of the gastrointestinal tract
Neurofibromatosis (von Recklinghausen's disease)	Café-au-lait spots Axillary freckling Multiple freckling Multiple neurofibromas Pheochromocytoma
Von Hippel–Lindau disease	Retinal hemanagiomatosis Cerebellar hemangioblastoma Pheochromocytoma Renal cell tumors

in excision of a malignant lesion that has not yet satisfied the requisite malignant criteria.

Functional pheochromocytomas secrete a variety of vasoactive compounds either continually or episodically. Norepinephrine is the most common.

Clinical Manifestations

The classic presentation of a symptomatic pheochromocytoma is episodic attacks of headaches, diaphoresis, and palpitations.[65,66] Although hypertension is commonly present during an attack, it is important to remember that between attacks approximately 50% of affected individuals are normotensive. The hypertension can result in stroke, renal insufficiency, and cardiac failure.[67]

DIAGNOSIS

The most commonly employed biochemical screening tests require 24-h urinary collections for the measurement of vanillymandelic acid (VMA), metanephrines, or fractionated catecholamines.[66] In addition, recent studies indicate that plasma levels of metanephrine and normetanephrine are sensitive and specific for pheochromocytoma. In select circumstances, additional pharmacological tests are required to yield an unequivocal biochemical diagnosis.[68] However, the clonidine suppression test and the glucagon stimulation test are not routinely required.[65,66,68,69]

Imaging

Once the diagnosis of a pheochromocytoma has been made, the next step is tumor localization using imaging studies including ultrasound, CT, MRI, and MIBG scans. MRI scans have several unique characteristics that make them the imaging study of choice. The MRI scan will enhance on T_2-weighted images, and administration of i.v. contrast agents are not required (see Adrenal Imaging).

Treatment

Because of chronic hypersecretion of catecholamines, patients with pheochromocytomas are often severely volume contracted. In the past, when these patients underwent general anesthesia, it was not uncommon for them to experience severe hemodynamic instability. Accordingly, it is necessary to initiate a 1- to 4-week period of preoperative alpha-adrenergic receptor blockade. The most commonly used agent is the selective alpha-1-adrenergic receptor blocker, phenoxybenzamine. Occasional patients will also require beta-adrenergic receptor blockade because of breakthrough tachycardia. However, beta receptor blockade should not be administered in the absence of prior alpha receptor blockade because of the risk of unopposed alpha receptor-induced malignant hypertension.[65,70]

The anesthestic and surgical care of these patients is critical and requires a concerted effort. Patients may experience both hypertension and hypotension (following tumor removal), and the anesthesiologist must be prepared to treat preciptious changes in blood pressure. Infusions of phentolamine and sodium nitroprusside are often required.[65] In addition, anesthestic agents that lower the threshold of catecholamine-induced arrhythmias (halothane) or histamine release (morphine) should be avoided.[71]

Surgical treatment in the past required an open laparotomy with early control of the main adrenal vein and bilateral as well as extraadrenal exploration. This practice has been changed by the exquisite sensitivity of current imaging techniques and the use of laparoscopic adrenalectomy. At many institutions, laparoscopic adrenalectomy has become the procedure of choice.[14]

Malignant Pheochromocytoma

Complete surgical excision is the only potentially curative therapy for malignant pheochromocytoma.[66,67] However, the criteria for malignancy, invasion into adjacent tissue or distant metastases, are not always demonstrable at the time of surgery or on pathological review of the specimen. It is for this reason that initial total tumor extirpation as well as long-term follow-up are essential.

Patients with malignant pheochromocytomas, even in the setting of metastatic disease, can have prolonged survival. The mean 5-year survival ranges from 30% to 40%.[72] Surgical resection is indicated whenever feasible. The most effective chemotherapeutic regiment includes cyclophosphamide, vincristine, and dacarbazine.[73] Although pheochromocytomas are not generally radiosensitive,[65] treatment with ^{131}I-MIBG has been shown to be of benefit in selected patients.[74,75]

Familial Pheochromocytoma

Pheochromocytomas occur in association with several genetic syndromes including MEN2, von Hippel–Lindau disease, and von Recklinghausen's disease (see Table 29.5). When individuals from an affected family are identified they should undergo screening. If they are found to have biochemical evidence of catecholamine excess, localization procedures are indicated. Bilateral adrenalectomy has been generally recommended in familial patients because at the time of biochemical abnormalities at least bilateral adrenal medullary hyperplasia has already developed.[76,77]

Recent evidence suggests that it may be prudent to perform a unilateral adrenalectomy for macroscopically normal glands in the setting of familial pheochromocytomas. Serial follow-up is required.

Adrenocortical Carcinoma

Adrenocortical carcinoma is rare, with an incidence of 0.6 to 2 cases per million individuals per year.[78–80] The prognosis is poor, and most series report a 5-year mortality between 55% and 90%.[81,82] It accounts for approximately 0.2% of cancer deaths.[83] Because of its rare incidence, controlled clinical trials have not addressed major issues in the diagnosis or treatment of this disease.

Presentation

The majority of patients (68%–80%) present with an endocrinopathy, most commonly Cushing's syndrome.[61,79] Patients often have advanced disease at the time of presentation with almost 40% presenting with metastatic disease.[79] The most common sites of distant metastases are the liver, lung, bone, and brain.[79,81] However, local invasion into adjacent organs including the kidney, liver, diaphragm, spleen, pancreas, and vena cava are common at the time of diagnostics.[50] A female predominance of at least 2:1 is noted in most series,[61,82,84] and the mean age at presentation ranges from 30 to 50 years.[61,80–82] The staging criteria for adrenocortical carcinoma are shown in Table 29.6. The majority of patients present with tumors greater than 5 cm in size with local invasion into adjacent organs with or without distant metastases (stage II or III).[50]

Surgery is the mainstay of therapy and remains the only potential for cure. Aggressive local resection is indicated whenever feasible. Adjacent organs including lymph nodes, kidney, spleen, diaphragm, distal pancreas, liver, and vena cava are often resected in continuity with the primary tumor. MRI scans, especially MRI "angiograms," are used when there is a suspicion of major vascular involvement.

The role of adjuvant chemotherapy is somewhat controversial.[61] The single most effective agent, mitotane (o,p'-DDD or 1,1-dichlorodiphenyldichloroethane), has been used since 1960[85] with moderate success. It is the only agent

associated with long-term remissions and regression of metastases.[61,82–84]

The overall prognosis for adrenal cortical carcinoma remains poor. Mean survival rates are approximately 22 to 47 months.[61,82,83] However, long-term survival can occur. Patients who develop locally recurrent disease can benefit from reoperative surgery.

Laparoscopic Adrenalectomy

There are multiple surgical approaches to the adrenal gland, including anterior transabdominal, flank, thoracoabdominal, supracostal, posterior, and the newer laparoscopic techniques via a transperitoneal or retroperitoneal approach. The traditional techniques of adrenalectomy are well described and are beyond the scope of this review.[86–89] Laparoscopic adrenalectomy has already had a major impact on the management of adrenal neoplasms. In skilled hands this technique is appropriate for virtually all nonmalignant adrenal tumors. Most, but not all, endocrine surgeons agree that large tumors and clearly malignant tumors should be excised using an open technique.[14,90–92]

Laparoscopic adrenalectomy appears to have distinct advantages compared to traditional open techniques. Avoidance of large incisions and decreased tissue trauma appears to decrease morbidity and mortality.[14,93–96] Interestingly, even pheochromocytomas have been successfully managed with this technique.[14,96–99]

Several investigations have compared various anatomical approaches with laparoscopic adrenalectomy.[14,90,100–103] It is now clear that in skilled hands laparoscopic adrenalectomy can be performed safely, resulting in decreased hospital stays, increased patient comfort, and a shorter interval until the resumption of normal activity.[101,102]

Although there are no randomized prospective trials comparing the results of laparoscopic and open adrenalectomy, the results obtained in several retrospective case-controlled studies are presented in Table 29.7. These data demonstrate that laparoscopic adrenalectomy is consistently associated with marked decreases in the postoperative length of stay and the interval until resumption of normal diet and activity.

Adrenal Insufficiency

Patients with overt or occult adrenal insufficiency pose significant management issues that have not yet been resolved. Primary adrenal insufficiency occurs when there is direct destruction of the adrenal glands, which occurs most commonly from autoimmune adrenal atrophy (Addison's disease) and infectious diseases (tuberculosis, histoplasmosis), as well as following adrenal hemorrhage, metastasis, and surgical resection. Secondary adrenal insufficiency occurs when there is an impairment of ACTH secretion at either the pituitary or hypothalamic level. The most common cause of adrenal insufficiency is iatrogenic administration of glucocorticoids, which results in suppression of ACTH. This population of adrenal-insufficient patients poses significant surgical ramifications.

It was estimated that in 1971 more than 5 million patients in the United States received glucocorticoids at doses

TABLE 29.6. Staging Criteria for Adrenocortical Carcinoma.

T_1	<5 cm, no local invasion
T_2	>5 cm, no local invasion
T_3	Any size, local invasion
N_0	No positive lymph nodes
N_1	Positive lymph nodes
M_0	No distant metastasis
M_1	Distant metastasis
Stage	
I	T_1, N_0, M_0
II	T_2, N_0, M_0
III	T_1, or T_2 N_1 M_0, or T_3 N_0 M_0
IV	Any T, any NM_1, or T_3 N_1 M_0

Source: Udelsman R. Tumors of the adrenal cortex. In: Cameron JL, ed. Current Surgical Therapy, 6th Ed. St. Louis: Mosby, 1998:579.

TABLE 29.7.

Laparoscopic versus Open Adrenalectomy.

Study	Laparoscopic	Open anterior	Level of evidence[a]
Prinz 1995[90]			
n:	10	11	II
OR time (min):	212	174	
Postoperative stay (days):	2.1	6.4	
Guazzoni et al. 1995[108]			
n:	20	20	II
OR time (min):	170	145	
Postoperative stay (days):	3.4	9	
Return to work activity (days):	9.7	16	
Brunt et al. 1996[92]			
n:	24	25	II
OR time (min):	183	242	
Postoperative stay (days):	3.2	8.7	
Resumption of regular diet (days):	1.6	6.0	
MacGillivray et al. 1996[109]			
n:	14	9	II
OR time (min):	289	201	
Postoperative stay (days):	3.0	7.9	
Resumption of regular activity (days):	8.9	14.6	
Vargas et al. 1997[110]			
n:	20	20	II
OR time (min):	193	178	
Postoperative stay (days):	3.1	7.2	
Convalescence (weeks):	3	7	
Korman et al. 1997[111]			
n:	10	10	II
OR time (min):	164	124	
Postoperative stay (days):	4.1	5.9	
Direct charges:	$3,645	$5,752	
Linos et al. 1997[112]			
n:	18	86	II
OR time (min):	116	155	
Postoperative stay (days):	2.2	8	
Winfield et al. 1998[113]			
n:	21	17	II
OR time (min):	309	233	
Postoperative stay (days):	2.7	6.2	
Resumption of regular diet (days):	1.7	4.6	
Shell et al. 1998[14]			
n:	22	17	II
OR time (min):	267	257	
Postoperative stay (days):	1.7	7.8	
Resumption of regular diet (days):	1.6	6.1	
Resumption of independent activity (days):	1.6	7.9	
Hospital charges:	$8,698	$12,610	

[a]Clinical studies are classified according to the design of study and the quality of the resulting data: class I, prospective randomized studies; class II, prospective, nonrandomized or case-controlled retrospective studies; class III, retrospective analyses without case controls.

sufficient to cause adrenal suppression.[104] Because of the known deleterious effects of adrenal cortical crisis, it had become the standard of care to administer large doses of perioperative glucocorticoids to obviate hemodynamic inability in this population. However, a series of clinical studies published in the 1970s suggested that physiological rather than pharmacological glucocorticoid supplementation may be sufficient for patients with adrenal insufficiency who require surgical intervention.[105–107] These studies suggest that the perioperative pharmacological doses that are often administered to adrenal-insufficient patients far exceed their physiological requirements.

References

1. Mihai R, Farndon JR. Surgical embryology and anatomy of the adrenal glands. In: Clark OH, Duh QY, eds. Textbook of Endocrine Surgery. Philadelphia: Saunders, 1997:447–459.
2. Kloss RT, Gross MD, Francis IR, et al. Incidentally discovered adrenal masses. Endocr Rev 1995;16(4):460–484.
3. Hamaji M, Harrison TS. Blood vessels and lymphatics of the

adrenal gland. In: Blood Vessels and Lymphatics in Organ Systems. New York: Academic Press, 1984:280–295.

4. Pohorecky L, Wortman R. Adrenocortical control of epinephrine synthesis. Pharmacol Rev 1971;2:1–35.

5. Hayashi K, Sala G, Catt KJ, et al. Regulation of steroidogenesis by adrenocorticotrophic hormone in isolated adrenal cells. J Biol Chem 1979;154:6678–6683.

6. Gill GN. ACTH regulation of the adrenal cortex. In: Gill GN, ed. Pharmacology of Adrenal Cortical Hormones. New York: Pergamon, 1979:35.

7. Udelsman R, Holbrook NJ. Endocrine and molecular responses to surgical stress. Curr Probl Surg 1994;31:653–728.

8. Munck A, Guyre PM, Holbrook NJ. Physiological functions of glucocorticoids in stress and their relation to pharmacological actions. Endocr Rev 1984;5:25–44.

9. Cryer PE. Physiology and pathophysiology of the human sympathoadrenal neuroendocrine system. N Engl J Med 1980;303:436–444.

10. Axelrod J, Weinshilboum R. Catecholamines. N Engl J Med 1972;287:237–242.

11. Badder EM, Santen R, Sasmojlik E, et al. Adrenal medullary epinephrine secretion: effects of cortisol alone and combined with aminoglutethimide. J Lab Med 1980;96:815–821.

12. Blaschko H. The specific action of L-dopa decarboxylase. J Physiol 1939;96:50P–51P.

13. Lefkowitz RJ, Hoffman BB, Taylor P. Neurohumoral transmission: the autonomic and somatic motor nervous systems. In: Gilman AG, Rall TW, Nies AS, et al, eds. Goodman and Gilman's: The Pharmacological Basis of Therapeutics, 8th Ed. New York: Pergamon Press, 1990:84–121.

14. Shell SR, Talamini MA, Udelsman R. Laparoscopic adrenalectomy for non-malignant disease: improved safety, morbidity and cost-effectiveness. Surg Endosc 1998;13:30–34.

15. Korobkin M, Brodeur FJ, Yutzy GG, et al. Differentiation of adrenal adenomas from nonadenomas using CT attenuation values. Am J Roentgenol 1996;166:531–536.

16. Lee MJ, Hahn PF, Papanicolaou N, et al. Benign and malignant adrenal masses: CT distinction with attenuation coefficients, size, and observer analysis. Radiology 1991;79:415–418.

17. Singer AA, Obuchowski NA, Einstein DM, et al. Metastasis or adenoma? Computed tomographic evaluation of the adrenal mass. Clevel Clin J Med 1994;18:432–438.

18. McNicholas MMJ, Lee MJ, Mayo-Smith WW, et al. An imaging algorithm for the differential diagnosis of adrenal adenomas and metastases. Am J Roentgenol 1995;165:1453–1459.

19. Boland GW, Hahn PF, Pena C, et al. Adrenal masses: characterization with delayed contrast-enhanced CT. Radiology 1997;202:693–696.

20. Thrall JH, Freitas JE, Beierwaltes WH. Adrenal scintigraphy. Semin Nucl Med 1978;8(1):23–41.

21. Herd GW, Semple PF, Parker D, et al. False localization of an aldosteronoma by dexamethasone-suppressed adrenal scintigraphy. Clin Endocrinol 1987;26(2):699–705.

22. Ackery DM, Tippett P, Condon B, et al. New approach to the localization of pheochromocytoma: imaging with 131-I-MIBG. Br Med J 1984;288:1587–1599.

23. Sisson JC, Frager MS, Balk TW, et al. Scintigraphic localization of pheochromocytoma. N Engl J Med 1981;305:12–17.

24. Arnold DR, Villemagne VI, Civelek AC, et al. FDG PET scan: a sensitive tool for the localization of MIBG negative pelvic pheochromocytomas. Endocrinologist 1998;8:295–298.

25. Sosano H, Shizawa S, Nagura H. Adrenocortical cytopathology. Am J Clin Pathol 1995;104:161–166.

26. Moulton JS. CT of the adrenal glands. Semin Rotentgenol 1988;23:288–303.

27. Ross NS, Aron DC. Hormonal evaluation of the patient with an incidentally discovered adrenal mass. New Engl J Med 1990;323:1401–1405.

28. Osella G, Terzol M, Borretta G, et al. Endocrine evaluation of incidentally discovered adrenal masses (incidentalomas). J Clin Endocrinol Metab 1994;79:1532–1539.

29. Staren ED, Prinz RA. Selection of patients with adrenal incidentalomas for operation. Surg Clin North Am 1995;75:499–509.

30. Terzolo M, Osella G, Ali A, et al. Subclinical Cushing's syndrome in adrenal incidentaloma. Clin Endocrinol 1998;48:89–97.

31. Herrera MF, Grant Cs, van Heerden JA, et al. Incidentally discovered adrenal tumors: an institutional perspective. Surger (St. Louis) 1991;110:1014–1021.

32. Kasperlik-Zaluska AA, Roslonowska E, Slowinska-Srzednicka J, et al. Incidentally discovered adrenal mass (incidentaloma): investigation and management of 208 patients. Clin Endocrinol 1997;46:29–37.

33. Corry DB, Tuck ML. Secondary aldosteronism. Endocrinol Metab Clin North Am 1995;24:511–528.

34. Gröndal S, Hamberger B. Primary aldosteronism. Br J Surg 1992;79:484–485.

35. Blevins LS Jr, Wand GC. Primary aldosteronism: an endocrine perspective. Radiology 1992;184:599–600.

36. Biglieri EG, Irony I, Kater CE. Identification and implications of new types of mineralocorticoid hypertension. J Steroid Biochem 1989;32:199–204.

37. Irony I, Kater CE, Biglieri EG, et al. Correctable subsets of primary aldosteronism: primary adrenal hyperplasia and renin responsive adenoma. Am J Hypertens 1990;3:576–582.

38. Taylor W, Carroll D, Bethwaite P. Adrenal carcinoma presenting as Conn's syndrome. Aust NZ J Med 1997;27:201–202.

39. Obara T, Ito Y, Okamato T, et al. Risk factors associated with postoperative persistent hypertension in patients with primary aldosteronism. Surgery (St. Louis) 1992;112:987–993.

40. Grant C, Carpenter P, van Heerden JA, et al. Primary aldosteronism. Clinical management. Arch Surg 1984;119:585–590.

41. Young WF Jr, Klee GG. Primary aldosteronism: diagnostic evaluation. Endocrinol Metab Clin North Am 1988;14:367–395.

42. Young WF Jr. Primary aldosteronism: update on diagnosis and treatment. Endocrinologist 1997;7:213–221.

43. Vallotton MB. Primary aldosteronism. Part I. Diagnosis of primary hyperaldosteronism. Clin Endocrinol 1996;45:47–52.

44. Kem DC, Weinberger MH, Gomez-Sanchez CE, et al. Circadian rhythms of plasma aldosterone concentration in normal subjects and patients with primary aldosteronism. J Clin Invest 1973;52:2272–2277.

45. Hiramatsu K, Yamada T, Yukimura Y, et al. A screening test to identify aldosterone-producing adenoma by measuring plasma renin activity. Results in hypertensive patients. Arch Intern Med 1981;141:1589–1593.

46. Gordon RD. Primary aldosteronism. J Endocrinol Invest 1995;18:495–511.

47. Gomez-Sanchez CE. Primary aldosteronism and its variants. Cardiovasc Res 1998;37:8–13.

48. Holland O, Brown H, Kuhnert L, et al. Further evaluation of saline infusion for the diagnosis of primary aldosteronism. Hypertension 1984;6:717–723.

49. Streeten DHP, Tomyez N, Anderson GH. Reliability of screening methods for the diagnosis of primary aldosteronism. Am J Med 1979;67:403–413.

50. Udelsman R. Tumors of the adrenal cortex. In: Cameron JL, ed. Current Surgical Therapy, 6th Ed. St. Louis: Mosby, 1998:577–580.

51. Dunnick NR, Leight GS, Roubidoux MA, et al. CT in the diagnosis of primary aldosteronism: sensitivity in 29 patients. Am J Radiol 1993;160:321–324.

52. Go H, Takeda M, Takahashi H, et al. Laparoscopic adrenalectomy for primary aldosteronism: a new operative method. J Laparoendosc Surg 1993;3:455–459.

53. Gagner M, Lacroix A, Prinz RA, et al. Early experience with laparoscopic approach for adrenalectomy. Surgery (St. Louis) 1993; 114:1120–1125.

54. Takeda M, Go H, Imai T, et al. Laparoscopic adrenalectomy for primary aldosteronism: report of initial ten cases. Surgery (St. Louis) 1994;115:621–625.

55. Horgan S, Sinanan M, Helton S, et al. Use of laparoscopic techniques improves outcome from adrenalectomy. Am J Surg 1997; 173:371–374.

56. Nakada T, Kobota Y, Sasagawa I, et al. Therapeutic outcome of primary aldosteronism: adrenalectomy versus enucleation of aldosterone-producing adenoma. J Urol 1995;153:1775–1780.

57. Walz MK, Peitgen K, Saller B, et al. Subtotal adrenalectomy by the posterior retroperitoneoscopic approach. World J Surg 1998; 22:621–627.

58. Lo CY, Tam PC, Kung AWC, et al. Primary aldosteronism: results of surgical treatment. Ann Surg 1996;224:125–130.

59. Favia G, Lumachi F, Scarpa V, et al. Adrenalectomy in primary aldosteronism: a long-term follow-up study in 52 patients. World J Surg 1992;16:680–684.

60. Cushing H. The basophil adenomas of the pituitary body and their clinical manifestations (pituitary basophilism). Bull Johns Hopkins Hosp 1932;50:137–195.

61. Luton JP, Cerdas S, Billaud L, et al. Clinical features of adrenocortical carcinoma, prognostic factors, and the effect of mitotane therapy. N Engl J Med 1990;322:1195–1201.

62. Van Heerden JA, Young WF Jr, Grant CS, et al. Adrenal surgery for hypercorticalism—surgical aspects. Surgery (St. Louis) 1995; 117:466–472.

63. Favia G, Boscaro M, Lumachi F, et al. Role of bilateral adrenalectomy in Cushing's disease. World J Surg 1994;18:462–466.

64. O'Riordain DS, Farley DR, Young WF Jr, et al. Long-term outcome of bilateral adrenalectomy in patients with Cushing's syndrome. Surgery (St. Louis) 1994;116:1088–1094.

65. Gifford RW Jr, Manger WM, Bravo EL. Pheochromocytoma. Endocrinol Metab Clin North Am 1994;23:387–404.

66. Bravo EL, Gifford RW Jr. Pheochromocytoma: diagnosis, localization and management. N Engl J Med 1984;311:1298–1303.

67. Shapiro B, Gross MD. Pheochromocytoma. Crit Care Clin 1991; 7:1–20.

68. Grossman E, Goldstein DS, Hoffman A, et al. Glucagon and clonidine testing in the diagnosis of pheochromocytoma. Hypertension 1991;17:733–741.

69. Sioberg RJ, Simcic KJ, Kidd GS. The clinidine suppression test for pheochromocytoma: a review of its utility and pitfalls. Arch Intern Med 1992;152:1193–1197.

70. Malone MJ, Liberetino JA, Tsapatsaris NP, et al. Preoperative and surgical management of pheochromocytoma. Urol Clin North Am 1989;6:567–582.

71. Jovenich JJ. Anesthesia in adrenal surgery. Urol Clin North Am 1998;16:583–587.

72. Grant CS. Pheochromoytoma. In: Clark OH, Duh QY, eds. Textbook of Endocrine Surgery. Philadelphia: Saunders, 1997;513–522.

73. Averbuch SD, Steakley CS, Young RC, et al. Malignant pheochromocytoma: effective treatment with a combination of cyclophosphamine, vincristine, and dacarbazine. Ann Intern Med 1988;109:267–273.

74. Thompson NW, Allo MD, Shapiro B, et al. Extra-adrenal and metastatic pheochromocytoma: the role of ^{131}I meta-iodobenzylguanidine (^{131}I MIBG) in localization and management. World J Surg 1984;8:605–611.

75. Krempf M, Lumbroso J, Mornex R, et al. Use of m-[^{131}]iodobenzylguanidine in the treatment of malignant pheochromocytoma. J Clin Endocrinol Metab 1991;72:455–461.

76. Webb TA, Sheps SG, Carney JA. Differences between sporadic pheochromocytoma and pheochromocytoma in multiple endocrine neoplasia, type 2. Am J Surg Pathol 1980;4:121–126.

77. Van Heerden JA, Sizemore GW, Carney JA, et al. Surgical management of the adrenal glands in the multiple endocrine neoplasia type II syndrome. World J Surg 1984;8:612–621.

78. Ross N, Aron D. Hormonal evaluation of the patient with an incidentally discovered adrenal mass. N Engl J Med 1990;323: 1401–1405.

79. Gicquel C, Audin E, Lebove Y, et al. Adrenocortical carcinoma. Ann Oncol 1997;8:423–427.

80. Schteingart DE. Treating adrenal cancer. Endocrinologist 1992;2: 149–157.

81. King DR, Lack EE. Adrenal cortical carcinoma: a clinical and pathologic study in 49 cases. Cancer (Phila) 1979;44:239–244.

82. Icard P, Louvel A, Chapuis Y. Survival rates and prognostic factors in adrenocortical carcinoma. World J Surg 1992;16:753–758.

83. Schteingart DE, Motazedi A, Noonan RA, et al. Treatment of adrenal carcinomas. Arch Surg 1982;17:1142–1146.

84. Kasperlik-Zahuska AA, Migdalska BM, Zgliczynski S. Adrenocortical carcinoma: a clinical study and treatment results in 52 patients. Cancer (Phila) 1995;75:2587–2591.

85. Bergenstal DM, Hertz R, Lipsett MB, et al. Chemotherapy of adrenocortical cancer with o,p-DDD. Ann Intern Med 1960;53: 672–682.

86. Guz BV, Straffon RA, Novick AC. Operative approaches to the adrenal gland. Urol Clin North Am 1989;16:527–534.

87. Gonzalez-Serva L, Glenn JF. Adrenal surgical techniques. Urol Clin North Am 1977;4:327–336.

88. Raynor RW, Del Guercio LRM. The eleventh rib transcostal incision: an extrapleural, transperitoneal approach to the upper abdomen. Surgery (St. Louis) 1985;99:95–100.

89. Vaughan ED Jr, Phillips H. Modified posterior approach for right adrenalectomy. Surg Gynecol Obstet 1987;165:453–455.

90. Prinz RA. A comparison of laparoscopic and open adrenalectomies. Arch Surg 1995;130:489–494.

91. Gagner M. Laparoscopic adrenalectomy. Surg Clin North Am 1996;76(3):523–537.

92. Brunt LM, Doherty Gm, Norton JA, et al. Laparoscopic adrenalectomy compared to open adrenalectomy for benign adrenal neoplasms [see comments]. J Am Coll Surg 1996;183(1):1–10.

93. Takeda M, Go H, Imai T, Komeyama T, et al. Experience with 17 cases of laparoscopic adrenalectomy: use of ultrasonic aspirator and argon beam coagulator. J Urol 1994;152(3):902–905.

94. Go H, Takeda M, Imai T. Laparoscopic adrenalectomy for Cushing's syndrome: comparison with primary aldosteronism. Surgery (St. Louis) 1995;117:11–17.

95. Fletcher DR, Beiles CB, Hardy KJ. Laparoscopic adrenalectomy. Aust N Z J Surg 1994;64(6):427–430.

96. Gagner M, Lacroix A, Bolte E, et al. Laparoscopic adrenalectomy. The importance of a flank approach in the lateral decubitus position. Surg Endosc 1994;8(2):135–138.

97. Miccoli P, Iacconi P, Conte M, et al. Laparoscopic adrenalectomy. J Laparoendosc Surg 1995;5(4):221–226.

98. Ganger M, Pomp A, Heniford BT. Laparoscopic adrenalectomy. Ann Surg 1997;226:238–247.

99. Fernandez-Cruz L, Taura P, Saenz A, et al. Laparoscopic approach to pheochromocytoma: hemodynamic changes and catecholamine secretion. World J Surg 1996;20:762–768.

100. Duh QY, Siperstein AE, Clark OH, et al. Laparoscopic adrenalectomy. Comparison of the lateral and posterior approaches. Arch Surg 1996;13(8):870–875.

101. Guazzoni G, Montorsi F, Bergamaschi F, et al. Effectiveness and safety of laparoscopic adrenalectomy. J Urol 1994;152(5 pt 1):1375–1378.

102. Rutherford JC, Stowasser M, Tunny TJ, et al. Laparoscopic adrenalectomy. World J Surg 1996;20(7):758–760; discussion 761.

103. Thompson GB, Grant CS, can Heerden JA, et al. Laparoscopic versus open posterior adrenalectomy: a case-controlled study in 100 patients. Surgery (St. Louis) 1997;122:1132–1136.

104. Christy NP. Iatrogenic Cushing's syndrome. In: Christy NP, ed. The Human Adrenal Cortex. New York: Harper & Row, 1971: 395–425.

105. Kehlet H, Binder C. Adrenocortical function and clinical course during and after surgery in unsupplemented glucocorticoid treated patients. Br J Anaesth 1973;45:1043–1048.

106. Kehlet H. A rational approach to dosage and preparation of parenteral glucocorticoid substitution therapy during surgical procedures. Acta Anaesthesiol Scand 1975;19:260–264.

107. Symreng T, Karlberg E, Kageldal B, et al. Physiological cortisol substitution of long-term steroid-treated patients undergoing major surgery. Br J Anaesth 1981;53:949–953.

108. Guazzoni G, Montorsi F, Bocciardi A, et al. Transperitoneal laparoscopic versus open adrenalectomy for benign hyperfunctioning adrenal tumors: a comparative study. J Urol 1995;153:1597–1600.

109. MacGillivray DC, Shichman SJ, Ferrer SJ, et al. A comparison of open vs laparoscopic adrenalectomy. Surg Endosc 1996;10:987–990.

110. Vargas HI, Kavoussi LR, Bartlett DL, et al. Laparoscopic adrenalectomy: a new standard of care. Urology 1997;49:673–678.

111. Korman JE, Ho T, Hiatt JR, et al. Comparison of laparoscopic and open adrenalectomy. Am Surg 1997;63:908–912.

112. Linos DA, Stylopoulos N, Boukis M, et al. Anterior, posterior, or laparoscopic approach for the management of adrenal diseases? Am J Surg 197;173:120–125.

113. Winfeld HN, Hamilton BD, Brovo EL, et al. Laparoscopic adrenalectomy: the preferred choice? A comparison to open adrenalectomy. Am J Urol 1998;160:325–329.

30

Neuroendocrine Tumors of the Pancreas and Gastrointestinal Tract and Carcinoid Disease

James P. Dolan and Jeffrey A. Norton

The neuroendocrine and carcinoid tumors of the pancreas and gastrointestinal tract are a group of similar neoplasms that, although they may behave clinically and biochemically in different ways, share a number of common features. Although originally thought to be of neural crest origin, these cells are now considered to originate from embryonic endoderm.[1] They are capable of taking up and decarboxylating aromatic amines or their precursors, giving rise to the term APUD (amine precursor uptake and decarboxylation) cells or *apudomas*. This term has largely been replaced by their designation as neuroendocrine neoplasms of the gastrointestinal tract.[2]

Epidemiology

Neuroendocrine tumors of the gastrointestinal tract are uncommon. Functional tumors are reported to have a prevalence of 10 per million population.[3] The incidence of clinically significant neuroendocrine tumors is around 3.6 to 4 per million population per year.[3,4] Nonfunctional tumors account for 15% to 30% of all neuroendocrine tumors.[5] Insulinoma is the most common islet cell tumor, with an approximate prevalence of 4 per 5 million population per year.[6] Gastrinoma or PPomas are the most common malignant islet cell tumors. The incidence of gastrinomas is estimated to be 0.1 to 3 persons per million each year.[7,8] The remaining neuroendocrine tumors occur less frequently.

Embryology and Anatomy

The gut and its associated organs develop between the third and eighth week of embryonic life.[9] During this period, the three germ layers undergo differentiation and give rise to the tissues and organ systems unique to each. During the fourth week of development, when the body of the developing embryo folds, the somatic mesoderm expands ventrally to form the intraembryonic coelomic cavity. Suspended within this cavity by the dorsal mesentery is the endodermal-lined primitive gut. This endoderm forms the epithelial lining of the digestive tract as well as giving rise to the liver and pancreas.

The embryonic epithelium of the pancreatic ducts contains the basic cell types for the development of the cells of the endocrine pancreas. During the twelfth to sixteenth week of development, endocrine glands migrate from the ductal system and aggregate around capillaries to form isolated clumps of cells scattered throughout the exocrine glandular tissue. These collections are known as the *islets of Langerhans* and contain at least five different types of secretory cells, namely *alpha, beta, delta, F,* and *enterochromaffin cells*, which secrete glucagon, insulin, somatostatin, pancreatic polypeptide, and serotonin, respectively. The epithelium of the primitive gut also gives rise to a number of other neuroendocrine-secreting cells that have a varied distribution within the adult gastrointestinal tract. Unregulated or ectopic secretion of any of these endocrine or exocrine products may result in one of several tumor syndromes (Table 30.1).

Because the foregut is supplied by the celiac artery and the midgut by the superior mesenteric artery, the duodenum and pancreas are supplied by branches of both arteries. The main arterial blood supply of the body and tail of the pancreas is derived from branches of the splenic artery, which include the dorsal or superior pancreatic artery and the great pancreatic artery, both of which communicate by means of the inferior or transverse pancreatic artery. The transverse pancreatic artery also communicates with the superior mesenteric artery. The pancreatic head and uncinate process share a common blood supply with the duodenum, a fact that underlies the need for a pancreaticoduodenectomy for a tumor involving this area. Both are supplied by branches of the anterior and posterior pancreaticoduodenal artery, which originate as superior branches from the gastroduodenal artery and common hepatic artery and as inferior branches from the

TABLE 30.1. Distribution and Actions of the Common Neuroendocrine Cells and Enteric Neuropeptides Involved in Neuroendocrine Pathology.

Designation[a]	Cell type	Distribution	Product(s)	Active product	Target organs	Actions
B	β cell	Pancreas	Insulin	51aa polypeptide	Muscle Liver Other	Stimulate glucose uptake by muscle cells Stimulate hepatic glycogenesis Stimulates muscle protein synthesis Stimulates triglyceride deposition Inhibits hepatic gluconeogenesis
G IG	G cell	Stomach Duodenum Jejunum	Gastrin (? ACTH, met-enkephalin, GH)	17aa "little" and 34aa "big" polypeptide	Stomach Pancreas (small effect)	Stimulates parietal cell H^+ secretion, pepsinogen secretion, gastric mucosal growth
	α cell	Pancreas	Glucagon	Linear polypeptide	Liver Pancreas Heart	Stimulates gluconeogenesis, glycogenolysis, lipolysis and ketogenesis; increases blood glucose Stimulates growth hormone and insulin secretion and positive cardiac inotropy
D_1	? δ cell	Small bowel Colon Pancreas Gallbladder CNS	VIP	28aa polypeptide	GI tract Vasculature	Stimulates intestinal, pancreatic and bilary secretion GI smooth muscle relaxation Splanchnic vasodilatation
D	δ cells	Pancreas Pylorus Duodenum	Somatostatin	14aa and 28aa polypeptide		Inhibition of gastrin release, blockade of glucagon action on jejunum Inhibition of release of most GI and pancreatic hormones
$EC_{1,2,n}$	Enterochromaffin cells	Stomach Small bowel Large bowel CNS	Serotonin Substance P ? Leuenkephalin ? Others	Neuropeptide ? Polypeptide	Smooth muscle Nerve cells	Vasomotor disturbance (flushing, diarrhea, nausea, and vomiting) Bronchospasm Right-sided valvular endocardial fibrosis
PP	F cells ? Other islet cells	Pancreas	Pancreatic polypeptide	36aa polypeptide	Pancreas	Inhibits pancreatic exocrine secretion
N	N cells	Ileum Jejunum Duodenum Colon CNS	Neurotensin	Tridecapeptide	? GI tract	? Inhibition of gastric secretion ? Modulation of GI tract motility
PYY	?	Terminal ileum Colon Rectum	Peptide YY	36aa polypeptide	GI tract Pancreas	Inhibits autonomic neuro-transmission in GI tract and prolongs small-bowel transit time Inhibits pancreatic exocrine secretion
L	L cell	Small intestine Large intestine	Enteroglucagon	Variety of peptides	? Liver ? Pancreas	? Complete with, and have similar actions to, glucagon
X	? Islet cell	Pancreas Lung Small intestines	Growth hormone-releasing factor (GRF)	Polypeptide	Bone Muscle Other	Stimulation of growth hormone release
	? Islet cell	Pancreas ? Other	ACTH	39aa polypeptide	Adrenal	Stimulation of release of glucocorticoids, mineralo-corticoids and androgenic steroids from adrenal cortex

aa, amino acid.

[a]Designations from O'Briain and Duyal (1981).[128]

superior mesenteric artery. The supraduodenal artery, the first branch of the gastroduodenal artery, provides additional arterial supply to the first part of the duodenum.

Neuroendocrine Tumors and the MEN-1 Syndrome

The multiple endocrine neoplasia syndromes (MEN) are a fascinating group of endocrine syndromes first reported by Wermer in 1963.[10] MEN-1 (Wermer's syndrome) describes a wide range of pathology including parathyroid hyperplasia, pituitary adenoma, and endocrine tumors of the duodenum and pancreas. MEN-1 patients may also develop multiple subcutaneous lipomas, adenomas of the thyroid gland, and adrenocortical adenomas or carcinoma. This familial disease has an autosomal dominant mode of transmission with incomplete penetrance. The initial manifestation of MEN-1 is primarily hyperparathyroidism.

Neuroendocrine tumors in patients with MEN-1 are characteristically multiple and often small.[6,11,12] Depending on the particular tumor, they may also have an increased propensity to occur at extrapancreatic sites and may be difficult to localize radiologically. The management of neuroendocrine tumors in the setting of MEN-1 is dependent on the clinical syndrome that results from hormone overproduction.[11] In general, surgical resection is the treatment of choice for insulinoma, glucagonoma and VIPoma, whereas the treatment for gastrinoma (medical versus surgical) is controversial. Nonfunctioning neuroendocrine tumors, which produce no symptoms, are generally treated surgically only in situations where the tumor is clearly imaged (2–3 cm) or when complications such as obstruction arise. Overall, the surgical treatment of a given tumor, when it occurs in the MEN-1 setting, is less successful than treatment of the same tumor when it occurs sporadically.[11]

Neuroendocrine Tumors

Insulinoma

Insulinoma is the most common pancreatic islet cell tumor. The mean age of patients with insulinoma is 45 years and the female to male ratio is around 1.5 to 2:1.[4,13] It generally occurs at a younger age in the context of MEN-1, in which patients usually present in the third decade of life.

TUMOR CHARACTERISTICS

Approximately 80% to 90% of insulinomas are small (<2 cm), solitary, benign tumors distributed with equal probability among the head, body, and tail of the pancreas. Approximately 5% to 10% occur as multiple islet cell tumors in the setting of MEN-1.[6,14] The presence of diffuse microadenomatosis, in which multiple small nonencapsulated tumors or nodules are distributed throughout the pancreas (nesidioblastosis), may occur in the neonatal and infant setting and cause neonatal hypoglycemia.

Most benign insulinomas are between 0.5 and 2 cm in diameter. Tumors appear reddish brown in color due to in-

creased vascularity. Microscopic examination cannot distinguish between benign and malignant insulinomas, although malignant lesions tend to be larger with an average size of 6.2 cm. The diagnosis of malignancy is made at the time of surgery by the identification of either lymph node or liver metastases.

PRESENTING SYMPTOMS AND SIGNS

In almost all cases, patients with insulinoma have symptoms that are caused by hypoglycemia, with rare cases causing symptoms due to the size of the tumor itself (see Table 30.2). Most commonly, patients have neuroglycopenic symptoms that include seizures, difficulty awakening, visual disturbances, confusion, lethargy, weakness, or transient motor deficits.[6,12] Hypoglycemia also causes catecholamine release with subsequent sympathetic discharge resulting in sweating, anxiety, and palpitations.[6] Erroneous psychiatric or neurological diagnoses are common and, on average, it may take up to 2 years before the correct diagnosis is made.[12,15] Symptoms tend to occur early in the morning after an overnight fast or during periods of fasting for religious or other observances. Patients come to learn that food relieves or avoids symptoms and thus most gain weight. A family history of hypoglycemia or other endocrine abnormalities should be sought to exclude the presence of MEN-1.

DIAGNOSIS

The measurement of severe hypoglycemia and inappropriately elevated levels of insulin is essential for the diagnosis (Table 30.2). Before the development of laboratory techniques to measure serum insulin levels, Whipple proposed the diagnostic triad of symptomatic hypoglycemia induced by fasting, a blood glucose level less than 45 mg/dl, and prompt relief of symptoms following administration of glucose.[16] Since that time, the development of a sensitive radioimmunoassay for serum insulin as well as several suppression and stimulation tests have simplified the diagnosis of insulinoma.[12,17] The diagnostic test of choice is a 72-h fast during which serum levels of glucose and insulin are measured every 6 h.[18,19] The fast is terminated at 72 h or when the patient develops neuroglycopenic symptoms. At that point serum levels of glucose, insulin, C-peptide, and proinsulin are measured and intravenous glucose administered.

In interpreting laboratory results it is important to understand the usual components of insulin secretion. Insulin is secreted from cells in secretory granules that contain both the inactive, or proinsulin, form of the hormone as well as a protease that cleaves the terminal C-peptide sequence of the molecule. This cleavage yields both active insulin as well as inactive C-peptide fragments in equimolar amounts. Patients with an insulinoma have an immunoreactive insulin to glucose ratio greater than 0.3 and an elevated serum level of proinsulin. These values are not found in normal individuals or in patients with factitious hypoglycemia. If factitious hypoglycemia is caused by the administration of exogenous insulin, appreciable amounts of C-peptide will not be detected and the proinsulin to insulin ratio is generally low. Urinary sulfonylurea and serum insulin antibodies should not be detectable (Table 30.3).

TABLE 30.2. Common Symptoms and Signs of the Main Neuroendocrine Tumor Syndromes.

Tumor	Syndrome	Main hormone(s)	Symptoms	Signs	Diagnostic study	Diagnostic criteria
Insulinoma	Insulinoma	Insulin	Neuro-glycopenic	Somnolence Seizures Coma Diaphoresis Tremulousness	Supervised 72-h fast	Serum glucose <45 mg/dl Serum insulin >5 μU/ml C-peptide >1.2 ng/ml Proinsulin >25%
Gastrinoma	Zollinger-Ellison	Gastrin	Heartburn Dysphagia Diarrhea	Peptic ulceration Esophagitis or strictures Weight loss	Serum gastrin Basal acid output (BAO) Secretin stimulation test	Serum gastrin >100 pg/ml BAO >15 mEq/h (>5 mEq/hr if prior operation for peptic ulcers) >200 pg/ml increase in gastrin levels after secretin stimulation
Glucagonoma	Glucagonoma	Glucagon	Skin rash Diarrhea Abdominal pain	Diabetes mellitus type II Weight loss/cachexia Venous thrombosis Pulmonary emboli	Fasting plasma glucagon Plasma amino acids	Plasma glucagon >500 pg/ml Decreased plasma amino acids
VIPoma	Verner-Morrison Pancreatic cholera Endocrine cholera WDHA	Vasoactive intestinal peptide (VIP)	Secretory diarrhea Abdominal colic Flushing	Hypokalemia Dehydration Weight loss	Serum potassium Fasting plasma VIP	Plasma VIP >500 pg/ml (potassium <2.5 mmol/l)
Somato-statinoma	Somato-statinoma	Somatostatin	Diarrhea Abdominal pain	Diabetes mellitus type II Cholelithiasis Steatorrhea Weight loss Hypochlorhydria	Fasting plasma somatostatin	Elevated plasma somatostatin
GRFoma	GRFoma	Growth hormone-releasing factor (GRF)		Acromegaly	Fasting Plasma GRF	Elevated plasma GRF
ACTHoma	Cushing's	Adrenocortico-tropic hormone (ACTH)	Easy bruisability Atrophied skin	Hypertension Centripetal obesity Skin/mucosal pigmentation	Urinary free cortisol Plasma ACTH Dexamethasone suppression test	Elevated urinary cortisol Elevated plasma ACTH Failure to suppress with dexamethasone
Neuro-tensinoma	Neuro-tensinoma	Neurotensin	Tachycardia Flushing Diarrhea	Hypotension Malabsorption Weight loss Cyanosis Diabetes mellitus	Fasting plasma neurotensin	Elevated plasma neurotensin
PTH-RPoma	PTH-RPoma	Parathyroid hormone-related peptide (PTH-RP)	Bone pain Renal colic Weakness	Decreased bone density Pathological fractures Nephrolithiasis Pseudogout Peptic ulcers Pancreatitis	Serum calcium Serum PTH Serum PTH-related peptide	Elevated serum calcium Low or nondetectable serum PTH Elevated serum PTH-related peptide
Nonfunctional	None	Neuron-specific enolase Pancreatic poly-peptide Chromogranin A	Abdominal pain Weakness Palpated mass	Bowel obstruction Gastrointestinal bleeding/anemia jaundice	None	Radiologic imaging
Carcinoid	Carcinoid	5-HT 5-HTP	Diarrhea Flushing Wheezing Pain	Flushing rash Anemia Bowel obstruction Recurrent pneumonia Heart failure Pellagra	Urinary 5-HIAA Urinary 5-HT Platelet 5-HT	Elevated urinary 5-HIAA Elevated urinary 5-HT Increased platelet 5-HT

Sources: Norton (1998)[6]; Meko and Norton (1994)[7]; Feldman (1989)[75]; Norheim et al. (1987)[129]; Thorson (1958).[130]

TABLE 30.3. Interpretation of Biochemical Studies in the Diagnosis of Insulinoma.

Patient type	Serum glucose (mg/dl)	Serum insulin (μU/ml)	Proinsulin (%)	C-peptide (ng/ml)	Antibodies to insulin	Sulfonylurea (blood or urine)
Normal	80–100	2–10	12–20	0.5–1	Absent	Absent
Insulinoma	<45	>5	>25	>1.2	Absent	Absent
Factitious hypoglycemia	<45	>5	12–20	≤0.5	Present	Present

LOCALIZATION

Because insulinomas are usually small and lack a high density of somatostatin receptors, the results of conventional, noninvasive, radiographic imaging studies are poor. Computed tomography, magnetic resonance imaging, and ultrasound identify only 17% to 26% of tumors. However, either MR or CT should be obtained to exclude liver metastases or the presence of a large malignant primary tumor.

Endoscopic ultrasound (EUS), is observer-dependent and is not available in all centers, but it has been found to have a sensitivity of 80% to 85% and a specificity of 95% in identifying intrapancreatic neuroendocrine tumors.[7] However, EUS cannot reliably localize extrapancreatic disease.[7,20]

Portal venous sampling (PVS) for insulin and the newer intraarterial calcium angiogram are invasive studies that may help with pancreatic regional localization. The latter of the two is currently favored, and has the potential to image tumor based on a characteristic vascular "blush." In general, if the surgeon wants confirmation of the pancreatic region within which the insulinoma is contained, calcium angiogram is the preoperative invasive study of choice.[19,21]

The single best modality in localizing insulinomas during surgery is intraoperative ultrasound (IOUS).[22,23] It is now apparent that surgical exploration with exposure and palpation of the pancreas combined with the use of IOUS is the most cost-effective therapy for insulinomas, even when other preoperative studies are negative (see Table 30.4).

Gastrinoma

It was Zollinger and Ellison who first reported the unusual occurrence of jejunal peptic ulcer disease in association with gastric acid hypersecretion and islet cell tumors of the pancreas.[24] We now know that the Zollinger–Ellison syndrome (ZES) is caused by a pancreatic or duodenal neuroendocrine tumor called a *gastrinoma* that elaborates excessive and unregulated amounts of the hormone gastrin which stimulates gastric acid secretion leading to peptic ulcer disease.

ZES is a functional neuroendocrine tumor syndrome. In 80% of cases it occurs in a sporadic form, while the familial or inherited form occurs in 20% of cases.[8,23] The familial form is associated with the multiple endocrine neoplasia type 1 (MEN-1) syndrome and, within this setting, most functional neuroendocrine tumors are gastrinomas.[11] ZES is the underlying cause in approximately 0.1% to 1% of patients with peptic ulcer disease.[25] Gastrinomas are slow growing but approximately 60% are malignant, with patients having lymph node, liver, or distant metastatic disease at diagnosis.[26]

The mean age at diagnosis of ZES is 50 years, although children as young as 7 years and adults as old as 90 have been reported. There is a slight male preponderance with a male to female ratio of approximately 2:1. In patients with the MEN-1 syndrome, ZES is usually diagnosed in the third decade of life.[26]

TUMOR CHARACTERISTICS

Gastrinomas may be single or multiple and may range in size from less than 1 cm to more than 3 cm. Multiple duodenal or pancreatic tumors are found in patients with the MEN-1 syndrome.[27,28] Although it has been suggested that the tumors found in MEN-1 patients may have a lower potential for metastases, they appear to metastasize with a similar frequency to their sporadic counterparts when evaluated in long-term follow-up.

Approximately 80% of gastrinomas are found within the *gastrinoma triangle*, an area that includes the first, second, and third portion of the duodenum and the head of the pancreas.[29] Although rare, primary gastrinomas have also been found in the jejunum, stomach, liver, spleen, mesentery, ovary, and heart.[30,31]

PRESENTING SYMPTOMS AND SIGNS

Clinical manifestations of the syndrome are related to the excessive secretion of gastric acid (see Table 30.2). The most common symptoms are epigastric pain, heartburn, diarrhea, and dysphagia. Approximately 90% of patients with ZES are found to have peptic ulceration, with the proximal duodenum as the most commonly involved site.[32] In 7% to 10% of patients, a perforated peptic ulcer may be the initial sign of the disease.[33] Gastric acid hypersecretion also leads to a secretory diarrhea, which is seen in up to 40% of patients with ZES, and may be the sole presenting complaint in 20% of individuals.[26] As the tumor develops and metastases occur, symptoms may be related to the size of the tumor itself.

DIAGNOSIS

In most cases, the diagnosis of ZES is not immediately considered. Many series report a mean period of 6 years from presentation of symptoms to diagnosis.[8] This delay may be the consequence of a number of factors. First, hypergastrinemia may occur as a manifestation of other diseases or conditions, most of which do not lead to excessive gastric acid secretion and ulcer formation (Table 30.5). Second, because ZES is rare and few clinicians have seen many cases, there may be a failure to consider the diagnosis of ZES initially.

ZES can be accurately diagnosed in all patients by measurement of an elevated fasting serum level of gastrin and an elevated basal acid output (BAO) (see Table 30.2). Patients should be off all antisecretory medications (H$_2$-receptor antagonists and proton pump inhibitors) for 3 to 7 days before the determination because medications that reduce gastric acid secretion cause a false elevation of serum gastrin levels. 100% of patients with ZES have a fasting serum gastrin level greater than 100 pg/ml.[26] A BAO greater than 15 mEq/h in most patients and above 5 mEq/h in patients with prior acid-reduction operations, in conjunction with an elevated fasting gastrin level, unequivocally establishes the diagnosis. If the

TABLE 30.4.
Outcome of Various Preoperative Localization Studies for Neuroendocrine Tumors.

Reference	Level of evidence[a]	n	MEN	True positive/total (%)									
				US	CT	MRI	SRS	PVS	Angiography	Provocative angiography	EUS	IOUS	Palpation
Insulinoma													
Norton et al. (1992)[62]	II	8	0									6/8 (75)	5/8 (63)
Böttger et al. (1990)[131]	III	43	1	13/21 (62)	11/15 (73)			10/13 (77)	20/30 (67)			12/16 (75)	40/42 (95)
Norton et al. (1990)[22]	II	12	0					9/12 (75)				10/12 (83)	5/12 (42)
Doherty et al. (1991)[57]	II	25	0	6/22 (27)	4/22 (18)	2/22 (9)		17/22 (77)	9/22 (41)			22/24 (92)	16/24 (67)
Kisker et al. (1997)[54]	II	6	0	4/6 (67)	4/6 (67)		0/6 (0)						
Brown et al. (1997)[132]	II	36	5	4/31 (13)	8/34 (24)	15/33 (45)	1/6 (17)		13/30 (43)	29/31 (94)		12/14 (86)	22/27 (81)
Lo et al. (1997)[59]	II	27	1	2/6 (33)	11/25 (44)			2/3 (67)	11/21 (52)	7/7 (100)	1/3 (33)	17/17 (100)	
Boukhman et al. (1998)[56]	III	67	11	4/6 (67)	13/35 (37)	6/14 (43)		7/10 (70)	14/30 (47)			9/11 (82)	42/56 (75)
Gastrinoma													
Norton et al. (1988)[63]	II	39	0									29/35 (83)	33/35 (94)
Kisker et al. (1997)[52]	II	17	NR	7/17 (41)	7/17 (41)		9/17 (53)						15/17 (88)
Cohen et al. (1997)[133]	II	8	4		2/8 (25)		1/3 (33)		7/9 (78)	8/9 (89)			
Krausz et al. (1998)[55]	II	5	0		2/5 (40)		4/5 (80)						
Alexander et al. (1998)[39]	II	37	4	6/37 (16)	18/37 (49)	21/37 (57)	29/37 (78)		21/37 (57)				
Kisker et al. (1998)[134]	II	25	2	11/25 (44)	14/25 (56)	1/4 (25)	9/17 (53)		1/10 (10)		4/6 (67)	14/15 (93)	24/25 (96)
Other NETs													
Krausz et al. (1998)[55]	II	6	NR		4/6 (67)		5/6 (83)						
Carcinoid													
Kisker et al. (1996)[93]	II	22	NR	8/22 (36)	12/22 (55)		9/22 (41)						11/11 (100)
Krausz et al. (1998)[55]	II	23	0	4/9 (44)	4/9 (44)		3/9 (33)						

aI, prospective, randomized; II, prospective; III, retrospective, review or anecdotal; NR, not reported.
Other NETs (neuroendocrine tumors): glucagonoma (n = 3), somatostatinoma (n = 1), VIPoma (n = 1), PTH-Rpoma (n = 1).

TABLE 30.5. Differential Diagnoses of Hypergastrinemia.

With excessive gastric acid secretion (ulcerogenic):
  ZES (Zollinger–Ellison syndrome)
  Gastric outlet obstruction
  Retained gastric antrum (after Bilroth II reconstruction)
  G-cell hyperplasia
  Medications for peptic ulcers or GERD (H_2 receptor antagonists
    or proton pump inhibitors)

No excessive gastric acid secretion (nonulcerogenic):
  Pernicious anemia
  Atrophic gastritis
  Renal failure
  Postvagotomy
  Short gut syndrome (after significant intestinal resection)

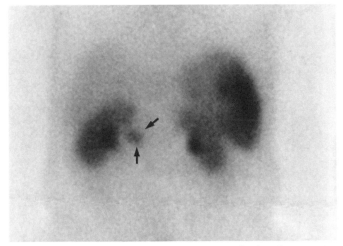

FIGURE 30.1. Somatostatin receptor scintigraphy (SRS) in a patient with Zollinger–Ellison syndrome (ZES) shows signal uptake in a lesion that is consistent with a gastrinoma (*arrows*) within the area of the gastrinoma triangle. On exploration, the lesion was found in the wall of the duodenum.

diagnosis remains uncertain, the secretin stimulation test is the test of choice as it has a sensitivity of 85% or greater.[34] Using this test, a 2 U/kg bolus of secretin is given intravenously, and serum levels of gastrin are measured before and at 2, 5, 10, and 15 min after administration. An increase of 200 pg/ml in the serum gastrin level following secretin administration is consistent with a diagnosis of ZES. This test may be of particular utility in patients who have undergone prior operations to reduce acid output.

RADIOLOGIC LOCALIZATION

As a first-line study, ultrasound has a sensitivity no greater than 30% but its specificity approaches 92%.[35] The accuracy of CT scanning is dependent on the size of the gastrinoma.[26,36] Tumors less than 1 cm in size are rarely visualized. Overall, CT imaging can identify approximately 80% of pancreatic and 35% of extrahepatic gastrinomas.[36] MRI is expensive and, on the basis of most studies, images only about 25% of primary gastrinomas.[35] EUS has a sensitivity of 50–75%, but is highly operator-dependent.

Somatostatin receptor scintigraphy (SRS) was first evaluated in 1993,[37] and is now regarded as the imaging test of choice for localizing both primary and metastatic gastrinomas (Fig. 30.1). 90% of tumors can be imaged by this modality with a specificity approaching 100%.[38] In the setting of ZES, when clinical suspicion of gastrinoma is high, it has a positive predictive value of 100% and can have a sensitivity exceeding all other imaging studies combined.[38,39] However, it still may be unable to identify small primary duodenal gastrinomas.

Invasive studies, such as PVS for gastrin and intraarterial secretion injections, have largely been supplanted by SRS.

Intraoperative studies, such as intraoperative ultrasound IOUS and intraoperative endoscopy (IOE), with and without transillumination, have proven utility.[40]

Other Neuroendocrine Tumors

GLUCAGONOMA

Glucagonoma is a malignant pancreatic islet cell tumor that usually presents during the fifth or sixth decade of life; 16% of cases occur in those less than 40 years old.[41] Patients have a characteristic raised red pruritic rash called necrolytic migratory erythema (NME) that typically involves the pretibial, perioral, and intertriginous areas. It is seen in approximately 64% to 90% of patients. Patients also have severe hypo-

aminoacidemia, weight loss, type 2 diabetes mellitus, and marked muscle wasting or cachexia (see Table 30.2).

NME can precede diagnosis or suspicion of a glucagonoma for many years, leading to patients being treated for dermatological findings. The biochemical diagnosis of glucagonoma is made by measuring elevated plasma levels of glucagon (>500 pg/ml) and decreased plasma levels of amino acids (Table 30.2). Because the cachexia is so severe, most patients are initially managed by total parenteral nutrition (TPN) with supplemental zinc, trace metals, and insulin. Long-term management of patients with metastatic glucagonoma has relied on the use of octreotide, which can reduce circulating plasma levels of glucagon and improve the rash and malnutrition.[42] At the time of diagnosis, most tumors are large (average size, 5–10 cm) and either locally advanced or metastatic and unresectable. For this reason, surgery for glucagonoma is seldom curative.[43]

VASOACTIVE INTESTINAL PEPTIDE TUMOR (VIPOMA)

The VIPoma syndrome was first reported by Verner and Morrison in 1958[44] and came to bear their names. Because of the associated severe diarrhea, it is also referred to as the pancreatic cholera syndrome,[45] endocrine cholera syndrome,[46] or WHDA (watery diarrhea, hypokalemia, and achlorhydria) syndrome.[47] The mean age at diagnosis is 50 years, and there is a slight female preponderance.[46,48]

VIPomas induce a severe secretory diarrhea, a form of diarrhea that is defined by persistence despite abstaining from oral intake. This leads to hypokalemia, hypochlorhydria, hypovolemia, and dehydration (Table 30.2). Patients with VIPoma commonly have 5 to 10 L of stool output per day and report abdominal cramping and flushing. Approximately 85% to 90% of VIPomas arise within the pancreas, but extrapancreatic duodenal VIPomas have also been described.[12,49] Elevated serum levels of pancreatic polypeptide have been used to distinguish pancreatic VIPomas from extrapancreatic tumors.[48] In children, a ganglioneuroma or ganglioneuroblastoma may also produce the syndrome.[49] The diagnosis of VIPoma is made when fasting plasma levels of vasoactive intestinal polypeptide (VIP) are above 500 pg/ml in the presence of secretory diarrhea (Table 30.2).

Because of the severe dehydration and electrolyte abnormalities, it is necessary to correct these abnormalities before surgery. Octreotide dramatically reduces serum VIP levels and secretory diarrhea in more than 80% of patients and greatly simplifies fluid and electrolyte resuscitation before surgery.[42,46] Although these tumors are malignant, surgery is often effective.

SOMATOSTINOMA

Somatostatinomas[50] are very rare malignant neuroendocrine tumors that arise in either the duodenum or pancreas. Pancreatic tumors are seen in about 50% of cases, and duodenal tumors may be associated with von Recklinghausen's disease. The somatostatinoma syndrome includes steatorrhea, cholelithiasis, diabetes mellitus type 2, and hypochlorhydria (Table 30.2). The mean age at presentation is 51 to 53 years.[51] Somatostatin-like activity can be measured by immunological assays and is the key to the diagnosis (Table 30.2). Most patients have unresectable metastatic tumor at the time of diagnosis.

NONFUNCTIONING ISLET CELL TUMORS

Nonfunctioning islet cell tumors or pancreatic polypeptide-producing tumors (PPoma) do not have a clinical syndrome related to the excessive hormone secretion.[6] These tumors usually present during the fourth or fifth decade of life.[51] They are usually malignant and large at the time of clinical diagnosis and produce symptoms secondary to the mass effects of the tumor. Most of these tumors are resectable but they often require pancreaticoduodenectomy (Whipple resection) or subtotal pancreatectomy.[52]

RARE ISLET CELL TUMORS

Islet cell tumors have been found to cause severe hypercalcemia secondary to parathyroid hormone–related peptide, Cushing's syndrome secondary to ectopic adrenocorticotropic hormone (ACTH) production, and acromegaly secondary to GRF production. Cushing's syndrome has been reported in a small number of ZES patients as the result of concomitant elaboration of ACTH.[53]

RADIOLOGIC LOCALIZATION OF RARE ISLET CELL TUMORS

Radiologic localization of the less frequent islet cell tumors such as somatostatinoma, VIPoma, glucagonoma, PPoma, and nonfunctional tumors is relatively simple. In contrast to insulinomas or gastrinomas, virtually all these tumors will be visible with current CT imaging. Somatostatin receptor scintigraphy (SRS) should also be used for these patients to detect occult distant metastases and to determine if the tumor has functional somatostatin receptors.[54] Approximately 80% to 90% of these rare islet cell tumors will image on octreoscan.[15,54,55] If an individual tumor can be detected by this modality, the hormonal syndrome will usually respond to octreotide.

Treatment of Neuroendocrine Tumors

Insulinoma

MEDICAL MANAGEMENT

Medical management is the initial treatment of patients diagnosed with insulinoma (Table 30.5).

SURGICAL MANAGEMENT

Surgery is the only curative treatment for patients with an insulinoma.[13,22,56,57] Often, medical control of the hypoglycemia is unsatisfactory, placing more emphasis on a successful surgical outcome. The presence of MEN-1 should be excluded by testing for other components of the syndrome, which may include primary hyperparathyroidism, nephrolithiasis, and the presence of other endocrine or pituitary tumors.[58]

Enucleation is the preferred surgical treatment for insulinoma[23] because most tumors are solitary and benign. IOUS is critical during surgery for insulinoma as it facilitates both identification and removal of these tumors. Occasionally, the surgeon is unable to remove these tumors by enucleation. In this case, lesions are resected by either distal pancreatectomy or Whipple pancreaticoduodenectomy. Many large series from different institutions have demonstrated that more than 90% of patients can have successful surgery with correction of the hypoglycemia.[22,57,59]

Gastrinoma

MEDICAL MANAGEMENT

With the advent of histamine H_2-receptor antagonists and, more importantly, proton pump inhibitors, all patients can experience control of acid hypersecretion and complete relief of symptoms (Table 30.6). Omeprazole and lansoprazole block gastric acid secretion by inhibiting the parietal cell apical H^+–K^+-ATPase. H_2-receptor antagonists are also effective, but progressively higher doses may be required to control

TABLE 30.6. Medical and Preoperative Treatment Modalities for Neuroendocrine Tumors.

Tumor	Treatment
Insulinoma	Frequent small meals
	Cornstarch
	Diazoxide
	Verapamil
	Octreotide
	Propanolol
	Phenytoin
Gastrinoma	Omeprazole or lansoprazole
	H_2-receptor antagonists
Glucagonoma	Octreotide
	Total parenteral nutrition with added trace elements
	Diabetes control
VIPoma	Octreotide
Somatostatinoma	Octreotide
	Fluids
	Diabetes control
PTH-RPoma	Fluids
	Lasix
	Mitramycin
	Diphosphonates
ACTHoma	Ketoconazole
	Aminoglutethimide
	Mifepristone
GRFoma	Octreotide
Carcinoid	Octreotide

symptoms. They may be associated with a long-term failure rate, making proton pump inhibitors the current drugs of choice. Periodic gastric surveillance endoscopy should be performed on all patients treated with proton pump inhibitors for long periods.

SURGICAL MANAGEMENT

Medical control of acid hypersecretion obviates the need for total gastrectomy.[26,60] Based on the results of a number of long-term studies, the malignant potential of the tumor itself is the main determinant of long-term survival.[29,61,62] Because of this, all patients with sporadic gastrinoma are candidates for tumor localization and surgery. The goals of surgery are twofold: resection of primary tumor for potential cure and prevention of malignant progression. In patients with the MEN-1 and primary hyperparathyroidism (HPT), it has been shown that successful neck exploration for resection of parathyroid hyperplasia can significantly lessen the end-organ effects of hypergastrinemia. Therefore, in patients with MEN-1 who have HPT in conjunction with ZES, neck exploration and subtotal or 4-gland parathyroidectomy with autotransplantation should be performed before attempting gastrinoma resection.[58]

At surgery, a tumor will be found in approximately 95% of sporadic gastrinoma patients, and 14% to 58% of patients will be cured immediately following resection.[11,63] The long-term cure rate, with surgery, is 34% to 81%. In patients with MEN-1 and gastrinoma; however, the identification of all tumor foci is imprecise, and surgery results in a significantly lower cure rate.[28,64]

Other Islet Cell Tumors

MEDICAL MANAGEMENT

Medical therapy may be used to control the signs and symptoms of excessive hormonal secretion, but it will seldom control the tumoral process (Table 30.5). Medical therapy is not curative, but it can provide symptomatic relief.

SURGICAL MANAGEMENT

Overall, surgical resection is the only potentially curative therapy for patients with islet cell tumors.[6,12] In general, surgery is indicated for all patients with islet cell tumors in whom all tumors can be imaged and removed with acceptable morbidity and mortality. Debulking surgery may also be indicated in any patient with a large tumor burden or metastatic disease in whom medical treatment does not control hormonal symptoms.[7] Similarly, other procedures such as bilateral adrenalectomy may be indicated because of the inability to effectively treat symptoms.[65]

In patients with MEN-1 and concomitant neuroendocrine tumors, resection should be pursued if the tumors are larger than 2 cm because size correlates with increased malignant potential. The major consideration in dealing with the tumors found in the setting of MEN-1 is that these tumors are usually multiple and it may be unclear which exact tumor is responsible for the excessive hormone production.[14] However, most patients will have a large dominant tumor that may be responsible for most, if not all, the symptoms.[23] Therefore,

in MEN-1 patients, surgery should be attempted for all large pancreatic islet cell tumors that are detected by conventional studies.

Metastatic Disease

Malignant Insulinoma

Surgery in patients with malignant insulinoma may be curative, but only if all tumor can be completely removed.[23,66] Resection of all identifiable tumor appears to improve survival and may even cure a subset of patients. Debulking and/or ablation may also lessen the signs and symptoms of hypoglycemia, especially in patients who do not respond adequately to medical management. Aggressive surgery may also be indicated in instances in which the tumor causes gastrointestinal hemorrhage or biliary or intestinal obstruction.

Chemotherapy for metastatic insulinoma has been largely ineffective. Chemoembolization, a combination of simultaneous hepatic artery occlusion and chemotherapy, has had some significant antitumor responses and may also be used to ameliorate symptoms.[67] However, side effects and complications may occur including life-threatening liver abscesses. Alcohol injection, radiofrequency ablation, and cryotherapy have also been used in the treatment of metastatic insulinoma without clear benefit, but can control individual lesions.

Malignant Gastrinoma

With successful control of gastric acid hypersecretion and the indolent growth pattern of the gastrinoma, distant metastatic disease becomes the most important determinant of mortality. The 5-year survival for patients with metastasis disease is, on average, approximately 40%.[26] Chemotherapy has been utilized in the treatment of metastatic gastrinomas but does not prolong survival. A combination of doxorubicin, 5-fluorouracil, and streptozotocin provides a 40% partial response rate but no survival benefit or complete responses.[68] Likewise, hepatic artery chemoembolization has minimal, and transient, efficacy and the use of octreotide or alpha-interferon as antitumor agents has also shown little effect on the malignant process.[69]

Surgery remains the major effective treatment for metastatic gastrinoma. Aggressive surgery in appropriate patients with hepatic metastases seems to demonstrate a survival advantage. Furthermore, although studies are ongoing, it appears that, even in those patients with unresectable disease, hepatic cryosurgery or radiofrequency ablation may serve to reduce symptoms, control tumor and prolong survival.

Other Islet Cell Tumors

Chemotherapy has been used in the treatment of metastatic islet cell tumors, with 40% partial but few documented complete responses.[68] Recently, chemoembolization, with simultaneous hepatic artery occlusion and doxorubicin infusion, has had dramatic antitumor responses in individuals with large hepatic tumor volumes.[67] However, side effects have been reported and complications may occur. Intralesional alcohol injection and cryotherapy have been also been used in a few patients without clear benefit.

Surgical Techniques

Enucleation of Insulinoma

Because insulinomas are usually benign, small, and uniformly distributed throughout the pancreas, the goal of surgery is precise localization of tumor and excision with preservation of normal pancreas and spleen. At the time of surgery, the pancreas is fully exposed to allow complete palpation and inspection of the gland. IOUS is performed with a high-resolution real-time transducer (7.5–10 MHz). Insulinomas appear sonolucent compared to the more echo-dense normal pancreas. IOUS has been useful in facilitating the enucleation of nonpalpable insulinomas within the pancreatic head. Recent reports have also suggested that insulinoma resection can be accomplished laparoscopically.[70,71]

Duodenotomy for Gastrinoma

During surgery for a gastrinoma, it is important to remember that these tumors can occur in extrapancreatic locations, particularly the duodenum. It is important to explore and palpate the liver, stomach, small bowel, and mesentery as well as the pancreas and pelvis. Once adequate exposure is accomplished, the duodenum and pancreas can be fully palpated and examined by IOUS. IOUS should also be used to image the liver. Tumors appear sonolucent and should be imaged in two dimensions. The duodenum can then be palpated between thumb and forefinger for the presence of mass lesions. IOE with duodenal transillumination may also be performed. A duodenal gastrinoma appears as a photopaque mass lesion within the wall of the duodenum upon transillumination. The endoscopist may occasionally also visualize the tumor as a raised mucosal defect.

Regardless of the results of IOUS or IOE, a duodenotomy is indicated in all cases (Fig. 30.2). This procedure allows for visualization as well as a more careful palpation of the entire duodenal wall, particularly its medial portion.

Reoperation for recurrent localized gastrinoma is indicated if the tumor is imageable and the patient is a suitable candidate for surgery. Reoperation can result in elimination of all tumor in nearly every patient and complete remission in 30%.[68]

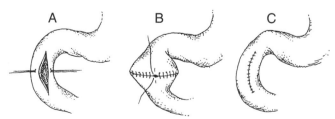

FIGURE 30.2. Illustration of the closure of a duodenotomy after examination and palpation for the presence of a duodenal gastrinoma. The duodenotomy (**A**), which is usually started at the junction of the first and second portion of the duodenum, is normally closed transversely (**B**) in two layers to minimize the risk of leakage or narrowing. In the case of a long duodenotomy, it may be necessary to close the incision longitudinally (**C**).

Carcinoid Disease

Epidemiology

The exact incidence of carcinoid disease is unknown because it differs considerably in different populations and with different study types. Overall, the estimated incidence is thought to be 1.5 per 100,000 of the general population.[72] The incidence seems to vary with regard to age and gender. The age of patients ranges from 8 to 93 years,[73–76] with a mean age at presentation of 55 to 60 years. The incidence in women seems to be slightly higher than in men.

Classification and Tumor Characteristics

Carcinoid tumors are derived from chromaffin or Kulchitsky cells,[77] which are ubiquitous throughout the gastrointestinal and urogenital tract as well as the bronchial epithelium.[78,79] This explains the occurrence of carcinoids in a wide range of anatomical sites. Importantly, malignancy cannot be identified on the basis of histology or cytochemical findings alone and, as with other neuroendocrine tumors, remains a clinical diagnosis after the finding of lymph node or distant metastases.

From a histological standpoint, carcinoid tumors generally cannot be differentiated from other neuroendocrine tumors when viewed under the light microscope with the usual stains. They are composed of homogenous sheets of small round cells with uniform cytoplasm and nuclei and rare mitotic figures.[80–82] Characteristically, carcinoid tumors may take up and reduce silver salts (argentaffin reaction of Masson) or may take up, but not reduce, silver unless exogenous reducing substances are added (argyrophilic reaction). The histochemical diagnosis of the tumor may be complimented by the use of monoclonal antibodies to serotonin.[80,81]

In the early 1960s, Williams and Sandler proposed a classification system based on the carcinoid tumor anatomical site of origin.[83] This system proposed that tumors be classified into foregut (including respiratory tract and thymus), midgut, and hindgut carcinoids. Foregut carcinoids are derived from the respiratory tract, stomach, proximal duodenum, and pancreas. They are generally argentaffin negative but argyrophilic. They occasionally secrete 5-hydroxytryptophan (5-HTP) or ACTH and other hormones, are associated with an atypical carcinoid syndrome, and have the potential to metastasize to bone.[83] Midgut carcinoids (jejunum, ileum, and right colon) are argentaffin positive. They rarely secrete 5-HTP or ACTH but do release 5-HT and tachykinins and do cause the classic carcinoid syndrome with liver metastases. They rarely metastasize to bone.[83] Hindgut (transverse colon, left colon, and anorectum) carcinoid tumors are described as being argentaffin negative, but argyrophilic. They hardly ever secrete 5-HTP or ACTH, but can contain numerous gastrointestinal hormones and rarely cause a classic carcinoid syndrome. Like, midgut carcinoids, they rarely metastasize to bone.[83]

Tumor Biology

The exact factors involved in carcinoid tumorigenesis are largely unknown. In general, they are slow-growing neoplasms. Clinical manifestation of the disease tends to increase with tumor size and metastatic behavior.[84,85] The most frequent site of occurrence is the appendix, where up to 40% of tumors are found.[86] These are usually small, and frequently asymptomatic. The next most common sites are the small intestine, rectum, and bronchus.[86] Small intestine carcinoids, especially those in the jejunoileum, seem to manifest the most aggressive clinical behavior.[76,84,87]

The release of 5-HT into systemic circulation has long been thought to be responsible for the symptoms of the carcinoid syndrome, and numerous studies have documented both an increase in serum and platelet serotonin levels as well as urinary levels of the serotonin metabolite 5-HIAA. The classic carcinoid syndrome is usually a consequence of disseminated midgut carcinoids. Foregut carcinoids, on the other hand, rarely cause the classic syndrome but may manifest an atypical carcinoid syndrome, mainly comprising a generalized flushing, headache, cutaneous edema, lacrimation, and bronchoconstriction.[75] Patients with an atypical carcinoid syndrome usually have significantly increased urinary levels of 5-HT and 5-HTP but normal or only slightly elevated levels of 5-HIAA.[75] However, there remains an inconsistent relationship between elevated 5-HT or 5-HTP levels and symptoms caused by carcinoid disease.

Signs and Symptoms

Approximately 40% to 60% of carcinoid tumors can be asymptomatic[87,88] and are only diagnosed after investigation of nonspecific complaints or after appendectomy. In those that are symptomatic, the presentation varies considerably according to tumor location. The most dramatic presentation is that of the carcinoid syndrome itself, and it is usually a consequence of tumor factors gaining access to the systemic circulation, thus circumventing metabolism in the portal or pulmonary arterial circulation.

As a general rule, patients with the classic syndrome present with diarrhea, flushing, localized, or generalized pain and right-sided endocardial involvement, ultimately producing valvular heart disease and heart failure (Tables 30.2 and 30.7).

Diagnosis

The presumptive diagnosis of carcinoid disease can be suspected in all patients with clinical symptoms or signs suggestive of a carcinoid tumor or carcinoid syndrome. However, the characteristic clinical presentation may not always be apparent. Because of nonspecific symptoms, the diagnosis of small intestinal carcinoids may be frequently delayed, sometimes with a median time from presentation to diagnosis of approximately 2 years.[84]

Biochemical testing remains the cornerstone of diagnosis for symptomatic carcinoid tumors (Table 30.2). The most widespread and inexpensive tests rely on the measurements of serotonin or its metabolites in urine. The measurement of the serotonin metabolite 5-HIAA in a 24-h urine sample is commonly used.[89] Patients with carcinoid tumors have increased urinary 5-HIAA excretion, in the range of 8 to 30 mg per day. When used alone, urinary 5-HIAA levels have a sensitivity of around 73% and a specificity of 88% to 100%.[75,89,90] Similarly, urinary 5-HT levels have sensitivities of 55%, 82%, and 60% for foregut, midgut, and hindgut carcinoid tumors, respectively.[91] It should be remembered that, in patients with an atypical carcinoid syndrome, urinary 5-HIAA levels may not be significantly elevated because the principal metabolite in this case is 5-HTP. In this case, measurement of urinary 5-HT, platelet serotonin levels, or urinary levels of tryptophan metabolites will contribute to the diagnosis.[92] Recently, serum levels of chromogranin A are found to be elevated in 90% of patients with carcinoid tumors, and thus provide a useful marker.

Localization

Up to 40% of primary and metastatic disease may not be visualized by usual techniques.[93] Chest radiography is usually the first imaging modality to detect bronchial carcinoids and is usually performed to investigate nonspecific respiratory complaints.[75,94] As the tumors are slow growing, they may compress airways and induce an obstructive pneumonia or atelectasis and may appear as opacities with notched margins.[95] CT scanning then allows for greater resolution of the lesion, and tissue for diagnosis may be obtained by bronchoscopy if the lesion is proximal in the respiratory tree. Gastric carcinoids are also usually asymptomatic and are usually diagnosed on endoscopy. Upper-gastrointestinal barium contrast studies are generally nonspecific or fail to visualize the lesion.[96,97] Likewise, lower gastrointestinal contrast studies have poor sensitivity and specificity for hindgut carcinoid tumors[98] but are more successful in localizing those in the cecum and ascending colon.[76,98]

Ultrasonography has received renewed interest in recent years in the localization of primary as well as metastatic disease. Transabdominal US can identify about 36% of small bowel carcinoids (Table 30.4) and 67% or more of liver metastases.[54] Ultrasound may also be of utility in guiding percutaneous liver biopsies of suspected lesions.[99] Endoscopic ultrasound has become increasingly important in the localization of tumors, particularly colorectal carcinoids. EUS may also be valuable in identifying local nodal involvement.[100]

The localization of midgut carcinoid disease remains a problem. The tumors are usually small and asymptomatic, or are larger and have metastasized at the time of symptomatic presentation. Usually barium studies fail to localize these lesions.[101] CT scanning has been use extensively in the localization of carcinoid tumors but images only about 44% to 55% of the primary lesions. Its greatest utility, and that of MR imaging, lies in the detection of metastatic disease and in monitoring medical therapy.[102]

Iodine-131 metaiodobenzylguanidine (^{131}I-MIBG) is concentrated by both pheochromocytomas and carcinoids. Scinti-

TABLE 30.7. Usual Presenting Symptoms in Patients with Classic Carcinoid Syndrome.

Symptom	Presenting (%)
Diarrhea	32–68
Flushing	23–74
Reactive airway disease	4–18
Heart disease	41
Pain	10
Pellagra	5

Sources: Norheim et al. (1987)[169]; Thorson (1958).[130]

graphic scans using this tracer localize about 68% of midgut and 38% of foregut carcinoids,[103] and have an average sensitivity of about 70% with a specificity of 95%[37] when using the iodine-123 isotope. The utility of ^{131}I-MIBG scanning seems to lie in its ability to localize metastatic tumor rather than as a first-line imaging modality.[103] SRS or octreoscan images approximately 90% of carcinoid tumors and metastases and is the imaging study of choice. Further, imageable tumors will respond to octreotide therapy. Technetium-99m bone scanning appears to be superior to other isotopic studies at imaging bony metastases.[104]

Metastatic Disease and Survival

Carcinoid tumors are malignant and the presence of metastasis directly influences survival. In one multivariate analysis of gastrointestinal carcinoids, gender and the presence of local or distant metastases were independently predictive of death.[105] A number of factors have been found to have an influence on the development of metastatic disease, the most important being size, location, and histological stage of the primary tumor.[84,98,105–107] 54% to 66% of patients with sporadic gastric carcinoid develop metastases.

Similarly, overall survival rates are dependent on tumor location and size. 94% 5-year survival with local disease and 18% 5-year survival with distant metastases has been reported. Appendiceal lesions showed the most favorable prognosis, with 76% to 100% 5-year survival, even with regional metastases, and 27% 5-year survival with distant involvement. For other tumor sites, 5-year survival ranges from 52%–96% for local disease, to 0%–44% for distant spread.

Treatment of Carcinoid Disease

Medical Management and Chemotherapy

The medical management of carcinoid disease is essentially the treatment of the carcinoid syndrome that may occasionally be precipitated by any number of stressors. Its immediate life-threatening manifestation is that of the carcinoid crisis with intense flushing, diarrhea, abdominal pain, altered mental status, and cardiovascular derangements, particularly hypertension or hypotension.[108]

Although a variety of agents have been employed to treat the carcinoid syndrome or crisis, octreotide is the only current agent that has been shown in a number of studies to have any value in treatment and prevention.[108–111]

Interferon-α has also been employed in treating the carcinoid syndrome and metastatic disease. Long-term follow-up has reported an objective response rate of the order of 12% to 48%.[112,113] The adverse side effects of interferon therapy, unlike those of octreotide, have limited its use. Currently, interferon therapy has utility in patients who have failed octreotide treatment, or in combination with hepatic embolization or certain chemotherapy regiments.

Other agents have been tried and evaluated on a sporadic basis. Antidiarrheal agents such as loperamide, selective bronchodilators, and diuretics have all been employed to control diarrhea, wheezing, or heart failure seen with advanced disease. 5-HT receptor antagonists have also been used to treat carcinoid syndrome with some success.[114]

There is no strong consensus on the type or timing of chemotherapy for malignant carcinoid tumors. Given the indolent growth pattern of the tumor, the generally poor efficacy of chemical agents, and the ability to control symptoms of the carcinoid syndrome with octreotide or interferon, chemotherapy is usually reserved for advanced tumors. Chemotherapy for metastatic carcinoid tumors has generally had poor results, with single-agent regimens producing no more than a 30% transient response rate.[115] Streptozotocin (STZ), dacarbazine (DTIC), or 5-fluorouracil (5-FU) showed the largest response.[111,115]

The introduction of hepatic artery embolization has allowed for the application of more aggressive multimodality therapy. Numerous studies[116–120] have evaluated selected embolization using both oil emulsions and gelfoam and found overall favorable biochemical (5-HIAA) and symptom response, but no significant increase in survival.[117] Embolization can have significant side effects in up to 12% of patients, including nausea, abscess formation, abdominal pain, fever, and ileus. In addition, the mortality rate may be as high as 3%.[119] It is usually contraindicated in patients with obstructive jaundice or in cases where the portal vein is occluded by tumor.

Multimodality therapy using hepatic embolization and chemotherapy (chemoembolization) has combined the use of gelfoam embolization with 5-FU, doxorubicin, STZ or dacarbazine (DTIC), and/or interferon-α. A number of large studies have documented improvement of carcinoid symptoms in virtually all patients with objective response, in terms of reduction in tumor size, seen in 35% to 100% of individuals.[84,121–123]

Radiation therapy is usually reserved for cases of advanced metastatic and unresectable carcinoid tumors whose symptoms have become resistant to maximal medical management. At present, it is particularly helpful in controlling symptomatic bone metastases.

Surgical Management

Surgery remains the only potentially curative treatment for patients with carcinoid disease.[124–127] However, surgery for cure is mainly dependent on the location and size of the primary tumor because these elements largely influence the potential for metastatic spread.[98,105–107] Even with regional lymph node metastases, surgery may still be curative in some patients,[125] and there is still a role for more aggressive surgical therapy in select patients with advanced disease.[126]

References

1. LeDouarin NM. The Embryological Origin of Cells Associated with the Digestive Tract. Edinburgh: Churchill Livingstone, 1978.
2. Kloppel G, Heitz PU. Classification of normal and neoplastic neuroendocrine cells. Ann N Y A Sci 1994;733:18–24.
3. Metz DC. Diagnosis and treatment of pancreatic neuroendocrine tumors. Semin Gastrointest Dis 1995;6:67–74.
4. Jensen RT, Norton JA. Endocrine tumors of the pancreas. In: Yamada T, et al., eds. Textbook of Gastroenterology, 2nd Ed. Philadelphia: Lippincott, 1995.
5. Dent RB. Nonfunctioning islet cell tumors. Ann Surg 1981;193: 185–189.
6. Norton JA. Pancreatic Islet Cell Tumors Excluding Gastrinomas. St. Louis: Mosby, 1998.
7. Meko JB, Norton JA. Endocrine tumors of the pancreas. Curr Opin Gen Surg 1994:186–194.

8. Meko JB, Norton JA. Management of patients with Zollinger-Ellison syndrome. Annu Rev Med 1995;46:395–411.

9. Sadler TW. Digestive System, 6th Ed. Baltimore: Williams & Wilkins, 1990.

10. Wermer P. Endocrine adenomatosis and peptic ulcer in a large kindred: inherited multiple tumors and mosaic pleiotropism in man. Am J Med 1963;35:205.

11. Veldhuis JD, Norton JA, Wells SA Jr, Vinik AI, Perry RR. Surgical versus medical management of multiple endocrine neoplasia (MEN) type I. J Clin Endocrinol Metab 1997;82(2):357–364.

12. Norton JA, Doherty GM, Fraker DL. Surgery for Endocrine Tumors of the Pancreas, 2nd Ed. New York: Raven Press, 1993.

13. Pasieka JL, McLeod MK, Thompson NW, Burney RE. Surgical approach to insulinomas. Assessing the need for preoperative localization. Arch Surg 1992;127(4):442–447.

14. Sheppard BC, Norton JA, Doppman JL, Maton PN, Gardner JD, Jensen RT. Management of islet cell tumors in patients with multiple endocrine neoplasia: a prospective study. Surgery (St. Louis) 1989;106(6):1108–1117; discussion 1117–1118.

15. Modlin IM, Tang LH. Approaches to the diagnosis of gut neuroendocrine tumors: the last word (today). Gastroenterology 1997;112(2):583–590.

16. Whipple AO. The surgical therapy of hyperinsulinism. J Int Chir 1938;3:237.

17. Comi RJ, Gorden P, Doppman JL, Norton JA. Insulinoma. New York: Raven Press, 1986.

18. Fajans SS, Vinik AI. Insulin-producing islet cell tumors. Endocrinol Metab Clin North Am 1989;18(1):45–74.

19. Norton JA, Whitman ED. Insulinoma. Endocrinologist 1993;3(4):258–267.

20. Palazzo L, Roseau G, Salmeron M. Endoscopic ultrasonography in the preoperative localization of pancreatic endocrine tumors. Endoscopy 1992;24(suppl 1):350–353.

21. Doppman JL, Chang R, Fraker DL, et al. Localization of insulinomas to regions of the pancreas by intra-arterial stimulation with calcium [see comments] [published erratum appears in Ann Intern Med 1995;123(9):734]. Ann Intern Med 1995;123(4):269–273.

22. Norton JA, Shawker TH, Doppman JL, et al. Localization and surgical treatment of occult insulinomas [see comments]. Ann Surg 1990;212(5):615–620.

23. Norton JA. Surgical treatment of islet cell tumors with special emphasis on operative ultrasound. In: Mignon M, Jensen RT, eds. Endocrine Tumors of the Pancreas: Recent Advances in Research and Management. Basel: Krager, 1995;309–332.

24. Zollinger RM, Ellison EH. Primary peptic ulceration of the jejunum associated with islet cell tumors of the pancreas. Ann Surg 1955;142:709–728.

25. Isenberg JI, Walsh JH, Grossman MI. Zollinger-Ellison syndrome. Gastroenterology 1973;65(1):140–165.

26. Norton JA. Gastrinoma: advances in localization and treatment. Surg Oncol Clin North Am 1998;7(4):845–861.

27. Thompson NW. Surgical treatment of the endocrine pancreas and Zollinger-Ellison syndrome in the MEN 1 syndrome. Henry Ford Hosp Med J 1992;40(3–4):195–198.

28. Norton JA, Fraker DL, Alexander HR, et al. Surgery for the cure of the Zollinger-Ellison Syndrome. N Engl J Med 1999;341:635–644.

29. Stabile BE, Morrow DJ, Passaro E Jr. The gastrinoma triangle: operative implications. Am J Surg 1984;147(1):25–31.

30. Gibril F, Curtis LT, Termanini B, et al. Primary cardiac gastrinoma causing Zollinger-Ellison syndrome. Gastroenterology 1997;112(2):567–574.

31. Maton PN, Mackem SM, Norton JA, Gardner JD, O'Dorisio TM, Jensen RT. Ovarian carcinoma as a cause of Zollinger-Ellison syndrome. Natural history, secretory products, and response to provocative tests. Gastroenterology 1989;97(2):468–471.

32. Deveney CW, Deveney KE. Zollinger-Ellison syndrome (gastrinoma). Current diagnosis and treatment. Surg Clin North Am 1987;67(2):411–422.

33. Norton JA. Advances in the management of Zollinger-Ellison syndrome. Adv Surg 1994;27:129–159.

34. Slaff JL, Howard JM, Maton PN, et al. Prospective assessment of provocative gastrin tests in 81 consecutive patients with Zollinger-Ellison syndrome. Gastroenterology 1986;90:1637–1643.

35. Frucht H, Doppman JL, Norton JA, et al. Gastrinomas: comparison of MR imaging with CT, angiography, and US. Radiology 1989;171(3):713–717.

36. Wank SA, Doppman JL, Miller DL, et al. Prospective study of the ability of computed axial tomography to localize gastrinomas in patients with Zollinger-Ellison syndrome. Gastroenterology 1987;92(4):905–912.

37. Krenning EP, Kwekkeboom DJ, Bakker WH, et al. Somatostatin receptor scintigraphy with [111In-DTPA-D-Phe1]- and [123I-Tyr3]-octreotide: the Rotterdam experience with more than 1000 patients. Eur J Nucl Med 1993;20(8):716–731.

38. Gibril F, Reynolds JC, Doppman JL, et al. Somatostatin receptor scintigraphy: its sensitivity compared with that of other imaging methods in detecting primary and metastatic gastrinomas. A prospective study [see comments]. Ann Intern Med 1996;125(1):26–34.

39. Alexander HR, Fraker DL, Norton JA, et al. Prospective study of somatostatin receptor scintigraphy and its effect on operative outcome in patients with Zollinger-Ellison syndrome. Ann Surg 1998;228(2):228–238.

40. Sugg SL, Norton JA, Fraker DL, et al. A prospective study of intraoperative methods to diagnose and resect duodenal gastrinomas. Ann Surg 1993;218(2):138–144.

41. Stacpoole PW. The glucagonoma syndrome: clinical features, diagnosis, and treatment. Endocr Rev 1981;2(3):347–361.

42. Maton PN. Use of octreotide acetate for control of symptoms in patients with islet cell tumors. World J Surg 1993;17(4):504–510.

43. Guillausseau PJ, Guillausseau-Scholer C. Glucagonomas: Clinical Presentation, Diagnosis, and Advances in Management. Basel: Karger, 1995.

44. Verner JV, Morrison AB. Islet cell tumor and a syndrome of refractory water diarrhea and hypokalemia. Am J Med 1958;29:529–533.

45. Matsumoto KK, Perer JB, Schultze RG, et al. Watery diarrhea and hypokalemia associated with a pancreatic islet cell adenoma. Gastroenterology 1967:52:695–699.

46. Matuchansky C, Rambaud JC. VIPomas and Endocrine Cholera: Clinical Presentation, Diagnosis, and Advances in Management. Basel: Karger, 1995.

47. Verner JV, Morrison AB. Non-B islet tumors and the syndrome of watery diarrhea, hypokalemia, and hypochlorhydria. Clin Gastroenterol 1974;3:595–600.

48. Mekhjian HS, O'Dorisio TM. VIPoma syndrome. Semin Oncol 1987;14(3):282–291.

49. Long RG, Bryant MG, Mitchell SJ, Adrian TE, Polak JM, Bloom SR. Clinicopathological study of pancreatic and ganglioneuroblastoma tumours secreting vasoactive intestinal polypeptide (vipomas). Br Med J (Clin Res Ed) 1981;282(6278):1767–1771.

50. Ganda OP, Weir GC, Soeldner JS, et al. "Somatostatinoma": a somatostatin-containing tumor of the endocrine pancreas. N Engl J Med 1977;296(17):963–967.

51. Vinik AI, Strodel WE, Eckhauser FE, Moattari AR, Lloyd R. Somatostatinomas, PPomas, neurotensinomas. Semin Oncol 1987;14(3):263–281.

52. Kent RBd, van Heerden JA, Weiland LH. Nonfunctioning islet cell tumors. Ann Surg 1981;193(2):185–190.

53. Maton PN, Gardner JD, Jensen RT. The incidence and etiology of Cushing's syndrome in patients with the Zollinger-Ellison syndrome. N Engl J Med 1986;315(1):1–5.

54. Kisker O, Bartsch D, Weinel RJ, et al. The value of somatostatin-receptor scintigraphy in newly diagnosed endocrine gastroenteropancreatic tumors. J Am Coll Surg 1997;184(5):487–492.

55. Krausz Y, Bar-Ziv J, de Jong RB, et al. Somatostatin-receptor

scintigraphy in the management of gastroenteropancreatic tumors. Am J Gastroenterol 1998;93(1):66–70.

56. Boukhman MP, Karam JH, Shaver J, Siperstein AE, Duh QY, Clark OH. Insulinoma—experience from 1950 to 1995. West J Med 1998;169(2):98–104.

57. Doherty GM, Doppman JL, Shawker TH, et al. Results of a prospective strategy to diagnose, localize, and resect insulinomas. Surgery (St. Louis) 1991;110(6):989–996; discussion 996–997.

58. Norton JA, Cornelius MJ, Doppman JL, Maton PN, Gardner JD, Jensen RT. Effect of parathyroidectomy in patients with hyperparathyroidism, Zollinger-Ellison syndrome, and multiple endocrine neoplasia type I: a prospective study. Surgery (St. Louis) 1987;102(6):958–966.

59. Lo CY, Lam KY, Kung AW, Lam KS, Tung PH, Fan ST. Pancreatic insulinomas. A 15-year experience. Arch Surg 1997;132(8):926–930.

60. Maton PN, Frucht H, Vinayek R, et al. Medical management of patients with Zollinger-Ellison syndrome. Gastroenterology 1988;94:294–299.

61. Sutliff VE, Doppman JL, Gibril F, et al. Growth of newly diagnosed, untreated metastatic gastrinomas and predictors of growth patterns. J Clin Oncol 1997;15(6):2420–2431.

62. Norton JA, Doppman JL, Jensen RT. Curative resection in Zollinger-Ellison syndrome. Results of a 10-year prospective study. Ann Surg 1992;215(1):8–18.

63. Norton JA, Cromack DT, Shawker TH, et al. Intraoperative ultrasonographic localization of the islet cell tumors. A prospective comparison to palpation. Ann Surg 1988;207(2):160–168.

64. MacFarlane MP, Fraker DL, Alexander HR, Norton JA, Lubensky I, Jensen RT. Prospective study of surgical resection of duodenal and pancreatic gastrinomas in multiple endocrine neoplasia type 1. Surgery (St. Louis) 1995;118(6):973–979; discussion 979–980.

65. Norton JA. Neuroendocrine tumors of the pancreas and duodenum. Curr Probl Surg 1994;31(2):77–156.

66. Fraker DL, Norton JA. The role of surgery in the management of islet cell tumors. Gastroenterol Clin North Am 1989;18(4):805–830.

67. Berwaerts J, Verhelst J, Hubens H, et al. Role of hepatic arterial embolisation in the treatment for metastatic insulinoma. Report of two cases and review of the literature. Acta Clin Belg 1997;52(5):263–274.

68. von Schrenck T, Howard JM, Doppman JL, et al. Prospective study of chemotherapy in patients with metastatic gastrinoma. Gastroenterology 1988;94:1326–1331.

69. Creutzfeldt W, Bartsch HH, Jacubaschke U, St Eöckmann F. Treatment of gastrointestinal endocrine tumours with interferon-alpha and octreotide. Acta Oncol 1991;30(4):529–535.

70. Sussman LA, Christie R, Whittle DE. Laparoscopic excision of distal pancreas including insulinoma. Aust N Z J Surg 1996;66(6):414–416.

71. Gagner M, Pomp A, Herrera MF. Early experience with laparoscopic resections of islet cell tumors. Surgery (St. Louis) 1996;120(6):1051–1054.

72. Buchanan KD, Johnston CF, O'Hare MM, et al. Neuroendocrine tumors. A European view. Am J Med 1986;81(6B):14–22.

73. Lu Cortez L, Clemente C, Puig V, Mirada A. [Carcinoid tumor. An analysis of 131 cases]. Rev Clin Esp 1994;194(4):291–293.

74. Parkes SE, Muir KR, al Sheyyab M, et al. Carcinoid tumours of the appendix in children 1957–1986: incidence, treatment and outcome [see comments]. Br J Surg 1993;80(4):502–504.

75. Feldman JM. Carcinoid tumors and the carcinoid syndrome. Curr Probl Surg 1989;26(12):835–885.

76. Vinik AI, McLeod MK, Fig LM, Shapiro B, Lloyd RV, Cho K. Clinical features, diagnosis, and localization of carcinoid tumors and their management. Gastroenterol Clin North Am 1989;18(4):865–896.

77. Masson P. Carcinoids (argentaffin-cell tumors) and nerve hyperplasia of appendicular mucosa. Am J Pathol 1928;4:181–212.

78. Zeitels J, Naunheim K, Kaplan EL, Straus F. Carcinoid tumors: a 37-year experience. Arch Surg 1982;117:732–737.

79. Todd TR, Cooper JD, Weissberg D, Delarue NC, Peason FG. Bronchial carcinoid tumors: twenty years experience. J Thorac Cardiovasc Surg 1980;71:532–536.

80. Wilander E, Scheibenpflug L, Ericksson B, Oberg K. Diagnostic criteria of classical carcinoids. Acta Oncol 1991;30:469–476.

81. Wilander E. Diagnostic pathology of gastrointestinal and pancreatic neuroendocrine tumors. Acta Oncol 1989;28:363.

82. Creutzfeldt W. Historical background and natural history of carcinoids. Digestion 1994;55:3–12.

83. Williams ED, Sandler M. The classification of carcinoid tumors. Lancet 1963;1:238–239.

84. Moertel CG. Karnofsky memorial lecture. An odyssey in the land of small tumors. J Clin Oncol 1987;5(10):1502–1522.

85. Davis Z, Moertel CG, McIlrath DC. The malignant carcinoid syndrome. Surg Gynecol Obstet 1973;137:637–642.

86. Godwin JD. Carcinoid tumors: an analysis of 2837 cases. Cancer (Phila) 1975;36:560–565.

87. Moertel CG, Suer WG, Docherty MG, et al. Life history of the carcinoid tumor of the small intestine. Cancer (Phila) 1961;14:901–905.

88. Eller R, Frazee R, Roberts J. Gastrointestinal carcinoid tumors. Am Surg 1991;57(7):434–437.

89. Tormey WP, Fitzgerald RJ. The clinical and laboratory correlates of an increased urinary 5-hydroxyindoleactic acid. Postgrad Med J 1995;71:542–545.

90. Feldman JM. Carcinoid tumors and syndrome. Semin Oncol 1987;14:237.

91. Kema IP, deVries GE, Sloof MJH, Biesma B, Muskiet FAJ. Serotonin, catecholamines, histamine, and their metabolites in urine, platelets, and tumor tissue of patients with carcinoid tumors. Clin Chem 1994;40:86–91.

92. Feldman JM. Urinary serotinin in the diagnosis of carcinoid tumors. Clin Chem 1986;32:840–845.

93. Kisker O, Weinel RJ, Geks J, Zacara F, Joseph K, Rothmund M. Value of somatostatin receptor scintigraphy for preoperative localization of carcinoids. World J Surg 1996;20:162–167.

94. Dusmet M, McNeally MF. Bronchial and thymic carcinoid tumors: a review. Digestion 1994;55:70–75.

95. Nessi R, Ricci D, Ricci SB, Bosco M, Blanc M. Bronchial carcinoid tumors: radiologic observations in 49 cases. J Thorac Imaging 1991;6:47–52.

96. Gough DB, Thompson GB, Crotty TB, et al. Diverse clinical and pathologic features of gastric carcinoid and the relevance of hypergastrinemia. World J Surg 1994;18:473–478.

97. Davies MG, O'Dowd GO, McEntee GP, Hennessey TPJ. Primary gastric carcinoid tumors: a view on management. Br J Surg 1990;77:1013.

98. Thompson GB, van Heerden JA, Martin JK, et al. Carcinoid tumors of the gastrointestinal tract: presentation, management and prognosis. Surgery (St. Louis) 1985;98:1054–1059.

99. Andersson T, Eriksson B, Lindgren PG, Wilander E, Oberg K. Percutaneous ultrasonography-guided cutting biopsy from liver metastases of endocrine gastrointestinal tumors. Ann Surg 1987;206:728–732.

100. Yoshikane H, Tsukamoto Y, Niwa Y, et al. Carcinoid tumors of the gastrointestinal tract: evaluation with endoscopic ultrasonography. Gastrointest Endosc 1993;39:375–383.

101. Sugimoto E, Lorelius LE, Eriksson B, Oberg K. Midgut carcinoid tumors. Acta Radiol 1995;36:367–374.

102. Makridis C, Oberg K, Juhlin C, et al. Surgical treatment of midgut carcinoid tumors. World J Surg 1990;14:377–383.

103. Hanson MW, Feldman JM, Blinder RH, Moore JO, Coleman RE. Carcinoid tumors: iodine[131]I MIBG scintigraphy. Radiology 1989;172:699.

104. Feldman JM, Plunk JW. ^{99m}Tc-pyrophosphate bone scans in patients with metastatic carcinoid tumors. J Med 1977;8:71.

105. McDermott EWM, Guduric B, Brennan MF. Prognostic variables in patients with gastrointestinal carcinoid tumors. Br J Surg 1994;81:1007–1009.

106. Agranovich AL, Anderson GH, Manji M, Acker BD, MacDonald WC, Threlfall WJ. Carcinoid tumor of the gastrointestinal tract: prognostic factors and disease outcome. J Surg Oncol 1991;47:45.

107. MacGillivary DG, Snyder DA, Druker W, Remine SR. Carcinoid tumors: the relationship between clinical presentation and the extent of disease. Surgery (St. Louis) 1991;110:68.

108. Warner RRP, Mani S, Profeta J, Grunstein E. Octreotide treatment of carcinoid hypertensive crisis. Mt Sinai Med J 1994;61:349–355.

109. Reichlin S. Somatostatin. N Engl J Med 1983;309:1495–1501.

110. Kvols LK, Martin JK, Marsh HM, Moertel CG. Rapid reversal of carcinoid crisis with a somatostatin analog [letter]. N Engl J Med 1985;313:1229.

111. Kvols LK. Therapy of malignant carcinoid syndrome. Endocrinol Metab Clin North Am 1989;18:557.

112. Obert K, Funa K, Alm G. Effects of leukocyte interferon on clinical symptoms and hormone levels in patients with midgut carcinoid tumors and the carcinoid syndrome. N Engl J Med 1983;309:129–133.

113. Hanssen LE, Schrumpf E, Klobenstiedt AN, Tausjo J, Dolva LO. Treatment of metastatic midgut carcinoid tumors with recombinant human alpha 2b interferon with or without prior hepatic artery embolization. Scand J Gastroenterol 1989;24:787–795.

114. Gregor M. Therapeutic principles in the management of metastasising carcinoid tumors: drugs for symptomatic treatment. Digestion 1994;55:60.

115. Maton PN, Hodgson HJF. Carcinoid tumours and the carcinoid syndrome. In: Bouchier IAD, Allan RN, Hodgson HJF, Keighly MRB, eds. Textbook of Gastroenterology. London: Balliere-Tindall, 1984:620.

116. Winkelbauer FW, Niederle B, Pietschmann F, et al. Hepatic artery embolectomy of hepatic metastases from carcinoid tumors: value of using a cranacrylate and ethiodized oil. Am J Roentgenol 1995;165:323–327.

117. Maton PN, Camilleri M, Griffin G, Allison DJ, Hodgson HJ, Chadwick VS. Role of hepatic artery embolization in the carcinoid syndrome. Br Med J 1983;287:932–935.

118. Mitty HA, Warner RR, Newman LH, Train J, Parnes IH. Control of carcinoid syndrome with hepatic artery embolization. Radiology 1985;155:623–626.

119. Marlink RG, Lakich JJ, Robins JR, Clouse ME. Hepatic arterial embolization for metastatic hormone secreting tumors. Cancer (Phila) 1991;65:2227–2231.

120. Norbin A, Mansson B, Lunderquist A. Evaluation of temporary liver dearterialization and embolization in patients with metastatic carcinoid tumors. Acta Oncol 1989;28:419.

121. Moertel CG, Johnson CM, McKusick MA, et al. The management of patients with advanced carcinoid tumors and islet cell carcinomas. Ann Intern Med 1994;120:302.

122. Stokes KR, Stuart K, Clouse ME. Hepatic arterial chemoembolization for metastatic endocrine tumors. J Vasc Interventional Radiol 1993;4:341.

123. Therasse E, Breittmayer F, Roche A, et al. Transcatheter chemoembolization of progressive carcinoid liver metastasis. Radiology 1993;189:541.

124. Loftus JP, van Heerden JA. Surgical management of gastrointestinal carcinoid tumors. Adv Surg 1995;28:317–336.

125. Rothmund M, Kister O. Surgical treatment of carcinoid tumors of the small bowel, appendix, colon and rectum. Digestion 1995;55:86.

126. Norton JA. Surgical management of carcinoid tumors: role of debulking and surgery in patients with advanced disease. Digestion 1995;55(suppl 3):98–103.

127. Stinner B, Kisker O, Zielke A, Rothmund M. Surgical management of carcinoid tumor of small bowel, appendix, colon and rectum. World J Surg 1996;20:183–188.

128. O'Briain DS, Duyal Y. The pathology of the gastrointestinal endocrine cells. In: Delellis RA, ed. Diagnostic Immunohistochemistry. New York: Masson, 1981:75.

129. Norheim I, Oberg K, Theodorsson-Norheim E, et al. Malignant carcinoid tumors. Ann Surg 1987;206:373–378.

130. Thorson AH. Studies on carcinoid disease. Acta Med Scand 1958;334:81–85.

131. Böttger TC, Weber W, Beyer J, Junginger T. Value of tumor localization in patients with insulinoma. World J Surg 1990;14(1):107–112; discussion 112–114.

132. Brown CK, Bartlett DL, Doppman JL, et al. Intraarterial calcium stimulation and intraoperative ultrasonography in the localization and resection of insulinomas. Surgery (St. Louis) 1997;122(6):1189–1193; discussion 1193–1194.

133. Cohen MS, Picus D, Lairmore TC, Strasberg SM, Doherty GM, Norton JA. Prospective study of provocative angiograms to localize functional islet cell tumors of the pancreas. Surgery (St. Louis) 1997;122(6):1091–1100.

134. Kisker O, Bastian D, Bartsch D, Nies C, Rothmund M. Localization, malignant potential, and surgical management of gastrinomas. World J Surg 1998;22(7):651–657; discussion 657–658.

Multiple Endocrine Neoplasia

Terry C. Lairmore

Multiple Endocrine Neoplasia Type 1

Clinical Features

Wermer in 1954[1] first described the features of MEN 1 in several members of a single kindred, and correctly reasoned that the disease was caused by an autosomal dominant gene with high penetrance. Multiple endocrine neoplasia (MEN) type 1 is characterized by the development of parathyroid hyperplasia (greater than 95% of patients), neuroendocrine tumors of the pancreas and duodenum (35–75%), and pituitary adenomas (16–65% of patients with MEN-1). In addition, bronchial and thymic carcinoids (8%) benign thyroid tumors, benign and malignant adrenocortical tumors, lipomas, and ependymomas of the CNS occur with increased frequency in patients with MEN 1.

HYPERPARATHYROIDISM

More than 95% of individuals with MEN 1 ultimately develop primary hyperparathyroidism as the result of multiglandular parathyroid hyperplasia. The clinical features of hyperparathyroidism in patients with MEN 1 are indistinguishable from those in patients with sporadic hyperparathyroidism, except for the development of hypercalcemia at a markedly earlier age in patients with MEN 1. The average age for onset of hypercalcemia in patients with MEN 1 is approximately 25 years.[2] Owing to the autosomal dominant pattern of inheritance for MEN 1, males and females are affected nearly equally, in contrast to the 3:1 female-to-male ratio in sporadic hyperparathyroidism.

NEUROENDOCRINE TUMORS OF THE PANCREAS AND DUODENUM

Depending on the method of study, 35% to 75% of patients with MEN 1 develop neuroendocrine tumors of the pancreas and duodenum. These tumors cause symptoms because of either hormone oversecretion or mass effects from the tumor growth itself. The pancreaticoduodenal tumors in patients with MEN 1 are characterized by a high malignant potential and aggressive biological behavior. Nonfunctioning or pancreatic polypeptide (PP-oma) producing tumors may be the most frequent neuroendocrine tumor of the pancreas that occurs in patients with MEN 1.

GASTRINOMA

Gastrinoma is the most common functional neuroendocrine tumor associated with the MEN 1 syndrome. The diagnosis of Zollinger–Ellison syndrome (ZES) is made by the finding of gastric acid hypersecretion (>15 mEq/h in patients with no history of gastric surgery or >5 mEq/h in patients with prior gastric surgery for peptic ulcer disease), in association with inappropriately elevated fasting serum gastrin levels (>100 pg/ml). The diagnosis is confirmed by an abnormal secretin stimulation test. A positive test is present when serum levels of gastrin rise more than 200 pg/ml following the intravenous administration of secretin (2 U/kg). The most common presenting symptom is pain in the epigastrium,[3–5] and some degree of peptic ulcer disease is identifiable in approximately 70% to 80% of patients. Control of the acid hypersecretion is usually achievable with medical treatment either with potent H_2-receptor antagonists or proton-pump inhibitors. The acid output should be maintained at levels less than 5 mEq/h at all times. Approximately 15% to 50% of patients with gastrinoma have liver metastases at the time of diagnosis.[6]

Patients with primary hyperparathyroidism should undergo parathyroidectomy because normalization of the serum calcium level improves the ZES.[7] Management of patients with ZES should also include intensive medical treatment to control the gastric acid hypersecretion. Although most evidence indicates that patients with ZES and MEN 1 are rarely cured by surgery, localized resection of a potentially malignant neuroendocrine tumor may be indicated in an attempt to control the tumoral process and prevent subsequent malignant dissemination.

INSULINOMA

The second most common functional pancreatic neuroendocrine tumor in patients with MEN 1 is insulinoma. The clinical elements needed for the diagnosis of insulinoma are the signs and symptoms of neuroglycopenia during fasting (anxiety, tremor, confusion, sweating, seizure, syncope), profound hypoglycemia, and alleviation of symptoms after the administration of glucose. The biochemical diagnosis is established during a supervised fast with the measurement of plasma levels of glucose, insulin, proinsulin, and C-peptide at frequent intervals. The treatment for insulinomas is accurate localization and resection to control the potentially life-threatening hyperinsulinemia. In patients with MEN 1 and insulinoma, despite the fact that these patients have multiple pancreatic neuroendocrine tumors, the insulinoma is generally a large identifiable tumor that is easy to find.[6]

Neuroendocrine tumors that secrete vasoactive intestinal peptide (VIP), glucagon, or somatostatin occur less frequently. These tumors produce characteristic syndromes depending on the specific hormone produced.

Genetics of MEN 1

The *MEN1* predisposition locus was assigned to chromosome band 11q13 by a combination of genetic linkage mapping and chromosome deletion studies in patients with MEN 1.[8] The *MEN1* tumor suppressor gene encodes a predicted 610-amino-acid protein product termed menin.[9] The precise role of menin in the regulation of cell growth has yet to be elucidated.

Evaluation and Management of Endocrine Neoplasia in Patients with MEN 1

Hyperparathyroidism

Because patients with MEN 1 have multiple gland involvement of the parathyroid glands, there is a significantly higher rate of recurrent or persistent hyperparathyroidism[10–14] after parathyroidectomy when compared to the results for the treatment of sporadic parathyroid adenoma. The appropriate initial surgical procedure for patients with MEN 1 is either total four-gland parathyroidectomy with intramuscular autotransplantation of parathyroid tissue to an accessible site in the forearm, or subtotal three-and-one-half-gland parathyroidectomy leaving the parathyroid tissue remnant in situ in the neck. Direct comparison of these two accepted surgical treatments awaits the performance of a prospective, randomized study.

Pancreaticoduodenal Neuroendocrine Tumors

The optimal management of the neuroendocrine tumors of the pancreas and duodenum in patients with MEN 1 remains controversial.

Multiple Endocrine Neoplasia Type 2

Clinical Features

The multiple endocrine neoplasia type 2 (MEN 2) syndromes are a group of clinically and genetically related autosomal dominant familial cancer syndromes in which the principal feature is medullary thyroid carcinoma (MTC). The diagnosis of MTC in a patient with a thyroid nodule should prompt a thorough family history and measurement of urinary catecholamines to exclude pheochromocytoma. Pathological features that suggest a familial form of MTC include multiple bilateral foci of MTC and the presence of a C-cell hyperplasia.

MEN 2A

Multiple endocrine neoplasia type 2A (MEN 2A) consists of MTC, pheochromocytomas, and parathyroid hyperplasia.[15,16] Virtually all patients with MEN 2A develop MTC in the second or third decade of life. Approximately 50% of patients[17] with MEN 2A develop pheochromocytomas, which may be bilateral. The most variable component of the syndrome is hyperparathyroidism, occurring in as many as 30% of patients.[17]

MEN 2B

The multiple endocrine neoplasia type 2B (MEN 2B) syndrome[18,19] is characterized by a slightly different complex of abnormalities. Affected individuals have a recognizable phenotype (Fig. 31.1) that includes thick "bumpy" lips caused by the development of multiple neuromas on the tongue and buccal mucosa, prognathism, skeletal abnormalities, and a "marfanoid" body habitus. Multiple ganglioneuromas of the gastrointestinal tract also occur in patients with MEN 2B, often resulting in the presence of disordered colonic motility associated with megacolon. Patients with MEN 2B do not develop hyperparathyroidism.

FAMILIAL MEDULLARY THYROID CARCINOMA

Familial medullary thyroid carcinoma (FMTC) consists of MTC inherited in an autosomal dominant pattern without

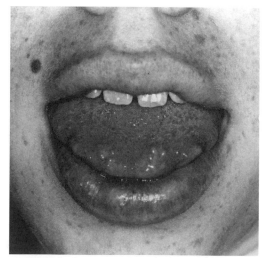

FIGURE 31.1. Characteristic appearance of multiple mucosal neuromas on the lips, tongue, and buccal mucosa of a patient with MEN 2B.

the presence of any associated endocrinopathies.[20] The MTC in patients with FMTC may not develop until the fifth or sixth decade and is relatively indolent.

Genetics of MEN 2

The *ret* proto-oncogene encodes a transmembrane receptor tyrosine kinase (RTK) that functions in signal transduction. The MEN 2A syndrome is associated with missense germline *ret* proto-oncogene mutations involving one of five codons in either exon 10 or 11 (codons 609, 611, 618, 620, 634) in over 95% of families.

Evaluation and Management of Endocrine Neoplasia in Patients with MEN 2

Calcitonin as a Tumor Marker for MTC

Calcitonin (CT), the hormone secreted by the thyroid C-cells, serves as a sensitive plasma tumor marker for the detection of MTC or C-cell hyperplasia.[21] The basal plasma calcitonin level is related to the extent of MTC and the frequency of regional and distant metastases.[22]

Early Thyroidectomy for Medullary Thyroid Carcinoma Based on Genetic Testing

MTC is the common feature of the MEN 2 syndromes and, more importantly, the consistently malignant neoplasm that is responsible for almost all of the disease-related morbidity and mortality. Therefore, early detection and effective treatment of the MTC is the key to improving outcome in patients with the MEN 2 syndromes. Total thyroidectomy before regional or distant metastasis of MTC is the preferred treatment. Patients with MEN 2B should undergo thyroidectomy as soon as the disease is recognized owing to the early onset and aggressive nature of the MTC in this syndrome.

Pheochromocytoma

Patients with MEN 2 are diagnosed with pheochromocytoma based on the findings of signs and symptoms of catecholamine excess, elevated 24-h urinary catecholamine excretion, and unilateral or bilateral adrenal masses on cross-sectional imaging tests. It is imperative that the presence of pheochromocytomas is excluded before performing thyroidectomy because of the anesthetic risks of unsuspected catecholamine excess.

Controversy exists concerning the optimal surgical management of the adrenal glands in patients with the MEN 2 syndromes. Preneoplastic (adrenal medullary hyperplasia) and neoplastic change of the adrenal medulla in patients with MEN 2A or MEN 2B is nearly always bilateral at the histopathological level.[23,24] For this reason, some experts advocate routine bilateral adrenalectomy for patients with MEN 2A or MEN 2B, whether or not both adrenal glands contain a macroscopic pheochromocytoma.[24-27] Others have recommended a selective approach[28,29] with excision of only those adrenal glands containing a grossly evident pheochromocytoma at the time of intervention. Although some studies have reported the occurrence of malignant pheochromocytomas in patients with MEN 2,[24] other series suggest that malignancy is very infrequent in this setting.[25,26,28,29] However, the risk of a malignant pheochromocytoma should not be totally dismissed, and bilateral adrenalectomy may be appropriate for members of families with a clear history of malignant pheochromocytoma.

Hyperparathyroidism

The appropriate management of the parathyroid glands in MEN 2 patients undergoing thyroidectomy for inherited MTC remains controversial. Our group has recommended total parathyroidectomy and autotransplantation of parathyroid tissue into the forearm muscle, especially in patients undergoing early thyroidectomy based on genetic testing.[11,30] Other experts argue that selective parathyroidectomy is effective in almost all patients and that routine total parathyroidectomy with autotransplantation results in an increased rate of permanent postoperative hypoparathyroidism.[31,32]

References

1. Wermer P. Genetic aspects of adenomatosis of the endocrine glands. Am J Med 1954;16:363–371.
2. Marx SJ, Vinik AI, Santen RJ, Floyd JCJ, Mills JL, Green J. Multiple endocrine neoplasia type I: assessment of laboratory tests to screen for the gene in a large kindred. Medicine (Baltimore) 1986;65:226–241.
3. Norton JA, Doppman JL, Jensen RT. Curative resection in Zollinger–Ellison syndrome: results of a 10-year prospective study. Ann Surg 1992;215:8–18.
4. Friesen SR. Treatment of the Zollinger–Ellison syndrome. Am J Surg 1982;143:331–338.
5. Cameron AJ, Hoffman HN. Zollinger–Ellison syndrome: clinical features and long-term follow-up. Mayo Clin Proc 1974;49:44–51.
6. Norton JA. Neuroendocrine tumors of the pancreas and duodenum. Curr Probl Surg 1994;31:11–164.
7. Norton JA, Cornelius MJ, Doppman JL. Effect of parathyroidectomy in patients with hyperparathyroidism and multiple endocrine neoplasia type I. Surgery (St. Louis) 1987;102:958–966.
8. Larsson C, Skogseid B, Öberg K, Nakamura Y, Nordenskjöld M. Multiple endocrine neoplasia type 1 gene maps to chromosome 11 and is lost in insulinoma. Nature (Lond) 1988;332:85–87.
9. Chandrasekharappa SC, Guru SC, Manickamp P, et al. Positional cloning of the gene for multiple endocrine neoplasia-type 1. Science 1997;276:404–407.
10. Rizzoli R, Green J, Marx SJ. Long-term follow-up of serum calcium levels after parathyroidectomy. Am J Med 1985;78:467–473.
11. Wells SA Jr, Farndon JR, Dale JK, Leight GS, Dilley WG. Long term evaluation of patients with primary parathyroid hyperplasia managed by total parathyroidectomy and heterotopic autotransplantation. Ann Surg 1980;192:451–458.
12. Hellman P, Skogseid B, Juhlin C, Akerstrom G, Rastad J. Findings and long-term results of parathyroid surgery in multiple endocrine neoplasia type 1. World J Surg 1992;16:718–723.
13. Kraimps JL, Duh Q-Y, Demeure M, Clark OH. Hyperparathyroidism in multiple endocrine neoplasia syndrome. Surgery (St. Louis) 1992;112:1080–1088.
14. van Heerden JA, Kent RB, Sizemore GW, Grant CS, ReMine WM. Primary hyperparathyroidism in patients with multiple endocrine neoplasia syndromes: surgical experience. Arch Surg 1983;118:533–536.
15. Sipple JH. The association of pheochromocytoma with carcinoma of the thyroid gland. Am J Med 1961;31:163–166.

16. Steiner AL, Goodman AD, Powers SR. Study of a kindred with pheochromocytoma, medullary thyroid carcinoma, hyperparathyroidism and Cushing's disease: Multiple endocrine neoplasia type 2. Medicine (Baltimore) 1968;47:371–409.

17. Howe JR, Norton JA, Wells SA Jr. Prevalence of pheochromocytoma and hyperparathyroidism in multiple endocrine neoplasia type 2A: results of long-term follow-up. Surgery (St. Louis) 1993;114:1070–1077.

18. Williams ED, Pollack DJ. Multiple mucosal neuromata with endocrine tumours: a syndrome allied to von Recklinghausen's disease. J Pathol Bacteriol 1966;91:71–80.

19. Schimke RN, Hartmann WH, Prout TE, Rimoin DL. Syndrome of bilateral pheochromocytoma, medullary thyroid carcinoma and multiple neuromas. N Engl J Med 1968;279:1–7.

20. Farndon JR, Leight GS, Dilley WG, et al. Familial medullary thyroid carcinoma without associated endocrinopathies: a distinct clinical entity. Br J Surg 1986;73:278–281.

21. Tashjian AH Jr, Howland BG, Melvin KEW, Hill CS Jr. Immunoassay of human calcitonin: clinical measurement, relation to serum calcium and studies in patients with medullary carcinoma. N Engl J Med 1970;283:890–895.

22. Wells SA Jr, Baylin SB, Leight GS, Dale JK, Dilley WG. Farndon JR. The importance of early diagnosis in patients with hereditary medullary thyroid carcinoma. Ann Surg 1982;195:595–599.

23. Carney JA, Sizemore GW, Tyce GM. Bilateral adrenal medullary hyperplasia in multiple endocrine neoplasia, type 2: the precursor of bilateral pheochromocytoma. Mayo Clin Proc 1975;50:3–10.

24. Carney JA, Sizemore GW, Sheps SG. Adrenal medullary disease in multiple endocrine neoplasia, type 2: pheochromocytoma and its precursors. Am J Clin Pathol 1976;66:279–290.

25. Freier DT, Thompson NW, Sisson JC, Nishiyama RH, Freitas JE. Dilemmas in the early diagnosis and treatment of multiple endocrine adenomatosis, type II. Surgery (St. Louis) 1977;82:407–413.

26. Lips KJM, van der Sluys Veer J, Struyvenberg A, et al. Bilateral occurrence of pheochromocytoma in patients with the multiple endocrine neoplasia syndrome type 2A (Sipple's syndrome). Am J Med 1981;70:1051–1060.

27. van Heerden JA, Sizemore GW, Carney JA, Grant CS, ReMine WH, Sheps SG. Surgical management of the adrenal glands in the multiple endocrine neoplasia type II syndrome. World J Surg 1984;8:612–621.

28. Tibblin S, Dymling J-F, Ingemansson S, Telenius-Berg M. Unilateral versus bilateral adrenalectomy in multiple endocrine neoplasia IIA. World J Surg 1983;7:201–208.

29. Lairmore TC, Ball DW, Baylin SB, Wells SA Jr. Management of pheochromocytomas in patients with multiple endocrine neoplasia type 2 syndromes. Ann Surg 1993;217:595–603.

30. Herfarth KK-F, Bartsch D, Doherty GM, Wells SA Jr, Lairmore TC. Surgical management of hyperparathyroidism in patients with multiple endocrine neoplasia type 2A. Surgery (St. Louis) 1996;120:966–974.

31. O'Riordain DS, O'Brien T, Grant CS, Weaver A, Gharib H, van Heerden JA. Surgical management of primary hyperparathyroidism in multiple endocrine neoplasia types 1 and 2. Surgery (St. Louis) 1993;114:1031–1039.

32. Raue F, Kraimps JL, Dralle H, et al. Primary hyperparathyroidism in multiple endocrine neoplasia type 2A. J Intern Med 1995;238:369–373.

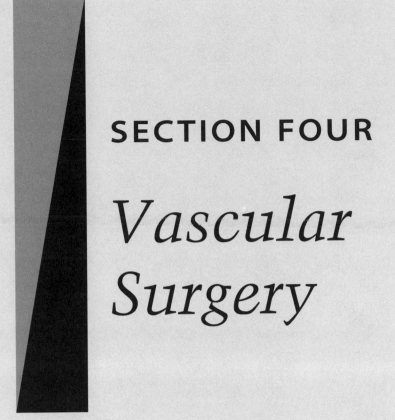

SECTION FOUR

Vascular Surgery

32

Cerebrovascular Disease

Sheela T. Patel and K. Craig Kent

Approximately 500,000 people in the United States develop new strokes each year; stroke is a leading cause of neurological disability and the third most common cause of death, preceded only by coronary artery disease and cancer. Carotid endarterectomy (CEA) is the most commonly performed peripheral vascular operation in the United States. In this chapter, the anatomy, pathophysiology, diagnosis, and treatment of cerebrovascular disease are reviewed.

Anatomy

Anterior Circulation

The brain is supplied anteriorly by paired internal carotid arteries, which provide approximately 80% to 90% of the total cerebral blood flow. The left common carotid artery originates directly from the aortic arch, whereas the right common carotid artery originates from the innominate artery. The common carotid arteries bifurcate at the angle of the mandible into external and internal branches. The external carotid artery has many divisions, several of which supply the cerebral circulation through collaterals. The internal carotid artery can be divided into the cervical (or extracranial), intrapetrosal, intracavernous, and supraclinoid segments. The intracavernous and supraclinoid segments of the internal carotid artery are referred to as the carotid siphon.

Posterior Circulation

The vertebral arteries supply 10% to 20% of the total cerebral circulation. Both vertebral arteries originate from the first portion of their respective subclavian arteries and then enter the vertebral canal at the transverse foramina of the sixth cervical vertebra. The vertebral arteries unite to form the basilar artery, which then branches into the right and left posterior cerebral arteries. The posterior circulation supplies the brainstem, cranial nerves, cerebellum, and the occipital and temporal lobes of the cerebrum.

Circle of Willis

The anterior communicating artery connects the two anterior cerebral arteries. The posterior communicating artery connects the internal carotid arteries (anterior circulation) to the posterior cerebral arteries (posterior circulation). This interconnecting network, which is termed the circle of Willis, is completely intact in 20% to 40% of individuals and allows for collateral flow between the hemispheres and the anterior and posterior circulations (Fig. 32.1).

Clinical Presentation and Pathophysiology

Atherosclerosis is the pathological process most often responsible for cerebrovascular insufficiency. The carotid bifurcation is the predominant location for atherosclerotic disease. Low shear stress in well-defined regions of the carotid bulb appear to stimulate the formation of atherosclerotic plaque.

Symptoms of cerebrovascular disease may be the consequence of distal embolization from an atherosclerotic plaque or hypoperfusion related to a flow-limiting lesion. The most common cause of a cerebral ischemic event, however, is embolization.

Hypoperfusion related to carotid artery stenosis is a less common source of symptoms because extensive collateral circulation is provided by the contralateral carotid and vertebral arteries via the circle of Willis and by the external carotid artery via transcranial connections. The fact that 90% to 95% of patients undergoing CEA do not develop cerebral insufficiency during clamping of the carotid artery confirms that, in the majority of individuals with progressive atherosclerotic disease, this collateral network is adequate to prevent cerebral ischemia.

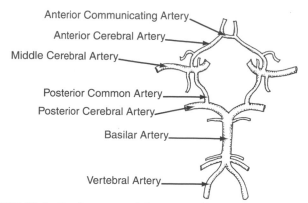

FIGURE 32.1. Configuration of the terminal branches of the vertebral and internal carotid arteries and their interconnections to form the circle of Willis.

Symptoms of cerebrovascular disease include hemispheric transient ischemic attacks (TIAs), amaurosis fugax, and stroke. A TIA is defined as an acute loss of cerebral function that persists for less than 24 h, although most events are brief, lasting 15 min or less. The specific clinical presentation depends on the anatomical location of the area of cerebral ischemia. Symptoms associated with anterior or carotid bifurcation disease include sensory or motor deficits affecting the contralateral face, arms, or legs, aphasia (if the dominant hemisphere is affected), or alterations in higher cortical dysfunction. Patients with posterior or vertebrobasilar ischemia may present with vertigo, dizziness, gait ataxia, dysarthria, nystagmus, diplopia, bilateral visual loss, drop attacks (collapse caused by loss of control of extremities without loss of consciousness), as well as bilateral or alternating motor or sensory impairment. Nonfocal symptoms, such as syncope, confusion, and "light-headedness" are rarely the result of cerebrovascular disease. Reversible ischemic neurological deficits (RINDs) are cerebral vascular symptoms that persist for more than 24 h but less than 7 days. Although the definitions can vary, deficits that persist more than 7 days are usually considered strokes. A stroke may or may not be associated with an obvious infarct identified by computed tomography (CT) or magnetic resonance imaging (MRI).

Transient unilateral loss of vision is referred to as amaurosis fugax. This symptom is classically described as the sensation of a shade coming down over the entire, half, or a quadrant of one eye. This event is the consequence of a microembolus lodging in the opthalmic artery or one of its retinal branches. A cholesterol crystal (Hollenhorst plaque) is occasionally observed on funduscopic examination as a bright refractile body in a branch of the retinal artery. Although amaurosis fugax is a temporary event, retinal artery occlusion may lead to permanent blindness.

There are several symptoms that suggest instability of a carotid lesion and the potential of an imminent stroke. The term crescendo TIAs is used to describe a series of transient neurological events that occur with increasing frequency, duration, or severity. A stroke-in-evolution is a neurological deficit that progressively worsens through a series of discrete exacerbations without intervening periods of normal neurological function. Patients with these clinical presentations should be treated with anticoagulation if there is no radiological evidence of hemorrhage and then urgent CEA so long

as the neurological deficit is not severe.[1] Although no randomized data are available, the outcome of urgent operation appears to be superior to the natural history of this disease process.[2,3]

Indications for Carotid Endarterectomy

Symptomatic Carotid Artery Disease

The North American Symptomatic Carotid Endarterectomy Trial (NASCET) was a large prospective randomized trial designed to test the efficacy of CEA in patients with symptomatic carotid stenosis.[4] From 50 centers in the United States and Canada, 659 patients with greater than 70% symptomatic carotid stenosis were randomized to CEA or best medical management. The cumulative 2-year risk of ipsilateral stroke was 26% in patients treated medically and 9% in patients treated with carotid endarterectomy, representing an absolute risk reduction of 17% and a relative risk reduction of 65%. Patients in this study who had surgical correction of high-grade carotid stenoses gained a durable benefit from their operation that persisted for at least 8 years.[5] In subset analysis, it was found that the degree of stenosis, clinical presentation, and the presence or absence of ulceration affected the efficacy of CEA. The benefit of CEA increased with the degree of carotid stenosis. Medically treated patients with stenoses of 70% to 79%, 80% to 89%, and 90% to 99% had a 2-year risk of stroke of 19.9%, 28.5%, and 34.6%, respectively. The 2-year risk of stroke in patients treated with CEA was 9% regardless of the degree of stenosis. Interestingly, the existence of comorbidities, such as diabetes, coronary artery disease, or hypertension, increased the incidence of stroke in medically treated patients.[4] However, the stroke rate was constant at 9% in the surgical group regardless of the number of comorbidities. These findings challenge the frequently expressed notion that patients with multiple comorbidities benefit less from surgical intervention.

A second cohort of patients, those with symptomatic 30% to 69% stenoses, were also studied as part of NASCET. Although patients with symptomatic moderate 50% to 69% stenoses benefit less from carotid endarterectomy than those with 70% to 99% lesions, in both groups surgery provided a more durable long-term benefit than did treatment with the best medical therapy. Thus, carotid endarterectomy has been shown in prospective randomized trials to be effective in treating symptomatic patients with greater than 50% carotid artery stenosis.

Asymptomatic Carotid Disease

The Asymptomatic Carotid Atherosclerosis Study (ACAS) is the largest available randomized trial of patients with asymptomatic carotid stenosis.[6] In this study, 1662 asymptomatic patients with 60% to 99% carotid stenoses were randomized to receive CEA or medical management. The 5-year risk of stroke was 5.1% in patients treated surgically and 11% in patients treated medically, yielding a statistically significant 5.9% absolute risk reduction. This beneficial effect of surgery in asymptomatic carotid disease was in large part the result of a low 30-day operative risk (2.3%) for CEA. The effect of degree of stenosis on the efficacy of CEA in asymptomatic patients was not adequately addressed by ACAS. Several non-randomized studies, however, have demonstrated an association in asymptomatic patients between increasing degrees of stenosis and the benefit of CEA.[7,8]

Although a statistical benefit for CEA in asymptomatic patients with 60% to 99% carotid stenoses was demonstrated by ACAS, skeptics argue that 17 operations were required to prevent one stroke over 5 years. This observation raised questions about the cost-effectiveness as well as the sensibility of treating asymptomatic patients with CEA.[9,10] Recent analyses, however, have demonstrated that CEA in the cohort of asymptomatic patients defined by ACAS is indeed cost effective[11,12] when certain factors are taken into account. First, longevity of a patient is an important criterion when selecting asymptomatic candidates for CEA because the benefit demonstrated by ACAS can only be achieved in patients who are expected to live at least an additional 5 years. Accordingly, CEA is rarely cost effective in individuals above the age of 80. Degree of stenosis may also be an important factor in patient selection. Several studies have shown an increased risk of stroke in medically managed patients with stenoses greater than 80%. Thus, patients with high-grade stenoses may comprise a subgroup of patients in whom CEA provides greater benefit.

Tandem Lesions/Contralateral Carotid Occlusion/"String Sign"

The carotid siphon is the second most common location for cerebrovascular atherosclerotic disease. Thus, the coexistence of tandem lesions in the carotid siphon and the ipsilateral carotid bifurcation is not unusual. Several retrospective studies have addressed the question of whether a carotid siphon lesion adversely affects the perioperative risk as well as the long-term benefit of CEA.[13–16] No significant difference in risk was found. Thus, under most circumstances, CEA is still indicated in patients with tandem siphon stenoses.

CEA can be performed contralateral to an occluded carotid artery with acceptable safety. Although some studies suggest that CEA in these patients is associated with an increased incidence of stroke, in many other studies the rate of stroke is equivalent to that of patients without contralateral disease.[17–20] Patients may present with a carotid "string sign" in which arteriography reveals only minimal flow in the internal carotid artery. The presence of a string sign may imply markedly diminished flow through a highly stenotic proximal carotid stenosis. In these patients urgent CEA can be performed with the usual morbidity and mortality.[21] A string sign may also be associated with a diffusely diseased and fibrotic carotid artery that is technically challenging to reconstruct.[22] The rate of stroke with CEA is increased under this circumstance.

Timing of Carotid Endarterectomy

The timing of CEA after an acute stroke is a critical issue that has been studied in some detail. Early reperfusion following endarterectomy of a large recently infarcted region of the brain can lead to cerebral hemorrhage and potentially devastating consequences. This observation led to the traditional dictum that CEA should be delayed a minimum of 4 to 6

weeks in patients presenting with completed strokes.[23] Unfortunately, if this policy is rigidly followed, some patients, because of instability of their carotid artery disease, will be vulnerable to a second stroke that occurs during this 4- to 6-week interval.[24] It has since been shown that, in patients with small fixed deficits or small infarcts seen by CT or MRI, the risk of early CEA is not increased.[25,26] Thus, patients with small strokes and significant carotid stenosis should be considered for early operative intervention.

Patients scheduled for elective coronary artery bypass grafting (CABG) may harbor significant carotid disease. Reports estimate that 4% to 12% of patients awaiting elective CABG will have, by duplex ultrasound, a carotid artery stenosis greater than 80%.[27] Conversely, up to 35% of patients with carotid disease will have significant coexisting coronary artery disease.[28] The appropriate treatment of patients with surgical lesions of both the carotid and coronary arteries remains controversial. A meta-analysis of more than 30 studies in which this question was addressed calculated the following mortality and stroke rates: CEA before CABG (9.4%, 5.3%), CABG before CEA (3.6%, 10%), and simultaneous CABG and CEA (5.6%, 6.2%). Until further data are available, the timing of CEA in patients requiring CABG should be individualized with consideration given to the severity of symptoms.

Preoperative Studies

Contrast Arteriography

Contrast arteriography is the traditional method for evaluating the carotid bifurcation before CEA. Angiography can provide complete and detailed images of the proximal (aortic arch and branches) and distal (intracranial) circulation as well as the carotid bifurcation. Unfortunately, the incidence of stroke associated with arteriography is not insignificant and this morbidity must be included when calculating the overall risk of intervention for carotid artery disease.

Duplex Ultrasonography

Duplex ultrasound (DU) can be an accurate, noninvasive preoperative method of imaging the carotid bifurcation. Peak systolic and end-diastolic velocities measured in the common and internal carotid arteries are used to determine the degree of stenosis. Accuracies for DU in the 90% range have been obtained in laboratories with appropriate expertise.[29] There are, however, several limitations to DU, including the need for experienced sonographers, the inability to accurately anatomically define intracranial or intrathoracic circulation, and the potential for misinterpretation of flow-related artifacts. Thus, validation of the accuracy of DU in individual laboratories is essential before DU can be used as the sole imaging modality before carotid endarterectomy.

Magnetic Resonance Angiography

Magnetic resonance angiography (MRA) is a variant of magnetic resonance imaging (MRI) that has been used increasingly in the evaluation of patients with cerebrovascular occlusive disease. The carotid bifurcation, because of its straight-line configuration and rapid blood flow, is especially

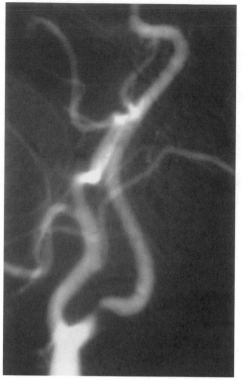

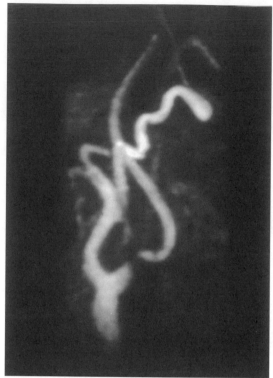

FIGURE 32.2. Contrast arteriogram (**A**) and (**B**) MRA (magnetic resonance angiography) of the carotid bifurcation. MRA can provide a precise anatomical depiction of carotid bifurcation disease.

well suited for evaluation by MRA. An appealing advantage of MRA over DU is that it anatomically displays the intracranial and extracranial circulation in a format strikingly similar to that of a conventional arteriogram (Fig. 32.2). DU and MRA can be complementary techniques for evaluating carotid artery disease; when there is agreement between both studies, contrast arteriography is rarely necessary.[30–32]

Carotid Endarterectomy

Although CEA is a conceptually simple operation, precision and attention to technical detail are required to achieve a low rate of stroke (Fig. 32.3). It has been demonstrated that the outcome of CEA is directly related to the frequency with which this operation is performed. Accordingly, it has been advised that CEA be performed by surgeons who perform 12 to 15 or more CEAs per year.[33–35] Also noteworthy is the technique of eversion endarterectomy (Fig. 32.4) which has been popularized in recent years. Because this technique avoids the need for a suture line in the distal internal carotid artery where the luminal diameter is small, it has been suggested that eversion endarterectomy reduces the incidence of occlusion and restenosis compared to the more conventional endarterectomy techniques.

Type of Anesthesia

Carotid endarterectomy may be performed under either general or regional anesthesia. The choice of anesthetic technique has been subject of intense debate. The risk of stroke/death or MI are 0–6.5% and 0.6–6.7% respectively in patients re-

ceiving general anesthesia, and 0–5.4% and 0–3.6% in patients receiving local anesthesia. Although both alternatives have been studied and compared on numerous occasions, no consistent benefit has been found with either approach.

Cerebral Protection

There is no consensus regarding the appropriate technique for cerebral protection during CEA. Options include routine shunting of all patients versus selective shunting, based upon measures of cerebral ischemia such as stump pressures, electroencephalography (EEG), or awake monitoring. Despite multiple prejudices, no method of cerebral protection has been proven to be superior. Maintainence of adequate cerebral flow, however, is an essential part of CEA because strokes related to hypoperfusion are usually major and devastating.

Patch Angioplasty

Although CEA has become a well-established and commonly performed procedure, there remains controversy as to the appropriate method of closing the arteriotomy (Table 32.1). Primary closure is the most expeditious. Alternatively, patch angioplasty with autogenous or prosthetic material serves to increase the luminal diameter of the endarterectomized vessel. Proponents of carotid patch angioplasty argue that this technique reduces the incidence of perioperative thrombosis and carotid occlusion. However, advantages of primary closure include its simplicity, technical ease, and a reduction in operative time. Moreover, primary closure does not involve complications inherent to patch angioplasty, such as vein patch "blowout," pseudoaneurysm formation, and prosthetic

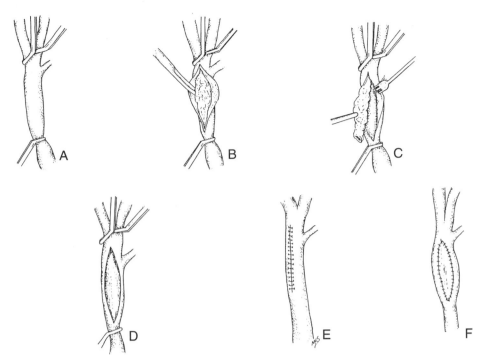

FIGURE 32.3. Technique of standard carotid endarterectomy. After adequate exposure is achieved, the internal, external, and common carotid arteries are clamped (**A**). A plane of dissection is created between the arterial wall and the atheromatous process (**B**). After the plaque is transected proximally, it can be reflected upward to aid in the distal portion of the endarterectomy (**C**). After completion of the endarterectomy, any remaining loose pieces of atheroma or strands of media are removed (**D**). The arteriotomy is closed primarily (**E**) or with a patch graft (**F**).

graft infection. Interestingly, a number of authors report no advantage in terms of either perioperative stroke or late restenosis rates in patients treated with patch angioplasty versus primary closure.[36–40]

Ultimately, both approaches, patch angioplasty and primary closure, have been associated with excellent short- and long-term outcomes following CEA. Surgeon experience and preference is the primary determinant of which technique is used.

Verification of Technical Result

Many surgeons have recommended intraoperative imaging of the reconstructed carotid artery with the presumption that immediate recognition of technical defects will decrease the incidence of postoperative stroke and late restenosis.[41–45]

There are no randomized studies available that address this question, nor is there a consensus. Currently, most surgeons evaluate the adequacy of CEA using a Doppler probe and palpation of the distal internal carotid artery pulse.

Postoperative Care

Current practice standards dictate that patients following CEA can be discharged to the ward after a brief stay in the recovery room if they are neurologically intact and hemodynamically stable. Only a small percentage of patients actually require intensive care unit monitoring.[46] Moreover, most patients can be discharged safely to home on the first postoperative day. These approaches, which have been successfully employed in many centers, substantially reduce the hospital cost of CEA and are well accepted by patients.[47–49]

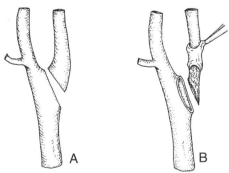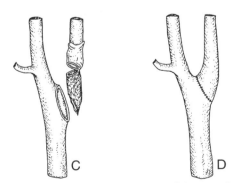

FIGURE 32.4. Technique of eversion carotid endarterectomy. Internal carotid artery is transected obliquely at the carotid bifurcation (**A**). Medial and adventitial layers of the internal carotid artery are everted over the atheromatous core (**B**). Completion of endarterectomy with the distal endpoint directly visualized (**C**). Internal carotid artery is reanastomosed to the common carotid artery (**D**).

TABLE 32.1.
Influence of Method of Arteriotomy Closure on Perioperative Complications and Restenosis in Patients Undergoing CEA.

Author	Year	Primary closure				Vein patch closure				Prosthetic patch closure			
		CEAs	Stroke/death (%)	Restenosis (%)	F/U (months)	CEAs	Stroke/death (%)	Restenosis (%)	F/U (months)	CEAs	Stroke/death (%)	Restenosis (%)	F/U (months)
Nene et al.[36]	1999	75	0	1.3	18					67	1.5	0	18
AbuRahma et al.[87]	1998	135	5.9*	34*	30	130	1.5*	9*	30	134	0.7*	2*	30
Desiron et al.[88]	1997	837		13*	69	1320		4.8*	35				
Allen et al.[89]	1997					287	1.7	1.0	29.3	110	4.5	2.7	27.6
Katz SG et al.[90]	1996					100	1.0	0	19	107	2.8	0.9	19
Goldman et al.[91]	1995					184	2.2	4.2	16.1	91	1.1	7.9	9.3
Katz D et al.[37]	1994	51	3.9	3.9	29.2					49	2.0	0	29.2
Myers et al.[38]	1994	64	1.6	7.8	57	61	0	14.8	59				
Gonzales-Fajardo et al.[92]	1994					45	0	0	29	50	4	4	29
Treiman et al.[39]	1993	1173	2.7			240	4.6	0		266	2.3		
Ranaboldo et al.[93]	1993	104	2.9	16.3*	12	109[b]	2.8	5.5*	12				
DeLetter et al.[94]	1993	62	6.5	27.4*	60	67	4.5	11.9*	60				
Whereatt et al.[95]	1990					75	4.0	5.3	29.3	16	12.5	6.3	29.3
Rosenthal et al.[40]	1990	250	1.6	4.1	37.8	250	0	0.9	37.8	500	1.8	4.8	37.8
Lord et al.[96]	1989	50	2	19.1*	<1	43	0	0*	<1	47	0	0*	<1
Katz MM et al.[97]	1987	47	4.3	19.1*	6–24	42	0	2.4*	6–24				
Ouriel and Green[98]	1987	82[c]	3.7	28.6*	17.2					70§	0	5.7*	16
Hertzer et al.[99]	1987	483	3.3*	14*	21	434	0.9*	4.8*	21				
Fode et al.[100]	1986	2714	6.6*			266	2.3*			257	7		

CEA, caroid endarterectomy; F/U, mean follow-up time.
[a]Only stroke rates given, death rates not specified.
[b]Patched group includes 52 vein and 56 prosthetic patches; rates not stratified although authors state that there was no significant difference between vein and prosthetic subgroups with respect to neurological complications or restenosi rates.
[c]Number of patients undergoing CEA (number of procedures performed not indicated).
*p value < 0.05 (primary versus patch closure).

Postoperative Complications

The most devastating consequence of CEA is stroke. Causes of intra- or postoperative stroke include (1) embolization that occurs during dissection of the carotid artery, (2) inadequate cerebral protection during carotid cross-clamping, (3) postoperative thrombosis, and (4) intracerebral hemorrhage (reperfusion syndrome). Before leaving the operating room, the patient is fully awakened and assessed for neurological deficits. The finding of a major neurological deficit warrants immediate reexploration with intraoperative imaging of the carotid reconstruction. A neurological deficit that occurs within the first 24 h should likewise lead to either an urgent duplex ultrasound or surgical reexploration. A hemorrhagic stroke may develop 3 to 7 days postoperatively as a consequence of a hyperperfusion syndrome. The initial symptom may be a severe unilateral throbbing headache. There is usually associated hypertension. Seizures may then occur, followed by a permanent neurological deficit that is usually associated with intracranial hemorrhage. Early recognition is essential and should be rapidly followed by precise blood pressure control, avoidance of anticoagulation, and anticonvulsants as necessary. If cerebral hemorrhage occurs, placement of an intraventricular pressure monitor or craniotomy with evacuation of the hematoma may be lifesaving, although the outcome once hemorrhage has developed is usually poor.[50–52]

Other than stroke, myocardial infarction is the most common major complication following CEA. Postoperative fluctuations in blood pressure, either hyper or hypotension, develop in 20% to 60% of patients.[53,54] Severe hypertension should be controlled with sodium nitroprusside and hypotension with fluid administration or phenylephrine. These fluctuations may be related to carotid sinus manipulation. Cranial nerve injury can complicate CEA, particularly if the carotid bifurcation is high and more cephalad exposure is required.[55–57] Most injuries result from traction rather than inadvertent division of the nerve and resolve completely within a few weeks. A wound hematoma is unusual, but if large may compromise either the arterial repair or a patient's airway. An early postoperative hematoma deserves close monitoring and urgent surgical evacuation if there is suspicion of airway compromise.

Postoperative Surveillance

CEA is a durable procedure; however, restenosis and occasionally recurrent symptoms may develop. Restenosis is the result of either myointimal hyperplasia, which tends to develop within the first 2 years following CEA, or recurrent atherosclerosis, which is most predominant after 2 years. Symptoms are relatively rare in patients who develop intimal hyperplasia because these lesions are smooth, nonulcerated, and do not act as a nidus for cholesterol or platelets. Beyond 2 years, symptoms are more frequent and are related to embolization from atherosclerotic plaque. Recurrent stenosis and symptoms are more frequent in women, in patients with atherosclerotic risk factors such as cigarette smoking and hypercholesterolemia, or if residual disease remains following the initial endarterectomy.[58–60] Postoperative surveillance protocols using duplex ultrasound are frequently employed in patients following CEA.

Although controversial, many authors have reported an increased rate of complication following CEA in patients with recurrent disease. Thus, "redo" CEA is usually reserved for symptomatic patients or those without symptoms who have preocclusive lesions. Patch angioplasty rather than endarterectomy is indicated in patients in whom intimal hyperplasia is the pathological lesion because a precise endarterectomy plane cannot usually be identified. For recurrent atherosclerotic lesions, CEA is the procedure of choice.

Vertebrobasilar Ischemia

Posterior ischemic symptoms may result from atherosclerotic disease involving the vertebral or proximal subclavian arteries. Symptoms of vertebrobasilar ischemia usually result from hypoperfusion and only rarely from embolization. A systemic process that decreases blood pressure, such as orthostatic hypotension, overaggressive treatment with antihypertensives, anemia, or arrhythmias, can precipitate symptoms. Symptoms may also be prompted by rotation of the neck if osteophytes arising from the cervical vertebrae compress the vertebral artery as it passes through the vertebral canal. Hypoperfusion-related vertebrobasilar ischemia seldom results in cerebral infarction, but can produce functional disability. Because the vertebral arteries unite to form the basilar artery, occlusive disease involving both vertebral arteries is required for symptoms of hypoperfusion to develop. The exception to this rule is in patients with subclavian steal.

There is little role for surgery in the treatment of asymptomatic vertebrobasilar insufficiency. It can be assumed that these patients are receiving adequate collateral flow from either the anterior circulation and/or the contralateral vertebral artery. In patients who have concomitant carotid and vertebral lesions, correction of the anterior circulation lesion should be the initial treatment and is usually effective in alleviating symptoms.

Carotid Artery Occlusion

The extracranial internal carotid artery has no branches. Thus, if a lesion at the origin of the internal carotid artery leads to occlusion, clot propagates distally to the next collateral, which is either the opthalmic or the middle cerebral arteries. Unless urgently addressed, this clot cannot be removed. Thus, CEA is not an option in patients with chronic internal carotid artery occlusion. The rate of stroke associated with carotid occlusion is as high as 5% per year.[61,62] Although treatment of symptomatic patients with carotid artery occlusion is usually with coumadin or antiplatelet agents, there are several surgical options that should be considered. If there is severe disease of the contralateral carotid artery, contralateral CEA should be performed. Extracranial–intracranial bypass was developed for the treatment of symptomatic patients with internal carotid occlusion and involves the anastomosis, through a craniotomy, of the superficial temporal artery branch of the external carotid artery to the ipsilateral middle cerebral artery. After a prospective randomized trial in 1985 demonstrated that extracranial–intracranial bypass was ineffective in preventing long-term stroke, enthusiasm for this procedure markedly diminished.[63] There has recently been a renewed interest in this technique in a subset of patients in whom hypoperfusion (rather than embolization) is the primary problem.

Extracranial Carotid Artery Aneurysms

Extracranial carotid artery aneurysms are uncommon lesions, accounting for less than 2% of all carotid interventions. Atherosclerosis, trauma, previous carotid surgery, dissection, and fibromuscular dysplasia are the usual etiologies. Patients may present with an asymptomatic pulsatile neck or pharyngeal mass or with symptoms, including neck pain, hoarseness, or dysphagia (the latter two related to compression of the vagus or glossopharyngeal nerves). TIAs or strokes are also common presenting symptoms and most often result from the distal embolization of atheromatous debris from the aneurysmal sac.[64,65] Rupture of carotid artery aneurysms is rare.

All aneurysms of the carotid artery should be repaired regardless of symptoms.[66] Resection of the aneurysm and restoration of arterial continuity is the procedure of choice.[67]

Nonatherosclerotic Cerebrovascular Disease

Carotid Body Tumors

The carotid body is a highly vascular chemoreceptor located in the adventitial layer of the carotid bifurcation. Carotid body tumors (or carotid paragangliomas) present as painless, pulsatile but not expansile, usually asymptomatic neck masses that are found just below the angle of the mandible. They lie between the internal and external carotid arteries, just cephalad to the carotid bifurcation, and may extend to the base of the skull. Symptoms occasionally develop (related to pressure on the adjacent cranial nerves or local structures) and include neck or ear pain, dysphagia, hoarseness, tinnitus, or dizziness. Although duplex ultrasound can be used to identify carotid body tumors, MRI/MRA, CT, and/or arteriography are usually necessary for diagnosis and preoperative planning. Typical arteriographic features include splaying of the internal and external carotid arteries by a vascular mass. The blood supply to the tumor is derived predominantly from the external carotid artery. Needle or open biopsy of these masses should be avoided. The recommended treatment for a carotid body tumor is surgical excision.[68–70]

Fibromuscular Dysplasia of the Extracranial Carotid Artery

Fibromuscular arterial dysplasia is an uncommon disorder that primarily affects the renal and carotid arteries of young women. Morphologically, lesions present as alternating stenoses and regions of dilatation involving the internal carotid artery distal to the bifurcation. Angiographically, this appears as a "string of beads," a finding that is pathognomonic for fibromuscular dysplasia. Associated intracranial aneurysms are found in 10% of patients.[71] Fibromuscular dysplasia has also been associated with spontaneous carotid dissection. The pathogenesis of fibromuscular dysplasia is unknown. Although natural history data are lacking, patients with asymptomatic lesions should probably be treated with antiplatelet agents and carefully observed. Intervention should be reserved for patients with symptoms.[72,73] Open surgery with graduated intraluminal dilatation is the most widely used procedure for treating fibromuscular dysplasia. Other treatment options include per-

cutaneous carotid angioplasty (although experience with this technique is limited) and resection with primary anastomosis or an interposition bypass.

Carotid Coils and Kinks

Coils (circular or exaggerated S-shape configurations) and kinks (sharp angulations) of the carotid artery may be congenital or acquired. The most common symptomatic lesion is the carotid kink. Atherosclerotic plaques are frequently found at the site of kinks and may be responsible for embolic symptoms. Turning of the head or twisting of the neck may accentuate a kink and also produce symptoms related to hypoperfusion. Operation should be considered only in patients with symptoms.[74–77] Options for treatment include patch angioplasty, resection of the redundant segment of the carotid artery with primary end-to-end anastomosis, resection of a segment of the common carotid artery with reduction of the kink and primary reanastomosis, or detachment of the internal carotid artery at its origin with translocation to a more proximal location on the common carotid artery.

Carotid Dissection

Carotid dissection is increasingly recognized as a major cause of cerebral infarction in young adults. An intimal tear or a ruptured vasa vasorum allows blood to penetrate and dissect into the arterial wall. This process may result in narrowing or occlusion of the arterial lumen. Carotid artery dissection may be either spontaneous or traumatic. The most commonly reported symptom is an abrupt neurological deficit preceded by a sudden, severe, ipsilateral headache or neck–face pain.[78] Patients may also develop an incomplete Horner's syndrome (ptosis and miosis without facial sweating) or a lower cranial nerve palsy, secondary to nerve compression by an intramural hematoma.[79]

Prompt recognition and timely treatment is of the utmost importance.[80,81] Systemic anticoagulation is the initial treatment for carotid dissection and is administered to patients who do not have radiographic evidence of intracranial bleeding or massive infarction. In the majority of patients, there is gradual restoration of the arterial lumen over time.[82] Anticoagulation is thought to reduce the risk of embolization and to prevent extension of thrombus and is usually continued for 3 to 6 months or until the carotid artery recanalizes.[83] Surgical treatment, such as carotid resection with graft interposition or carotid ligation with or without extracranial–intracranial bypass, is indicated only in patients who develop progressive or recurrent neurological symptoms despite adequate anticoagulation.

Arteriopathies Affecting the Carotid Vessels

Takayasu's Arteritis

Takayasu's disease is an arteriopathy of unknown etiology that affects the major branches of the aorta and the pulmonary artery. Patients are typically young to middle-aged females, often of Asian descent. The early phase of Takayasu's disease is characterized by nonspecific symptoms such as headache, malaise, myalgia, and fever. As the disease progresses, segmental stenoses or occlusions occur in the arteries branching from the aortic arch.

It is generally agreed that corticosteroids should be administered as the initial therapy for symptomatic disease. One-third of symptomatic patients require surgery for ischemic complications. Bypass is considered the procedure of choice.

TEMPORAL ARTERITIS

Temporal arteritis, also known as giant cell arteritis, is a disease of unknown etiology affecting predominantly older women. Symptoms associated with temporal arteritis result from the gradual occlusion of the branches of the carotid and vertebral arteries. The most serious complication of temporal arteritis is loss of vision. The erythrocyte sedimentation rate is almost always elevated and provides an accurate measure of disease activity. Once the diagnosis of temporal arteritis is made, usually by temporal artery biopsy, steroids should be immediately administered. Unlike Takayasu's disease, steroids are highly effective in treating the complications of temporal arteritis and surgical intervention is almost never required.

RADIATION-INDUCED ARTERITIS

Patients who have received irradiation for treatment of malignancies are at risk for the later development of radiation-induced carotid artery occlusive disease.[84] Lesions related to a radiation injury are morphologically indistinguishable from those of atherosclerosis and are frequently associated with cerebrovascular symptoms. Extensive changes occur in the entire arterial wall, particularly if the radiation injury is more than 5 years old. As such, it may be difficult to establish a plane in the vessel wall, thereby precluding endarterectomy. Still, although technically demanding, CEA has been successfully used to treat irradiated stenotic carotid arteries.[85,86]

Carotid Angioplasty and Stenting

With the emergence of endovascular technology to treat peripheral vascular occlusive disease, there has been considerable interest in the technique of angioplasty and stenting as a treatment of carotid artery stenosis. A multicenter prospective, randomized trial, the Carotid Revascularization Endarterectomy versus Stent Trial (CREST), has been instituted to evaluate the safety and efficacy of carotid angioplasty and stenting compared to carotid endarterectomy. This study will provide the most valid and accurate data regarding the relative morbidity and mortality of these two interventions.

References

1. Wilson SE, Mayberg MR, Yatsu F, et al. Crescendo transient ischemic attacks: a surgical imperative. J Vasc Surg 1993;17: 249–256.
2. Gertler JP, Blankensteijn JD, Brewster DC, et al. Carotid endarterectomy for unstable and compelling neurologic conditions: do results justify an aggressive approach? J Vasc Surg 1994;19:32–42.
3. Mentzer RM Jr, Finkelmeier BA, Crosby IK, et al. Emergency carotid endarterectomy for fluctuating neurologic deficits. Surgery (St. Louis) 1981;89:60–66.
4. North American Symptomatic Carotid Endarterectomy Trial Collaborators. Beneficial effect of carotid endarterectomy in symptomatic patients with high-grade carotid stenosis. N Engl J Med 1991;325:445–453.
5. Barnett HJ, Taylor DW, Eliasziw M, et al. Benefit of carotid endarterectomy in patients with symptomatic moderate or severe stenosis. North American Symptomatic Carotid Endarterectomy Trial Collaborators. N Engl J Med 1998;339:1415–1425.
6. Executive Committee for the Asymptomatic Carotid Atherosclerosis Study. Endarterectomy for asymptomatic carotid artery stenosis. JAMA 1995;273:1421–1428.
7. Norris JW, Zhu CZ, Bornstein NM, et al. Vascular risks of asymptomatic carotid stenosis. Stroke 1991;22:1485–1490.
8. Moore DJ, Miles RD, Gooley NA, et al. Noninvasive assessment of stroke risk in asymptomatic and nonhemispheric patients with suspected carotid disease: five-year follow-up of 294 unoperated and 81 operated patients. Ann Surg 1985;202: 491–504.
9. Perry JR, Szalai JP, Norris JW. Consensus against both endarterectomy and routine screening for asymptomatic carotid artery stenosis. Arch Neurol 1997;54:25–28.
10. Barnett HJM, Meldrum HE, Eliasziw M. The dilemma of surgical treatment for patients with asymptomatic carotid disease. Ann Intern Med 1995;123:723–725.
11. Cronenwett JL, Birkmeyer JD, Nackman GB, et al. Cost-effectiveness of carotid endarterectomy in asymptomatic patients. J Vasc Surg 1997;25:298–311.
12. Kuntz KM, Kent KC. Is carotid endarterectomy cost-effective? An analysis of symptomatic and asymptomatic patients. Circulation 1996;94:II-194–II-198.
13. Mattos MA, van Bemmelen PS, Hodgson KJ, et al. The influence of carotid siphon stenosis on short- and long-term outcome after carotid endarterectomy. J Vasc Surg 1993;17:902–911.
14. Mackey WC, O'Donnell TF Jr, Callow AD. Carotid endarterectomy in patients with intracranial vascular disease: short-term risk and long-term outcome. J Vasc Surg 1989;10:432–438.
15. Lord RS, Raj TB, Graham AR. Carotid endarterectomy, siphon stenosis, collateral hemispheric pressure, and perioperative cerebral infarction. J Vasc Surg 1987;6:391–397.
16. Schuler JJ, Flanigan DP, Lim LT, et al. The effect of carotid siphon stenosis on stroke rate, death, and relief of symptoms following elective carotid endarterectomy. Surgery (St. Louis) 1982;92:1058–1067.
17. Mackey WC, O'Donnell TF, Callow AD. Carotid endarterectomy contralateral to an occluded carotid artery: perioperative risk and late results. J Vasc Surg 1990;11:778–785.
18. Perler BA, Burdick JF, Williams GM. Does contralateral internal carotid artery occlusion increase the risk of carotid endarterectomy? J Vasc Surg 1992;16:347–353.
19. Aungst M, Gahtan V, Berkowitz H, et al. Carotid endarterectomy outcome is not affected in patients with a contralateral carotid artery occlusion. Am J Surg 1998;176:30–33.
20. Mattos MA, Barkmeier LD, Hodgson KJ, et al. Internal carotid artery occlusion: operative risks and long-term stroke rates after contralateral carotid endarterectomy. Surgery (St. Louis) 1992;112:670–680.
21. Morgenstern LB, Fox AJ, Sharpe BL, et al. The risks and benefits of carotid endarterectomy in patients with near occlusion of the carotid artery. Neurology 1997;48:911–915.
22. Archie JP Jr. Carotid endarterectomy when the distal internal carotid artery is small or poorly visualized. J Vasc Surg 1994; 19:23–31.
23. Giordano JM, Trout HH III, Kozloff L, et al. Timing of carotid artery endarterectomy after stroke. J Vasc Surg 1985;2:250–255.
24. Dosick SM, Whalen RC, Gale SS, et al. Carotid endarterectomy in the stroke patient: computerized axial tomography to determine timing. J Vasc Surg 1985;2:214–219.
25. Whittemore AD, Mannick JA. Surgical treatment of carotid disease in patients with neurologic deficits. J Vasc Surg 1987;5: 910–913.

26. Piotrowski JJ, Bernhard VM, Rubin JR, et al. Timing of carotid endarterectomy after acute stroke. J Vasc Surg 1990;11:45–52.

27. Salasidis GC, Latter DA, Steinmetz OK, et al. Carotid artery duplex scanning in preoperative assessment for coronary artery revascularization: the association between peripheral vascular disease, carotid artery stenosis, and stroke. J Vasc Surg 1995; 21:154–162.

28. Hertzer NR, Beven EG, Young JR, et al. Coronary artery disease in peripheral vascular patients: a classification of 1000 coronary angiograms and results of surgical management. Ann Surg 1984; 199:223–333.

29. Fillinger MF, Baker RJ Jr, Zwolak RM, et al. Carotid duplex criteria for a 60% or greater angiographic stenosis: variation according to equipment. J Vasc Surg 1996;24:856–864.

30. Turnipseed WD, Kennell TW, Turski PA, et al. Combined use of duplex imaging and magnetic resonance angiography for evaluation of patients with symptomatic ipsilateral high-grade carotid stenosis. J Vasc Surg 1993;17:832–840.

31. Patel MR, Kuntz KM, Klufas RA, et al. Preoperative assessment of the carotid bifurcation: can magnetic resonance angiography and duplex ultrasonography replace contrast arteriography? Stroke 1995;26:1753–1758.

32. Kent KC, Kuntz KM, Patel MR, et al. Perioperative imaging strategies for carotid endarterectomy: an analysis of morbidity and cost-effectiveness in symptomatic patients. JAMA 1995;274: 888–893.

33. Kucey DS, Bowyer B, Iron K, et al. Determinants of outcome after carotid endarterectomy. J Vasc Surg 1998;28:1051–1058.

34. Rubin JR, Pitluk HC, King TA, et al. Carotid endarterectomy in a metropolitan community: the early results after 8535 operations. J Vasc Surg 1988;7:256–260.

35. Mattos MA, Modi JR, Mansour AM, et al. Evolution of carotid endarterectomy in two community hospitals: Springfield revisited—seventeen years and 2243 operations later. J Vasc Surg 1995;21:719–728.

36. Nene S, Moore W. The role of patch angioplasty in prevention of early recurrent carotid stenosis. Ann Vasc Surg 1999;13: 169–171.

37. Katz D, Snyder SO, Gandhi RH, et al. Long-term follow-up for recurrent stenosis: a prospective randomized study of expanded polytetrafluoroethylene patch angioplasty versus primary closure after carotid endarterectomy. J Vasc Surg 1994;19:198–205.

38. Myers SI, Valentine RJ, Chervu A, et al. Saphenous vein patch versus primary closure for carotid endarterectomy: long-term assessment of a randomized prospective study. J Vasc Surg 1994; 19:15–22.

39. Treiman RL, Foran RF, Wagner WH, et al. Does routine patch angioplasty after carotid endarterectomy lessen the risk of perioperative stroke? Ann Vasc Surg 1993;7:317–319.

40. Rosenthal D, Archie JP, Garcia-Rinaldi R, et al. Carotid patch angioplasty: immediate and long-term results. J Vasc Surg 1990;12:326–333.

41. Courbier R, Jausseran J, Reggi M, et al. Routine intraoperative carotid angiography: its impact on operative morbidity and carotid restenosis. J Vasc Surg 1986;3:343–350.

42. Donaldson MC, Ivarsson BL, Mannick JA, et al. Impact of completion angiography on operative conduct and results of carotid endarterectomy. Ann Surg 1993;217:682–687.

43. Baker WH, Koustas G, Burke K, et al. Intraoperative duplex scanning and late carotid artery stenosis. J Vasc Surg 1994;19: 829–833.

44. Westerband A, Mills JL, Berman SS, et al. The influence of routine completion arteriography on outcome following carotid endarterectomy. Ann Vasc Surg 1997;11:14–19.

45. Scott SM, Sethi GK, Bridgman AH. Perioperative stroke during carotid endarterectomy: the value of intraoperative angiography. J Cardiovasc Surg (Torino) 1982;23:353–358.

46. O'Brien MS, Ricotta JJ. Conserving resources after carotid endarterectomy: selective use of the intensive care unit. J Vasc Surg 1991;14:796–802.

47. Hirko MK, Morasch MD, Burke K, et al. The changing face of carotid endarterectomy. J Vasc Surg 1996;23:622–627.

48. Kraiss LW, Kilberg L, Critch S, et al. Short-stay carotid endarterectomy is safe and cost-effective. Am J Surg 1995;169: 512–515.

49. Back MR, Harward TRS, Huber TS, et al. Improving the cost-effectiveness of carotid endarterectomy. J Vasc Surg 1997;26: 456–464.

50. Ouriel K, Shortell CK, Illig KA, et al. Intracerebral hemorrhage after carotid endarterectomy: incidence, contribution to neurologic morbidity, and predictive factors. J Vasc Surg 1999;29:82–89.

51. Hafner DH, Smith RB III, King OW, et al. Massive intracerebral hemorrhage following carotid endarterectomy. Arch Surg 1987; 122:305–307.

52. Pomposelli FB, Lamparello PJ, Riles TS, et al. Intracranial hemorrhage after carotid endarterectomy. J Vasc Surg 1988;7:248–255.

53. Skydell JL, Machleder HI, Baker JD, et al. Incidence and mechanism of post-carotid endarterectomy hypertension. Arch Surg 1987;122:1153–1155.

54. Wong JH, Findlay JM, Suarez-Almazor ME. Hemodynamic instability after carotid endarterectomy: risk factors and associations with operaive complications. Neurosurgery 1997;41:35–43.

55. Schauber MD, Fontenelle LJ, Solomon JW, et al. Cranial/cervical nerve dysfunction after carotid endarterectomy. J Vasc Surg 1997;25:481–487.

56. Zannetti S, Parente B, De Rango P, et al. Role of surgical techniques and operative findings in cranial and cervical nerve injuries during carotid endarterectomy. Eur J Vasc Endovasc Surg 1998;15:528–531.

57. Ballotta E, Da Giau G, Renon L, et al. Cranial and cervical nerve injuries after carotid endarterectomy: a prospective study. Surgery (St. Louis) 1999;125:85–91.

58. Barnes RW, Nix ML, Wingo JP, et al. Recurrent versus residual carotid stenosis: incidence detected by doppler ultrasound. Ann Surg 1986;203:652–660.

59. Clagett GP, Rich NM, McDonald PT, et al. Etiologic factors for recurrent carotid artery stenosis. Surgery (St. Louis) 1983;93: 313–318.

60. Reilly LM, Okuhn SP, Rapp JH, et al. Recurrent carotid stenosis: a consequence of local or systemic factors? The influence of unrepaired defects. J Vasc Surg 1990;11:448–460.

61. Cote R, et al. Internal carotid occlusion: a prospective study. Stroke 1983;14:898–902.

62. Nicholls SC, Kohler TR, Bergelin RO, et al. Carotid artery occlusion: natural history. J Vasc Surg 1986;4:479–485.

63. The EC/IC Bypass Study Group. Failure of extracranial-intracranial arterial bypass to reduce the risk of ischemic stroke: results of an international randomized trial. N Engl J Med 1985; 313:1191–1200.

64. de Jong KP, Zondervan PE, van Urk H. Extracranial carotid artery aneurysms. Eur J Vasc Surg 1989;3:557–562.

65. Painter TA, Hertzer NR, Beven EG, et al. Extracranial carotid aneurysms: report of six cases and review of the literature. J Vasc Surg 1985;2:312–318.

66. Zwolak RM, Whitehouse WM Jr, Knake JE, et al. Atherosclerotic extracranial carotid artery aneurysms. J Vasc Surg 1984;1: 415–422.

67. Faggioli G, Freyrie A, Stella A, et al. Extracranial internal carotid artery aneurysms: results of a surgical series with long-term follow-up. J Vasc Surg 1996;23:587–595.

68. Westerband A, Hunter GC, Cintora I, et al. Current trends in the detection and management of carotid body tumors. J Vasc Surg 1998;28:84–93.

69. Muhm M, Polterauer P, Gstottner W, et al. Diagnostic and therapeutic approaches to carotid body tumors: review of 24 patients. Arch Surg 1997;132:279–284.

70. Hallett JW, Nora JD, Hollier LH, et al. Trends in neurovascular complications of surgical management for carotid body and cervical paragangliomas: a fifty-year experience with 153 tumors. J Vasc Surg 1988;7:284–291.

71. Cloft HJ, Kallmes DF, Kallmes MH, et al. Prevalence of cerebral aneurysms in patients with fibromuscular dysplasia: a reassessment. J Neurosurg 1998;88:436–440.

72. Moreau P, Albat B, Thevenet A. Fibromuscular dysplasia of the internal carotid artery: long-term surgical results. J Cardiovasc Surg 1993;34:465–472.

73. Effeney DJ, Ehrenfeld WK, Stoney RJ, et al. Why operate on carotid fibromuscular dysplasia? Arch Surg 1980;115:1261–1265.

74. Ballotta E, Abbruzzese E, Thiene G, et al. The elongation of the internal carotid artery: early and long-term results of patients having surgery compared with unoperated controls. Ann Vasc Surg 1997;11:120–128.

75. Fearn SJ, McCollum CN. Shortening and reimplantation for tortuous internal carotid arteries. J Vasc Surg 1998;27:936–939.

76. Poindexter JM, Patel KR, Clauss RH. Management of kinked extracranial cerebral arteries. J Vasc Surg 1987;6:127–133.

77. Coyle KA, Smith RB, Chapman RL, et al. Carotid artery shortening: a safe adjunct to carotid endarterectomy. J Vasc Surg 1995;22:257–263.

78. Silbert PL, Mokri B, Schievink WI. Headache and neck pain in spontaneous internal carotid and vertebral artery dissections. Neurology 1995;45:1517–1522.

79. Mokri B, Silbert PL, Schievink WI, et al. Cranial nerve palsy in spontaneous dissection of the extracranial internal carotid artery. Neurology 1996;46:356–359.

80. Biousse V, D'Anglejan-Chatillon J, Touboul PJ, et al. Time course of symptoms in extracranial carotid artery dissections: a series of 80 patients. Stroke 1995;26:235–239.

81. Sturzenegger M. Spontaneous internal carotid artery dissection: early diagnosis and management in 44 patients. J Neurol 1995;242:231–238.

82. Treiman GS, Treiman RL, Foran RF, et al. Spontaneous dissection of the internal carotid artery: a nineteen-year clinical experience. J Vasc Surg 1996;24:597–607.

83. Lucas C, Moulin T, Deplanque D, et al. Stroke patterns of internal carotid artery dissection in 40 patients. Stroke 1998;29:2646–2648.

84. Moritz MW, Higgins RF, Jacobs JR. Duplex imaging and incidence of carotid radiation injury after high-dose radiotherapy for tumors of the head and neck. Arch Surg 1990;125:1181–1183.

85. Kashyap VS, Moore WS, Quinones-Baldrich WJ. Carotid artery repair for radiation-associated atherosclerosis is a safe and durable procedure. J Vasc Surg 1999;29:90–99.

86. Rockman CB, Riles TS, Fisher FS, et al. The surgical management of carotid artery stenosis in patients with previous neck irradiation. Am J Surg 1996;172:191–195.

87. AbuRahma AF, Robinson PA, Saiedy S, et al. Prospective randomized trial of carotid endarterectomy with primary closure and patch angioplasty with saphenous vein, jugular vein, and polytetrafluoroethylene: long-term follow-up. J Vasc Surg 1998;27:222–234.

88. Desiron Q, Detry O, Van Damme H, et al. Comparison of results of carotid artery surgery after either direct closure or use of a vein patch. Cardiovasc Surg 1997;5:295–303.

89. Allen PJ, Jackson MR, O'Donnell SD, et al. Saphenous vein versus polytetrafluoroethylene carotid patch angioplasty. Am J Surg 1997;174:115–117.

90. Katz SG, Kohl RD. Does the choice of material influence early morbidity in patients undergoing carotid patch angioplasty? Surgery (St. Louis) 1996;119:297–301.

91. Goldman KA, Su WT, Riles TS, et al. A comparative study of saphenous vein, internal jugular vein, and knitted Dacron patches for carotid artery endarterectomy. Ann Vasc Surg 1995;9:71–79.

92. Gonzalez-Fajardo JA, Perez JL, Mateo AM. Saphenous vein patch versus polytetrafluoroethylene patch after carotid endarterectomy. J Cardiovasc Surg 1994;35:523–528.

93. Ranaboldo CJ, Barros D'Sa AAB, Bell PRF, et al. Randomized controlled trial of patch angioplasty for carotid endarterectomy. Br J Surg 1993;80:1528–1530.

94. De Letter JAM, Moll FL, Welten RJT, et al. Benefits of carotid patching: a prospective randomized study with long-term follow-up. Ann Vasc Surg 1993;8:54–58.

95. Whereatt N, Burke K, Littooy FN, et al. An evaluation of external jugular vein patch angioplasty after carotid endarterectomy. Am Surg 1990;56:455–459.

96. Lord RSA, Raj TB, Stary DL, et al. Comparison of saphenous vein patch, polytetrafluorocthylene patch, and direct arteriotomy closure after carotid endarterectomy. Part I: perioperative results. J Vasc Surg 1989;9:521–529.

97. Katz MM, Jones GT, Degenhardt J, et al. The use of patch angioplasty to alter the incidence of carotid restenosis following thromboendarterectomy. J Cardiovasc Surg 1987;28:2–8.

98. Ouriel K, Green RM. Clinical and technical factors influencing recurrent carotid stenosis and occlusion after endarterectomy. J Vasc Surg 1987;5:702–706.

99. Hertzer NR, Beven EG, O'Hara PJ, et al. A prospective study of vein patch angioplasty during carotid endarterectomy: three-year results for 801 patients and 917 operations. Ann Surg 1987;206:628–635.

100. Fode NC, Sundt TM, Robertson JT, et al. Multicenter retrospective review of results and complications of carotid endarterectomy in 1981. Stroke 1986;17:370–376.

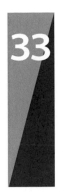

Diseases of the Thoracic Aorta and Great Vessels

Thoralf M. Sundt and Robert W. Thompson

Aneurysmal Disease

Aortic Dissection

Acute aortic dissection is the most common catastrophe of the thoracic aorta.[1–3] Population-based studies indicate that aortic dissection exceeds rupture of abdominal aortic aneurysms as a cause of death by as much as twofold.[3] The acute onset and potentially rapid progression of the disease to fatal rupture or visceral malperfusion dominates the clinical picture, mandating rapid diagnosis and aggressive institution of medical or surgical therapy. Accordingly, the condition is considered first.

ETIOLOGY

Little is known with certainty about the etiological factors responsible for aortic dissection despite its common occurrence. The term Erdheim's cystic medial necrosis has become nearly synonymous with aortic dissection, but this is a bit of a misnomer, as neither necrosis nor cystic lesions are typical of dissection.[4]

Degenerative changes in collagen and elastin are commonly observed in dissected aorta. Because such changes are typical with aging, their causal relationship has been questioned.[5,6]

Genetic factors may play a role in acute dissection. Marfan's syndrome has been recognized as a risk factor for aortic aneurysmal disease, with dissection occurring in approximately one-third of Marfan patients even in the absence of significant aneurysmal dilatation.[7] Individuals with Ehlers–Danlos syndrome, Noonan's syndrome, and Turner's syndrome are also at higher risk for dissection.[2] Familial predisposition to dissection even in the absence of known collagen–vascular conditions is also well documented.[8] Bicuspid aortic valve,[9] aortic coarctation,[10] and pregnancy[2] are also associated with dissection.

Atherosclerotic vascular disease does not appear to predispose to dissection, although chronic hypertension is strongly associated with the disease,[11] particularly of the descending thoracic and thoracoabdominal aorta.[12] The causative mechanism remains speculative; chronic hemodynamic stress is presumed to accelerate degenerative medial changes.[13]

PATHOPHYSIOLOGY

Pathologically, aortic dissection is defined by the presence of blood within the layers of the tunica media. There is, however, uncertainty about the initiating event. An obvious intimal disruption is present in most instances,[11] leading to the hypothesis that an intimal tear occurs first, permitting entry of blood into the media. An intimal tear is not identifiable in approximately 5% of cases,[11] however, suggesting that rupture of the vasa vasora into a diseased media is the primary event, with progression to free rupture into the lumen in the majority of patients. When no entry site is apparent, the condition has been termed an intramural hematoma. Clinically, such lesions behave like acute dissections.[14,15]

In the acute phase, dissection is thought to rapidly progress distally from the site of intimal disruption, ending either in a blind pouch or with a reentry tear into the true lumen. The pathology may be limited to the ascending or descending aorta only, or may involve both, with—of necessity—dissection of the arch as well. The natural history of acute dissection is dismal without treatment, as shown in Figure 33.1. Early studies demonstrated mortality of one-third of patients within 24 h and 80% within 1 week when the ascending aorta was involved.[16] Those with distal dissection have a more favorable natural history, with three-quarters surviving more than 1 month from the acute event.[16] Rupture of the aorta into the pleural or pericardial space is responsible for three-quarters of mortalities,[17] with free rupture occurring most often adjacent to the intimal tear.[18] Myocardial infarction may occur secondary to involvement of the right coronary sinus with compression of the right coronary artery. Distal progression may create a malperfusion syndrome in as many as 30% of patients by compression of the true lumen

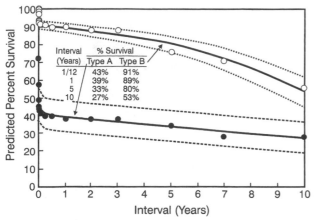

FIGURE 33.1. The natural history of acute aortic dissection involving the ascending aorta (type A) or limited to the descending aorta (type B). (Adapted from Kirklin JW, Barratt-Boyes BG. Cardiac Surgery, 2nd Ed. New York: Churchill Livingstone, 1993.)

by the false lumen.[19] The mortality rate for patients with stroke or visceral infarction secondary to malperfusion is particularly high, whether treated surgically or medically.[20]

Two schemes for the classification of aortic dissections are in common use (Fig. 33.2). The more descriptive and hence complex scheme is that proposed by DeBakey in 1965.[21] The type I is most common, and is considered most often to originate with a tear in the ascending aorta with progression through the arch into the descending thoracoabdominal aorta. DeBakey type II dissection is limited to the ascending aorta and is the least common, whereas type III is limited to the descending thoracic or thoracoabdominal aorta. An alternative classification scheme has been proposed by the group at Stanford University on the basis of the natural history of the disease and the treatment strategies that have evolved.[17] Those dissections involving the ascending aorta, whether DeBakey type I or II, are designated type A, while those limited to the descending aorta are type B. The unusual dissections

involving the arch and descending aorta, but not the ascending aorta, are designated type A.[22]

CLINICAL PRESENTATION

Intense pain, often described as tearing or ripping, is almost universally present when acute dissection occurs, although occasional patients have chronic dissection without history of such an episode. The pain may be migratory, typically anterior when the ascending aorta is involved and moving to the back as the dissection progresses distally. On examination, patients may be hypertensive or hypotensive.[11] Extremity blood pressures may be quite disparate, and peripheral pulses may be absent as the false lumen compresses the true. Pulses may reappear as distal reentry restores flow via the false lumen. Malperfusion may also result in stroke, intestinal ischemia, or rarely paraplegia. Auscultation of the heart may reveal aortic regurgitation which, if known to be acute in onset, is a highly reliable sign.

DIAGNOSTIC EVALUATION

Diagnostic evaluation should include electrocardiography, which may show left-ventricular hypertrophy or acute inferior myocardial ischemia. Simple chest radiography may demonstrate widening of the mediastinum, blurring of the aortic nob, or a left pleural effusion, or may be entirely normal. The definitive diagnosis of acute aortic dissection relies on advanced imaging techniques.

Aortography was the traditional mode of diagnosis and remains the "gold standard" in the opinion of many. It offers the advantage of demonstrating the origins of important branches and their perfusion by the true or false lumen, and remains particularly useful in the preoperative evaluation of chronic dissection.

Transesophageal echocardiography (TEE) is fast becoming the technique of choice in many centers as it is noninvasive, highly sensitive, and provides important information regarding ventricular function and aortic valve function.

Acute dissection is frequently diagnosed by computerized

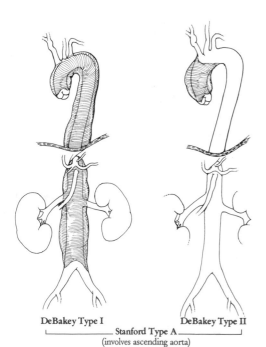

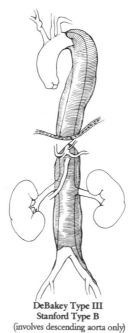

DeBakey Type I   DeBakey Type II

├─────── Stanford Type A ───────┤
(involves ascending aorta)

DeBakey Type III
Stanford Type B
(involves descending aorta only)

FIGURE 33.2. The DeBakey and Stanford classifications of aortic dissection according to extent of involvement.

tomographic (CT) scanning (Fig. 33.3), likely because of its widespread availability. It is less operator dependent than other modalities, but is still subject to misinterpretation from streak artifact. Images can be obtained rapidly and, with the advent of spiral CT scanning, with remarkable accuracy.

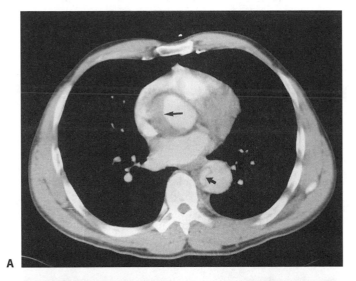

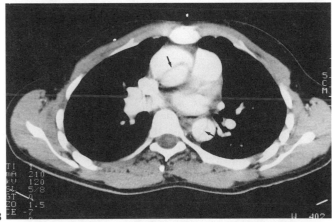

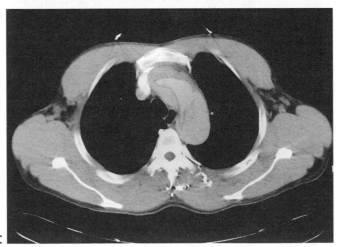

FIGURE 33.3. Computerized tomography of acute dissection. **A.** Thrombosis of the false lumen in the ascending aorta (*thin arrow*) and compression of the true lumen in the descending aorta (*thick arrow*). **B.** Patency of true and false lumen with an intimal flap visible in both the ascending and descending aorta (*arrows*). **C.** Complex dissection involving the arch.

Magnetic resonance imaging (MRI) can provide enhanced definition over CT scanning in some instances, and may be better able to distinguish between blood and other fluid in and around the dissection aorta. Sagittal reconstructions of the aorta can easily be obtained as well, and the technique can provide information regarding aortic valve function. Its use is greatest in ruling out dissection among patients with complex aortic anatomy who are hemodynamically stable.

Choice amongst these modalities may be difficult. Many studies have been published in recent years comparing angiography, TEE, CT, and MRI,[23] but the optimal diagnostic strategy in any particular institution will depend upon the locally available technology and expertise.

MEDICAL AND SURGICAL MANAGEMENT

Pharmacological intervention to reduce both the mean blood pressure and the rate of rise of the pulse wave (dp/dt) should be instituted as soon as the diagnosis of acute dissection is suspected. Initially, beta-blockade should be instituted to decrease both blood pressure and myocardial contractility. Additional blood pressure control may require nitroprusside. Once the diagnosis has been established, immediate surgical intervention is indicated if the ascending aorta is involved.[24,25]

In contrast, continuation of medical therapy is the standard of care in most institutions for DeBakey type III/Stanford type B dissection unless there is uncontrolled recurrent pain suggestive of ongoing dissection, evidence of a malperfusion syndrome, uncontrollable hypertension, or rupture. Unfortunately, no prospective randomized trials have been performed examining this treatment strategy.

Chronic dissection, by definition, is one continuing more than 14 days from the index event. More often, however, chronic dissection is discovered incidentally many months or years after the event, when calcification of the wall may make the diagnosis obvious even on plain chest radiography. Expeditious operative repair is indicated when the ascending aorta is involved because the risk of rupture is significant and the operative risk is, in most instances, low.[4] Chronic type B dissection should be monitored by periodic (annual or semiannual) imaging studies with surgery indicated on the basis of the onset of symptoms or size criteria identical to those for chronic degenerative aneurysms of the descending thoracic and thoracoabdominal aorta (see following).

Degenerative Aneurysmal Disease

ETIOLOGY

Histologically, disruption of the elastic lamellae with thinning of the media and loss of smooth muscle cells is typically present in aneurysms of degenerative origin. Degradation of elastin is likely central to the development of degenerative aneurysms, although its biochemical basis remains incompletely defined.

As is the case for aortic dissection, the association between hypertension and degenerative aneurysmal disease is clear but the mechanism is not. Genetic factors likely play a significant role here as well. Apart from the recognized collagen vascular diseases such as Marfan syndrome and Ehlers–Danlos syndrome, familial clustering has been recognized.[26] Furthermore, a family history of aneurysmal disease is present in 10% to 15% of patients with abdominal aortic aneurysms.[27,28] Abnormalities in type II procollagen have been identified in some of these cases.[29]

PATHOPHYSIOLOGY

Degenerative aneurysms are heterogeneous in their location and gross appearance. Aneurysms of the ascending aorta may produce insufficiency of the aortic valve despite structurally normal valve leaflets because of loss of central leaflet coaptation. Alternatively, the ascending aorta and arch may be spared with dilatation only of the descending thoracic aorta. Crawford established a classification scheme, as shown in Figure 33.4.

The natural history of thoracic aortic aneurysmal disease has been defined. Progressive dilatation to eventual rupture is common for thoracic aneurysms.[30] Large aneurysms are particularly prone to rupture,[31] although even those less than 5 cm in diameter may do so.[2] Once symptoms occur, the mean interval to rupture is 2 years.[30] The majority of degenerative aneurysms are fusiform, but saccular aneurysms do occur, and are probably at higher risk of rupture.[4] Those caused by chronic dissection also appear to be at higher risk of rupture.[4]

CLINICAL PRESENTATION

Degenerative aneurysms are often asymptomatic, being discovered incidentally during an imaging study performed for another purpose. Rapid expansion, particularly of the thoracoabdominal aorta, may produce pain that may be mistaken for arthritic symptoms. Involvement of the aortic root with resultant aortic regurgitation may result in heart failure. Distal embolization with the resulting "blue toe syndrome" may also occur. Physical examination may reveal aortic regurgitation, a palpable pulsatile abdominal mass, or abdominal bruits. Most often, however, the diagnosis is made via advanced imaging modalities.

DIAGNOSTIC EVALUATION

Chest radiography often offers the first clue to the presence of a thoracic aortic aneurysm. A widened mediastinum or apparent mass may lead to other studies that make the diagnosis. Calcification of the wall of aneurysm will occasionally make the diagnosis clear on the basis of the plain film alone.

Aortography is less often the initial diagnostic test today than it was previously, although it continues to provide use-ful information, particularly in the preoperative evaluation of thoracoabdominal aneurysmal disease. Transesophageal echo may be virtually diagnostic when aneurysmal dilatation of the ascending aorta is questioned, but is less useful in the assessment of descending thoracic aneurysms and those involving the aortic arch. Computerized tomography (with contrast) offers accuracy and accessibility, and can rule out other intrathoracic pathology. Images so obtained define the external size, the longitudinal extent, the presence of intraluminal thrombus, ulceration, or atheroma. As is the case for acute dissection, MRI can provide excellent detail in any plane, but is limited by its time-consuming nature. Its utility is greatest in evaluating complex anatomy in detail.

MEDICAL AND SURGICAL MANAGEMENT

Medical therapy is of limited utility in the management of most aneurysms of degenerative etiology. While aggressive antihypertensive therapy is clearly protective in patients with chronic dissection,[4] it is less so for degenerative aneurysms. Instead, the emphasis of nonoperative treatment is on the close monitoring of aneurysm size. Surgical intervention on aneurysms exceeding 5 cm in maximum diameter has been advocated.

Posttraumatic Thoracic Aortic Aneurysms

Acute aortic transection is the most common traumatic process resulting in aneurysmal dilatation or, more properly, pseudoaneurysm formation of the thoracic aorta.

ETIOLOGY

Blunt trauma characterized by a rapid deceleration injury is the most common cause of aortic transection. Although the ascending aorta may be involved, the most common location is the aortic isthmus just distal to the left subclavian artery at the ligamentum arteriosum. The exact mechanism remains unclear.

PATHOPHYSIOLOGY

Approximately 15% of traffic fatalities are associated with aortic transection, and 85% of individuals suffering this injury die at the scene.[32] The fortunate minority of individuals surviving this insult will have partial or complete disruption

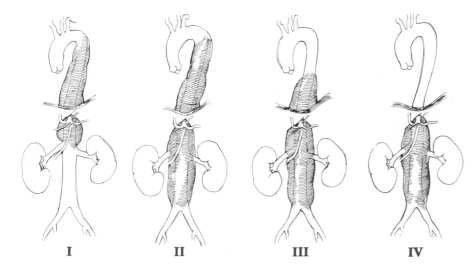

I   II   III   IV

FIGURE 33.4. The Crawford classification of thoracoabdominal aortic aneurysms.

of the intima and media with preservation of vascular continuity by virtue of the aortic adventitia alone.

CLINICAL PRESENTATION

The principles of the evaluation and management of the trauma patient are discussed elsewhere. Acute transection is often clinically remarkably silent if the rupture has been contained by the aortic adventitia. Hence its diagnosis depends heavily on a high index of suspicion in an appropriate clinical setting. Chronic pseudoaneurysms are most often similarly subtle, although occasional airway or esophageal compression may be noted. Despite the proximity of the recurrent laryngeal nerve, hoarseness is uncommon.

DIAGNOSTIC EVALUATION

The optimal diagnostic strategy for acute transection is controversial and is primarily within the purview of the trauma management team. Although transesophageal echo is gaining popularity, aortography remains the "gold standard," providing valuable information about the status of the other great vessels.

Chronic pseudoaneurysms are most often identified by computerized tomography (CT) of the chest during the evaluation of a mass of uncertain etiology identified on plain chest radiography. Magnetic resonance imaging (MRI) provides similar information and offers the capability of reconstruction in multiple planes such that the arch and descending aorta may be visualized in continuity. Aortography continues to be used by some, particularly when surgical intervention is planned and coronary arteriography is desired.

MEDICAL AND SURGICAL MANAGEMENT

As with aortic dissection, antiimpulse therapy with beta-blockade and aggressive blood pressure control should be instituted as soon as the diagnosis is entertained. Once the diagnosis is made, immediate aortic repair has traditionally taken priority over other injuries.

The indications for repair of chronic pseudoaneurysms are also undergoing reevaluation. Early studies[33–35] suggested that such aneurysms should be repaired once identified. However, with recent radiologic advances, a number of authors have argued in favor of serial imaging studies, reserving surgery for those with symptoms or evidence of enlargement.[36,37] The advent of intraluminal stents may lay many of these issues aside as both acute and chronic transections may be readily correctable with this technology.[38]

Surgical Approach

The surgical approach to aneurysmal disease is dictated primarily by the anatomical extent of involvement rather than the etiological basis of the condition. Indeed, not infrequently the etiology remains uncertain until the aorta has been opened at surgery.

ANEURYSMS OF THE ASCENDING AORTA

PREOPERATIVE EVALUATION

Once aneurysmal disease of the ascending aorta requiring surgical intervention has been identified, the extent of aortic involvement proximally and distally and the presence of coexisting cardiac valve disease or coronary artery disease requiring concomitant correction must be determined. The extent of aortic pathology impacts on the technical approach as well as the preoperative assessment of risk. Often the initial diagnostic studies reveal involvement of the aortic arch that will dictate the use of profound hypothermic cardiopulmonary bypass and circulatory arrest. Proximal involvement of the aortic root may mandate root replacement with a valved conduit.

SURGICAL TECHNIQUE

Aneurysms of the ascending aorta are most conveniently approached via median sternotomy. Arterial cannulation for cardiopulmonary bypass is via the femoral artery in the setting of acute dissection. In degenerative disease, cannulation of the aortic arch or even the aneurysm itself will spare the patient the morbidity of a groin wound. If the disease is limited to the ascending aorta with sufficient room to cross-clamp the aorta below the inominant artery, the operation can be performed with only mild hypothermia (28°–32°C) or even normothermic cardiopulmonary bypass. If the aneurysm extends to the innominate artery, an episode of circulatory arrest under profound hypothermia (13°–18°C) may be required to perform the distal anastomosis. Liberal use of circulatory arrest in cases of acute dissection is also gaining popularity. Anastomotic options are shown in Figure 33.5.

ANEURYSMS OF THE AORTIC ARCH

PREOPERATIVE EVALUATION.

The use of profound hypothermia and circulatory arrest in acute dissection permits open distal anastomosis and provides an opportunity for direct inspection of the aortic arch for intimal disruption intraoperatively. This approach lessens the importance of excessive preoperative imaging studies in this potentially unstable subset of patients. Patients with chronic dissection or degenerative disease that appears to involve the arch should, however, generally undergo aortography or magnetic resonance imaging to precisely define the anatomy of the brachiocephalic vessels.

SURGICAL TECHNIQUE

Repair of aneurysms of the aortic arch continues to represent a major surgical challenge. Neurological function must be preserved by continued cerebral perfusion, or protected by a combination of hypothermia and pharmacological agents, while arch reconstruction is underway. The former may be accomplished by selective antegrade perfusion of the brachiocephalic vessels, while the latter is most often accomplished via the induction of profound hypothermia on bypass before initiating circulatory arrest. Arch replacement may be accomplished via a variety of techniques depending on the extent of disease proximally and distally (see Fig. 33.5).

ANEURYSMS OF THE THORACIC AND THORACOABDOMINAL AORTA

PREOPERATIVE EVALUATION

Every attempt should be made to manage acute distal dissection pharmacologically. Should pain persist or malperfusion ensue, operative intervention may be indicated urgently. Preoperative evaluation should be directed toward clear definition of the proximal extent of the dissection as involvement of the arch will make proximal control with clamps

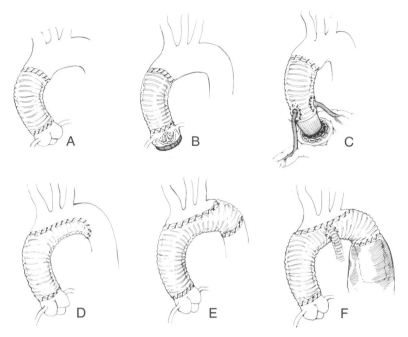

FIGURE 33.5. Repair of aneurysms of the ascending aorta and arch. **A.** Tube graft ascending aortic replacement. **B.** Separate tube graft and aortic valve replacement when the sinuses are normal. **C.** Composite graft repair with reimplantation of the coronary arteries when the sinuses are diseased. **D.** Hemiarch replacement. **E.** Total arch replacement. **F.** Elephant trunk arch replacement.

difficult and may direct the surgeon to employ profound hypothermia and circulatory arrest. If time permits, aortography to demonstrate the origins of visceral vessels from the true or false lumen and any malperfusion is helpful when the dissection extends below the diaphragm.

The presence of ischemic heart disease before elective procedures may be sought noninvasively by thallium-201 scintigraphy[39–41] or by using echocardiography with dobutamine infusion.[42] Preoperative echocardiography may reveal significant left-ventricular hypertrophy or aortic regurgitation, either of which would discourage the use of circulatory arrest as subendocardial myocardial perfusion may be impaired once ventricular fibrillation ensues.

Pulmonary function tests may be helpful in the estimation of operative risk as history of smoking and chronic obstructive pulmonary disease are independent predictors of prolonged ventilatory support following thoracoabdominal aortic aneurysm repair.

SURGICAL TECHNIQUE

Surgical procedures on thoracic and thoracoabdominal aneurysms continue to carry significant risk of death and complications. In addition to risks of renal and respiratory failure, paraplegia may occur because of the tenuous blood supply to the anterior spinal cord. Enormous efforts have been directed toward the development of techniques to reduce the incidence of this devastating complication. Although a variety of surgical approaches to such aneurysms have been championed, none have proven clearly superior.

Congenital Abnormalities

Coarctation of the Aorta

The most common congenital anomaly of the aorta is coarctation, occurring in 40 to 50 of 100,000 live births.[4] The majority of such lesions are identified and treated in infancy and childhood. As such their diagnosis and treatment fall within the purview of the pediatric cardiac surgeon. Occasionally, however, coarctation or even aortic interruption remains undetected until adulthood during evaluation of hypertension, when delayed or diminished femoral pulsation is found, or a routine chest X-ray demonstrates rib notching or an abnormal cardiomediastinal silhouette.

The natural history of coarctation is well established.[10] Left untreated, 80% of adults will die of complications of proximal hypertension, most often in the second, third, or fourth decades of life. Correction is indicated when the condition is diagnosed. Even with late repair, postoperative normotension or only mild hypertension can be anticipated in the majority of patients.[43] Long-term postoperative follow-up is indicated.

Aberrant Subclavian Artery

As in coarctation, the majority of clinically significant congenital abnormalities related to aortic arch development, such as double aortic arch with vascular ring, become apparent in infancy and childhood. Occasionally, however, adults may present with dysphagia secondary to an aberrant right subclavian artery from a left-sided arch, or an aberrant left subclavian artery from a right-sided arch. The origin of the aberrant vessel is usually dilated and is known as a Kommerell's diverticulum. This anomaly results in compression of surrounding structures, most often the esophagus behind which the aberrant vessel most often passes.

Diagnostic evaluation may begin with CT or MRI scanning. These studies often provide all the required information, although aortography may also be helpful. Surgical correction can be accomplished simply by carotid–subclavian bypass and oversewing of the origin of the aberrant vessel, most often via a left thoracotomy.

Occlusive Disease of the Aortic Arch Branches

Atherosclerosis

ETIOLOGY AND PATHOPHYSIOLOGY

The aortic arch and its branches are a common location for the development of atherosclerosis. Like atherosclerosis in other areas of the arterial tree, the pathology ranges from mild, nonocclusive intimal thickening to complex atheromata. Complex atheromatous plaques may evolve to a size large enough to encroach upon the lumen, thereby restricting flow, or they may be complicated by intraplaque hemorrhage, ulceration and discharge of atheromatous debris, and surface thrombosis. Well-established clinical risk factors for atherosclerosis include family history, aging, cigarette smoking, hypertension, hyperlipidemia, and diabetes.

CLINICAL PRESENTATION AND DIAGNOSIS

Symptoms caused by atherosclerotic lesions of the innominate artery may be either acute or chronic. Acute symptoms include either stroke or transient ischemic attacks, caused by atheroembolization. With gradual occlusion, innominate lesions may lead to chronic or intermittent ischemia of the arm, particularly during active use or when the arm is used in an overhead position, with symptoms analogous to intermittent calf claudication caused by lower-extremity occlusive disease.

Occlusive lesions of the proximal subclavian artery are responsible for the "subclavian steal" syndrome. In this situation, low flow to the upper extremity is compensated by collateral flow through the intracranial circulation via the ipsilateral vertebral artery. When exacerbated by arm exercise, retrograde flow in the vertebral artery may transiently lower perfusion pressure in the posterior vertebrobasilar circuit, leading to sudden episodes known as "drop attacks." These episodes are characterized by a near loss of consciousness and collapse, without antecedent cortical symptoms; typically, consciousness is quickly regained without sequelae.

MANAGEMENT

The medical management of atherosclerosis is discussed in more detail elsewhere. In general, this consists of lifestyle modifications and medical control of risk factors such as diabetes and hypertension. Treatment for symptomatic atherosclerotic lesions may include regular administration of aspirin or other platelet antagonists; in some circumstances, anticoagulation is also used. These approaches are of limited value, however, in preventing the cerebrovascular or limb-threatening complications of complex atheromatous plaques in this location. Thus, surgical or endoluminal interventions remain the mainstay of treatment for atherosclerotic lesions affecting the aortic arch branches.

INNOMINATE ARTERY RECONSTRUCTION

Symptomatic lesions of the innominate artery may be treated by either innominate thromboendarterectomy (TEA) or bypass grafting. The surgical approach for either of these options requires direct exposure through a median sternotomy. Although no prospective clinical studies are available, a number of clinical series have demonstrated that excellent results can be achieved by direct innominate artery reconstruction with either thromboendarterectomy or prosthetic bypass grafting.[44–49] In addition, four particularly large studies have been published in the past decade that offer detailed analysis of perioperative and long-term results for a total of nearly 400 patients (Table 33.1).[50-53] The 10-year patency rates for innominate reconstruction were 88% to 97%, with similar figures reported for long-term relief of symptoms. These results demonstrate that direct innominate artery reconstruction is safe and durable when either endarterectomy or prosthetic bypass is used.

SUBCLAVIAN ARTERY TRANSPOSITION AND CAROTID–SUBCLAVIAN ARTERY BYPASS

The most widely utilized approach to subclavian reconstruction is direct transposition of the subclavian artery to the side of the common carotid artery. This repair can be accomplished with relative ease on either side using a supraclavicular incision. Carotid–subclavian bypass is also commonly utilized for symptomatic lesions of the proximal subclavian artery. This procedure is performed through a supraclavicular exposure similar to that for subclavian artery transposition.

Clinical experience demonstrates excellent long-term results for extraanatomical subclavian artery reconstruction.[54–60] Patency rates of 99%–100% for transposition and 52%–95% for bypass have been reported at 4–10 year follow-up.

AXILLO–AXILLARY ARTERY BYPASS

Axillo–axillary artery crossover bypass offers another alternative for extraanatomical revascularization of the aortic arch

TABLE 33.1.

Results of Innominate Artery Reconstruction (Level III Evidence).

Source	Patients (n)	TEA/BPG/Ex	Mortality (%)	Neuro Cx (%)	Patency (f/u)
Reul et al. 1991[50]	54	11/27/16	0	1.8	92.6% (10)
Kieffer et al. 1995[51]	148	32/116	5.4	5.4	96.3% (10)
Berguer et al. 1998[52]	100	8/92	8	8	88% (10)
Azakie et al. 1998[53]	94	72/22	3	6	97% (10)
Totals	396	123/257	2.8	5.8	93.8

TEA, thromboendarterectomy; BPG, innominate artery bypass graft; Ex, extrathoracic reconstruction; f/u, follow-up.

branch vessels. Operative mortality and complication rates for axillo–axillary artery bypass are generally less than 2%, in contrast to other approaches that may involve thoracotomy, sternotomy, or carotid dissection and clamping. The long-term patency rate is approximately 90%.

ENDOVASCULAR REPAIR

Recent advances in endovascular technology have provided an alternative means of therapy for the treatment of occlusive lesions in the innominate, subclavian, and axillary arteries. Innovations in imaging, guidewire, catheter, stent, and balloon technology allow one to obtain percutaneous access and perform therapeutic procedures in a relatively safe manner. Despite the appeal of these less-invasive techniques, the morbidity, mortality, and durability of novel treatments remain largely unknown.[61] Nonetheless, it can be expected that in the next decade endovascular approaches will assume an increasingly prominent role in the management of these lesions.

Large Vessel Arteritides

A number of inflammatory disorders have a predilection for affecting the thoracic aorta and its branches. The most important of these conditions are giant cell (temporal) arteritis and Takayasu's arteritis, each of which is much less common than atherosclerosis (Table 33.2). Although the etiology of large vessel arteritides is largely unknown and specific diagnosis may be difficult, clinical recognition of these conditions is important because they usually require alternative approaches to treatment than those used for occlusive atherosclerosis.[62,63]

ETIOLOGY AND PATHOPHYSIOLOGY

The etiology of large vessel vasculitides is unknown, but each of these disorders appears to be characterized by cell-mediated immune or inflammatory responses localized to the arterial wall. In turn, soluble factors released by inflammatory cells are thought to play a significant role in thrombosis, vessel occlusion, and ischemic complications.[64]

GIANT CELL (TEMPORAL) ARTERITIS

CLINICAL PRESENTATION AND DIAGNOSIS

Giant cell arteritis is a disorder of small and medium-sized blood vessels that commonly presents in elderly Caucasian women.[65] It may occur in association with polymyalgia rheumatica or as isolated temporal arteritis, but both types are thought to represent variants of the same disease. The annual incidence of giant cell arteritis is 7 per 100,000, but this rises to approximately 15 per 100,000 in populations over 50 years of age.[66,67] It is rare

before the age of 50 and typically occurs between 65 and 75 years of age; there is a 2:1 predominance of women over men.

Giant cell arteritis appears to have a unique predilection for the temporal and ophthalmic arteries, and it only rarely involves the aortic arch or carotid arteries. Symptoms typically occur with rapid onset (within 1 month). The classical symptoms of temporal arteritis are headache, scalp and temporal tenderness, visual symptoms, and jaw claudication.[68] Ocular symptoms may include blurred vision, diplopia, visual hallucinations, or amaurosis fugax. These symptoms are particularly important because failure to promptly initiate treatment may lead to permanent loss of vision.[69]

The erythrocyte sedimentation rate (ESR) is almost always markedly elevated in patients with giant cell arteritis, as a reflection of a systemic acute-phase response.[70,71] Elevated levels of C-reactive protein and interleukin-6 have also been reported.[71,72] Some patients with giant cell arteritis have anticardiolipin antibodies, an alteration associated with vascular complications.[73,74]

The diagnosis of giant cell arteritis is usually suggested by a characteristic clinical history and supplemented by physical findings, but it can only be confirmed by a positive tissue biopsy. Problems are encountered when the history is atypical or the biopsy is negative; thus, the American College of Rheumatology has outlined a series of five diagnostic criteria when the diagnosis of giant cell arteritis is in question (Table 33.3).

MEDICAL MANAGEMENT

Large vessel vasculitides often respond favorably to treatment with glucocorticosteroids. Prompt steroid treatment is particularly important in temporal arteritis, because the response is often rapid and dramatic, and because early intervention may prevent the progression to loss of vision.

SURGICAL MANAGEMENT

There is no direct role for surgical treatment in giant cell (temporal) arteritis other than that of obtaining appropriate biopsy material.

TAKAYASU'S ARTERITIS (PULSELESS DISEASE)

CLINICAL PRESENTATION AND DIAGNOSIS

Takayasu's arteritis exhibits a more varied and nonspecific pattern of clinical presentation than temporal arteritis.[75,76] Although it remains a rare disorder, it is most commonly seen in young women from South America, India, or Asia.[77–79] The inflammatory and occlusive aspects of the disease can affect the thoracic or abdominal aorta, the brachiocephalic vessels, or other aortic branches and their tributaries. Symptoms and

TABLE 33.2. Features Distinguishing Temporal Arteritis and Takayasu's Disease.

	Giant cell (temporal) arteritis	Takayasu's arteritis
Prevalence	Common	Rare
Age/gender	Elderly women	Young women
Descent	Caucasian	South American, Asian, Indian
Vessels	Small and medium	Large
Defin Dx	Histology	Arteriography
Steroids	Curative	Palliative (active phase)
Surgery	Diagnosis	Definitive (quiescent phase)

TABLE 33.3. Diagnostic Criteria for Giant Cell (Temporal) Arteritis.

1. Age at onset >50 years
2. New onset of localized headache
3. Temporal artery abnormality (tenderness or reduced pulsation) unrelated to arteriosclerosis
4. Erythrocyte sedimentation rate (ESR) >50 mm in first hour
5. Abnormal arterial biopsy

At least three of five features are required for diagnosis.
Source: American College of Rheumatology.[110]

clinical findings of Takayasu's arteritis are most often related to cerebrovascular disease, branciocephalic occlusions, or renovascular hypertension; although ophthalmological manifestations may also occur, they are usually seen only late in the course of the disease. There is a distinct female predominance at a ratio of 5:1, and the onset is usually at 15 to 40 years of age. The condition is characterized by a biphasic illness, with an initial inflammatory phase and a late stage when vascular stenosis and occlusion predominate. Systemic features often predominate in the inflammatory phase, consisting of fever, malaise, and other nonspecific symptoms. Symptoms localize in the late phase according to the specific pattern of vessel involvement; symptoms may therefore include headache, limb fatiguability, dizziness, palpitations, dyspnea, or visual disturbances.

In contrast to giant cell (temporal) arteritis, arterial wall biopsies play little role in the diagnosis or management of Takayasu's arteritis. There have been a number of attempts to establish diagnostic criteria for this disease (Table 33.4), with the most widely used criteria known as the Ishikawa classification.[80] This system was found to have a diagnostic sensitivity of 92.5%.

It is notable that arteriography plays a major role in the diagnosis of Takayasu's arteritis. In addition to the clinical criteria just discussed, angiography provides specific information on the location and extent of occlusive or aneurysmal lesions, and it is especially helpful in planning treatment. In some instances, arteriographic interventions may also be utilized as the primary form of treatment.

MEDICAL MANAGEMENT

In Takayasu's arteritis, steroid therapy is usually considered only palliative for active phases of disease. For patients refractory to steroids, additional treatment options include cyclophosphamide or methotrexate. For patients with renovascular hypertension, treatment with angiotensin-converting enzyme (ACE) inhibitors may be deleterious.

SURGICAL MANAGEMENT

Interventional techniques may be used in patients with symptoms related to specific occlusive lesions caused by Takayasu's arteritis, but they have a high rate of recurrence and are usually considered only a secondary or temporizing method of treatment for this disease. Surgical reconstruction is therefore the preferred method for managing symptomatic occlusive or aneurysmal lesions in patients who have had remission into an inactive phase of the disease.[82–88]

Surgical reconstruction for Takayasu's arteritis consists of various forms of bypass procedures, as thromboendarterectomy is precluded by the obliterative or aneurysmal nature of the disease process. Surgical reconstruction is reserved for patients in an inactive phase of the disease to limit the risk of graft occlusion by disease progression. The most common locations of disease requiring surgical reconstruction are cerebrovascular lesions, brachiocephalic lesions, and those causing renovascular hypertension.

Disorders of the Thoracic Outlet

The thoracic outlet encompasses a unique region dominated by the first rib, the anterior and middle scalene muscles, and their associated structures (Fig. 33.6). The subclavian artery, the subclavian vein, and the five nerve roots of the brachial plexus are all potentially subject to extrinsic compression within this relatively confined space; thus, thoracic outlet syndrome (TOS) represents a complex array of clinical conditions characterized by one or more of the following: occlusive or aneurysmal lesions of the subclavian artery (arterial TOS), "effort thrombosis" of the subclavian vein (venous TOS), or symptoms related to compression and irritation of the brachial plexus nerve roots (neurogenic TOS).[89,90]

Diagnosis

Although vascular lesions associated with thoracic outlet compression typically give rise to easily recognized syndromes, the diagnosis of neurogenic TOS often remains difficult, confusing, and elusive. Uncertainties in diagnosis and disappointing results of treatment have led some to question the existence of neurogenic TOS, adding to the many controversies surrounding this condition.[91]

Neurogenic TOS

Patients with TOS frequently describe previous trauma to the head, neck, or upper extremity, followed by a variable in-

TABLE 33.4. Diagnostic Criteria for Takayasu's Arteritis.

Ishikawa Criteria[150]: Age <40 years plus 2 major or 1 major/2 minor or 4 minor criteria
  Major criteria: (1) left midsubclavian artery lesion; (2) right midsubclavian artery lesion
  Minor criteria: (1) elevated ESR; (2) carotid artery tenderness; (3) hypertension; (4) aortic regurgitation or annuloaortic ectasia; (5) pulmonary artery lesion; (6) left midcommon carotid artery lesion; (7) distal brachiocephalic lesion; (8) descending thoracic aorta lesion; (9) abdominal aortic lesion

American College of Rheumatology[151]: at least 3 of 6 features are required for Dx
  1. Age at onset ≤40 years
  2. Extremity claudication
  3. Reduced brachial artery pressure
  4. >10 mmHg difference in systolic BP between arms
  5. Subclavian or aortic bruit
  6. Abnormal arteriogram

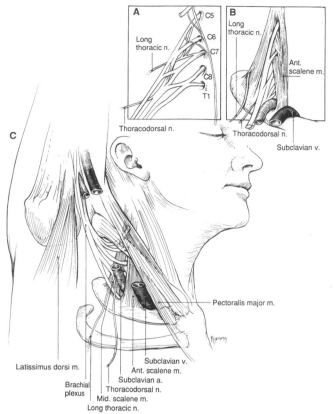

FIGURE 33.6. The surgical anatomy of the thoracic outlet. **A.** The brachial plexus arises from nerves roots C5, C6, C7, C8, and T1. The phrenic nerve arises from the upper cervical roots, including a contribution from C5. **B.** The thoracic outlet is conceptualized as a triangle bordered by the anterior scalene muscle, the middle scalene muscle, and the first rib. The subclavian artery and nerve roots of the brachial plexus course through this triangle, whereas the subclavian vein crosses the first rib just in front of the anterior scalene muscle. Each of these structures is potentially subject to extrinsic compression at several different levels by the musculoskeletal components of the scalene triangle. **C.** The anatomy of the thoracic outlet as viewed with the arm elevated. The long thoracic and thoracodorsal nerves pass vertically along the lateral chest wall, where they may be readily identified during transaxillary exposures. The second intercostal brachial cutaneous nerve courses in a transverse orientation through the midportion of the axilla (not shown). (From Thompson and Petrinec,[90] with permission.)

terval before the onset of progressively disabling upper-extremity symptoms.[89,90] The interval between traumatic injury and the onset of symptoms may range from days to weeks, or even several years. It is thought that scalene muscle spasm and persistent inflammation can lead to delayed healing, with fibrosis and nerve root irritation that eventually result in compressive neurological symptoms.

Symptoms of TOS include hand or arm pain, dysesthesias, numbness, and weakness. The symptoms may be bilateral, but they most commonly have their greatest effect on the dominant upper extremity. The distribution of symptoms does not follow typical patterns referable to a single peripheral nerve. Headache is a common complaint associated with TOS, most likely caused by secondary spasm within the trapezius and paraspinous muscles. Symptoms of TOS are typically reproduced or exacerbated by activity requiring elevation or sustained use of the arms or hands, such as reaching for objects overhead, lifting, prolonged typing or work at computer consoles, driving, speaking on the telephone, shaving, and combing or brushing the hair. Positional complaints may also be brought on by lying supine, resulting in pain and difficulty sleeping.

Physical examination is directed toward eliciting the degree of neurogenic disability and particular factors that exacerbate hand and arm complaints. A thorough peripheral nerve examination is performed to exclude ulnar nerve entrapment, carpal tunnel syndrome, and other etiologies. The neck is examined to identify the extent of local muscle spasm and to localize areas where focal digital compression reproduces the individual patient's symptom pattern. The presence of "trigger points" over the scalene triangle serves to reinforce the diagnosis of TOS. The Adson maneuver is used to identify any degree of subclavian artery compression, by detecting ablation of the radial pulse when the patient elevates the arm, inspires deeply, and turns the neck away from the affected extremity. Although this maneuver does not specifically reveal nerve root compression, positive findings are often associated with neurogenic TOS. Perhaps the most useful component of physical examination is the elevated arm stress test ("EAST"), in which the patient is asked to repetitively open and close the hands with the arms elevated in a "surrender" position. Most patients with neurogenic TOS report the rapid reproduction of upper-extremity symptoms with EAST, often being unable to complete the exercise beyond 30 to 60 s.

There are no specific diagnostic tests or imaging studies that can replace the clinical diagnosis of neurogenic TOS. Plain radiographs of the neck are helpful in determining if an osseous cervical rib is present, although this is relatively uncommon. The results of computed tomography, magnetic resonance imaging, electromyography/nerve conduction studies, and other examinations are usually negative, even in patients with pronounced disability. Nonetheless, these tests are often important to exclude other conditions, such as degenerative cervical spine disease, neoplasms or other masses, and intracranial pathology.

ARTERIAL TOS

Extrinsic compression of the subclavian artery may occur between the anterior scalene muscle and the first rib, leading to pathological changes in the arterial wall. This leads to complications related to the development of mural thrombus and acute thromboembolism to the upper extremity.

Patients with arterial TOS may present with acute ischemia of the hand or digits, with pain, paresthesias, and weakness of the affected upper extremity. The brachial and axillary artery pulses may be absent with extensive thromboembolism; however, palpable pulses suggest a proximal source of atheroembolism. One should also seek additional evidence of arterial compromise to the upper extremity, such as sympathetic overactivity with vasospasm, digital or hand ischemia, cutaneous ulceration or emboli, forearm claudication, or the pulsatile supraclavicular mass or bruit characteristic of a subclavian artery aneurysm. Because the anatomical abnormalities underlying TOS are often bilateral, it may also be informative to examine the contralateral extremity.

Patients with features suggesting arterial TOS may be evaluated by positional noninvasive vascular laboratory studies (segmental arterial pressures, waveform analysis, and duplex imaging), but it is often difficult to visualize the subclavian artery behind the clavicle. The definitive examination necessary to completely exclude or prove the existence of a fixed arterial lesion is provided by contrast arteriography.

VENOUS TOS

Venous TOS is caused by compression of the subclavian vein immediately anterior to the scalene muscle. This condition typically occurs in young, otherwise healthy patients, who are often involved in vigorous occupational or recreational use of the upper extremity. This habit is thought to cause repetitive venous trauma between the first rib and clavicle, resulting in the evolution of fibrosis and encasement of the vein by scar tissue, as well as eventual venous thrombosis. Patients with venous TOS most commonly present with the "effort thrombosis" syndrome, an acute event characterized by the sudden development of hand and arm edema, upper-extremity cyanosis, enlarged subcutaneous collateral veins, and early forearm fatigue in the absence of arterial compromise.

Patients in whom venous TOS is suspected should be studied promptly by contrast venography, particularly in the context of an effort thrombosis event.

Treatment

INITIAL MANAGEMENT

NEUROGENIC TOS

Conservative approaches serve as the initial treatment for neurogenic TOS.[92–94] These therapeutic efforts are focused on relaxing the scalene muscles and strengthening the muscles of posture through physical therapy, combined with hydrotherapy and massage. Pain medications, nonsteroidal antiinflammatory agents, and muscle relaxants are often useful adjuncts in treatment.

ARTERIAL TOS

The initial treatment of arterial TOS is focused on revascularization for acute ischemia, if necessary. This step is typically performed via brachial artery thromboembolectomy, with the hope of restoring sufficient inflow to the hand and digits to permit salvage. The demonstration of a fixed arterial lesion, either occlusive or aneurysmal in nature, is an indication for surgical reconstruction. Given that these lesions occur secondary to extrinsic compression rather than atherosclerosis or other forms of intrinsic arterial disease, there is no significant role for endovascular approaches to their management.

VENOUS TOS

As discussed earlier, the initial treatment of effort thrombosis generally involves contrast venography and catheter-directed thrombolytic therapy; this frequently results in restoration of venous drainage and resolution of the acute symptoms. Patients are then maintained on intravenous heparin and converted to oral anticoagulation with warfarin. Most patients with venous TOS are candidates for surgical decompression.

SURGICAL STRATEGIES

Transaxillary first rib resection has been the mainstay of surgical treatment for TOS for many years.[95–98] However, this approach has several significant limitations when used as a single strategy for all patients with TOS.[90,99] Efforts to overcome these limitations led to the introduction of combined approaches in which transaxillary first rib resection was performed concomitantly with supraclavicular exploration.[100] This approach subsequently led many groups to adopt the supraclavicular approach as the predominant treatment strategy.[101–103] Some have more recently adopted a highly selective approach in which supraclavicular scalenectomy is the principal operative strategy and first rib resection is reserved solely for vascular forms of TOS.[104,105]

First rib resection and subclavian artery reconstruction are required for any degree of aneurysmal degeneration, particularly if the patient has had preoperative symptoms of digital thromboembolism, as well as for persistent occlusive lesions of the arterial wall that are still evident after scalenectomy. Although prosthetic materials such as ringed PTFE are most commonly used, autologous conduits are sometimes preferable.

Patients with disabling neurogenic or arterial TOS may present with symptoms characteristic of sympathetic overactivity resulting in painful vasospasm, delayed healing of digital skin lesions, and, at times, even reflex sympathetic dystrophy. In these situations, cervical sympathectomy is a useful adjunct to thoracic outlet decompression, helping to alleviate vasospastic complaints and to facilitate healing of digital lesions caused by atheroemboli or ischemic injury.

Thoracic outlet decompression for venous TOS involves several additional considerations to the standard supraclavicular exploration for neurogenic TOS.[106,107] Although the initial steps of the procedure are conducted as for neurogenic TOS (anterior and middle scalenectomy and brachial plexus neurolysis), resection of the first rib is always indicated for venous TOS. Two additional aspects of the procedure are then specifically directed toward the venous problem: circumferential venolysis and resection of the medial first rib. In situations where external venolysis and paraclavicular first rib resection has been insufficient to relieve venous obstruction, additional venous reconstruction may be required. All patients undergoing operation for venous TOS are maintained on anticoagulation for at least 4 to 6 weeks in the postoperative period.

POSTOPERATIVE CARE

Postoperative care includes continued use of pain medications, muscle relaxants, and antiinflammatory agents. The expected recovery from thoracic outlet decompression is approximately 2 days in the hospital and 4 to 6 weeks at home, during which physical therapy remains an important component of treatment. Patients with venous TOS undergo predischarge contrast venography, both to assess the adequacy of venous decompression on the operative side and, if not previously determined, to assess the possibility that symmetrical venous compression may exist on the contralateral side. Any residual venous stenoses may be safely treated at this time by transluminal balloon angioplasty, a therapeutic option that is strongly contraindicated before surgical decompression. In patients with bilateral TOS, it is essential to ensure that any degree of phrenic nerve paresis has completely resolved before a second operation on the contralateral side.

The overall results of surgical treatment for neurogenic TOS remain difficult to define. In the hands of those performing these procedures with frequency, good to excellent results are reported in approximately 80% of patients, with complication rates as low as 5%.[89,108] In long-term follow-up, there appears to be no demonstrable difference in outcomes following the appropriate use of transaxillary or supraclavicular approaches, with recurrent symptoms occurring in up to 20% to 50% of patients.[89,109] Despite the persistence or recurrence of mild neurogenic symptoms, many of these patients experience a degree of improvement sufficient to permit daily activities and a higher degree of function than they had before surgical treatment.

References

1. Sorenson HR, Olsen H. Ruptured and dissecting aneurysms of the aorta: incidence and prospects of surgery. Acta Chir Scand 1964;128:644–650.
2. Svensson LG, Crawford ES. Aortic dissection and aortic aneurysm surgery: clinical observations, experimental investigations, and statistical analyses. Part II. Curr Probl Surg 1992;29:915–1057.
3. Ponraj P, Pepper J. Aortic dissection. Br J Clin Pract 1992;46:127–131.
4. Svensson LG, Crawford ES. Cardiovascular and Vascular Diseases of the Aorta, Philadelphia: Saunders, 1997.
5. Schlatmann TJM, Becker AE. Histologic changes in the normal aging aorta: implications for dissecting aortic aneurysm. Am J Cardiol 1977;39:13–20.
6. Schlatmann TJ, Becker AE. Pathogenesis of dissecting aneurysm of aorta: comparative histopathologic study of significance of medial changes. Am J Cardiol 1977;39(1):21–26.
7. Marsalese DL, Moodie DS, Vacante M. et al. Marfan's syndrome: natural history and long-term follow-up of cardiovascular involvement. J Am Coll Cardiol 1989;14:422–428.
8. Nicod P, Bloor C, Godfrey M, et al. Familial aortic dissecting aneurysms. J Am Coll Cardiol 1989;13:811–819.
9. Edwards WD, Leaf DS, Edwards JE. Dissecting aortic aneurysm associated with congenital bicuspid aortic valve. Circulation 1978;57:1022–1025.
10. Abbott ME. Coarctation of the aorta of the adult type, II. Am Heart J 1928;3:574–618.
11. Hirst AE Jr, Johns VJ Jr, Kime SW. Dissecting aneurysm of the aorta: a review of 505 cases. Medicine (Baltimore) 1958;37:217–279.
12. Larson EW, Edwards WD. Risk factors for aortic dissection: a necropsy study of 161 cases. Am J Cardiol 1984;53:849–855.
13. Carlson RG, Lillehei CW, Edwards JE. Cystic medial necrosis of the ascending aorta in relation to age and hypertension. Am J Cardiol 1970;25:411–415.
14. Harris KM, Braverman AC, Guitierrez FR, et al. Transesophageal echocardiographic and clinical features of aortic intramural hematoma. J Thorac Cardiovasc Surg 1997;114(4):619–626.
15. Robbins RC, McManus RP, Mitchell RS, et al. Management of patients with intramural hematoma of the thoracic aorta. Circulation 1993;88(5 pt 2):II1–II0.
16. Lindsay J Jr, Hurst JW. Clinical features and prognosis in dissecting aneurysms of the aorta: a re-appraisal. Circulation 1967;35:880–888.
17. Daily PO, Trueblood W, Stinson EB, et al. Management of acute aortic dissections. Ann Thorac Surg 1970;10:237–247.
18. Ergin MA, Griepp RB. Dissections of the aorta. In: Baue AE, Geha AS, Hammond GL, et al, eds. Glenn's Thoracic and Cardiovascular Surgery. Stamford, CT: Appleton & Lange, 1996;2273–2298.
19. Fann JI, Sarris GE, Mitchell RS, et al. Treatment of patients with aortic dissection presenting with peripheral vascular complications. Ann Surg 1990;212:705.
20. Deeb GM, Williams DM, Bolling SF, et al. Surgical delay for acute type A dissection with malperfusion. Ann Thorac Surg 1997;64(6):1669–1675.
21. DeBakey ME, Henly WS, Cooley DA, et al. Surgical management of dissecting aneurysms of the aorta. J Thorac Cardiovasc Surg 1965;49:130–149.
22. Miller DC, Mitchell RS, Oyer PE, et al. Independent determinants of operative mortality for patients with aortic dissections. Circulation 1984;70(suppl I):I-153–I-164.
23. Sommer T, Fehske W, Holzknecht N, et al. Aortic dissection: a comparative study of diagnosis with spiral CT, multiplanar transesophageal echocardiography, and MR imaging. Radiology 1996;199(2):347–352.
24. Miller DC. Surgical management of aortic dissections: indications, perioperative management, and long-term results. In: Doroghazi RM, Slater EE, eds. Aortic Dissection. New York: McGraw-Hill, 1983:193–243.
25. Masuda Y, Yamada Z, Morooka N, et al. Prognosis of patients with medically treated aortic dissections. Circulation 1991;84(suppl 5):III-7–III-13.
26. Clifton MA. Familial abdominal aortic aneurysm. Br J Surg 1977;64:765–766.
27. Bengtsson H, Norrgard O, Angquist KA, et al. Ultrasonographic screening of the abdominal aorta among siblings of patients with abdominal aortic aneurysms. Br J Surg 1989;76:589–591.
28. Majumber PP, St. Jean PL, Ferrell RE, et al. On the inheritance of abdominal aortic aneurysm. Am J Hum Genet 1991;48:164–170.
29. Kontusaari S, Tromp G, Kuivaniemi H, et al. A mutation in the gene for type III procollagen (COL3A1) in a family with aortic aneurysms. J Clin Invest 1990;86:1465–1473.
30. Bickerstaff LK, Pairolero PC, Hollier LH, et al. Thoracic aortic aneurysms: a population-based study. Surgery (St. Louis) 1982;92:1103–1109.
31. McNamara JJ, Pressler VM. Natural history of arteriosclerotic thoracic aortic aneurysms. Ann Thorac Surg 1978;26:468–473.
32. Warren RL, Hilgenberg AD, McCabe CJ. Blunt and penetrating trauma to the great vessels. In: Baue AE, Geha AS, Hammond GL, et al, eds. Glenn's Thoracic and Cardiovascular Surgery. Stamford, CT: Appleton & Lange, 1996:2213–2224.
33. Bennett DE, Cherry JK. The natural history of traumatic aneurysms of the aorta. Surgery (St. Louis) 1967;61:516–523.
34. McCollum CH, Graham JM, Noon GP, et al. Chronic traumatic aneurysms of the thoracic aorta: an analysis of 50 patients. J Trauma 1979;19:248–252.
35. Finkelmeier BA, Mentzer RM, Kaiser DL, et al. Chronic traumatic thoracic aneurysm. Influence of operative treatment on natural history: an analysis of reported cases, 1950–1980. J Thorac Cardiovasc Surg 1982;84:257–266.
36. Bacharach JM, Garratt KN, Rooke TW. Chronic traumatic thoracic aneurysm: report of two cases with the question of timing for surgical intervention. J Vasc Surg 1993;17(4):780–783.
37. Katsumata T, Shinfeld A, Westaby S. Operation for chronic traumatic aortic aneurysm: when and how? Ann Thorac Surg 1998;66:774–778.
38. Semba CP, Kato N, Kee ST, et al. Acute rupture of the descending thoracic aorta: repair with use of endovascular stent-grafts. J Vasc Intervent Radiol 1997;8(3):337–342.
39. Eagle KA, Coley CM, Newell JB, et al. Combining clinical and thallium data optimizes preoperative assessment of cardiac risk before major vascular surgery. Ann Intern Med 1989;110:859–866.
40. Boucher CA, Brewster DC, Darling RC, et al. Determination of cardiac risk by dipyridamole-thallium imaging before peripheral vascular surgery. N Engl J Med 1985;1312:389–394.

41. Cutler BS, Leppo JA. Dipyridamole thallium 201 scintigraphy to detect coronary artery disease before abdominal aortic surgery. J Vasc Surg 1987;5:91–100.

42. Lalka SG, Sawada SG, Dalsing MC, et al. Dobutamine stress echocardiography as a predictor of cardiac events associated with aortic surgery. J Vasc Surg 1992;15:831–842.

43. Lawrie GM, DeBakey ME, Morris GC Jr, et al. Late repair of coarctation of the descending thoracic aorta in 190 patients. Arch Surg 1981;116:1557–1560.

44. Carlson RE, Ehrenfeld WK, Stoney RJ, et al. Innominate artery endarterectomy: a 16-year experience. Arch Surg 1977;112:1389–1393.

45. Vogt DP, Hertzer NR, O'Hara PJ, Beven EG. Brachiocephalic arterial reconstruction. Ann Surg 1982;196:541–552.

46. Crawford ES, Stone CL, Powers RW Jr. Occlusion of the innominate, common carotid, and subclavian arteries: long-term results of surgical treatment. Surgery (St. Louis) 1983;94:781–791.

47. Zelenock GB, Cronenwett JL, Graham LM, et al. Brachiocephalic arterial occlusions and stenoses: manifestations and management of complex lesions. Arch Surg 1985;120:370–376.

48. Brewster DC, Moncure AC, Darling RC, et al. Innominate artery lesions: problems encountered and lessons learned. J Vasc Surg 1985;2:99–112.

49. Cherry KJ, McCullough JL, Hallett JW Jr, et al. Technical principles of direct innominate artery revascularization: a comparison of endarterectomy and bypass grafts. J Vasc Surg 1989;9:718–724.

50. Reul GJ, Jacobs MJ, Gregoric ID, et al. Innominate artery occlusive disease: surgical approach and long-term results. J Vasc Surg 1991;14(3):405–412.

51. Kieffer E, Sabatier J, Koskas F, Bahnini A. Atherosclerotic innominate artery occlusive disease: early and long-term results of surgical reconstruction. J Vasc Surg 1995;21(2):326–336, discussion 336–337.

52. Berguer R, Morasch MD, Kline RA. Transthoracic repair of innominate and common carotid artery disease: immediate and long-term outcome for 100 consecutive surgical reconstructions. J Vasc Surg 1998;27(1):34–41.

53. Azakie A, McElhinney DB, Higashima R, Messina LM, Stoney RJ. Innominate artery reconstruction: over 3 decades of experience. Ann Surg 1998;228(3):402–410.

54. Salam TA, Lumsden AB, Smith RB III. Subclavian artery revascularization: a decade of experience with extrathoracic bypass procedures. J Surg Res 1994;56(5):387–392.

55. Edwards WH Jr, Tapper SS, Edwards WH Sr, Mulherin JL Jr, Martin RS III, Jenkins JM. Subclavian revascularization. A quarter century experience. Ann Surg 1994;219(6):673–677, discussion 677–678.

56. van der Vliet JA, Palamba HW, Scharn DM, van Roye SF, Buskens FG. Arterial reconstruction for subclavian obstructive disease: a comparison of extrathoracic procedures. Eur J Vasc Endovasc Surg 1995;9(4):454–458.

57. Law MM, Colburn MD, Moore WS, Quinones-Baldrich WJ, Machleder HI, Gelabert HA. Carotid-subclavian bypass for brachiocephalic occlusive disease. Choice of conduit and long-term follow-up. Stroke 1995;26(9):1565–1571.

58. Schardey HM, Meyer G, Rau HG, Gradl G, Jauch KW, Lauterjung L. Subclavian carotid transposition: an analysis of a clinical series and a review of the literature. Eur J Vasc Endovasc Surg 1996;12(4):431–436.

59. Toursarkissian B, Rubin BG, Reilly JM, Thompson RW, Allen BT, Sicard GA. Surgical treatment of patients with symptomatic vertebrobasiliar insufficiency. Ann Vasc Surg 1998;12(1):28–33.

60. Deriu GP, Milite D, Verlato F, et al. Surgical treatment of atherosclerotic lesions of subclavian artery: carotid-subclavian bypass versus subclavian-carotid transposition. J Cardiovasc Surg (Torino) 1998;39(6):729–734.

61. Greenberg RK, Waldman D. Endovascular and open surgical treatment of brachiocephalic arterial disease. Semin Vasc Surg 1998;11(2):77–90.

62. Cid MC, Font C, Coll-Vinent B, Grau JM. Large vessel vasculitides. Curr Opin Rheumatol 1998;10:18–28.

63. Giordano JM. Takayasu's disease and temporal arteritis. Semin Vasc Surg 1995;8(4):335–341.

64. Weyand CM, Goronzy JJ. Molecular approaches toward pathologic mechanisms in giant cell arteritis and Takayasu's arteritis. Curr Opin Rheumatol 1995;7(1):30–36.

65. AbuRrahma AF, Thaxton L. Temporal arteritis: diagnostic and therapeutic considerations. Am Surg 1996;62(6):449–451.

66. Nordborg E, Bengtsson BA. Epidemiology of biopsy-proven giant cell arteritis (GCA). J Intern Med 1990;227:233–236.

67. Huston KA, Hunder GG, Lie JT, et al. Temporal arteritis: a 25 year epidemiologic, clinical and pathologic study. Ann Intern Med 1978;88:162–167.

68. Desmet GD, Knockaert DC, Bobbaers HJ. Temporal arteritis: the silent presentation and delay in diagnosis. J Intern Med 1990; 227:237–240.

69. Clearkin LG, Watts MT. Ocular involvement in giant cell arteritis. Br J Hosp Med 1990;43:373–376.

70. Andersson R, Malmvall BE, Bengtsson BA. Acute phase reactants in the initial phase of giant cell arteritis. Acta Med Scand 1986;220:365–367.

71. Kyle V, Cawston TE, Hazleman BL. Erythrocyte sedimentation rate and C-reactive protein in the assessment of polymyalgia rheumatica/giant cell arteritis on presentation and during follow-up. Ann Rheum Dis 1989;48:667–671.

72. Dasgupta B, Panayi GS. Interleukin-6 in serum of patients with polymyalgia rheumatica and giant cell arteritis. Br J Rheumatol 1990;29:456–458.

73. Espinoza LR, Jara LJ, Silveira LH, et al. Anticardiolipin antibodies in polymyalgia rheumatica and giant cell arteritis: association with severe vascular complications. Am J Med 1991;90:474–478.

74. McHugh NJ, James IE, Plant GT. Anticardiolipin and antineutrophil antibodies in giant cell arteritis. J Rheumatol 1990; 17:916–922.

75. Pariser KM. Takayasu's arteritis. Curr Opin Cardiol 1994;9:575–580.

76. Procter CD, Hollier LH. Takayasu's arteritis and temporal arteritis. Ann Vasc Surg 1992;6(2):195–198.

77. Robles M, Reyes PA. Takayasu's arteritis in Mexico: a clinical review of 44 consecutive cases. Clin Exp Rheumatol 1994;12(4): 381–388.

78. Moriwaki R, Noda M, Yajima M, Sharma BK, Numano F. Clinical manifestations of Takayasu arteritis in India and Japan—new classification of angiographic findings. Angiology 1997; 48(5):369–379.

79. Kerr G. Takayasu's arteritis. Curr Opin Rheumatol 1994; 6(1):32–38. Numano F. Differences in clinical presentation and outcome in different countries for Takayasu's arteritis. Curr Opin Rheumatol 1997;9(1):12–15.

80. Ishikawa K. Diagnostic approach and proposed criteria for the clinical diagnosis of Takayasu's arteriopathy. J Am Coll Cardiol 1988;12:964–972.

81. Hoffman GS. Takayasu arteritis: lessons from the American National Institutes of Health experience. Int J Cardiol 1996; 54(suppl):S99–S102.

82. Sharma S, Rajani M, Kaul U, et al. Initial experience with percutaneous transluminal angioplasty in the management of Takayasu's arteritis. Br J Radiol 1990;63:517–522.

83. Takagi A, Tada Y, Sato O, Miyata T. Surgical treatment for Takayasu's arteritis. A long-term follow-up study. J Cardiovasc Surg (Torino) 1989;30(4):553–558.

84. Kieffer E, Piquois A, Bertal A, Bletry O, Godeau P. Reconstructive surgery of the renal arteries in Takayasu's disease. Ann Vasc Surg 1990;4(2):156–165.

85. Weaver FA, Yellin AE, Campen DH, et al. Surgical procedures in the management of Takayasu's arteritis. J Vasc Surg 1990; 12(4):429–437; discussion 438–439.

86. Giordano JM, Leavitt RY, Hoffman G, Fauci AS. Experience with

surgical treatment of Takayasu's disease. Surgery (St. Louis) 1991;109(3 pt 1):252–258.

87. Robbs JV, Abdool-Carrim AT, Kadwa AM. Arterial reconstruction for non-specific arteritis (Takayasu's disease): medium to long term results. Eur J Vasc Surg 1994;8(4):401–407.

88. Miyata T, Sato O, Deguchi J, et al. Anastomotic aneurysms after surgical treatment of Takayasu's arteritis: a 40-year experience. J Vasc Surg 1998;27(3):438–445.

89. Sanders RJ. Thoracic Outlet Syndrome: A Common Sequelae of Neck Injuries. Philadelphia: Lippincott, 1991.

90. Thompson RW, Petrinec D. Surgical treatment of thoracic outlet compression syndromes. I. Diagnostic considerations and transaxillary first rib resection. Ann Vasc Surg 1997;11:315–323.

91. Wilbourn AJ. Thoracic outlet syndromes—plea for conservatism. Neurosurg Clin North Am 1991;2:235–245.

92. Walsh MT. Therapist management of thoracic outlet syndrome. J Hand Ther 1994;7:131–144.

93. Novak CB. Conservative management of thoracic outlet syndrome. Semin Thorac Cardiovasc Surg 1996;8:201–207.

94. Aligne C, Barral X. Rehabilitation of patients with thoracic outlet syndrome. Ann Vasc Surg 1992;6:381–389.

95. Roos DB. Transaxillary approach for first rib resection to relieve thoracic outlet syndrome. Ann Surg 1966;163:354–358.

96. Roos DB. Experience with first rib resection for thoracic outlet syndrome. Ann Surg 1971;173:429–433.

97. Machleder HI. Transaxillary operative management of thoracic outlet syndrome. In: Ernst CB, Stanley JC, eds. Current Therapy in Vascular Surgery, 2nd ed. Philadelphia: Decker; 1991:227–230.

98. Urschel HC Jr. The transaxillary approach for treatment of thoracic outlet syndromes. Semin Thorac Cardiovasc Surg 1996; 8:214–220.

99. Sanders RJ, Monsour JW, Gerber WF, et al. Scalenectomy versus first rib resection for treatment of the thoracic outlet syndrome. Surgery (St. Louis) 1979;85:109–121.

100. Qvarfordt PG, Ehrenfeld WK, Stoney RJ. Supraclavicular radical scalenectomy and transaxillary first rib resection for the thoracic outlet syndrome: a combined approach. Am J Surg 1984; 148:111–116.

101. Hempel GK, Rucher AH Jr, Wheeler CG, Hunt DG, Bukhari HI. Supraclavicular resection of the first rib for thoracic outlet syndrome. Am J Surg 1981;141:213–215.

102. Sanders RJ, Raymer S. The supraclavicular approach to scalenectomy and first rib resection: description of technique. J Vasc Surg 1985;2:751–756.

103. Reilly LM, Stoney RJ. Supraclavicular approach for thoracic outlet decompression. J Vasc Surg 1988;8:329–334.

104. Cheng SW, Reilly LM, Nelken NA, Ellis WV, Stoney RJ. Neurogenic thoracic outlet decompression: rationale for sparing the first rib. Cardiovasc Surg 1995;3:617–624.

105. Fantini GA. Reserving supraclavicular first rib resection for vascular complications of thoracic outlet syndrome. Am J Surg 1996;172:200–204.

106. Thompson RW, Schneider PA, Nelken NA, Skioldebrand CG, Stoney RJ. Circumferential venolysis and paraclavicular thoracic outlet decompression for "effort thrombosis" of the subclavian vein. J Vasc Surg 1992;16:723–732.

107. Azakie A, McElhinney DB, Thompson RW, Raven RB, Messina LM, Stoney RJ. Surgical management of subclavian-vein effort thrombosis as a result of thoracic outlet compression. J Vasc Surg 1998;28:777–786.

108. Hempel GK, Shutze WP, Anderson JF, Bukhari HI. 770 Consecutive supraclavicular first rib resections for thoracic outlet syndrome. Ann Vasc Surg 1996;10:456–463.

109. Lindgren KA, Oksala I. Long-term outcome of surgery for thoracic outlet syndrome. Am J Surg 1995;169:358–360.

110. Hunder GG, Bloch DA, Michel BA, et al. The American College of Rheumatology 1990 criteria for the classification of giant cell arteritis. Arth Rheum 1990;33:1122–1128.

34

Diseases of the Abdominal Aorta and Its Branches

Brad A. Winterstein and B. Timothy Baxter

Abdominal Aortic Aneurysms (AAA)

Definition, Incidence, and Significance

Normal aortic diameter decreases from the heart to the iliac bifurcation and is affected by age, gender, and body surface area. The diameter of the infrarenal aorta, the most aneurysm-prone segment of the circulation, is normally less than 2 cm. A number of definitions have been used to distinguish an aneurysm from mild dilatation. One generally accepted definition is a 50% increase above the expected normal diameter of the artery.[1] Embolization, compression, fistula formation, and occlusion can occur, but rupture is the gravest and most common complication of aortic aneurysm. Exsanguination following AAA rupture is reported to be the fifteenth most common cause of death in the United States. The actual death rate likely exceeds the 15,000 deaths[2] attributed to AAA each year, because sudden death in the elderly is often attributed to myocardial infarction and autopsy verification is rare.[3] The prevalence of AAA in screening studies is approximately 5%.[4,5] The overall incidence of AAA is greater in men than in women, but the rate of death from rupture is equivalent in the eighth decade, suggesting that if women live long enough they "catch up" with their male counterparts. Aneurysms can occur throughout the aorta, although the most common location by far is the distal aorta (95% of all aortic aneurysms), and their location is more precisely defined by the relationship to the renal arteries (infrarenal, juxtarenal, suprarenal). We focus here on the most common presenting aneurysm of the aorta, the infrarenal AAA.

Pathogenesis, Expansion, and Rupture Risk

The modern-day biochemical investigation of the pathogenesis of AAA began with reports demonstrating increased protease activity in aneurysm tissue.[6,7] Since these reports, the application of more sophisticated molecular and biochemical techniques has suggested a pivotal role for invading inflammatory cells that appear to regulate the activity of matrix-degrading enzymes. Current focus is on understanding underlying factors predisposing to AAA and the regulation of matrix degradation with a long-term goal of identifying AAA-prone individuals and using pharmacological approaches to target and inhibit aneurysm development and growth.

The normal aorta consists of three layers: the tunica intima, tunica media, and tunica adventitia. The major matrix proteins within the aortic wall are elastin and fibrillar collagen, providing the necessary compliance and strength, respectively. All layers contain varying amounts of collagen and elastin, but the media undergoes the most significant changes during aneurysm formation[8] (see Fig. 34.1).

Because AAA is a treatable disease that is asymptomatic until rupture occurs, clinical management is predicated on our understanding of its natural history. The natural history of aortic aneurysms is to progressively increase in size. Several studies in the past decade have helped to more precisely define mean and median expansion rates.[9–13] These reports and previous studies have been consistent in demonstrating that expansion rate increases with increasing aneurysm size, with an average growth rate of 0.42 cm/year for a 3.0–3.9 cm initial aneurysm size to 0.54 cm/year rate for a 4.0–5.9 cm initial aneurysm size.

These studies have also demonstrated a consistent relationship between aneurysm size and rupture rate. The risk of rupture of aneurysms that are less than 4 cm in greatest diameter at the time of diagnosis is less than 3% over the ensuing 5-year period.[10,12] Aneurysms 4 to 5 cm in diameter at the time of diagnosis have a 5-year rupture rate of 3% to 12%.[14,15] Those aneurysms larger than 5 cm at detection have a rupture rate of 25% at 5 years.[12]

Factors shown to increase the risk of expansion and rupture are shown in Table 34.1.[9,10,13,16] The observations regarding AAA growth, most recently from a randomized control study, have led to recommendations for regular 3- or

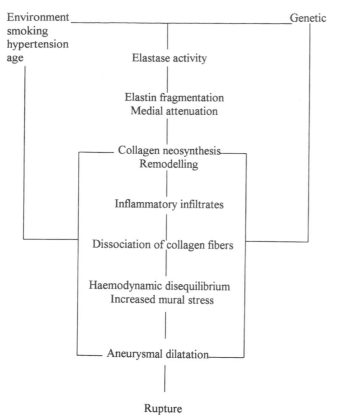

FIGURE 34.1. Proteolytic enzymes involved in aortic adventitial dilation. (From Wilson,[8] with permission.)

6-month evaluation of aneurysm size by ultrasound or CT scan in patients with AAA that are less than 5.5 cm.[17]

Treatment

Many selected studies have shown that elective AAA repair can be performed with mortality rates of less than 2%, citing data from single-center reports.[18–20] The mortality rate for AAA as reported in multicenter trials rises to 4.2%.[21] Age, myocardial ischemia, and pulmonary and renal insufficiency are the comorbidities associated with increased mortality rates.[22–24]

Operative survival after rupture of AAA has not improved over the last decade and remains dismal. Overall mortality after rupture may exceed 90%, although this rate is decreased to 50% for the select group of patients who reach the hospital.[25] Poor prognostic indicators following rupture are similar to those for elective repair.[23]

TABLE 34.1. Risk Factors Associated with Aneurysm Expansion and Rupture.

Initial size of aneurysm
Hypertension
Cigarette smoking
Chronic obstructive pulmonary disease
Severe cardiac disease
Advanced age
Previous stroke
Family history of AAA

Advances in endoluminal techniques have followed from the introduction of stents and the next logical step, covered stent grafts. Endovascular interposition of grafts in AAA is now possible. A recent multicenter trial has demonstrated that the endovascular treatment of AAA is safe and effective in a select group of patients in the short term.[26] The mid- and long-term prognosis for endografts remains unknown.

The treatment of AAA is complicated. Current recommendations are for elective repair of AAA between 5 and 6 cm in diameter. This decision obviously requires the clinical skill and judgment to factor in operative mortality versus longevity without repair.

Visceral Artery Aneurysms

As with AAA, visceral artery aneurysms also cause death by rupture. Most are asymptomatic and detected as incidental findings on imaging studies. Surgical intervention is usually the best approach, although the location and size may warrant observation in some cases. Repair typically involves interposition grafting, although surgical and radiological exclusion can be performed selectively.

Splenic Artery Aneurysms

Splenic artery aneurysms (SAA) are the most commonly recognized visceral artery aneurysm. The incidence of SAA in autopsy reports has varied from 1.6% to 10.4% and SAA account for almost 60% of all visceral artery aneurysms.[27] In distinction to AAA, they are found more often in women (4:1 women:men). They are saccular in nature and usually appear in the distal third of the artery.[28]

Splenic artery aneurysms occur more frequently in patients with medical fibrodysplasia, multiple pregnancies, portal hypertension, splenomegaly, local inflammation from pancreatitis, and after trauma or orthotopic liver transplants.[29,30]

As is true with AAA, most patients are asymptomatic at the time of diagnosis of a splenic artery aneurysm. When symptoms do occur, patients report pain in the epigastrium, left upper quadrant, and flank.[31] Plain films may be diagnostic in up to two-thirds of patients because of the extensive calcification in the wall of the aneurysm.[27] Other modes for diagnosis include ultrasound, computed tomography, and visceral angiography. Unfortunately, most patients are unaware of the problem and are diagnosed at the time of rupture. The risk of rupture is reported to be between 3.0% and 10.0%.[27,31]

The indication for surgical intervention of SAA corresponds to the natural progression of the aneurysm. Surgical treatment obviously should be undertaken for symptomatic, expanding, or ruptured aneurysms. Splenic artery aneurysms discovered in women of childbearing age should be repaired regardless of size because of risk of expansion and rupture peripartum. All healthy patients with splenic artery aneurysms should be offered surgical treatment.[27] Expectant management is reasonable in elderly patients with small (<2 cm) aneurysms and for those with larger aneurysms (2–3 cm) who have contraindications to surgery.

The surgical treatment options for SAA includes aneurysm resection or ligation. Splenic viability should be assessed intraoperatively because splenectomy is not routinely required. Isolated percutaneous splenic artery embolization is another effective treatment option although long-term follow-up is insufficient to ensure that recanalization and rupture cannot occur.

Hepatic Artery Aneurysms

Hepatic artery (HA) aneurysms, are the second most common splanchnic artery aneurysm, accounting for one-fifth of all splanchnic aneurysms.[32] They can involve the intrahepatic artery or be extrahepatic, which is four times as common.[27,33] The aneurysms are usually saccular.[35] The mean age at presentation is 40 with a male predominance (2:1 men:women).[32,34]

In the past, HA aneurysms were usually associated with infection. Today, mycotic aneurysms are rare and often are the result of intravenous drug abuse.[29] Most HA are associated with localized atherosclerosis (32%); it is unclear if atherosclerosis has a causal role. Other etiologies include medial degeneration (24%), trauma that includes iatrogenic injuries (22%), polyarteritis nodosa, and periarterial inflammation.[28,30,34]

Clinical symptoms of HA aneurysms may be absent or vague. The most common presenting feature is right upper quadrant or epigastric pain, which may prompt evaluation for cholecystitis. A pulsatile mass or bruit is uncommon on physical examination. Ultrasonography, computed tomography, or selective angiography is diagnostic. Unfortunately, 44% to 80% of patients first present with rupture.[27,28,35] Mortality associated with rupture is high (80%),[36] especially with free rupture into the peritoneal cavity.

Treatment of HA aneurysms must be considered in all low-risk patients and any patient with a symptomatic aneurysm. Before performing surgical resection, selective celiac and superior mesenteric artery (SMA) angiography must detail the aneurysm location and hepatic blood supply. Excision or ligation of the aneurysm, with or without revascularization, are treatment options for extrahepatic aneurysms depending on the location.

Intrahepatic aneurysms require special consideration as to location, size, and overall liver function before treatment can be instituted. Larger, peripherally oriented aneurysms can be treated with liver resection. Percutaneous catheter embolization of intrahepatic HA aneurysms has become the most popular mode of treatment over the last decade.[29]

Superior Mesenteric Artery Aneurysms

Superior mesenteric artery (SMA) aneurysms are the third most common splanchnic artery aneurysm, accounting for approximately 5% of all splanchnic aneurysms.[29] The etiology of most SMA aneurysms is infection secondary to subacute bacterial endocarditis. SMA aneurysms differ from other splanchnic artery aneurysms in that most (90%) are symptomatic. Severe, progressive abdominal pain is the most common presenting symptom. Approximately half of patients have a palpable pulsatile abdominal mass.

Treatment via ligation without revascularization can be achieved because of the extensive collaterals (Fig. 34.2). The decision to revascularize the SMA must be based on careful examination of the small bowel to ensure adequate perfusion.

Celiac Artery Aneurysms

Celiac artery aneurysms account for approximately 4% of visceral artery aneurysms. Celiac artery aneurysms can be diag-

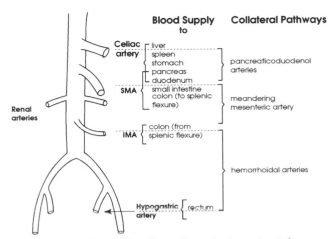

FIGURE 34.2. Collateral blood supply to the intestine. The pancreaticoduodenal arteries are the major collateral pathway between the celiac and superior mesenteric arteries (SMA). The meandering mesenteric connects the SMA to the inferior mesenteric. The hemorrhoidal arteries are the major communicating pathways between the inferior mesenteric and internal iliac (hypogastric) arteries.

nosed by plain radiograph when calcified, or by ultrasound, CT, or angiography. Unfortunately, the majority are diagnosed after rupture.[29] The mortality associated with rupture still remains close to 100%.[37]

Because of the high mortality associated with rupture, surgical intervention should be offered to all low-risk patients when diagnosed. Options for repair include aneurysmectomy and bypass, reimplantation, and ligation.[38,39]

Renal Artery Aneurysms

Renal artery aneurysms (RAA) were once considered a rare disease process. However, angiographic studies that included the renal arteries have shown the incidence to be between 0.3% and 1.0%.[40,41] The incidence may be as high as 2.5% when studies are performed for presumed renovascular hypertension.[42] Renal artery aneurysms are described slightly more often in women than in men. These aneurysms have also been reported to occur more commonly on the right side than the left.[43] Most RAA are saccular. Multiple aneurysms occur in approximately 20% of patients, and they are usually bilateral.[42]

Renal artery aneurysms have been classified into four distinct categories including (1) fusiform dilatations associated with medial fibrodysplastic disease, (2) aneurysmal dissections, (3) microaneurysms because of an inflammatory process, and (4) macroaneurysms of undetermined etiology.[42] The distinction between these groups of aneurysms is related to differences in etiology, which result in varying natural histories. Macroaneurysms and dissecting aneurysms are most amenable to surgical treatment.

The reported risk of rupture from renal artery aneurysms varies between 0% and 14.2%. Noncalcified aneurysms have been shown to have a higher propensity toward rupture.[44,45] Another important risk factor for renal artery aneurysm rupture is pregnancy. There has been no correlation made between risk of rupture and the size of the aneurysm; this is difficult to interpret given that large aneurysms are currently treated surgically due to the concern of rupture.

Most renal artery aneurysms are asymptomatic at the time of diagnosis. Symptomatic aneurysms may present with flank or abdominal pain, hematuria, or even renal insufficiency from distal embolization of thrombus from within the aneurysm. The diagnosis may be made by calcification seen on abdominal flatplate, ultrasound, or computed tomography. Angiography is the means by which the majority of small RAA are diagnosed.

Treatment of renal artery aneurysms should be tailored to the type of aneurysm. Small aneurysms, especially if calcified, usually do not require surgical treatment unless they become symptomatic; they should be followed on an annual basis with either CT scan or ultrasound. Surgical therapy is the best option in women of childbearing age regardless of aneurysm size. Patients with noncalcified aneurysms greater than 2.0 cm with hypertension, renal insufficiency, abdominal or flank pain, or hematuria or those with a solitary kidney or bilateral aneurysms should be advised to undergo elective aneurysm repair.[46]

Aortoiliac Occlusive Disease

The infrarenal aorta and iliac vessels are prone to atherosclerotic lesions leading to ischemia of the lower extremities. These lesions often extend into the infrainguinal vessels because of the generalized nature of atherosclerosis. Leriche[47] described the triad of bilateral claudication, sexual impotence, and absent common femoral pulses caused by infrarenal aortic occlusion.

Pathophysiology

Atherosclerosis causes progressive narrowing of the distal aorta and iliac vessels. Risk factors for aortoiliac occlusive disease are the same as for generalized atherosclerosis, including cigarette smoking, diabetes, hypertension, hyperlipidemia, and hyperhomocytenemia.[48] The plaque is usually more extensive on the posterior wall and is worst at the bifurcation of the aorta.

Although atherosclerosis is a diffuse process, its severity is greater in the infrarenal aorta, and the severity decreases at or above the renal arteries. This consideration is important in the surgical treatment of aortoiliac disease because adequate inflow can usually be obtained just below the renal arteries, eliminating concerns about renal ischemia.

The natural history of aortoiliac atherosclerosis is chronic progression to severe ischemia.[49] The development of large collateral pathways is critical in maintaining viability of the lower extremities as the process advances. Important collateral pathways include (1) the internal mammary artery to inferior epigastric artery, (2) the hypogastric and gluteal branches to the common femoral and profunda branches, (3) the superior mesenteric artery and inferior mesenteric artery to the middle and inferior hemorrhoidal arteries, and (4) the lumbar artery branches to the circumflex iliac and internal iliac arteries.

Clinical Manifestations

The initial manifestation of moderate aortoiliac disease is lower-extremity ischemia. The initial symptom is intermittent claudication causing external pain in the muscle groups of the thigh, hip, and buttock region. Symptoms can also occur in the calf but these are usually caused by more extensive disease involving the superficial femoral artery. Men may also experience erectile dysfunction.

Diagnosis

The diagnosis of aortoiliac disease is usually straightforward. Complaints of thigh, hip, or buttock pain with exertion are suggestive of the disease.

Inspection of the legs may be normal or reveal slight atrophy. A marked decrease or absence of palpable femoral pulses is a good indication of significant disease. The presence of femoral or pedal pulses at rest does not exclude stenosis, which becomes significant with increased flow during exertion.[50] Femoral bruits may also be present.

Noninvasive assessment of ischemic disease of the lower extremities starts with measurements of ankle brachial indices (ABIs), which measure the pressures at the ankles and compare them to that of the brachial artery. A ratio of 1.0 to 1.2 is normal. Ratios less than 1.0 signify atherosclerotic disease of the arteries of the lower extremities.

Duplex ultrasonography may provide additional information regarding disease location and severity. Duplex ultrasonography allows direct evaluation of aortoiliac disease by identifying areas of disturbed flow, especially increased peak systolic velocity.[51,52] Duplex scanning has been shown to have 95% sensitivity, 80% specificity, and 87% accuracy in predicting significant aortoiliac disease when compared to angiography.[53] Angiography should only be performed when symptoms are significant enough to warrant intervention. The goal of arteriography is not only to diagnose and determine the significance of lesions but also to plan therapy and, in some cases, to proceed with angioplasty.

Treatment

There are several options available to treat aortoiliac occlusive disease. Absolute indications for treatment are ischemic rest pain and tissue loss. Claudication is a relative indication. The type of procedure performed is based on the extent of the disease and overall patient condition.

Aortic Reconstruction

The current gold standard for aortoiliac disease is aortobifemoral bypass. The proximal anastamosis can be end to end or end to side. The end-to-end anastamosis is clearly indicated in patients with aneurysmal disease or complete aortic occlusion and is preferable in most other cases because of a slightly better long-term patency. The end-to-side anastamosis is indicated when retrograde flow from the femoral arteries would not provide adequate flow to the internal iliac arteries.

Extraanatomical Bypass

The role for extraanatomical bypasses has been debated because patency rates are compromised in favor of less morbidity with the operative procedure. The use of femoral–femoral bypass in unilateral iliac disease is an accepted alternative. Axillounifemoral and axillobifemoral bypasses are two other procedures that can be used for limb-threatening ischemia associated with aortoiliac disease. The use of these procedures should be limited to those individuals in whom a transabdominal approach places them at an increased risk. However, these bypasses are still inferior to aortobifemoral bypass. The 5-year primary patency rate for axillobifemoral bypass ranges from 50% to 70%, with secondary patency at 70% to 80%.

ENDOVASCULAR TREATMENT

The use of endovascular techniques such as percutaneous transluminal balloon angioplasty with or without stent placement has become an important component in the management of aortoiliac disease. Several variables help to predict the success of angioplasty. These variables include (1) performing angioplasty in patients who have claudication symptoms rather than for limb salvage; (2) lesions that are limited to the common iliac arteries; (3) stenotic rather than occlusive lesions; and (4) patients with good distal runoff.[54] Results of iliac angioplasty are quite good with a 5-year patency rate of approximately 70%.[55]

Mesenteric Ischemia

Mesenteric ischemia offers a difficult and challenging problem in both diagnosis and treatment. Mortality associated with mesenteric ischemia remains high and in direct relationship to the extent of bowel infarction. Although time is of the essence, delays in diagnosis are common and usually result from failure to consider mesenteric ischemia in the differential diagnosis of abdominal pain.

There is a wide spectrum of bowel ischemia, ranging from focal areas of ischemia to global transmural necrosis with a systemic inflammatory response resulting in bacterial translocation, endotoxemia, and sepsis.[56] These processes do not necessarily subside when perfusion is restored. Reperfusion injures tissues both locally and systemically by producing harmful free radicals after oxygen is reintroduced to ischemic areas,[57] which can lead to acute complications such as cardiac arrest or more gradual pathological activation of the immune response, resulting in multiorgan failure. Mesenteric ischemia has historically been divided into two broad categories: acute and chronic mesenteric ischemia.

Acute Mesenteric Ischemia

Acute mesenteric ischemia is caused by four distinct problems that compromise blood flow, including (1) acute embolic occlusion, (2) acute thrombotic occlusion, (3) nonocclusive mesenteric ischemia, and (4) mesenteric vein thrombosis. Early in the clinical course of an acute ischemic event, abdominal pain is typically severe and out of proportion to the findings on physical examination. This pain is associated with diffuse intestinal spasm that is manifest as vomiting, diarrhea, or both. On physical exam, the abdomen is soft and bowel sounds are hyperactive. As ischemia progresses bowel dilatation occurs, bowel activity decreases, and inflammation moves to the parietal peritoneum, resulting in peritoneal signs. At this point the ischemia is fairly advanced.

Diagnosis of Acute Forms of Mesenteric Ischemia

Because of the rarity of mesenteric ischemia, it may not be considered in the differential diagnosis of patients presenting with abdominal pain. Specific laboratory tests are not available, partly because of the ability of the liver to clear many of the products of ischemia released by the gut. Leukocytosis is usually present but is, obviously, nonspecific.

During the past decade, technological improvements in duplex ultrasonography have made it more reliable in imaging the mesenteric circulation and identifying flow disturbances. When visualization is adequate, this is a useful screening test, especially in acute thrombotic ischemia and mesenteric venous thrombosis.

Computed tomography also provides important clues to acute mesenteric ischemia and is diagnostic for mesenteric venous thrombosis. Atherosclerosis of the aorta and mesenteric ostia, lack of contrast in the proximal celiac or SMA, and bowel wall thickening may all suggest the diagnosis.

Aortography is the gold standard for acute embolic, acute thrombotic, and nonocclusive mesenteric ischemia. Initial films should include *lateral* aortogram to view the ostia of the celiac and SMA. Catheters can be positioned to selectively infuse therapeutic levels of vasodilators into the SMA in patients with nonocclusive mesenteric ischemia.

Treatment of Acute Mesenteric Ischemia

Once the diagnosis is made, treatment consists of correcting any underlying medical conditions that may be contributing such as myocardial dysfunction or hypovolemia. Provided that the patient is not in heart failure, fluid resuscitation should be started and heparin anticoagulation began to prevent propagation of thrombus.

There are nonsurgical options for treatment of mesenteric ischemia if the patient does not have signs of bowel infarction. Catheter-directed thrombolytic therapy has been used successfully in the treatment of early acute embolic occlusion.[58] Angioplasty can also be performed at the time of diagnostic angiography to dilate ostial lesions of the celiac and superior mesenteric arteries.[59,60] Local infusion of vasodilators into the SMA using selective catheterization is also important. Even when perfusion can be restored, the duration of ischemia may result in infarcted bowel, requiring resection.

Treatment of mesenteric venous thrombosis is nonsurgical and relies on anticoagulation as a means of reversing the hypercoaguability.

There are several clear indications for surgical intervention for acute mesenteric ischemia: (1) mesenteric embolization requiring embolectomy, (2) peritonitis, (3) other clinical signs suggestive of bowel infarction, and (4) thrombotic occlusion requiring revascularization. The goals of surgery are to restore blood flow when possible and resect any bowel that is obviously necrotic. To this end, "second-look" operations may be advisable.

Chronic Mesenteric Ischemia

Chronic mesenteric ischemia is a rare disease, although the incidence may be rising with the increase in the aged population. The typical patient is elderly and vasculopathic, usually having had multiple procedures for coronary, cerebral, and peripheral vascular disease. The disease history includes weight loss, postprandial pain, and food fear.[61,62]

The etiology of chronic mesenteric ischemia is progressive atherosclerotic occlusion of the ostia of the mesenteric arteries near the aorta. The slowly progressive nature of this disease allows collateral circulation to compensate during the initial stages.

Duplex ultrasound, the preferred screening test when the diagnosis is suspected, can usually demonstrate occlusion or stenosis of the ostia with collateral flow patterns. When duplex studies are positive or equivocal, angiography should be performed in anticipation of identifying occlusion or preocclusive stenosis of all mesenteric vessels.

There are two treatment options for chronic mesenteric ischemia, with the decision based on the surgeon's estimated surgical risk for that patient. If the patient has extensive comorbidities and is not a surgical candidate, mesenteric angioplasty can be performed with the expectation of a good rate of initial technical success and relief of symptoms in the majority of patients.[59] The downside of angioplasty is its lack of durability. Surgical revascularization is the treatment of choice.

Renal Artery Occlusive Disease

Renal artery occlusive disease is the most common form of surgically correctable hypertension. Renovascular hypertension has been increasingly diagnosed as a result of the increasing population at risk and improved diagnostic techniques.[63] The prevalence of renovascular hypertension in the general population is estimated to be 0.13%.[64]

Pathology

There are two important causes of stenosis of the renal arteries. The most common cause is atherosclerosis, followed by fibrodysplasia of the arterial wall. Other uncommon causes are congenital aortic malformations, arterial dissections, and renal artery emboli.

Pathophysiology

Hypertension can be caused by the narrowing of the renal arteries. The decrease in renal perfusion activates the renin-angiotensin system; this is mediated by the juxtaglomerular apparatus, which, in response to decreased renal perfusion, secretes renin. Renin is a proteolytic enzyme that acts on angiotensinogin to produce angiotensin I. Angiotensin I has very little direct vasoactive property. When the two C-terminal peptides are cleaved from angiotensin I by angiotensin-converting enzyme, angiotensin II is formed. Angiotensin II has properties that affect both the acute phase of hypertension and a chronic phase. The acute phase is mediated by direct, potent vasoconstriction. Angiotensin II also activates the adrenal cortex, increasing aldosterone secretion. This, in turn, increases sodium retention and intravascular volume. Angiotensin II normally exerts a negative feedback on renin release by increasing blood pressure. With severe renal artery stenosis, renal perfusion will not increase appropriately, perpetuating systemic hypertension.

Diagnosis

To properly diagnose the presence of renal artery occlusive disease, the anatomical lesion as well as its physiological significance must be demonstrated. Renal artery duplex scanning provides important information about kidney size and blood flow in the renal artery. Two parameters have been proposed to identify significant stenosis, including a systolic velocity greater than 200 cm/s[65] or a ratio of renal to aortic systolic velocity greater than 3.5. Sensitivity of duplex scanning is from 75% to 98% with specificity in a range between 90% and 100%.[65–67]

With technological improvements, magnetic resonance angiography (MRA) is becoming more reliable in detection of significant renal artery disease. The benefits that MRA has over arteriography are that it is noninvasive and uses no nephrotoxic contrast agents. Its sensitivities and specificity appear to be similar to duplex ultrasonography.[68,69] Dynamic CT scanning may also prove to be a useful screening tool.

Angiography remains the gold standard to evaluate stenosis in the renal arteries. Angiography also allows measurements of the gradient across the stenosis, and angioplasty can be performed at the same time. The current recommendations are for arteriography for any patient who is being considered for a revascularization. This approach could change in the next decade with continued improvement in duplex ultrasonography, MRA, and dynamic CT scanning.

Several functional studies are available to assess whether hypertension is caused by renovascular disease; these rely on measurements of renin activity. The advent of angiotensin-converting enzyme (ACE) inhibitors has increased the value of these tests in documenting renovascular hypertension. Captopril is given orally and combined with radionuclide renography. These studies are highly sensitive for hemodynamically significant unilateral renal artery stenosis.[70]

The renal vein renin ratio is another test that can help determine the significance and response to intervention of unilateral renal artery stenosis. It is calculated by dividing the renin activity of the affected kidney by the contralateral kidney. A ratio of 1.5 or more is believed to be of significance and correlates with a good response to revascularization.[71]

Treatment

MEDICAL MANAGEMENT

Within the last 20 years, successful treatment of renal hypertension has been easier with the advent of such classes of drugs as beta blockers and ACE inhibitors. The first-line therapy for treatment should be a beta blocker. A diuretic, either thiazide or loop, may be used if the hypertension is refractory to the beta blockers. The most effective drugs in the treatment of renovascular hypertension are the ACE inhibitors. Unfortunately, the use of ACE inhibitors may be associated with deterioration in renal function.

PERCUTANEOUS TRANSLUMINAL RENAL ANGIOPLASTY

The benefits of percutaneous transluminal renal artery angioplasty (PTRA) as a treatment of renovascular hypertension are that it is less invasive and does not require general anesthesia, resulting in a shorter hospital stay. Complications of this procedure are usually limited to the site of catheter in-

TABLE 34.2.
Arteriosclerotic Renovascular Hypertension.

Institution	Number of patients	Operative outcome (%)			Surgical mortality (%)
		Cured	Improved	Failed	
Bowman Gray	152	15	75	10	1.3
University of Michigan	135	29	52	19	4.4
University of California, San Francisco	84	39	23	38	2.4
Cleveland Clinic	78	40	51	9	2

Source: Stanley,[87] with permission.

sertion, although major events such as renal artery rupture and dissection can occur and renal salvage can be difficult.

Results of renal artery angioplasty for control of renovascular hypertension related to fibrodysplasia are excellent and angioplasty should be considered the first line of treatment. Complete resolution of hypertension occurs in 22% to 50% of patients, with improvements seen in 63% to 91%. Results for patients treated for atherosclerotic lesions are not as favorable, with 19% of patients obtaining complete resolution and 70% to 71% being improved.[72–74] The worst results are obtained with ostial lesions. Stent placement may improve the durability of these results, but this remains to be verified. Close clinical follow-up and ultrasonography are needed after PTRA to monitor for recurrent disease. Repeat PTRA can be considered if initial results demonstrated reasonable durability.

SURGICAL MANAGEMENT

The largest experience in the treatment of renovascular hypertension is surgical. Operative treatment must consider not only the risk of surgery to the patient but also the long-term effects of the disease process. Factors that suggest a relatively poor long-term prognosis for revascularization include a chronically elevated serum creatinine, male gender, increasing age, bilateral stenosis, and previous vascular operation.[75,76]

The most common surgical procedure for revascularization of the renal artery is aortorenal bypass, with saphenous vein graft being the most common conduit. Dacron or polytetrafluoroethylene (PTFE) can also be used, and these conduits are preferable in young patients where vein graft aneurysm formation is problematic.[77,78]

Nonanatomical renal artery revascularization can also be performed with excellent results. Splenorenal and hepatorenal bypasses are the two most common procedures.[79,80]

Endarterectomy with or without a vein patch provides good results for atherosclerotic lesions of the proximal renal arteries. The adequacy of the revascularization should be documented by intraoperative ultrasonography, especially when blind endarterectomy is performed.

Ex vivo reconstruction of the renal arteries can be performed for more complicated disease in the hilar areas. The downside of this procedure is the need for cold ischemia, long operative time, and most importantly the loss of established collateral networks, which may be critical if revascularization fails.

Results of surgical revascularization for renovascular hypertension vary with the underlying etiology of the disease (Table 34.2). Cure rates for the surgical treatment of fibrodysplasia are superior to those for treating atherosclerosis. Long-term results show a benefit to surgical revascularization in the treatment of renovascular hypertension.[81] Surgical revascularization for renal dysfunction is also clearly beneficial. Improvements in renal function are seen in 22% to 58% of patients, while deterioration occurs in 11% to 25%.[76,82–86]

References

1. Johnston K, Rutherford RB, Tilson MD, et al. Suggested standards for reporting on arterial aneurysms. J Vasc Surg 1991;3: 452–458.
2. Sliverberg E, Boring C, Squires T. Cancer statistics 1990. Cancer J Clin 1990;40:9–26.
3. Lundberg GD. Low-tech autopsies in the era of high-tech medicine: continued value for quality assurance and patient safety. JAMA 1998;280:1273–1274.
4. Collin J, Araujo L, Walton J, et al. Oxford screening programme for abdominal aortic aneurysm in men aged 65 to 74 years. Lancet 1988;ii:613–615.
5. Scott R, Ashton H, Sutton G. Ultrasound screening of a general practice population for aortic aneurysm. Br J Surg 1986;73:318.
6. Busuttil R, Abou-Zamzam AM, Machleder HI. Collagenase activity of the human aorta: a comparison of patients with and without abdominal aortic aneurysms. Arch Surg 1980;115:1373–1378.
7. Cannon DJ, Read RC. Blood elastolytic activity in patients with aortic aneurysm. Ann Thorac Surg 1982;34:10–15.
8. Wilson K, et al. Expansion rates of abdominal aortic aneurysm: current limitations in evaluation. Eur J Endovasc Surg 1997;13: 521–526.
9. Englund R, Hudson P, Hanel K, et al. Expansion rates of small abdominal aortic aneurysms. Aust N Z J Surg 1998;68:21–24.
10. Cronenwett J, Murphy TF, Belenock GB, et al. Actuarial analysis of variables associated with rupture of small abdominal aortic aneurysms. Surgery (St. Louis) 1985;98:472–483.
11. Cronenwett J, Sargent SK, Wall MH, et al. Variables that effect the expansion rate and outcome of small abdominal aortic aneurysms. J Vasc Surg 1990;11:260–269.
12. Nevitt M, Ballard D, et al. Prognosis of abdominal aortic aneurysms: a population-based study. N Engl J Med 1989; 321:1009–1014.
13. Guirguis E, Barber G. The natural history of abdominal aortic aneurysms. Am J Surg 1991;162:481–483.
14. Limet R, Sakalihassan N, Albert A. Determination of the expansion rate and incidence of rupture of abdominal aortic aneurysms. J Vasc Surg 1991;14:540–548.

15. Glimaker H, Holmberg L, Elvin A, et al. Natural history of patients with abdominal aortic aneurysm. Eur J Vasc Surg 1991; 5:125–130.

16. Chang J, Stein TA, Liu JP, et al. Risk factors associated with rapid growth of small abdominal aortic aneurysms. Surgery (St. Louis) 1997;121:117–122.

17. Powell JT, et al. Mortality results for randomised controlled trial of early elective surgery or ultrasonographic surveillance for small abdominal aortic aneurysms. Lancet 1998;352:1649–1655.

18. Bernstein EF, Dilley RB, Randolph HF. The improving long term outlook for patients over 70 years of age with abdominal aortic aneurysms. Ann Surg 1988;207:318–322.

19. Golden MH, Whittemore AD, Donaldson MC, et al. Selective evaluation and management of coronary artery disease in patients undergoing repair of abdominal aortic aneurysms: a 16 year experience. Ann Surg 1990;212:415–423.

20. Perry M, Calcagno D. Abdominal aortic aneurysm surgery: the basic evaluation of cardiac risk. Ann Surg 1988;208:738–742.

21. Zarins C, Harris EJ. Operative repair for aortic aneurysms: the gold standard. J Endovasc Surg 1997;4:232–241.

22. Richardson J, Main K. Repair of abdominal aortic aneurysms: a statewide experience. Arch Surg 1991;126:614–616.

23. Katz D, Stanley J, Zelenock G. Operative mortality rates for intact and ruptured abdominal aortic aneurysms in Michigan: an eleven year statewide experience. J Vasc Surg 1994;19:804–817.

24. Hollier LH, Taylor LM, Ochsner J. Recommended indications for operative treatment of abdominal aortic aneurysms. J Vasc Surg 1992;15:1046–1056.

25. Ernst C. Abdominal aortic aneurysm. N Engl J Med 1993; 328(16):1167–1172.

26. Moore W, Rutherford R. Transfemoral endovascular repair of abdominal aortic aneurysm: results of the North American EVT phase 1 trial. J Vasc Surg 1996;23:543–553.

27. Stanley J, Thompson N, Fry W. Splanchnic artery aneurysms. Arch Surg 1970;101:689.

28. Graham J, McCollum C, DeBakey M. Aneurysms of the splanchnic arteries. Am J Surg 1980;140:797–801.

29. Messina L, Shanley C. Visceral artery aneurysms. Surg Clin North Am 1997;77(2):425–442.

30. Busuttil R, Brin B. The diagnosis and management of visceral artery aneurysms. Surgery (St. Louis) 1980;88:619–624.

31. Trastek V, Pairolero PC, Joyce JW, et al. Splenic artery aneurysms. Surgery (St. Louis) 1982;91:694–699.

32. Countryman D, et al. Hepatic artery aneurysm: report of an unusual case and review of the literature. Am Surg 1983;49:51–54.

33. Zachary K, Geier S, Pellecchia C, et al. Jaundice secondary to hepatic artery aneurysm: radiological appearance and clinical features. Am J Gastroenterol 1986;81:295–298.

34. Schroeyers P, Lismonde M, Vermonden J, et al. Management of hepatic artery aneurysm: case report and literature review. Acta Chir Belg 1995;95:89–91.

35. Lal RB, Strohl JA, Piazza S, et al. Hepatic artery aneurysm. J Cardiovasc Surg 1989;30:509–513.

36. Dougherty M, et al. Hepatic artery aneurysms: evaluation and current management. Int Angiol 1993;12:178–184.

37. Shanley C, Shah N, Messina L. Common splanchnic artery aneurysms: splenic, hepatic, and celiac. Ann Vasc Surg 1996; 10:315.

38. Graham LM, Stanley JC, Whitehouse WM Jr, et al. Celiac artery aneurysms: historic (1745–1949) versus contemporary (1950–1984) differences in etiology and clinical importance. J Vasc Surg 1985;5:757.

39. Risher W, Hollier L, Bolton J. Celiac artery aneurysm. Ann Vasc Surg 1991;5:392–395.

40. Hageman JH, Smith RF, Szilagyi E, et al. Aneurysms of the renal artery: problems of prognosis and surgical management. Surgery (St. Louis) 1978;84:563–571.

41. Tham G, Ekelund L, Herrlin K, et al. Renal artery aneurysms. Natural history and prognosis. Ann Surg 1983;197:348–352.

42. Stanley JC, Rhodes EL, Gewertz BL, et al. Renal artery aneurysms: significance of macroaneurysms exclusive of dissections and fibrodysplastic mural dilations. Arch Surg 1975;110:1327–1333.

43. Lumsden AB, Salam TA, Walton KG. Renal artery aneurysm: a report of 28 cases. Cardiovasc Surg 1996;4:185–189.

44. Harrow BR, Sloan JA. Aneurysm of renal artery: report of five cases. J Urol 1959;81:35–41.

45. Cerny JC, Chang CY, Fry WJ. Renal artery aneurysms. Arch Surg 1968;96:653–663.

46. Dzsinich C, Gloviczki P, McKusick MA, et al. Surgical management of renal artery aneurysm. Cardiovasc Surg 1993;1:2 43–247.

47. Leriche R, Morel A. The syndrome of thrombotic obliteration of the aortic bifurcation. Ann Surg 1948;127:193.

48. Cacoub P, Godeau P. Risk factors for atherosclerotic aortoiliac occlusive disease. Ann Vasc Surg 1993;7:394–405.

49. Duprez D. Natural history and evolution of peripheral obstructive arterial disease. Int Angiol 1992;11:165–168.

50. Sobinsky KR, Borozan PG, Gray B, et al. Is femoral pulse palpation accurate in assessing the hemodynamic significance of aortoiliac occlusive disease? Am J Surg 1984;148:214–216.

51. deSmet AA, Kitslaar PJ. A duplex criterion for aorto-iliac stenosis. Eur J Vasc Surg 1990;4:275–278.

52. Rosfors S, Eriksson M, Hoglund N, et al. Duplex ultrasound in patients with suspected aorto-iliac occlusive disease. Eur J Vasc Surg 1993;7:513–517.

53. Sensier Y, Bell PR, London NJ. The ability of qualitative assessment of the common femoral Doppler waveform to screen for significant aortoiliac disease. Eur J Vasc Endovasc Surg 1998;15:357–364.

54. Johnston KW, et al. 5-Year results of a prospective study of percutaneous transluminal angioplasty. Ann Surg 1987;206:403–412.

55. Becker G, Katzen B, Dake M. Noncoronary angioplasty. Radiology 1989;170:921–940.

56. Turnage RH, Guice KS, Oldham KT. Endotoxemia and remote organ injury following intestinal reperfusion. J Surg Res 1994;56: 571–578.

57. Zimmerman BJ, Granger DN. Reperfusion injury. Surg Clin North Am 1992;72:65–84.

58. Rivitz SM, Geller SC, Hahn C, et al. Treatment of acute mesenteric venous thrombosis with transjugular intramesenteric urokinase infusion. J Vasc Interventional Radiol 1995;6:219–223.

59. Allen RC, Martin GH, Rees CR, et al. Mesenteric angioplasty in the treatment of chronic intestinal ischemia. J Vasc Surg 1996;24:415–423.

60. Hallisey MJ, Deschaine J, Illescas FF, et al. Angioplasty for the treatment of visceral ischemia. J Vasc Interventional Radiol 1995;6:785–791.

61. Cunningham CG, Reilly LM, Stoney R. Chronic visceral ischemia. Surg Clin North Am 1992;72:231–244.

62. Moawad J, Gewertz BL. Chronic mesenteric ischemia: clinical presentation and diagnosis. Surg Clin North Am 1997;77:357–370.

63. Textor SC. Renovascular hypertension. Endocrinol Metab Clin North Am 1994;23:235–253.

64. Lewin A, Blaufox MD, Castle H, et al. Apparent prevalence of curable hypertension in the hypertension detection and follow-up program. Arch Intern Med 1985;245:424–427.

65. Mollo M, Pelet V, Mouawad J, et al. Evaluation of colour duplex ultrasound scanning in diagnosis of renal artery stenosis, compared to angiography: a prospective study on 53 patients. Eur J Vasc Endovasc Surg 1997;14:305–309.

66. Hansen KJ, Tribble RW, Reavis SW, et al. Renal duplex sonography: evaluation of clinical utility. J Vasc Surg 1990;12:227–236.

67. Olin JW, Piedmonte MR, Young JR, et al. The utility of duplex ultrasound scanning of the renal arteries for diagnosing significant renal artery stenosis. Ann Intern Med 1995;122:833–838.

68. Kim D, et al. Abdominal aorta and renal artery stenosis: evaluation with MR angiography. Radiology 1990;174:727–731.

69. Hertz SM, Holland GA, Baum RA, et al. Evaluation of renal artery stenosis by magnetic resonance angiography. Am J Surg 1994;168:140–143.

70. Meier GH, Sumpio B, Setaro JF, et al. Captopril renal scintigraphy: a new standard for predicting outcome after renal revascularization. J Vasc Surg 1993;17:280.

71. Stanley J, Gecse A, Erdos E. Renal: systemic renin indices and renal vein renin ratios as prognostic indicators in remedial renovascular hypertension. J Surg Res 1976;20:149.

72. Weibull H, Bergqvist D, Jonsson K. Long-term results after percutaneous transluminal angioplasty of atherosclerotic renal artery stenosis—the importance of intensive follow-up. Eur J Vasc Surg 1991;5:291–301.

73. Ramsay LE, Waller PC. Blood pressure response to percutaneous transluminal angioplasty for renovascular hypertension. An overview of published series. Br Med J 1990;300:569–572.

74. Bonnelli FS, et al. Renal artery angioplasty: technical results and clinical outcome in 320 patients. Mayo Clin Proc 1995;70: 1041–1052.

75. Lawrie GM, Morris GC Jr, Glaeser DH, et al. Renovascular reconstruction: factors affecting long-term prognosis in 919 patients followed up to 31 years. Am J Cardiol 1989;63:1085–1092.

76. VanDamme H, et al. The impact of renal revascularization on renal dysfunction. Eur J Vasc Surg 1995;10:330–337.

77. Stanley JC, Zelenock GB, Messina LM, et al. Pediatric renovascular hypertension: a thirty-year experience of operative treatment. J Vasc Surg 1995;21:212.

78. Stoney RJ, De Luccia N, Ehrenfeld WK, et al. Aortorenal arterial autografts: long-term assessment. Arch Surg 1981;116:1416–1422.

79. Moncure AC, Brewster DC, Darling RC, et al. Use of the splenic and hepatic arteries for renal revascularization. J Vasc Surg 1986;3:196–203.

80. Khauli RB, Novick AC, Ziegelbaum M. Splenorenal bypass in the treatment of renal artery stenosis: experience with sixty-nine cases. J Vasc Surg 1985;2:547–551.

81. vanBockel JH, et al. Long-term results of renal artery reconstruction with autogenous artery in patients with renovascular hypertension. Eur J Vasc Surg 1989;3:515–521.

82. Novick A, et al. Trends in surgical revascularization for renal artery disease: ten years' experience. JAMA 1987;257:498–501.

83. Libertino JA, Bosco PJ, Ying CY, et al. Renal revascularization to preserve and restore renal function. J Urol 1992;147:1485–1487.

84. Bredenberg C, Sampson LN, Ray FS, et al. Changing patterns in surgery for chronic renal artery occlusive diseases. J Vasc Surg 1992;15:1018–1024.

85. Hansen KJ, Starr SM, Sands RE, et al. Contemporary surgical management of renovascular disease. J Vasc Surg 1992;16:319–331.

86. Hallett JW Jr, Fowl R, O'Brien PC, et al. Renovascular operations in patients with chronic renal insufficiency: do the benefits justify the risks? J Vasc Surg 1987;5:622–627.

87. Stanley JC. Surgical treatment of renovascular hypertension. Am J Surg 1997;174:102–110.

Arterial Disease of the Lower Extremity

David G. Neschis and Michael A. Golden

The overwhelming majority of vascular disease of the lower extremities is secondary to atherosclerosis. Depending on the severity of the vascular lesions and the existing collateral circulation, symptoms generally follow a continuum ranging from claudication, to rest pain, to frank gangrene with tissue loss. A primary goal of the vascular surgeon is the preservation of limb function by appropriate timing of vascular reconstruction.

The term claudication is from the Latin word, *claudico*, meaning to limp. Claudication is defined as a reproducible pain in a muscle group, usually in the calf or thigh depending on the level of vascular disease. The pain is brought on by exercise; usually a specific distance walked is enough to elicit the pain, which is generally relieved by a brief period of rest.

Rest pain is not merely claudication while at rest; rather, it is pain, usually in the forefoot, that occurs at rest and is often relieved by dependency of the affected limb. Rest pain indicates inadequate perfusion of the extremity even at rest and portends eventual progression to frank tissue loss.

Nonhealing ischemic ulcers or gangrene indicate insufficient perfusion to maintain viability of the affected limb, and progression to limb loss in the absence of intervention is almost certain.

Epidemiology of Lower-Extremity Ischemia

Prevalence

The prevalence of vascular disease is dependent on the definition used. Lower-extremity arterial disease can be classified as (1) asymptomatic, (2) symptomatic disease presenting as intermittent claudication confirmed by noninvasive testing, and (3) critical leg ischemia.

Asymptomatic arterial insufficiency is defined by a low ankle–brachial index (ABI). This index is acquired by measuring Doppler occlusion pressures of the lower extremity and comparing this to an upper-extremity occlusion pressure as a fraction. A normal ABI is approximately 1.1; a low ABI is generally defined as below 0.9. When this value is used as a standard, the incidence of asymptomatic lower-extremity arterial disease is about 10% in the 55- to 74-year-old age group.[1]

To summarize the available data for patients older than 50, approximately 15% to 20% have some form of lower-extremity arterial disease. Of these, 20% to 30% will eventually require some intervention, with 10% eventually requiring amputation. Alternatively, a full 70% of patients with lower-extremity arterial disease will not experience a significant progression of their disease.

Risk Factors

AGE

For males younger than 50, the prevalence of intermittent claudication is 1% to 2%, and this rises to 5% for those over 50 years of age.[2,3] This trend is similar in women as well.

MALE GENDER

The prevalence of intermittent claudication in women over 50 is about half that of males; however, by age 70, the rates are similar.[3]

DIABETES

Diabetics have comprised up to 25% of patients in series of lower-extremity revascularization.[4] The amputation rate in diabetics is about seven times that of nondiabetics.[5]

SMOKING

The association between smoking and peripheral vascular disease has been well documented.[6] Additionally, smokers are diagnosed with peripheral vascular disease a full decade earlier than nonsmokers.[7]

HYPERTENSION

Hypertension seems to have a greater impact on females than males, with a relative risk ratio of approximately 4 in female hypertensives and 2 in males.[8]

HYPERLIPIDEMIA

A fasting cholesterol level greater than 270 mg/dl has been associated with a doubled incidence of intermittent claudication.[9]

Patient Evaluation

Patient evaluation should begin with a complete history, focusing on the symptoms and risk factors just described. The physical exam should include a complete assessment of the pulses, as well as evaluation for pallor, cyanosis, dependent rubor, ulceration, gangrene, atrophy, infection, temperature, and trophic changes such as thickened nails and loss of hair on dorsum of foot. Ischemic ulcers are generally painful, do not bleed, and are located on the heel, toes, or forefoot, in distinction from venous ulcers, which are usually not painful, may bleed, and are located above the medial malleolus. A careful neurological exam is important as well, particularly because occasionally symptoms of neurological origin may mimic vascular insufficiency.

The most common conflicting diagnosis is that of neurogenic leg pain. As this condition can occur concomitantly with vascular occlusion, the absence of distal pulses does not rule it out. Symptoms that begin with a change in position and are relieved only by assuming the recumbent position must be suspected to be of spinal origin.[10] Additionally, a normal systolic pressure response to exercise, despite the occurrence of symptoms with exercise, effectively excludes vascular claudication.[10] Further studies to evaluate patients with atypical symptoms thought likely neurogenic in origin include lumbosacral spine films, electromyography, lumbosacral spinal MRI or CT, and myelography. In addition, patients in whom symptoms do not resolve following revascularization should be evaluated for a neurogenic process.

Patients with signs and symptoms suggestive of vascular disease should first undergo noninvasive testing of the arterial system. Two simple tests include the measurement of segmental systolic pressures and the ankle brachial index (ABI). Normally, Doppler segmental pressures increase 20 mmHg from the brachial artery to the proximal femoral artery. Any change less than a 20-mmHg increase suggests aortoiliac disease. A pressure drop of more than 30 mmHg between any two successive cuffs normally placed at the arm, proximal thigh, distal thigh, proximal calf, and distal calf signifies a significant arterial obstruction.[11] The ABI is also a helpful test. An ABI greater than 0.9 is considered normal. An ABI between 0.5 and 0.85 suggests the degree of arterial obstruction often associated with claudication, and an ABI less than 0.50 suggests severe arterial obstruction often associated with critical ischemia.[11]

A more rigid objective determination of claudication severity utilizes exercise testing. Severe claudication can be defined as an inability to complete the treadmill exercise because of leg symptoms and ankle pressures below 50 mmHg following exercise.[12] Although angiography remains the gold standard for anatomical evaluation of vascular lesions, its use

should be limited to only those patients who are to undergo intervention.

TOE SYSTOLIC PRESSURE INDEX

The prevalence of peripheral disease has been reported to be as much as 20-fold higher in diabetics than in age- and sex-matched controls.[13] In diabetics, calcification of the media often makes their vessels noncompressible, leading to artifactually high ankle pressures. However, this medial calcification generally does not extend into the digital arteries. Therefore, it is possible to measure toe pressure using a strain-gauge sensor or photoplethysmograph.[14] Toe systolic pressure index (TSPI) value is normally greater than 0.60. If the absolute toe systolic pressure is less than 30 mmHg, healing without intervention is unlikely.[14]

DUPLEX ULTRASOUND

Duplex ultrasound is the combination of B-mode imaging and Doppler ultrasound. Although B-mode imaging can demonstrate a stenotic vessel segment, the degree of stenosis cannot be accurately measured. Doppler ultrasound however allows accurate measurement of blood velocity. In normal volunteers, the normal peak systolic velocity is 100 ± 20 cm/s in the aorta, 119 ± 22 cm/s in the external iliac artery, and 69 ± 14 cm/s in the popliteal artery. In general, a 20% to 49% stenosis is indicated by an increase in peak systolic velocity more than 30% but less than 100% from the preceding vessel segment. A critical (50%–99%) stenosis is indicated by an increase in peak systolic velocity greater than 100%. No flow, obviously, indicates occlusion.[15] Duplex scanning has been reported to be able to detect significant stenoses with an average 82% sensitivity and 92% specificity, depending on the vessels studied.[16]

ANGIOGRAPHY

Magnetic resonance angiography (MRA) is becoming increasingly popular in the evaluation of lower-extremity ischemia, particularly for patients who have a contraindication to standard contrast angiography. Its safe use as a replacement for angiography requires careful evaluation and significant experience with MRA.

Contrast angiography should be reserved for patients without a contraindication who are expected to undergo revascularization. Currently, antiography remains the gold standard in the evaluation of lower-extremity ischemia.

Lower-Extremity Occlusive Disease

Natural History

In studies of patients with claudication followed for a mean of 2.5 years and up to 8 years, 79% remained stable or improved, with only 21% worsening. Only 5.8% had progression to gangrene and required an amputation. These studies have established the safety of treating most patients with claudication nonoperatively with programs of exercise, risk management, including smoking cessation and control of lipid, glucose and blood pressure levels, medication with antiplatelet and rheologic agents, and meticulous care of the lower extremity. These studies have also provided the basis for considering claudication as only a relative indication for revascularization, warranting careful selection of low-risk patients with disabling symptoms for such procedures. It is well accepted that ischemic rest pain and certainly tissue loss are signs of limb-threatening ischemia, the natural history of which is progression to amputation unless intervention with improvement of arterial perfusion occurs.

Aortoiliac Occlusive Disease

Atherosclerotic lesions in the aortoiliac location generally begin at the bifurcation of the aorta or the common iliac arteries and can progress in either direction. In general, patients complaining of claudication as a result of isolated aortoiliac disease tend to be younger than those whose claudication is caused by disease of the femoropopliteal system. Additionally, the fact that lesions of the aortoiliac system are less likely to cause symptoms is a tribute to the excellent collateral system in this area. However, due to the larger number of muscle groups directly perfused by these vessels, claudication as a result of aortoiliac disease may result in greater disability. In addition, lesions of the aortoiliac system, regardless of lumen diameter, are at risk for distal embolization. It is for these reasons, as well as the excellent long-term results obtained with this patient population, that a more aggressive approach to claudication is taken as a result of aortoiliac disease.

Operative Alternatives for Patients with Aortoiliac Occlusive Disease

A number of surgical options are available for the treatment of aortoiliac disease. Over the last decade, however, percutaneous techniques have become more frequently employed. Details of the various options are described in Chapter 34.

Infrainguinal Arterial Occlusive Disease

Atherosclerotic lesions often affect the major arteries below the inguinal ligament. The most common lesion is a short-segment occlusion of the distal superficial femoral artery, especially in the region of Hunter's canal. Other vessels commonly involved include the above- and below-knee popliteal artery, the anterior and posterior tibial arteries, and the peroneal artery. Additionally, the common and deep femoral arteries may be affected as well. Evidence of disease is probably present in early adult life and progresses gradually until becoming symptomatic. Due to the large potential for collateral flow, a single lesion is often asymptomatic or at least not limb threatening. In general, to produce significantly severe symptoms or limb-threatening ischemia, lesions at multiple levels must be present. This then is called combined segment disease and involves any combination of aortoiliac, femoropopliteal, and infrapopliteal lesions.

As discussed earlier, the great majority of patients complaining of intermittent calf claudication can be safely observed until symptoms of critical ischemia provide an absolute indication for revascularization. However, it is quite reasonable to consider a good-risk patient with incapacitating claudication for revascularization as well.

A 1980 review of femoropopliteal reconstructions for disabling claudication showed that all patients experienced relief of their symptoms after surgery. Cumulative graft patency was 93% at 2 years and 88% at 5 years, with no operative mortality. These patency rates are clearly superior to collective results of femoropopliteal graft patency performed for limb salvage.[17] More contemporary series have shown similar results.

Surgical Alternatives for Patients with Limb-Threatening Ischemia and Infrainguinal Occlusive Disease

Femoropopliteal bypass is indicated when the superficial femoral artery or proximal popliteal artery is occluded and the patent popliteal artery has luminal continuity on arteriogram with any of its three terminal branches. In the case of a popliteal occlusion, bypass to an isolated segment of popliteal artery is effective if the segment is more than 7 cm long. If the isolated popliteal segment is less than 7 cm, or if there is severe gangrene of the foot, a sequential bypass to the popliteal and then to a more distal vessel should be considered.[18] Femoropopliteal bypass grafts are categorized as either above knee or below knee (Tables 35.1, 35.2). Based on these data, prosthetic material is avoided whenever possible for infrageniculate bypass.

The use of PTFE in the above-knee position is a far more viable alternative. Proponents of its use as the material of choice in the above-knee position cite early patency rates similar to those for autologous vein,[19] and the frequent need of saphenous vein for future coronary bypass or more distal peripheral arterial bypass revision. However, the argument for future vein requirements does not appear justified. A policy of the preferential use of autologous vein graft in any position is followed by most vascular surgeons.

Infrapopliteal bypass should be performed only in situations of lower-extremity ischemia in which femoropopliteal bypass is not feasible (Table 35.3). These data are the basis for the avoidance of the use of prosthetic material to bypass to infrapopliteal arteries if at all possible.

The selection of the posterior tibial artery, the anterior tibial artery, or the peroneal artery for the infrapopliteal anastomosis is important. A retrospective review showed no difference in hemodynamic parameters among the different outflow groups.[20] Therefore the choice of outflow vessel should be based on the overall quality of the vessel. If two vessels of excellent quality are available, the preference probably should go to the vessel with the greatest degree of direct continuity with the foot.

One of many unanswered questions in vascular surgery is

TABLE 35.1.

Above-Knee Femoropopliteal Grafts[42]: A Review of Series Published Since 1981

	Primary patency		
	1 Year	3 Year	4 Year
Autologous Vein[19,43–48]	84%		69%
PTFE[19,44–46,48–50]	79%	57%	60%
Dacron[49]		62%	

TABLE 35.2.

Below-Knee Femoropopliteal Grafts[42]: A Review of Series Published Since 1981

	Primary patency/ secondary patency	
	1 Year	4 Year
Autologous Vein[19,43–48,51–55]	82%/96%	72%/81%
PTFE (secondary patency only)[44–46,48,50,52]	68%	40%
Limb Salvage (autologous vein only)[19,43,51]	92%	75%

which operation is best for infrapopliteal reconstruction. There is general agreement that autologous vein is currently the best conduit. However, this can be used as a reversed graft, requiring complete excision from its bed, or left in situ, requiring ablation of all valves, and side-branch ligation but allowing the vein to remain, for the most part, in its bed, theoretically preventing ischemic damage to the vein graft wall and avoiding significant size mismatch at the proximal and distal anastomoses. In a prospective, randomized comparison of reversed and in situ vein grafts, there was no significant difference between the types of bypass, particularly when the veins were greater than 3.5 mm in diameter.[21] For veins of 3.5 mm in diameter, there was a trend toward improved results in the in situ group.

In a situation where extensive disease involves multiple levels of the lower extremity, a long bypass from groin to ankle may be required. In a study of in situ grafts for this situation, there is a 73% cumulative patency rate at 5 years with an 89% limb salvage rate.[22]

In popliteal to distal artery bypass for limb-threatening ischemia, there is a 55% and 60% primary and secondary patency at 5 years and 73% limb salvage. Factors that were noted to be associated with a decrease in graft patency included small-diameter grafts, a dorsalis pedis outflow site, and poor-quality outflow.

Finally, bypass to inframaleolar sites such as the dorsalis pedis artery has proven to be a durable procedure. When compared to peroneal bypass in a large series, no significant differences were found, with 5-year secondary patency rates of 76% and 68% in the peroneal and dorsalis pedis arteries, respectively. Limb salvage rates in the same groups were 93% and 87%, respectively, at 5 years.[23]

Clearly all forms of bypass benefit when good-quality, large-diameter autologous greater saphenous vein is available. However, that is often not the case. As a rule of thumb, the shortest graft to adequate inflow and outflow vessels is advisable.

USE OF THE DEEP FEMORAL ARTERY IN LIMB SALVAGE

Profundaplasty is a procedure consisting of endarterectomy of the origin and proximal portion of the deep femoral artery. It is most useful when combined with an inflow procedure such as an aortobifemoral bypass or axillofemoral bypass. On occasion it is performed as an isolated procedure, usually following graft failure, in attempt to achieve limb salvage by less than maximal improvement in limb perfusion.

Axillopopliteal bypass is generally used as a final effort to prevent amputation. It is usually performed in a situation in which the usual options are not available, whether this is the result of groin infection with or without graft infection, extensive operative scaring, or extensive involvement of the iliac and femoral systems.

POSTOPERATIVE GRAFT SURVEILLANCE

There are three major causes of graft failure. Failure in the immediate postoperative period (<30 days) is most often due to technical or judgmental error. Other causes include inadequate inflow or outflow, poor conduit, infection, or an unrecognized hypercoagulable state. Failure between 30 days and 2 years is most often the result of myointimal hyperplasia within the vein graft or at anastomotic sites. Late graft failure is usually caused by the natural progression of atherosclerotic disease. It is estimated that strictures develop in 20% to 30% of infrainguinal vein bypasses during the first year.[24] Careful surveillance is justified in that intervention based on a duplex surveillance protocol has resulted in 5-year assisted patency rates of 82% to 93% for all infrainguinal grafts studied, significantly higher than the 30% to 50% secondary patency rates of thrombosed vein grafts. A typical surveillance protocol would include duplex ultrasonography to measure flow velocity and the velocity ratio across a stenosis. Further workup would be indicated in vein grafts with flow velocity less than 45 cm/s and a velocity ratio greater than 3.5 across a stenosis. In addition, ABIs can be easily measured, with decrease more than 0.15 between exams considered significant. Exams should be performed perioperatively and at 6 weeks, at 3-month intervals for 2 years, and every 6 months thereafter.

The Role of Percutaneous Transluminal Angioplasty and Stenting in the Management of Lower-Extremity Occlusive Disease

Since the earliest reports in 1964,[25] PTA has become an important tool in the management of patients with lower-extremity occlusive disease (Table 35.4). More recently, the use of intravascular stents has increased the number of lesions amenable to endovascular therapy and has been shown to improve on results of PTA alone.[26] The more common indications for iliac PTA are focal concentric stenosis of the common and/or external iliac arteries, to increase flow (1) in

TABLE 35.3.

Infrapopliteal Grafts[42]: A Review of Series Published Since 1981

	1 Year	4 Year
Primary Patency		
Reverse saphenous vein[19,43–45,51,52,56–62]	76%	62%
In situ vein bypass[46,53–56]	81%	68%
Secondary Patency		
Reverse saphenous vein[43,56,57,60,62]	83%	76%
In situ vein bypass[54–56]	87%	81%
PTFE[19,45,56,61,63]	47%	21%
Limb Salvage		
Reverse saphenous vein[19,52,58–61,64]	85%	82%
In situ, vein bypass[53,65]	91%	83%
PTFE[19,52,61]	68%	48%

TABLE 35.4.
Percutaneous Transluminal Angioplasty Patency.[66]

	1 Year	4 Year
Aortoiliac[67–70]	88%	75%
Femoropopliteal[67–69,71]	81%	63%

patients with claudication from aortoiliac disease, (2) in patients in whom either PTA or surgical bypass is considered for infrainguinal arterial occlusive disease, and to increase flow for limb salvage (3) in the patient with severe infrainguinal arterial disease. Relative contraindications include diffuse iliac artery stenoses and heavily calcified lesions.

Current indications for iliac artery stent placement include atherosclerotic stenosis with ulcerated plaques, iliac artery occlusion, post-PTA arterial dissection, failure of balloon angioplasty (defined as a residual stenosis of 30% or greater or a pressure gradient greater than 5 mmHg), and recurrent stenosis following PTA.

Predictors of improved long-term success include PTA for claudication as opposed to limb salvage, an ABI above 0.57, stenosis versus occlusion, and good runoff. Factors that do not seem to significantly affect late results include site of PTA, diabetes, number of sites treated, and pressure gradient across the lesion. Overall, the best results seem to have been in stenotic lesions with good runoff. Occlusions with poor runoff were associated with a 16% success rate at 5 years. PTA is a satisfactory option for lower-extremity revascularization, particularly in patients at high risk for surgery with good runoff and stenotic lesions.

Lumbar Sympathectomy

In a small number of cases, reconstructive arterial surgery is not feasible in a patient with severe lower-extremity ischemia. Lumbar sympathectomy may be a reasonable alternative to improve rest pain and avoid amputation. In a review of 60 consecutive patients undergoing lumbar sympathectomy, there was a zero mortality rate and minimal morbidity.[27] It was concluded that lumbar sympathectomy is a useful procedure in patients with lower-extremity ischemia presenting only as rest pain without gangrenous changes and having an ABI greater than 0.30. In addition, lumbar sympathectomy may be useful in patients with nonreconstructable disease and focal tissue loss, with an ABI greater than 0.30, but with transcutaneous oxygen tensions less than 30 mmHg that increase by more than 20 mmHg with limb dependency. Endoscopic approaches to lumbar sympathectomy should be considered.[28]

Amputation

Fortunately, the vast majority of patients presenting with even critical ischemia can be offered a reasonable attempt at limb salvage. However, there are situations in which the best option remains primary amputation. Some specific indications of lower-extremity amputation include nonsalvageable dry or wet gangrene, unremitting and unreconstructable rest pain, nonhealing ulcers, chronic infection, neuroma, frostbite, malignancy, chronic pain, congenital deformity, and unsalvageable venous insufficiency.

The selection of amputation levels should consider the objectives of removing all nonviable tissue while ensuring primary wound healing and an acceptable functional result. The outcome following below-knee amputation is far better than that following amputation at the ankle despite the higher level. In cases where the patient has severe depression of mental status such that he or she is unable to ambulate, communicate, or provide self-care, an above-knee primary amputation should be considered. Severe, long-standing contractures can occur with below-knee amputations in this bedridden patient group, and often local trauma may make the below-knee amputation less likely to heal than an amputation at the more proximal level.

Clearly, therefore, selection of the correct level of amputation is critical to ensure maximum rehabilitation potential and avoid multiple procedures. A useful algorithm is described by Dwars and colleagues.[29] The authors analyzed a series of 85 lower-extremity amputations and determined that the presence of a palpable pulse immediately above the level of amputation correlated well with primary wound healing and a 100% negative predictive value. The absence of palpable pulses was of no use in selecting an amputation level. They found a skin perfusion pressure greater than 20 mmHg to be highly predictive of primary amputation healing, with a positive predictive value of 89% and a negative predictive value of 99%. The authors suggest if there is no palpable pulse immediately proximal to the level of amputation, and the skin perfusion pressure at that level is less than 20 mmHg, a higher amputation level should be selected.

The indications for toe amputation include gangrene, infection, ulceration, or osteomyelitis confined to the mid- or distal phalanx. If gangrene is dry, consideration can be made toward expectant management allowing autoamputation as this would allow for maximal retention of viable tissue. The downside to this approach is that it could take months for autoamputation to be complete. Contraindications to toe amputation include cellulitis proximal to the site, presence of dependent rubor, forefoot infection, and involvement of the metatarsalphalangeal joint or distal metatarsal head. Skin flaps should be reapproximated without tension; 100% rehabilitation potential should be expected.

If gangrene or infection approaches the phalangeal–metatarsal crease or involves the metatarsal head, a partial distal forefoot amputation in the form of a ray amputation can be performed by extending the toe amputation to include the distal metatarsal shaft and head. As in toe amputations, infection or gangrene proximal to the involved site is a contraindication to ray amputation. Again, with the proper postoperative footwear, 100% rehabilitation should be expected.

Transmetatarsal amputation is indicated when gangrene or infection involves multiple toes. It is contraindicated when deep forefoot infection, cellulitis, lymphangitis, or dependent rubor involve the dorsal forefoot proximal to the metatarsal–phalangeal crease. If the wound heals successfully, transmetatarsal amputation affords an excellent functional result, particularly with proper shoe modification.

The Syme's amputation involves disarticulation at the ankle. It has generally fallen into disfavor in that it is technically demanding and, more importantly, it is more difficult to create a well fitting prosthetic for a Syme's amputation than for a below-knee amputation.

The below-knee amputation is a commonly performed procedure indicated when gangrene, infection, or ischemic lesions are present that preclude a more distal amputation. If objective criteria are used, primary healing of below-knee amputations should approach 95%. Contraindications to below-knee amputation include situations wherein the gangrenous or infectious process extends to involve the anterior portion of the lower extremity within 4 or 5 cm of the tibial tuberosity or would involve the posterior skin flap, a flexion contracture greater than 20°, or neurological dysfunction creating muscle spasticity or rigidity on the affected side. The energy requirement for a unilateral below-knee amputee is increased approximately 40% to 60% compared to normal. Most patients who were ambulatory before hospitalization can expect to have a reasonable degree of function with a well-fitted below-knee prosthesis.

An above-knee amputation is indicated when a more distal amputation is contraindicated, or in an elderly or disabled patient who is not expected to be ambulatory or stand and pivot. Energy expenditure is increased 80% to 120%, and only 40% to 50% of patients can be expected to ambulate after above-knee amputation.

Acute Arterial Obstruction

The manifestations of acute arterial occlusion vary greatly, depending on the level and severity of the obstruction, timing from onset to presentation, and degree of chronic vascular disease and collateral circulation. The classic signs and symptoms of acute arterial occlusion include pain, pallor, pulselessness, paresthesias, and paralysis.

Cutaneous manifestations are among the earliest in an acute occlusion. Pallor is seen initially and occurs with the loss of pulses. If timely revascularization does not take place, blistering of the skin may develop, followed by frank gangrene.

Sensorimotor manifestations are among the most common symptoms in acute ischemia. Pain is noted early in the course of events; however, this may progress to numbness, which should not be mistaken as improvement. As ischemia progresses, nerve dysfunction may lead to sensory loss, followed by paralysis and muscle destruction resulting in paralysis; a late manifestation of ischemia in muscle is rigor, suggesting muscle death.

The quality of pulses in the contralateral extremity can be very informative. It is uncommon for a patient with chronic vascular disease in one extremity to have full, strong, distal pulses in the other. A normal pulse exam in the contralateral leg suggests that the patient has had an acute event in the absence of chronic disease. This patient is unlikely to have developed significant collaterals, and expediency in obtaining revascularization is vital.

The two major causes of acute arterial occlusion are emboli and thrombosis. An embolic source accounts for 80% of cases. The most common sites in the lower extremity for emboli to become lodged are, in descending order, the femoral, iliac, aorta, and popliteal arteries.

Acute thrombosis, usually of a previously stenotic area in the setting of atherosclerosis, is the second most common cause of acute arterial occlusion. Thrombosis may also occur in the setting of low flow states such as congestive heart failure or hypotension, in hypercoagulable states, and in vascular grafts.

The management of the patient with acute lower-extremity ischemia includes a thorough but expeditious history and physical, followed by optimization of hemodynamics and fluid balance. Unless a contraindication exists, most patients are heparinized. If the patient is thought to have potentially viable extremities, the lesion can be further delineated with arteriography.

At this point a decision is made whether to treat the patient operatively or with an attempt at thrombolysis. If open surgery is chosen, the most common procedure is a catheter embolectomy, usually via a cutdown at the femoral or below-knee popliteal location. Alternatively, particularly in the setting of a thrombosed bypass graft, bypass reconstruction may be necessary. In an analysis of multiple series, the mortality and limb salvage rates were 12.6% and 78%, respectively, for the use of heparin alone in the setting of acute ischemia, 17% and 84% for thromboembolectomy alone, and 10.2% and 92% when the combination of perioperative heparin and catheter embolectomy was used.[30] Postoperatively one should consider long-term anticoagulation as it may reduce the incidence of recurrent embolization from 21% to 7%.[30]

The comparison of lytic therapy and surgical therapy in the initial management of acute lower-extremity ischemia has been carefully studied in several multiinstitutional studies. In one study there was a significantly increased number of major adverse events in the thrombolysis group at 1 month as compared to the surgery-alone group. However, when patients were stratified to duration of ischemia, there were clear trends in favor of lysis in patients whose onset of ischemic symptoms was less than 14 days before presentation.[31] An optimal situation in the setting of acute ischemia would be that of a patient with evidence of an acute thrombotic event who undergoes thrombolysis that clears the thrombus and reestablishes flow nonoperatively and also uncovers a culpable lesion which would be angioplastied or surgically reconstructed electively.

Other principles of management of the patient with acute lower-extremity ischemia include careful monitoring postoperatively for metabolic derangements related to reperfusion such as acidosis and hyperkalemia, evaluation of the urine for myoglobin, and, if present, treatment with hydration, manitol, and bicarbonate to induce an alkaline diuresis. Additionally, if a limb has been ischemic for a significant time or develops elevated compartment pressures, one should have a low threshold for performing fasciotomy.

Embolic events can also take the form of atheroemboli as atherosclerotic debris in a proximal artery dislodges and occludes distal arteries. The most common manifestation of this event is the blue toe syndrome. Blue toe syndrome consists of the sudden appearance of a cool, painful, cyanotic toe or forefoot in the often perplexing presence of strong pedal pulses and a warm foot. By far the most common source is the distal aorta, but atheromatous debris can embolize from anywhere along the aorta as well as from peripheral arteries such as the femoral or popliteal. These episodes portend both similar and more severe episodes in the future. Therefore, location and eradication of the embolic source is usually indicated.[32]

Lower-Extremity Aneurysms

Aneurysms of the lower extremity are not uncommon, and share similar risk factors with their abdominal counterparts, as discussed elsewhere. It is clear that patients with aneurysmal disease have a propensity for aneurysmal degeneration in other locations. In a series of 100 patients with femoral artery aneurysms, 72% of patients had a contralateral femoral artery aneurysm, 85% had a concomitant aortoiliac aneurysm, and 44% had a concurrent popliteal aneurysm.[33] Conversely, a patient with an AAA (abdominal aortic aneurysm) has a 3% chance of a concomitant femoral artery aneurysm. There is a strong predilection of peripheral artery aneurysms in males as compared to females.

In recent times, the majority of femoral artery aneurysms present while asymptomatic. However, these lesions can present with a variety of symptoms. Acute thrombosis, which occurs approximately 8% of the time, is manifest as sudden onset of ischemic symptoms such as coolness, hypesthesia, and pain. Chronic thrombosis, which occurs about 8% of the time, is similar in presentation to the more common occlusion of the superficial femoral artery (SFA), causing calf claudication or ischemic rest pain. In both the acute and chronic situation, the presence of a mass at the level of the femoral artery should help distinguish the diagnoses.

Ultrasound is the modality of choice for diameter size assessment of peripheral arterial aneurysms. In general, it is recommended that asymptomatic femoral artery aneurysms greater than two times the diameter of the external iliac artery be repaired in good-risk patients. Additionally, all symptomatic femoral artery aneurysms should be considered for repair. If treatment is elective, most patients should undergo preoperative angiography, and all should have a search for other aneurysms, particularly in the aortic and popliteal locations. Repair can be accomplished by either aneurysm excision or interposition graft, depending on the size or location of the lesion. It is important to remember that all patients treated for femoral artery aneurysms need to be followed for life for aneurysms in other locations. Successful cases of management of femoral artery aneurysms with endoluminally placed covered stents have been reported.[34,35]

The popliteal artery is the most common site for peripheral aneurysmal disease. Similar to femoral artery aneurysms, the danger of popliteal artery aneurysms is their propensity to thrombose, embolize, or rupture. A patient with a unilateral popliteal artery aneurysm has an approximately 50% chance of a contralateral aneurysm, and a greater than 30% chance of having an AAA. As with most peripheral artery aneurysms, most popliteal artery aneurysms occur in men. The average age at time of diagnosis is between 50 and 70 years of age.

Approximately half of popliteal artery aneurysms are detected while asymptomatic. A popliteal artery is considered aneurysmal if its diameter exceeds 2 cm or is 1.5 times the diameter of the proximal nonaneurysmal arterial segment.[36] In general patients should undergo ultrasound examination for size assessment, and arteriography to evaluate the proximal and distal vasculature before reconstruction.

Based on the available data, it is recommended to repair all popliteal aneurysms electively in good-risk patients. Additionally, patients presenting with popliteal artery aneurysm and limb-threatening ischemia secondary to thrombosis or distal emboli should be treated with initial angiography and lytic therapy before surgical revascularization. Endoluminal repair of popliteal artery aneurysms with covered stents has been reported.[37]

Pseudoaneurysms

The majority of pseudoaneurysms encountered by the vascular surgeon are the result of percutaneous catheterization procedures. In a large series of cardiac catheterizations, the incidence of vascular injury requiring repair was approximately 1%.[38] Most complications of catheterization involve some degree of extravasation of blood, leading to ecchymosis and hematoma formation. The majority of these resolve without surgical intervention. However, if a large amount of blood accumulates to the point that the thigh becomes tense, painful, or blistered, operative intervention with evacuation of the hematoma and repair of the affected vessel should be considered. In some cases where the puncture site fails to heal, a cavity lined by thrombus and soft tissue may form. If blood flow persists within this cavity, it is considered a pseudoaneurysm. In general, small pseudoaneurysms less than 2 to 3 cm in diameter may resolve spontaneously. If a pseudoaneurysm persists, increases in size, or is more than 3 cm in diameter, some form of obliteration is indicated. The conventional approach is operative exploration of the site of injury with suture repair of the defect. More recently, reasonable success with ultrasound-guided compression therapy has been reported. Additionally, the injection of thrombin in the pseudoaneurysm sac under ultrasound guidance has produced impressive results.[39] Based on these experiences, it would seem appropriate to attempt thrombosis of pseudoaneurysms via ultrasound-guided techniques, reserving operative repair for pseudoaneurysms that are particularly large or have large necks.

Unfortunately, femoral artery pseudoaneurysms also occur as a result of drug abuse. The patient usually presents with a painful groin mass, which is pulsatile only half the time. A major error would be to treat this as merely an abscess and attempt blind incision and drainage. Angiography should be obtained in most patients with a history of self-injection and a groin mass and will distinguish pseudoaneurysm from simple abscess. The definitive treatment of an infected pseudoaneurysm relies on principles of debridement of all affected tissue including artery to healthy vessel, proximal ligation, and distal revascularization if needed. Revascularization should be attempted with autologous tissue if possible and should be tunneled in such a way to avoid contact with potentially infected sites.

Popliteal Entrapment Syndrome

Popliteal entrapment usually occurs because of an abnormal relationship between the popliteal artery and the medial head of the gastrocnemius muscle. The normal position of the popliteal artery is in the popliteal fossa, running between the medial and lateral heads of the gastrocnemius muscle. The most common anatomical abnormality is that of medial deviation of the popliteal artery around the medial head of the gastrocnemius, although other anatomical configurations can lead to potential popliteal entrapment.

Patients are most commonly male, presenting before the age of 40 years. In the absence of acute thrombosis or occlusion, the most common presentation is that of intermittent claudication, which often occurs with walking, more so than with running. The diagnosis of popliteal entrapment is suggested by disappearance or weakening of tibial pulses with forced plantar flexion and knee extension. If suspected on the basis of history and physical and initial noninvasive studies, the best study to evaluate for popliteal entrapment syndrome is an MRI. Additionally, duplex imaging may demonstrate popliteal artery impingement with plantar flexion.

Surgical treatment is almost always indicated for patients with intermittent claudication with evidence of popliteal entrapment. Surgical correction of asymptomatic functional entrapment is generally not warranted.

Adventitial Cystic Disease of the Popliteal Artery and Buerger's Disease

Adventitial cystic disease almost always affects the popliteal artery. This entity is relatively rare, but must be considered, particularly in cases of young males presenting with intermittent claudication. Additionally, patients with this disorder are generally nonsmokers and have no other evidence of atherosclerotic disease. Surgical correction generally involves evacuation of the cyst contents and excision of the wall.[40] In cases of complete occlusion, resection of the involved popliteal artery followed by vein interposition grafting is warranted.

A variety of hypercoagulable states and local and systemic vasculidities may cause lower extremity ischemia, the extent of which is beyond the scope of this chapter. Although uncommon, cases of Buerger's disease will be encountered by most surgeons, and is worthy of further discussion. Buerger's disease, or thromboangiitis obliterans, is an inflammatory, occlusive vascular disease that involves both small and medium-sized arteries and veins. This process usually affects both the upper and lower extremities. Buerger's disease most commonly affects male smokers under the age of 40.

Most often patients present with intermittent claudication, but 90% will eventually develop upper extremity manifestations as well. Progression to tissue loss and amputation is very common. Arteriographic findings of smooth tapered segmental narrowing of peripheral arteries without evidence of more proximal atherosclerotic disease may suggest the diagnosis.[41] Although bypass of larger vessels is possible, treatment depends almost completely on cessation of smoking, with potential for a remarkable recovery.

References

1. Fowkes FG, Housley E, Cawood EH, Macintyre CC, Ruckley CV, Prescott RJ. Edinburgh Artery Study: prevalence of asymptomatic and symptomatic peripheral arterial disease in the general population. Int J Epidemiol 1991;20:384–392.
2. Dormandy J, Mahir M, Ascady G, et al. Fate of the patient with chronic leg ischaemia. A review article. J Cardiovasc Surg 1989;30:50–57.
3. Vogt MT, Wolfson SK, Kuller LH. Lower extremity arterial disease and the aging process: a review. J Clin Epidemiol 1992;45:529–542.
4. Farkouh ME, Rihal CS, Gersh BJ, et al. Influence of coronary heart disease on morbidity and mortality after lower extremity revascularization surgery: a population-based study in Olmsted County, Minnesota (1970–1987). J Am Coll Cardiol 1994;24:1290–1296.
5. Jonason T, Ringqvist I. Factors of prognostic importance for subsequent rest pain in patients with intermittent claudication. Acta Med Scand 1985;218:27–33.
6. Gordon T, Kannel WB. Predisposition to atherosclerosis in the head, heart, and legs. The Framingham study. JAMA 1972;221:661–666.
7. Kannel WB, Shurtleff D. The Framingham Study. Cigarettes and the development of intermittent claudication. Geriatrics 1973;28:61–68.
8. Hughson WG, Mann JI, Garrod A. Intermittent claudication: prevalence and risk factors. Br Med J 1978;1:1379–1381.
9. Kannel WB, Skinner JJ Jr, Schwartz MJ, Shurtleff D. Intermittent claudication. Incidence in the Framingham Study. Circulation 1970;41:875–883.
10. Goodreau JJ, Creasy JK, Flanigan P, et al. Rational approach to the differentiation of vascular and neurogenic claudication. Surgery (St. Louis) 1978;84:749–757.
11. Barnes RW. Noninvasive diagnostic assessment of peripheral vascular disease. Circulation 1991;83(suppl):I20–I27.
12. Anonymous. Suggested standards for reports dealing with lower extremity ischemia. Prepared by the Ad Hoc Committee on Reporting Standards, Society for Vascular Surgery/North American Chapter, International Society for Cardiovascular Surgery [published erratum appears in J Vasc Surg 1986;4(4):350]. J Vasc Surg 1986;4:80–94.
13. Beach KW, Brunzell JD, Strandness DE Jr. Prevalence of severe arteriosclerosis obliterans in patients with diabetes mellitus. Relation to smoking and form of therapy. Arteriosclerosis 1982;2:275–280.
14. Orchard TJ, Strandness DE Jr. Assessment of peripheral vascular disease in diabetes. Report and recommendations of an international workshop sponsored by the American Diabetes Association and the American Heart Association September 18–20, 1992, New Orleans, Louisiana [see comments]. Circulation 1993;88:819–828.
15. Strandness DE Jr. Peripheral arterial system. In: Duplex Scanning in Vascular Disorders. New York: Raven Press, 1993:159–195.
16. Kohler TR, Nance DR, Cramer MM, Vandenburghe N, Strandness DE Jr. Duplex scanning for diagnosis of aortoiliac and femoropopliteal disease: a prospective study. Circulation 1987;76:1074–1080.
17. Dalman RL, Taylor LM Jr. Infrainguinal revascularization procedures. In: Porter JM, Taylor LM Jr, eds. Basic Data Underlying Clinical Decision Making in Vascular Surgery. St. Louis: Quality Medical, 1994:141–143.
18. Veith FJ, Gupta SK, Wengerter KR, Rivers SP. Femoral-popliteal-tibeal occlusive disease. In: Moore WS, ed. Vascular Surgery: A Comprehensive Review. Philadelphia: Saunders, 1991:364–389.
19. Veith FJ, Gupta SK, Ascer E, et al. Six-year prospective multicenter randomized comparison of autologous saphenous vein and expanded polytetrafluoroethylene grafts in infrainguinal arterial reconstructions. J Vasc Surg 1986;3:104–114.
20. Raftery KB, Belkin M, Mackey WC, O'Donnell TF. Are peroneal artery bypass grafts hemodynamically inferior to other tibial artery bypass grafts? J Vasc Surg 1994;19:964–968; discussion 968–969.
21. Harris PL, Veith FJ, Shanik GD, Nott D, Wengerter KR, Moore DJ. Prospective randomized comparison of in situ and reversed infrapopliteal vein grafts [see comments]. Br J Surg 1993;80:173–176.
22. Shah DM, Darling RC III, Chang BB, Kaufman JL, Fitzgerald

KM, Leather RP. Is long vein bypass from groin to ankle a durable procedure? An analysis of a ten-year experience. J Vasc Surg 1992;15:402–407; discussion 407–408.

23. Wengerter KR, Yang PM, Veith FJ, Gupta SK, Panetta TF. A twelve-year experience with the popliteal-to-distal artery bypass: the significance and management of proximal disease. J Vasc Surg 1992;15:143–149; discussion 150–151.

24. Bandyk DF. Surveillance of lower extremity bypass grafts. In: Ernst CB, Stanley JC, eds. Current Therapy in Vascular Surgery. St. Louis: Mosby-Year Book, 1995:492–499.

25. Dotter CT, Judkins MP. Transluminal treatment of arteriosclerotic obstruction. Description of a technique and a preliminary report of its application. Circulation 1964;30:654–670.

26. Bosch JL, Hunink MG. Meta-analysis of the results of percutaneous transluminal angioplasty and stent placement for aortoiliac occlusive disease [published erratum appears in Radiology 1997;205(2):584]. Radiology 1997;204:87–96.

27. Johnson WC, Watkins MT, Baldwin D, Hamilton J. Foot TcPO$_2$ response to lumbar sympathectomy in patients with focal ischemic necrosis. Ann Vasc Surg 1998;12:70–74.

28. Hourlay P, Vangertruyden G, Verduyckt F, Trimpeneers F, Hendrickx J. Endoscopic extraperitoneal lumbar sympathectomy. Surg Endosc 1995;9:530–533.

29. Dwars BJ, van den Broek TA, Rauwerda JA, Bakker FC. Criteria for reliable selection of the lowest level of amputation in peripheral vascular disease. J Vasc Surg 1992;15:536–542.

30. Mills JL, Porter JM. Acute limb ischemia. In: Porter JM, Taylor LM Jr, eds. Basic Data Underlying Clinical Decision Making in Vascular Surgery. St. Louis: Quality Medical, 1994:134–136.

31. Anonymous. Results of a prospective randomized trial evaluating surgery versus thrombolysis for ischemia of the lower extremity. The STILE trial. Ann Surg 1994;220:251–266; discussion 266–268.

32. Karmody AM, Powers SR, Monaco VJ, Leather RP. "Blue toe" syndrome. An indication for limb salvage surgery. Arch Surg 1976;111:1263–1268.

33. Graham LM, Zelenock GB, Whitehouse WM Jr, et al. Clinical significance of arteriosclerotic femoral artery aneurysms. Arch Surg 1980;115:502–507.

34. Michel C, Laffy PY, Leblanc G, et al. [Percutaneous treatment of a superficial femoral artery aneurysm using an intravascular stent-prosthesis]. [in French.] J Radiol 1999;80:473–476.

35. Schneider PA. Abcarian PW, Leduc JR, Ogawa DY. Stent-graft repair of mycotic superficial femoral artery aneurysm using a Palmaz stent and autologous saphenous vein. Ann Vasc Surg 1998;12:282–285.

36. Szilagyi DE, Schwartz RL, Reddy DJ. Popliteal arterial aneurysms. Their natural history and management. Arch Surg 1981;116:724–728.

37. Kudelko PE Jr, Alfaro-Franco C, Diethrich EB, Krajcer Z. Successful endoluminal repair of a popliteal artery aneurysm using the Wallgraft endoprosthesis. J Endovasc Surg 1998;5:373–377.

38. McCann RL, Schwartz LB, Pieper KS. Vascular complications of cardiac catheterization. J Vasc Surg 1991;14:375–381.

39. Liau CS, Ho FM, Chen MF, Lee YT. Treatment of iatrogenic femoral artery pseudoaneurysm with percutaneous thrombin injection. J Vasc Surg 1997;26:18–23.

40. Melliere D, Ecollan P, Kassab M, Becqemin JP. Adventitial cystic disease of the popliteal artery: treatment by cyst removal. J Vasc Surg 1988;8:638–642.

41. Rivera R. Roentgenographic diagnosis of Buerger's disease. J Cardiovasc Surg 1973;14:40–46.

42. McCann RL. Peripheral artery aneurysms. In: Porter JM, Taylor LM Jr, eds. Basic Data Underlying Clinical Decision Making in Vascular Surgery. St. Louis: Quality Medical, 1994:137–140.

43. Taylor LM Jr, Edwards JM, Porter JM. Present status of reversed vein bypass grafting: five-year results of a modern series. J Vasc Surg 1990;11:193–205.

44. Bergan JJ, Veith FJ, Bernhard VM, et al. Randomization of autogenous vein and polytetrafluoroethylene grafts in femoral-distal reconstruction. Surgery (St. Louis) 1982;92:921–930.

45. Rutherford RB, Jones DN, Bergentz SE, et al. Factors affecting the patency of infrainguinal bypass. J Vasc Surg 1988;8:236–246.

46. Kent KC, Whittemore AD, Mannick JA. Short-term and midterm results of an all-autogenous tissue policy for infrainguinal reconstruction. J Vasc Surg 1989;9:107–114.

47. Brewster DC, LaSalle AJ, Darling RC. Comparison of above-knee and below-knee anastomosis in femoropopliteal bypass grafts. Arch Surg 1981;116:1013–1018.

48. Hall RG, Coupland GA, Lane R, Delbridge L, Appleberg M. Vein, Gore-Tex or a composite graft for femoropopliteal bypass. Surg Gynecol Obstet 1985;161.308–312.

49. Davies MG, Dalen H, Svendsen E, Hagen PO. The functional and morphological consequences of balloon catheter injury in veins. J Surg Res 1994;57:122–132.

50. Quinones-Baldrich WJ, Busuttil RW, Baker JD, et al. Is the preferential use of polytetrafluoroethylene grafts for femoropopliteal bypass justified? [see comments]. J Vasc Surg 1988;8:219–228.

51. Anonymous. Comparative evaluation of prosthetic, reversed, and in situ vein bypass grafts in distal popliteal and tibial-peroneal revascularization. Veterans Administration Cooperative Study Group 141. Arch Surg 1988;123:434–438.

52. Hobson RW Jr, Lynch TG, Jamil Z, et al. Results of revascularization and amputation in severe lower extremity ischemia: a five-year clinical experience. J Vasc Surg 1985;2:174–185.

53. Harris RW, Andros G, Dulawa LB, Oblath RW, Apyan R, Salles-Cunha S. The transition to "in situ" vein bypass grafts. Surg Gynecol Obstet 1986;163:21–28.

54. Leather RP, Shah DM, Chang BB, Kaufman JL. Resurrection of the in situ saphenous vein bypass. 1000 cases later [see comments]. Ann Surg 1988;208:435–442.

55. Bandyk DF, Kaebnick HW, Stewart GW, Towne JB. Durability of the in situ saphenous vein arterial bypass: a comparison of primary and secondary patency. J Vasc Surg 1987;5:256–268.

56. Varty K, Allen KE, Jones L, Sayers RD, Bell PR, London NJ. Influence of Losartan, an angiotensin receptor antagonist, on neointimal proliferation in cultured human saphenous vein. Br J Surg 1994;81:819–822.

57. Barry R, Satiani B, Mohan B, Smead WL, Vaccaro PS. Prognostic indicators in femoropopliteal and distal bypass grafts. Surg Gynecol Obstet 1985;161:129–132.

58. Cantelmo NL, Snow JR, Menzoian JO, LoGerfo FW. Successful vein bypass in patients with an ischemic limb and a palpable popliteal pulse. Arch Surg 1986;121:217–220.

59. Schuler JJ, Flanigan DP, Williams LR, Ryan TJ, Castronuovo JJ. Early experience with popliteal to infrapopliteal bypass for limb salvage. Arch Surg 1983;118:472–476.

60. Berkowitz HD, Greenstein SM. Improved patency in reversed femoral-infrapopliteal autogenous vein grafts by early detection and treatment of the failing graft. J Vasc Surg 1987;5:755–761.

61. Dalsing MC, White JV, Yao JS, Podrazik R, Flinn WR, Bergan JJ. Infrapopliteal bypass for established gangrene of the forefoot or toes. J Vasc Surg 1985;2:669–677.

62. Rosenbloom MS, Walsh JJ, Schuler JJ, et al. Long-term results of infragenicular bypasses with autogenous vein originating from the distal superficial femoral and popliteal arteries. J Vasc Surg 1988;7:691–696.

63. Flinn WR, Rohrer MJ, Yao JS, McCarthy WJ III, Fahey VA, Bergan JJ. Improved long-term patency of infragenicular polytetrafluoroethylene grafts. J Vasc Surg 1988;7:685–690.

64. Taylor LM Jr, Edwards JM, Brant B, Phinney ES, Porter JM. Autogenous reversed vein bypass for lower extremity ischemia in patients with absent or inadequate greater saphenous vein. Am J Surg 1987;153:505–510.

65. Leather RP, Shan DM, Karmody AM. Infrapopliteal arterial by-

pass for limb salvage: increased patency and utilization of the saphenous vein used "in situ." Surgery 1981;90:1000–1008.

66. Wilson SE, Sheppard B. Results of percutaneous transluminal angioplasty for peripheral vascular occlusive disease. In: Porter JM, Taylor LM Jr, eds. Basic Data Underlying Clinical Decision Making in Vascular Surgery. St. Louis: Quality Medical, 1994: 144–148.

67. Johnston KW, Rae M, Hogg-Johnston SA, et al. 5-year results of a prospective study of percutaneous transluminal angioplasty. Ann Surg 1987;206:403–413.

68. Gallino A, Mahler F, Probst P, Nachbur B. Percutaneous trans-

luminal angioplasty of the arteries of the lower limbs: a 5 year follow-up. Circulation 1984;70:619–623.

69. Hewes RC, White RI, Jr., Murray RR, et al. Long-term results of superficial femoral artery angioplasty. AJR Am Roentgenol 1986; 146:1025–1029.

70. Spence RK, Freiman DB, Gatenby R, et al. Long-term results of transluminal angioplasty of the iliac and femoral arteries. Arch Surg 1981;116:1377–1386.

71. Krepel VM, van Andel GJ, van Erp WF, Breslau PJ. Percutaneous transluminal angioplasty of the femoropopliteal artery: initial and long-term results. Radiology 1985;156:325–328.

Venous Disease and Pulmonary Embolism

Matthew I. Foley and Gregory L. Moneta

Venous Thromboembolism

Epidemiology

Venous thromboembolism (VTE) is an important cause of preventable morbidity and mortality in the United States. Although precise figures are difficult to obtain as a result of undiagnosed cases, the annual incidence of VTE has been estimated at 71 and 117 per 100,000. Deep venous thrombosis (DVT) poses not only the immediate threat of pulmonary embolus (PE) but chronic disability secondary to venous insufficiency as well. PE is estimated to be responsible for the deaths of 50,000 to 100,000 persons per year in U.S. hospitals who would not otherwise be expected to die of their underlying disease process.[1–3] Despite this awareness and evidence for the efficacy of various forms of prophylaxis, attention toward prevention remains inadequate.[4]

Pathophysiology

The complexities of the coagulation system are beyond the scope of this chapter and are detailed elsewhere. Suffice it to say the coagulation system exists in a state of homeostasis. Unbalance in this system may result in thrombus formation. Rudolf Virchow, a pathologist, identified three conditions that tended toward thrombosis. His well-known triad consists of intimal injury, stasis of blood flow, and a hypercoaguable state. All risk factors relate back to one of the conditions described by Virchow.

Risk Factors

HISTORY OF VTE

A previous history of VTE was found to be the strongest "intrinsic factor" contributing to a new objectively determined DVT with an odds ratio of 7.9 (95% CI, 4.4–14.19).[5]

AGE

Increased age is consistently associated with increased incidence of VTE. U.S. population-based studies demonstrate dramatic increases after age 40 that continue exponentially until death.[6,7] However, the number of risk factors does also increase with age.

MAJOR SURGERY

Depending on the procedure, VTE incidence ranges from 18%–57% in patients undergoing major surgery.

MALIGNANCY

Meta-analysis of general surgery patients distinguished patients with malignancy in 16 studies and found a 4% higher incidence of VTE. At least two prospective studies have shown an increased incidence of occult malignant neoplasm in patients with DVT.[8,9]

OBESITY

When specifically assessing obesity as a risk factor for VTE, it seems at worst to provide only a small incremental risk of VTE.[10]

TRAUMA

The risk factors for VTE in trauma patients have been difficult to discern secondary to the variety of injury patterns. In a prospective study of 716 consecutive trauma patients admitted to a regional trauma unit with an Injury Severity Score (ISS) of at least 9, 58 percent had DVT, of which 18% were in a proximal location. These authors identified five independent risk factors by multivariate analysis (Table 36.1). Surprisingly, less than 2% of patients with DVT confirmed by venography had clinical symptoms. Another study identified four patterns of injury that were independent predictors of PE (Table 36.2)

TABLE 36.1. Risk Factors for Venous Thromboembolism in 349 Trauma Patients.

Risk factor	Odds ratio (95% confidence interval)
Age (each 1-year increment)	1.05 (1.03–1.06)
Blood transfusion	1.74 (1.03–2.93)
Surgery	2.30 (1.08–4.89)
Fracture of femur or tibia	4.82 (2.79–8.33)
Spinal cord injury	8.59 (2.92–25.28)

[a]Determined by multivariate logistic regression.

Source: From Geerts WH, Code KI, Jay RM, et al.,[107] with permission. Copyright ©1994 Massachusetts Medical Society. All rights reserved.

compared to a control group who had neither PE nor inferior vena cava (IVC) filters placed.

Varicose Veins/Superficial Thrombophlebitis

Varicose veins (VVs) appear to be an associated but not an independent risk factor for VTE.

Cardiac Disease

Patients with cardiac disease are likely to have associated risk factors for DVT (i.e., age, immobilization). Older studies looking for DVT in patients with acute myocardial infarction using radiofibrinogen leg scanning showed an incidence as high as 40%.[11,12] It has been shown that this rate can be reduced using low-dose heparin as prophylaxis.[13,14]

Hormones

There has been controversy regarding the risks of VTE with oral contraceptive (OC) use. There does seem to be some increased risk that must be weighed against the benefits of OC use. However, estrogen replacement therapy has not been shown to carry an increased risk of VTE.[15,16]

Prolonged Immobilization/Paralysis

A study using data from the National Spinal Cord Injury Statistical Center discovered an incidence of 14.5% for DVT and 4.6% for PE in patients with acute spinal cord injury.[17] These risks seem to diminish with time.[18,19]

Pregnancy

Two recent cohort studies examining venous thrombosis during pregnancy emphasize that DVT can occur during any trimester, that symptoms in the first semester are more likely to be confirmed as DVT, and that the left leg is by far most often involved.

Central Venous Catheterization

The incidence of central venous catheter (CVC)-associated DVT and its sequelae are probably underappreciated. The incidence has been demonstrated in children requiring long-term access for parenteral nutrition.[20] CVC-associated DVT is more common at the femoral site.

Hypercoaguable States

Numerous blood protein and platelet defects have been implicated in venous thrombosis (Table 36.3).[21] The most prevalent appears to be resistance to activated protein C.[22]

Natural History

DVT and PE are not pathologically distinct entities; they lie along the continuum of VTE. Since it was shown that there is improved survival in patients diagnosed with PE treated with anticoagulation compared to no treatment,[23] the natural history of VTE has been obscured by intervention. What information exists is largely based on trials in which patients were undertreated.

It has been shown in a recent large study using duplex ultrasound that patients who present with symptomatic DVT may have thrombus located anywhere within the deep system (even within the contralateral leg).[24] The majority of DVT originate in the infrapopliteal veins or muscular sinuses of the calf.[25,26] Studies suggest that between 10 and 25% propagate proximally. Because they are virtually always treated, little is really known about the natural history of proximal vein DVT (PDVT).

Two recent studies found that between 40% and 50% of patients with venographically proven DVT and no respiratory symptoms had high-probability V/Q scans for PE at presentation.[27,28] In an ambulatory population randomized to receive or not to receive anticoagulant therapy, there was no difference in progression of PE or development of PE symptoms at 2 months.

Resolution of DVT by DUS 6 months after diagnosis occurs in 70% for all lower-extremity veins affected by DVT, with damage to the vessel wall or valves occurring in 44% of patients by this time.[29] Chronic venous insufficiency can eventually be demonstrated in a large percentage of persons with a history of DVT.

The greatest risk of death from PE and incidence of recurrent PE appears to be within the first few hours[30] to weeks of the initial event. Beyond this period, most patients who die do so of their underlying illnesses. Like DVT, PE has been objectively shown to resolve.

TABLE 36.2. Pattern of Injury Analysis: Pulmonary Embolus (PE) vs. Control.

Injury pattern	Number	Number (%) of pulmonary emboli	Odds ratio
Head + spinal cord injury	195	3 (1.5)	4.5*
Head + long bone fracture	471	11 (2.3)	8.8%
Severe pelvis + long bone fracture	106	4 (3.8)	12*
Multiple long bone fracture	275	8 (2.9)	10*

*p < 0.05 compared with control group.

Source: From Winchell RJ, Hoyt DB, Walsh JC, et al.,[108] with permission.

TABLE 36.3. Hypercoaguable States.

Antiphospholipid syndrome
Activated protein C resistance (factor V Leiden)
Sticky platelet syndrome
Protein S defects
Protein C defects
Antithrombin defects
Heparin cofactor II defects
Plasminogen defects
Tissue plasminogen activator defects
Plasminogen activator inhibitor defects
Factor XII defects
Dysfibrinogenemia
Homocystinemia

Source: From Bick RL, Kaplan H,[21] with permission.

Prophylaxis

The primary goal of prophylaxis is to prevent the morbidity and mortality of VTE. DVT is frequently asymptomatic, so the first evidence of VTE may be a life-threatening PE. The high incidence of VTE without prophylaxis and the ability to significantly reduce this incidence with treatment speaks strongly in favor of prophylaxis.

The general surgery population has been the most extensively studied. Low-dose heparin (LDH) with or without dihydroergotamine (DHE), low molecular weight heparin (LMWH), warfarin, intermittent pneumatic compression (IPC), and elastic stockings (ES) all reduce the incidence of DVT from 25% to 10% or less. In recent, randomized, prospective studies LMWH is shown to be at least as efficacious as LDH with perhaps a lower incidence of major bleeding complications, although this finding is not consistent.[31–33]

It should be noted that the risk of VTE does not disappear at the time of hospital discharge and that perhaps some patients should continue to receive prophylaxis at home. In a retrospective study, the rate of postoperative PE increased by 30% when including PEs that occurred within 30 days of discharge from a digestive surgery hospital. Specific risk factors for postdischarge DVT were not identified. Further trials are necessary before definite conclusions can be drawn.

Finally, cost-effectiveness must be a concern. It has been estimated that $59 to $118 million spent on VTE prophylaxis in 1.18 million major abdominal surgery patients over age 40 would save $59.3 to $118.5 million in DVT diagnosis and treatment and $60 to $120 million on fatal PE each year. See Table 19.5 for usage guidelines.

Diagnosis of Deep Venous Thrombosis

Signs and symptoms of DVT include swelling, pain, tenderness, warmth, discoloration, and a palpable cord. In extreme cases, phlegmasia alba dolens (pain, pitting edema, and blanching) or phlegmasia cerulea dolens (loss of sensory and motor function) may occur. Unfortunately, signs and symptoms of DVT are not reliable for diagnosis. In large studies using either DUS or venography, DVT was found in 50% or less of patients in whom it was clinically suspected.[24,26] However, these signs and symptoms cannot be ignored and generally merit consideration for the presence of DVT.

Contrast Venography

Contrast venography is considered the "gold standard" for the diagnosis of DVT. The procedure involves placement of a needle in the dorsum of the foot and injection of a radioopaque contrast medium. X-Rays are then obtained in at least two projections. Studies are determined to be positive when a persistent filling defect is present. However, not all patients are candidates for venography based on previous history of contrast reactions or renal insufficiency, and contrast venography has largely been replaced by noninvasive techniques.

Iodine-125 Fibrinogen Uptake (FUT)

FUT is based on the idea that by radiolabeling fibrinogen and injecting it into a peripheral vein, DVT can be identified by scanning the legs for "hot spots." Hot spots represent fibrinogen being incorporated into fibrin clots. At this time, FUT has, however, been replaced by other diagnostic tests.

Impedance Plethysmography (IPG)

IPG involves obstructing the venous outflow of the leg with some external device, removing the device, and then quantifying changes in electrical resistance resulting from changes in calf blood volume. Serial IPG has been shown as safe when applied to an outpatient or inpatient population suspected of having DVT with a venogram-documented positive predictive value of approximately 90% and a low incidence of subsequent clinical DVT or PE in patients with serially negative IPG exams.[34–36] More recent evidence, however, has shown that IPG with or without FUT is not acceptable for the purpose of surveillance of high-risk asymptomatic patients.

Duplex Ultrasound (DUS)

DUS is now considered by many to be the new "gold standard" for diagnosing PDVT. DUS combines real-time B-mode ultrasound (US) with pulsed Doppler capability. This combination allows determination of vein compressibility as well as flow characteristics. Veins that are incompressible with firm pressure applied by the ultrasound scanhead are considered to be thrombosed. Prospective studies comparing B-mode US to venography using lack of vein compression as the sole determinant of a positive ultrasound study show sensitivities of at least 91% and specificities of 97% or better.[37–41] Detection of calf vein DVT (CDVT) is generally regarded as poor but may be improved with the addition of duplex scanning in which flowing blood is color coded on the gray-scale B-mode image (color flow). DUS is reliable, noninvasive, and portable but does require experienced personnel to obtain results similar to those reported.

D-Dimers

The most studied serological marker for VTE is the D-dimer (DD). DD is a specific derivative of cross-linked fibrin that is released when fibrin is lysed by plasmin. It is indicative of thrombosis but can be falsely elevated postoperatively and in the setting of sepsis, ARDS, and myocardial infarction. It may be helpful as a screening exam in outpatients suspected of having DVT as the sensitivity of a positive DD assay was found to be 93% for PDVT and 70% for CDVT.

Diagnosis of Pulmonary Embolism (PE)

Signs and symptoms of PE include dyspnea, tachypnea, chest pain, tachycardia, cyanosis, hemoptysis, hypotension, syncope, evidence of right-sided heart failure, and a pleural rub or rales. Investigators involved in the Prospective Investigation of Pulmonary Embolism Diagnosis (PIOPED) trial found that 90% of patients without a history of cardiac or pulmonary disease and who had a PE confirmed by pulmonary angiography (PA) had either dyspnea or tachycardia.[42] However, there were no statistically significant differences in signs and symptoms between patients who did or did not subsequently have PE diagnosed by PA.[42] Patients with PE may also present with coexisting signs and symptoms of DVT.

NONSPECIFIC TESTS

An arterial blood gas (ABG), chest X-ray (CXR), and electrocardiogram (EKG) are usually obtained in cases in which the diagnosis of PE is considered. Characteristic early ABG findings include respiratory alkalosis, decreased CO_2, and decreased O_2, which results in an increased alveolar–arterial gradient (A-a). In more severe cases, or during progression of PE, acidosis and worsening hypoxia may develop.

Suggestive CXR findings of PE include Westermark's sign (prominent central pulmonary artery and decreased pulmonary vascularity) and a pleural-based, wedge-shaped pulmonary density. These findings are, however, infrequent and present in both patients with and without PE. The most common EKG findings in the PIOPED trial in patients with PE

were nonspecific ST segment or T-wave changes.[42] The importance of these nonspecific tests is to rule out other pathological processes with similar signs and symptoms as PE.

PULMONARY ANGIOGRAPHY (PA)

Pulmonary angiography is the "gold standard" for diagnosing PE.[43] A catheter is placed into the pulmonary artery, usually via a femoral vein puncture, and a contrast agent is injected into both lungs. Either complete obstruction of, or filling defects within, the vessels are the basis for diagnosis. Nondiagnostic angiograms are uncommon (5% or less),[44,45] and a negative PA effectively rules out a PE.

VENTILATION/PERFUSION (V/Q) SCANNING

Perfusion scans involve injection of radiolabeled colloid through a peripheral vein followed by lung scanning in several views. Although perfusion scans alone are sensitive for PE, they lack specificity because many conditions other than PE cause perfusion defects (pneumonia, bronchospasm, COPD, cancer). In an attempt to improve specificity, ventilation studies (using radiolabeled aerosol) have been added, producing the V/Q scan. In the presence of PE, a perfusion defect should be present without a corresponding ventilation defect (V/Q mismatch). The PIOPED trial developed well-defined V/Q scan interpretation criteria defining five categories (Table 36.4). Combining scans of high, intermediate, and low probability, the V/Q scan had a sensitivity of 98%, but specificity was only 10% for diagnosis of PE. A high-

TABLE 36.4.
PIOPED[a] Central Scan Interpretation Categories and Criteria.

High probability

≥2 Large (>75% of a segment) segmental perfusion defects without corresponding ventilation or roentgenographic abnormalities or substantially larger than either matching ventilation or chest roentgenogram abnormalities
≥2 Moderate segmental (≥25% and ≤75% of a segment) perfusion defects without matching ventilation or chest roentgenogram abnormalities and 1 large mismatched segmental defect
≥4 Moderate segmental perfusion defects without ventilation or chest roentgenogram abnormalities

Intermediate probability (indeterminate)

Not falling into normal, very low, low-, or high-probability categories
Borderline high or borderline low
Difficult to categorize as high or low

Low probability

Nonsegmental perfusion defects (e.g., very small effusion causing blunting of the costophrenic angle, cardiomegaly, enlarged aorta, hila and mediastinum, and elevated diaphragm)
Single moderate mismatched segmental perfusion defect with normal chest roentgenogram
Any perfusion defect with a substantially larger chest roentgenogram abnormality
Large or moderated segmental perfusion defects involving no more than 4 segments in 1 lung and no more than 3 segments in 1 lung region with matching ventilation defects either equal to or larger in size and chest roentgenogram either normal or with abnormalities substantially smaller than perfusion defects
>3 Small segmental perfusion defects (<25% of a segment) with a normal chest roentgenogram

Very low probability

≤3 Small segmental perfusion defects with a normal chest roentgenogram

Normal

No perfusion defects seen
Perfusion outlines exactly the shape of the lungs as seen on the chest roentgenogram (hilar and aortic impressions may be seen, chest roentgenogram and/or ventilation study may be abnormal)

[a]Prospective Investigation of Pulmonary Embolism Diagnosis.
Source: The PIOPED Investigators,[109] with permission.

probability scan was quite specific (97%) but missed more than half of PA-determined PE (sensitivity, 41%). V/Q scans were diagnostic in only 27% of patients (either high probability or normal/near normal), but improved with the support of clinical judgement. Overall, a high-probability scan in a suspicious clinical setting is highly suggestive of PE. Low-probability V/Q scans combined with low clinical suspicion or normal/near-normal scans effectively ruled out PE.

D-DIMERS

D-Dimers (DD) can be used for the detection of PE as well as DVT. They are most useful as a screening test in the outpatient setting.

ADDITIONAL NONINVASIVE TESTING

When V/Q scanning is nondiagnostic, some investigators have evaluated the lower-extremity veins where the majority of PE are believed to originate. In a small study, the combination of V/Q scanning and DUS yielded only a sensitivity of 62% and a specificity of 78% for diagnosing PE using PIOPED criteria.[46]

ON THE HORIZON

Helical CT and MR angiography are being studied in some centers, but they may prove to be inadequate for small periphera subsegmental PE.

Treatment

THROMBOLYSIS

Ideally, treatment of DVT would result in early dissolution of thrombus, thereby eliminating the risk of PE and theoretically reducing the incidence of the postphlebitic syndrome. Unfortunately, only a minority (<10%) of patients with VTE are candidates for thrombolytic therapy. Contraindications to lytic therapy are listed in Table 36.5.

Three potential thrombolytic agents are available: strep-

TABLE 36.5. Contraindications to Systemic Lytic Therapy.

Absolute
  Active internal bleeding
  Recent (<2 months) cerebrovascular accident
  Intracranial pathology
Relatively major
  Recent (<10 days) major surgery, obstetrical delivery, or organ biopsy
  Active peptic ulcer or gastrointestinal pathology
  Recent major trauma
  Uncontrolled hypertension
Relatively minor
  Minor surgery or trauma
  Recent cardiopulmonary resuscitation
  High likelihood of left heart thrombus (i.e., atrial fibrillation with mitral valve disease)
  Bacterial endocarditis
  Hemostatic defects (i.e., renal or liver disease)
  Pregnancy
  Diabetic hemorrhagic retinopathy

Source: From Quinones-Baldrich,[110] with permission.

tokinase, urokinase, and recombinant tissue plasminogen activator (rtPA). All convert plasminogen to plasmin. Streptokinase is antigenic, can induce allergic reactions, is not specific for fibrin-bound plasminogen, and requires plasminogen as a cofactor. Urokinase is not antigenic but is still nonspecific and can produce febrile reactions. rtPA is found in all human tissues and it has the advantage of being more specific for fibrin-bound plasminogen compared to the other agents but has not been shown to be superior in terms of ultimate thrombolysis of documented thrombi or reducing bleeding complications of thrombolytic therapy.

Currently, there is no clear benefit for thrombolytic therapy in the large majority of patients with DVT. Nevertheless, thrombolytic therapy for DVT may be appropriate in highly selected cases of massive iliofemoral DVT. A large prospective randomized trial to determine PE recurrence, death, and chronic pulmonary hypertension is necessary before definite recommendations are possible.

HEPARIN

Unfractionated heparin (UFH) has been the initial pharmacological treatment of choice for VTE. UFH functions by two mechanisms; (1) it binds to antithrombin III (ATIII) and amplifies the inhibition of thrombin and activated factor X by ATIII, and (2) it catalyzes the inhibition of thrombin by heparin cofactor II. The half-life of UFH is approximately 90 min. The level of anticoagulation produced by the administration of UFH can be monitored by the activated prothrombin time (aPTT), which is usually evaluated at 6-h intervals until a steady state has been reached. The lower limit for the aPTT when treating VTE is 1.5 times control. The incidence of both recurrence and extension have been shown to be unacceptably high when either levels are subtherapeutic (as with subcutaneous heparin)[47] or when oral anticoagulation is initiated alone.[48] In contrast, there does not appear to be an increased risk of hemorrhagic complications in patients with supratherapeutic levels (aPTT > 2.5).[49] Treatment typically is continued until the patient has become therapeutic on oral anticoagulation.

WARFARIN

Warfarin acts by interfering with the production of both the procoagulant (II, VII, IX, X) and anticoagulant (proteins C and S) vitamin K-dependent cofactors. Patient response to warfarin is variable depending on liver function, diet, age, and concomitant medications. The level of anticoagulation produced by warfarin can be monitored with prothrombin time (PT). The PT is determined using commercially available thromboplastin reagents. Secondary to a wide variability of thromboplastin reagents used, the International Normalized Ratio was created (INR). An INR of 2.0 to 3.0 is generally accepted to be therapeutic in most patients with VTE.[50]

It was initially thought that several days of heparin were necessary before initiating warfarin therapy. However, several prospective randomized trials have shown that starting warfarin therapy in addition to heparin within the first few days of VTE diagnosis is safe, effective, and permits earlier discharge from the hospital.[51–53] Patients should not be started on warfarin if any invasive procedures are planned. Warfarin has a long half-life and must be withheld for several days for the INR to normalize. Fresh frozen plasma may be administered to provide vitamin K–dependent cofactors when rapid reversal is necessary.

Warfarin has been shown to reduce the recurrence of VTE after an initial event.[54,55] What has been less clear is how long to treat a patient with warfarin after an initial event or recurrence. Based on available data, patients with an initial episode of VTE should receive 3 to 6 months of warfarin therapy depending upon their risk factors, and patients with a recurrence should be treated indefinitely.

LOW MOLECULAR WEIGHT HEPARINS (LMWHs)

Perhaps the most notable advance in the treatment of DVT in the past several decades has been the use of LMWHs. LMWHs have been shown to differ from UFH in significant ways. LMWHs have increased bioavailability, greater than 90% after a subcutaneous injection.[56,57] They have a much longer half-life than UFH[56,58] and predictable elimination rates,[59] allowing once or twice daily dosing. LMWHs also have a predictable anticoagulant effect based upon body weight, so that laboratory monitoring is unnecessary.[60] It has also been hoped that LMWHs would lack some of the complications seen with UFH such as hemorrhage, heparin-induced thrombocytopenia, and osteoporosis. It is important to note that the different LMWHs differ in their anti-X_a and anti-II_a activities. For this reason data from one LMWH may not be extrapolated to another. Early trials using LMWHs suggested that LMWHs may be as effective as UFH (Table 36.6).

INFERIOR VENA CAVA (IVC) FILTERS

Numerous different IVC filters are available today. A contraindication to, or a failure of anticoagulation, are the main indications for IVC filter placement in the treatment of lower-extremity DVT. Percutaneous techniques allow placement via percutaneous venotomy, usually through the right femoral vein.

Evidence for the efficacy of IVC filters is scarce; there are no randomized, prospective trials. Because the data on IVC filter efficacy are poor and the data on medical treatment are well established, the role of the IVC filter in the treatment of DVT should be limited to cases in which anticoagulation is contraindicated or has failed.

SURGICAL TREATMENT

There is little role for surgical management of DVT, although greater saphenous vein ligation, venous thrombectomy, creation of a temporary AV fistula, and pulmonary embolectomy have been used with varying degrees of success. Randomized data are lacking.

Chronic Venous Insufficiency/Venous Ulceration

Twenty-seven percent of the adult U.S. population has some form of detectable lower-extremity venous abnormality,[61] usually superficial varicosities and/or telangiectasis. Up to 1.5% of European adults develop venous stasis ulceration at some point.[62]

Symptoms of chronic venous insufficiency (CVI) include leg fatigue, discomfort, and heaviness. Signs include venous telangiectasias and varicose veins as well as lipodermatosclerosis and venous ulceration. Risk factors associated with varicose veins may include prolonged standing,[61] heredity,[63] female sex,[63,64] parity,[65] and history of phlebitis.[64]

Risk factors for venous ulceration are different. The prevalence of venous disease increases with age and many risk factors for venous ulceration are associated with older age. The median age for patients with venous ulcers may be as high as 70 to 77 years.[66,67] Estimated incidence of venous ulcer in patients over 45 years is 3.5 per thousand per year.[68] Multivariant analysis suggests, in addition to age, the primary risk factors for venous ulceration are a history of deep venous thrombosis, a history of severe lower-extremity trauma, male sex, and obesity.[64]

Patients with venous ulceration have a severely impaired quality of life. Feelings of anger, depression, isolation, and/or diminished self-image are present in nearly 70%, and 80% have decreased mobility.[69] As many as 2 million workdays are lost per year in the United States secondary to venous ulceration,[70] and 5% of patients with venous ulcers lose jobs as a result of their venous ulcer.[71] The cost of treatment for venous ulceration alone is staggering, with annual health care costs estimated at $1 billion in the United States.[72]

TABLE 36.6.

Randomized Trials of LMWH[a] versus UFH[b] for Treatment of Deep Venous Thrombosis (DVT) (Level I Evidence).

Agent	Dose	Recurrent DVT (%); LMWH vs. UFH	Major bleeding (%); LMWH vs. UFH
Fraxiparine[111]	<55 kg 12,500 XaIU[c] >55 kg <80 kg 15,000 XaIU >80 kg 17,500 XaIU (Q 12 h)	7 vs. 14 (p = ns)	1 vs. 4 (p = ns)
Dalteparin[112]	200 XaIU/kg (Q 24 h)	5 vs. 3 (p = ns)	None, either group
Enoxaparin[113]	100 XaIU/kg (Q 12 h)	1 vs. 10 (p < 0.02)	None, either group
Logiparin[114]	175 XaIU/kg (Q 24 h)	3 vs. 7 (p = 0.07)	0.5 vs. 5 (p = 0.06)

[a]Low molecular weight heparin.
[b]Adjusted dose unfractionated heparin.
[c]Factor Xa inhibitory units.

Pathophysiology

MACROCIRCULATION

Venous reflux, venous obstruction, and calf muscle pump dysfunction contribute singularly or in combination to the signs and symptoms of chronic venous insufficiency. Of these, reflux is probably the most important. Venous reflux can be described as primary or secondary and results from abnormalities of the venous valve. Primary valvular reflux (incompetence) is diagnosed when there is no known underlying etiology of valvular dysfunction. Most cases of what clinically appears to be isolated superficial venous insufficiency are secondary to primary venous incompetence.[73]

An obvious identifiable antecedent condition is required for valvular incompetence to be described as secondary. Most frequently this is a deep venous thrombosis (DVT). The presence of thrombus within the vein is thought to have led to destruction or dysfunction of the venous valves.

EVALUATION OF VENOUS INSUFFICIENCY

Evaluation of the macrocirculation in chronic venous insufficiency initially utilized invasive measurements of ambulatory venous pressure (AVP) and venous recovery times (VRT). On the other hand, photoplethysmography (PPG) is a noninvasive alternative to the performance of direct ambulatory venous pressure measurements. In limbs with venous insufficiency the calf veins will refill from capillary inflow as well as from axial reflux. In such extremities, the venous recovery time will be shortened compared to normals. In most vascular laboratories, a PPG VRT less than 17 to 20 s is considered to indicate the presence of venous reflux in that extremity. Most cases of venous ulceration are associated with VRTs of less than 10 s. Unfortunately, invasive measurements of AVP and its noninvasive alternative, PPG VRT, do not completely characterize the function of the lower-extremity venous system. These tests do not distinguish the combined effects of reflux and obstruction, localize the site of reflux, or evaluate the role of the calf muscle pump in venous insufficiency.

The air plethysmograph (APG) theoretically permits assessment of calf muscle pump function, venous reflux, and overall lower-extremity venous function. When corrected for location and magnitude of lower-extremity venous reflux, calf muscle pump function as measured by APG appears to have an independent effect on the severity of chronic venous insufficiency.[74] Information obtained from the APG may allow for more precise preoperative assessment of patients before deep venous reconstruction or ablative superficial vein procedures.

Duplex ultrasound has also now achieved considerable importance in the evaluation of patients with chronic venous insufficiency. In addition to ruling out the presence of acute venous thrombosis, duplex ultrasound can be used to evaluate venous reflux in individual venous segments of the lower extremity. Knowledge of the relative contribution of individual venous segments to overall venous reflux may prove to be useful in planning venous reconstructive procedures.

Clearly, location of venous reflux is important. Reflux in popliteal and infrapopliteal veins is more significant than more proximal reflux in the development of skin changes and ulcers associated with severe venous insufficiency.[75–77] Venous ulceration can, however, also occur with reflux isolated to the superficial veins.[78,79] Up to 17% of patients with venous ulceration have reflux isolated to the superficial veins alone.[75–79]

Less than 5% of limbs initially involved with the deep venous thrombosis develop a venous ulcer.[80–82] Currently, one of the most intense areas of investigation related to chronic venous insufficiency (CVI) is the relationship between the development of CVI symptoms and the location of valvular dysfunction with respect to extent and location of thrombus following an acute episode of deep venous thrombosis. Using duplex ultrasound, detailed follow-up studies of the development of venous reflux have been performed in patients with an acute deep venous thrombosis. These studies indicate that some degree of recanalization of thrombosed veins occurs by 3 months in almost all lower extremities involved with deep venous thrombosis and treated with standard intravenous heparin and follow-up warfarin therapy.[80–82] In fact, by 90 days approximately half the lower extremities involved with deep venous thrombosis show recanalization of all segments initially noted to be thrombosed.[82]

As noted, an estimated 50% of above-knee deep venous thrombi and the great majority of isolated calf vein thrombi are asymptomatic.[83] This fact, combined with the fact that many patients who clearly have venous insufficiency have never had a documented episode of deep venous thrombosis,[75–79] suggests that subclinical venous thrombi may play a role in the development of chronic venous insufficiency.

MICROCIRCULATORY CONSIDERATIONS

Skin and subcutaneous tissue are the end organs of chronic venous insufficiency. Functional and morphological abnormalities of the cutaneous capillaries and lymphatics characterize advanced chronic venous insufficiency. Several theories seek to link these abnormalities with venous reflux.

Therapy for Chronic Venous Insufficiency

Nonoperative therapy has long been the basic treatment for venous ulceration and chronic venous insufficiency. It is highly effective in controlling symptoms of chronic venous insufficiency and promoting healing of venous ulcers. However, healing can be prolonged and painful and recurrence of ulceration post healing is a significant problem. Although lower-extremity elevation (feet above the thighs when sitting and above the heart when supine) is very effective treatment, enforced inactivity is impractical for most patients. Ideally, nonoperative therapy for chronic venous insufficiency should control symptoms while promoting healing of existing ulcers and preventing recurrence of ulceration. At the same time the patient should be allowed to maintain a normal ambulatory status.

COMPRESSION THERAPY

Compression therapy is the primary treatment for chronic venous insufficiency and remains so despite progress in both ablative[84] and reconstructive venous surgery (see following).[85,86] Compression therapy is usually delivered in the form of elastic stockings, paste boots, or elastic wraps. Results obtained with elastic wraps in general have, however, been inferior to those achieved with elastic stockings or past boots.[87–90]

There are significant problems with compression therapy. Most noteworthy is poor patient compliance.[91] Patients may be initially intolerant of the sensation of compression. Frequently, stockings can initially be worn only for brief periods. At the beginning of therapy, patients need to be instructed to wear elastic stockings only for so long as tolerable and then increase gradually the time wearing the stockings. Patients also may initially need to be fitted with lesser strength of compression (20–30 mmHg) and many elderly, weak, or arthritic patients cannot apply elastic stockings.

Paste gauze compression dressings were developed in 1896.[92] The current Unna's boot consists of dome paste dressing containing calamine, zinc oxide, glycerine, sorbitol, gelatin, and magnesium aluminum silicate. This dressing provides both compression and topical therapy and is preferentially applied by trained personnel. The dome paste gauze bandage is first applied with graded compression from the forefoot to the knee. A second layer consists of a 4-in.-wide continuous gauze dressing. The final layer is an elastic wrap applied with graded compression. The bandage stiffens with drying and is generally changed weekly. Studies evaluating the effectiveness of Unna boot therapy indicate about 70% of ulcers can be healed with Unna boot treatment.[93–95] After healing, lifetime compression therapy with elastic compression stockings is required to minimize recurrence.

Circ-Aid is a legging orthosis consisting of multiple pliable, rigid, adjustable compression bands.[96] These bands wrap around the leg from the ankle to the knee and are held in place with Velcro. The device provides rigid compression similar to an Unna boot with increased ease of application. A preliminary study suggests this legging orthosis may be superior to elastic stockings in preventing limb swelling in patients with advanced venous insufficiency.[97]

External pneumatic compression devices can serve as adjunctive measures in the treatment of lower-extremity lymphedema, venous ulceration, or both. These devices may be particularly applicable to patients who have severe edema or morbid obesity. Relative contraindications to external pneumatic compression are arterial insufficiency and uncontrolled congestive heart failure.

PHARMACOLOGICAL THERAPY

There are multiple pharmacological strategies to treat lipodermatosclerosis and venous ulceration. With the exception of diuretics, these agents are relatively unknown in the United States. Diuretics have, in fact, little role in the treatment of chronic venous insufficiency. They may be appropriate for short periods in patients with severe edema, but must be used judiciously.

Other pharmacological agents for treatment of chronic venous insufficiency are widely used in Europe. In 1993, a German study indicated that 11% of people in Germany 15 years of age and older received a medication for venous disease in the previous 12 months.[98]

ORAL AND INTRAVENOUS THERAPIES

Zinc, fibrinolytic agents and phlebotrophic agents have not shown any major benefits in venous ulcer healing.

Use of the hemorrheological agent pentoxifylline resulted in significant reduction in ulcer size after 6 months when combined with compression stockings. Aspirin may also accelerate ulcer healing. Prostaglandin E may also be beneficial.

TOPICAL THERAPIES

Without evidence of invasive infection, wound bacteriology appears to have little impact on healing of venous ulcers.[99] Use of topical antibiotics on a routine basis is therefore not recommended. Application of antiseptics is also counterproductive to wound healing.

The serotonin II antagonist ketanserin increases fibroblast collagen synthesis. A double-blind study of venous ulcers comparing the use of topical 2% ketanserin and compressive bandage use with bandage use alone indicated a 91% improvement in the ketanserin-treated group compared with 50% of controls.[100]

Hydrocolloid occlusive dressings (DuoDERM) maintain a moist wound environment. Such dressings are often comfortable for the patient and may produce more rapid epithelialization of granulating wounds.[101] However, although occlusive dressings are comfortable, they have not been conclusively demonstrated to produce more rapid healing and may lead to an increased number of local infectious complications.[94]

SKIN SUBSTITUTES

Human skin substitutes to promote permanent closure of open wounds. These products vary from simple acellular skin substitutes to complete living bioengineered, bilayered human skin equivalents with allogenic epidermal and dermal layers. They may possibly serve as delivery vehicles for various growth factors and cytokines important in wound healing.

Surgical Therapy

Procedures designed to treat chronic venous insufficiency can be classified as ablative or reconstructive. Ablative procedures are generally applicable only to disease of the superficial veins. Reconstructive procedures are designed to treat either reflux or obstruction of the deep veins.

VENOUS SCLEROTHERAPY

Venous sclerotherapy is the most widespread method for treatment of venous telangiectasias and small superficial varicose veins. Both telangiectatic vessels and small varicose veins may be associated with symptoms of leg heaviness, as well as localized pain or burning sensation. Many, of course, are asymptomatic and are treated primarily for cosmetic purposes.

There are many reported techniques for sclerotherapy treatment of different-sized varicosities and telangiectatic vessels. Although the specifics of these techniques vary, there are a number of underlying principles. The first is treatment of larger varicosities initially, followed by treatment of smaller varicosities, and then reticular veins, and finally telangiectatic veins. Varicosities greater than 4 to 5 mm in size with the patient in the upright position generally respond poorly to sclerotherapy and should be treated by a direct surgical approach (see following).

VEIN STRIPPING

Varicose veins not suitable for treatment by injection sclerotherapy may be treated by surgical removal. Branch varicosities are treated by the so-called stab-avulsion technique. In this technique, 2-mm incisions are made directly over branch varicosities, and the varicosity is teased away from surrounding subcutaneous tissue so far proximally and distally as possible through the small incision. The vein is then avulsed and no attempt is made to ligate the vessel. If the patient has significant greater saphenous reflux, the greater saphenous vein should also be removed. Surgical removal of varicose veins is very well tolerated and effective.

PERFORATOR LIGATION

Incompetence of the perforating veins connecting the superficial and deep venous systems of the lower extremities may play a role in the development of venous ulceration.[102–105] Ligation of these perforating veins for treatment of CVI,[105] however, had a high incidence of wound complications. In addition, isolated perforating vein incompetence is uncommon. A newer technique, subfascial endoscopic perforator vein surgery (SEPS), has evolved with the advent of the endoscope and may cause this strategy to be revisited.

VENOUS RECONSTRUCTION

In the absence of deep venous valvular incompetence, saphenous vein stripping and perforator ligation can be effective in treating CVI. However, in patients with a combination of superficial and deep venous valvular incompetence, the addition of deep venous valve correction improved the ulcer healing rate from 43% (14 of 33) to 79% (34 of 43) during an average 43 months of follow-up.[106]

Numerous techniques of deep venous valve correction exist for treatment of CVI. These techniques consist of repair of existing valves, transplant of venous segments from the arm, and transposition of an incompetent vein onto an adjacent competent vein. Success rates range from 40%–80% depending on the nature of the disease and the procedure performed.

References

1. Dalen JE, Albert JS. Natural history of pulmonary embolism. Prog Cardiovasc Dis 1975;17:257–270.
2. Dismuke SE, Wagner EH. Pulmonary embolism as a cause of death; the changing mortality in hospitalized patients. JAMA 1986;255(15):2039–2042.
3. Salzman EW, Hirsh J. The epidemiology, pathogenesis, and natural history of venous thromboembolism. In: Colman RW, Hirsh J, Marder VJ, Salzman EW, eds. Hemostasis and Thrombosis. Philadelphia: Lippincott, 1994:1275–1296.
4. Anderson FA Jr, Wheeler HB. Physician practices in the management of venous thromboembolism: a community wide survey. J Vasc Surg 1992;16:707–714.
5. Samama MM, Simmoneau G, Wainstein JP, et al. SIRIUS study: epidemiology of risk factors of deep venous thrombosis of the lower limbs in community practice. Thromb Haemostasis 1993;69(6):763.
6. Anderson FA Jr, Wheeler HB, Goldberg RJ, et al. A population-based perspective of the hospital incidence and case-fatality rates of deep venous thrombosis and pulmonary embolus. Arch Intern Med 1991;151:933–938.
7. Silverstein MD, Heit JA, Mohr DN, Petterson TM, O'Fallon WM, Melton LJ III. Trends in the incidence of deep vein thrombosis and pulmonary embolism; a 25-year population-based study. Arch Intern Med 1998;158:585–593.
8. Goldberg RJ, Seneff M, Gore JM, et al. Occult malignant neoplasm in patients with deep venous thrombosis. Arch Intern Med 1987;147:251–253.
9. Prandoni P, Lensing AWA, Buller HR, et al. Deep-vein thrombosis and the incidence of subsequent cancer. N Engl J Med 1992;327:1128–1133.
10. Priten KJ, Miller EV, Mason E, et al. Venous thrombosis in the morbidly obese. Surg Gynecol Obstet 1978;147:63–64.
11. Mauer BJ, Wray R, Shillingford JP. Frequency of venous thrombosis after myocardial infarction. Lancet 1971;ii:1385–1387.
12. Kotilainen M, Ristola P, Ikkala E, Pyorala K. Leg vein thrombosis diagnosed by ^{125}I-fibrinogen test after acute myocardial infarction. Ann Clin Res 1973;5:365–368.
13. Handley AJ, Emerson PA, Fleming PR. Heparin in the prevention of deep vein thrombosis after myocardial infarction. Br Med J 1972;2:436–438.
14. Warlow C, Terry G, Kenmure ACF, et al. A double-blind trial of low-dose subcutaneous heparin in the prevention of deep vein thrombosis after myocardial infarction. Lancet 1973;2:934–937.
15. Devor M, Barrett-Connor E, Renvall M, et al. Estrogen replacement therapy and the risk of venous thrombosis. Am J Med 1991;92:275–282.
16. Boston Collaborative Drug Surveillance Program. Surgically confirmed gall bladder disease, venous thromboembolism, and breast tumours in relation to post-menopausal estrogen therapy. N Engl J Med 1974;290:15–19.
17. Waring WP, Karunas RS. Acute spinal cord injuries and the incidence of clinically occuring thromboembolic disease. Paraplegia 1991;29:8–16.
18. Green D, Lee Y, Ito VY, et al. Fixed- vs adjusted-dose heparin in the prophylaxis of thromboembolism in spinal cord injury. JAMA 1988;260:1255–1258.
19. Green D, Lee MY, Lim AC, et al. Prevention of thromboembolism after spinal cord injury using low-molecular weight heparin. Ann Intern Med 1990;113:571–574.
20. Dollery CM, Sullivan ID, Bauraind O, et al. Thrombosis and embolism in long-term central venous access for parenteral nutrition. Lancet 1994;344:1043–1045.
21. Bick RL, Kaplan H. Syndromes of thrombosis and hypercoagulability, congenital and acquired causes of thrombosis. Med Clin North Am 1998;82(3):409–458.
22. Svensson PJ, Dahlback B. Resistance to activated protein c as a basis for thrombosis. N Engl J Med 1994;330:517–522.
23. Barritt DW, Jordan SC. Anticoagulant drugs in the treatment of pulmonary embolism: a controlled trial. Lancet 1960;1:1309–1312.
24. Markel A, Manzo RA, Bergelin RO, Strandness DE Jr. Pattern and distribution of thrombi in acute venous thrombosis. Arch Surg 1992;127:305–309.
25. Kakkar VV, Howe CT, Franc C, Clarke MB. Natural history of postoperative deep venous thrombosis. Lancet 1969;2:230–232.
26. Nicolaides AN, Kakkar VV, Field ES, Renney JTG. The origin of deep venous thrombosis: a venographic study. Br J Radiol 1971;44:653–663.
27. Moser KM, Fedullo PF, LitteJohn JK, Crawford R. Frequent asymptomatic pulmonary embolism in patients with deep venous thrombosis. JAMA 1994;271:223–225.
28. Nielsen HK, Husted SE, Kursell LR, et al. Silent pulmonary embolism in patients with deep venous thrombosis. Incidence and fate in a randomized, controlled trial of anticoagulation versus no anticoagulation. J Intern Med 1994;235:457–461.
29. Caprinin JA, Arcelus JI, Hoffman KN, et al. Venous duplex imaging follow-up of acute symptomatic deep vein thrombosis of the leg. J Vasc Surg 1995;21:472–476.
30. Donaldson GA, Williams C, Scannel JG, et al. A reappraisal of

the application of the Trendelenburg operation to massive fatal embolism: report of a successful pulmonary-artery thrombectomy using cardiopulmonary bypass. N Engl J Med 1963;268: 171–174.

31. Kakkar VV, Cohen AT, Edmonson RA, et al. Low molecular weight versus standard heparin for prevention of venous thromboembolism after major abdominal surgery. Lancet 1993;341: 259–265.

32. Nurmohamed MT, Verhaeghe R, Haas S, et al. A comparative trial of a low molecular weight heparin (enoxaparin) versus standard heparin for the prophylaxis of postoperative deep vein thrombosis in general surgery. Am J Surg 1995;169:567–571.

33. Koppenhagen K, Adolf J, Matthes M, et al. Low molecular weight heparin and prevention of postoperative thrombosis in abdominal surgery. Thromb Haemostasis 1992;67(6):627–630.

34. Hull RD, Hirsh J, Carter CJ, et al. Diagnostic efficacy of impedance plethysmography for clinically suspected deep-vein thrombosis; a randomized trial. Ann Intern Med 1985;102:21–28.

35. Huisman MV, Buller HR, ten Cate JW, Vreeken J. Serial impedance plethysmography for suspected deep venous thrombosis in outpatients; the Amsterdam general practitioner study. N Engl J Med 1986;314:823–828.

36. Huisman MV, Buller HR, ten Cate JW, et al. Management of clinically suspected acute venous thrombosis in outpatients with serial impedance plethysmography in a community hospital setting. Arch Intern Med 1989;149:511–513.

37. Lensing AWA, Prandoni P, Brandjes D, et al. Detection of deep-vein thrombosis by real-time B-mode ultrasonography. N Engl J Med 1989;320:342–345.

38. Cronan JJ, Dorfman GS, Scola FH, et al. Deep venous thrombosis: US assessment using vein compression. Radiology 1987; 162:191–194.

39. Appelman PT, De Jong TE, Lampmann LE. Deep venous thrombosis of the leg: US findings. Radiology 1987;163:743–746.

40. Vogel P, Laing FC, Jeffrey RB Jr, Wing VW. Deep venous thrombosis of the lower extremity: US evaluation. Radiology 1987;163: 747–751.

41. O'Leary DH, Kane RA, Chase BM. A prospective study of the efficacy of B-scan sonography in the detection of deep venous thrombosis in the lower extremities. J Clin Ultrasound 1988; 16:1–8.

42. Stein PD, Terrin ML, Hales CA, et al. Clinical, laboratory, roentgenographic, and electrographic findings in patients with acute pulmonary embolism and no pre-existing cardiac or pulmonary disease. Chest 1991;100:598–603.

43. Sasahara AA, Stein M, Simon M, Littmann D. Pulmonary angiography in the diagnosis of thromboembolic disease. N Engl J Med 1964;270:1075–1081.

44. Stein PD, Athanasoulis C, Alavi A, et al. Complications and validity of pulmonary angiography in acute pulmonary embolism. Circulation 1992;85:462–468.

45. Dalen JE, Brooks HL, Johnson LW, et al. Pulmonary angiography in acute pulmonary embolism; indications, techniques, and results in 367 patients. Am Heart J 1971;81:175–185.

46. Killewich LA, Nunnelee JD, Auer AI. Value of lower extremity venous duplex examination in the diagnosis of pulmonary embolism. J Vac Surg 1993;17:934–939.

47. Hull RD, Raskob GE, Hirsh J, et al. Continuous intravenous heparin compared with intermittent subcutaneous heparin in the initial treatment of proximal-vein thrombosis. N Engl J Med 1986;315:1109–1114.

48. Brandjes DPM, Heijboer H, Buller HR, et al. Acenocoumarol and heparin compared with acenocoumarol alone in the initial treatment of proximal-vein thrombosis. N Engl J Med 1992;327: 1485–1489.

49. Hull RD, Raskob GE, Rosenbloom D, et al. Optimal therapeutic level of heparin therapy in patients with venous thrombosis. Arch Intern Med 1992;152:1589–1595.

50. Hirsh J, Dalen JE, Deykin D, et al. Oral anticoagulants: mechanism of action, clinical effectiveness, and optimal therapeutic range. Chest 1995;108(suppl 4):231–465.

51. Hull RD, Raskob GE, Rosenbloom D, et al. Heparin for 5 days as compared with 10 days in the initial treatment of proximal venous thrombosis. N Engl J Med 1990;322:1260–1264.

52. Mohiuddin SM, Hilleman DE, Destache CJ, et al. Efficacy and safety of early versus late initiation of warfarin during therapy in acute thromboembolism. Am Heart J 1992;123:729–732.

53. Safety and efficacy of warfarin started early after submassive venous thrombosis of pulmonary embolism. Lancet 1986:1293–1296.

54. Coon WW, Willis PW III, Symons MJ. Assessment of anticoagulant treatment of venous thromboembolism. Ann Surg 1969; 170:559–568.

55. Hull R, Delmore T, Genton E, et al. Warfarin versus low-dose heparin in the long-term treatment of venous thrombosis. N Engl J Med 1979;301:855–858.

56. Anderson LO, Barrowcliffe TW, Holmer E, et al. Molecular weight dependency of the heparin potentiated inhibition of thrombin and activated factor X: effect of heparin neutralization in plasma. Thromb Res 1979;115:531–538.

57. Fareed J, Walenga JM, Racanelli A, et al. Validity of the newly established low molecular weight heparin standard in cross referencing low molecular weight heparins. Haemostasis 1988; 3(suppl):33–47.

58. Fareed J, Walenga JM, Hoppensteadt D, et al. Comparative study on the in vitro and in vivo activities of seven low-molecular weight heparins. Haemostasis 1988;18(suppl):3–15.

59. Boneu B, Caranobe C, Cadroy Y, et al. Pharmacokinetic studies of standard unfractionated heparin, and low molecular weight heparins in the rabbit. Semin Thromb Hemostasis 1988;14: 18–27.

60. Matzsch T, Bergqvist D, Hedner U, et al. Effects of low molecular weight heparin and unfragmented heparin on induction of osteoporosis in rats. Thromb Haemostasis 1990;63:505–509.

61. Brand FN, Dannenberg AL, Abbott RD, Kannel WB. The epidemiology of varicose veins: the Framingham study. Am J Prev Med 1988;4:96.

62. Madar G, Widmer LK, Zemp E, Maggs M. Varicose veins and chronic venous insufficiency—a disorder or disease? A critical epidemiological review. Vasa 1986;15:126.

63. Jamieson WG. State of the art of venous investigation and treatment. Can J Surg 1993;36:119.

64. Scott TE, La Morte WW, Gorin DR, et al. Risk factors for chronic venous insufficiency: a dual case-control study. J Vasc Surg 1995;22:622.

65. Criado E, Johnson G Jr. Venous disease. Curr Probl 1991;28:339.

66. Baker SR, Stacey MC, Jopp-McKay AG, et al. Ulcers. Br J Surg 1991;78:864.

67. Cornwall JV, Dore CJ, Lewis JD. Leg ulcers: epidemiology and aetiology. Br J Surg 1986;73:693.

68. Lees TA, Lambert D. Prevalence of lower limb ulcers in an urban health district. Br J Surg 1992;79:1032.

69. Phillips T, Stanton B, Provan A, et al. A study of the impact of leg ulcers on quality of life: financial, social, and psychologic implications. J Am Acad Dermatol 1994;31:49.

70. Browse NL, Burnand KG, Thomas ML. Diseases of the Veins. Pathology, Diagnosis and Treatment. London: Hodder and Stoughton, 1988.

71. Callam MJ, Harper DR, Dale JJ, Ruckley CV. Chronic leg ulceration: socioeconomic aspects. Scott Med J 1988;33:358.

72. Abenhaim L, Kurx X, VEINES Study Collaborators. The VEINES Study: an international cohort study on chronic venous disorders of the leg. Angiology 1997;48:59.

73. Clarke H, Smith SR, Vasdekis SN, et al. Role of venous elasticity in the development of varicose veins. Br J Surg 1989;76:577.

74. Araki CT, Back TL, Padberg FT, et al. The significance of calf

muscle pump function in venous ulceration. J Vasc Surg 1994;20: 872.

75. Rosfors S, Lamke LO, Nordstrom E, Bygdeman S. Severity and location of venous valvular insufficiency: the importance of distal valve function. Acta Chir Scand 1990;156:689.

76. Hanrahan LM, Araki CT, Rodriguez AA, et al. Distribution of valvular incompetence in patients with venous stasis ulceration. J Vasc Surg 1991;13:805.

77. Moore DJ, Himmel PD, Summer DS. Distribution of venous valvular incompetence in patients with the postphlebitic syndrome. J Vasc Surg 1986;3:49.

78. Sethia KK, Darke SG. Long saphenous incompetence as a cause of venous ulceration. Br J Surg 1984;71:754.

79. Hoare MC, Nicolaides AN, Miles CR, et al. The role of primary varicose veins in venous ulceration. Surgery (St. Louis) 1982; 92:450.

80. Lohr JM, McDevitt DT, Lutter KS, et al. Operative management of greater saphenous thrombophlebitis involving the saphenofemoral junction. Am J Surg 1992;164:269–275.

81. Strandness DE, Langlois Y, Cramer M, et al: Long-term sequelae of acute venous thrombosis. JAMA 1983;250:1289.

82. Killewich LA, Bedford GR, Beach KW, Strandness DE. Spontaneous lysis of deep venous thrombi: rate and outcome. J Vasc Surg 1989;9:89.

83. Langerstedt CI, Olsson CG, Fagher BO, et al. Need for longterm anticoagulant treatment in symptomatic calf-vein thrombosis. Lancet 1985;2:515–518.

84. Cikrit DF, Nichols WK, Silver D. Surgical management of refractory venous stasis ulceration. J Vasc Surg 1988;7:473.

85. Raju S, Fredericks R. Valve reconstruction procedures for nonobstructive venous insufficiency: rationale, techniques, and results in 107 procedures with two- to eight-year followup. J Vasc Surg 1988;7:301.

86. Bergan JJ, Yao JST, Flinn WR, McCarthy WJ. Surgical treatment of venous obstruction and insufficiency. J Vasc Surg 1986;3:174.

87. Stewart AJ, Leaper DJ. Treatment of chronic leg ulcers in the community: a comparative trial of Scherisorb and Iodosorb. Phlebology 1987;2:115.

88. Ormiston MC, Seymour MT, Venn GE, et al. Controlled trial of Iodosorb in chronic venous ulcers. Br Med J 1985;291:308.

89. Ryan TJ, Biven HF, Murphy JJ, et al. The use of a new occlusive dressing in the management of venous stasis ulceration. In: Ryan TJ, ed. An Environment for Healing: The Role of Occlusion. London: Royal Society of Medicine, 1984:99–103.

90. Eriksson G. Comparative study of hydrocolloid dressing and double layer bandage in treatment of venous stasis ulceration. In: Ryan TJ, ed. An Environment for Healing: The Role of Occlusion. London: Royal Society of Medicine, 1984:111–113.

91. Chant AD, Davies LJ, Pike JM, Sparks MJ. Support stockings in practical management of varicose veins. Phlebology 1989;4:167.

92. Unna PG. Ueber Paraplaste, eine neue Form medikamentoser Pflaster. Wien Med Wochenschr 1896;43:1854.

93. Rubin JR, Alexander J, Plecha EJ, Marman C. Unna's boots vs polyurethane foam dressings for the treatment of venous ulceration. Arch Surg 1990;125:489.

94. Kitka MJ, Schuler JJ, Meyer JP, et al. A prospective, randomized trial of Unna's boots versus hydroactive dressing in the treatment of venous stasis ulcers. J Vasc Surg 1988;7:478.

95. Cordts PR, Hanrahan LM, Rodriguez AA, et al. A prospective, randomized trial of Unna's boot versus DuoDERM CGF hydroactive dressing plus compression in the management of venous leg ulcers. J Vasc Surg 1992;15:480.

96. Vernick SH, Shapiro D, Shaw FD. Legging orthosis for venous and lymphatic insufficiency. Arch Phys Med Rehabil 1987;68: 459.

97. Spence RK, Cahall E. Inelastic versus elastic leg compression in chronic venous insufficiency: a comparison of limb size and venous hemodynamics. J Vasc Surg 1996;24:783–787.

98. Uber A. The socioeconomic profile of patients treated by phlebotropic drugs in Germany. Angiology 1997;48:595–607.

99. Gilchrist B, Reed C. The bacteriology of chronic venous ulcers treated with occlusive hydrocolloid dressings. Br J Dermatol 1989;121:337.

100. Roelens P. Double-blind placebo-controlled study with topical 2% ketanserin ointment in the treatment of venous ulcers. Dermatologica 1989;178:98.

101. Alvarez OM, Mertz PM, Eaglstein WH. The effect of occlusive dressings on collagen synthesis and re-epithelialization in superficial wounds. J Surg Res 1983;35:142.

102. Linton RR. The communicating veins of the lower leg and the operative technique for their ligation. Ann Surg 1938;107:582–593.

103. Gay J. Lettsonian Lectures 1867. Varicose Disease of the Lower Extremities. London: Churchill, 1868.

104. Homans J. The operative treatment of varicose veins and ulcers, based upon a classification of these lesions. Surg Gynecol Obstet 1916;22:143–158.

105. Linton RR. The post-thrombotic ulceration of the lower extremity: its etiology and surgical treatment. Ann Surg 1953;138: 415–432.

106. Sottiurai VS. Surgical correction of recurrent venous ulcer. J Cardiovasc Surg 1991;32:104–109.

107. Geerts WH, Code KI, Jay RM, et al. A prospective study of venous thromboembolism after major trauma. N Engl J Med 1994;331:1601–1606.

108. Winchell RJ, Hoyt DB, Walsh JC, et al. Risk factors associated with pulmonary embolism despite routine prophylaxis: implications for improved protection. J Trauma 1994;37(4):600–606.

109. The PIOPED Investigators. Value of the ventilation/perfusion scan in acute pulmonary embolism; results of the prospective investigation of pulmonary embolism diagnosis (PIOPED). JAMA 1990;263:2753–2759.

110. Quinones-Baldrich WT. Thrombolytic therapy for vascular disease. In: Moore WS, editor. Vascular Surgery: A Comprehensive Review. Philadelphia: Saunders, 1998:361–389.

111. Prandoni P, Lensing AWA, Buller HR, et al. Comparison of subcutaneous low-molecular-weight heparin with intravenous standard heparin in proximal deep-vein thrombosis. Lancet 1992; 339:441–445.

112. Lindmarker P, Holstrom M, Granqvist S, et al. Comparison of once-daily subcutaneous fragmin with continuous intravenous unfractionated heparin in the treatment of deep vein thrombosis. Thromb Haemostasis 1994;72(2):186–190.

113. Simmonneau G, Charbonnier B, Decousus H, et al. Subcutaneous low-molecular-weight heparin compared with continuous intravenous unfractionated heparin in the treatment of proximal deep vein thrombosis. Arch Intern Med 1993;153:1541–1546.

114. Hull RD, Raskob GE, Pineo GF, et al. Subcutaneous low-molecular-weight heparin compared with continuous intravenous heparin in the treatment of proximal-vein thrombosis. N Engl J Med 1992;326:975–982.

Vascular Trauma

Paul E. Bankey

Vascular Trauma Priorities

The priorities in the management of the patient with vascular trauma are to treat immediately life-threatening injuries by maintaining a patient airway, supporting respiration, restoring circulation, and evaluating neurological disability. Many types of vascular injuries require a multidisciplinary approach with treatment from orthopedic surgeons for concurrent fracture management, plastic surgeons for wound coverage, interventional radiologists for diagnosis and endovascular management, and cardiac or neurosurgeons for selected types of injuries. It is critical that the trauma vascular surgeon maintains control of the patient and establishes the priorities during the evaluation and treatment.

Pathology

Two large series of vascular injuries from urban trauma centers indicate that the most common injury mechanism is penetrating, with about 50% of the injuries as a result of gunshot wounds.[1,2] Extremities are the most frequently injured site with a roughly equal distribution between the arms and legs. The abdomen is the next most common site of injury, with visceral vessels injured most frequently. Combined, the incidence of chest and abdominal vascular injuries makes up about 45% of the total and is equal to the number of extremity injuries.

Arteries and veins may be injured in several ways, each with different clinical manifestations and consequences (Fig. 37.1). Laceration and transection account for the majority of injuries, with incomplete transections hemorrhaging to a greater extent than complete transections because the vessel cannot spasm and retract to the same degree to reduce blood loss. Pseudoaneurysms, arteriovenous fistula, and intimal disruption or flaps may result from penetrating or blunt mechanisms of injury. These injuries may manifest in a variety of ways clinically: exsanguination and hemorrhagic shock; complete thrombosis and distal ischemia; compression of adjacent structures and compartment syndrome; partial thrombus formation and distal embolization; or, infrequently, chronic arterial or venous insufficiency.

Interruption of arterial flow produces regional ischemia in the organ or extremity distal to the injury. Tissues vary in their tolerance to reduced arterial flow and irreversible ischemic damage. Nerves are extremely sensitive to ischemia whereas skeletal muscle is relatively tolerant of reduced arterial flow. Muscle that has been ischemic for 4 h may demonstrate no histological changes; however, restoration of flow is uniformly associated with a reperfusion injury that exacerbates the insult to local tissues and can produce systemic inflammation, acute lung injury, and renal failure.

Prolonged ischemia without collateral flow will cause muscle necrosis or rhabdomyolysis with the release of potassium and myoglobin into the circulation. Reperfusion exacerbates muscle injury[3] (Fig. 37.2). Myoglobin is filtered in the kidney and can precipitate in the tubules, resulting in acute renal failure. Maintaining high urine output, which flushes the pigment from the tubules (that is, more than 100 ml/h), using osmotic or loop diuretics prevents precipitation. Alkalization of the urine by adding sodium bicarbonate to the resuscitation fluids also helps prevent precipitation of myoglobin in the tubules.

Evaluation

History and Physical Exam

The mechanism of injury and a history derived from prehospital personnel provide valuable information. Historical clues that raise suspicion of vascular injury include the report of extensive blood loss at the scene or during transport, bleeding from a puncture site that is either bright red or dark, and head-on vehicular collision with deformation of the steering wheel, which is associated with cardiac and thoracic aortic

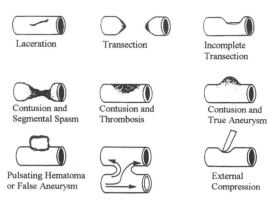

Laceration   Transection   Incomplete Transection

Contusion and Segmental Spasm   Contusion and Thrombosis   Contusion and True Aneurysm

Pulsating Hematoma or False Aneurysm   Arteriovenous Fistula   External Compression

FIGURE 37.1. Types of vascular trauma pathology. Each injury may manifest clinically in a variety of ways. (From Shackford SR, Rich NH.[1])

TABLE 37.1. Physical Findings Indicating Vascular Injury.

Hard signs	*Soft signs*
Absent distal pulse	Proximity of injury to artery
Obvious arterial bleeding	History of arterial bleeding at scene of accident
Expanding or pulsatile hematoma	
Bruit or thrill at injury	Diminished distal pulse
Six P's of vascular injury:	Small nonpulsatile hematoma
Pulselessness	Questionable neurological deficit
Pallor	
Pain	Fracture
Poikilothermia	Knee dislocation
Paresthesia	
Paralysis	

Source: Adapted from Mattox et al.[2]

injury. Falls from significant height can result in aortic or renal artery intimal tear, ligamentous instability of the knee (with a posterior knee dislocation is associated with popliteal vascular injury, and supracondylar fractures of the humerous, are associated with brachial arterial injuries, especially in the pediatric population.

Physical findings indicating vascular injury have been categorized as hard signs or soft signs[4] (Table 37.1). Before this designation, recommendations from most major trauma centers dealing with penetrating injuries were for the routine exploration of all vessels in anatomic proximity to the wound. Subsequent reports indicated that this approach resulted in a low diagnostic yield.[5,6]

Based on the mechanism, history, and physical findings, further observation, immediate operation, or additional diagnostic tests may be appropriate. In general, patients with hard signs of vascular injury do not require preoperative arteriography. In fact, formal arteriography may delay restoration of flow in a marginally perfused extremity, leading to irreversible ischemia. Patients with hard signs should be taken directly to the operating room for exploration and definitive treatment.

Possible exceptions to this recommendation are when angiography is critical for incision planning, such as in zone 1 of the neck, or when definitive therapy can be provided via interventional techniques with a high degree of success.

Interventional angiography is the preferred procedure in selected vascular injuries where surgical intervention is excessively hazardous, such as pelvic fracture, or technically difficult, such as vertebral artery injury.[7] Interventional angiography also allows the placement of intravascular stents that show promise in the treatment of certain arterial injuries.[8] Occasionally, angiography assists in the retrieval of foreign bodies, usually intracardiac or intravascular bullets and fragments.[9]

Arteriography

Arteriography to exclude vascular injury is highly reliable, with a sensitivity of 97% to 100%, specificity of 90% to 98%, and accuracy of 92% to 98%.[10] However, false positives are reported at 2% to 8%, and the procedure is invasive with an incidence of serious complication such as occlusion or pseudoaneurysm reported as 0.6%.[11] A formal arteriogram even in the best of centers takes a minimum of 2 h to complete, and this time factor must be considered in the overall management of the patient's injuries.

The use of digital subtraction angiography (DSA) reduces time, cost, and contrast medium requirements.[12] This technique uses computerized subtraction and enhancement of the image after arterial injection; however, motion artifacts may limit subtraction enhancements and concurrent injuries may prevent use of paralytic agents.

The most common soft sign of vascular injury is a penetrating wound in proximity to an artery in an otherwise asymptomatic patient. Proximity is defined as any wound or missile track located within 1 to 5 cm of a major vessel and excludes patients with pulse deficit, bruit, thrill, history of arterial hemorrhage, fracture, large soft tissue deficit, or neurological finding. The workup of penetrating injuries requires the complete evaluation of the tract of the missile with plain films, including areas not amenable to physical examination even in asymptomatic patients. A bullet's path can be altered by direct contact, temporary cavitation, and fragmentation such that a straight line cannot be assumed and vascular structures may be at risk. Stab wound tracts and impaled objects are frequently in proximity to vascular structures.[13] Despite these risks, proximity as the only indication for arteriography in otherwise asymptomatic patients has a low yield of clini-

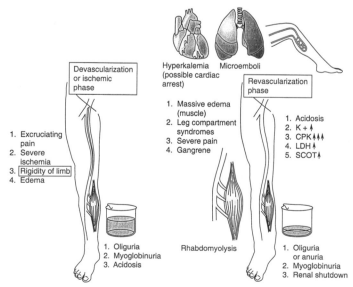

Devascularization or ischemic phase

1. Excruciating pain
2. Severe ischemia
3. Rigidity of limb
4. Edema

Hyperkalemia (possible cardiac arrest)   Microemboli

1. Massive edema (muscle)
2. Leg compartment syndromes
3. Severe pain
4. Gangrene

Revascularization phase

1. Acidosis
2. K + ↑
3. CPK ↑↑↑
4. LDH ↑
5. SCOT ↑

1. Oliguria
2. Myoglobinuria
3. Acidosis

Rhabdomyolysis

1. Oliguria or anuria
2. Myoglobinuria
3. Renal shutdown

FIGURE 37.2. Clinical and metabolic effects of muscle ischemia-reperfusion after vascular trauma. (From Haimovici H, ed. Vascular Surgery. Norwalk: Appleton & Lange, 1989, with permission.[3])

cally significant injury. This approach is not cost effective in screening patients without additional clinical signs of injury and should no longer be the only indication for arteriography. Careful physical examination has now replaced both surgery andangiography in the asymptomatic patient with a solitary penetrating injury to the extremity distal to the axilla or groin.[14–16] Current recommendations are for all shotgun wounds and multiple penetrating injuries to extremities to be evaluated by angiography even if asymptomatic.

Noninvasive Studies

Noninvasive vascular assessment using ultrasonic Doppler signals or duplex ultrasonography is another useful diagnostic approach in the patient with soft signs of vascular injury. These modalities have reported high sensitivities in the detection of vascular injury, making them useful for the low prevalence of significant injury in this group of patients.[17] Evaluation of Doppler signals with a handheld ultrasonic flow detector can be performed in the trauma resuscitation bay. Absence of flow confirms a hard sign of injury and the necessity for operative intervention. Triphasic signals are reassuring that no significant obstruction is present, whereas a monophasic signal suggests an obstruction requiring further evaluation. A Doppler-derived ankle-brachial index (ABI) or arterial pressure index (API) has been proposed as a noninvasive approach to screen and triage patients with soft signs of injury to arteriography. The technique is limited in patients with preexisting peripheral vascular disease and when injuries are present at the wrist, ankle, or bilaterally. Another limitation is that pressure determinations are successful in identifying obstruction secondary to injury; however, significant vascular injuries such as intimal flaps or pseudoaneurysms may not present with obstruction initially. Even so, this technique has been reported as sensitive and cost effective.[18]

Duplex ultrasonography combines real-time ultrasound imaging with a Doppler flow detector. Its sensitivity, specificity, and accuracy compare favorably with arteriography (Table 37.2). On the down side, duplex scanning presents logistical and resource considerations. The technology is sophisticated and requires skill in operation and interpretation that may not always be immediately available.

Other diagnostic modalities may be considered in the evaluation of vascular injury. Plain film radiography is still the best way to visualize the skeleton during initial evalua-

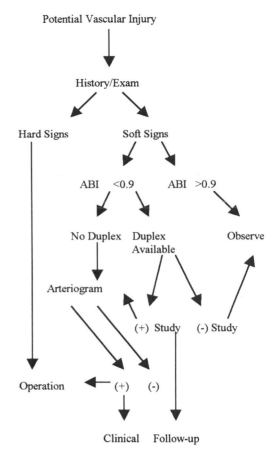

FIGURE 37.3. Diagnostic approach for extremity vascular injury. Physical exam, noninvasive testing, and arteriography each contribute to the evaluation. *ABI*, ankle-brachial index.

tion and is the mainstay for diagnosing associated orthopedic injuries. It is also useful for identification of retained foreign bodies such as missiles. The utility of plain films in vascular trauma is limited because of the high rate of false-positive and false-negative findings. The advent of helical and spiral computed tomography (CT) has greatly enhanced the resolution, speed of acquisition, and ability to reconstruct and manipulate images, including three-dimensional (3-D) vascular images.[19] The role of CT angiography in the setting of trauma is uncertain. From an imaging viewpoint, CT angiography can produce images sharp enough to allow diagnosis of vascular injury. However, CT does not allow intervention such as the ability to control or prevent hemorrhage with embolization or balloon deployment or treatment of injuries such as the placement of endovascular stents. Magnetic resonance imaging (MRI) is rapidly evolving but at the current time its applications to vascular trauma are limited.

A summary of a recommended approach for the evaluation of vascular injury primarily for extremity trauma is shown in Figure 37.3.

Management

Vascular Control

The operative management of all types of vascular injury has common elements. The immediate requirement is to stop bleeding. A firm compression bandage over the site of injury

TABLE 37.2.

Experience with Duplex Scanning in Trauma.

Authors	Total patients	Sensitivity	Specificity	Accuracy
Bynoe et al. 1991[68]	198 (20 injuries)	95	99	98
Fry et al. 1993[69]	175 (18 injuries)	100	97	97
Bergstein et al. 1992[70]	67 (4 injuries)	50	99	96
Knudson et al. 1993[71]	77 (4 injuries)	100	100	100

is helpful, but direct digital compression of the bleeding point is most effective. Tourniquet control of hemorrhage is rarely indicated and increases the risk of ischemic necrosis. The blind placement of clamps within a wound for hemostasis should also be avoided as these frequently exacerbate the injury or cause additional damage. Penetrating wounds in proximity to vessels should not be probed. Removing the clot on a vessel can turn a temporized, stable condition to an unstable, emergency situation.

The operative management of vascular trauma requires a generous incision to gain control proximally and distally of the injured vessel. The preparation of skin and draping of the patient should also be generous and include preparation for a number of contingencies. The vascular trauma patient must be prepped to allow rapid exposure to the chest and abdomen for resuscitation or control of inflow, harvest of autologous vein from an uninjured extremity to serve as a conduit, and direct observation of the distal hand or foot to assess pulses during the operation. In addition, the preparation and draping must allow the ability to perform intraoperative angiograms for diagnosis and assessment of reconstruction and fasciotomies in the setting of a compartment syndrome. Wounds with vascular injuries in the neck or groin at times require a sternotomy or laparotomy for proximal control and these are best planned for and performed at the outset of the operation.

Although achieving proximal and distal control of the injury is ideal before exposing the vascular injury, this is not practical when there is ongoing hemorrhage. In this situation the initial maneuver is isolation of the injury with more generous proximal and distal control for repair performed after control.

A variety of autotransfusion devices have been developed for use in the operating room. This device may be applied to many types of vascular injury as well as blood loss from a hemothorax, mediastinal hemorrhage, or nonenteric-contaminated abdominal hemorrhage. Care must be used to make sure the patient does not become coagulopathic as a result of heparin in the system. Gastrointestinal injuries contraindicate the use of autotransfusion.

Reconstruction

A bloodless, dry vascular field is achieved in preparation for repair by the application of specially designed noncrushing vascular occluding clamps. Clamps of appropriate size and angle are applied to provide an unobstructed field with enough pressure to stop bleeding. Vascular control may also be achieved with the placement of Fogarty-type balloon catheters into the open end of the vessel or injury.

The preferred method of arterial reconstruction is an end-to-end anastomosis. Lateral arteriorrhaphy may be appropriate for small puncture wounds or small lacerations from a knife wound. Constriction at the site of lateral arteriorrhaphy may be prevented with an autologous vein patch. The damaged vessel must be sharply debrided and contused segments excised if the intima is damaged. Additional vessels may have to be mobilized to accomplish a tension-free repair.

Depending on the size and location of the artery involved, a number of conduits both autologous and synthetic have been utilized to bridge the gap when an end-to-end anastomosis without tension cannot be performed. Popular substitute conduits for an interposition graft include Dacron tube grafts, polytetrafluroethylene (PTFE), and autogenous saphenous vein. Autologous greater saphenous vein from an unin-

jured lower extremity has been used successfully for many years and remains the conduit of choice for extremity trauma or vessels less than 6 mm in diameter.[20,21]

The majority of vascular repairs after trauma can be performed with local heparin rather than systemic heparinization. Systemic heparin may be contraindicated with concomitant injuries or coagulopathy. It is important to include a completion angiogram which should include the area of clamp application, anastomosis, and distal circulation to identify spasm, narrowing, clot, and additional injury.

Wound Management

Vascular repairs should be covered at the initial operation to prevent desiccation and infection, which cause thrombosis or anastomotic breakdown. Debridement of devitalized tissue and foreign material are important components of preventing late complications after a successful revascularization. Copious irrigation of the wound with a pulsatile, low-pressure spray reduces bacterial counts and should be standard to wound management.

Antibiotics should be administered parenterally and started as soon as possible after trauma has occurred. Tetanus and diphtheria toxoid or tetanus immunoglobulin should be administered as indicated. The ideal duration of antibiotic therapy in wounds with vascular injury has not been established, but administration for a minimum of 24 h would appear appropriate. Irrigation of the wound with antibiotic-containing lavage has been reported but has not been studied to determine if it reduces wound or graft infection rates.

Tissue coverage of the vascular reconstruction can usually be achieved by mobilization of adjacent soft tissue. In large tissue defects, a transposed muscle flap or free tissue transfer may be required.[22] Another option is an extraanatomical bypass to avoid the wound. Drains should be avoided near a vascular repair as it may erode into or infect the anastomosis.

Use of Shunts

Rapid restoration of perfusion distal to a vascular injury is even more critical in complex wounds, in major orthopedic injuries, and in the patient in shock from multiple injuries. Occasionally, definitive treatment of the vascular injury, orthopedic injury, and wound or soft tissue injury will compromise the patient's survival because of concurrent injuries and systemic acidosis, hypothermia, and coagulopathy. In these cases, the placement of a temporary intraluminal shunt in the injured artery has restored perfusion and allowed resuscitation of the patient. The placement of a shunt also allows a more controlled evaluation and treatment of orthopedic and soft tissue injuries without ongoing ischemia.[23]

Observation of Injuries

Clinical and experimental evidence exists suggesting that angiographically identified arterial lesions in patent vessels can heal without surgical intervention.[24,25] The natural history of intimal injury in a patent vessel is not clearly known, and the incidence of progression to thrombosis or becoming a source of distal embolization is unknown. The selective use of nonoperative observation and serial follow-up has been applied to angiographically documented intimal flaps, segmental arterial narrowing, and pseudoaneurysms. Although arteriovenous fistulas have been reported to close spontaneously, significant late sequelae including edema of the extremity, cutaneous ulceration, and high-output congestive heart failure have been reported, making them less optimal for observation.[26,27]

The observational management of clinically occult segmental narrowing, intimal flap, or pseudoaneurysm is safe provided the patients have close follow-up until complete resolution. A smaller percentage of patients with these findings will progress to symptomatic vascular problems even several years later.[28] As many as 61% will go on to complete resolution and 18% will progress to requiring surgery at some time in the future. The ideal criteria for observational management include intact distal circulation, a complaint patient willing to participate in regular follow-up, small lesion on angiogram (<5 mm), a low-velocity injury such as a stab wound, and an injury in a vessel difficult to expose or control such as the vertebral artery. It is imperative that the treating surgeon direct the plan of management and be familiar with the initial angiogram interpretation, duplex examinations in follow-up, and decisions for endovascular or antiplatelet therapies.

Endovascular Approaches

Endovascular treatment of vascular trauma includes the placement of embolization coils and intravascular stents or the employment of stented grafts.[29–31] The potential advantages include decreased blood loss, less invasive insertion procedure, reduced anesthesia requirements, and limited need for an extensive dissection in a traumatic wound. This approach is appealing in the critically ill trauma victim. Initial reports are encouraging for patency; however, documentation of longer-term effectiveness must be obtained before generalized use can be recommended[32–35] (Table 37.3). In a review of 15 cases there was 100% patency with follow-up from 2 months to 1 year.

Issues Based on Location of Injury

Cervical Vascular Injury

The neck is commonly divided into three anatomical areas as an aid to workup and operative planning. Zone I is the thoracic outlet extending from clavicle/sternal notch to cricoid cartilage. Injuries here usually require proximal control

through the chest via a sternotomy or thoracotomy. Zone II is from cricoid to angle of mandible and is the easiest region to expose surgically. Zone III is above the angle of the mandible to the base of the skull and a much more difficult area for exposure of the carotid or vertebral artery.

In stable patients with penetrating neck injury, the selective workup of injuries has gained popularity by virtue of its safety and cost-effectiveness.[36,37] Angiography is of the greatest value in assessing possible injuries to the vertebral arteries and trauma in zones I and III.[38] In zone II, physical examination resulted in a 0.9% (1/110) missed injury rate, similar to that of angiography. Clinical evaluation is highly accurate in determining which patients with zone II injuries need surgical intervention; however, there is a significant incidence of occult, asymptomatic vascular injuries.[39,40]

The vast majority of carotid artery injuries are from penetrating trauma. Exposure of the carotid in zones II and III is through an incision anterior to the sternocleidomastoid muscle from the angle of the mandible to just above the clavicle. Injuries at the thoracic outlet are approached via a median sternotomy and ipsilateral anterior neck incision.

The technical aspects of reconstruction of carotid injuries follow the same principles as other vascular injuries. For carotid injuries that require an interposition graft, mobilization of the external carotid artery and for an autologous conduit has been used successfully.[41]

The incidence of carotid injury after blunt trauma is small (0.08%–0.86%); however, the neurological consequences can be devastating.[42] Most injuries are identified only after neurological events or when the brain CT scan does not correlate with the patient's neurological exam. Currently, the mainstay of therapy is anticoagulation to prevent clot propagation and embolic stroke.

Vertebral artery injuries have been diagnosed with increasing frequency with the more liberal use of helical scanning, MRI, and arteriography. Ligation of the vessel is readily accomplished proximally at its takeoff from the subclavian artery. Before ligation, the contralateral vertebral artery and circle of Willis should be studied by arteriography to assure collateral circulation. Therapeutic embolization of the vertebral artery may also be used to control bleeding or treat other injuries at the time of arteriography.

Thoracic Vascular Injuries

Injuries to vessels at the base of the neck or thoracic outlet require aggressive management and many necessitate emergency thoracotomy for definitive treatment in the unstable patient. Vessels at risk include the innominate artery, proximal carotid arteries, subclavian arteries, aortic arch, superior vena cava, innominate vein, and azygos vein. A critical decision in the management of injuries in this region is performance of an appropriate incision (Fig. 37.4). A preoperative arteriogram can assist in incision planning if the patient is stable. The proximal right subclavian, proximal left common carotid, and innominate artery and vein can be exposed through a median sternotomy.[43] The distal right subclavian and distal left subclavian arteries can be exposed supraclavicularly. The proximal left subclavian requires a trapdoor incision, a supraclavicular incision with subperiosteal removal of the middle one-third of the clavicle, or a formal left thoracotomy. Clavicular resection has the advantages of being extracavitary and resulting in minimal sequelae provided a subperiosteal resection is performed for re-

TABLE 37.3.
Endovascular Stents in Arterial and Venous Trauma.

Author	Patients	Location	Patency (%)	Follow-up
Marin et al. 1994[32]	7	Varied	100	6.5 months
Duke et al. 1997[33]	6	Carotid	100	
Goodman et al. 1998[34]	1	Renal	100	9 months
Denton et al. 1997[35]	1	Vena cava	100	2 months
Babatasi et al. 1998[72]	1	Subclavian	100	1 year
Total	15		100	

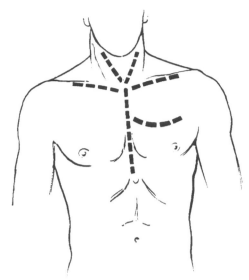

FIGURE 37.4. Incision options for the exposure of thoracic vascular injuries. Not shown is the posterolateral thoracotomy used for descending aortic injury. (From Mattox K. Vascular trauma. In: Haimovici H., ed. Vascular Surgery. Norwalk: Appleton & Lange, 1989, with permission.[4])

generation; however, it may not provide adequate proximal exposure in all injuries.[44]

Most patients with major vascular injuries of the base of the neck or thoracic outlet die before arrival at the hospital (71%). For those patients in whom operative intervention is attempted, median sternotomy with cervical extension is the incision of choice.

Thoracic Aortic Injury

Blunt thoracic aortic injury is a highly lethal injury that may present with no external signs of injury in up to 50% of cases.[4] The mechanism of injury may provide information to heighten awareness to the existence of this injury. Acute deceleration injuries result in shear and bending stress that tear the aorta at the isthmus. Most commonly this occurs following head-on motor vehicle collisions, especially if there is associated ejection or associated fatalities. Falls from height are also the type of mechanism to result in this injury; however, the distance cannot be quantified that assures risk. Physical signs of chest trauma, sternal and scapular fractures, supraclavicular bruit, diminished femoral pulses, or upper-extremity hypertension are suggestive of aortic injury. Death occurs immediately in 80% to 90% of victims and within 24 h in 30% of those who survive the initial injury.[45] A diagnostic approach is suggested in Figure 37.5.

A portable anteroposterior 40-in. chest radiograph in the trauma bay is the first study to assist in the diagnosis. The most reliable sign is loss of the aortic knob.[46] A widened mediastinum (>8 cm) has a sensitivity of 90% but a very low specificity. Chest X-ray findings associated with aortic tear are listed in Table 37.4. Cases of aortic injury have been documented in the setting of a normal initial chest film so that with the appropriate mechanism one should not be reluctant to pursue additional diagnostic workup.

The standard examination for the diagnosis of blunt injury to the aorta is aortography. Oblique views are used to

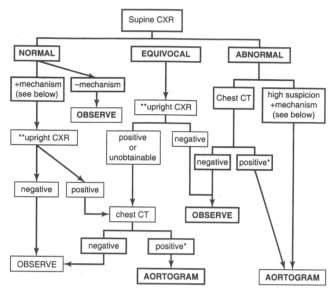

Criteria for (+) Chest CT
1. blood in posterior or middle mediastinum
2. abnormal aortic contour

+Mechanism of injury (suggested)
1. ejection from vehicle
2. fall>20ft
3. high speed MVC
4. steering wheel damage

**Must have CTLS spine cleared prior to upright CXR

FIGURE 37.5. Diagnostic imaging approach to the patient with possible thoracic aortic injury. Chest CT scan implies helical scanner with experienced physician available for interpretation.

identify intimal flap, subadvential hematoma, or false aneurysm. False-positive studies occur in 2% of studies.[47]

Recent literature supports the use of contrast-enhanced spiral or helical CT as a screening test for the diagnosis of thoracic aortic injury.[48] Diagnosis of aortic injury is based on the findings of mediastinal hematoma or direct aortic abnormality such as pseudoaneurysm, irregular border, intimal flap, or pseudocoarctation.

Transesophageal echocardiography (TEE) has also been used as a screening modality for the presence of aortic injury.

TABLE 37.4. Radiologic Signs Suggesting Aortic Rupture.

1. Transverse width of the mediastinum at the aortic knob equal to 8 cm or greater
2. Mediastinal-to-chest-width (M-C) ratio greater than 0.25 at the level of the aortic arch
3. Abnormality of the aortic contour
4. Aortopulmonary window opacification
5. Deviation of an opaque nasogastric tube to the right of the spinous process of T4
6. Deviation of the trachea or endotracheal tube to the right of midline
7. Depression of the left mainstem bronchus greater than 40° below the horizontal
8. Widening of the right paratracheal stripe to 5 mm or greater
9. Widening of the right or left paraspinal line
10. Right or left apical cap
11. The presence of left hemothorax, without associated rib fractures

Source: Reprinted from Pezzella et al. Injuries of the thoracic aorta and great vessels. In: Current Problems in Surgery: Cardiothoracic Trauma. St. Louis: Mosby, 1998, with permission.[45]

It is a more rapid, less expensive test than aortography; however, it is extremely dependent on the skill of the person operating the equipment. In many institutions these are cardiologists, although recently trauma surgeons have taken more interest in hands-on ultrasound techniques. In recent reports, the sensitivity of this technique has ranged from 63–91%. An additional advantage of TEE is the ability to perform the exam in the trauma resuscitation bay or in the operating room while the patient is undergoing other procedures.[49] The neck should be cleared of cervical spine injury before the study.

Once the diagnosis is made, emergency operation is mandated with few exceptions. Before surgical intervention, medical management to control hypertension and shearing forces can successfully temporize the patient for confirmation of the diagnosis and tolerance for the thoracotomy.[50]

Approximately 15% of injuries observed at operation can be successfully managed with primary repair, but the majority of injuries require an interposition graft. In a meta-analysis of patients with aortic injury arriving at the hospital alive, overall mortality was 32%, one-third died before surgical intervention, and among those reaching the OR in relatively stable condition, 9.9% were complicated by paraplegia.

Abdominal Vascular Injuries

Penetrating truncal wounds from the nipples to the upper thighs are the most common cause of abdominal vascular injuries, with the vessel injured related to the track of the missile or stab. Less commonly blunt injuries associated with a direct crush, posterior blow to spine, or rapid deceleration with avulsion result in major abdominal vascular injuries.[51] Physical findings may be obvious with peritoneal signs and shock or much more subtle. Femoral pulse deficits suggest major vascular injury in the abdomen. A plain abdominal X-ray should be performed in all penetrating injuries along the missile or knife tract.

Patients are explored through a midline incision, and inspection for areas of hematoma and active hemorrhage is performed with packing as needed for hemostasis. The finding of black small intestine on opening the abdomen is diagnostic of a proximal superior mesenteric artery injury.[52] Frequently there is associated gastrointestinal perforation and soilage of the abdomen with bowel contents. These enterotomies should be controlled with clamps and an assessment for ongoing hemorrhage and the presence of a major vascular injury performed before bowel repair.

Hematoma or hemorrhage associated with abdominal vascular injury occurs in the following regions: midline superior to the mesocolon, midline inferior to the mesocolon, perirenal, pelvic, and subhepatic or porta hepatitis. With appropriate visceral mobilization, aortic, caval, or other vascular control can be achieved accordingly. Damage may be controlled by repair, interposition grafting, shunting, or ligation as needed (Table 37.5).

Extremity Vascular Trauma

Upper-extremity vascular injuries are equally as common as lower-extremity vascular injuries. Injuries to the brachial artery are the most commonly reported upper-extremity injury. Upper-extremity limb loss is the exception unless there is associated major nervous and soft tissue injury. General

TABLE 37.5. Location and Survival after Abdominal Vascular Injuries.

Site of hematoma or hemorrhage	Injury	Survival rate (%)
Supramesocolic	Aorta/celiac axis	35
Supramesocolic	Superior mesenteric artery	57
Supramesocolic	Proximal renal artery	86
Inframesocolic	Aorta	45
Inframesocolic	Supra- or renal inferior vena cava	59
	Infrarenal vena cava	77
Lateral perirenal	Renal artery or vein	86–88
Pelvic	Iliac artery	61–80
	Iliac vein	70–90
Portal	Hepatic artery	No data
	Portal vein	50
Retrohepatic	Vena cava	20–40

Source: Adapted from Feliciano D. Injuries to the Great Vessels of the Abdomen. In: Scientific American Surgery, 1998–1999. New York: Scientific American, Inc., by permission.

principles are followed in approaching these injuries. Documentation of hand function is critical preoperatively, including examination of all major nerves. Functional outcome is more dependent on the associated nerve injuries than the vascular injury.[53,54] Isolated injuries to the radial or ulnar artery are best managed with ligation unless the hand shows signs of inadequate perfusion. Patency following repair of the radial or ulnar artery is only 50%, and the collateral flow through the palmar arches is satisfactory in more than 90% of individuals.[55,56]

The incidence of associated nerve injury is lower in vascular injuries to the legs. In a series of patients with femoral vascular injuries, the amputation rate was only 4.7% however, only 74% of the patients reported normal or good limb function, indicating a significant number of patients with morbidity caused by soft tissue, venous, bone, or nerve dysfunction despite a viable lower extremity. Patients with venous injuries treated with repair had a higher incidence of significant morbidity (34%) than those treated with venous ligation.[57]

The incidence of amputation after popliteal artery injury ranges from 10% to 25%.[58] When hard signs of injury such as severe ischemia are present, arteriography in the radiology department should not be performed as it delays restoration of perfusion and contributes to limb loss. Early aggressive monitoring for repair thrombosis such as with duplex ultrasonography should be done because delayed recognition of thrombosis can lead to amputation. A low threshold for performance of a prophylactic fasciotomy should be practiced and compartment pressures closely monitored. In the setting of a repair of the popliteal artery and vein together or delayed arterial repair, a fasciotomy is highly recommended.

Knee dislocation is associated with an increased incidence (23%) of popliteal vascular injury. Clinical evaluation with ABI and noninvasive testing with a duplex ultrasound is adequate to diagnose significant injuries. Arteriography is recommended on a selective basis with the majority of patients diagnosed with early duplex ultrasonography and managed with close follow-up.

In injuries below the knee, amputation is rare. Significant

morbidity does occur from hemorrhage, compartment syndrome, and associated nerve or bone injury.

A small group of patients present with a "mangled extremity" from the combination of an open, comminuted fracture, large soft tissue loss, vascular injury, and nerve injury. Crush injuries, industrial or farm accidents, or close-range shotgun wounds are reported mechanisms. These combined injuries require a multidisciplinary approach with an orthopedic surgeon and a plastic and reconstructive surgeon. The central problem is that despite the technology to revascularize and reconstruct the limb, late or secondary amputation rates remain very high. The high amputation rate is the result of prolonged functional impairment, infection, or nerve deficits.[59] The time to achieve a functional outcome may take months to more than a year in many of these types of cases.

The goal in the management of patients with a mangled extremity is to define the patient population that is best served by primary or immediate amputation and those best served by salvage and reconstruction. Compounding the problem is that patients are very reluctant to accept amputation under any circumstances.

Extremity injury severity scores have been developed to help provide objective criteria for the decision to perform an amputation. The MESS or Mangled Extremity Severity Score is one such score; it is based on skeletal/soft tissue damage, limb ischemia, shock, and age (Table 37.6).

Compartment Syndrome

Extremity musculature is divided into distinct groups or compartments by a tough layer of noncompliant fascia (Fig. 37.6). A compartment syndrome occurs when there is increased interstitial pressure within a myofascial compartment that compromises capillary perfusion and neurological function. The pressure may be the result of edema from fluid resuscitation, muscle swelling from an ischemia-reperfusion insult, or direct hemorrhage into the compartment. Unrecognized compartment syndromes lead to nerve destruction and mus-

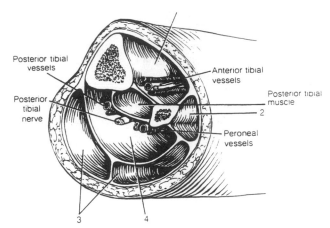

FIGURE 37.6. Cross section of calf shows location of neurovascular bundles and four fascial compartments: anterior, lateral, superficial posterior, deep posterior. (From Haimovici H. The lower extremity. In: Haimovici, ed. Vascular Surgery. Norwalk: Appleton & Lange, 1989, with permission.)

cle necrosis that result in limb loss, myoglobinuria, acute renal failure, and adult respiratory distress syndrome.

Normal capillary pressures are 15 to 25 mmHg, and normal compartment pressure is less than 10 mmHg.[60] Complete cessation of tissue perfusion in extremities has been documented when compartment pressure exceeds 35 mmHg in the calf; this is well below mean arterial pressure and indicates that cell death from lack of perfusion can occur in compartment syndrome despite the presence of palpable pulses. Anaerobic metabolism starts when the gradient between mean arterial pressure and compartmental pressure is reduced to less than 40 mmHg in traumatized muscle.[61] Ischemic neuronal injury is evident after only 15 min of anaerobic metabolism; however, if perfusion is restored the changes are entirely reversible. Irreversible damage to nerves and muscles occurs within 4 to 6 h of ischemia.

Compartment syndromes can occur in the buttock,[62] thigh, calf, forearm, hand, and foot. The calf is most frequently involved because of the lack of compliancy of the fascia. The diagnosis of compartment syndrome can be made clinically. The physical findings are pain, tenderness, hypoesthesia, weakness, and a tense compartment. Passive stretch of the compartment muscles produces pain out of proportion to the situation. Hypoesthesia in the interdigit space between the first and second toes is an early finding of an anterior compartment syndrome associated with dysfunction of the deep peroneal nerve. The diagnosis is more difficult in the sedated or unconscious patient because clinical signs may be absent.

Direct measurement of compartment pressures is the most practical and widely used diagnostic test. A straightforward technique is to use the strain gauge transducer-amplifier that is used to measure arterial pressure in the intensive care unit. The transducer is attached to noncompliant tubing and a 20-gauge needle in a closed system. The needle is directly passed into the compartment through prepped and anesthetized skin. Care must be taken to measure pressures in all four compartments in the calf, including the deep posterior compartment, which can easily be missed (see Fig. 37.6). Measured pressures less than 30 mmHg are unlikely to produce neuromuscular injury and can be observed. Fas-

TABLE 37.6. MESS: Mangled Extremity Severity Score.

Diagnosis	Points
Skeletal/soft tissue injury	
Low-energy (stab, simple fracture)	1
Medium energy (open/multiple fracture)	2
High energy (shotgun or crush)	3
Limb ischemia	
Reduced pulse but normal perfusion	1[a]
Pulseless, parasthesias	2[a]
Cool, paralyzed, insensate	3[a]
Shock	
Blood pressure always >90	0
Hypotensive transiently	1
Persistent hypotension	2
Age (years)	
<30	0
>30 but <50	1
>50	2

Sum individual diagnoses for MESS; MESS >7 suggests amputation.

[a]Score is doubled for ischemia >6 h.

Source: Johansen J, Daines M, Howley T, et al. J Trauma, 1990.[73]

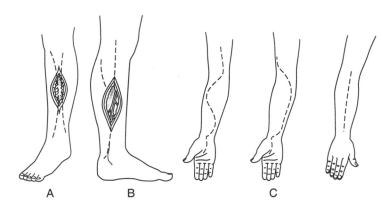

FIGURE 37.7. Incisions used for upper and lower fasciotomies. Incision extends full length of *dashed lines*. (From Omert X, Rich X. Peripheral vascular complications. In: Maull, Rodriguez, Wiles, eds. Complications in Trauma and Critical Care. Philadelphia: Saunders, 1996, with permission.)

ciotomy should be performed for compartment pressures greater than 35 to 40 mmHg, although some have advocated even higher pressures.[63]

Fasciotomy of the calf is performed using either of two techniques. All four compartments must be decompressed. Fibulectomy accomplishes this through a single lateral incision and is associated with no long-term morbidity. It is an extensive dissection that puts the peroneal artery and veins at risk. A two-incision, four-compartment fasciotomy also accomplishes the decompression and is used most frequently (Fig. 37.7). A long anteriolateral incision is made 2 cm anterior to the shaft of the fibula to open the anterior and lateral compartments. A second long posteromedial incision is made 2 cm posterior to the tibia to decompress the superficial and deep posterior compartments. The thigh contains three compartments and the forearm two compartments. At the time of fasciotomy nonviable muscle should be debrided, and tissue that is questionable be reinspected in the operating room 24 h later. A high index of suspicion is required to avoid the devastating consequences of this entirely preventable problem. Liberal use of prophylactic fasciotomy is recommended in the trauma population with vascular injuries and concurrent injuries that distract from the clinical evaluation of the leg.

Venous Injuries

The true incidence of venous injuries in the extremities is unknown because workup of extremity vascular injury focuses on arterial injury and literature on venous trauma examines primarily the patient population with concurrent arterial injury. Furthermore, there is little documentation of adverse consequences of a missed isolated venous injury.[64]

Venous injuries encountered during exploration for arterial injury should be repaired unless repair will delay treatment of associated injuries or destabilize the patient's condition. Repair provides the theoretical advantages of decreased soft tissue bleeding, improved patency of the arterial repair, and reduced severity of postphlebitic syndrome.[65] Despite this recommendation, there are equal clinical and retrospective data to indicate that treatment with ligation and leg elevation, compression stockings, and liberal use of fasciotomy provide similar results.[1]

Venous Thromboembolism After Trauma

A recent large prospective study has helped define the incidence of venous thromboembolism in trauma patients.[66] Geerts and coworkers reported that 201 of 349 (58%) patients with Injury Severity Scores (ISS) greater than 9 developed deep-vein thrombosis (DVT) as diagnosed by bilateral contrast venography. No mechanical or pharmacological antithrombotic prophylaxis was used during the study. Proximal deep-vein thrombosis was diagnosed in 63 patients (18%). Only 3 of the 201 patients had clinical signs of DVT before the diagnosis by venography. In the group of 63 patients with proximal DVT, 3 died of massive pulmonary embolism. Multivariate analysis revealed five statistically significant factors that were independent predictors of DVT: older age (odds ratio, 1.05 per year of age); blood transfusion; surgery, fracture of femur or tibia; and spinal cord injury. Clearly DVT is a significant problem in trauma patients who require prophylaxis. Greenfield and coworkers have developed a risk assessment profile for thromboembolism (RAPT) (Table 37.7) in which a score of 5 or greater indicates a threefold greater incidence of DVT.[67] See Chapter 49 for a complete discussion on prophylaxis and treatment of DVT.

TABLE 37.7. Risk Assessment Profile for Thromboembolism (RAPT).

Diagnosis	Weight
Underlying conditions	
Obese (>120% Metropolitan Life Table)	2
Abnormal coagulation factors	2
Iatrogenic factors	
Central femoral line >24 h	2
Transfusions >4 in first 24 h	2
Surgical procedure >2 h	2
Repair or ligation major venous injury	3
Injury-related factors	
AIS >2 for chest or abdomen	2
Spinal fractures	2
Coma (GCS <8 for >4 h)	3
Complex lower-extremity fracture	4
Pelvic fracture	4
Paraplegia or quadriplegia	4
Age (years)	
>40	2
>60	3
>75	4

Sum individual diagnoses. RAPT >5 indicates high-risk group.

Source: Greenfield L, Proctor M, Rodriguez J, et al. Posttrauma thromboembolism prophylaxis. J Trauma 1997;42:100–103.[67]

References

1. Shackford SR, Rich NH. Peripheral vascular injury. In: Moore E, Mattox K, Feliciano D, eds. Trauma Stamford: Appleton & Lange, 1996:819–851.

2. Mattox KL, Feliciano DV, Burch J, et al. Five thousand seven hundred sixty cardiovascular injuries in 4459 patients: epidemiologic evolution 1958 to 1987. Ann Surg 1989;209:698–707.

3. Haimovici H. Metabolic complications of acute arterial occlusions and related conditions: role of free radicals. In: Haimovici H, ed. Vascular Surgery. Norwalk: Appleton & Lange, 1989:386–408.

4. Mattox K. Vascular trauma. In: Haimovici H, ed. Vascular Surgery. Norwalk: Appleton & Lange, 1989:370–385.

5. Richardson JD, Vitale GC, Flint LM Jr. Penetrating arterial trauma. Arch Surg 1987;122:678.

6. Sirinek K, Levine B, Gaskill H, et al. Reassessment of the role of routine operative exploration in vascular trauma. J Trauma 1981;21:339–344.

7. Higashida RT, Halbach VV, Tsai FY, et al. Interventional neurovascular treatment of traumatic carotid and vertebral artery lesions: results in 234 cases. Am J Radiol 1989;153:577.

8. Becker GJ, Benenati JF, Zemel G, et al. Percutaneous placement of a balloon-expandable intraluminal graft for life-threatening subclavian arterial hemorrhage. J Vasc Interventional Radiol 1991;2:225.

9. Sclafani SJA, Shatzker D, Scalea T. The removal of intravascular bullets by interventional radiology: the prevention of central migration by balloon occlusion—case report. J Trauma 1991;31:1423.

10. McDonald EJ, Goodman PC, Winestock DP. The clinical indications for arteriography in trauma to the extremity. Radiology 1975;116:45.

11. Reid JDS, Weigelt JA, Thal ER, et al. Assessment of proximity of a wound to major vascular structures as an indication for arteriography. Arch Surg 1988;123:942.

12. Ben-Menachem Y, Fisher R. Radiology. In: Feliciano D, Moore E, Mattox K, eds. Trauma. Stamford: Appleton & Lange, 1996:207–236.

13. Frykberg ER, Feliciano DV. Arteriography of the injured extremity: are we in proximity to an answer? J Trauma 1992;32:551.

14. Kaufman JA, Parker JE, Gillespie DL, et al. Arteriography for proximity of injury in penetrating extremity trauma. J Vasc Interventional Radiol 1992;3:719.

15. Weaver PA, Yellin AE, Bauer M, et al. Is arterial proximity a valid indication for arteriography in penetrating extremity trauma? Arch Surg 1990;125:1256.

16. Francis H, Thal ER, Weigelt JA, et al. Vascular proximity: is it a valid indication for arteriography in asymptomatic patients? J Trauma 1991;31:512.

17. Schwartz M, Weaver F, Yellin A. The utility of color flow doppler examination in penetrating extremity arterial trauma. Am Surg 1993;59:375–378.

18. Johansen K, Lynch K, Paun M, et al. Non-invasive vascular tests reliably exclude occult arterial trauma in injured extremities. J Trauma 1991;31:515–522.

19. Dillon EH, van Leeuwen MS, Fernandez MA, et al. Spiral CT angiography. Am J Radiol 1993;160:1273.

20. McCready RA, Logan NM, Daugherty ME, et al. Long term results with autogenous tissue repair of traumatic extremity vascular injuries. Ann Surg 1987;206:804.

21. Mitchell FL III, Thal ER. Results of venous interposition grafts in arterial injuries. J Trauma 1990;30:336.

22. Melissinos EG, Parks DH. Post-trauma reconstruction with free tissue-transfer-analysis of 442 consecutive cases. J Trauma 1989;29:1095.

23. Johansen K, Bandyk D, Thiele B, et al. Temporary intraluminal shunts: resolution of management dilemma in complex vascular injuries. J Trauma 1982;22:395.

24. Frykberg ER, Vines FS, Alexander RH. The natural history of clinically occult arterial injuries: a prospective evaluation. J Trauma 1989;29:577–583.

25. Frykberg ER, Crump JM, Dennis JW, et al. Nonoperative observation of clinically occult arterial injuries: a prospective evaluation. Surgery (St. Louis) 1991;109:85–96.

26. Mills JL, Wiedeman JE, Robinson JG, et al. Minimizing mortality and morbidity from iatrogenic arterial injuries: the need for early recognition and prompt repair. J Vasc Surg 1986;4:22.

27. Perry MO. Complications of missed arterial injuries. J Vasc Surg 1993;17:399–407.

28. Stain S, Yellin A, Weaver F, et al. Selective management of nonocclusive arterial injuries. Arch Surg 1989;124:1136–1140.

29. Ohki. Endovascular approaches for traumatic arterial lesions. Semin Vasc Surg 1997;10:272–285.

30. Whigham C, Bodenhamer J, Miller J. Use of the palmaz stent in primary treatment of renal artery intimal injury secondary to blunt trauma. J Vasc Interventional Radiol 1995;6:175–178.

31. Reber P, Patel A, Do D, et al. Surgical implications of failed endovascular therapy for postraumatic femoral arteriovenous fistula repair. J Trauma 1999;46:352–354.

32. Marin ML, Veith FJ, Panetta TF, et al. Transluminally placed endovascular stented graft repair for arterial trauma. J Vasc Surg 1994;3:466–473.

33. Duke BJ, Ryu RK, Coldwell DM, et al. Treatment of blunt injury to the carotid artery by using endovascular stents: an early experience. J Neurosurg 1997;6:825–829.

34. Goodman DN, Saibil EA, Kodama RT. Traumatic intimal tear of the renal artery treated by insertion of a Palmaz stent. Cardiovasc Interventional Radiol 1998;1:69–72.

35. Denton JR, Moore EE, Coldwell DM. Multimodality treatment for grade V hepatic injuries: perihepatic packing, arterial embolization, and venous stenting. J Trauma 19975;5:964–968.

36. Jurkovich GJ, Zingarelli W, Wallace J, Curreri PW. Penetrating neck trauma: diagnostic studies in the asymptomatic patient. J Trauma 1985;25:819.

37. Wood J, Fabian TC, Mangiante EC. Penetrating neck injuries: recommendations for selective management. J Trauma 1989;29:602–605.

38. Sclafani SJA, Panetta T, Goldstein AS, et al. The management of arterial injuries caused by penetration of Zone III of neck. J Trauma 1985;25:871.

39. Beitsch P, Weigelt J, Flynn E, et al. Physical examination and arteriography in patients with penetrating zone II neck wounds. Arch Surg 1994;129:577–581.

40. Biffl W, Moore E, Rehse D, et al. Selective management of penetrating neck trauma based on cervical level of injury. Am J Surg 1997;174:678–682.

41. Thal E. Injury to the neck. In: Moore E, Mattox K, Feliciano D, eds. Trauma. Stamford: Appleton & Lange, 1996:329–343.

42. Biffl W, Moore E, Ryu R, et al. The unrecognized epidemic of blunt carotid arterial injuries: early diagnosis improves neurologic outcome. Ann Surg 1998;4:462–470.

43. Graham JM, Feliciano DV, et al. Innominate vascular injury. J Trauma 1982;22:647.

44. Demetriades D, Rabinowitz B, Pezikis A, et al. Subclavian vascular injuries. Br J Surg 1987;74:1001.

45. Pezzella AT, Silva WE, Lancey RA. Injuries of the thoracic aorta and great vessels. In: Pezzella AT, Silva WE, Lancey RA, eds. Current Problems in Surgery: Cardiothoracic Trauma. St. Louis: Mosby, 1998:762–771.

46. Miller F, Richardson J, Thomas H. Role of CT in the diagnosis of major arterial injury after blunt thoracic trauma. Surgery (St. Louis) 1989;106:596.

47. Sturm J, Hankins D, Young G. Thoracic aortography following blunt chest trauma. Am J Emerg Med 1980;8:92–96.

48. Dyer DS, Moore EE, Mestek M, et al. Thoracic aortic injury: how predictive is mechanism and is chest CT a reliable screening tool? A prospective study of 1000 patients (abstract). J Trauma 1998;45:190.

49. Cohn SM, Burns GA, Jaffee C, Milner KA. Exclusion of aortic tear in the unstable trauma patient: the utility of transesophageal echocardiography. J Trauma 1995;39:1087–1090.

50. Pate JW, Gavant ML, Weiman DS, et al. Traumatic rupture of the aortic isthmus: program of selective management. World J Surg 1999;23:59–63.

51. Roth SM, Wheeler JR, Gregory RT, et al. Blunt injury of the abdominal aorta: a review. J Trauma 1997;42:748–755.

52. Feliciano D, Burch J, Graham J. Abdominal vascular injury. In: Moore E, Mattox K, Feliciano D, eds. Trauma. Stamford: Appleton & Lange, 1996:615–633.

53. Borman KR, Snyder WH III, Weigelt JA. Civilian arterial trauma of the upper extremity. An 11 year experience in 267 patients. Am J Surg 1984;6:796–799.

54. Orcutt MB, Levine BA, Gaskill HV, et al. Civilian vascular trauma of the upper extremity. J Trauma 1986;26:63–67.

55. Johnson M, Ford M, Johansen K, Combined Hand Surgery Service. Radial or ulnar artery laceration: repair or ligate? Arch Surg 1992;128:971–975.

56. Ballard JL, Bunt TJ, Malone JM. Management of small artery vascular trauma. Am J Surg 1992;4:316–319.

57. Cargile JS III, Hunt JL, Purdue GF. Acute trauma of the femoral artery and vein. J Trauma 1992;3:364–371.

58. Melton SM, Croce MA, Patton JH Jr, et al. Popliteal artery trauma. Systemic anticoagulation and intraoperative thrombolysis improves limb salvage. Ann Surg 1997;5:518–529.

59. Lin C, Wei F, Levin S, et al. The functional outcome of lower-extremity fractures with vascular injury. J Trauma 1997;43:480–485.

60. Rohrer MJ. Compartment syndromes. In: Irwin, Cerra, Rippe, eds. Intensive Care Medicine. Philadelphia: Lippincott, 1999:2058–2065.

61. Heppenstall R, Sapega A, Scott R, et al. The compartment syndrome. An experimental and clinical study of muscular energy metabolism using phosphorus nuclear magnetic spectroscopy. Clin Orthop 1988;226:138–155.

62. Bleicher R, Sherman H, Latenser B. Bilateral gluteal compartment syndrome. 1997;42:118–122.

63. Matsen F, Winquist R, Krugmire R. Diagnosis and management of compartmental syndromes. J Bone Joint Surg 1980;62:286–291.

64. Arrillaga A, Nagy K, Frykberg E. Practice management guidelines for management of penetrating trauma to the lower extremity. EAST web page. http://www.eat.org/tpg.html 1998:2–8.

65. Arrillaga A, Taylor S. Natural history of penetrating lower extremity venous injuries: a case report of recanalization after nonoperative treatment. J Trauma 1999;46:1126–1129.

66. Geerts W, Code K, Jay R, et al. A prospective study of venous thromboembolism after major trauma. N Engl J Med 1994;331:1601–1606.

67. Greenfield L, Proctor M, Rodriguez J, et al. Posttrauma thromboembolism prophylaxis. J Trauma 1997;42:100–103.

68. Bynoe R, Miles W, Bell R, et al. Noninvasive diagnosis of vascular trauma by duplex ultrasonography. J Vasc Surg 1991;14:346–352.

69. Fry W, Smith R, Sayers D, et al. The success of duplex ultrasonographic scanning in diagnosis of extremity vascular proximity trauma. Arch Surg 1993;128:1368–1372.

70. Bergstein J, Blair J, Edwards J, et al. Pitfalls in the use of color-flow duplex ultrasound for screening of suspected arterial injuries in penetrated extremities. J Trauma 1992;33:395–402.

71. Knudson M, Lewis F, Atkinson K, et al. The role of duplex ultrasound arterial imaging in patients with penetrating extremity trauma. Arch Surg 1993;128:1033–1038.

72. Babataski G, Massetti M, Le Page O, et al. Endovascular treatment of a traumatic subclavian artery aneurysm. J Trauma 1998;44:545–547.

73. Johansen J, Daines M, Howley T, et al. Objective criteria accurately predict amputation following lower extremity trauma. J Trauma 1990;30:568–573.

Minimally Invasive Approaches to Vascular Disease

Rishad M. Faruqi and Timothy A.M. Chuter

General Considerations

The concept of improving arterial blood flow by dilating a stenotic lesion and the development of the catheter-based balloon revolutionized the field. These two contributions, along with the development of improved imaging modalities, have been the foundation on which the field of endovascular intervention has developed.

Initially, it was thought that percutaneous transluminal angioplasty (PTA) worked by plaque compression and redistribution.[1] However, this is not the case. Plaque fracture with medial and adventitial stretching is largely responsible for the success of PTA[2]; also, a *localized dissection* of the media is *necessary* for PTA and stenting to be effective.[3,4] A "controlled" injury is needed for the PTA to be optimal, although obviously overstretching the vessel to the point of adventitial disruption or extensive dissection is to be avoided.

The technical success of PTA is related to the morphology of the lesion, its location, and the disease process that caused the lesion. The clinical indication for PTA is also an important determinant of outcome. Limb-threatening ischemia is often associated with advanced disease and hence a poorer outcome. Short stenotic lesions yield better results than longer lesions or occlusions. Concentric lesions are easier to treat than eccentric ones. Lesions located near the origin of the vessel or at branch points are more likely to have a suboptimal outcome compared to lesions further along the vessel. In cases of fibromuscular dysplasia of the renal arteries, PTA is often curative, whereas atherosclerotic lesions are less likely to have similar rates of long-term cure. Conversely, myointimal hyperplasia of vein grafts seldom respond well to PTA. A heavily calcified plaque is less amenable to PTA and often requires higher inflation pressures, and the extent of lesion calcification is directly related to the incidence of overdistension-related injuries.[5] Finally, the extent of distal disease is also considered an important determinant for the long-term success of the procedure because poor runoff is often associated with a high failure rate.

Unfortunately, data review is problematic because reporting guidelines have not been universally standardized. As a result, it is sometimes difficult to perform an objective comparison between the results of various groups reporting on the same procedure, let alone compare endovascular procedures with surgery.

Technique

Vascular Access

All procedures are performed under sterile conditions. Percutaneous access to the target vessel is usually obtained via the femoral artery, although the brachial artery has also been used for this purpose. After infiltration of the subcutaneous tissue with a local anesthetic agent. The cannule is exchanged over a guidewire for a catheter or sheath.

Arteriography

The catheter, having been appropriately positioned, is connected to a power injector filled with contrast. After ensuring that the column of contrast is free of air, a series of angiograms are obtained to visualize the lesion(s), the state of the rest of the vascular tree, and the runoff. The lesion is visualized in at least two projections, and a detailed assessment, including the type of lesion, the presence of a pressure gradient, the degree of calcification, and the presence of aneurysmal disease or ulceration, is made.

Measurements

A calibration device is used to assess the extent of lumen compromised, the length of the lesion, and the caliber of the normal vessel proximal and distal to the lesion. Hemodynamic measurements are made to assess the pressure gradient across the lesion. A peak systolic gradient greater than 10 to 15 mmHg is considered hemodynamically significant.

PTA

An appropriate balloon is selected based on the measurements made as just described. With the wire in place through the lesion, the balloon catheter is threaded into position and inflated gently with dilute contrast. Although inflation pressures of 10 to 12 atm may be required to achieve the desired result, lower pressures are used during the initial inflation. The inflation is usually continued until there is no longer a waist in the balloon.

Completion

If angiographic appearances and the absence of a significant pressure gradient suggest a satisfactory result, the angiographic catheter is removed along with the sheath. Compression to the puncture site is applied for 15 to 20 min either manually or with specially constructed closure devices. The patient is instructed to lie supine for 4 to 6 h before ambulating and to keep well hydrated to minimize the nephrotoxic effects of the contrast medium. Antiplatelet agents such as aspirin, ticlopidine, or clopidogrel are often given after PTA.

Stents

The advent of intravascular stents has clearly expanded the indications for percutaneous interventions in vascular disease. Stents buttress the arterial wall and resist the elastic recoil of the artery, thereby preventing immediate restenosis; they are also used to treat post-PTA dissection. Stents do not necessarily improve the long-term patency following PTA, because they do not prevent neointimal hyperplasia.

Balloon-Expandable Stents

The advantages of these types of stents are that they have excellent radial strength and are consequently designed to resist the elastic recoil of the artery. Moreover, they can be sequentially expanded with progressively larger balloons until there is no residual stenosis or pressure gradient present.

Self-Expanding Stents

These stents expand by elastic recoil without the aid of balloon inflation until they reach their resting diameter or the diameter of the artery. Self-expanding stents are more compliant than balloon-expanded stents. This lack of "radial strength" makes them unsuitable for heavily calcified lesions.

Complications

Puncture site complications include bleeding, with hematoma or pseudoaneurysm, dissection, acute thrombosis, embolization, arteriovenous fistula, and nerve injury. Careful local-

ization of the puncture site and single wall puncture technique help to minimize bleeding complications. A high femoral puncture can cause a retroperitoneal hematoma, which may be missed on clinical examination. The risk of bleeding complications is also increased by postprocedure anticoagulation, thrombolysis, and large-bore arterial access. If the route of leakage persists, a false aneurysm develops. Most false aneurysms resolve spontaneously; others can be treated by ultrasound-guided compression or thrombin injection. Continuing hemorrhage, aneurysm expansion, and signs of femoral nerve compression are indications for urgent surgical repair.

Distal embolization is more common when manipulating severely diseased vessels. It is important to compare pre- and postprocedure angiograms to allow early recognition of the emboli, which can then be aspirated or lysed. Massive embolization can lead to limb loss, stroke, blindness, renal failure, and even death depending on the site of obstruction.

The use of nonionic contrast materials has diminished the incidence of contrast-related complications. Predisposing factors include age, diabetes, and preexisting renal impairment. Such patients should be well hydrated before and after the procedure.

Iliac Artery PTA and Stenting

Indications

Several studies question the need for iliac artery PTA in patients with mild to moderate claudication and suggest that PTA should be reserved for those with truly disabling or lifestyle-limiting claudication, rest pain, limb-threatening ischemia, or tissue loss (ischemic ulceration or gangrene). Another indication for PTA of the iliac arteries with or without stenting is to improve inflow before an infrainguinal or femoro–femoral bypass procedure. This approach is based on the untested assumption that the progression of iliac disease will jeopardize the patency of the bypass graft. Also, improvement in inflow alone may alleviate the symptoms and obviate the need for surgery.

Recanalization of Occluded Iliac Arteries

Until quite recently, an occluded iliac artery was considered a relative contraindication for PTA and stenting because manipulation might shower emboli distally. However, in recent series the embolization rate was less than 5% to 7%. Recanalization of occluded iliac arteries is not only feasible but appears to have acceptable long-term patency rates (Fig. 38.1).[6–11]

Results

When comparing results of different reports, one needs to take into account differences in the indication for treatment, the type of lesion, the method of determining patency, and the method of statistical analysis. The effect of patency assesment was well illustrated in a Dutch study in which primary patency at 2 years was 85% using hemodynamic criteria (ABI),

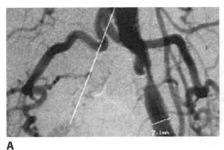
A
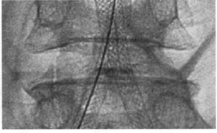
B
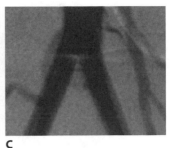
C

FIGURE 38.1. The use of "kissing stents" in the revascularization of both common iliac arteries. **A.** Occluded right common iliac artery with stenotic left common iliac artery. **B.** Recanalization of right common iliac artery with primary stenting of the left common iliac artery. **C.** Final result.

77% using clinical criteria, and only 70% using duplex scanning.[12] The indication for intervention is also a determinant of short- and long-term success. Patients treated for claudication do better than those treated for rest pain, critical ischemia, or tissue loss. The latter are almost invariably associated with more extensive disease, longer and more complex lesions, occlusions, and poorer distal runoff, all of which result in poorer outcome. Differing methods of statistical analysis also alter the results.

Most studies report a high technical success rate with acceptable primary and secondary patency rates. In one meta-analysis, there was a 91% and 96% initial technical success rate, a 64% and 77% primary patency rate, and an 80% and 88% secondary patency rate in patients treated with PTA and stenting, respectively.[13] However, if technical failures are included in the meta-analysis, the secondary patency rate at 4 years drops from 80% and 88% to 58% and 74% for PTA and stenting, respectively.[13]

Complications and Predictors of Outcome

The complication rate following iliac angioplasty varies from 1% to 52% (Fig. 38.2).[4,6,8,9,12,14–22] Most groups report major complications under 7% with an embolization rate of less than 5%.

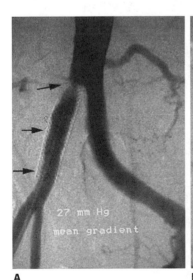
A
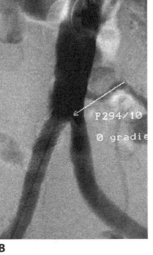
B

FIGURE 38.2. Restenosis of right common iliac artery following stent deployment. **A.** Angiogram demonstrates myointimal hyperplasia (arrows) 9 months following stent placement. **B.** Final result after using PTA for rescue.

As discussed earlier, occlusions, long-segment stenoses, tandem lesions, female gender, and the need for multiple stents are all associated with poorer outcome.[21,23] In addition, superficial femoral artery (SFA) occlusion, smoking, stent diameter less than 8 mm, a higher level of baseline ischemia, and younger age normotensive patients have a worse long-term outlook.[24] SFA occlusions are associated with a lower poorer initial technical success rate and a poorer long-term outcome.[25]

Open Surgery Versus Percutaneous Intervention

The less invasive nature of percutaneous intervention is a clear advantage that has led to a steady decline in the number of patients undergoing open surgical reconstruction of the aortoiliac circulation. Nevertheless, there is still some debate whether the results of interventional treatment are as durable as those of surgery. Most studies demonstrating excellent patency rates for percutaneous intervention have a relatively short follow-up period. Comparisons between these two treatment modalities are often difficult because patients who undergo surgery often have more extensive disease with more severe symptoms.[26] The Veterans Administrations Cooperative Study no. 199 was a prospective, randomized trial comparing PTA with surgery.[27] The study demonstrated that if early failures were excluded from the analysis, the two forms of treatment offered equivalent results over a 3-year period; if early treatment failures were included, surgery was significantly superior. The main indication for treatment in this study was claudication. The results of PTA might have been worse in patients with more severe disease, who typically undergo surgical repair. Whether there is truly a cost-savings benefit of PTA over conventional surgery remains to be seen.

Renal PTA and Stenting

Indications

The prevalence of renovascular hypertension is estimated to be 0.13% in the United States,[1] while renovascular disease is responsible for only 3% to 5% of all patients with hypertension.[2] The most common causes of renal artery stenosis are atherosclerosis and fibromuscular dysplasia. Other rarer causes include Takayasu's arteritis (nonspecific aortoarteritis), transplant renal artery stenosis, middle aortic syndrome, William's syndrome, and neurofibromatosis. The morbidity associated with the treatment and the chances of long-term success must be viewed in the context of the patient's phys-

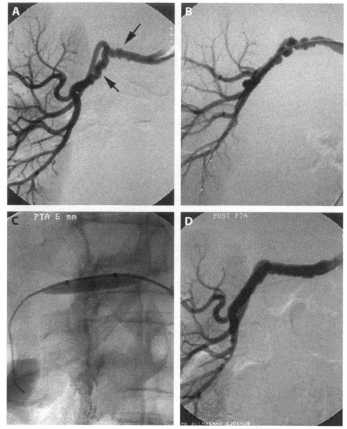

FIGURE 38.3. Percutaneous transluminal renal angioplasty (PTRA) for fibromuscular dysplasia (FMD) in a 41-year-old woman with uncontrollable hypertension. **A.** Diagnostic angiogram shows pathognomonic "string of beads" appearance. **B.** Lesion is crossed with a wire. **C.** PTA using a 6-mm balloon. **D.** Final result with excellent clinical outcome.

iological condition and life expectancy before an informed decision regarding the best treatment option is made for each individual patient. The mere presence of a renal artery stenosis is not in itself an indication for treatment. Most lesions neither produce hypertension nor imperil renal function. In patients with renal stenosis who are being managed medically, renal function needs to be regularly monitored. When these parameters change, the indications for treatment must be reassessed.[1]

The indications for percutaneous transluminal renal angioplasty (PTRA) and/or stent insertion are the presence of a hemodynamically significant renal artery lesion in the face of accelerated or "difficult to control" hypertension (with or without renal insufficiency) (Fig. 38.3), noncompliance or intolerance of antihypertensive medication, and loss of renal mass or worsening of renal function while on antihypertensive medication.

Results

Follow-up data has varied greatly as to the mode of assessment of outcome. Some have used clinical criteria, such as blood pressure and serum creatinine, while others have used anatomical criteria based on either Duplex imaging or angiography. Patency rates are calculated based on patient numbers by some, while others use the number of arteries or number of lesions as their denominator. Definitions of hy-

pertension and renal insufficiency are not uniform in the published literature; neither is the definition of cure or improvement. There is a paucity of data from prospective randomized trials. Follow-up has tended to be limited, making it difficult to ascertain the durability of these procedures. Comparing early series with more recent ones suggests improvement over time. Despite these varied and disparate definitions of significant disease and outcome criteria, the general trend has been toward increasing use of renal angioplasty and decreasing use of surgical reconstruction to treat renovascular hypertension and ischemic nephropathy.

Factors that affect the outcome of PTRA include the pathology of the lesion [fibromuscular dysplasia (FMD) versus atherosclerotic occlusive disease (ASOD)], the presence of renal dysfunction, the location of the stenosis (ostial or nonostial), and unilateral or bilateral disease. Although early studies suggested that PTRA was most beneficial in cases of fibromuscular dysplasia (FMD) and nonostial lesions,[3,4] recent data show acceptable results in ostial atherosclerotic lesions.[5–11]

Patients with renal dysfunction and unilateral lesions often have renal disease and tend to do worse compared with those with bilateral lesions.[7] On the other hand, the technical results of PTRA are better in patients with unilateral lesions or FMD lesions than in patients with bilateral lesions.[12] In p*atients without renal insufficiency*, unilateral lesions fare better.[13]

Technical success can usually be achieved in more than 90% of cases. Failure is usually a result of failure to cross the lesion, insufficient dilatation, the creation of an intimal flap, or thrombosis of the renal artery. These are rare occurrences, many of which can be handled by endovascular means. Most interventionalists would consider a residual stenosis of 30% or greater to be unacceptable and would either redilate the lesion or stent it. Technical success is usually associated with functional improvement. "Improvement" is defined as a 15% decrease in diastolic pressure (DP) to 90 to 110 mmHg,[14] with improved blood pressure control on the same medications as before PTRA.[5] "Benefit" is defined as cure and improvement.[5,16] It is apparent that "benefit" can be achieved in about 75% of the patients undergoing PTRA. If initial failures are included and the results analyzed on an "intention to treat basis," the results are worse.[9]

The long-term benefits of PTRA can be described in terms of patency and clinical outcome. Unfortunately, long-term follow-up data are lacking in most series published to date.

The effect of PTRA on renal function continues to be controversial. It is worth noting that only 4% of patients with renal failure have renal artery stenosis.[13] The rationale for performing PTRA for renal insufficiency is to improve renal function or prevent further deterioration and avoid the need for hemodialysis. Most studies have defined an improvement in renal function to be a decrease in serum creatinine or an increase in the glomerular filtration rate or creatinine clearance. Although numerous studies have reported an improvement or stabilization of renal function, none of these were prospective randomized trials.[4–8,10] In two separate meta-analyses, renal function was improved in 46% and 44% of patients, respectively.[5,14] Other studies that demonstrated no change in serum creatinine following PTRA reported the procedure as having "stabilized" renal function.[9,11] A carefully designed prospective, randomized, multicenter trial comparing angioplasty with medical therapy showed no difference in renal function following PTRA,[15] mainly because there was no deterioration in renal function in the medically treated arm. This result suggests a benign natural history of renal artery stenosis, but the explanation may only reflect the number of patients with a lesser degree of renal artery stenosis. Others have shown progression of the disease and deterioration of renal function with a stenosis of 60% or more.[6,16]

The reported incidence of restenosis following PTRA is 25% to 30%.[6,14] Restenosis can occur immediately following PTRA, as the result of elastic recoil, within 6 to 12 months from myointimal hyperplasia and after 2 years because of progression of disease. Certain risk factors predispose to the development of restenosis. Ostial lesions are particularly prone to elastic recoil, as are lesions with very thick aortic plaques. A residual post-PTRA stenosis of 30% or more appears to be more prone to restenosis.[5,6,12,14,17] Others have noted a higher incidence in females, who have smaller arteries.[18] When to intervene in the presence of restenosis is a difficult problem because anatomical lesions often do not correlate with functional abnormality and vice versa. Most interventionalists would intervene when restenosis exceeds 60%.

The development of intravascular stents has changed both the indications and results of PTRA. The usual indications for stent placement have been ostial lesions, a residual stenosis of 30% or more following PTRA, restenosis, dissection, or intimal flap and in the management of "difficult and complex" lesions or failed PTRA. Both balloon-expandable and self-expanding stents have been used with equivalent results.[19–21] The technical results of renal stenting have tended to be better than PTRA alone, although this may not be valid to compare recent series with stents with older series of PTRA alone. The technical success rate of renal stenting approaches 100% in more recent series.[19,20,22] Unfortunately, follow-up data with stent placement are limited, as are prospective randomized studies to determine its place in the management of renovascular hypertension and ischemic nephropathy.

The complication rates of renal angioplasty tend to be low and are usually related to puncture sites. Contrast-induced renal failure can be minimized with the use of carbon dioxide arteriography and judicious hydration. Atheroembolism is another potential cause of procedure–related declines in renal functions. Other complications include intimal flaps, vessel thrombosis, arterial rupture, and renal embolism and infarction. In a recent meta-analysis of 1118 patients, the complication rate was 9.3%.[14]

Surgery versus PTRA With or Without Stent

Operative intervention has dominated the management of renovascular disease for several decades. Only recently has its dominance has been challenged by the less invasive methods of PTRA or stenting. Although it is clear that angioplasty should be the treatment of choice for renal lesions secondary to FMD and possibly other localized, short-segment lesions, it is still a matter of debate as to the best treatment for atherosclerotic ostial lesions secondary to ASOD. Complicating the issue is the fact that most patients requiring surgery are elderly and have multiple comorbid conditions that make them less likely to tolerate the physiological consequences of surgical revascularization. Despite this, there are several reports in the surgical literature demonstrating an acceptably low perioperative mortality rate of less than 3%.[23,24] Longevity data also support the role for surgery in the man-

agement of renovascular disease.[25–27] Most of these reports, however, do not address the issue of how many patients were denied operative intervention in the face of a prohibitive operative risk. In this patient population a minimally invasive procedure is most appealing, despite the lack of long-term patency data. Patients with diffuse or branch vessel disease are best treated surgically. Patients unfit for surgery and those with FMD are best treated with PTRA.

The management of the patient with localized atherosclerotic disease who is also a surgical candidate depends on local experience. For these patients we usually recommend PTRA with selective stenting, with surgical intervention being reserved for situations where this approach is either not technically feasible or fails. Careful patient selection and experience of the surgeon/interventionalist are probably the most important determinants of outcome.

Extracranial Carotid Artery Angioplasty and Stenting

PTA and stenting are particularly appealing in cases of reoperative surgery or operations on an irradiated neck, which have increased rates of complications such as neck hematoma, respiratory compromise, wound infection, and cranial nerve injury. Occlusion time with PTA and stenting is less compared to surgery, even if the operation is performed with a shunt in place. Furthermore, PTA and stenting can treat lesions that are inaccessible surgically.

On the other hand, there are also some inherent risks associated with angioplasty and stenting of the carotid artery. The lack of distal control exposes the patient to the hazard of cerebral embolism. Current cerebral protection devices can reduce embolism associated with balloon inflation, but they do not protect against embolism during initial instrumentation of the lesion. Moreover, PTA is not always free of cardiac complications. Balloon inflation in the carotid bifurcation is often associated with profound reflex bradycardia.

Carotid artery PTA is still a relatively new technique and is still in a state of evolution. Most interventionalists would now agree that routine stenting is not necessary following PTA for FMD. There is less of a consensus regarding the role of stents following PTA for atherosclerosis. Any stent implanted in the neck should be of the self-expanding variety, because the neck is a mobile region and balloon-expandable stents are likely to deform or collapse.[1,2]

The main drawback of PTA is embolism. The risk is higher for heavily calcified lesions, symptomatic lesions and for lesions that require higher inflation pressures. Due to the embologenic potential of this procedure, several workers have suggested that in the case of carotid PTA and stenting, "less is more," and one should accept a less than perfect result, rather than strive for an angiographically perfect outcome. The presence of emboli has been detected using transcranial Doppler ultrasound[3,4] and has led to the development of cerebral protection devices that are designed to trap the debris released during the procedure.[5]

Many authors recommend that patients undergoing carotid PTA and stenting procedures should be started on an antiplatelet agent 48 h before the procedure and continued on it for at least 4 weeks following the procedure. The patient is also given 0.4 to 0.6 mg atropine i.v. to counteract baroreceptor-mediated responses to the balloon dilatation of the carotid bifurcation.

What the Published Literature Tells Us

CAROTID ENDARTERECTOMY (CEA)

The publication of several prospective multicenter trials, both in Europe and the United States, has caused a resurgence in the use of CEA.[6–19] These well-structured trials provide "level 1" evidence establishing the superiority of CEA over "best medical therapy" in the prevention of stroke in both symptomatic and asymptomatic patients with a high-grade stenosis of the carotid artery. These studies have demonstrated that CEA is a well-tolerated, safe, and durable operation, allowing patients to be discharged home free of the risk of embolic stroke within 48 h of operation. The evidence supporting its use is indisputable.

CAROTID PTA AND STENTING (PTA + S)

In a recent review it was concluded that the complication rate of PTA was unacceptably high, compared to surgery, and that most studies of PTA failed to observe standard reporting guidelines and few had much follow-up.[20] Other authors have reached similar conclusions.[21,22] Still, some studies report very promising results with PTA alone.[23]

In a 1998 publication, Wholey undertook a survey of all the carotid PTA + S performed globally.[28] He reported a technical success rate of 98.6%, with a 5.77% stroke and death rate and a 4.8% restenosis rate at 6 months.

The potential cost savings from PTA have not been demonstrated. We know from previous studies that CEA is a highly cost-effective form of treatment.[24,25] The only cost comparison showed that CEA was more cost-effective than carotid PTA + S.[26,27]

The advent of cerebral protection devices may prove to be an important development in the prevention of embolic complications during angioplasty and stenting of the carotid arteries. One report demonstrated a dramatic reduction in embolic complications with use of a coaxial cerebral protection device.[29] However, in another recent study, 6.25% of patients that did have cerebral protection did develop major neurological complications, showing the limitations of current devices.

Randomized Trials Comparing CEA with Carotid PTA + S

Six multicenter, randomized trials are currently recruiting patients. These include the *Carotid Revascularization Endarterectomy versus Stent Trial (CREST)* and the *Carotid Artery Stent versus Endarterectomy Trial (CASET)*.[30]

Current Indications for Carotid Angioplasty and Stenting

The clearest indication for carotid PTA is in a patient for whom surgery carries too high a risk of complications and medical therapy carries too high a risk of stroke. Carotid

PTA + S in the high-risk patient has been recommended under the following circumstances:

  Contralateral occlusion
  Restenosis following CEA
  Synchronous carotid and coronary disease
  Preexisting cranial nerve palsy
  Very distal and very proximal lesions
  Unusual cervical anatomy or scarring (previous neck surgery or radiation)

Endovascular Repair of Abdominal Aortic Aneurysms

Although 10 years have passed since endovascular repair of abdominal aortic aneurysm (AAA) was first reported,[1] we still lack the kind of controlled, prospective, randomized comparisons to alternative forms of therapy with which to perform an evidence-based assessment of the new technique.

Aneurysm repair is a prophylactic operation, intended to eliminate the risk of death from rupture.[2] Most of what we know about endovascular repair of AAA relates to the short term, and most of what we do not know relates to the long term. A selection of issues is listed in Table 38.1 under the headings "Known" and "Unknown," although there is clearly significant overlap between the two columns. Some of the arguments for and against each of these points are admittedly based on relatively low-level evidence. A selection of these points is discussed in further detail below.

DISTAL ATTACHMENT

The first reported cases of endovascular aneurysm repair were performed using a tube of graft fabric attached to the aorta by a single proximal stent.[1] The distal end of the graft was left free. The result was continued aneurysm perfusion and growth, even after the addition of a second stent. The inadequacy of distal aortic implantation has since been confirmed in several series. The initial computed tomography (CT) may show no leak, but subsequent CT often shows stent-graft migration, leakage around the distal end of the stent-graft (type I endoleak), or aneurysm growth.[3]

Experience has shown that the distal aortic "neck" is rarely long enough, straight enough, healthy enough, or stable enough for stent-graft implantation.[4] Angiographic appearances may be misleading in this regard because of the presence of mural thrombus. Implantation in a bed of mural thrombus is a well-recognized cause of late failure in the form of secondary leak, aneurysm growth, or aneurysm rupture. Types of distal attachment are illustrated in Figures 38.4–38.6.

PROXIMAL ATTACHMENT

The proximal stent performs two functions, fixation and sealing. Fixation is important because aortic flow generates large forces at any point where the graft changes size or direction. Self-expanding stents generate insufficient friction to prevent

TABLE 38.1. What Is Known and Unknown About Endovascular Repair of Abdominal Aortic Aneurysms.

A. Known	B. Unknown
1. Endovascular repair avoids abdominal operation.	1. Can endovascular repair be accomplished percutaneously?
2. Endovascular repair produces less physiological derangement than open repair.	2. Will new techniques allow treatment of pararenal and thoraco-abdominal aneurysms?
3. The mortality, morbidity, and length of stay are less for endovascular repair than for open repair, particularly in high-risk patients.	3. Does endovascular repair cost less than open repair?
4. Endovascular repair has particular advantages in the treatment of traumatic, inflammatory, anastomotic, and ruptured aneurysms.	4. Should high-risk patients be treated by endovascular repair?
5. It is rarely possible to obtain secure, hemostatic stent-graft implantation between the aortic aneurysm and the aortic bifurcation.	5. Should low-risk patients be treated by endovascular repair?
6. The proximal end of the stent-graft will migrate if it is not attached to nondilated aorta with barbs or supported from below by a structural framework (column strength).	6. Should small aneurysms be treated by endovascular repair?
7. Pararenal stents cause very few problems in the short term.	7. Will the implantation sites dilate over time?
8. Iliac tortuosity rarely prevents delivery system insertion.	8. What is the relationship between endoleak and aneurysm dilatation?
9. Unilateral iliac aneurysm rarely precludes endovascular aneurysm repair.	9. What is the relationship between endoleak and aneurysm rupture?
10. The iliac segment of an unsupported stent-graft is prone to kinking, folding, and thrombosis.	10. What is the potential for hematogenous stent-graft infection, and does it ever decline?
11. Successful endovascular aneurysm repair usually prevents aneurysm dilatation.	11. How durable are stent-grafts?
12. Leakage of blood directly into the aneurysm (endoleak, type I or III) represents failed repair.	12. Why do fully stented grafts sometimes kink?
13. Many patients with aortic aneurysms lack the anatomical substrate for endovascular repair.	13. What is the proper long-term follow-up?
14. Patient selection and stent-graft sizing both depend on detailed preoperative imaging.	14. Why do many patients have a fever following endovascular aneurysm repair?
15. Infection of a stent-graft is rare in the short to medium term.	
16. Clinically significant embolism is rare.	

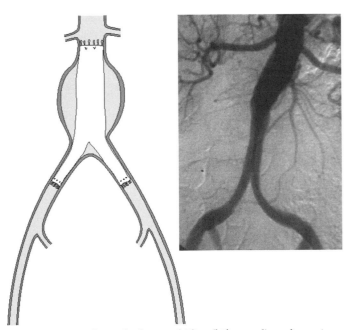

FIGURE 38.4. The unibody aortobiiliac (bifurcated) configuration.

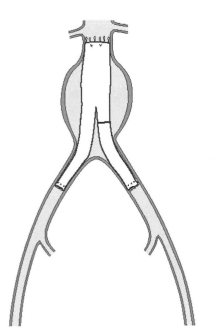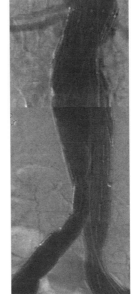

FIGURE 38.5. The modular aortobiiliac (bifurcated) stent-graft.

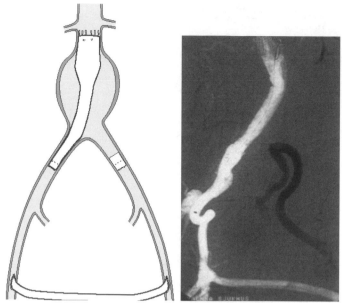

FIGURE 38.6. The aortomonoiliac (tapered) stent-graft, femoral–femoral bypass, and common iliac artery occluder.

migration.[5] Current stent-grafts employ a variety of strategies to provide additional stability. Caudally directed barbs have been shown to resist very high displacement forces.

Fully stented systems have an intrinsic "column strength" that provides the proximal stent with support from below. In addition to hanging from the aorta, these stent-grafts can be said to stand on the iliac arteries.[6] However, the stability provided by column strength comes at a price. Unless the stent-graft is absolutely straight, high column strength implies high rigidity. Rigid stent-grafts cannot accommodate aortic tortuosity and angulated implantation sites.

In the short/medium migration rates are all less than 5%.[6–10] However, recent reports suggest that in the absence of proximal barbs, the rate rises progressively, leading to reintervention in almost half of those followed for more than 4 years.

Iliac Aneurysm

Approximately 30% of patients with aortic aneurysms also have a common iliac aneurysm, most of which extend all the way to the iliac bifurcation, leaving no suitable site for stent-graft implantation in the common iliac artery. The external iliac artery is rarely involved and can be used as the site of distal stent-graft implantation. However, this approach has several disadvantages, of which the most important is internal iliac artery occlusion with potential consequences such as impotence, buttock claudication, colon ischemia, and paralysis.

Of course, all these complications are more common if both internal iliac arteries are occluded during the same procedure. For this reason, bilateral iliac aneurysm is often considered to be an exclusion criterion for endovascular aneurysm repair.

The Natural History of Endoleak

Aneurysm shrinkage does not occur in the presence of type I (leak around the proximal or distal attachment site) or type

III endoleaks (leak via tears in the fabric or component disruption), both of which allow blood to flow directly into the aneurysm. In type I, blood flows around the end of the stent-graft, and in type III blood flows through the holes in the stent-graft. Under these circumstances the aneurysm remains at risk for rupture.

Type II (retrograde collateral perfusion of AAA sac via lumbar arteries or the inferior mesenteric artery) and type IV endoleaks (graft porosity) appear to be more benign, although their natural history is not yet well defined. In the presence of a type II leak the aneurysm is less pulsatile than an untreated aneurysm[11] and less prone to dilatation.[12–14] Type IV leaks occur through tiny holes in the fabric of the graft, which seals spontaneously, resulting in cessation of leakage and a corresponding reduction in aneurysm diameter and rupture risk.

Although these broad generalizations seem to make sense, exceptions are common. Some aneurysms increase in diameter, or even rupture, despite the lack of any endoleak on CT. The term "endopressure" or "endotension" has been coined to describe such cases.

Preoperative Imaging

Endovascular repair is neither as versatile nor as flexible as conventional repair; hence, the need for detailed preoperative evaluation of arterial anatomy. One needs this information to determine the feasibility of endovascular repair and the appropriate size of the stent-graft. Most centers rely on a combination of CT, MR, and angiography. Others have substituted three-dimensional reconstruction of spiral CT data for angiography.[15,16] However, this trend toward ever more sophisticated preoperative imaging become unnecessary with newer devices which allow for intraoperative adjustment to accommodate minor inaccuracies in preoperative measurement.

The Cost of Endovascular Aneurysm Repair

Given its lower morbidity and hospital stay, one would expect that endovascular repair would be less expensive than conventional open repair. The few studies that have addressed this question, however, have produced conflicting conclusions.[17] One reason is that endovascular repair generates a series of costs not normally associated with open repair, including imaging equipment, preoperative angiography, angiographic supplies, stent-grafts, and lifelong image-based follow-up. Some studies include these costs, others do not. The source of cost data also varies. Some studies rely on patient charges; others examine costs.

In our study of short-term perioperative costs (unpublished data), we used a hospital-wide system that prospectively assigned "variable, fixed, direct, and indirect" costs to every patient who spent time in each of the "cost centers." We found that the cost of endovascular repair in high-risk patients was 57% of the cost of open repair in normal-risk patients. However, the costs of preoperative angiography and follow-up studies (mainly CT) beyond 1 month were not included for two reasons. First, pre- and postoperative imaging studies were performed at outside hospitals, so their costs were more difficult to assess reliably. Second, the role of pre- and postoperative imaging is likely to change. Many centers already perform endovascular aneurysm repair without angiography.[15,16] One might argue that serial CT is also unnecessary. At present every patient who undergoes endovascular repair can expect to be followed for life by serial CT, because the technique is experimental; this may change.

ENDOVASCULAR ANEURYSM REPAIR IN HIGH-RISK PATIENTS

The long-term benefit of endovascular repair depends on the risk of aneurysm rupture, the patient's life expectancy, and the durability of endovascular repair. Although the long-term durability of endovascular repair is as yet unknown, it is possible to estimate both rupture risk and life expectancy. We believe that endovascular aneurysm repair in a high-risk patient with a reduced life expectancy is only justified if the aneurysm is large and the risk of rupture correspondingly high.

ENDOVASCULAR ANEURYSM REPAIR IN LOW-RISK PATIENTS

In low-risk patients, the mortality rate of conventional open repair is so low that one would need a very large study to demonstrate a mortality advantage of endovascular repair. As no such studies exist, the choice of endovascular repair over open repair is based upon the anticipated reduction in pain, hospital stay, and debility and upon the assumption that conversion to open repair would carry little risk. Although there are conflicting data on this point, this assumption would appear to be valid. Conversion carries little additional risk[18,19] unless the patient is too sick to tolerate open operation or conversion to the open operation is performed for aneurysm rupture.

Low-risk patients generally have sufficient life expectancy to justify repair. However, the longer a patient lives, the more one has to worry about the durability of the endovascular technique. There are enough unanswered questions regarding the mechanical integrity of the prosthesis and the stability of the implantation sites (see following) to cast doubt on the long-term durability of endovascular repair.

ENDOPRESSURE OR ENDOTENSION

Few aneurysms rupture following endovascular repair in the absence of endoleak or aneurysm dilatation. Nevertheless, we still do not know why some aneurysms dilate without any demonstrable endoleak, why some aneurysms shrink even in the presence of an endoleak, which endoleaks are dangerous, and whether they can be prevented or treated.

The phenomenon of aneurysm dilatation in the absence of endoleak (endopressure or endotension) is troubling because we have come to rely on the presence or absence of endoleak on CT as a criterion of failure or success. Early findings suggest that aneurysms with type I endoleaks behave like untreated aneurysms. In contrast, type II endoleaks are associated with an intermediate degree of aneurysm pulsatility and that these aneurysms do not dilate.

Conclusion

Despite the limitations of the current studies, it is clear that endovascular aneurysm repair of abdominal aortic aneurysm is a reasonably safe and effective in properly selected patients. Its ultimate role in the management of patients with abdominal aortic aneurysms will depend on the answers to many of the questions discussed here.

References

Iliac Artery PTA and Stenting

1. Zeitler E, Schoop W, Zahnow W. The treatment of occlusive arterial disease by transluminal catheter angioplasty. Radiology 1971;99:19.
2. Becker G, Katzen B, Dake M. Noncoronary angioplasty. Radiology 1989;170:921–940.
3. Ahn SS, Obrand DI, Moore WS. Transluminal balloon angioplasty, stents, and atherectomy. Semin Vasc Surg 1997;10:286–296.
4. Long A, Sapoval M, Beyssen B, et al. Strecker stent implantation in iliac arteries: patency and predictive factors for long-term success. Radiology 1995;194:739–744.
5. Waller B, Miller J, Morgan R, Tejada E. Atherosclerotic plaque calcific deposits: an important factor in success or failure of transluminal coronary angioplasty (TCA). Circulation 1988;78:I1–I376.
6. Long AL, Page PE, Raynaud AC, et al. Percutaneous iliac artery stent: angiographic long-term follow-up. Radiology 1991;180:771–778.
7. Colapinto R, Stronell R, Johnston W. Transluminal angioplasty of complete iliac obstructions. AJR 1985;146:859–862.
8. Murphy TP, Webb MS, Lambiase RE, et al. Percutaneous revascularization of complex iliac artery stenoses and occlusions with use of Wallstents: three-year experience. J Vasc International Radiol 1996;7:21–27.
9. Gupta A, Ravimandalam K, Rao V, et al. Total occlusion of iliac arteries: results of balloon angioplasty. J Cardiovasc Interventional Radiol 1993;16:165–177.
10. Blum U, Gabelmann A, Redecker M, et al. Percutaneous recanalization of iliac artery occlusions: results of a prospective study. Radiology 1993;189:536–540.
11. Henry M, Amor M, Ethevenot G, Henry I, Mentre B, Tzvetanov K. Percutaneous endoluminal treatment of iliac occlusions: long-term follow-up in 105 patients. J Endovasc Surg 1998;5:228–235.
12. Tetteroo E, van der Graaf Y, Bosch JL, et al. Randomised comparison of primary stent placement versus primary angioplasty followed by selective stent placement in patients with iliac-artery occlusive disease. Dutch Iliac Stent Trial Study Group. Lancet 1998;351:1153–1159.
13. Bosch JL, Hunink MG. Meta-analysis of the results of percutaneous transluminal angioplasty and stent placement for aortoiliac occlusive disease [published erratum appears in Radiology 1997;205(2):584]. Radiology 1997;204:87–96.
14. Tegtmeyer CJ, Hartwell GD, Selby JB, Robertson R Jr, Kron IL, Tribble CG. Results and complications of angioplasty in aortoiliac disease [see comments]. Circulation 1991;83:I53–I60.
15. Vorwerk D, Gunther RW, Schurmann K, Wendt G. Aortic and iliac stenoses: follow-up results of stent placement after insufficient balloon angioplasty in 118 cases. Radiology 1996;198:45–48.
16. Vorwerk D, Gunther RW. Stent placement in iliac arterial lesions: three years of clinical experience with the Wallstent. Cardiovasc Interventional Radiol 1992;15:285–290.
17. Martin EC, Katzen BT, Benenati JF, et al. Multicenter trial of the wallstent in the iliac and femoral arteries [see comments]. J Vasc International Radiol 1995;6:843–849.
18. Palmza J, Laborde J, Rivera F, Encarnacion C, Lutz J, Moss J. Stenting of the iliac arteries with the Palmaz Stent: experience from a multicenter trial. Cardiovasc Interventional Radiol 1992;15:291–297.
19. Cikrit DF, Gustafson PA, Dalsing MC, et al. Long-term follow-up of the Palmaz stent for iliac occlusive disease. Surgery (St. Louis) 1995;118:608–13; discussion 613–614.
20. Vorwerk D, Guenther RW, Schurmann K, Wendt G, Peters I. Primary stent placement for chronic iliac occlusions: follow-up results in 103 patients. Radiology 1995;194:745–749.
21. Henry H, Amor M, Ethevenot G, et al. Palmaz stent placement in iliac and femoropopliteal arteries: primary and secondary pa-

tency in 310 patients with 2–4 year follow-up. Radiology 1995;197:167–174.

22. van Andel G, WFM vE, Krepel V, Breslau P. Percutaneous transluminal dilatation of the iliac artery: long-term results. Radiology 1985;156:321–323.

23. Johnston K. Iliac arteries: Reanalysis of results of balloon angioplasty. Radiology 1993;186:207–212.

24. Sapoval MR, Long AL, Pagny JY, et al. Outcome of percutaneous intervention in iliac artery stenosis. Radiology 1996;198:481–486.

25. Sullivan TM, Childs MB, Bacharach JM, Gray BH, Piedmonte MR. Percutaneous transluminal angioplasty and primary stenting of the iliac arteries in 288 patients. J Vasc Surg 1997; 25:829–38; discussion 838–839.

26. Becquemin J-P, Cavillon A, Allaire E, Haiduc F, Desgranges P. Iliac and femoropopliteal lesions: Evaluation of balloon angioplasty and classical surgery. J Endovasc Surg 1995;2:42–50.

27. Wilson SE, GL W, Cross AP, et al. Percutaneous transluminal angioplasty versus operation for peripheral arteriosclerosis. J Vasc Surg 1989;9:1–9.

Renal PTA and Stenting

1. Working Group on Renovascular Hypertension: Final report: detection, evaluation, and treatment of renovascular hypertension. Arch Intern Med 1987;147:820.

2. Gifford R Jr. Evaluation of the hypertensive patient with emphasis on detecting curable causes. Millbank Mem Fund Q 1969;47:170–186.

3. Ramsay L, Waller P. Blood pressure response to percutaneous transluminal angioplasty for renovascular hypertension: an overview of published series. Br Med J 1990;300:569–572.

4. Tegtmeyer CJ, Selby JB, Hartwell GD, Ayers C, Tegtmeyer V. Results and complicationis of angioplasty in fibromuscular disease. Circulation 1991;83:I155–I161.

5. Tegtmeyer CJ, Matsumoto AH, Johnson AH. Renal angioplasty. In: Baum S, Pentecost MJ, eds. Abrams' Angiography: Interventional Radiology, Vol. III. New York: Churchill-Livingstone, 1997:294–325.

6. Sos T. Angioplasty for the treatment of azotemia and renovascular hypertension in atherosclerotic renal artery disease. Circulation 1991;83:I-162–I-166.

7. Losinno F, Zuccala A, Busato F, Zucchelli P. Renal artery angioplasty for renovascular hypertension and preservation of renal function: long-term angiographic and clinical follow-up. AJR 1994;162:853–857.

8. Jensen G, Zachrisson B, Delin K, Volkmann R, Aurell M. Treatment of renovascular hypertension: One year results of renal angioplasty. Kidney Int 1995;48:1936–1945.

9. Eldrup-Jorgensen J, Harvey H, Sampson L, Amberson S, Bredenberg C. Should percutaneous transluminal renal artery angioplasty be applied to ostial renal artery atherosclerosis. J Vasc Surg 1995;21:909–915.

10. Baumgartner I, Triller J, Mahler F. Patency of transluminal renal angioplasty: a prospective sonographic study. Kidney International 1997;51:798–803.

11. Hoffman O, Carreres T, Sapoval MR, et al. Ostial renal artery stenosis angioplasty: immediate and mid-term angiographic and clinical results. J Vasc International Radiol 1998;9:65–73.

12. Sos T, Pickering T, Sniderman K, et al. Percutaneous transluminal angioplasty in renovascular hypertension due to atheroma or fibromuscular dysplasia. N Engl J Med 1983;309:274–279.

13. Kidney DD, Deutsch LS. The indications and results of percutaneous transluminal angioplasty and stenting in renal artery stenosis. Semin Vasc Surg 1996;9:188–197.

14. Martin L, Rees C, O'Bryant T. Percutaneous angioplasty of the renal arteries. In: Strandness DE Jr, Van Breda A, eds. Vascular Diseases: Surgical & Interventional Therapy, Vol. 2. New York: Churchill Livingstone, 1994:721–741.

15. Webster J, Marshall F, Abdalla M, et al. Randomized comparison of percutaneous angioplasty vs continued medical therapy for hypertensive patients with atheromatous renal artery stenosis. J Hum Hypertens 1998;12:329–335.

16. Tollefson D, Ernst C. Natural history of atherosclerotic renal artery stenosis associated with aortic disease. J Vasc Surg 1991; 14:327–331.

17. Tegtmeyer C, Kellum C, Ayers C. Percutaneous transluminal angioplasty of the renal arteries: results and long-term follow-up. Radiology 1984;153:77–84.

18. Tullis MJ, Zierler RE, Glickerman DJ, Bergelin RO, Cantwell-Gab K, Strandness DE Jr. Results of percutaneous transluminal angioplasty for atherosclerotic renal artery stenosis: a follow-up study with duplex ultrasonography. J Vasc Surg 1997;25:46–54.

19. Rodriguez-Lopez JA, Werner A, Ray LI, et al. Renal artery stenosis treated with stent deployment: indications, technique, and outcome for 108 patients. J Vasc Surg 1999;29:617–624.

20. Henry M, Amor M, Henry I, et al. Stents in the treatment of renal artery stenosis: long-term follow-up. J Endovasc Surg 1999;6: 42–51.

21. Hennequin LM, Joffre FG, Rousseau HP, et al. Renal artery stent placement: long-term results with the Wallstent endoprosthesis [see comments]. Radiology 1994;191:713–719.

22. White CJ, Ramee SR, Collins TJ, Jenkins JS. Renal artery stent placement. J Endovasc Surg 1998;5:71–77.

23. Hansen K, Starr S, Sands R, Burkart J, Plonk G, Dean R. Contemporary surgical management of renovascular disease. J Vasc Surg 1992;16:319–331.

24. Novick A, Ziegelbaum M, Vidt D, Gifford R, Pohl M, Goormastic M. Trends in surgical revascularization for renal artery disease: ten years' experience. JAMA 1987;257:498–501.

25. Steinbach F, Novick A, Campbell S, Dykstra D. Long-term survival after surgical revascularization for atherosclerotic renal artery disease. J Urol 1997;158:38–41.

26. Cambria R, Brewster D, L'Italien G, et al. The durability of different reconstructive techniques for atherosclerotic renal artery disease. J Vasc Surg 1994;20:76–87.

27. Cambria R, Brewster D, L'Italien G, et al. Simultaneous aortic and renal artery reconstruction: evolution of an eighteen-year experience. J Vasc Surg 1995;21:916–925.

Extracranial Carotid Artery Angioplasty and Stenting

1. Mathur A, Dorros G, Iyer SS, Vitek JJ, Yadav SS, Roubin GS. Palmaz stent compression in patients following carotid artery stenting. Catheterization Cardiovasc Diagn 1997;41:137–140.

2. Roubin GS, Yadav S, Iyer SS, Vitek J. Carotid stent-supported angioplasty: a neurovascular intervention to prevent stroke. Am J Cardiol 1996;78:8–12.

3. Benichou H, Bergeron P. Carotid angioplasty and stenting: will periprocedural transcranial Doppler monitoring be important? J Endovasc Surg 1996;3:217–223.

4. Jordan WD Jr, Voellinger DC, Doblar DD, Plyushcheva NP, Fisher WS, McDowell HA. Microemboli detected by transcranial Doppler monitoring in patients during carotid angioplasty versus carotid endarterectomy. Cardiovasc Surg 1999;7:33–38.

5. Theron J. [Protected carotid angioplasty and carotid stents]. J Mal Vasc 1996;21:113–122.

6. Beneficial effect of carotid endarterectomy in symptomatic patiens with high-grade carotid stenosis. North American Symptomatic Carotid Endarterectomy Trial Collaborators [see comments]. N Engl J Med 1991;325:445–453.

7. National Institute of Neurological Disorders and Stroke and Trauma Division. Clinical alert: benefit of carotid endarterctomy for patients with high-grade stenosis of the internal carotid artery. North American Symptomatic Carotid Endarterectomy Trial (NASCET) investigators. Stroke 1991;22:816–817.

8. Mayberg MR, Wilson SE, Yatsu F, et al. Carotid endarterectomy and prevention of cerebral ischemia in symptomatic carotid

stenosis. Veterans Affairs Cooperative Studies Program 309 Trialist Group [see comments]. JAMA 1991;266:3289–3294.

9. Hobson RW, Weiss DG, Fields WS, et al. Efficacy of carotid endarterectomy for asymptomatic carotid stenosis. The Veterans Affairs Cooperative Study Group [see comments]. N Engl J Med 1993;328:221–227.

10. Clinical advisory: carotid endarterectomy for patients with asymptomatic internal carotid artery stenosis. Stroke 1994;25:2523–2524.

11. Barnett HJ. Progress in stroke prevention: an overview [see comments]. Health Rep 1994;6:132–138.

12. Coyne TJ, Wallace MC. Surgical referral for carotid artery stenosis—the influence of NASCET. North American Symptomatic Carotid Endarterectomy Trial [see comments]. Can J Neurol Sci 1994;21:129–132.

13. Hobson RW Jr. Randomized clinical trial results define operative indications in symptomatic and asymptomatic carotid endarterectomy patients. Curr Opin Gen Surg 1994:265–271.

14. Fox AJ. Carotid endarterectomy trials. Neuroimaging Clin N Am 1996;6:931–938.

15. Moore WS, Young B, Baker WH, et al. Surgical results: a justification of the surgeon selection process for the ACAS trial. The ACAS Investigators. J Vasc Surg 1996;23:323–328.

16. Randomised trial of endarterectomy for recently symptomatic carotid stenosis: final results of the MRC European Carotid Surgery Trial (ECST) [see comments]. Lancet 1998;351:1379–1387.

17. Barnett HJ, Taylor DW, Eliasziw M, et al. Benefit of carotid endarterectomy in patients with symptomatic moderate or severe stenosis. North American Symptomatic Carotid Endarterectomy Trial Collaborators [see comments]. N Engl J Med 1998;339:1415–1425.

18. Hallett JW Jr, Pietropaoli JA Jr, Ilstrup DM, Gayari MM, Williams JA, Meyer FB. Comparison of North American Symptomatic Carotid Endarterectomy Trial and population-based outcomes for carotid endarterectomy. J Vasc Surg 1998;27:845–850; discussion 851.

19. Mayo SW, Eldrup-Jorgensen J, Lucas FL, Wennberg DE, Bredenberg CE. Carotid endarterectomy after NASCET and ACAS: a statewide study. North American Symptomatic Carotid Endarterectomy Trial. Asymptomatic Carotid Artery Stenosis Study. J Vasc Surg 1998;27:1017–1022; discussion 1022–1023.

20. Becquemin JP, Qvarfordt P, Castier Y, Melliere D. Carotid angioplasty: is it safe? [see comments]. J Endovasc Surg 1996;3:35–41.

21. Bergeron P, Chambran P, Hartung O, Bianca S. Cervical carotid artery stenosis: which technique, balloon angioplasty or surgery? J Cardiovasc Surg (Torino) 1996;37(suppl 1):73–75.

22. Motarjeme A. Percutaneous transluminal angioplasty of supraaortic vessels. J Endovasc Surg 1996;3:171–181.

23. Kachel R. Results of balloon angioplasty in the carotid arteries. J Endovasc Surg 1996;3:22–30.

24. Kuntz KM, Kent KC. Is carotid endarterectomy cost-effective? An analysis of symptomatic and asymptomatic patients. Circulation 1996;94:II194–III198.

25. Nussbaum ES, Heros RC, Erickson DL. Cost-effectiveness of carotid endarterectomy. Neurosurgery (Baltim) 1996;38:237–244.

26. Fisher WS, 3rd, Jordan WD. Carotid angioplasty. Surg Neurol 1998;50:295–298; discussion 298–299.

27. Jordan WD, Jr., Roye GD, Fisher WS, 3rd, Redden D, McDowell HA. A cost comparison of balloon angioplasty and stenting versus endarterectomy for the treatment of carotid artery stenosis. J Vasc Surg 1998;27:16–22; discussion 22–24.

28. Wholey MH, Wholey M, Bergeron P, et al. Current global status of carotid artery stent placement [see comments]. Catheterization Cardiovasc Diagn 1998;44:1–6.

29. Theron JG, Payelle GG, Coskun O, Huet HF, Guimaraens L. Carotid artery stenosis: treatment with protected balloon angioplasty and stent placement [see comments]. Radiology 1996;201:627–636.

30. Hobson RW Jr. Status of carotid angioplasty and stenting trials [comment]. J Vasc Surg 1998;27:791.

Endovascular Repair of Abdominal Aortic Aneurysms

1. Parodi JC, Palmaz JC, Barone HD. Transfemoral intraluminal graft implantation for abdominal aortic aneurysms. Ann Vasc Surg 1991;5:491–499.

2. Katz DA, Littenberg B, Cronenwett JL. Management of small abdominal aortic aneurysms: early surgery versus watchful waiting. JAMA 1992;268:2678–2686.

3. Parodi JC. Endovascular repair of abdominal aortic aneurysms and other arterial lesions. J Vasc Surg 1995;21:549–557.

4. Chuter TAM, Green RM, Ouriel K, De Weese JA. Infrarenal aortic aneurysm morphology: implications for transfemoral repair. J Vasc Surg 1993;1994;20:44–50.

5. Malina M, Lindblad, Ivancev K, Lindh M, Malina J, Brunkwall J. Endovascular AA exclusion: will stents with hooks and barbs prevent stent-graft migration? J Endovasc Surg 1998;5:310–317.

6. Zarins C, White RA, Schwarten D, Kinney E, Dietrich EB, Hodgson KJ, Fogarty TJ. AneuRx stent graft versus open surgical repair of abdominal aortic aneurysm: Multicenter prospective clinical trial. J Vasc Surg 1999;29:292–308.

7. May J, White GH, Yu W, et al. Concurrent comparison of endoluminal versus open repair in the treatment of abdominal aortic aneurysm: analysis of 303 patients by life table method. J Vasc Surg 1998;27:213–221.

8. Stelter W, Umscheid T, Siegler P. Three-year experience with modular stent-graft devices for endovascular AAA treatment. J Endovasc Surg 1997;4:362–369.

9. May J, White GH, Waugh R, et al. Adverse events after endoluminal repair of abdominal aortic aneurysms: a comparison during two successive periods of time. J Vasc Surg 1999;29:32–39.

10. Chuter TAM, Gordon RL, Reilly LM, et al. Abdominal aortic aneurysm in high-risk patients: short- to intermediate-term results of endovascular repair. Radiology 1999;210:316–365.

11. Malina M, Lanne T, Ivancev K, Lindblad B, Brunkwall J. Reduced pulsatile wall motion of abdominal aortic aneurysm after endovascular repair. J Vasc Surg 1998;27:624–631.

12. Matsumura JS, Moore WS. Clinical consequences of periprosthetic leak after endovascular repair of abdominal aortic aneurysm. Endovascular Technologies Investigators. J Vasc Surg 1998;27:606–613.

13. Resch T, Ivancev K, Lindh M, et al. Persistent collateral perfusion of abdominal aortic aneurysm after endovascular repair does not lead to progressive change in aneurysm diameter. J Vasc Surg 1998;28:242–249.

14. Armon MP, Yusuf SW, Whitaker SC, Gregson RH, Wenham PW, Hopkinson BR. Thrombus distribution and changes in aneurysm size following endovascular aortic aneurysm repair. Eur J Vasc Endovasc Surg 1998;16:472–476.

15. Armon MP, Whitaker SC, Gregson RH, Wenham PW, Hopkinson BR. Spiral CT angiography versus aortography in the assessment of aortoiliac lengths in patients undergoing endovascular abdominal aortic aneurysm repair. J Endovasc Surg 1998;5:222–227.

16. Diethrich EB. Will contrast aortography become obsolete in the preoperative evaluation of abdominal aortic aneurysm for endovascular exclusion? J Endovasc Surg 1997;4:5–12.

17. Raithel D. Surveillance of patients after abdominal aortic aneurysm repair with endovascular grafting or conventional treatment. J Mal Vasc 1998;23:390–392.

18. Jacobowitz GR, Lee AM, Riles TS. Immediate and late explantation of endovascular aortic grafts: the Endovascular Technologies experience. J Vasc Surg 1999;29:309–316.

19. May J, White GH, Yu W, et al. Conversion from endoluminal to open repair of abdominal aortic aneurysms: a hazardous procedure. Eur J Vasc Endovasc Surg 1997;14:4–11.

Cardiothoracic Surgery

Lung Neoplasms

Christine L. Lau and David H. Harpole, Jr.

Lung cancer is the leading cause of cancer-related death among women and men. In women, lung cancer is second only to breast cancer in incidence, and in males, it is the most prevalent type of cancer diagnosed. The average age at diagnosis of lung cancer is 60 years. One-year survival has increased from 32% in 1973 to 40%, but the overall 5-year survival remains only 14% despite continued research.[1]

The major cause of lung cancer in the world is tobacco smoking, the majority being from cigarette use. The biology of lung cancer is being elucidated as understanding of oncogenes, tumor suppressor genes, and molecular pathways are better defined. Despite multiple therapeutic modalities therapies, the long-term survival rate for non-small cell lung cancer (NSCLC) has not significantly changed over recent years.

Pathology

The histological classification of lung tumors according to the World Health Organization is seen in Table 39.1.[2] The overwhelming majority of lung tumors are malignant (95%). Approximately 5% are bronchial carcinoids and the rest are mesenchymal tumors and miscellaneous neoplasms.[3] More than 90% of malignant tumors are one of four types: (1) squamous cell carcinoma, (2) adenocarcinoma, (3) large cell carcinoma, or (4) small cell carcinoma. The first three are collectively referred to as non-small cell lung cancer (NSCLC) and account for approximately 80% of the lung cancers. All four types probably share a common precursor, arising from malignant transformation of bronchial basal cells; therefore, mixed tumor types are not uncommon, for example, the finding of squamous cell carcinoma and small cell carcinoma in the same tumor.

Non-Small Cell Lung Cancer

SQUAMOUS CELL OR EPIDERMOID CARCINOMA

Until recently, squamous cell carcinoma was the most common type of NSCLC, having been replaced now by adeno-

carcinoma.[4,5] The majority of these tumors are centrally located, although 20% are found peripherally; 80% of squamous cell carcinomas have an endobronchial component.[6] As these tumors grow they have a tendency to develop central necrosis, which may be evident. Often these tumors grow and obstruct the bronchus. Squamous cell carcinomas may obtain large sizes before metastasizing. When they do metastasize, often they spread only to the peribronchial or hilar lymph nodes. Microscopically these tumors may be well, moderately, or poorly differentiated.

ADENOCARCINOMA

Adenocarcinomas (Fig. 39.1) are the most common histological type of lung cancer seen, representing 46% of cases. Adenocarcinomas are often located in the periphery, arising from subsegmental bronchioles and not major bronchi. They may appear as a solitary pulmonary nodule on radiographic studies (Fig. 39.2). These tumors have a tendency to spread lymphatogenously and hematogenously. In 20% of cases, metastatic disease by a hematogenous route occurs before lymph node metastasis.

LARGE CELL CARCINOMA

This tumor is an undifferentiated, aggressive tumor that may be difficult to distinguish from poorly differentiated adenosquamous or small cell carcinomas. Specific immunoperoxidase stains may be helpful in this regard. Like adenocarcinoma, these tumors often present in a peripheral location and show early lymphatogenous and hematogenous spread. Histologically these tumors are comprised of large, polygonal cells with vesicular nuclei. The giant cell type has large multinucleated cells, while clear cells make up the other variant.

Small Cell Carcinoma

Of patients presenting with lung cancer, 10% to 15% are diagnosed with this aggressive tumor type. Small cell carcinoma (SCLC) is characterized usually by a central or hilar location.

TABLE 39.1. Histological Classification of Malignant Epithelial Lung Tumors.

Squamous cell carcinoma
  Variant:
    Papillary
    Clear cell
    Small cell
    Basaloid
Small cell carcinoma
  Variant:
    Combined small cell carcinoma
Adenocarcinoma
  Acinar
  Papillary
  Bronchioloalveolar carcinoma
  Solid adenocarcinoma with mucin
Large cell carcinoma

Source: World Health Organization. Histological typing of lung and pleural tumours, 3 ed, 1999:21–22. Reprinted with permission.

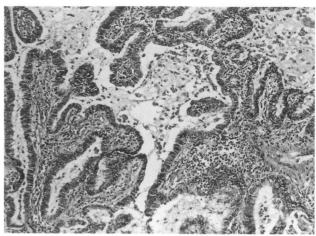

FIGURE 39.1. Histopathological examination of adenocarcinoma (papillary subtype) of the lung. Hematoxylin and eosin, ×100.

Histologically, these tumors are composed of small cells approximately twice the size but similar in appearance to lymphocytes. These tumors have classically been referred to as "oat cell" carcinomas (see Table 39.1). Small cell carcinomas are most commonly the tumors associated with ectopic hormone production.[19]

Pathogenesis

Epidemiology

Early case-control studies indicated tobacco, largely cigarette smoking, as the cause of lung cancer. Confirmation came from several cohort studies, the best known of which was the British Doctors Study by Doll and Peto.[7] In this large study of 34,440 male physicians followed for 20 years, it was concluded that cancers of the lung, esophagus, and other respiratory sites were a direct result of smoking. The female doctor follow-up study was reported in 1980 by Doll.[8] In this cohort study of 6,194 female doctors it was concluded that cigarette smoking was associated with lung cancer, chronic obstructive pulmonary disease (COPD), and heart disease.

It is now known that 80% to 90% of lung cancers result from tobacco usage, and that the risk of developing lung cancer is 4 to 10 times greater in smokers than nonsmokers. While duration of tobacco use is the most important factor, the amount and type are also important. Additionally, the age when smoking began is important. Initially it was thought that tobacco smoking caused only small cell and squamous cell carcinomas of the lung, but now adenocarcinoma is known to be related to smoking.[9]

Other factors that may less commonly be the cause of lung cancers include radiation, chemicals, and mineral exposures. There are multiple carcinogens involved in causing lung cancer including various chemical carcinogens (chloromethyl methyl ether, polycyclic aromatic hydrocarbons); ionizing radiation (survivors of Hiroshima, uranium miners, and radon gas exposure); various minerals (asbestos, fiberglass, glass wool, and alumina); and also various metals (chromium, nickel, lead, arsenic, iron and iron oxides).

More recently, exposure to environmental smoke, also known as secondhand or passive smoke, has been explored as a cause of lung cancer. In one case-control study, there was a 30% increased risk of lung cancer in women exposed to secondhand smoke from a spouse. A 50% increase was observed for adenocarcinoma of the lung. In a review of 10 case controls and 3 prospective studies, there was an overall 35% increased risk of lung cancer among nonsmokers living with a smoker or a relative risk of 1.35.

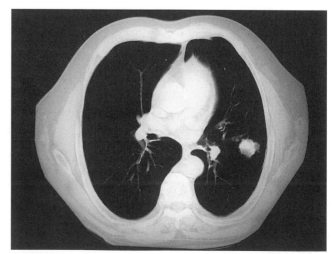

FIGURE 39.2. CT scan of chest shows peripheral nodule found at resection to be adenocarcinoma of the lung.

Genetic

The genetic steps involved in transforming normal bronchial epithelium to a dysplastic tumor are multiple, and include mutations, altered expression of critical regulatory genes in a cell, and chromosomal deletions and rearrangements. Common proto-oncogenes involved in NSCLC are K-*ras*, erbB-1 (EGFr), and erbB-2 (*Her2/neu*). The most common activated proto-oncogene found in non-small cell lung cancer is K-*ras*. The tumor suppressor genes implicated in NSCLC include p53, retinoblastoma susceptibility gene (Rb), and bcl-2. In more than half of all non-small cell lung cancers, p53 is either overexpressed or mutated.

A genetic predisposition to the development of lung cancer is suggested by the development of cancer in some patients who are nonsmokers and the fact that only 20% of patients who are smokers eventually develop cancer. Current belief, supported by epidemiological studies, is that lung cancer is associated with codominant inheritance of an autosomal dominant gene, especially in patients developing lung cancer before the age of 50. The most common chromosomal abnormalities involve deletions of the short arm of chromosomes 1, 3, 9, and 17, and polysomy of chromosome 7. Other deletions and rearrangements of chromosomes are also commonly seen, and even in early-stage tumors multiple abnormalities can potentially exist.[10]

Clinical Manifestations

Approximately 95% of patients with lung cancer present with symptoms from disease and the remaining 5% present asymptomatically with abnormal chest radiographs. Symptoms may arise from primary tumors, distant metastatic disease, systemic symptoms, or paraneoplastic syndromes.[5] Figure 39.3 notes the risk factors and symptoms to be evaluated in suspected or proven lung cancer.[6] Table 39.2 lists the initial symptoms at presentation of lung cancer in one series of 2000 patients.[11]

Extrathoracic Manifestations from Metastatic Disease

Distant metastatic disease is the first presentation of lung cancer in 32% of cases.[12] Common locations of distant metastatic spread including adrenals, liver, bone, lung, and brain have been documented in autopsy series (Table 39.3).[13,14] Multiple other sites of metastatic spread including the diaphragm, skin, pleura, pericardium, spinal cord, kidney, soft tissues, and heart can also occur, although these sites of spread are less common. Extrathoracic nodal involvement, especially the supraclavicular and anterior cervical nodes, occurs in up to 30% of presentation.[5,6]

PARANEOPLASTIC SYNDROMES

Ten percent to 20% of patients with lung carcinomas have paraneoplastic syndromes; these syndromes occur most commonly with small cell and squamous cell carcinomas (Table 39.4).[6,9] Common paraneoplastic syndromes include hyper-

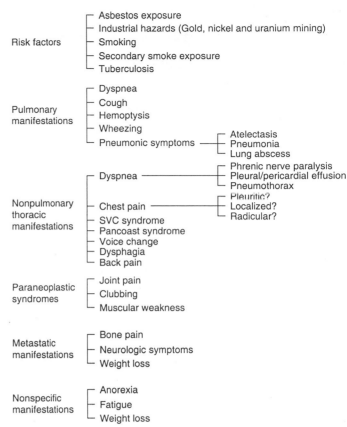

FIGURE 39.3. Risk factors and symptoms to be evaluated in patients with suspected or proven lung cancer. (From Maddaus M, Ginsberg RJ. Cancer/diagnosis and staging. In: Pearson FG, Deslauriers J, Ginsberg RJ, et al., eds. Thoracic Surgery. New York: Churchill Livingstone, 1995:672. Reprinted with permission.)

trophic pulmonary osteoarthropathy, syndrome of inappropriate antidiuretic hormone secretion, and hypercalcemia. Hypertrophic pulmonary osteoarthropathy is characterized by a proliferating periositis, resulting in bone and joint pain. The syndrome of inappropriate antidiuretic hormone (ADH) secretion is seen primarily with small cell carcinoma. Although

TABLE 39.2. Initial Symptoms at Presentation of Lung Cancer.

Symptoms	Percentage (%)
Cough	74
Weight loss	68
Dyspnea	58
Chest Pain	49
Hemoptysis	29
Lymphadenopathy	23
Bone pain	25
Hepatomegaly	21
Clubbing	20
Intracranial	12
Superior vena cava syndrome	4
Hoarseness	18

Source: Hyde L, Hyde CI. Clinical manifestations of lung cancer. Chest 1974;65:300.[11]

TABLE 39.3. Common Metastatic Sites Found at Autopsy in NSCLC.

Site of metastases	Percentage (%)
Mediastinal lymph nodes	83
Lung	47
Brain	43
Liver	40
Adrenal	36
Bone	33

NSCLC, non-small cell lung cancer.

Source: Abrams HL, Spiro R, Goldstein N. Metastases in carcinoma: analysis of 1000 autopsied cases. Cancer 1950; 3:77.[13]

up to 70% of lung cancers are found to have elevated ADH, symptomatic presentation is unusual. Hypercalcemia is seen in 10% of lung cancer patients, but of these only 15% have hypercalcemia as a result of a paraneoplastic syndrome caused by production of either a parathyroid hormone or hormone-like substance. This syndrome is most commonly associated with squamous cell carcinomas. Cushing's syndrome from secretion of ectopic adrenocorticotropin is most commonly related to small cell lung cancer.[5,6] Neurological and myopathic syndromes are also associated with lung cancer.

Diagnosis and Staging

The goals of diagnosis and staging of lung cancer are early identification and treatment of patients potentially curable by surgical resection. Following a through history and physical examination, radiologic films should be carefully reviewed and compared with priors if available.

Noninvasive Diagnostic Techniques

CHEST RADIOGRAPHY

The posteroanterior and lateral chest radiographs are carefully inspected for primary tumor size and evidence of more advanced disease including pleural or pericardial effusions, evidence of nodal involvement, evidence of bony involvement, and areas of consolidation. If previous films are available, these should be used for comparison. Chest radiography, however, lacks sensitivity in detection of mediastinal adenopathy and in detailing the primary tumor involvement with mediastinal structures or the chest wall.[5]

COMPUTED TOMOGRAPHY

A CT scan of the chest and upper abdomen should be performed to provide additional information about tumor size, possible lymph node involvement, other intrathoracic structure involvement, and possible metastatic spread. Intravenous contrast administration is not necessary, but may provide more detail regarding invasion of mediastinal structures and help differentiate vascular structures from mediastinal adenopathy. Assessment of the lung lesion may differentiate benign from malignant nodules based on fat and calcium patterns. In evaluation of the primary tumor, a CT scan is neither sensitive nor specific in detection of chest wall or parietal pleural involvement by the tumor.[5]

TABLE 39.4. Paraneoplastic Syndromes in Lung Cancer Patients.

Metabolic
  Hypercalcemia
  Cushing's syndrome
  Inappropriate antidiuretic hormone production
  Carcinoid syndrome
  Gynecomastia
  Hypercalcitonemia
  Elevated growth hormone level
  Elevated prolactin, follicle-stimulating hormone, luteinizing
    hormone levels
  Hypoglycemia
  Hyperthyroidism
Neurological
  Encephalopathy
  Subacute cerebellar degeneration
  Peripheral neuropathy
  Polymyositis
  Autonomic neuropathy
  Lambert–Eaton syndrome
  Opsoclonus and myoclonus
Skeletal
  Clubbing
  Pulmonary hypertrophic osteoarthropathy
Hematological
  Anemia
  Leukemoid reactions
  Thrombocytosis
  Thrombocytopenia
  Eosinophilia
  Pure red cell aplasia
  Leukoerythroblastosis
  Disseminated intravascular coagulation
Cutaneous and muscular
  Hyperkeratosis
  Dermatomyositis
  Acanthosis nigricans
  Hyperpigmentation
  Erythema gyratum repens
  Hypertrichosis lanuginosa acquisita
Other
  Nephrotic syndrome
  Hypouricemia
  Secretion of vasoactive intestinal peptide with diarrhea
  Hyperamylasemia
  Anorexia-cachexia

Source: Shields, TW. Presentation, diagnosis, and staging of bronchial carcinoma and of the asymptomatic solitary pulmonary nodule. In: Shields TW, ed. General Thoracic Surgery. Malvern, PA: Williams & Wilkins, 1994:1123.[55] Reprinted with permission.

The chest CT scan should include cuts through the upper abdomen to assess the liver and adrenals for asymptomatic metastatic disease. Intravenous contrast is not required or routinely performed to evaluate the adrenals, but differentiation of benign from metastatic liver disease cannot be made without intravenous contrast administration. Suspicious lesions may require percutaneous biopsy for diagnosis.[5]

MAGNETIC RESONANCE IMAGING

Magnetic resonance imaging (MRI) is slightly more sensitive than CT scanning in detecting mediastinal invasion and chest wall involvement, and is most useful in evaluation of superior sulcus tumors. Nonetheless, MRI has not proven to be particularly useful in the diagnosis of lung cancer.

POSITRON EMISSION TOMOGRAPHY

Positron emission tomography (PET) detects increased rates of glucose metabolism, which is commonly seen in malignant tissues. Measurement of a positron-emitting glucose analogue (2-^{18}F) fluoro-2-deoxy-D-glucose (FDG) can be detected by PET. FDG-PET can detect primary lung cancers and metastases to mediastinal and scalene lymph nodes.[15–18] Importantly, anatomical detail is not provided as well with PET as it is with CT. CT scanning and PET are complementary, as CT aids in the anatomical detail. More recently, PET scanning is being used to help evaluate for possible metastatic disease, with great promise in this regard.[19,20] Using whole-body PET imaging for staging lung cancer, unsuspected distant metastatic disease is seen in 11% to 14% of patients.[19,20]

LABORATORY VALUES

The essential initial laboratory tests include a complete blood count, chemistries including electrolytes, liver function panel (SGOT/SGPT/alkaline phosphatase/and total bilirubin), albumin, urea, creatinine, and calcium. Although liver enzymes are rarely abnormal in the absence of extensive liver metastases, they should be obtained as a screen. Abnormalities in creatinine, blood urea nitrogen, and electrolytes may suggest a small cell carcinoma with associated syndrome of inappropriate antidiuretic hormone secretion. Elevated calcium and alkaline phosphatase should raise suspicion of bony involvement. The patient's nutritional status can be evaluated by albumin, which has been proven to be a prognostic factor.[5]

SERUM TUMOR MARKERS

Several tumor markers are currently being investigated and are known to be associated with different types of lung cancers.[5] At the present time none have been shown to be useful.

BRAIN AND BONE SCANS

Brain CT scans and radionuclide bone scans should be performed for certain indications but not in every case. Current recommendations are to perform head CT and radionuclide bone scans in patients with specific neurological or bony symptoms, in patients with nonspecific symptoms suggestive of metastatic disease, clinically stage I or II but marginally operative candidates, and patients with clinically stage IIIA disease that are potential operative candidates or potentially candidates for curative chemoradiation.[6]

Pathological Diagnosis

When an otherwise healthy patient presents with a new pulmonary nodule suspicious for lung cancer, a biopsy is not an absolute requirement before exploration, but histological confirmation is desirable. If nonsurgical treatment is being considered either as neoadjuvant or in lieu of surgery because of the apparent extent of disease, a tissue diagnosis is required before initiation of such therapy. Cytological specimens may be initially attempted before surgical biopsy techniques, and the ability to make the diagnosis using cytological techniques depends on the quality of the specimen, including number of cells and viability of cells. Six different types of cytological specimens may be collected, including sputum, bronchial washings, bronchial brushings, transbronchial needle aspirates, bronchoalveolar lavage, and transthoracic fine-needle aspiration. If a diagnosis is not provided by these cytological techniques, tissue may be obtained by endobronchial biopsy, transbronchial biopsy, transthoracic biopsy, or by thoracoscopy or thoracotomy for wedge resection.

BRONCHOSCOPY

Flexible fiberoptic bronchoscopy is a routine part of preoperative evaluation of lung cancer patients, although it may be performed at the time of more definitive surgical treatment. It is valuable in the diagnosis and staging of lung cancer and for assessment of the bronchial tree. For diagnosis of central lesions, the yield with SCLC and NSCLC using bronchial forceps to biopsy and brushings is greater than 70%, increasing to more than 90% if an endobronchial component is appreciated.[21] Because mediastinal lymph nodes can be biopsied by this technique, it is useful in staging. The sensitivity of this procedure in mediastinal staging is only 50% but the specificity in 96%.[22] Complications from this procedure are infrequent, but include bleeding and pneumothorax.[5] For peripheral lesions the diagnostic yields from bronchoscopy and transbronchial needle biopsies and washings are only 40% to 80%.

TRANSTHORACIC NEEDLE ASPIRATION

Transthoracic needle aspiration (TTNA) is performed by radiologists with expertise in the area in close collaboration with a pathologist with the obtainment of either cytological or histological material for evaluation. This is the procedure of choice if a diagnosis of a small peripheral nodule is desired. CT or fluoroscopic guidance of transthoracic needle aspiration can detect malignancy with an accuracy of 80% to 95%.[23] Patients with indeterminate studies have a 20% to 30% chance of having cancer.[23] Therefore, a negative or nondiagnostic study does not preclude proceeding with surgical intervention if suspicion is high that the lesion is cancerous.

THORACOSCOPY/THORACOTOMY FOR WEDGE RESECTION

Usually thoracoscopy or thoracotomy for wedge resection is performed at the time definitive treatment is planned. Close collaboration between surgeon and pathologist is essential.[5] The presence of a pleural or pericardial effusion likewise requires cytological proof of the presence of malignant cells in the effusion before presuming inoperability, and thoracoscopic techniques may aid in the diagnosis. Thoracentesis may also be used to obtain cytological diagnosis in malignant pleural effusions.

CERVICAL MEDIASTINOSCOPY

Enlarged mediastinal lymph nodes on CT scan in the absence of other more accessible evidence of disease necessitates mediastinoscopy for lymph node biopsy before surgical or alternative therapy initiation. It should be performed before thoracotomy in a patient with a CT scanning showing enlarged mediastinal lymph nodes greater than 1 cm because the CT scan is only 70% accurate in this case. If mediastinal lymph nodes are not enlarged, the decision to proceed with mediastinoscopy may be individualized. Cervical mediastinoscopy allows access to the paratracheal lymph nodes, the subcarinal lymph nodes, and occasionally tracheobronchial angle lymph nodes. This technique can be performed before planned resective surgery, or at the time of thoracotomy.[5]

EXTENDED CERVICAL MEDIASTINOSCOPY

Extended cervical mediastinoscopy, left anterior mediastinotomy (Chamberlain procedure), or thoracoscopy can be used to biopsy an enlarged aortopulmonary window and paraaortic lymph nodes. Extended cervical mediastinoscopy is particularly useful if a standard cervical mediastinoscopy is negative for metastatic disease and the CT scan shows enlargement of the aortopulmonary and paraaortic lymph nodes, commonly seen in left upper lobe lung tumors. If standard mediastinoscopy is negative and CT scanning does not show enlargement in anterior mediastinal lymph nodes, extended cervical mediastinoscopy is not recommended.

SCALENE NODE BIOPSY

Scalene lymph node biopsying during mediastinoscopy may be valuable in N2 or N3 staged patients with centrally located, nonsquamous lung cancers to identify those who would not be helped by aggressive surgical intervention in combination with multimodal therapy.[24]

Staging of Non-Small Cell Lung Cancer

The TNM descriptors are shown in Table 39.5, and the modified staging system is shown in Table 39.6. Stages I through IIIB are depicted schematically in Figure 39.4.

Surgical Management of Non-Small Cell Lung Carcinoma

The most effective treatment for NSCLC remains surgical resection. When surgical cure is not possible because of the extent of disease, chemotherapy and radiotherapy may provide palliation. The best indicator that surgical therapy will provide cure is the stage of the lung cancer at diagnosis. All the primary lung tumor and surrounding intrapulmonary lymphatics must be removed. The removal must be complete. Lobectomy is the procedure of choice, but pneumonectomy may be required for negative surgical margins. Mediastinal lymph nodes should be dissected or sampled for the most accurate staging. Utilizing these surgical principles, stage I and II and a subset of stage III non-small cell lung cancers are treated best by complete resection.[6] New solitary pulmonary nodules should be resected in any patient medically fit to undergo surgical removal. Optimization of preoperative pulmonary and overall medical status will result in less postop-

TABLE 39.5. Lung Cancer TNM Descriptors.

Primary tumor (T)
TX	Primary tumor cannot be assessed, or tumor proven by the presence of malignant cells in sputum or bronchial washings but not visualized by imaging or bronchoscopy
T0	No evidence of primary tumor
Tis	Carcinoma *in situ*
T1	Tumor ≤3 cm in greatest dimension, surrounded by lung or visceral pleura, without bronchoscopic evidence of invasion more proximal than the lobar bronchus* (i.e., not in the main bronchus)
T2	Tumor with any of the following features of size or extent: >3 cm in greatest dimension Involves main bronchus, ≥2 cm distal to the carina Invades the visceral pleura Association with atelectasis or obstructive pneumonitis that extends to the hilar region but does not involve the entire lung.
T3	Tumor of any size that directly invades any of the following: chest wall (including superior sulcus tumors), diaphragm, mediastinal pleura, parietal pericardium; or tumor in the main bronchus <2 cm distal to the carina, but without involvement of the carina; or associated atelectasis or obstructive pneumonitis of the entire lung
T4	Tumor of any size that invades any of the following: mediastinum, heart, great vessels, trachea, esophagus, vertebral body, carina; or tumor with a malignant pleural or pericardial effusion,† or with satellite tumor nodule(s) within the ipsilateral primary tumor lobe of the lung

Regional lymph nodes (N)
NX	Regional lymph nodes cannot be assessed
N0	No regional lymph node metastasis
N1	Metastasis to ipsilateral peribronchial and/or ipsilateral hilar lymph nodes, and intrapulmonary nodes involved by direct extension of the primary tumor
N2	Metastasis to ipsilateral mediastinal and/or subcarinal lymph node(s)
N3	Metastasis to contralateral mediastinal, contralateral hilar, ipsilateral or contralateral scalene, or supraclavicular lymph node(s)

Distant metastasis (M)
MX	Presence of distant metastasis cannot be assessed
M0	No distant metastasis
M1	Distant metastasis present‡

*The uncommon superficial tumor of any size with its invasive component limited to the bronchial wall, which may extend proximal to the main bronchus, is also classified T1.

†Most pleural effusions associated with lung cancer are due to tumor. However, there are a few patients in whom multiple cytopathologic examinations of pleural fluid show no tumor. In these cases, the fluid is nonbloody and is not an exudate. When these elements and clinical judgment dictate that the effusion is not related to the tumor, the effusion should be excluded as a staging element and the patient's disease should be staged T1, T2, or T3. Pericardial effusion is classified according to the same rules.

‡Separate metastatic tumor nodule(s) in the ipsilateral nonprimary tumor lobe(s) of the lung also are classified M1.

Source: Mountain CF. Revisions in the international system for staging lung cancer. Chest 1997;111:1711.[32] Reprinted with permission.

TABLE 39.6. Stage Grouping: TNM Subsets.

Stage	TNM Subset
0	Carcinoma *in situ*
IA	T1N0M0
IB	T2N0M0
IIA	T1N1M0
IIB	T2N1M0
	T3N0M0
IIIA	T3N1M0
	T1N2M0
	T2N2M0
	T3N2M0
IIIB	T4N0M0
	T4N1M0
	T4N2M0
	T1N3M0
	T2N3M0
	T3N3M0
	T4N3M0
IV	Any T Any N M1

*Staging is not relevant for occult carcinoma, designated TXN0M0.

Source: Mountain CF. Revisions in the international system for staging lung cancer. Chest 1997;111:1712.[32] Reprinted with permission.

erative morbidity and mortality. Patients should be counseled in smoking cessation before surgical resection, and ideally be smoke free for several weeks before surgery.

Determination of Operability

PREOPERATIVE LUNG FUNCTION ASSESSMENT

Patients thought to be resectable need pulmonary function tests before major lung resections. Routine pulmonary function tests and an arterial blood gas provide the necessary information in most instances, but borderline pulmonary function may require radionuclide scanning or exercise testing. If on spirometry testing the FEV_1 is greater than 2.0 l or greater than 60% of predicted normal value, pneumonectomy is thought to be safe in an otherwise healthy patient.[25] Maximal voluntary ventilation above 50% of predicted normal, a ratio of residual volume to total lung capacity below 50%, and a diffusing capacity greater than 60% of predicted are further indicators a patient can tolerate a pneumonectomy. Arterial hypoxemia ($PaO_2 < 50$–60 torr on room air), and hypercapnia ($PaCO_2 > 45$ torr) are relative contraindications.[5,25]

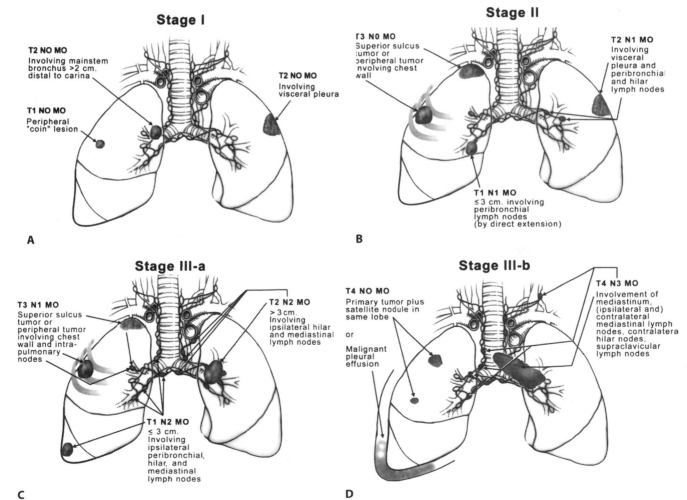

FIGURE 39.4. A. Schematic of stage I disease. **B.** Stage II disease. **C.** Stage IIIA disease. **D.** Stage IIIB disease. [Adapted from Mountain CF. A new international staging system for lung cancer. Chest 1986;89:225S–233S, and updated to reflect revisions in the international system for staging lung cancer (Mountain CF. Revisions in the international system for staging lung cancer. Chest 1997;111:1710–1717[32]).]

MEDICAL CONTRAINDICATIONS

A patient's overall medical health must be assessed before consideration of surgical resection. Attention must be given to patient's age, pulmonary function (as discussed above), and extent of resection necessary.[26] Coexisting diseases and weight loss (10%) before surgery place a patient at increased risk for postoperative complications. A history of angina or abnormal preoperative EKG requires a radionuclide cardiac study to assess perfusion or function and, if positive, a cardiac catherization should be performed before lung resection. Recent myocardial infarction, stroke, severe congestive heart failure, or refractory arrhythmias make a patient inoperable for medical reasons.

Surgical Procedures

LOBECTOMY

Lobectomy is the preferred and most frequently performed operative procedure for early-stage lung cancer. The Lung Cancer Study Group (LCSG) conducted a prospective, randomized trial comparing lobectomy to segmentectomy or wedge resection in patients not able to tolerate a lobectomy with stage I (T1N0M0) lung cancer and found no differences in morbidity, mortality, or postoperative pulmonary function between the groups. Locoregional recurrence was significantly higher in patients undergoing conservative pulmonary resections (15%) compared to patients who underwent lobectomy (5%).[27] Mortality after lobectomy is less than 3%.[28]

PNEUMONECTOMY

Often intraoperatively a patient is found to have a cancer completely resectable only by a pneumonectomy. Cases in which a pneumonectomy is usually required include central lesions at the orifices of lobar bronchi, lymph node involvement by cancer proximal to the upper lobe takeoff, involvement of "sump" lymph nodes located on the pulmonary artery between lobes (except when involvement is of sump nodes between right middle and lower lobes, where a bilobectomy can be performed), and involvement of lymph nodes along the main pulmonary artery.[6] Careful patient selection in cases of lung cancer requiring pneumonectomy for complete resections is necessary. Mortality after pneumonectomy should be less than 7%.[28]

WEDGE RESECTION/SEGMENTECTOMY

These procedures should be performed for lung cancer only in patients with limited pulmonary function. As noted, the high local–regional recurrence rate requires close follow-up for patients treated by these operations.

THORACOSCOPIC PROCEDURES

The use of thoracoscopy before thoracotomy to confirm the diagnosis of lung cancer or evaluate a pleural effusion is well established, but its use in performing lobectomies and mediastinal lymph node dissection is being investigated.

SLEEVE RESECTION

Sleeve lobectomy may be considered as an alternative to pneumonectomy, and may be performed on all five lobes. The procedure entails resection of the mainstem bronchus and lobar orifice of the lobe involved, lobectomy, and reanastomosis of other lobar bronchi to the remaining larger proximal bronchus. Patients over the age of 65, those with chronic obstructive pulmonary disease, and those with second primary lung cancers should be considered for sleeve resections when they present with tumors precluding lobectomy, as these patients poorly tolerate extensive pulmonary resections.

MEDIASTINAL LYMPH NODE DISSECTION

Mediastinal lymph node dissection is an integral part of surgical treatment of patients with lung cancer if it allows the most accurate staging. The normal number of nodes removed in a mediastinal lymph node dissection is 25 to 40, and more nodes are removed by dissection versus sampling. For stage I or II lung cancers, mediastinal lymph node dissection confirms the absence of mediastinal node involvement. For stage IIIA, the value of mediastinal lymph node dissection is in further defining extent of disease and potentially improving survival.[29–31]

Results of Surgical Resection

Survival curves based on clinical staging of NSCLC are shown in Figure 39.5.

Stage I

Following surgical resection for stage I NSCLC the 1-year survival rate is between 72% and 94% and the 5-year survival rate is between 38% and 67%. The presence of symptoms, vascular invasion, pleural invasion, and tumor size greater than 3 cm are significant multivariate independent variables for early recurrence and cancer death in stage I NSCLC.

Stage II

Following surgical resection, patients diagnosed with stage II NSCLC experience 1-year survival rates between 55% and

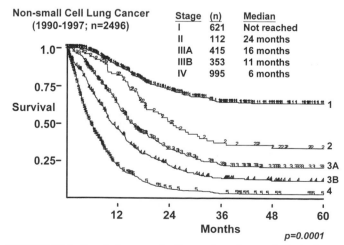

FIGURE 39.5. Survival curves for 5 years based on pathological staging through stage IIIB. Some IIIB–IV were staged radiographically with biopsy proven metastases. Overall median survival, 10 months. *Number symbol* (#) denote censored data.

89% and 5-year survival rates between 22% and 55%. Favorable prognostic indicators were tumors smaller than 3 cm and single N1 node involvement. Either distant metastases or locoregional recurrences occurred in 53% of patients. Overall distant metastases were the most common type of recurrence, with the most frequent site or relapse being the brain.

Stage IIIA

Improved survival is seen in the subset of stage IIIA NSCLC that is amenable to complete surgical resection. Following definitive multimodality therapy including surgical resection, 5-year survival of 23% to 25% is seen in this stage of disease as staged surgically and pathologically.[32]

Stage IIIB–IV

The role of surgical treatment in stage IIIB–IV is currently controversial. Clinically staged IIIB NSCLC patients have 1-year survival rates between 32% and 37% and 5-year survival rates between 3% and 7%. Occasional cures have been seen with resections of T4 lesions, and carinal pneumonectomy may result in long-term survivors in carefully selected patients with T4 lesions invading the carina. Patients with clinically stage IV disease have a 1-year survival rate of 20% and 5-year survival rate of 1%.[32] Selected patients with stage IV disease may be candidates for surgical resection.

Superior Sulcus Tumor

These tumors, arising in the apex of the lung (Pancoast tumors), are currently best treated initially by radiotherapy. A pathological diagnosis is a prerequisite to treatment and fine-needle aspiration is the procedure of choice for confirmation of lung cancer.[33] The majority of superior sulcus tumors are adenocarcinomas. Palliation of the characteristic arm pain may be achieved with radiation treatment alone or combined radiation and surgery with good to excellent success. Curative treatment of superior sulcus tumors can consist of radiotherapy and resection or combination of chemotherapy, radiotherapy, and resection. Five-year survival after curative treatment with radiotherapy followed by surgery is approximately 40% compared to 20% after radiotherapy alone (50–60 Gy).[33]

Other Pulmonary Cancers

Multiple primary lung cancers are seen in approximately 0.8% to 7.6% of patients, occurring synchronously in 0.26% to 1.33% and metachronously in 0.5% of all lung cancer cases.[34] This low number of synchronous primary lesions necessitates evaluation of two lesions for the possibility of (1) two benign lesions; (2) two cancers metastatic from extrathoracic sites; (3) one benign and one malignant pulmonary lesion; (4) two primary lung cancers; and (5) one primary lung cancer and one metastatic lesion. Treatment of synchronous and metachronous primaries is surgical resection if possible; pulmonary compromise after resection needs preoperative evaluation.

Induction and Adjuvant Therapies

Stage I through IIIA NSCLC

Four randomized, prospective adjuvant therapy trials have been reported evaluating patients with stage I lung cancer (Table 39.7). From these studies, recommendation for adjuvant therapy after resection for stage I cancers cannot be made.

The Lung Cancer Study Group has reported three completed adjuvant therapy trials for stage II or III lung cancer (Table 39.8).[35–37] None showed a significant survival advantage with adjuvant therapy administration.

The role of postoperative radiotherapy in treatment of patients with completely resected non-small cell lung cancer was recently evaluated in a meta-analysis from nine randomized trials[38] comparing postoperative radiotherapy versus surgery alone. The findings from this meta-analysis were surprising, showing a significantly adverse effect of postoperative radiotherapy on survival.

There have been five recently completed randomized trials evaluating neoadjuvant treatment of patients with stage II or III NSCLC (Table 39.9).[39–43] Though not conclusive, there was some evidence that induction/preoperative chemotherapy or chemoradiotherapy may offer a survival benefit.

TABLE 39.7.
Randomized, Prospective Adjuvant Stage I NSCLC Trials (Level I Evidence).

Study	Patients (n)	Treatment	Eligibility	Survival
LCSG (1981)[56]	425	S + Intrapleural BCG/S + Saline	T1N0, T2N0, T1N1 resected	NS
Niiranen et al. (1992)[57]	99	S + C/S	T1-3N0 resected	$p = 0.05$
LCSG (1993)[58]	269	S + C/S	T2N0-T1N1 resected	NS
Japan (1995)[59]	309	S + C/S	Stage I-III resected	NS (adjusted survival, $p = 0.044$)

LCSG, Lung Cancer Study Group.

TABLE 39.8.

Randomized, Prospective Adjuvant Therapy in Stage II–III NSCLC (Level I Evidence).

Study	Patients (n)	Treatment	Eligibility	Survival
LCSG (1986)[37]	130	S + C/S + BCG + levamisole	Resected stage II/III adeno- and large cell carcinomas	NS
LCSG (1986)[36]	210	S + RT/S	Resected stage II/III squamous cell carcinoma	NS
LCSG (1988)[35]	164	S + C + RT/ S + RT	Incompletely resected NSCLC	NS
Japan (1993)[60]	181	S + C/S	Resected stage III (any T3 or N2)	NS
Dautzenberg (1995)[61]	267	S + C + RT/S + RT	Resected stage I–III (71% stage III)	NS

In summary, for lung cancer patients with stage II to IIIA tumors, there appears to be a trend toward improved survival with multimodality treatment. Newer chemotherapeutic agents will most likely convert this trend into significance. Whether postinduction surgery is the standard of care in patients with stage IIIA disease remains debated[44] and will be answered only by further randomized, controlled trials with careful subset selections.

Stage IIIB

At the current time resection of N3 disease can not be routinely recommended. Patients with T4N0-1 stage IIIB disease may benefit from postinduction surgery.

Stage IV

Stage IV disease is, for the most part, considered incurable and is treated with palliative chemotherapy and radiation.

ADRENAL METASTASES

At presentation 5% to 10% of patients with non-small cell lung cancer have adrenal metastases.[45] The percentage of patients with operable lung cancer and solitary adrenal metastases, however, is lower, ranging from 1.62% to 3.5%.[45,46] When a patient with potentially curable NSCLC is found to have an adrenal mass, a diagnosis of benign versus malignant needs to be made. In a treatment protocol, resection of isolated adrenal metastasis can be undertaken.

BRAIN METASTASES

Surgical removal of brain metastases for NSCLC is the best treatment for both palliation and possible long-term survival.[47] Without treatment of brain metastasis, the survival is only 1 month.[34] Treatment of brain metastases with steroids palliates symptoms and extends the median survival to 2 months. Radiation treatment also extends survival, on the order of 3 to 6 months. Five-year survival of approximately 30% is seen after complete resection of solitary brain metastases.[34]

TABLE 39.9.

Randomized, Prospective Induction Therapy in Stage II–III NSCLC (Level I Evidence).

Study	# of patients	Treatment	Eligibility	Survival
NCI[39]	28	C + S + C/ S + RT	Stage IIIA (N2 disease biopsy proven)	$p = 0.12$
M.D. Anderson[40]	60	C + S ± C/S	Stage IIIA (mixed, N2 not required) some IIIB	$p < 0.008$
Spain[41]	60	C + S + RT/ S + RT	Stage IIIA (mixed, N2 not required)	$p < 0.001$
Japan[42]	83	C + RT + S/ S	Clinical IIIA Select IIIB	NS
CALGB, 1997[43]	57	C + S + C + RT/ RT + S + RT	Stage IIIA (N2 disease biopsy proven)	NS

Follow-Up of Lung Cancer Patients

There are no definitive guidelines for follow-up of lung cancer patients following surgical resection. Although frequency of follow-up remains debated, examination including chest radiograph every 3 months to 4 months for the first year, followed by every 6 months afterward, is commonly practiced by thoracic surgeons. Although not recommended, an annual chest CT scan can be obtained.

Small Cell Lung Cancer

Small cell lung cancer represents approximately 15% of all lung cancers and has the poorest 5-year survival of all histological types. The approach to treatment is different, and in general a significantly larger role is played by the medical oncologist than the thoracic surgeon. Exposure to tobacco smoke and environmental risk factors such as ionizing radiation play a high risk in the development of SCLC. Current 5-year survival for SCLC is 5% to 10%.

Treatment of SCLC

The treatment of SCLC depends on stage at diagnosis. There have been multiple reports of surgery followed by chemotherapy with or without radiotherapy in the treatment of pathological stage I or II SCLC. The results have been quite encouraging for surgical treatment in this group of patients, with an overall 5-year survival rate of 54%.[48–53] Unfortunately, stage I/II disease represents only 1% of SCLC patients at diagnosis. For patients with stage IIIA/IIIB (limited stage) SCLC, the results of surgery after chemotherapy and radiotherapy do not suggest a significant survival benefit for patients treated with surgery after chemotherapy with or without radiotherapy compared to patients treated with chemotherapy with or without radiotherapy without surgery.[54] Therefore surgical treatment of limited stage IIIA/IIIB SCLC is currently not recommended, and chemotherapy with concurrent or alternating radiotherapy is the preferred treatment. Palliative chemotherapy is the cornerstone of treatment of patients with extensive (stage IV) SCLC.

References

1. American Cancer Society: 1998 Cancer Facts and Figures. Atlanta: American Cancer Society, 1998.
2. World Health Organization. Histological typing of lung tumors. International Histological Classification of Tumors, No. 1. Geneva: World Health Organization, 1981.
3. Cotran RS. The respiratory system: lung. In: Cotran RS, Kumar V, Robbins SL, eds. Robbins Pathologic Basis of Disease. Philadelphia: Saunders, 1989;755–810.
4. Melamed MR, Flehinger BJ, Zaman MB. Impact of early detection on the clinical course of lung cancer. Surg Clin North Am 1987;67:909.
5. American Thoracic Society ERS. Pretreatment evaluation of non-small cell-lung cancer. Am J Respir Crit Care Med 1997;156:320–332.
6. Lung cancer. In: Pearson FG, Deslauriers J, Ginsberg RJ, Hiebert CA, McKneally MF, Urschel HC, eds. Thoracic Surgery. New York: Churchill Livingstone, 1995;637–706.
7. Doll R, Peto R. Mortality in relation to smoking: 20 years' observations on male British doctors. Br Med J 1976;2:1525–1536.
8. Doll R, Gray R, Hafner B, Peto R. Mortality in relation to smoking: 22 years' observations on female British doctors. Br Med J 1980:967–971.
9. Carcinoma of the lung. In: Shields TW, ed. General Thoracic Surgery, Vol. 1. Baltimore: Williams & Wilkins, 1994:1095–1286.
10. Rusch VW, Dmitrovsky E. Molecular biologic features of non-small cell lung cancer: clinical implications. Chest Surg Clin N Am 1995;5:39–55.
11. Hyde L, Hyde CI. Clinical manifestations of lung cancer. Chest 1974;65:299.
12. Carbone PP, Frost JK, Feinstein AR, et al. Lung cancer: perspective and prospects. Ann Internal Med 1970;73:1024.
13. Abrams HL, Spiro R, Goldstein N. Metastases in carcinoma: analysis of 1000 autopsied cases. Cancer (Phila) 1950;3:74–85.
14. Ochsner A, DeBakey M. Carcinoma of the lung. Arch Surg 1941;42:209–258S.
15. Patz EF, Lowe VL, Hoffman JM, et al. Focal pulmonary abnormalities: evaluation with F-18 fluorodeoxyglucose PET scanning. Radiology 1993;188:487–490.
16. Scott WJ, Schwabe JL, Gupta NC, et al. Positron emission tomography of lung tumors and mediastinal lymph nodes using (18F) fluorodeoxyglucose. Ann Thorac Surg 1994;58:698–703.
17. Scott WJ, Gobar LS, Hauser LG, Sunderland JJ, Dewan NA, Sugimoto JT. Detection of scalene lymph node metastases from lung cancer: positron emission tomography. Chest 1995;107:1174–1176.
18. Wahl RL, Quint LE, Greenough RL, Meyer CR, White RI, Orringer MB. Staging of mediastinal non-small cell lung cancer with FDG-PET, CT, and fusion images: preliminary prospective evaluation. Radiology 1994;191:371–377.
19. Valk PE, Pounds TR, Hopkins DM, et al. Staging non-small cell lung cancer by whole-body-positron emission tomographic imaging. Ann Thorac Surg 1995;60:1573–1582.
20. Weder W, Schmid RA, Bruchhaus H, Hillinger S, Schulthess GKv, Steinert HC. Detection of extrathoracic metastases by positron emission tomography in lung cancer. Ann Thorac Surg 1998;66:886–893.
21. Arroliga AC, Matthay RA. The role of bronchoscopy in lung cancer. Clin Chest Med 1993;14:87–98.
22. Harrow EM, Wang KP. The staging of lung cancer by bronchoscopic transbronchial needle aspiration. Chest Surg Clin North Am 1996;6:223–235.
23. Salazar AM, Westcott JL. The role of transthoracic needle biopsy for the diagnosis and staging of lung cancer. Clin Chest Med 1993;14:99–110.
24. Lee JD, Ginsberg RJ. Lung cancer staging: the value of ipsilateral scalene lymph node biopsy performed at mediastinoscopy. Ann Thorac Surg 1996;62:338–341.
25. Dunn WF, Scanlon PD. Preoperative pulmonary function testing for patients with lung cancer. Mayo Clin Proc 1993;68:371–377.
26. Deslauriers J, Ginsberg RJ, Dubois P, Beaulieu M, Goldberg M, Piraux M. Current operative morbidity associated with elective surgical resection for lung cancer. Can J Surg 1989;32:335–339.
27. Ginsberg R, Rubinstein L, LCSG. A randomized trial of lobectomy versus limited resection in patients with T1N0 non-small cell lung cancer (abstract). Lung Cancer 1991;7:83.
28. Ginsberg RJ, Hill LD, Eagan RT, et al. Modern thirty-day operative mortality for surgical resections in lung cancer. J Thorac Cardiovasc Surg 1983;86:654–658.
29. Naruke T, Suemasu K, Ishikawa S. Lymph node mapping and curability at various levels of metastasis in resected lung cancer. J Thorac Cardiovasc Surg 1978;76:832–839.
30. Naruke T, Goya T, Tsuchiya R, et al. The importance of surgery to non-small cell carcinoma of the lung with mediastinal lymph node metastases. Ann Thorac Surg 1988a;46:603–610.
31. Watanabe Y, Shimizu J, Oda M, et al. Aggressive surgical inter-

vention in N2 non-small cell cancer of the lung. Ann Thorac Surg 1991;51:253–261.

32. Mountain CF. Revisions in the international system for staging lung cancer. Chest 1997;111:1710–1717.

33. Detterbeck FC. Pancoast (superior sulcus) tumors. Ann Thorac Surg 1997;63:1810–1818.

34. Olak J, Ferguson MK. Surgical management of metastatic lung cancer. In: Pass HI, Mitchell JB, Johnson DH, Turrisi AT, eds. Lung Cancer: Principles and Practice. Philadelphia: Lippincott-Raven, 1996;603–613.

35. Lad T, Rubinstein L, Sadeghi A. The benefit of adjuvant treatment for resected locally advanced non-small-cell lung cancer. J Clin Oncol 1988;6:9–17.

36. LCSG. Effects of postoperative mediastinal radiation on completely resected stage II and stage III epidermoid cancer of the lung. N Engl J Med 1986;315:1377–1381.

37. Holmes C, Gail M, LCSG. Surgical adjuvant therapy for stage II and stage III adenocarcinoma and large-cell undifferentiated carcinoma. J Clin Oncol 1986;4:710–715.

38. PORT Meta-analysis Trialist Group. Postoperative radiotherapy in non-small cell lung cancer: systematic review and meta-analysis of individual patient data from nine randomized controlled trials. Lancet 1998;352:257–263.

39. Pass HI, Pogrebniak HW, Steinberg SM, Mulshine J, Minna J. Randomized trial of neoadjuvant therapy for lung cancer: interim analysis. Ann Thorac Surg 1992;53:992–998.

40. Roth JA, Fossella F, Komaki R, et al. A randomized trial comparing perioperative chemotherapy and surgery with surgery alone in resectable stage IIIA non-small-cell lung cancer. J Natl Cancer Inst 1994;86:673–680.

41. Rosell R, Gomez-Codina J, Camps C, et al. A randomized trial comparing preoperative chemotherapy plus surgery with surgery alone in patients with non-small-cell lung cancer. N Engl J Med 1994;330:153–158.

42. Yoneda S, Hibino S, Gotoh I, et al. A comparative trial of induction chemoradiotherapy followed by surgery or immediate surgery for stage III NSCLC (Abstract 1128). Proc Am Soc Clin Oncol 1995;14:367.

43. Elias AD, Herndon J, Kumar P, et al. A phase III comparison of "best local-regional therapy" with or without chemotherapy (CT) for stage IIIA T1-3N2 non-small cell lung cancer (NSCLC): preliminary results (abstract 1611S). Proc Am Soc Clin Oncol 1997;16:448a.

44. Albain KS. Induction chemotherapy with/without radiation followed by surgery in stage III non-small-cell lung cancer. Oncology 1997;11:51–57.

45. Porte HL, Roumilhac D, Graziana J-P, et al. Adrenalectomy for a solitary adrenal metastasis from lung cancer. Ann Thorac Surg 1998;331–335.

46. Ettinghausen SE, Burt ME. Prospective evaluation of unilateral adrenal masses in patients with operable non-small cell lung cancer. J Clin Oncol 1991;9:1462–1466.

47. Burt M, Wronski M, Arbit E, et al. Resection of brain metastases from non-small-cell lung carcinoma. J Thorac Cardiovasc Surg 1992;103:399–411.

48. Cook RM, Miller YE, Paul A, Bunn J. Small cell lung cancer: etiology, biology, clinical features, staging, and treatment. Curr Probl Cancer 1993;17:69–141.

49. Karrer K, Shields TW, Denck H, et al. The importance of surgical and multimodality treatment for small cell bronchial carcinoma. J Thorac Cardiovasc Surg 1986;97:168–176.

50. Salzer GM, Muller LC, Huber H, et al. Operation for N2 small cell lung carcinoma. Ann Thorac Surg 1990;49:759–762.

51. Ginsberg RJ. Surgery and small cell lung cancer—an overview. Lung Cancer 1989;5:232–236.

52. Ohta M, Hara N, Ichinose Y, et al. The role of surgical resection in the management of small cell carcinoma of the lung. Jpn J Clin Oncol 1986;16:289–296.

53. Meyer JA, Gullo JJ, Ikins PM, et al. Adverse prognostic effect of N2 disease in treated small cell carcinoma of the lung. J Thorac Cardiovasc Surg 1984;88:495–501.

54. Lad T, Thomas P, Piantadosi S. Surgical resection of small cell lung cancer—a prospective randomized evaluation (abstract). Proc ASCO 1991;10:244.

55. Shields TW. Presentation, diagnosis, and staging of bronchial carcinoma and of the asymptomatic solitary pulmonary nodule. In: Shields TW, ed. General Thoracic Surgery. Vol. 1. Baltimore: Williams & Wilkins, 1994:1122–1154.

56. Mountain CF, Gail MH, LCSG. Surgical adjuvant intrapleural BCG treatment for stage I non-small cell lung cancer. J Thorac Cardiovasc Surg 1981;82:649–657.

57. Niiranen A, Niitamo-Korhonen S, Kouri M, Assendelft A, Mattson K, Pyrhonen S. Adjuvant chemotherapy after radical surgery or non-small-cell lung cancer: a randomized study. J Clin Oncol 1992;10:1927–1932.

58. Feld R, Rubinstein L, Thomas PA, LCSG. Adjuvant chemotherapy with cyclophosphamide, doxorubicin, and cisplatin in patients with completely resected stage I non-small cell lung cancer. J Natl Cancer Inst 1993;85:299–306.

59. SGACLC. A randomized trial of postoperative adjuvant chemotherapy in non-small cell lung cancer (the second cooperative study). Eur J Surg Oncol 1995;21:69–77.

60. Ohta M, Tsuchiya R, Shimoyama M, et al. Adjuvant chemotherapy for completely resected stage III non-small-cell lung cancer: results of a randomized prospective study. J Thorac Cardiovasc Surg 1993;106:703–708.

61. Dautzenberg B, Chastang C, Arriagada R, et al. Adjuvant radiotherapy versus combined sequential chemotherapy followed by radiotherapy in the treatment of resected nonsmall cell lung carcinoma. Cancer 1995;76:779–786.

40

Lung Infections and Trauma

R. Lawrence Reed

Thoracic Trauma

Trauma to the chest is a common occurrence in modern society, with chest trauma causing one of every four trauma deaths in North America. Overall mortality for thoracic trauma is roughly 10%, with about 15% of patients with thoracic trauma requiring operative therapy. The most common intervention provided to thoracic trauma patients is insertion of a thoracostomy tube.

The standard evaluation of the acutely injured patient has been defined by the Advanced Trauma Life Support Course of the American College of Surgeons. Because of the vital cardiorespiratory organs housed in the thoracic cavity, the initial assessment of the trauma patient should identify any immediately life-threatening injuries. Such injuries include airway obstruction, open pneumothorax, tension pneumothorax, flail chest, massive hemothorax, and cardiac tamponade. The primary survey undertaken in the acutely injured patient goes through the "ABC" evaluation of airway, breathing, and circulation. Although usually not immediately life threatening, there are several other intrathoracic injuries that are potentially lethal if not effectively treated, including various ruptures (aortic, diaphragmatic, esophageal, or tracheobronchial) and contusions (pulmonary and myocardial). These injuries are usually detected during the secondary survey, including the use of adjunct diagnostic procedures such as chest radiography.

Early management of the injured patient with intrathoracic injuries is identical with that of any injured patient. An adequate airway must first be established or maintained, which may sometimes require endotracheal intubation. Effective ventilation must be instituted by whatever means necessary: this may require the placement of a thoracostomy tube in the case of a pneumothorax or a hemothorax. Circulatory support for patients in shock is initially provided by placement of two large-bore intravenous catheters and the rapid infusion of warmed Ringer's lactate. Blood transfusion is warranted in patients who have sustained a class III or a class IV hemorrhage as defined by the American College of Surgeons.

Chest radiographs are invaluable in the assessment and management of the injured patient with thoracic trauma. Findings on chest X-rays can often lead to a suspicion or diagnosis of a variety of traumatic conditions (Table 40.1).

It is infrequently necessary to perform a thoracotomy on injured patients. However, there are some clear acute indications for a thoracotomy in the traumatic setting. These include cardiac tamponade, great vessel injury or vascular injury at the thoracic outlet, traumatic thoracotomy (i.e., loss of chest wall substance), tracheal or bronchial injury (e.g., massive air leak), esophageal injury, massive or continuing hemothorax, thoracic penetration with industrial liquids (especially coal tar products), bullet embolism to the heart or pulmonary artery, the transcardiac placement of an inferior vena cava shunt for retrohepatic vascular wounds, and recent cardiac arrest in patients with penetrating truncal trauma. In less acute settings, thoracotomies are performed in trauma for indications including unevacuated clotted hemothorax, chronic traumatic diaphragmatic hernia, traumatic cardiac septal or valvular lesions, chronic traumatic aortic thoracic pseudoaneurysm, nonclosing thoracic duct fistula, chronic posttraumatic empyema, traumatic lung abscess, tracheoesophageal fistula, innominate artery–tracheal fistula, and traumatic arteriovenous fistula.

Tension Pneumothorax

A tension pneumothorax is an acute life-threatening condition that results when air pressure progressively accumulates in the pleural space. It can be caused during mechanical ventilation with positive end-expiratory pressure, with a spontaneous pneumothorax in which ruptured emphysematous bullae fail to seal, or blunt chest trauma with failure of the lung parenchymal injury to seal. In the acutely traumatic setting, a common mechanism for tension pneumothorax is the development of a simple pneumothorax from a lung laceration. If the patient subsequently requires intubation and mechanical ventilation, air will then enter the pleural space under positive pressure but cannot exit.

TABLE 40.1. Association Between Abnormal Findings on Chest X-Ray and Associated Traumatic Conditions.

Abnormal finding	Potentially associated traumatic condition
Any rib fracture	Pneumothorax
Fracture, first 3 ribs	Airway or great vessel injury
Fracture, ribs 9–12	Abdominal injury
2 or more rib fractures in 2 or more places	Flail chest, pulmonary contusion
GI gas pattern in chest	Diaphragmatic rupture
Nasogastric tube in chest	Diaphragmatic rupture, ruptured esophagus
Air–fluid level in chest	Hemothorax, diaphragmatic rupture
Sternal fracture	Myocardial contusion, head injury, cervical spine injury
Mediastinal hematoma	Great vessel injury, sternal fracture
Disrupted diaphragm	Abdominal visceral injury
Respiratory distress	CNS injury, aspiration
Persistent large pneumothorax after chest tube insertion	Bronchial tear, esophageal disruption
Mediastinal air	Esophageal disruption, pneumoperitoneum, tracheal injury
Scapular fracture	Airway or great vessel injury, pulmonary contusion
Subdiaphragmatic air	Ruptured hollow abdominal viscus

The consequences of tension pneumothorax are parenchymal compression of the lung, shift of the mediastinum, and impaired venous return to the heart because of the elevated intrathoracic pressure. Hemodynamic instability is the sine qua non of tension pneumothorax in the acute trauma setting, and it poses an immediate threat to life. The diagnosis should typically be purely a clinical diagnosis, as there is usually insufficient time for diagnostic studies. Diagnostic clues are provided by the presence of respiratory distress with hypotension, jugular venous distension, unilateral percussive hyperresonance, and tracheal deviation. Needle decompression of the chest can be diagnostic and therapeutic, performed by placing a large-bore (12- to 14-gauge) needle over the superior edge of the second or third rib of the hyperresonant side in the midclavicular line. A subsequent chest tube insertion is mandatory as the needle decompression is only a temporizing maneuver.

Open Pneumothorax

Open pneumothoraces result from larger chest wall defects. Usually the defect must be at least two-thirds of the tracheal diameter for the pathway of least resistance for airflow to be through the defect; this results in what is commonly called a "sucking chest wound." Ventilatory insufficiency develops as a result of disruption of the bellows mechanism provided by the intact chest wall; negative pressure cannot adequately develop to expand the lung. Initial ventilatory assistance can be provided by applying an occlusive dressing taped securely on three sides; this provides a temporary one-way valve, allowing air to exit the chest but not reenter. This process converts the open pneumothorax to a closed pneumothorax. Because evacuation of air can sometimes be compromised, there is a danger of developing a tension pneumothorax. If a tension pneumothorax develops, it can be relieved temporarily by lifting the dressing and allowing the accumulated intrapleural air to escape. A chest tube must be inserted to effectively complete the arrangement by facilitating reestablishment of negative intrapleural pressure. Surgical debridement and closure is required in most cases of open pneumothorax, sometimes requiring chest wall reconstruction to handle the defect.

Massive Hemothorax

Massive is typically defined as more than 1500 ml of bloody output after placement of a chest tube or more than 200 ml/h output for more than 2 to 4 h. It is most commonly caused by major systemic or pulmonary vessel disruption and usually results from penetrating forms of trauma. The neck veins may be flat because of the severe hypovolemia or they may be distended from elevated intrathoracic pressure resulting from blood accumulation in the chest. The diagnosis should be suspected in a patient who is in shock with unilateral percussive dullness and the absence of breath sounds in one hemithorax. The condition is managed by the simultaneous restoration of blood volume and chest decompression with at least one large-bore (36-French) chest tube insertion. All patients with massive hemothorax should be taken promptly to the operating room for definitive control of their hemorrhage. Animal studies suggest that clamping the chest tube to help tamponade bleeding (to "buy time" while getting the patient to the operating room) does not offer a physiologic advantage and is therefore not recommended.

Flail Chest

Flail chest is defined as paradoxical movement of a portion of the chest wall, usually produced by a fracture of two or more ribs or the sternum in two or more places. In other words, a significant length of chest wall must be involved with the injury to produce an instability sufficient to be noticeable. Flail chest is typically associated with chest wall pain, dyspnea, hypoxia, and pulmonary failure.

Based upon a number of clinical studies, nonventilatory therapy of flail chest has emerged as the standard method for treatment. Endotracheal intubation and mechanical ventilation are reserved for cases of flail chest associated with true respiratory failure. This method of management has generally been shown to reduce morbidity, mortality, and hospital cost over mandatory ventilatory support for all flail chest patients.

Still controversial is the issue of the need for chest wall stabilization. Multiple studies suggest that there is a marked improvement seen in those patients who have undergone operative chest wall stabilization, allowing for more rapid weaning from mechanical ventilation and fewer associated complications. Unfortunately, no prospective, randomized trial exists concerning the issue. Based upon the available evidence, however, operative stabilization of chest wall should be considered when extensive flail chest is present.

From the experience and study of flail chest and pulmonary contusion, it has become apparent that aggressive pulmonary toilet is essential for good clinical outcomes to occur. Generally, it appears that epidural and intrapleural anesthesia or analgesia benefit patient care from the standpoint of pain relief and pulmonary function with minimal side effects or complications.

Cardiac Tamponade

Cardiac tamponade can result from either penetrating or blunt injuries. As the result of injury, blood leaks into the pericardial sac, impeding further ventricular filling and thereby depressing cardiac output. Because of the fixed fibrous nature of the pericardium, very little fluid is required to produce hemodynamic changes. As little as 60 to 100 ml of blood and clots in the pericardium are necessary to produce tamponade physiology. Thus, clinical relief may be achieved with removal of as little as 15 to 20 ml.

Ideally, the clinical diagnosis is made by detecting Beck's triad, consisting of hypotension, jugular venous distension, and muffled heart sounds. However, Beck's triad is detectable in only 10% to 40% of cases, Thus, myocardial tamponade is usually suspected by the presence of persistent hypotension and the finding of an elevated central venous pressure. This same constellation of findings, however, can be associated with tension pneumothorax, shivering, or straining. Moreover, volume infusion can temporize and maintain a patient's blood pressure in a state of compensated tamponade. However, there is a critical level of intrapericardial volume that will produce severe unrelenting hypotension.

The diagnosis of cardiac tamponade is confirmed by performing subxyphoid pericardiocentesis, although a 23% false-negative rate has been reported.[1] Aspiration of the contained blood will usually ameliorate the patient's circulatory problem. However, recurrence can occur. Therefore, it is important to leave a catheter in place to allow for the performance of repeated aspiration as necessary. Ultimately, pericardiocentesis should always be considered only a temporizing maneuver while preparing the patient for thoracotomy and definitive control of the source of hemorrhage. Subxiphoid, subdiaphragmatic, and transdiaphragmatic pericardiotomy may also have a role in evaluation, diagnosis, and temporization.

Aortic Rupture

Aortic rupture can occur following blunt trauma, usually following a deceleration event. Most believe that the aorta is torn as a result of an avulsion mechanism. Segments of the aorta are relatively mobile within the mediastinum. These mobile areas are partitioned by specific points of fixation, namely, the pericardium at the aortic root, the ligamentum arteriosum, and the crus of the diaphragm. With a sudden deceleration event, shear forces develop between the areas of relative mobility and the areas of fixation, tearing the aortic wall at the fixation points.

The prehospital mortality of aortic rupture is 85% because the most common anatomical location for rupture is at the aortic root. A tear in this location uniformly produces an immediate and massive pericardial tamponade with nearly instantaneous death. The next most common location for injury is at the isthmus below the ligamentum arteriosum; as a result of the near-100% mortality for aortic root injuries, injuries at the ligamentum become the type most commonly observed clinically. This type of injury is responsible for 80% to 90% of those patients arriving alive. Other locations for aortic injury that have been observed include the ascending aorta (proximal to the innominate), the aorta at the origin of the innominate, the aortic arch, and the descending aorta.

The diagnosis of blunt thoracic aortic injury requires a high level of suspicion; 30% of patients with this injury will have no external evidence of chest trauma. The chest radiograph is usually crucial to making the diagnosis, but injury may exist without any obvious signs on the initial chest radiograph. The role of serial chest radiographs has not been adequately evaluated, although it has clearly been useful in every trauma surgeon's experience.

There are several radiological clues to thoracic great vessel injury on chest radiograph (Table 40.2). In general, these signs represent evidence of a mediastinal hematoma and are thus not specific for aortic rupture, as injuries to several other vessels in the mediastinum (usually venous) can produce the findings. Nevertheless, these findings should prompt a more thorough evaluation of the aorta for evidence of rupture, usually performed with an aortogram. However, in recent years, computerized tomography (CT) of the chest has been increasingly employed to evaluate the mediastinum for potential aortic injury. The CT scan can certainly detect the presence of a mediastinal hematoma much more accurately than plain chest radiographs. In one study, for aortic injury and mediastinal hemorrhage, respectively, specificity for traumatic aortic injury was 99% and 87% and sensitivity was 90% and 100%.

As previously mentioned, 80% to 85% of patients with blunt aortic rupture die at the scene. Of those who survive to hospital arrival, 21% die within 6 h of admission. Without operative treatment, 32% are dead within 24 h, and without operative therapy mortality is 50% in the initial 48 h fol-

TABLE 40.2. **Radiological Signs of Mediastinal Hematoma or Thoracic Great Vessel Injury.**

Widened mediastinum (>8 cm)

Depressed left mainstem bronchus (>140°)

Loss of aortic knob contour

Lateral tracheal deviation

Deviation of nasogastric tube in esophagus

Anterior tracheal displacement

Calcium "layering" in the aortic arch

Massive left-sided hemothorax

Fracture of thoracic spine, clavicle, sternum, or scapula

Loss of parasternal "stripe"

Loss of aorticopulmonary "window"

Left apical pleural hematoma "cap"

lowing injury. If no surgery is performed, 75% are dead from rupture within less than a month.

Surgical management of aortic rupture is through a left posterolateral thoracotomy and typically requires an interposition woven or knitted graft. The potential for paraplegia exists because of temporary ischemia of the spinal cord. It has been argued that shunting may either ameliorate or worsen this risk. Unfortunately, no randomized comparative trials have ever been performed, and the issue of shunting appears to depend solely on the individual surgeon's preference and experience.

Diaphragmatic Rupture

The diaphragm can be injured through either blunt or penetrating mechanisms. Blunt trauma can produce radial tears in the diaphragm, leading to herniation of abdominal viscera through the resulting defect. Penetrating injuries can produce small defects that may be initially undetectable by all methods except laparoscopy or laparotomy; however, over weeks, months, or even years, the defect can enlarge sufficiently to allow visceral herniation. Because the liver tends to protect against visceral herniation, diaphragmatic rupture is more commonly diagnosed on the left side. Chest radiographs are usually the key diagnostic tool provoking a suspicion for diaphragmatic rupture, although misinterpretation is often possible. Findings that make one suspicious for the presence of a diaphragmatic rupture include an elevated left hemidiaphragm, acute gastric dilatation, a loculated pneumohemothorax, or a subpulmonic hematoma. Placement of a nasogastric tube can be diagnostic, as this will often reveal the radiopaque strip of the tube to be coiled up in the left hemithorax and not in its normal vertical midline position. Diaphragmatic ruptures require surgical repair.

Esophageal Trauma

Because of its narrow dimension and protected location, the esophagus is rarely injured in the chest. Both blunt and penetrating mechanisms are possible. Esophageal rupture following blunt injury can result from a forceful expulsion of gastric contents into the esophagus from a severe blow in the upper abdomen. An increasingly common mechanism for esophageal injury is that resulting from instrumentation mishaps, such as the placement of nasogastric tubes, endoscopes, Sengstaken–Blakemore (also known as Minnesota) tubes to tamponade esophageal and gastric varices, and dilators.

The potential for esophageal injury should be suspected in cases of a pneumohemothorax without rib fractures. The presence of mediastinal air should also provoke a suspicion for esophageal trauma. A definite indication of esophageal disruption is the placement of a chest tube that returns particulate matter. A contrast swallowing study can define the location of the injury to help plan the surgical approach. Dilute barium is considered the contrast solution of choice, although Hypaque may also be used. While gastrografin (diatrizoate meglumine) may seem to be a reasonable solution given its water solubility and the lack of the contamination and suffusion problems provide by barium, gastrografin may be a problem if any of the solution is aspirated because it provokes a severe pneumonitis.[2,3]

False-negative rates for esophagography are reported to range from 0% to 50%.[4–8] Rigid or fiberoptic esophagoscopy can also be used to detect the presence of esophageal injury, carrying false-negative rates ranging from 0% to 40%.[9,10] However, the combination of esophagography and esophagoscopy provides the highest sensitivity, with false-negative rates typically less than 10%.[11–13]

Esophageal injuries should be repaired promptly to minimize the potential for contamination to produce a severe infection such as mediastinitis or empyema. If operative intervention is early enough and the tissues appear healthy and viable, then primary closure is the procedure of choice; one or two layers of closure may be used. Nasogastric suction is established with the nasogastric tube placed in its proper position by the surgeon during operative repair. Extensive wound drainage, typically with closed suction catheters, is routinely employed to control any potential leak. With extensive injury or soilage, esophageal exclusion or diversion may be beneficial, employing a pharyngostomy and an operative or percutaneous gastrostomy.

Tracheobronchial Rupture

Tracheal injuries usually result from penetrating trauma. The majority of bronchial injuries occur within 1 in. of the carina. Most patients with this injury die at the scene of rapid suffocation. There is a 30% mortality among those who reach the hospital, often the result of associated injuries.

The diagnosis of tracheobronchial rupture is frequently missed. The condition can be suggested by hemoptysis, subcutaneous emphysema, or a tension pneumothorax, although these conditions are certainly common without the presence of tracheobronchial rupture. However, a strong suspicion for the presence of tracheobronchial rupture should be provoked with the finding of a persistent and continuous (i.e., during both inspiration and expiration) air leak. Bronchoscopy can often be useful in confirming the presence of tracheobronchial rupture. A patient who presents with noisy breathing indicates partial airway obstruction that could suddenly become complete. Such a situation requires immediate operative repair.

Pulmonary Contusion

Pulmonary contusion represents the most common potentially lethal chest injury in North America. Rupture of the pulmonary microvasculature results in alveolar hemorrhage and interstitial and alveolar flooding. Areas of microvascular occlusion develop through the thrombotic process. Yet, the more physiologically damaging condition occurs in those areas where blood is flowing around flooded alveoli, producing intrapulmonary shunting and low ventilation/perfusion regions. The physiological consequences of a sufficient volume of such alveolocapillary complexes are hypoxia and respiratory distress.

Endotracheal intubation should be selective, based on the patient's oxygenation and ventilation requirements. Primary treatment for pulmonary contusion consists of pulmonary toilet, regional pain control, and judicious fluid maintenance. Pulmonary contusions may predispose to infection in patients who are intubated.

Myocardial Contusion

Myocardial contusion results from blunt chest trauma that has caused a direct blow to the sternum, often pinning the heart between the sternum and the spinal column. The adverse consequences of myocardial contusion are primarily those of pump failure and dysrhythmias, with the latter being the much more common occurrence. Overall, between 2.6% and 4.5% of patients with myocardial contusion suffer clinically significant cardiac complications.[14] Significant pump failure usually becomes evident early in the initial trauma assessment and resuscitation during the primary survey. Arrhythmias, however, may not show up immediately, although they usually do present within several hours of injury.

Because of the potential for subsequent cardiac complications such as arrhythmias, early detection of myocardial contusion is desired. The most important diagnostic element for myocardial contusion is suspicion for injury based upon the history of blunt chest trauma, especially if there is a report of a "broken steering wheel."

Physical examination may reveal the presence of precordial tenderness, bruising, and ecchymosis. A sternal fracture is often a strong clue for the presence of myocardial contusion. The presence or absence of pericardial friction rubs should be assessed. A variety of tests and studies have been employed to help detect the presence or absence of myocardial contusion. Typically, these include electrocardiography, cardiac enzyme levels (primarily CPK-MB), echocardiography, and radionuclide studies.

Electrocardiography (EKG) appears to be the single most sensitive test for the presence of significant myocardial contusion. Most of the EKG changes that require treatment will occur within 24 h, especially in those patients without other major injuries. There are no "classic" changes on the EKG that are diagnostic of myocardial contusion. ST-segment and T-wave changes may occur, but the clinical significance of these changes is usually unclear. Of dysrhythmias, both atrial and ventricular forms occur; it is these dysrhythmias that represent the most common indications for any specific treatment for myocardial contusion.

Because of their value in the diagnostic evaluation of potential myocardial infarction, cardiac enzymes have been evaluated in the workup of potential myocardial contusion. Unfortunately, their use can be problematic in the setting of multiple trauma. The relatively small muscle mass of the myocardium can be obscured by the larger muscle mass of the rest of the body. It has been estimated that cardiac enzyme analysis can be insensitive for myocardial injury as much as 40% of the time. The utility of troponin levels in the setting of blunt trauma is not yet clear.

Echocardiography has also been used to evaluate patients with potential mycardial contusion. The appearance is typically that of increased echocardiographic brightness, increased end-diastolic wall thickness, and local systolic hypofunction.

The ability for any of these and other diagnostic modalities (such as radioisotope scanning) to identify those blunt trauma patients at risk for developing myocardial contusion has been the source of a great deal of controversy. While both EKG and CPK-MB appear to correlate well with the potential for cardiac complications, EKG is less problematic in the setting of diffuse blunt trauma. Because the major complication likely to develop from myocardial contusion is an arrhythmia, determination of an initial EKG and monitoring the patient for 12 to 24 h appears likely to identify those patients seriously at risk to develop significant cardiac complications.[15–17]

Emergency Department Thoracotomy

The use of thoracotomy in the emergency department was originally described for penetrating cardiac injuries associated with cardiac tamponade and other bleeding cardiopulmonary wounds. The reports of successful cardiorrhaphy led to an extension of the indication for immediate thoracotomy to include other injuries.

Overall, best survival statistics following emergency department thoracotomy exist for penetrating cardiac injuries. Other penetrating thoracic injuries (i.e., noncardiac) may also benefit from emergency department thoracotomy. In general, stab wounds appear to have a better prognosis than gunshot wounds.

Pooled analysis from 24 studies concerning emergency department thoracotomy indicates that penetrating trauma victims are much more likely to survive than blunt trauma patients.[18] The highest chances of survival (26%) are seen in those patients who have vital signs at the scene as well as in the emergency department; of course, these data raise the question how necessary the thoracotomy was if vital signs (and not merely electrical activity) were present in the emergency department. When the issue of cost-effectiveness has been evaluated, studies suggest that each survivor (regardless of functional status) costs in excess of $100,000.[19,20]

In summary, emergency thoracotomy is best reserved for penetrating thoracic trauma victims who have recently (i.e., within minutes) lost their vital signs. The use of this technique for blunt trauma victims and for patients with no vital signs at the scene appears to be futile, expensive, and potentially hazardous.

Lung Infections

Pneumonia

ETIOLOGY AND PATHOGENESIS

In the surgical patient, pneumonia nearly always occurs as a nosocomial process. It is a rare situation in which a patient presents with community-acquired pneumonia who also requires an operative procedure. In nearly every case, the pneumonia is related to intubation of the trachea, usually in association with mechanical ventilation. Pneumonia remains one of the leading types of infections complicating the course of ICU patients, with the reported incidence ranging from 12% to 63% of ICU patients developing the condition.[21–25] Mortality rates for ventilator-associated pneumonia ranges from 13% to 55%.[26]

DIAGNOSIS

The diagnosis of nosocomial pneumonia is typically made when a patient exhibits the combination of an abnormal temperature, an abnormal white blood cell count, an infiltrate on chest radiographs, and the presence of white blood cells in the sputum. These diagnostic criteria are accurate, at best, roughly 60% to 70% of the time in critically ill patients. The diagnosis of nosocomial pneumonia is especially difficult in the critically ill patient, who may be febrile and have an abnormal white blood cell count for a variety of reasons other than a pneumonia. Moreover, such patients can often have pulmonary infiltrates from the adult respiratory distress syndrome (ARDS), aspiration pneumonitis, or pulmonary contusions. Effusions and atelectasis can obscure or confuse the radiological image sufficiently to make the diagnosis difficult. The sensitivity of portable chest radiography in making the diagnosis of nosocomial pneumonia is only 0.62, and the specificity is low at 0.28.[27]

Because of these inherent problems in diagnosing pneumonia in intubated patients, adjunctive techniques have been evaluated to help in confirming the diagnosis. Criteria for a positive Gram stain have been increasingly refined. First, the sputum contains more than 25 polymorphonuclear cells and less than 10 epithelial cells per low-power field. These criteria tend to ensure that purulence is actually present and to minimize the likelihood that the specimen merely represents mouth secretions. Bronchoalveolar lavage has been determined to have a sensitivity for the diagnosis of pneumonia ranging from 72% to 100%.[28]

PREVENTION

Patients can be positioned to minimize aspiration by keeping the head and chest well elevated above the abdomen if this is not contraindicated by the patient's clinical condition; this position may also improve ventilation-perfusion relationships and minimize atelectasis in comparison to that which develops in the recumbent position. Nasogastric tubes could be avoided; if gastric decompression is necessary, surgical gastrostomy or percutaneous endoscopic gastrostomy (PEG) can be employed. Enteral feedings should be supplied to the small intestine when possible, thus minimizing gastric distension and bacterial growth from intragastric feedings in a poorly emptying stomach. Avoidance of gastric neutralization has been proposed as an effective preventative measure, using sucralfate to protect against stress gastritis while maintaining gastric acidity,[29,30] although there is a suggestion that H_2-blockers may not promote pneumonia as much as do the antacids.[31]

The concept of prophylactic antibiotics in intubated patients has been advanced as a method to potentially prevent the development of pneumonia in this high-risk group. However, the use of systemic intravenous antibiotics for prophylaxis of pneumonia appears to offer no benefit.[32]

A more reasonable approach would be to target the organisms where they are living. Because the colonies responsible for pneumonia are lining the throat and gastrointestinal tract, the defenses in those areas should be enhanced.[33] Selective decontamination of the digestive tract (SDD) indicates a method designed to prevent infection by eradicating and preventing carriage of aerobic potentially pathogenic microorganisms from the oropharynx, stomach, and gut. It consists of antimicrobials applied topically to the oropharynx and through a nasogastric tube. In some trials systemic antibiotic therapy has been added in the first days after patient admission to prevent "early" infections. Unfortunately, there is no standard SDD regimen that has been consistently applied in all these studies. Evidence to date indicates that SDD can reduce infection rates, but it has not been shown to reduce mortality. However, it has been estimated that to demonstrate a reduction in mortality of 10% to 20%, a study would have to include between 2000 and 3000 patients.[34] Between 1991 and 1995, five different meta-analyses[34–38] on the effect of SDD on respiratory tract infections and mortality were published. Their results are summarized in Table 40.3.

Moreover, despite evidence of efficacy, concern about the risk of emergence of antimicrobial resistance and increased costs have kept SDD from becoming a standard therapy.

TREATMENT

As with any localized infection, drainage is necessary to help control the process. Thus, pulmonary toilet, especially including deep breathing and coughing, is crucial to help eliminate the contaminated pulmonary secretions. Because pneumonia in the postoperative patient is usually related to endotracheal intubation, efforts to move the intubated patient toward extubation are generally regarded as key to effective therapy. Conversion to a tracheostomy in those patients who are not easily weaned can make pulmonary toilet more effective.

Antibiotic administration is specific therapy designed to eliminate the invasive microbes. Upon making the clinical diagnosis of pneumonia and obtaining a reliable sputum specimen for culture and antibiotic sensitivity analysis, empiric initial antibiotic therapy can be instituted.

Exactly which antibiotics to use for empiric initial treatment is often a difficult issue. Studies and recommendations

TABLE 40.3.

Meta-Analysis Performed on Studies Evaluating Selective Decontamination of the Digestive Tract.

	Number		Mortality		Infections	
Study	Studies	Patients	Odds ratio	95% confidence interval (CI)	Odds ratio	95% confidence interval (CI)
Vandenbroucke-Grauls[35]	6	49	0.70	0.45–1.09	0.12	0.08–0.19
SDD Trialists' Group[34]	22	4142	0.90	0.79–1.04	0.37	0.31–0.43
Heyland[36]	24	3312	0.87[a]	0.79–0.97[a]	0.46[a]	0.39–0.56[a]
Kollef[37]	16	2270	0.019[b]	−0.016 to 0.054[b]	Pneumonia: 0.145[b] Tracheobronchitis: 0.052[b]	0.116 to 0.174[b] 0.017 to 0.087[b]
Hurley[38]	26	3768	0.86	0.74–0.99	0.35	0.30–0.42

[a]Relative risk.
[b]Risk difference.

have been inconsistent. Thus, clinicians are currently presented with a difficult dilemma: effective empiric antibiotic treatment appears important in ensuring a successful outcome, yet there are no globally acceptable guidelines directing the appropriate selection of antibiotics. Knowledge of the ambient sensitivity of the microbiologic flora in one's own institution is crucial to selecting the optimal agents for empiric treatment of nosocomial pneumonia. Subsequent culture data should be used to refine the antibiotic regimen. Ensuring that adequate doses are administered to achieve effective tissue levels are also essential in controlling the infectious process.[39]

Lung Abscess

On occasion, infecting organisms involved in a pneumonic process in the lung will promote abscess formation through fibroblastic proliferation, walling off the infectious process. If the abscess cavity erodes into a bronchoalveolar space sufficiently to drain its contents, cavitation can occur. The resulting cavity can become secondarily infected. Usually, however, lung abscesses occur in patients with oral or dental infections who sustained a depression in their level of consciousness and aspirated their oral secretions. Most lung abscesses occur in the superior segment of the lower lobes of both lungs and the posterior segment of the right upper lobe. The most common organisms responsible for aspiration-induced abscesses are anaerobic bacteria.

The diagnosis is suspected in an individual with cough and fever. Hemoptysis or purulent, foul-smelling sputum may be produced. The diagnosis is confirmed with a chest radiograph, which can demonstrate an air–fluid level on an upright film. However, other conditions can often obscure the appearance, making it impossible to detect with any study short of a CT scan.

Most lung abscesses will respond and resolve with appropriate antibiotic therapy and pulmonary toilet. Surgical therapy is reserved for those cases that fail to resolve with nonoperative management or for those patients who develop severe hemoptysis, bronchopleural fistula, or empyema. Pulmonary resection is warranted if the abscess cavity is larger than 6 cm in diameter for more than 8 weeks of aggressive antibiotic therapy.

Initial treatment of lung abscess is with the use of antibiotics effective against the offending organism. Therefore, accurate culture material from the lung is imperative to prescribe appropriate therapy. This may require bronchoscopy, to determine the bacterial identity and sensitivities.

References

1. Sugg WL, Rea WJ, Ecker RR, Webb WR, Rose EF, Shaw RR. Penetrating wounds of the heart. An analysis of 459 cases. J Thorac Cardiovasc Surg 1968;56(4):531–545.
2. Trulzsch DV, Penmetsa A, Karim A, Evans DA. Gastrografin-induced aspiration pneumonia: a lethal complication of computed tomography. South Med J 1992;85(12):1255–1256.
3. Wells HD, Hyrnchak MA, Burbridge BE. Direct effects of contrast media on rat lungs. Can Assoc Radiol J 1991;42(4):261–264.
4. Feliciano DV Jr, Bitondo CG, Mattox KL, et al. Combined tracheoesophageal injuries. Am J Surg 1985;150:710–715.
5. Glatterer MS Jr, Toon RS, Ellestad C, et al. Management of blunt and penetrating external esophageal trauma. J Trauma 1985;25:784–792.
6. Splenler CW, Benfield JR. Esophageal disruption from blunt and penetrating external trauma. Arch Surg 1976;111:663–667.
7. Weaver AW, Sankaran S, Fromm SH, et al. The management of penetrating wounds of the neck. Surg Gynecol Obstet 1971;133:49–52.
8. Kelly JP, Webb WR, Moulder PV, Moustouakas NM, Lirtzman M. Management of airway trauma. II: Combined injuries of the trachea and esophagus. Ann Thorac Surg 1987;43(2):160–163.
9. Flowers JL, Graham SM, Ugarte MA, et al. Flexible endoscopy for the diagnosis of esophageal trauma. J Trauma 1996;40(2):261–265.
10. Horwitz B, Krevsky B, Buckman RF Jr, Fisher RS, Dabezies MA. Endoscopic evaluation of penetrating esophageal injuries. Am J Gastroenterol 1993;88(8):1249–1253.
11. Mizutani K, Makuuchi H, Tajima T, Mitomi T. The diagnosis and treatment of esophageal perforations resulting from nonmalignant causes. Surg Today 1997;27(9):793–800.
12. Yugueros P, Sarmiento JM, Garcia AF, Ferrada R. Conservative management of penetrating hypopharyngeal wounds. J Trauma 1996;40(2):267–269.
13. Weigelt JA, Thal ER, Snyder WH III, Fry RE, Meier DE, Kilman WJ. Diagnosis of penetrating cervical esophageal injuries. Am J Surg 1987;154(6):619–622.
14. Maenza RL, Seaberg D, D'Amico F. A meta-analysis of blunt cardiac trauma: ending myocardial contusion. Am J Emerg Med 1996;14:237–241.
15. Baxter BT, Moore EE, Moore FA, McCroskey BL, Ammons LA. A plea for sensible management of myocardial contusion. Am J Surg 1989;158(6):557–561.
16. Fabian TC, Cicala RS, Croce MA, et al. A prospective evaluation of myocardial contusion: correlation of significant arrhythmias and cardiac output with CPK-MB measurements. J Trauma 1991;31(5):653–659.
17. Miller FB, Shumate CR, Richardson JD. Myocardial contusion. When can the diagnosis be eliminated? Arch Surg 1989;124(7):805–807.
18. Boyd M, Vanek VW, Bourguet CC. Emergency room resuscitative thoracotomy: when is it indicated? J Trauma 1992;33(5):714–721.
19. Esposito TJ, Jurkovich GJ, Rice CL, Maier RV, Copass MK, Ashbaugh DG. Reappraisal of emergency room thoracotomy in a changing environment. J Trauma 1991;31(7):881–885.
20. Hoyt DB, Shackford SR, Davis JW, Mackersie RC, Hollingsworth-Fridlund P. Thoracotomy during trauma resuscitations—an appraisal by board-certified general surgeons. J Trauma 1989;29(10):1318–1321.
21. Ashbaugh DG, Petty TL. Sepsis complicating the acute respiratory distress syndrome. Surg Gynecol Obstet 1972;135:865.
22. Johanson WG, Pierce AK, Sanford JP, et al. Nosocomial respiratory infections with gram-negative bacilli. Ann Intern Med 1972;77:701.
23. Sanford JP. Infection control in critical care units. Crit Care Med 1974;2:211.
24. Stevens RM, Teres D, Skillman JJ, et al. Pneumonia in an intensive care unit. Arch Intern Med 1974;134:106.
25. Zapol WM, Snider MT, Hill JD, et al. Extracorporeal membrane oxygenation in severe acute respiratory failure: A randomized prospective study. JAMA 1979;242:2193.
26. Cook DJ, Brun-Buisson C, Guyatt GH, Sibbald WJ. Evaluation of new diagnostic technologies: bronchoalveolar lavage and the diagnosis of ventilator-associated pneumonia. Crit Care Med 1994;22(8):1314–1322.
27. Lefcoe MS, Fox GA, Leasa DJ, Sparrow RK, McCormack DG. Accuracy of portable chest radiography in the critical care setting. Chest 1994;105:885–887.
28. Cook DJ, Brun-Buisson C, Guyatt GH, Sibbald WJ. Evaluation of new diagnostic technologies: bronchoalveolar lavage and the

diagnosis of ventilator-associated pneumonia. Crit Care Med 1994;22:1314–1322.

29. Tryba M. Risk of acute stress bleeding and nosocomial pneumonia in ventilated intensive care unit patients: sucralfate versus antacids. Am J Med 1987;83(Suppl 3B):117.

30. Driks MR, Craven DE, Celli BR, et al. Nosocomial pneumonia in intubated patients given sucralfate as compared with antacids or histamine type 2 blockers. N Engl J Med 1987;317:1376.

31. Palmer RH, Gachot B, Jebrak G, et al. Nosocomial pneumonia in intubated patients. N Engl J Med 1988;318:1465.

32. Mandelli M, Mosconi P, Langer M, et al. Prevention of pneumonia in an intensive care unit: a randomized multicenter trial. Crit Care Med 1989;17:501.

33. van Saene HKF, Stoutenbeek CP, Miranda DR, et al. A novel approach to infection control in the intensive care unit. Acta Anaesthesiol Belg 1983;3:193–208.

34. SDD Trialists' Collaborative Group. Meta-analysis of randomised controlled trials of selective decontamination of the digestive tract. Br Med J 1993;307:525–532.

35. Vanderbrouk-Grauls CM, Vanderbrouke-Grauls JP. Effect of selective decontamination of the digestive tract on respiratory tract infections and mortality in intensive care unit. Lancet 1991;338:859–862.

36. Heyland DK, Cook DJ, Jaeschke R, Griffith L, Lee HN, Guyatt GH. Selective decontamination of the digestive tract. An overview. Chest 1994;105(4):1221–1229.

37. Kollef MH. The role of selective digestive tract decontamination on mortality and respiratory tract infections. A meta-analysis. Chest 1994;105(4):1101–1108.

38. Hurley JC. Prophylaxis with enteral antibiotics in ventilated patients: selective decontamination or selective cross-infection? Antimicrob Agents Chemother 1995;39(4):941–947.

39. Reed RL. Antibiotic choices in surgical intensive care unit patients. Surg Clin North Am 1991;71(4):765–789.

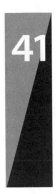

41

Pleura: Anatomy, Physiology, and Disorders

Joseph S. Friedberg

Anatomy

Embryology and Microscopic Anatomy

Embryologically, the pleural cavity is created during a month, starting in the third week of gestation. Eventually, the visceral pleura surrounds the lung and the parietal pleura lines the remainder of the chest cavity. The different embryological origins of the visceral and parietal pleura are responsible for the separate vascular, lymphatic, and neural supplies of these two structures as seen in the adult. By the end of the seventh week of gestation, the diaphragm has separated the thoracic cavity from the peritoneal cavity, and by the third month of gestation the two pleural cavities have expanded sufficiently to encase the pericardium.[1]

In the adult, both pleural surfaces are approximately 30 to 40 μm thick and are composed of a single layer of mesothelial cells with an underlying layer of connective tissue. It is these apposing layers of mesothelial cells that form the potential space of the pleural cavity and which glide over each other during respiration.[2-4]

The connective tissue layer contains the neurovascular and lymphatic supply of the pleura. There are certain important differences in this layer between the visceral and parietal pleura. For the visceral pleura, the connective tissue layer is functionally continuous with the fibroelastic network of the lung itself. Pathological disruption of this connection, however, may result in subpleural air collections known as blebs.[5] The connective tissue layer for the parietal pleura may also be tightly adherent to the underlying structures, as is characteristic of the diaphragmatic pleura. Around the skeletal portion of the thorax, however, the pleura is bound to the underlying tissue by another connective tissue layer called the endothoracic fascia, which forms a natural cleavage plane. It is this plane that the surgeon develops when performing an "extrapleural" dissection.[5,6]

The blood supply to the visceral pleura in humans is thought to reflect that of the lung itself, with a dual arterial supply from both the pulmonary and bronchial arteries and singular venous drainage into the pulmonary veins. The blood supply to the parietal pleura is from systemic arteries only and drains, predominantly, into peribronchial and intercostal veins, but it may also drain directly into the azygous vein and vena cava.[7-9]

The visceral pleura is innervated by vagal and sympathetic fibers, but has no somatic innervation and is therefore insensate. The parietal pleura is also innervated with sympathetic and parasympathetic fibers, but it is also somatically innervated. Thus, the parietal pleura is capable of sensing and transmitting the sensation of pain. "Pleurisy" from inflammation and pain from chest tubes, during insertion and subsequently as well, are attributable to the somatic intervention of the parietal pleura.

There are also differences in the lymphatic drainage between the two pleural layers. The visceral pleura drains through a lymphatic network into the pulmonary lymphatics, which eventually flow toward the pulmonary hilum. The parietal pleural lymphatics drain to different locations. The mediastinal pleura drains to the mediastinal and tracheobronchial nodes. The chest wall drains anteriorly to the internal thoracic chain and posteriorly toward the intercostal nodes near the heads of the ribs. The diaphragmatic pleura drains to the parasternal, middle phrenic, and posterior mediastinal lymph nodes.[7] There are also transdiaphragmatic lymphatic communications that allow some degree of lymphatic flow from the peritoneum to the pleural space.

The parietal pleura also differs from the visceral pleura by virtue of the presence of Kampmeier foci and stomata. Stomata are 2- to 6-μm pores that communicate directly with the parietal pleural lymphatics. During inspiration these pores have the capacity to stretch, and their architecture is such that they form functional one-way valves. Thus, they provide for a very effective system for draining both fluid and particles, including both red blood cells and macrophages.

527

Gross Anatomy

In each hemithorax, the visceral pleura is a continuous surface that completely envelops the entire lung, including the fissures. At the pulmonary hilum, it continues on as the parietal pleura to line the mediastinum, chest wall, diaphragm, and cupola of the chest cavity. In humans the pleural cavities are completely separate, coming into contact with each other for a short distance behind the upper half of the body of the sternum. It is this pleural separation of the right and left chest cavities that prevents bilateral pneumothoraces from occurring as the result of a unilateral chest injury. At the costophrenic and costomediastinal sinuses the parietal pleura folds back on itself, providing a potential space into which the lungs can expand during inspiration.

Superiorly, the pleura extends above the bony thorax into the base of the neck (Fig. 41.1). This fact explains why pneumothorax may complicate internal jugular central line placement as well as subclavian central line placement.[10] Anteriorly the pleura extends to the sixth rib, to the ninth rib laterally, and to the twelfth rib posteriorly (Fig. 41.1).

The pulmonary ligament is a double fold of the mediastinal pleura that tapers down from the root of the lung, where it is in continuity with the visceral pleura, to the caudal mediastinum. This ligament is one of the structures that must be divided to perform a pneumonectomy or lower lobectomy. It is also routinely divided to its superior border, the inferior pulmonary vein, when attempting to provide mobility to the lower lobe after resecting the upper and/or middle lobes. The lymph nodes within the pulmonary ligament are the level 9 nodes, which are N2 lymph nodes, and are routinely harvested when performing a resection for lung cancer.

Physiology

The pleura has both mechanical and physiological functions. It transmits negative pressure from the thorax to the lung, thereby opposing the lung's natural elastic recoil and maintaining pulmonary expansion. The pleura also controls the environment of the chest cavity by maintaining fluid homeostasis, preventing or removing air collections and keeping the space sterile.

Under normal conditions, the pleural cavity is a potential space with a thickness ranging from 10 to 20 μm. The lung is maintained in an expanded state by the maintenance of a negative pressure in the pleural space. The resting pressure in the pleural space, when the lung is at its functional residual capacity, is slightly negative at -2 to -5 cm H_2O. The negative pressure continues to increase through inspiration with the pressure ranging from -25 to -35 cm H_2O at the vital capacity. Disorders that decrease the compliance of the lung or increase airway resistance further increase the negative pressure in the pleural space with inspiration.[5,11]

Under normal conditions the pleural space contains very little fluid, estimated at approximately 0.3 ml/kg. The fluid is generally hypooncotic with a protein content of approximately 1 g/dl. The mechanisms of fluid production and reabsorption are complicated and not completely understood. The predominant factor, however, is thought to be the uptake of fluid into the parietal pleural lymphatics. Under normal conditions, this flow rate has been estimated at 0.1 to 0.15 ml/kg/h. The lymphatic flow rate has the capacity to increase and has been estimated to reach as high as 30 ml/h, approximately 700 ml/day in an average-size individual. When the dynamics of this equilibrium are unbalanced beyond the rate at which the lymphatics are able to compensate, pleural effusion accumulates.[3,4,11–14]

Disorders of the Pleura

Gas-Phase Disorders of the Pleural Space

PNEUMOTHORAX

Pneumothorax is defined as air in the pleural space. It may occur traumatically, iatrogenically, or spontaneously. Spontaneous pneumothorax may be subclassified as primary or secondary, with primary spontaneous pneumothorax arising in an otherwise healthy patient and secondary spontaneous pneumothorax arising as a complication in a patient with known underlying pulmonary disease. Essentially any pneumothorax resulting from pleural disruption can present as a tension pneumothorax. This condition represents a true emergency and is discussed separately.

PNEUMOTHORAX PRESENTATION AND DIAGNOSIS

Pneumothorax may cause pain or dyspnea, or it may be asymptomatic, depending on its size and the underlying pulmonary function of the patient. Physical findings may range from none to the classic findings seen with a tension pneumothorax: contralateral tracheal deviation, ipsilateral absent breath sounds, and percussive hyperresonance. Electrocardiographic changes may be present, including diminished voltage, right-axis deviation, or T-wave changes that may mimic a subendocardial myocardial infarction.[15]

Except for tension pneumothorax, most cases require an upright chest radiograph to establish the diagnosis. As the pneumothorax occupies a greater proportion of the chest cavity at expiration than inspiration, the former is more sensi-

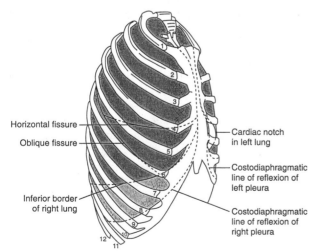

FIGURE 41.1. Relationship of the lung (dark gray) and the parietal pleural envelope, which extends down beyond the edge of the lung (light gray). (Reprinted with permission from Gray's Anatomy, 36th edition, ©1980, W.B. Saunders Co.)

Horizontal fissure

Oblique fissure

Inferior border of right lung

Cardiac notch in left lung

Costodiaphragmatic line of reflexion of left pleura

Costodiaphragmatic line of reflexion of right pleura

tive for detecting the diagnostic pleural line.[16] Although rarely indicated for a patient able to obtain an upright chest X-ray, a CT scan of the chest is the most sensitive test and may demonstrate a small amount of air in the pleural space that is not visible on the plain radiograph.[17,18]

PNEUMOTHORAX TREATMENT OPTIONS

For all pneumothoraces, the common goal is removal of air from the pleural space. Depending upon the etiology, however, prevention of recurrence may also be an objective of the treatment.

In practice, many physicians estimate the size of a pneumothorax by the area of the hemithorax that it appears to occupy in an anteroposterior radiograph of the chest. This practice generally underestimates the size of the pneumothorax. There are a number of formulas to better estimate the size of a pneumothorax, the simplest of which estimates the fractional volume occupied by a pneumothorax to be approximately equal to three times the fractional decrease in the linear dimensions of the lung.[19–21] The most accurate noninvasive estimate, however, is likely obtained by chest CT.

PNEUMOTHORAX TREATMENT OPTIONS: OBSERVATION

Observation is generally reserved for patients who are asymptomatic and are diagnosed with a small primary spontaneous pneumothorax or a simple iatrogenic pneumothorax. In such situations, the patient is followed with serial radiographs to ensure that the pneumothorax is decreasing in size. When a patient is breathing room air, gas is absorbed from the pleural cavity at approximately 1.25% of the pleural volume/day, approximately 50 to 70 ml/day.[22] Supplemental oxygen can increase this rate up to 4.2%/day.[23,24] As it is a minimal intervention, it is reasonable to place all hospitalized patients on supplemental oxygen if they are being observed for a pneumothorax.

It is recommended that observation be considered only for patients with a simple pneumothorax less than approximately 15%.[25] If the pneumothorax has not resolved within 1 to 2 weeks, intervention to achieve full expansion should be instituted. Another factor to consider, particularly with primary spontaneous pneumothorax, is that observation alone does nothing to decrease the chance of recurrence. Last, in this age of economic constraints, it may be more cost-effective to definitively treat a pneumothorax upon presentation.

PNEUMOTHORAX TREATMENT OPTIONS: SIMPLE ASPIRATION

Simple aspiration can be considered in the case of a simple pneumothorax in which there is no suspicion of an ongoing air leak and the patient is not on positive pressure ventilation. Some authors believe that in select situations aspiration is the treatment of choice.[26] The procedure is performed in a manner similar to that used for decompressing a tension pneumothorax. After sterilely preparing the skin and infiltrating with a local anesthetic, a 16-gauge intravenous catheter is placed into the pleural space in the midclavicular line over the superior surface of the second rib. The needle is then withdrawn and the catheter is connected to a short length of intravenous tubing capped with a three-way stopcock. A 60-ml syringe is then used to aspirate air from the chest cavity. When air can no longer be aspirated, the catheter is withdrawn and the first chest X-ray is obtained. If 4 l of air is aspirated and no resistance is met, there is an ongoing air leak and a chest tube should be placed.[7]

PNEUMOTHORAX TREATMENT OPTIONS: PERCUTANEOUS TUBE THORACOSTOMY

Percutaneous tube thoracostomy is a good option for a simple pneumothorax. Some authors consider this the procedure of choice for simple pneumothoraces. Depending upon the size and etiology of the pneumothorax, success rates for these catheters are reported in the 85% to 90% range.[27–30] The catheters range in size from 9 to 16 French and are placed using a catheter-over-needle or Seldinger technique. These tubes are limited by their size and would be a poor choice for a patient with a large air leak. The principal factor in determining the flow rate through a tube is the diameter of the tube. Thus, a patient with a massive air leak, especially on positive pressure ventilation, should have a standard chest tube placed. As a general guide, it takes at least a 28-Fr. tube to accommodate approximately 15 l/min of flow at −10 cm of H_2O suction.[31]

PNEUMOTHORAX TREATMENT OPTIONS: TUBE THORACOSTOMY

A standard chest tube should be placed for failure of a percutaneous tube, a pneumothorax associated with a significant fluid collection, or a pneumothorax where the leak is expected to overwhelm a small-caliber tube, more likely in the setting of positive pressure ventilation. Such tubes are generally placed under local anesthesia and sedation, employing sterile technique. Apical tubes, as employed for drainage of air, are best placed in the mid- or anterior axillary line in the third or fourth intercostal space.[32] The tube can then be placed for passive or active drainage. Passive drainage may be achieved by connecting the tube to a Heimlich flutter valve or waterseal on a PleurEvac. For active drainage, most surgeons use a three-bottle system (Fig. 41.2), generally unified as a commercially available unit such as PleurEvac. Active drainage expedites and facilitates full expansion of the lung. Although also reported with passive drainage, the rare complication of reexpansion pulmonary edema appears to be more common with active suction.[33,34]

PNEUMOTHORAX TREATMENT OPTIONS: SURGERY

With the exception of those with a large open pneumothorax, essentially all patients being considered for surgical treatment for a pneumothorax already have a chest tube in place. With a progressive air leak, tension physiology is imminent once positive pressure ventilation is instituted unless there is a pathway for egress of air from the pleural space or intubation is performed directly with a double-lumen endotracheal tube such that the leaking lung can be immediately isolated. Specific surgical procedures are discussed under the appropriate sections, but it is worth noting that there are two surgical approaches available, video-assisted thoracoscopic surgery (VATS) or standard thoracotomy.

General indications for surgical intervention for a pneumothorax are failure of less invasive therapy or occurrence of the pneumothorax in the context of additional indications for chest exploration. A VATS approach can be employed, at least

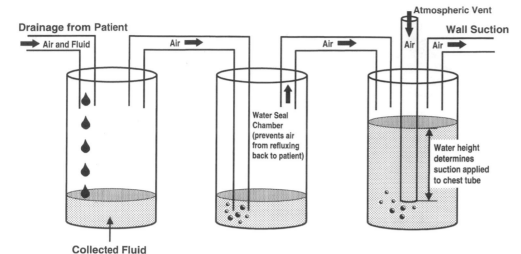

FIGURE 41.2. Three-bottle suction setup for pleural drainage.

initially, for most pneumothoraces. Examples of contraindications to a VATS approach are a pneumothorax secondary to an esophageal perforation, major airway disruption, or a pneumothorax accompanied by significant ongoing bleeding or concomitant trauma to other thoracic organs.

TYPES OF PNEUMOTHORAX

PRIMARY SPONTANEOUS PNEUMOTHORAX
Primary spontaneous pneumothorax most commonly occurs in tall young men, but may occur in anyone at any age. The peak incidence has been reported to occur for both men and women age 25 to 34 years old. It is approximately six times more common in men than women, with approximately 10,000 new cases per year in the United States.[7,35,36]

It is thought that the final common pathway for most primary spontaneous pneumothoraces is rupture of subpleural blebs.[37,38] It is also thought that inflammation of the distal airways plays a significant role in the pathogenesis of this disorder. The lack of communication between these blebs and the distal airways, and hence the inability to rapidly decompress, may explain the increased incidence of primary spontaneous pneumothorax associated with significant drops in atmospheric pressure.[39,40] The role of inflammation may explain why spontaneous pneumothorax is much more common in smokers.[41,42] In fact, there appears to be a dose–response relationship, with light smokers (fewer than 13 cigarettes/day) running a risk 7 times that of nonsmokers and those smoking more than 22 cigarettes/day at least 100 times more likely to have a spontaneous pneumothorax than nonsmokers.[43]

It is generally accepted that recurrent spontaneous pneumothoraces become increasingly likely with each successive occurrence. Cessation of smoking decreases the risk of recurrence. Although the literature reports many different recurrence rates, a reasonable estimation of recurrence following different treatments is observation alone, 30%; aspiration, 20% to 50%, tube thoracostomy drainage, 20% to 50%; tetracycline pleurodesis, 10% to 25%; talc pleurodesis, 7%; and surgical treatment, 0% to 2%.[5,44]

Selection of treatment remains an area of controversy. Observation alone should be reserved for the initial presentation of a small asymptomatic primary pneumothorax without any associated comorbidities. It should be reserved for patients who have no barotrauma risks and have ready access to medical help. This treatment may be particularly appropriate for patients who present with heavy cigarette abuse and are willing to stop smoking.

Aspiration is another option, but confers no significant protection from recurrence. Once the decision has been made to violate the pleura for aspiration, it is probably worthwhile leaving a catheter through which air can be continuously aspirated and subsequent pleurodesis can be performed. If a large air leak is anticipated or if there is significant effusion associated with the pneumothorax, then a standard 28-Fr. chest tube should be placed. Neither technique, without pleurodesis, seems to convey significant protection from recurrence.

Surgical treatment remains the gold standard in preventing recurrence of spontaneous pneumothorax. Some of the indications for surgical treatment of a spontaneous pneumothorax include a second pneumothorax (ipsilateral recurrence or a new pneumothorax on the contralateral side), tension physiology, synchronous bilateral pneumothoraces (rare but reported[45]), associated hemothorax (likely secondary to a torn adhesion and complicating approximately 5% of spontaneous pneumothoraces[46]), failure of tube thoracostomy, and lifestyle factors. Surgery should be considered if a leak persists for more than 3 to 4 days because most leaks seal within 48 h of instituting tube decompression and only a small additional fraction seal with further tube treatment, even after another week.[47] Lifestyle issues that are accepted indications for surgical therapy at the initial presentation of a primary spontaneous pneumothorax include occupational exposure to barotrauma (scuba diving or flying) and poor accessibility to medical care.[5]

The surgical procedure for spontaneous pneumothorax is resection of the blebs that are usually present, most commonly located in the apex of the upper lobe or the superior segment of the lower lobe. Resection of the blebs is performed with a pulmonary stapling device. Most surgeons also perform a mechanical pleurodesis of the pleura, utilizing an abrasive material. Currently, VATS is considered by many thoracic surgeons to be the preferred surgical approach.[48–51]

Secondary spontaneous pneumothorax is a more serious condition than primary spontaneous pneumothorax because of its occurrence in patients who likely have significantly less pulmonary reserve than the typical patient presenting with a primary spontaneous pneumothorax. As opposed to primary spontaneous pneumothoraces, secondary spontaneous pneumothoraces are associated with a significant mortality.[52] Historically, the most common cause of secondary spontaneous pneumothorax has been chronic obstructive pulmonary disease (COPD). More recently, at least in urban centers, there is an increase in secondary pneumothoraces presenting as complications of *Pneumocystis carinii* infections in patients with acquired immunodeficiency syndrome (AIDS).[53,54] There are many other causes of secondary spontaneous pneumothorax including, but not limited to, cystic fibrosis, asthma, cancer, many types of infection, sarcoid, collagen vascular diseases, and catamenial.

The recurrence rates for secondary primary pneumothoraces have been reported to be similar or slightly greater than those that are seen with primary spontaneous pneumothoraces.[55,56] Thus, the principal factor affecting choice of treatment in this setting is the more serious nature of a pneumothorax in a patient with underlying pulmonary disease. If the patient is symptomatic, which is far more likely with this patient population, then there is no role for observation. Furthermore, an increase in the pneumothorax could possibly place the patient's life in jeopardy. Therefore, observation of a secondary spontaneous pneumothorax is recommended only in very select and highly monitored situations. Any consideration of employing positive pressure ventilation in a patient with a secondary pneumothorax should be considered an automatic indication for thoracostomy tube placement.

Earnest consideration should be given to sclerosis for prevention in most of these cases. If the pneumothorax occurs in the setting of a disease, such as certain malignancies or infections, it may not be possible to staple the lung or to achieve total lung expansion. In these cases, particularly if the patient is terminally ill, consideration should be given to sending the patient home with a chest tube and a Heimlich valve if this provides adequate palliation.

TRAUMATIC PNEUMOTHORAX

Please refer to Chapter 54 on thoracic trauma.

IATROGENIC PNEUMOTHORAX

Iatrogenic pneumothorax may be the most common cause of pneumothorax.[57] The most common causes include transthoracic needle biopsy, subclavian central line placement, thoracentesis, transbronchial pulmonary biopsy, and positive pressure ventilation.

The development of a pneumothorax as a result of barotrauma is an indication for immediate placement of a standard chest tube.[58–60] This indication is also true for a procedure-induced pneumothorax in a ventilated patient because positive pressure ventilation could rapidly lead to a tension pneumothorax. The clinician should always consider pneumothorax as a cause for instability in a ventilated patient who recently underwent thoracentesis or central line placement.

Iatrogenic pneumothoraces differ from spontaneous pneumothoraces in that the patient is not at an increased risk for recurrence. For small asymptomatic pneumothoraces, observation is appropriate and thoracostomy tube placement and sclerosis are not indicated. For larger pneumothoraces or symptomatic pneumothoraces in ambulatory patients, simple aspiration or temporary placement of a small percutaneous catheter is the preferred approach of many clinicians.[61–64]

Last, it is worth remembering that an esophageal perforation, most commonly from endoscopy or dilatation, can present with a pneumothorax, usually accompanied by a pleural effusion. As with traumatic pneumothorax, if the diagnosis is seriously entertained, then it must be investigated with a contrast study or endoscopy.

TENSION PNEUMOTHORAX

Any closed pneumothorax arising from visceral pleural disruption has the potential to develop into a tension pneumothorax. Tension pneumothorax occurs when air accumulates in the pleural space in excess of atmospheric pressure and actively compresses the ipsilateral lung. This tension physiology will eventually lead to contralateral mediastinal shift and, in addition to pulmonary embarrassment, can severely limit venous return and compromise cardiac output. Untreated, tension pneumothorax may lead to cardiopulmonary arrest and, for this reason, is a life-threatening emergency. If the patient is in distress and the diagnosis is suspected, placement of a 16-gauge intravenous catheter through the second interspace, in the midclavicular line, will convert the tension pneumothorax to an open pneumothorax. After decompression has been achieved, a chest tube can then be placed in the usual manner. This procedure should always be performed immediately in any patient who is decompensating and for whom tension pneumothorax is in the differential diagnosis. It is a mistake to wait for a confirmatory chest X-ray in such a situation.

BLEBS AND BULLAE

Simply stated, blebs are subpleural collections of air.[65] They are usually small, less than 2 cm, and tend to occur at the apex of the upper lobe or the apex of the superior segment. The significance of blebs is uncertain. By themselves, it is doubtful that they cause any significant effect on pulmonary function. Their primary clinical significance lies in the fact that they appear to be involved in the pathogenesis of spontaneous pneumothorax.

No specific treatment is indicated for the finding of pulmonary blebs in the absence of pneumothorax. Cessation of smoking, as always, is recommended.

Bullae are air collections measuring at least 1 cm, but may become so large as to occupy the greater part of the hemithorax. As opposed to blebs, bullae are formed by destruction and coalescence of alveoli. They may demonstrate trabeculated lumens formed by the residual structural elements from the lung parenchyma they replaced. Blebs may be an incidental finding in patients with otherwise normal lungs, but bullae are likely to be associated with some form of pulmonary disease, most likely emphysema.[65]

Bullous disease is also frequently asymptomatic. In such cases, cessation of smoking and annual chest X-rays are sufficient. In the setting of known underlying lung disease, treat-

TABLE 41.1. Differential Diagnoses of Pleural Effusion.

Transudative Pleural Effusions	Drug-induced lupus
Congestive heart failure	Immunoblastic lymphadenopathy
Cirrhosis	Sjögren's syndrome
Nephrotic syndrome	Familial Mediterranean fever
Superior vena cava obstruction	Churg-Strauss syndrome
Fontan procedure	Wegener's granulomatosis
Urinothorax	Drug-induced pleural disease
Peritoneal dialysis	Nitrofurantoin
Glomerulonephritis	Dantrolene
Myxedema	Methysergide
Pulmonary emboli	Bromocriptine
Sarcoidosis	Amiodarone
	Procarbazine
Exudative Pleural Effusions	Methotrexate
Neoplastic disease	Miscellaneous diseases and conditions
Metastatic disease	Asbestos exposure
Mesothelioma	Postpericardiectomy or postmyocardial infarction
Infectious diseases	syndrome
Bacterial infections	Meig's syndrome
Tuberculosis	Yellow nail syndrome
Fungal infections	Sarcoidosis
Parasitic infections	Pericardial disease
Viral infections	After coronary artery bypass surgery
Pulmonary embolization	After lung transplant
Gastrointestinal disease	Fetal pleural effusion
Pancreatic disease	Uremia
Subphrenic abscess	Trapped lung
Intrahepatic abscess	Radiation therapy
Intrasplenic abscess	Ovarian hyperstimulation syndrome
Esophageal perforation	Postpartum pleural effusion
After abdominal surgery	Amyloidosis
Diaphragmatic hernia	Electrical burns
Endoscopic variceal sclerosis	Iatrogenic injury
After liver transplant	Hemothorax
Collagen vascular diseases	Chylothorax
Rheumatoid pleuritis	
Systemic lupus erythematosus	

Source: Reprinted with permission from Pleural Diseases, edited by RW Light, © 1995 Lippincott Williams & Wilkins.

ment of that disorder is the priority. Pneumothorax, infection, or hemoptysis can prompt surgical intervention.

Liquid-Phase Disorders of the Pleural Space

Pleural effusions are a very common disorder encountered by the clinician. There are many potential causes of effusions (Table 41.1). Occasionally it is possible to deduce the etiology in the context of the patient's chest radiograph and concurrent morbidities. Frequently, however, the fluid must be sampled to yield a diagnosis. There is a normal composition

TABLE 41.2. Normal Composition of Pleural Fluid.

Volume	0.1–0.2 ml/kg
Cells/mm^3	1000–5000
% mesothelial cells	3%–70%
% monocytes	30%–75%
% lymphocytes	2%–30%
% granulocytes	10%
Protein	1–2 g/dl
% albumin	50%–70%
Glucose	≈ plasma level
LDH	<50% plasma level
pH	≥ plasma

Data from humans and animals.

Source: Reprinted with permission from Pulmonary Diseases and Disorders, Alfred P. Fishman, editor. ©1998 McGraw Hill.

of pleural fluid (Table 41.2) and a host of tests that can be performed on the fluid in pursuit of a diagnosis (Table 41.3). Once the fluid is sampled, it will fall into one of two categories, transudative or exudative, and 99% of exudative effusions will demonstrate at least one of the following characteristics: pleural fluid protein/serum protein ratio greater than 0.5, pleural fluid LDH/serum LDH greater than 0.6, or pleural fluid LDH more than two-thirds of the upper normal limit for serum LDH.[66]

Transudative effusions result from a perturbation in the hydrostatic or oncotic forces that affect fluid formation and turnover in the pleural space. This imbalance results in fluid accumulation in the pleural space. For transudative effusions the goal is to drain the effusion for symptomatic relief, if necessary, but to focus on the systemic disease.

Exudative effusions result from diseases that involve the pleura and may be broadly grouped as benign or malignant. The treatment of an exudative effusion is disease specific.

Pleural effusions may be asymptomatic or may cause the patient to present with shortness of breath, secondary to compression of pulmonary parenchyma, as well as other symptoms. A nonspecific sign that is compatible with an effusion is the presence of a nonproductive cough. If the disorder causing the effusion has provoked an inflammatory response in the parietal pleura, the patient may complain of pain, known as pleuritic chest pain.

Plain radiographs of the chest remain the most common test obtained to evaluate a suspected effusion.[67] If the effu-

TABLE 41.3. Useful Tests in the Evaluation of Pleural Effusion.

Test	Abnormal value	Frequently associated condition
Red blood cells/mm³	>100,000	Malignancy, trauma, pulmonary embolism
White blood cells/mm³	>10,000	Pyogenic infection
Neutrophils, %	>50	Acute pleuritis
Lymphocytes, %	>90	Tuberculosis, malignancy
Eosinophilia, %	>10	Asbestos effusion, pneumothorax, resolving infection
Mesothelial cells	Absent	Tuberculosis
Protein, PF/S[a]	>0.5	Exudate
LDH, PF/S	>0.6	Exudate
LDH, IU[b]	>200	Exudate
Glucose, mg/dl	<60	Empyema, TB, malignancy, rheumatoid arthritis
pH	<7.20	Complicated parapneumonic effusion, empyema, esophageal rupture, TB, malignancy, rheumatoid arthritis
Amylase, PF/S	>1	Pancreatitis
Bacteriological	Positive	Cause of infection
Cytology	Positive	Diagnostic of malignancy

[a]PF/S, pleural fluid to serum ratio.

[b]IU, concentration in International Units.

sion is free flowing, the lateral costophrenic angle may be blunted on an upright posteroanterior radiograph if the effusion is greater than 175 ml. Sometimes more than 500 ml is required to achieve this effect.[68] The lateral radiograph is more sensitive than the posteroanterior view, but neither is as sensitive as the lateral decubitus projection, which can detect as little as 25 to 50 ml of fluid.[65]

For a free-flowing effusion that layers on a lateral decubitus film, additional radiographic studies are seldom indicated. Additional studies that are commonly used to obtain more information about a suspected effusion include ultrasound and CT scan. Ultrasound is very helpful in distinguishing pleural thickening from pleural fluid, determining if an effusion is complex or simple, and has the advantage of being portable. It can be used to help direct the clinician to the best area to perform a thoracentesis at the bedside. CT scans give the most information with respect to exact location of an effusion and may be particularly helpful in distinguishing effusion from pleural disease or parenchymal disease.[18,67] At this time, magnetic resonance imaging (MRI) scans are rarely indicated in the diagnosis or assessment of pleural effusions.

If the clinical scenario warrants diagnosis of the effusion, then the next step is to perform a thoracentesis to obtain a specimen for analysis and, possibly, to drain the effusion for relief of symptoms. It is generally recommended that not more than 1 l of fluid should be aspirated at one time as this increases the chances of developing reexpansion pulmonary edema.[7] The exact etiology of this syndrome is not fully understood and may be accompanied by a 20% mortality.[33] Treatment for reexpansion edema is similar to treatment for other causes of pulmonary edema; upright posture, diuresis, supplemental oxygen and, if necessary, intubation.

TRANSUDATIVE EFFUSIONS

If the effusion is transudative, then it is most likely to be secondary to congestive heart failure, hepatic insufficiency, or renal insufficiency. Pleural effusions secondary to congestive failure are the most common transudative effusions.[69] Most of these effusions are bilateral. In all cases, treatment should be aimed at the primary disorder. In severely symptomatic patients, drainage and sclerosis can be considered. Other conditions that may provoke a transudative effusion include, but are not limited to, pulmonary embolism, superior vena cava obstruction, peritoneal dialysis, myxedema, glomerulonephritis, Meigs' syndrome, and sarcoidosis.[7,65]

EXUDATIVE EFFUSIONS

Exudative effusions can be broadly grouped into benign and malignant effusions. The malignant effusions arise most commonly from metastatic disease, but can also herald the presence of a primary malignancy of the pleura. The benign causes of exudative effusion include a very long list of conditions including but not limited to infectious diseases, pulmonary embolism, collagen vascular diseases, drug-induced disorders, bleeding, chyle leak, subdiaphragmatic infections, pancreatitis, and esophageal perforation. If the cause is not obvious, then a thoracentesis should be the next step in diagnosing the etiology of the effusion.

EXUDATIVE EFFUSIONS: MALIGNANT

Malignant effusions represent one of the most common indications for chest tube placement. The diagnosis can frequently be established by cytological demonstration of cancer cells in the fluid although up to 40% of effusions yield nondiagnostic cytology.[70,71] Thus, if malignancy is suspected and the fluid cytology is nondiagnostic, a closed pleural biopsy should be considered. Depending on the patient's surgical risk and the expertise available, it may be in the patient's best interest to proceed to thoracoscopy if the thoracentesis is nondiagnostic. If such services are not readily available then closed pleural biopsy is clearly indicated. If, after both closed biopsy and thoracentesis, a diagnosis remains elusive, a surgical biopsy is the only remaining option.

Once the etiology of the malignant effusion is established,

a treatment strategy can be formulated. Surgical debulking of metastatic pleural tumor is generally not part of the treatment algorithm outside an experimental protocol. Most patients are relegated to chemotherapy and/or radiation therapy, or palliative measures directed at preventing further fluid accumulation.

If the patient is not receiving treatment for the underlying malignancy, or reaccumulates the effusion in spite of treatment, an alternative strategy must be considered if the effusion is causing symptoms. The options include chemical or surgical pleurodesis to prevent fluid accumulation or to provide a route for continuous drainage. Drainage may be accomplished by internal shunting of the fluid from the pleural cavity to the peritoneum or external drainage with a catheter connected to a collection bag.

EXUDATIVE EFFUSIONS: BENIGN

Effusions associated with pneumonia (parapneumonic effusions) are the most common cause of benign exudative effusions. They result from visceral pleural inflammation that alters the normal fluid balance of the pleural space.[7] These effusions may initially be sterile, but if the parenchymal infection spreads to the effusion, an empyema results.

There is a continuum that reflects the natural history of untreated parapneumonic effusions, from a thin, clear sterile collection to an infected fibrous peel encasing the lung. The first stage is the "exudative stage" characterized by fluid exuding from the lung into the pleural space, likely from the pulmonary interstitial space. This stage should resolve with antibiotic therapy and generally does not require drainage. Normal pH and glucose with a low LDH and white blood cell count are characteristic of the fluid at this stage.

Untreated, the effusion is likely to progress to the "fibropurulent stage," characterized by increased fluid that is heavily laden with white blood cells, microorganisms, and cellular debris. Fibrin is deposited on the pleural surfaces and the stage is set for pulmonary entrapment. At this point, the fluid pH and glucose fall and the LDH rises. Chest tube drainage is indicated, but becomes more difficult as the effusion loculates. The final stage is the "organizational stage" during which fibroblasts grow into the effusion, laying down a thick fibrous peel that encases the lung and results in entrapment. The remaining effusion is thick and infected and may necessitate through the chest wall or into the lung.[7,72]

The presentation of a parapneumonic effusion or empyema depends, to a certain extent, on the organism causing the infection. For aerobic organisms the presence of the effusion has little impact on the clinical picture, which is that of a bacterial pneumonia: fever, chest pain, and a productive cough. An anaerobic infection, frequently as a result of aspiration, is more likely to present in a subacute manner. A patient with an anaerobic empyema may have symptoms for more than a week before seeking medical help, and significant weight loss may be a chief component of their presentation.[7]

There are several surgical options for patients with an empyema. The goals of surgical therapy are to establish drainage and, depending upon the situation, to eliminate space in the pleural cavity. Space elimination can be accomplished by decortication to allow the lung to expand, collapsing the chest wall with a thoracoplasty or by transposing muscle flaps to fill the space. A critical component is to always establish drainage. The least invasive option is to thoracoscopically explore the chest cavity, disrupt loculations, debride the visceral pleura, and strategically place chest tubes. Frequently it is possible to accomplish this procedure utilizing the patient's already existing chest tube sites as video ports. This option is most likely to be successful if performed in the exudative or early fibrinopurulent stages.[73]

Once in the organizational stage, the lung is encased in a fibrous peel that most often requires an open thoracotomy to adequately remove. If the patient is able to tolerate such a procedure, then this represents the most effective treatment of the problem. The goal in such a situation is to drain the infection and obliterate any space with reexpanded lung tissue.

After a drainage procedure the clinician is faced with the management of the chest tubes. The classic treatment of a chest tube placed into an empyema is to leave it to closed suction drainage for 2 to 3 weeks. Thereafter, the tubes are taken off suction and converted to open drainage, slowly withdrawing them over the course of several more weeks.[5] The critical point is that the lung must be fully expanded.

For patients with chronic empyema, empyema with bronchopleural fistula, or patients unable to tolerate thoracotomy, an open drainage procedure may represent the best option.

EXUDATIVE EFFUSIONS: BENIGN, OTHER CAUSES

INFECTIOUS, NONBACTERIAL

Almost any organism can cause an infection with which a pleural effusion is associated. Tuberculosis may cause a pleural effusion that tends to be unilateral and of moderate size. The effusion usually responds to appropriate antibiotic therapy and, unless symptomatic or part of a mixed empyema, usually does not require drainage or surgery. Viral effusions usually elude diagnosis and are self-limited. Effusions may accompany any of a number of fungal pulmonary infections. The primary treatment is appropriate antibiotic therapy and, depending upon the infection, drainage. Finally, although relatively uncommon in the United States, the clinician should be aware that pleural effusions commonly accompany a number of parasitic infections. Again, appropriate drug therapy is essential.

PULMONARY EMBOLI

Pleural effusions may accompany pulmonary emboli in 30% to 50% of cases. Although the majority of these effusions are exudative, approximately one-quarter may be transudative. The treatment for pulmonary emboli with effusion is the same as for pulmonary emboli without effusion.

SUBDIAPHRAGMATIC PATHOLOGY

Inflammation or malignancy below the diaphragm can cause exudative pleural effusions as well as transudative effusions secondary to hepatic or renal dysfunction. Acute pancreatitis generally leads to a left-sided effusion, likely as a result of transdiaphragmatic transfer of exudative ascites arising from pancreatic inflammation. The fluid almost always has an elevated amylase, and that amylase is frequently higher than the serum amylase. The fluid generally resolves with resolution of the pancreatic inflammation. Pancreatic abscess can also cause a pleural effusion and, again, the treatment is the usual treatment of a pancreatic abscess. A pancreatic pseudocyst can decompress into the pleural space, forming a pancreaticopleural fistula. Treatment of this disorder is conservative, the same as the initial treatment of any pancreatic pseudocyst. Should conservative treatment fail, a percutaneous or surgical drainage procedure should be planned.

Subphrenic abscess from any number of intraabdominal sources can lead to an exudative effusion. The effusions rarely are culture positive and tend to have a very high WBC, yet the pH is usually above 7.20 and the glucose is usually greater than 60 mg/dl. Treatment of the effusion should be symptomatic, as the approach is treatment of the abscess and its underlying cause. The effusion usually resolves with these measures.

The clinician is advised to always consider esophageal perforation in the diagnosis of a pleural effusion, particularly after instrumentation of the esophagus or retching. Iatrogenic injury accounts for two-thirds of these injuries, and the patient frequently complains of chest pain. Treatment depends upon how early the disruption is diagnosed, and ranges from primary repair to esophageal exclusion. Pleural drainage and antibiotics are almost always necessary components of the treatment strategy.

CHYLOTHORAX

Chylothorax is an exudative effusion caused by disruption of the thoracic duct and subsequent drainage of chyle into the pleural space. Once a chest tube is in place, the symptoms are determined by the persistence of the drainage. The longer the drainage continues, the more dangerous it becomes with the consequences being dehydration, nutritional depletion, and immunocompromise.[74] More than 50% of chylothoraces are secondary to ductal obstruction and disruption by tumor, with lymphoma accounting for 75% of these cases. Approximately 25% of chyle leaks are traumatic, with iatrogenic trauma being the most common. Of the iat-rogenic causes, esophageal resection appears to be the leading cause. The remainders are idiopathic and thought to be related to minor trauma.[65]

The diagnosis is established by analysis of the fluid. Although classically viewed as milky in appearance, chyle may frequently appear serosanguinous, particularly in the fasting state. A triglyceride level in the fluid greater than 110 mg/dl is highly suggestive of chyle whereas a level below 50 mg/dl essentially excludes the diagnosis of chylothorax.

The treatment of chylothorax remains controversial; some authors advocate a generous period of conservative treatment while others recommend early intervention.[75–77] Conservative therapy involves pleural drainage and a no-fat diet or total parenteral nutrition. If the leak is secondary to a malignancy, then chemotherapy and/or radiation therapy may be the treatment of choice. For other chylothoraces, surgical intervention is indicated when conservative measures have failed.

At the time of surgery, heavy cream is administered via nasogastric tube immediately after intubation; this makes the duct more visible and may also identify the area of leak. A number of surgical options are available, including parietal pleurectomy, direct ligation of the leak, and mass ligation of the duct. In cases where surgery fails or the patient is at prohibitive risk for a major procedure, other options include pleuroperitoneal shunting or sclerosis.

HEMOTHORAX

The overwhelming majority of hemothoraces are caused by trauma, including iatrogenic trauma. There are other, signif-icantly less common, causes including bleeding from metastatic tumors involving the pleura, hemorrhage during anticoagulation therapy for pulmonary emboli, and catamenial hemothorax. The potential consequences of an undrained hemothorax include conversion to an empyema, provocation of a pleural effusion, and conversion to a fibrothorax with lung entrapment. The initial treatment of any hemothorax should be pleural drainage with a large-bore (32- or 36-French) chest tube. If the tube becomes clogged or is inadequate, additional tubes should be strategically placed.

MISCELLANEOUS

Collagen vascular disorders may be associated with pleural effusions. In each case, the treatment of the effusion is symptomatic with the primary goal being treatment of the underlying disorder.

Although many drugs can cause pleural effusions, it is not a common cause. Some of the more commonly used drugs that may cause an effusion include amiodarone, methotrexate, nitrofurantoin, dantrolene, and metronidazole. Early discontinuation of the offending agent usually results in resolution of the syndrome.[7,65]

There are numerous other causes of exudative effusions. These include but are not limited to cardiac surgery, lung transplantation, asbestos exposure, Dressler's syndrome, Meigs' syndrome, yellow nail syndrome, sarcoid, postpartum state, trapped lung, radiation exposure, ovarian hyperstimulation, amyloidosis, ARDS, electrical burns, and uremia.[7]

Solid Disorders of the Pleural Space

BENIGN DISORDERS

Fibrothorax results from deposition of a thick fibrous layer along the pleural surface. This layer may cause entrapment of the lung as well as contraction and immobility of the skeletal hemithorax. The most common causes of fibrothorax are hemothorax, tuberculosis, and bacterial pneumonia. Other causes include pancreatitis, collagen vascular diseases, and uremia.[7] The treatment of fibrothorax is decortication, which in this setting is generally a major operation requiring a full thoracotomy. Patients who are being considered for decortication should be low-risk surgical candidates and should have pulmonary parenchyma that is anticipated to be able to expand upon release. Generally, the indication is significant pulmonary compromise in a patient whose fibrothorax is stable or worsening for at least several months (Fig. 41.3).[7]

Pleural plaques are hard, raised discrete areas involving the parietal pleura, particularly in the lateral, posterior portion of the hemithorax; 80% of pleural plaques that are due to asbestos are bilateral, with the majority of unilateral plaques thought to be secondary to other causes such as previous trauma, tuberculosis, or collagen vascular disorders.[65] Generally, there is no therapy indicated for pleural plaques. Pleural plaques do not appear to be predecessors of mesothelioma.[7]

Diffuse pleural thickening, like pleural plaques, appears to be predominantly related to asbestos exposure. Other causes such as drug reaction, hemothorax, and tuberculosis have been reported. Unlike pleural plaques, however, diffuse pleural thickening affects the visceral pleura. Again, there is no specific treatment recommended, just routine surveil-

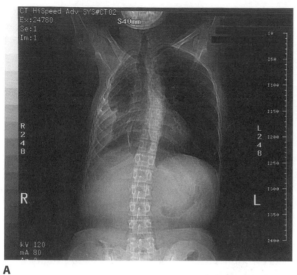
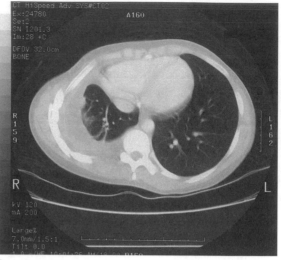

FIGURE 41.3. Anteroposterior radiograph of the chest (**A**) demonstrates scoliosis and volume loss resulting from a fibrothorax caused by a tuberculous empyema. CT cross section (**B**) demonstrates the thick parietal pleural peel entrapping healthy lung parenchyma. Notice contraction and overlapping of ribs in both radiographs. The patient underwent a decortication with dramatic improvement of her scoliosis and pulmonary function.

lance. In severe cases, pleurectomy has been performed, the results of which were poor secondary to concomitant pulmonary fibrosis.[7,65,78,79]

A rare primary, benign tumor of the pleura is the benign fibrous tumor of the pleura, previously called benign mesothelioma. These tumors arise from the visceral pleura, are not associated with asbestos, and are frequently discovered incidentally on chest X-ray. These tumors may reach enormous size, thereby causing symptoms by virtue of compression of other structures (Fig. 41.3). Surgery is the treatment of choice and is almost always curative.[65]

SOLID MALIGNANCIES OF THE PLEURA

The most common malignancies of the pleura are metastatic, predominantly from lung, breast, or colonic carcinomas. There are extremely rare primary sarcomas arising from the connective tissue elements of the pleura. The most common primary malignancy of the pleura is mesothelioma. Mesothelioma is almost always unilateral and is diagnosed either by cytology or pleural biopsy. From the time of diagnosis, the median survival is 4 to 12 months. The incidence of the disease has increased during the past decade, likely because legislation to curb asbestos exposure has only recently been widely adopted.[80–82]

Currently, mesothelioma continues to defy any single treatment modality including surgery, chemotherapy, and radiation therapy. Utilizing a trimodality approach of surgery, chemotherapy, and radiation therapy, survivals up to 39% at 5 years have been reported.[81]

References

1. Nebut M, Hirsch A, Chretien J. Embryology and anatomy of the Pleura. In: Chretien J, Hirsch A, eds. Diseases of the pleura. New York: Masson, 1982.
2. Wang N. Morphological data of pleura—normal conditions. In: Chretien J, Hirsch A, eds. Diseases of Pleura. New York: Masson, 1982:10.
3. Wang NS. Anatomy and physiology of the pleural space. Clin Chest Med 1985;6(1):3–16.
4. Miserocchi G. Physiology and pathophysiology of pleural fluid turnover. Eur Resp J 1997;10(1):219–225.
5. Pearson F, et al., eds. Thoracic Surgery. New York: Churchill Livingstone, 1995.
6. Williams P, Warwick R., eds. Gray's Anatomy, 36th ed. Philadelphia: Saunders, 1980.
7. Light R. Pleural Diseases, 3rd ed. 1980. Baltimore: Williams & Wilkins, 1995.
8. Albertine KH, et al. Structure, blood supply, and lymphatic vessels of the sheep's visceral pleura. Am J Anat 1982;165(3): 277–294.
9. Albertine KH, Wiener-Kronish JP, Staub NC. The structure of the parietal pleura and its relationship to pleural liquid dynamics in sheep. Anat Record 1984;208(3):401–409.
10. Chang TC, Funaki B, Szymski GX. Are routine chest radiographs necessary after image-guided placement of internal jugular central venous access devices? AJR 1998;170(2):335–337.
11. West J. 1981. Respiratory Physiology: The Essentials, 2nd ed. Baltimore: Waverly Press, 1981.
12. Shinohara H. Distribution of lymphatic stomata on the pleural surface of the thoracic cavity and the surface topography of the pleural mesothelium in the golden hamster. Anat Rec 1997; 249(1):16–23.
13. Stewart P. The rate of formation and lymphatic removal of fluid in pleural effusions. J Clin Invest 1963;42:258–262.
14. Leckie W, Tothill P. Albumin turnover in pleural effusions. Clin Sci 1965;29:339–352.
15. Walston A, et al. The electrocardiographic manifestations of spontaneous left pneumothorax. Ann Int Med 1974;80(3):p. 375–379.
16. Aitchison F, et al. Detection of pneumothorax by accident and emergency officers and radiologists on single chest films. Arch Emerg Med 1993;10(4):343–346.
17. Kiev J, Kerstein MD. Role of three hour roentgenogram of the chest in penetrating and nonpenetrating injuries of the chest. Surg Gynecol Obstet 1992;175(3):p. 249–253.
18. Maffessanti M, Bortolotto P, Grotto M. Imaging of pleural diseases. Monaldi Arch Chest Dis 1996;51(2):138–144.
19. Rhea JT, DeLuca SA, Greene RE. Determining the size of pneumothorax in the upright patient. Radiology 1982;144(4):733–736.

20. Choi BG, et al. Pneumothorax size: correlation of supine anteroposterior with erect posteroanterior chest radiographs. Radiology 1998;209(2):567–579.

21. Axel L. A simple way to estimate the size of a pneumothorax. Invest Radiol 1981;16(2):165–166.

22. Kircher LJ, Swartzel R. Spontaneous pneumothorax and its treatment. JAMA 1954;155:24–29.

23. Northfield TC. Oxygen therapy for spontaneous pneumothorax. Br Med J 1971;4(779):86–88.

24. Chadha TS, Cohn MA. Noninvasive treatment of pneumothorax with oxygen inhalation. Respiration 1983;44(2):147–152.

25. Light RW. Management of spontaneous pneumothorax. Am Rev Resp Dis 1993;148(1):245–248.

26. Andrivet P, et al. Spontaneous pneumothorax. Comparison of thoracic drainage vs. immediate or delayed needle aspiration. Chest 1995;108(2):335–339.

27. Conces DJ Jr, et al. Treatment of pneumothoraces utilizing small caliber chest tubes. Chest 1988;94(1):55–57.

28. Casola G, et al. Pneumothorax: radiologic treatment with small catheters. Radiology 1988;166(1 Pt 1):89–91.

29. Vallee P, et al. Sequential treatment of a simple pneumothorax. Ann Emerg Med 1988;17(9):936–942.

30. Minami H, et al. Small caliber catheter drainage for spontaneous pneumothorax. Am J Med Sci 1992;304(6):345–347.

31. Rusch VW, et al. The performance of four pleural drainage systems in an animal model of bronchopleural fistula. Chest 1988;93(4):859–863.

32. Kovarik JL, Brown RK. Tube and trocar thoracostomy. Surg Clin North Am 1969;49(6):1455–1460.

33. Woodring JH. Focal reexpansion pulmonary edema after drainage of large pleural effusions: clinical evidence suggesting hypoxic injury to the lung as the cause of edema. S Med J 1997;90(12):1176–1182.

34. Tarver RD, Broderick LS, Conces DJ Jr. Reexpansion pulmonary edema. J Thorac Imag 1996;11(3):198–209.

35. Melton LJD, Hepper NG, Offord KP. Influence of height on the risk of spontaneous pneumothorax. Mayo Clin Proc 1981;56(11):678–682.

36. Melton LJD, Hepper NG, Offord KP. Incidence of spontaneous pneumothorax in Olmsted County, Minnesota: 1950 to 1974. Am Rev Resp Dis 1979;120(6):1379–1382.

37. Lesur O, et al. Computed tomography in the etiologic assessment of idopathic spontaneous pneumothorax. Chest 1990;98(2):341–347.

38. Gobbel WJ, et al. Spontaneous pneumothorax. J Thorac Cardiovasc Surg 1963;46:331–345.

39. Smit HJ, et al. Spontaneous pneumothorax: predictable miniepidemics? Lancet 1997;350(9089):1450.

40. Bense L. Spontaneous pneumothorax related to falls in atmospheric pressure. Eur J Resp Dis 1984;65(7):p. 544–546.

41. Fox JT, Sawyer MA. Primary spontaneous pneumothorax and smoking. Military Med 1996;161(8):489–490.

42. Schramel FM, Postmus PE, Vanderschueren RG. Current aspects of spontaneous pneumothorax. Eur Resp J 1997;10(6):1372–1379.

43. Bense L, Eklund G, Wiman LG. Smoking and the increased risk of contracting spontaneous pneumothorax. Chest 1987;92(6):1009–1012.

44. Alfageme I, et al. Spontaneous pneumothorax. Long-term results with tetracycline pleurodesis. Chest 1994;106(2):347–50.

45. Hatta T, et al. A case of simultaneous bilateral spontaneous pneumothorax. Kyobu Geka (Jpn J Thorac Surg) 1993;46(3):287–289.

46. Rusch V. Pleural diseases. In: Faber L, ed. Chest Surgery Clinics of North America, Vol. 4. Philadelphia: Saunders, 1994.

47. Schoenenberger RA, et al. Timing of invasive procedures in therapy for primary and secondary spontaneous pneumothorax. Arch Surg 1991;126(6):764–766.

48. Waller DA, Forty J, Morritt GN. Video-assisted thoracoscopic surgery versus thoracotomy for spontaneous pneumothorax. Ann Thorac Surg 1994;58(2):372–376; discussion 376–377.

49. Freixinet J, et al. Surgical treatment of primary spontaneous pneumothorax with video-assisted thoracic surgery. Eur Resp J 1997;10(2):409–411.

50. Atta HM, et al. Thoracotomy versus video-assisted thoracoscopic pleurectomy for spontaneous pneumothorax. Am Surg 1997;63(3):209–212.

51. Dumont P, et al. Does a thoracoscopic approach for surgical treatment of spontaneous pneumothorax represent progress? Eur J Cardiothorac Surg 1997;11(1):27–31.

52. Tanaka F, et al. Secondary spontaneous pneumothorax. Ann Thorac Surg 1993;55(2):372–376.

53. Sassoon CS. The etiology and treatment of spontaneous pneumothorax. Curr Opin Pulmon Med 1995;1(4):331–338.

54. Wait MA, Estrera A. Changing clinical spectrum of spontaneous pneumothorax. Am J Surg 1992;164(5):528–531.

55. Light RW, et al. Intrapleural tetracycline for the prevention of recurrent spontaneous pneumothorax. Results of a Department of Veterans Affairs cooperative study. JAMA 1990;264(17):2224–2230.

56. Ferraro P, et al. Spontaneous primary and secondary pneumothorax: a 10-year study of management alternatives. Can J Surg 1994;37(3):197–202.

57. Despars JA, Sassoon CS, Light RW. Significance of iatrogenic pneumothoraces. Chest 1994;105(4):1147–1150.

58. Tocino I, Westcott JL. Barotrauma. Radiol Clin North Am 1996;34(1):59–81.

59. Schotland H. Images in clinical medicine. Barotrauma. N Engl J Med 1998;338(6):372.

60. Weg JG, et al. The relation of pneumothorax and other air leaks to mortality in the acute respiratory distress syndrome. N Engl J Med 1998;338(6):341–346.

61. Ng AW, Chan KW, Lee SK. Simple aspiration of pneumothorax. Sing Med J 1994;35(1):50–52.

62. Laub M, et al. Role of small caliber chest tube drainage for iatrogenic pneumothorax. Thorax 1990;45(10):748–749.

63. Brown KT, et al. Outpatient treatment of iatrogenic pneumothorax after needle biopsy. Radiology 1997;205(1):249–252.

64. Delius RE, et al. Catheter aspiration for simple pneumothorax. Experience with 114 patients. Arch Surg 1989;124(7):833–836.

65. Fishman A, ed. Pulmonary Diseases and Disorders, 3rd Ed. New York: McGraw-Hill, 1998.

66. Light RW, et al. Pleural effusions: the diagnostic separation of transudates and exudates. Ann Int Med 1972;77(4):507–513.

67. McLoud TC, Flower CD. Imaging the pleura: sonography, CT, and MR imaging. AJR 1991;156(6):1145–1153.

68. Colins JD, et al. Minimal detectable pleural effusions. A roentgen pathology model. Radiology 1972;105(1):51–53.

69. Kinasewitz GT. Transudative effusions. Eur Resp J 1997;10(3):714–718.

70. Assi Z, et al. Cytologically proved malignant pleural effusions: distribution of transudates and exudates. Chest 1998;113(5):1302–1304.

71. Landreneau RJ, et al. The role of thoracoscopy in lung cancer management. Chest 1998;113(1 Suppl):6S–12S.

72. Sasse SA. Parapneumonic effusions and empyema. Curr Opin Pulmon Med 1996;2(4):320–326.

73. Striffeler H, et al. Video-assisted thoracoscopic surgery for fibrinopurulent pleural empyema in 67 patients. Ann Thorac Surg 1998;65(2):319–323.

74. Merrigan BA, Winter DC, O'Sullivan GC. Chylothorax. Br J Surg 1997;84(1):15–20.

75. Milsom JW, et al. Chylothorax: an assessment of current surgical management. J Thorac Cardiovasc Surg 1985;89(2):221–227.

76. Johnstone DW, Feins RH. Chylothorax. Chest Surg Clin North Am 1994;4(3):617–628.

77. Selle JG, Snyder WHD, Schreiber JT. Chylothorax: indications for surgery. Ann Surg 1973;177(2):245–249.

78. Shih JF, et al. Asbestos-induced pleural fibrosis and impaired exercise physiology. Chest 1994;105(5):1370–1376.

79. Yates DH, et al. Asbestos-related bilateral diffuse pleural thickening: natural history of radiographic and lung function abnormalities [see comments]. Am J Resp Crit Care Med 1996;153(1):301–306.

80. Ryan CW, Herndon J, Vogelzang NJ. A review of chemotherapy trials for malignant mesothelioma. Chest 1998;113(1 Suppl):66S–73S.

81. Sugarbaker DJ, Norberto JJ. Multimodality management of malignant pleural mesothelioma. Chest 1998;113(1 Suppl):61S–65S.

82. Curran D, et al. Prognostic factors in patients with pleural mesothelioma: the European Organization for Research and Treatment of Cancer experience. J Clin Oncol 1998;16(1):145–152.

42

Pericardium

Rayman W. Lee and Joseph B. Zwischenberger

Anatomy

The pericardium is a strong, rather inelastic sac enclosing the heart. It is composed of two layers. The outer fibrous parietal pericardium is commonly referred to as "the pericardium." The thin inner serosal layer is the visceral pericardium, also called the epicardium. These two layers form a small space that usually contains only 15 to 50 ml of fluid. The parietal pericardium has ligamentous attachments to the manubrium, xiphoid process, vertebral bodies, and the central tendon of the diaphragm, which limit the movement of the heart with positional changes. The arterial blood supply is from small branches of the aorta, internal mammary, and musculophrenic arteries. Innervation is via the vagus nerve, left recurrent laryngeal nerve, esophageal plexus, and a rich sympathetic plexus. The phrenic nerves run along the pericardium to the diaphragm and can carry afferent pain perception to C4–C5. Microscopically, the pericardium has abundant microvilli that decrease friction and increase the surface area for reabsorption. The parietal lymphatics drain preferentially to the anterior and posterior mediastinal nodes,[1] whereas the visceral lymphatics drain to the tracheal and bronchial mid-mediastinal lymph nodes.[2]

Properties and Functions

The pericardial pressure–volume curve has an initial flat section followed by a knee and then a steep slope (Fig. 42.1).[3] The flat portion reflects the pericardial space reserve volume available. Pericardial constraint contributes to atrial and ventricular pressures[4] and limits the distension of the heart with acute volume overload. Constraint also plays a role in ventricular interdependence, when one ventricle dilates, causing the intrapericardial pressures to increase and limit filling of the other ventricle. This interdependence is more pronounced during cardiac tamponade. The pericardium mainly functions to reduce friction between the heart and surrounding tissues. Other functions include providing a mechanical barrier and producing prostaglandins and prostacyclin, which may have a role in coronary vasodilatation or fibrinolytic activity.

Acute Pericarditis

Acute pericarditis is simply inflammation of the pericardium characterized by chest pain, a pericardial friction rub, and electrocardiographic changes. Pericarditis is caused by myriad different entities. The most common etiologies are idiopathic or viral, uremic, postinfarct, neoplastic, and traumatic.

Clinical Presentation

The chest pain is sharp and pleuritic in nature and is commonly localized retrosternally or along the left precordial regions, radiating to the left trapezius ridge and neck. Trapezius ridge pain is transmitted via the phrenic nerves and is almost pathognomonic for pericardial irritation. The discomfort can be exacerbated by lying supine, breathing deeply, swallowing, or coughing, and patients frequently sit up and lean forward for relief. Dyspnea is also common usually because of splinting of the pain. Symptoms, however, may mimic a pulmonic, gastrointestinal, or cardiac source. The differentiation from ischemic pain may be especially difficult in the patient with cardiac risk factors. Fever, chills, weakness, cough, palpitations, nausea, and anorexia are other presenting symptoms.

A *pericardial friction rub* is the hallmark physical finding of acute pericarditis, with an unmistakable high-pitched grating or scratching sound. The classic rub is composed of three components, correlating to cardiac motion in atrial systole, ventricular systole, and ventricular diastole. These rubs can be transient and intermittent, so careful auscultation is needed. The best position to appreciate the sound is along the

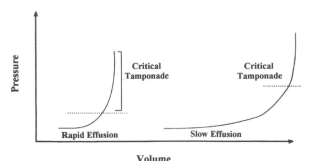

FIGURE 42.1. Pericardial pressure–volume curves. *Left:* Rapidly increasing pericardial fluid first fills the pericardial reserve volume (*initial flat segment*) then rises steeply to exceed the limit of parietal pericardium resulting in cardiac tamponade. *Right:* Slower rate of pericardial filling allows the pericardium to stretch and accommodate larger volumes. (Adapted from Spodick,[3] with permission.)

left sternal border with the patient leaning forward. Frequently the rub is loudest with inspiration.

Laboratory

The electrocardiogram can undergo four evolutionary stages, which are pathognomonic of acute pericarditis with the appropriate clinical history. Stage I changes are the most diagnostic of pericarditis. ST segments are elevated with diffuse upward concavity and reciprocal changes in leads V1 and aVR, PR intervals are depressed, and T waves are upright. Stage II starts several days later with the ST segments returning to baseline and the T waves flattening. Stage III is characterized by diffuse T-wave inversion, with stage IV showing reversion of the T waves back to normal. These changes may take several weeks or months to evolve and they may persist indefinitely. About one-half of patients with acute pericarditis will have all four stages, with most having at least PR segment depression. Atrial tachyarrhythmias are also prevalent.

Other diagnostic tests are usually nonspecific for pericarditis. The echocardiogram may show a small effusion or a "sunburst" appearance along the cardiac perimeters. Leukocytosis and a high sedimentation rate are common. The cardiac enzymes can be modestly elevated, probably because of subpericardial myocarditis.

Management

The usual course of acute idiopathic pericarditis is mild and self-limited, with initial management being bed rest. The chest pain can be treated with nonsteroidal antiinflammatory drugs (NSAIDs) such as aspirin (325–650 mg orally every 4–6 h) or ibuprofen (300–800 mg every 6–8 h). Patients are frequently admitted to the hospital to rule out a more serious condition such as myocardial infarction, pyogenic infection, or development of tamponade, which can occur in about 15% of patients. In cases unremitting despite medical therapy, large doses of corticosteroids (prednisone 60–80 mg/day) can be used, but tuberculous and infectious pericarditis should be excluded. Potential complications of acute pericarditis include cardiac tamponade, recurrent episodes of pericarditis, and progression to chronic constrictive pericarditis. The rate of recurrent pericarditis can be up to 30% of patients.

Pericardial Effusion

A pericardial effusion may develop from practically any cause of pericarditis. If the fluid accumulation is slow, the pericardial volume can expand to quite remarkable sizes, up to 3 to 4 l, and may be clinically silent. With faster development of fluid, cardiac tamponade may occur.

Clinical Presentation

Patients with a simple pericardial effusion may or may not have symptoms, depending on the degree of inflammation, intrapericardial pressure, and compression of adjacent organs. A dull chest pain or ache is the most frequent complaint. Cough and dyspnea can occur with atelectasis or tracheal compression, dysphagia can result from esophageal irritation, hiccups can be caused by phrenic nerve impingement, and nausea, vomiting, and fullness can be due to abdominal pressure. The physical exam in small effusions without pericarditis can be unremarkable. With larger effusions, the heart sounds become distant or muffled. An area of dullness and bronchial breathing below the left scapula caused by compression of the left lung base, called Ewert's sign, is an indication of a large effusion.

Laboratory

The chest X-ray is usually the first clue of a pericardial effusion in the asymptomatic patient. About 250 ml of fluid needs to be present before it can be appreciated on the plain films. With chronic pericardial effusions, the classic "water bottle heart" with a large globular cardiac silhouette and a thin neck may be seen. Mediastinal widening or a pericardial fat stripe may also be present on the chest X-ray. The electrocardiogram is nonspecific and insensitive[5] but can have reduced QRS voltage, flattened T waves, or PR segment depression with larger effusions.[6] Whenever a pericardial effusion is suspected, a transthoracic echocardiogram (ECHO) should be ordered. ECHO can easily, rapidly, and accurately detect even small amounts of fluid, as little as 20 ml, and assess the development of tamponade.[7] If the ECHO is indeterminate, CT and MRI may be helpful, especially with loculated effusions, pericardial thickening, calcifications, blood, fat, or chyle. Pericardial fluid analysis can be diagnostic and should be sent for cell count, glucose, protein, lactate dehydrogenase, bacterial culture, and cytology.[8] Depending on the clinical situation, other possible tests include AFB (acid-fast bacillus) culture and smear, fungal culture and smear, viral cultures, rheumatoid factor, complement, cholesterol, and triglyceride levels.

Management

Management of pericardial effusion depends on the patient's clinical course and suspected etiology. Most effusions are small, have a benign clinical course, and respond to treatment of the underlying systemic process, such as with congestive heart failure. Invasive diagnostic or therapeutic interventions are not needed in these cases, but further workup may be beneficial for symptomatic patients. With a bacterial process, pericardial fluid culture and Gram stain are required, and a pericardial biopsy may be needed for tuberculous or fungal infections. Pericardial fluid cytology can be diagnostic for malignant pericardial effusions. If patients are symptomatic with an idiopathic chronic effusion, good long-term relief[9] can be achieved with subxiphoid pericardial drainage.

Cardiac Tamponade

Cardiac tamponade can arise from any process that causes pericarditis or pericardial effusion. Expeditious diagnosis and intervention are essential because hemodynamic consequences can be fatal. Ordinarily fluid or blood causes tamponade, but air, mediastinal hematoma, or even large pleural effusions[10] can result in similar physiological compromise. Usually thought of as an acute problem, tamponade can be chronic. On a surgical service, trauma is responsible for the majority of cases, but on a medical service, malignancy is the cause of tamponade in more than one-half of patients.[11]

Clinical Presentation

Patients presenting with acute cardiac tamponade are typically in extremis with marked agitation and confusion, tachycardia, and tachypnea. In this setting, the classic clinical syndrome of *Beck's triad* can be seen with (1) elevation of systemic venous pressures, (2) systemic arterial hypotension, and (3) a small, quiet heart. With gradual development of tamponade, the presentation can be subtle. The main complaint is usually dyspnea on exertion, accompanied by anorexia, lethargy, edema, or weight loss. In these patients, there is almost always jugular venous distension and a paradoxical pulse. Also common are tachypnea and tachycardia; less common are diminished heart sounds and a pericardial rub. Interestingly, only about 25% of medical patients with tamponade have hypotension.[11,12]

Pulsus paradoxus, a characteristic finding in cardiac tamponade, was first described as the disappearance of the radial pulse despite a palpable heartbeat. Pulsus is not really paradoxical, but an exaggeration of the normal inspiratory drop in systolic pressure. It can be measured with a sphygmomanometer by inflating the cuff above the arterial pressure and very slowly deflating until the first Korotkoff sound is just heard. At this point, the Korotkoff sound will disappear with inspiration. With further slow deflation of the cuff, a continuous pulsation is heard. The difference in the systolic pressure of these two points is the amount of pulsus. A fall in the systolic blood pressure greater than 10 mmHg with inspiration signifies a pulsus paradox. Pulsus is not specific for tamponade and is frequently seen in chronic obstructive pulmonary disease (COPD) or asthma exacerbations. It can also occur with pulmonary embolus, cardiac constriction, or hypovolemia.

Laboratory

The chest X-ray appearance may vary depending on the time course of the tamponade. In acute situations, the cardiac shadow is normal because the pericardium cannot expand rapidly, but in chronic effusions, the classic water bottle heart may be seen, usually with clear lung fields. The electrocardiogram may show signs of pericarditis or decreased amplitude of the QRS complexes. A finding highly suggestive of tamponade is *electrical alternans*, representing the pendular swinging of the heart within the fluid-filled pericardium. This symp-

tom usually only involves the QRS complex in a 2:1 or 3:1 pattern, but when it involves the P, QRS, and T wave, it is pathognomonic for a severe tamponade. Electrical alternans, however, may also occur in pneumothorax, congestive heart failure, myocardial infarction, or constrictive pericarditis. An echocardiogram should be obtained whenever tamponade is suspected in the stable patient. The ECHO will verify a pericardial effusion and may have findings of tamponade such as a swinging pendular heart, right atrial diastolic collapse, and right ventricular collapse in early diastole. Other findings include an inspiratory increase in the right ventricular dimension and tricuspid valve flow, with a decrease in the left ventricular size and mitral valve flow and an inferior vena cava diameter greater than 20 mm with loss of normal inspiratory collapse.

CARDIAC CATHETERIZATION

Although the diagnosis of tamponade is mainly a clinical one[13] based on elevated venous pressures, tachycardia, dyspnea, and a pulsus paradoxus, cardiac catheterization is confirmatory. In the relatively stable patient, catheterization quantifies the hemodynamic compromise and guides pericardiocentesis. With tamponade, atrial, ventricular diastolic, and pericardial pressures all are elevated and virtually equal, which is sometimes referred to as *equalization of pressures.* Because there is no pressure gradient, there is no flow or filling causing an absent or small y descent, correlating with diastolic right atrial or ventricular collapse seen on ECHO.

SPECIAL CASES

Low-pressure cardiac tamponade occurs in the setting of hypovolemia such as with tuberculous or neoplastic pericarditis complicated by dehydration. Jugular venous distension is absent and right atrial pressure is normal, with the classic signs manifesting with volume administration. An elevated blood pressure can also accompany tamponade in the patient with underlying hypertension.[14] After pericardiocentesis, the arterial blood pressure may interestingly fall, but the cardiac output and systemic vascular resistance improve. Tension pneumopericardium is rare but can result from penetrating trauma or perforation.

Treatment

In the patient near death from tamponade, prompt drainage is vital. A blind pericardiocentesis can be done at the bedside, but this approach runs the risk of cardiac laceration. ECHO-guided aspiration is preferred if possible. Subxiphoid pericardiotomy can also be promptly accomplished under local anesthesia if necessary. In thoracic trauma, acute tamponade should probably be managed with thoracotomy and repair of the cardiac injury. Medical therapy with volume infusion and vasopressors is mainly supportive and temporary until a more definitive treatment can be rendered. In the stable patient, a combined procedure of cardiac catheterization or ECHO with pericardiocentesis can be done.

Constrictive Pericarditis

Constrictive pericarditis results from the healing of pericarditis with granulation tissue and obliteration of the pericardial cavity. The pericardium subsequently stiffens, forming a hard outer shell. The hemodynamic profile is very similar to cardiac tamponade because the pericardium restricts and impairs diastolic filling of the heart. It can also occur in concert with tamponade, causing an effusive-constrictive pericarditis. Any cause of pericarditis can produce constriction. The diagnosis can be difficult because the chronic nonspecific symptoms can mimic congestive heart failure, cirrhosis, or other organ dysfunction. Restrictive cardiomyopathy has a clinical presentation similar to constriction, and the differentiation between these two entities can be very challenging.

Clinical Presentation

The clinical course is usually gradual and often insidious. Weakness, fatigue, weight loss, and anorexia are common. Patients often appear chronically ill. Signs and symptoms of systemic venous congestion predominate, such as peripheral edema, hepatic congestion, exertional dyspnea, orthopnea, and pleural effusions. Hepatomegaly is present in about 70% of patients, and some may have evidence of severe hepatic congestion. Other symptoms include fatigue, weight loss, anorexia, cachexia, and cough. The hallmark finding of constrictive pericarditis is elevated jugular venous pressures. With close examination, a prominent y descent on the jugular venous pulsations can be appreciated. The apical pulse is typically reduced, and heart sounds may be distant. A distinguishing finding of constrictive pericarditis is the *pericardial knock*, a distinct, early-diastolic third heart sound caused by the abrupt cessation of ventricular filling by the rigid pericardium. The knock can be easily confused with an S3 or an opening snap of mitral stenosis. A widened split S2 may also occur. In contrast to pulsus paradoxus, *Kussmaul's sign* is the rise in venous pressure with inspiration because respiratory changes are minimized.

Laboratory

The chest X-ray cardiac silhouette in constrictive pericarditis is variable with a normal-size heart in one-half of cases. Pleural effusions are present in 60% of patients, but pulmonary edema is uncommon and implies concomitant heart or lung disease or a localized process. A useful marker is pericardial calcification, which can have unusual configurations, but calcification is not a frequent or specific finding for constrictive pericarditis. The electrocardiogram usually is nonspecific but may show reduced voltage, left atrial enlargement, or generalized ST–T wave changes. Atrial fibrillation is common.

Echocardiography findings include pericardial thickening, bilateral enlargement with good left ventricular function, and a dilated inferior vena cava without significant respiratory variation.[15] With transesophageal echocardiography, a thickened pericardium of constriction can be detected with 95% sensitivity and 86% specificity.[16] Doppler may also prove valuable with respiratory variation of transvalvular flow.[17] CT or MRI also can assess pericardial calcification and thickness in addition to examining myocardial atrophy or fibrosis in restrictive cardiomyopathy.

Hemodynamics

The diagnosis of constrictive pericarditis relies heavily on its characteristic hemodynamic profile (Fig. 42.2).[18] As in tam-

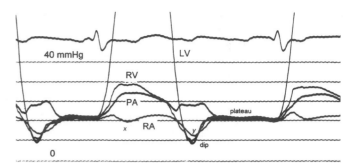

FIGURE 42.2. Constrictive pericarditis. Simultaneous left ventricular (*LV*), right ventricular (*RV*), pulmonary artery (*PA*), and right atrial (*RA*) pressures. Note equalization of pressures in end diastole. The *dip* and *plateau* of the ventricular waveforms are seen with the dip occurring in early diastole and the plateau in mid- to late diastole. A prominent y and normal x descent of the atrial waveform causes a characteristic M or W configuration. (Adapted from Reddy et al.[18])

ponade, there is marked elevation of venous and equalization of diastolic pressures. In addition, cardiac output and stroke volumes are low normal to reduced, resulting in a compensatory tachycardia and elevation of the systemic vascular resistance. In constriction, however, the pericardium acts as a shell allowing the ventricles to contract normally in systole, but limits filling in mid- to late diastole. Ventricular filling is followed by an abrupt halt when the cardiac volume expands to the volume set by the pericardium. This transition results in the *dip-and-plateau* or *square-root sign* seen in the ventricular waveforms.

DIFFERENTIAL

Constrictive pericarditis should be suspected in any patient with unexplained jugular venous distension, edema, or pleural effusion. It is often mistaken for hepatic disease, cirrhosis, Budd–Chiari syndrome, protein-losing enteropathy, superior vena cava syndrome, intraabdominal malignancy, or nephrotic syndrome. Constrictive physiology may also be seen in acute and massive right ventricular infarct with right ventricular dilatation, subacute tricuspid regurgitation, and rarely acute mitral regurgitation.

The primary diagnostic challenge is differentiating constriction from restrictive cardiomyopathy. In equivocal cases, an endomyocardial biopsy is needed for diagnosis. An accurate diagnosis is needed because pericardiectomy is not warranted in restriction, but it can be curative in constrictive pericarditis.

Management

This progressive disease process can be fatal if not treated. Medical management with diuretics is usually only a temporizing measure. Complete pericardial resection is the definitive treatment for constrictive pericarditis.[19]

Specific Pericardial Diseases

Infectious

Acute idiopathic pericarditis probably represents an acute viral process. Coxsackie virus group B and echovirus type B are the most common offenders. A prodrome of an upper respiratory illness or flu-like syndrome usually occurs several days or weeks before the pericarditis. The diagnosis is based on the clinical presentation of mild symptoms and a self-limited course.

Tuberculous pericarditis is still very common in developing countries, but with effective primary treatment of tuberculosis, the incidence has markedly diminished in the United States and industrialized countries. Unlike that of acute pericarditis, the clinical course is usually indolent, but it can also manifest rapidly. Nonspecific symptoms include fever, night sweats, and lethargy. The diagnosis can be made with isolation of tuberculosis from sputum, pleural fluid, or other tissue if available, but concomitant active pulmonary tuberculosis is the exception. A calcific pericardium is a common feature with tuberculous constriction.

Bacterial or purulent pericarditis is usually a result of direct contamination from adjacent infection, such as pneumonia or empyema, trauma, or hematogenous spread. It presents as an acute, severe illness with high fevers and shaking chills. Pneumococci, staphylococci, and streptococci remain likely causes, especially if community acquired.[20] The choice of antibiotics depends on the organism cultured and the sensitivity results. Although the pericardium can achieve high tissue and fluid concentrations of antibiotics, systemic antibiotics alone are not adequate and drainage procedure is necessary.

Neoplastic

Metastatic lesions to the heart are fairly common, with the pericardium involved in about 5% to 10% of cancer deaths.[21] The neoplasms most commonly metastatic to the pericardium are lung cancers, followed by breast.[22] Other malignancies include lymphoma, leukemia, melanoma, GI tumors, and sarcomas. The median survival for all malignant pericardial effusions is only 2 to 4 months with a 1-year survival of 25%.[23] The clinical presentation can vary from asymptomatic small effusions to acute, florid tamponade. Patients may have vague symptoms of dyspnea, cough, or chest pain. Once a malignant pericardial effusion is suspected, a pericardiocentesis should be done.

Management of malignant pericardial effusion is based on the patient's symptoms, prognosis, and general condition. Palliative care only should be considered in those patients with a poor prognosis and poor medical condition. The goal of therapy should be to alleviate symptoms, relieve cardiac tamponade, and prevent recurrence. A general algorithm for management and treatment of a malignant pericardial effusion is presented in Figure 42.3.

Primary neoplasms of the pericardium are rare, with the majority benign. Teratomas are the most common tumor followed by lipomas, fibromas, and angiomas. Of the malignant primary pericardial neoplasms, mesothelioma is the most frequent. Many times asbestos exposure cannot be elicited from the patient history. Mesothelioma can envelop the heart and has a poor prognosis.

Cardiac-Associated Pericarditis

Postinfarction pericarditis occurs in an early and late form, sometimes called infarct pericarditis and Dressler's syndrome, respectively. Infarct pericarditis tends to be localized to the area of injury. It usually has mild symptoms and responds to aspirin (up to 650 mg every 4 h for 5–10 days). In resistant cases, other NSAIDs and corticosteroids can be used. Dressler's syndrome presents weeks to months after the

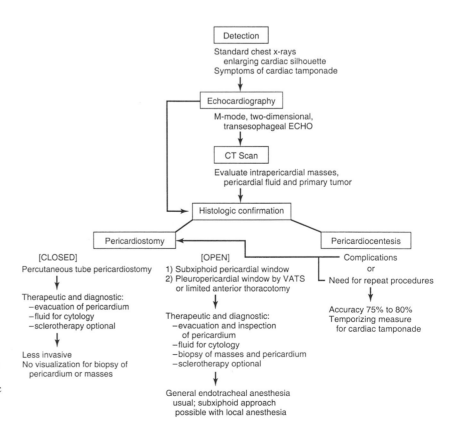

FIGURE 42.3. Algorithm for the diagnosis and treatment of malignant pericardial effusion. ECHO, echocardiography; VATS, video-assisted thoracoscopic surgery. (From Zwischenberger and Bradford,[2] with permission.)

TABLE 42.1. Comparison of Pericardial Procedures.

Procedure	Position	Anesthesia	Incision	Biopsy/window/ resection size	Pain	Advantages	Disadvantages
Pericardiocentesis	Supine	Local	Percutaneous	None	Minimal	Can be done emergently at bedside Fluid drainage/analysis Catheter for prolonged drainage or sclerosis	Drainage may be inadequate Blind approach associated with higher risk Higher recurrence rate
Balloon pericardi- otomy	Supine	Local	Percutaneous	Small window No biopsy	Minimal	Low morbidity Can be done in the catheterization lab	Limited availability
Subxiphoid peri- cardiotomy	Supine	Local or single lumen	Small incision	Small window 4×4 cm anterior sample	Mild	Good drainage Low morbidity	Limited access
VATS pericardi- otomy	Lateral decubitus	Double lumen Single-lung anesthesia	Three-port video equipment	Larger	Mild	Good drainage Low morbidity Access to pleura and lung	Surgeon unable to feel tissue
Anterolateral peri- cardiotomy or pericardiectomy	Lateral decubitus	Double lumen Single-lung anesthesia	Anterolateral thoracotomy	Larger	Most	Limited pericardiectomy Surgeon able to feel tissue Access to pleura and lung	Higher morbidity than with subxiphoid pericardiotomy
Radical pericardi- otomy	Supine	Single lumen	Median stern- otomy	Largest	Moderate	Complete pericardial resection Access for cardiopulmonary bypass	Pain/morbidity Operative risk

infarct and occurs in less than 3% of patients. The cause is unclear, but an autoimmune process is theorized, given the appearance of antimyocardial antibodies. The course is generally self-limited but the syndrome may be recurrent. Treatment is the same as with infarct pericarditis with bed rest and aspiration being the first choices, but other NSAIDs, colchicine, and corticosteroids are alternatives.

Pericardial effusions after cardiac surgery are very common, occurring in nearly two-thirds of patients. Frequently they are small, but are loculated in about 60% of patients and are significantly more common after valve replacement. Postpericardiotomy and postcardiac injury syndromes resemble Dressler's because of similar elevations of antimyocardial antibodies, thought to be an autoimmune reaction. Symptoms include fever, pleuritic chest pain, and malaise that start about 1 week after cardiac surgery or injury. Steroids may be used if severe symptoms do not abate within 48 h.

Traumatic

Exsanguination or pericardial tamponade are the principal immediate causes of death from cardiac trauma. Whenever traumatic injury to the pericardium occurs, whether blunt or penetrating, the heart and great vessels along with other vital organs are also frequently involved. The usual signs and symptoms of "medical" tamponade such as pulsus or rub are absent or variable in traumatic "surgical" tamponade. In addition, other serious concomitant wounds and shock may mask pericardial damage. In blunt trauma, pericardial rupture can result in cardiac herniation with displacement of cardiac and vascular structures. Although this may be immediately fatal, sometimes it does not occur until several hours after the injury. A chest X-ray can be diagnostic,[24] but pericardial rupture may not be found until surgery is performed.

In penetrating trauma, pericardial lacerations seldom occur alone, and their clinical significance depends on the underlying cardiac injury. Hemopericardium and tamponade are the main concerns. If the patient is in extremis, quick diagnosis and drainage are essential. Pericardiocentesis may not be possible because of clot formation. A subxiphoid pericardiotomy can be performed expeditiously and, if bleeding is found, be followed by median sternotomy with operative repair of the injury.[25]

Miscellaneous

Uremia is one of the most common causes of pericarditis on a medical service. The primary concern with uremic pericarditis is the development of cardiac tamponade, which can occur in 20% of patients,[26] especially those with new-onset renal failure or in underdialyzed patients. Management consists of intensive daily dialysis with regional or limited heparinization to minimize the risk of pericardial bleeding.[27] In resistant cases of recurrent effusion, drainage by a pigtail catheter, a subxiphoid pericardiotomy, or pericardiectomy may be needed.[28]

Chylopericardium is a rare condition usually resulting from the obstruction of the thoracic duct by trauma, cardiac surgery, or mechanical blockage, such as with neoplasms. These effusions are frequently idiopathic and tend to be large and chronic. Conservative treatment consists of a low-fat and high medium-chain triglyceride diet. For resistant cases, pericardiotomy following oral cream ingestion for exploration of source leak and thoracic duct ligation with or without pericardiectomy may be needed.[29,30]

Radiation therapy to the thorax is used commonly such as with breast cancer and lymphoma. Up to 20% of patients develop complications of radiation pericarditis. Radiation pericarditis usually occurs several months or sometimes years after the course of therapy[31] and can be difficult to distinguish from recurrent malignancy or pericardial effusion caused by radiation-induced hypothyroidism. For large recurrent effusions or constrictive pericarditis, an extensive pericardiectomy may be needed.

There is a high incidence and prevalence of pericardial effusion in AIDS. In one study, pericardial effusions developed at a rate of 11% per year. Most of these were small and rarely progressive, but patients had a significantly shortened survival.[32]

Pericardial Procedures

Procedures involving the pericardium are generally safe and effective, and most can be both diagnostic and therapeutic (Table 42.1).

Congenital Abnormalities

Congenital absence of the pericardium is uncommon. The defect can be partial or complete. In one-third of these cases, there are associated cardiac, valvular, pulmonary, or diaphragmatic anomalies. CT and MRI are very helpful in the diagnosis.[33] Isolated complete right or left pericardial defects are usually asymptomatic and can simply be observed. With partial absence of the pericardium, herniation of myocardium, great vessels, coronary arteries, and even the phrenic nerve can result in chest pain, syncope, or even sudden death. To relieve or prevent strangulation, pericardiotomy, pericardioplasty, or excision of the atrial appendage can be performed.[34]

Pericardial cysts are frequently asymptomatic and found on routine chest X-ray, ordinarily in the right cardiodiaphragmatic angle. Their clinical course is most often benign, but they can become infected or cause chest pain due to torsion. Surgery is generally not needed; however, excision may be helpful in diagnostically difficult cases or in the symptomatic patient.

Pericardium as Biomaterial

The pericardium has been used extensively as a biomaterial because of its strong, thin, but pliable properties. Heterograft, homograft, and autologous material have all been used as patches or bioprostheses.

References

1. Eliskova M, Eliska O, Miller AJ. The lymphatic drainage of the parietal pericardium in man. Lymphology 1995;28:208–217.
2. Zwischenberger JB, Bradford DW. Management of malignant pericardial effusion. In: Pass HI, Mitchell JB, Johnson DH, et al, eds. Lung Cancer: Principles and Practice. Philadelphia: Lippincott-Raven, 1996:655–662.

3. Spodick DH. The pericardium: a comprehensive textbook. New York: Dekker, 1997.
4. Hamilton DR, Dani RS, Semlacher RA, et al. Right atrial and right ventricular transmural pressures in dogs and humans. Effects of the pericardium. Circulation 1194;90:2492–2500.
5. Meyers DG, Bagin RG, Levene JF. Electrocardiographic changes in pericardial effusion. Chest 1993;104:1422–1426.
6. Eisenberg MJ, de Romeral LM, Heidenreich PA, et al. The diagnosis of pericardial effusion and cardiac tamponade by 12-lead ECG. A technology assessment. Chest 1996;110:318–324.
7. Schutzman JJ, Obarski TP, Pearce GL, et al. Comparison of Doppler and two-dimensional echocardiography for assessment of pericardial effusion. Am J Cardiol 1992;70;1353–1357.
8. Meyers DG, Meyers RE, Prendergast TW. The usefulness of diagnostic tests on pericardial fluid. Chest 1997;111:1213–1221.
9. Loire R, Goineau P, Fareh S, et al. Apparently idiopathic chronic pericardial effusion. Long-term outcome in 71 cases. Arch Mal Coeur Vaiss 1996;89:835–841.
10. Kaplan LM, Epstein SK, Schwartz SL, et al. Clinical, echocardiographic, and hemodynamic evidence of cardiac tamponade caused by large pleural effusions. Am J Respir Cell Mol Biol 1995;151:904–908.
11. Wang ML, Liao WB, Bullard MJ, et al. Cardiac tamponade in Taiwan. Jpn Circ J 1997;61:767–771.
12. Guberman BA, Fowler NO, Engel PJ, et al. Cardiac tamponade in medical patients. Circulation 1981;64:633–640.
13. Fowler NO. Cardiac tamponade: a clinical or echocardiographic diagnosis? Circulation 1993;87:1738–1741.
14. Brown J, MacKinnon D, King A, et al. Elevated arterial blood pressure in cardiac tamponade. N Engl J Med 1992;327:463–466.
15. Chandraratna PA. Echocardiography and Doppler ultrasound in the evaluation of pericardial disease. Circulation 1991;84(suppl 3):I303–I310.
16. Ling LH, Oh JK, Click RL, et al. Pericardial thickness measured with transesophageal echocardiography: feasibility and potential clinical usefulness. J Am Coll Cardiol 1997;29:1317–1323.
17. Oh JK, Hatle LK, Seward JB, et al. Diagnostic role of Doppler echocardiography in constrictive pericarditis. J Am Coll Cardiol 1994;23:154–162.
18. Reddy PS, Leon DF, Shaver JA, eds. Pericardial Disease. New York: Raven Press, 1982.
19. Culliford AT, Lipton M, Spencer FC, et al. Operation for chronic constrictive pericarditis: do the surgical approach and degree of pericardial resection influence the outcome significantly? Ann Thorac Surg 1980;29:146–152.
20. Sagristà-Sauleda J, Barrabes JA, Permanyer-Miralda G. Purulent pericarditis: review of a 20-year experience in a general hospital. J Am Coll Cardiol 1993;22:1661–1665.
21. Mukai K, Shinkai T, Tominaga K, et al. The incidence of secondary tumors of the heart and pericardium: a ten-year study. Jpn J Clin Oncol 1988;18:195–201.
22. Liu G, Crump M, Goss PE, et al. Prospective comparison of the sclerosing agents doxycycline and bleomycin for the primary management of malignant pericardial effusion and cardiac tamponade. J Clin Oncol 1996;14:3141–3147.
23. Posner MR, Cohen GI, Skarkin AT. Pericardial disease in patients with cancer. Am J Med 1981;71:407–413.
24. Carrillo EH, Heniford BT, Dykes JR, et al. Cardiac herniation producing tamponade: the critical role of early diagnosis. J Trauma 1997;43:19–23.
25. Johnson SB, Nielsen JL, Sako EY, et al. Penetrating intrapericardial wounds: clinical experience with a surgical protocol. Ann Thorac Surg 1995;60:117–120.
26. Rutsky EA, Rostrand SG. Treatment of uremic pericarditis and pericardial effusion. Am J Kidney Dis 1987;10:2–8.
27. Frommer JP, Young JB, Ayus JC. Asymptomatic pericardial effusion in uremic patients: effect of long-term dialysis. Nephron 1985;39:296–301.
28. Frame JR, Lucas SK, Pederson JA, et al. Surgical treatment of pericarditis in the dialysis patient. Am J Surg 1983;146:800–803.
29. Svedjeholm R, Jansson K, Olin C. Primary idiopathic chylopericardium: a case report and review of the literature. Eur J Cardiothorac Surg 1997;11:387–390.
30. Akamatsu H, Amano J, Sakamoto T, et al. Primary chylopericardium. Ann Thorac Surg 1994;58:262–266.
31. Martin RG, Ruckdeschel JC, Chang P, et al. Radiation-related pericarditis. Am J Cardiol 1975;35:216–220.
32. Heidenreich PA, Eisenberg MJ, Kee LL, et al. Pericardial effusion in AIDS: incidence and survival. Circulation 1995;92:3229–3234.
33. Gutierrez FR, Shackelford GD, McKnight CR, et al. Diagnosis of congenital absence of left pericardium by MR imaging. J Comput Assist Tomogr 1985;9:551–553.
34. Van Son JA, Danielson GK, Schaff HV, et al. Congenital partial and complete absence of the pericardium. Mayo Clin Proc 1993;68:743–747.

43

Mediastinum

Mark I. Block

Descending Necrotizing Mediastinitis

Descending necrotizing mediastinitis (DNM) is an uncommon but virulent form of mediastinal infection that arises from infectious sources in the head and neck and descends rapidly through cervical fascial planes to involve the mediastinum. It is distinguished from other forms of mediastinal infection not only by its unique pathophysiology but also by its potential for rapid progression to overwhelming sepsis and death, often within 24 to 48 h from the onset of symptoms. Recent large reviews document mortality rates persistently in cxccss of 30%.[1] However, a strategy of early and aggressive surgical debridement has been shown to reduce this figure to less than 20%.[2,3]

Epidemiology

More than half of all cases of DNM are odontogenic, arising most commonly from infections of the mandibular molars.[1,4] Less common sources of infection include retropharyngeal abscesses, iatrogenic pharyngeal injuries, cervical lymphadenitis, parotitis, and thyroiditis.[1,4,5] The mean age of patients is 32 to 36 years and most are men, with a ratio of men to women as high as 6:1.[1,2,6]

Anatomy

Infections that arise in the neck can descend into the mediastinum through planes defined by the three layers of deep cervical fascia—superficial, visceral, and prevertebral (Fig. 43.1).[5–7] These layers divide the neck into three potential spaces. (1) The *pretracheal* space is bordered by the strap muscles anteriorly and the trachea posteriorly. (2) The *retrovisceral* space is defined by the prevertebral fascia posteriorly and the esophagus anteriorly, and extends from the skull base down to the diaphragm. (3) The *perivascular* space is surrounded by the carotid sheath and contains the carotid artery, jugular vein, and vagus nerve. The retrovisceral space is the

most common avenue for descension of infection into the mediastinum, accounting for approximately 70% of cases.[3,8]

Microbiology

Multiple organisms have been isolated from patients with DNM. More than half are found to have a mixed aerobic/anaerobic infection,[1,3,4] with the most common organisms being *Staphylococcus*, β-hemolytic *Streptococcus*, *Pseudomonas*, and *Bacteroides*.[1,3–6,9] *Peptostreptococcus* has also been found relatively frequently.[9,10] Although fungal organisms are uncommon, species of *Aspergillus* and *Candida*[3] are occasionally isolated and should be a consideration in planning empiric antibiotic therapy.

Diagnosis

Because DNM can progress rapidly, successful management of patients requires early initiation of therapy based on a presumptive diagnosis. Definitive diagnosis is of primarily academic interest and is based on four criteria: (1) clinical manifestations of severe infection; (2) characteristic radiographic features; (3) documentation of necrotizing mediastinal infection at operation or autopsy; and (4) establishment of a relationship between oropharyngeal infection and the development of the necrotizing mediastinal process. It is emphasized, however, that because of the rapid progression and high mortality associated with DNM, appropriate treatment should not await definitive diagnosis. Clinical findings suspicious for DNM include fever, localized cervical or oropharyngeal pain, and respiratory distress.[5] Occasionally erythema and swelling in the submandibular or cervical region can be identified, while crepitus can be the result of either hollow viscus injury (trachea or esophagus) or advancing anaerobic infection. A recent history of dental work or dental infection combined with signs of infection outside the mouth should prompt immediate initiation of therapy. Respiratory distress is a particularly ominous finding and signals impending airway obstruction from progressive

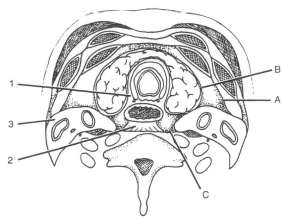

FIGURE 43.1. Tissue planes and spaces in the neck. Superficial (*A*), visceral (*B*), and prevertebral (*C*) cervical fascial planes create three potential spaces: pretracheal (*1*), retrovisceral (*2*), and perivascular (*3*). The retrovisceral space is the most common route for descending infection.

laryngeal edema. Features of DNM appreciable on plain X-rays include widening of the retrovisceral space with or without air–fluid levels, anterior displacement of the tracheal air column, loss of normal cervical spine lordosis, and mediastinal emphysema.[4] However, because these findings may not be apparent until late in the course of the illness, patients in whom the diagnosis is suspected should undergo immediate evaluation by computed tomography (CT). Findings such as soft tissue edema, fluid collections, pleural effusions, and cervical and mediastinal emphysema will establish the diagnosis early and define the extent of infection.[2,4]

Management

Treatment should be initiated as soon as the diagnosis of DNM is suspected and should address three considerations: airway maintenance, antibiotic therapy, and surgical debridement. Once antibiotics have been initiated, it is essential to monitor clinical response and results of antibiotic sensitivity testing, making appropriate changes as indicated. Concern over the continued high mortality associated with DNM has led to the recommendation that routine mediastinal debridement via thoracotomy should be considered the standard of care for all patients.[1,2,6] The decision not to directly debride and drain the mediastinum must be justified by clear and early signs of the patient's clinical improvement. It is likely that the worse the patient's condition, the greater is the extent of debridement required.

Postoperative Mediastinitis

Epidemiology

Mediastinitis complicating cardiac surgical procedures is associated with an in-hospital mortality of up to 35%,[11–17] a fourfold increase in long-term mortality,[14] and an increase in hospital costs of as much as 4.5 times.[13,18] *Staphylococcus* species are the most common causative organisms, with *Staphylococcus aureus* and *Staphylococcus epidermidis* responsible for more than 50% of cases in most reported series.[11,13,16,19–22]

Other important pathogens often recovered include *Pseudomonas*, *Enterobacter*, *Escherichia coli*, and *Serratia*.

Diagnosis

Establishing the diagnosis of postoperative mediastinitis can be challenging. Suspicious findings include increased incisional pain, sternal instability manifest as a "click" with coughing or palpation, dyspnea, fever, and incisional erythema and drainage. These signs and symptoms usually appear between 5 and 10 days postoperatively, but may not become apparent for several months.[11,23] Diagnosis is made difficult because many patients develop fever and leukocytosis without the finding of sternal instability, and minor sternal instability is not always a consequence of mediastinal infection. Diagnostic evaluation most commonly includes CT. Although the absence of suspicious findings on CT does not rule out mediastinitis, the presence of soft tissue swelling and fluid and air collections can be important indicators of ongoing infection.[24,25] Some authors have advocated radiolabeled leukocyte scintigraphy for early diagnosis.[26,27]

Risk Factors

Factors contributing to the development of postoperative mediastinitis can be grouped broadly into categories relating to the patient's preexisting conditions, the conduct of the operation, and the postoperative environment of the patient's care. Preexisting conditions such as obesity, chronic obstructive lung disease, prior cardiac surgery, diabetes, and heart failure have been identified as significant independent predictors of increased risk.[16,17,20,28–30] Similarly, studies identified urgency of the procedure, duration of cardiopulmonary bypass, and overall duration of the procedure as important intraoperative factors. Bilateral internal mammary artery (BIMA) use is generally accepted as an important risk factor, but the data are inconsistent.

Management

As with infected incisions elsewhere in the body, debridement followed by open or closed drainage can control infection and lead to complete wound healing. Definitive therapy for postoperative mediastinitis requires debridement of the infected sternum and costal cartilages and reconstruction with flaps made from pectoralis major, rectus abdominus, or omentum. Failure to debride all infected bone and cartilage can lead to reoperation and increased morbidity and mortality.

Long-Term Sequelae

Aggressive management of postoperative mediastinitis has led to a substantial decrease in mortality and requires early involvement of plastic surgery. Closed irrigation techniques may be associated with higher mortality,[11,12] but are more likely to preserve chest wall stability and function. Although follow-up studies have suggested minimal to no loss of muscle strength and function with tissue flap reconstruction,[31,32] surveyed patients report a high incidence of persistent pain or discomfort and half did not return to work.[31] Lack of prospective data and complete follow-up prevent drawing definitive conclusion, but their results are provocative and suggest that although associated with lower mortality, more aggressive treatment may lead to a significant decrement in quality of life.

Fibrosing Mediastinitis

Fibrosing mediastinitis, also known as sclerosing mediastinitis, is a rare disorder that is characterized by acute and chronic inflammation and progressive fibrosis within the mediastinum. The fibrosis can proceed relentlessly to compromise patency of the superior vena cava, major and minor airways, pulmonary arteries and veins, and the esophagus. Although the precise etiology remains unclear, it is now thought that an abnormal inflammatory response to fungal antigens is the most common cause.

Epidemiology and Clinical Features

Fibrosing mediastinitis usually presents in the second, third, or fourth decade of life, and men are affected slightly more often than are women.[33–36] Although some patients are asymptomatic at the time of diagnosis, more than 60% present with symptoms caused by compression of mediastinal structures.[37] Cough, dyspnea, wheezing, and the sequelae of superior vena caval obstruction are the most common symptoms.

Diagnosis

Fibrosing mediastinitis is often a diagnosis of exclusion. Plain chest X-ray may demonstrate an abnormal mediastinal contour or changes in pulmonary vasculature that indicate pulmonary arterial or venous compromise. CT is the study of choice for initial evaluation.[38] It readily identifies the extent of fibrosis, the presence of granulomas and calcification, and compression of mediastinal structures. Vascular anatomy is best assessed by combining venography with contrast-enhanced CT. Bronchoscopy should be performed to evaluate for the presence of broncholiths and distortion of bronchial anatomy. In general broncholiths should be left alone, as they are often densely adherent to the pulmonary artery and any attempt to remove them may result in massive hemoptysis.

The decision to pursue additional specific studies such as barium swallow, esophagoscopy, and cardiac catheterization should be guided by clinical signs and symptoms. Although not definitive, serological testing can be suggestive of the diagnosis and may be helpful for planning therapy. Ultimately however, because fibrosing mediastinitis is often a diagnosis of exclusion, biopsy may be necessary to rule out other disorders such as malignancy.

Therapy

Medical therapy for this disease has met with limited success. Steroids are of no proven benefit,[34,39] but for those patients in whom fungal infection has been implicated, therapy with antifungal agents has been shown effective.[35,36] Despite some success with antifungal therapy, many patients require surgical intervention for bypass of the superior vena cava or decompression of central airways and pulmonary vasculature. Airway

involvement can lead to distortion and obstruction with chronic postobstructive pneumonia; this is most frequent in the right middle lobe and is known as middle lobe syndrome. Treatment may require pulmonary resection.[40] Because surgery is likely to be difficult and hazardous, it should only be considered as an appropriate option for patients with progressive disease and severely limiting symptoms. Patients with stable disease and without severe disability may be managed expectantly.

Superior Vena Cava Syndrome

Obstruction of the superior vena cava (SVC) produces an unmistakable constellation of signs and symptoms known as SVC syndrome. The severity of symptoms is determined by the adequacy of collateral venous drainage, which is in turn a function of the rapidity with which the SVC obstruction progresses. As a general rule, the more rapid the process, the less time there is for development of collaterals and the more severe the symptoms. Although most patients are symptomatic, in unusual cases where obstruction develops over a prolonged period of time there may be minimal to no symptoms. Therapy is directed at palliation and, if possible, treatment of the underlying condition.

Epidemiology

Located in the middle mediastinum, the SVC is vulnerable to compression by mediastinal tumors, enlarging paratracheal lymph nodes, and aneurysms of the ascending aorta. Bronchogenic cancer is the most common malignant cause of SVC syndrome (70%–85%), lymphoma is second (5%–15%), and metastases from extrathoracic malignancies account for most of the rest (5%–10%).[41] The most common benign cause of SVC syndrome is thrombosis.

Clinical Presentation and Diagnosis

Clinical findings alone often establish the diagnosis of SVC syndrome. Approximately two-thirds of patients present with facial swelling, dyspnea at rest, orthopnea, and cough. Physical examination usually reveals a characteristic plethoric appearance with facial, neck, and arm swelling as well as prominent subcutaneous veins across the neck and upper torso.

Once the diagnosis of SVC syndrome has been made, it is essential to determine the underlying cause and, in some cases, the precise venous anatomy. CT and magnetic resonance imaging (MRI) are equally valuable for demonstrating the anatomical characteristics of the mediastinum and great vessels and for identifying the existence of synchronous disease elsewhere in the chest. Furthermore, these studies can also assess vessel patency and collateral circulation by demonstrating either opacification with contrast-enhanced CT (Fig. 43.2) or signal loss with MRI. Although CT and MRI can identify collateral vessels, bilateral upper extremity venography is essential if thrombolysis, surgical bypass, or percutaneous stenting of the SVC is contemplated.[42]

Therapy

The management of patients with SVC syndrome should be designed both to treat the underlying cause of the obstruc-

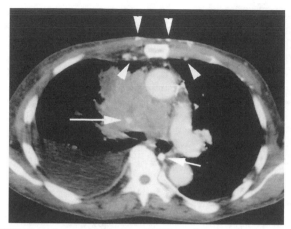

FIGURE 43.2. Superior vena cava (SVC) syndrome shown by CT with intravenous contrast of a patient who presented with SVC syndrome from small cell lung cancer. Note contrast in the narrowed SVC lumen (*long arrow*) and the large right pleural effusion. Collateral circulation can be seen in the prominent azygous (*short arrow*), subcutaneous (*arrowheads*), and internal mammary (*arrowheads*) veins. (Courtesy of M. McCowin, M.D., Department of Radiology, San Francisco Veterans Affairs Medical Center, San Francisco, CA.)

tion and to palliate symptoms. Although definitive therapy may require surgical bypass of the obstructed SVC, medical therapy, such as with thrombolytics, or, in the case of malignancy, chemo- and radiotherapy, may be adequate to achieve significant relief of symptoms. Simple measures such as elevation of the head and administration of diuretics should be initiated for all patients, regardless of the cause of the obstruction. Diuretics decrease edema generally, decrease the production of cerebrospinal fluid, and decrease cardiac output. Unfortunately, steroids are of no proven benefit for the treatment of laryngeal and cerebral edema in this setting.[42]

Mediastinal Lesions

The wide variety and diverse origins of tissues normally found within the mediastinum accounts for the extraordinary assortment of tumors and cysts that arise from them. These lesions are collectively referred to as primary mediastinal lesions (Table 43.1). Secondary lesions of the mediastinum are derived from extramediastinal tissues, such as thyroid, bone, or lung, and either migrate into or metastasize to the mediastinum. Many benign lesions are asymptomatic and are discovered incidentally, whereas malignant lesions are more likely to produce symptoms from compression and invasion of adjacent structures. Mediastinal tumors may also present as a consequence of systemic syndromes caused by the production of bioactive peptides and hormones. The diagnosis is usually suggested by the patient's age, the location of the lesion within the mediastinum, the presence or absence of symptoms, and its radiographic features. Ultimately however, definitive diagnosis rests on obtaining tissue, either through biopsy or excision.

Mediastinal Compartments

Although anatomists divide the mediastinum into four compartments, it is most helpful for discussions of mediastinal lesions to divide the region into only three: anterior, middle,

TABLE 43.1. Types of Primary Mediastinal Lesions.

Neurogenic tumors
  Neurilemoma (Schwannoma)
  Neurofibroma
  Ganglioneuroma
  Ganglioneuroblastoma
  Neuroblastoma
  Paraganglioma (pheochromocytoma)
    Chemodectoma

Cysts
  Foregut cysts
    Bronchogenic cyst
    Duplication (enteric) cyst
  Mesothelial cysts
    Pleuropericardial cyst
  Neurenteric cyst
  Thymic cyst
  Unclassified

Thymus
  Thymoma
  Thymic cyst
  Thymic carcinoma
  Thymolipoma

Lymphoma
  Hodgkin's disease
  Non-Hodgkin's lymphoma
    Primary mediastinal B-cell lymphoma
    Lymphoblastic
    Large cell diffuse
    Other

Germ cell tumors
  Benign
    Epidermoid cyst
    Dermoid cyst
    Mature teratoma
  Malignant
    Seminoma
  Nonseminomatous germ cell tumor

Mesenchymal tumors
  Lipoma/liposarcoma
  Fibroma/fibrosarcoma
  Leiomyoma/leiomyosarcoma
  Myxoma
  Mesothelioma
  Rhabdomyoma/rhabdomyosarcoma
  Hemangioma/hemangiosarcoma
  Hemangiopericytoma
  Lymphangioma (cystic hygroma)
  Lymphangiomyoma
  Lymphangiopericytoma

Endocrine
  Ectopic parathyroid
  Mediastinal thyroid
  Carcinoid

Other
  Giant lymph node hyperplasia (Castleman's disease)
  Granuloma

Source: Adapted from Davis et al. 1995,[89] with permission.

and posterior (Fig. 43.3). The anterior compartment, also known as the anterosuperior or prevascular compartment, extends from the posterior surface of the sternum to the anterior surface of the pericardium and great vessels. It can be readily identified on lateral chest X-ray and contains the thymus and surrounding lymphatic and connective tissues. A line drawn along the border between the esophagus and the anterior longitudinal spinal ligament separates the middle and posterior compartments. The posterior compartment extends

3. A paravertebral mass in an infant is most likely to be a neuroblastoma (malignant), in a child it is most likely to be a ganglioneuroma (benign), and in an adult it is most likely to be a neurilemmoma.

Clinical Presentation

Up to half of all mediastinal lesions are incidental discoveries on chest X-ray or CT scan. Symptoms can be caused by local mass effects, systemic effects of tumor-derived hormones and peptides, or infection. Local effects are dependent on the size and location of the lesion and result from compression of adjacent structures. Examples include cough, stridor, dyspnea, chest pain, and dysphagia. It has been generally accepted that symptoms are more likely to occur in children.[43] They are also more common with malignant tumors that, unlike benign lesions, are more likely to fix, encase, and invade adjacent structures. Many mediastinal tumors are associated with a variety of clinical syndromes. In some cases, tumor-derived hormones or peptides are directly causative.

Evaluation of the Patient with a Mediastinal Lesion

The primary goals of evaluation are to determine the correct diagnosis and to establish the tumor's anatomical relationships and resectability should surgery be indicated. In some circumstances, a precise tissue diagnosis is not required before proceeding to surgery, but in no case should an extensive resection be undertaken without one.

RADIOLOGY

Imaging is an essential part of the workup of all mediastinal lesions, and is often the only investigation needed before initiating therapy. CT scanning is typically the first step. As an alternative to CT, MRI has several advantages. Because it demonstrates flowing blood and the spinal cord exceptionally

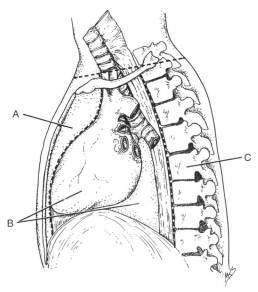

FIGURE 43.3. Mediastinal compartments: *A*, anterior; *B*, visceral; *C*, paravertebral (posterior).

posteriorly from the anterior longitudinal spinal ligament to the costovertebral junction and is equivalent to the bilateral paravertebral sulci. Division of the mediastinum into three compartments facilitates diagnosis because most lesions have a predilection for one of the three (Table 43.2).

Patient Age

The relative prevalence of specific primary lesions varies with the age of the patient population (Table 43.3). This information is thus most helpful in the following circumstances:

1. An anterior mediastinal mass in an adult is most likely to be a thymoma.
2. An anterior mediastinal mass in a child or young adult is most likely to be a lymphoma or a germ cell tumor.

TABLE 43.2. Usual Location of Mediastinal Lesions.

Type of lesion	Mediastinal compartment		
	Anterior	*Visceral*	*Paravertebral sulci*
Primary			
More common	Thymoma	Foregut cyst	Neurilemoma (schwannoma)
	Benign and malignant germ cell tumors	Pleuropericardial cyst	Neurofibroma
	Lymphoma	Lymphoma	Neuroblastoma
		Mediastinal granuloma	Malignant schwannoma
			Ganglioneuroma
			Ganglioneuroblastoma
			Foregut cyst
Less common	Mesenchymal tumors	Paraganglioma	Paraganglioma
	Thymic cyst	Neurenteric cyst	Pheochromocytoma
	Parathyroid adenoma	Thoracic duct cyst	Mesenchymal tumors
			Lymphoma
Secondary	Thyroid goiter	Thyroid goiter	Extramedullary hematopoiesis
	Bony tumors	Metastatic carcinoma	Bony tumors
		Foramen of Morgagni hernia	
		Hiatal hernia	
		Pancreatic pseudocyst	

Source: Adapted from Shields 1994,[90] with permission.

TABLE 43.3. Common Primary Lesions of the Mediastinum by Patient Age.

Children	Adults
40% Neurogenic tumors	20% Neurogenic tumors
Neuroblastoma (<2 years)	Neurilemmoma
Ganglioneuroma (2–10 years)	20% Thymoma
20% Lymphoma[a]	20% Congenital cyst
17% Congenital cyst	13% Lymphoma[a]
13% Germ cell tumor	12% Germ cell tumor

[a]Approximately two-thirds of mediastinal lymphomas are non-Hodgkin's disease in both pediatric and adult age groups.

Source: Adapted from Shields 1994[90] and Davis et al. 1995.[89]

well, it is the preferred study for evaluation of suspected vascular lesions and for lesions that may extend into the spinal canal. MRI is also indicated for those patients who should not receive contrast.

Ultrasonography has an evolving role in the evaluation of mediastinal lesions. Transesophageal echocardiography can be an invaluable tool for assessing the relationship of mediastinal lesions to the heart. A more recent development has been the use of esophageal endoscopic ultrasound (EUS) guided fine-needle aspiration biopsy.[44] This technique facilitates biopsy of lesions that may be difficult to reach through more traditional percutaneous approaches.

Nuclear medicine offers a variety of functional imaging studies to complement the anatomical imaging of CT, MRI, and ultrasound and can provide definitive diagnostic information in certain circumstances.

SEROLOGY

For most patients with mediastinal lesions, serological examination for the presence of tumor-specific biochemical markers is not routine. Important exceptions are the measurement of serum α-fetoprotein (AFP) and β-HCG levels in suspected nonseminomatous germ cell tumor (NSGCT), and the measurement of serum catecholamines in suspected catecholamine-producing neurogenic tumors.

BIOPSY

Tissue diagnosis is often, but not always, required before proceeding with therapy. As outlined, some imaging and serological information may be diagnostic. Furthermore, resection may be indicated regardless of the results of tissue biopsy. Circumstances in which biopsy is indicated include (1) suspicion of a tumor that is treated primarily with nonoperative therapy (e.g., lymphoma, NSGCT, or seminoma); (2) evidence of local invasion that would require resection and reconstruction of vital structures (e.g., involvement of the superior vena cava by a large anterior mediastinal mass); and (3) evidence of metastatic disease rendering resection inappropriate. The available techniques for biopsy include fine-needle aspiration cytology (FNA), cervical and anterior mediastinoscopy, and thoracoscopy. FNA is preferred as the least invasive and often simplest approach. Recent series report an accuracy at cytological diagnosis between 80% and 90%[45–48] and an accuracy at distinguishing benign from malignant that approaches 100%.[46]

Secondary Mediastinal Lesions

SUBSTERNAL GOITER

Substernal goiters are the most common mediastinal lesion of extramediastinal origin. Most patients present with an asymptomatic neck mass, but as many as half of patients with a partial or complete substernal goiter have symptoms such as dyspnea, cough, dysphagia, or stridor.[49–52] Thyrotoxicosis is rare, and hoarseness, an uncommon symptom, is highly suggestive of malignancy. Histologically, most lesions are nontoxic multinodular goiters but as many as 44% may be follicular adenomas.[51] Reports of the prevalence of malignancy vary from 2% to 21%.[49,51–53]

Both history and physical exam may suggest the diagnosis of substernal goiter, as up to 20% of patients have had a thyroidectomy and almost two-thirds have a palpable low cervical mass.[49–51] Imaging with plain films, CT, or MRI may be helpful. Although asymptomatic patients with a definitive diagnosis and a small lesion may be observed in selected circumstances, resection is usually indicated to prevent development of acute airway obstruction and because of the potential for malignancy. Radioactive iodine is contraindicated not only because it is ineffective in treating these large tumors, but also because it may initially aggravate airway compression.

LESIONS OF SKELETAL ORIGIN

A variety of lesions that arise in the thoracic skeleton can grow into the mediastinum. Sternal tumors usually are easily distinguished from true mediastinal masses, but lesions that arise from the vertebral bodies may be more difficult to differentiate. These lesions include chordomas, anterior meningoceles, and ectopic extramedullary hematopoietic tissue.

VASCULAR LESIONS

Although they arise from mediastinal structures, vascular abnormalities typically are not included within the spectrum of primary mediastinal lesions. Nevertheless, they should be considered in the differential diagnosis. They may originate from any of the major arteries or veins in the mediastinum and may be either congenital or acquired. Examples include the wide variety of aortic arch and pulmonary arterial anomalies, vascular rings, and aneurysms of the aorta and ductus arteriosus. Angiography is diagnostic, but MRI can be an effective noninvasive substitute.

LESIONS OF INTRAABDOMINAL ORIGIN

Herniation of abdominal viscera through the foramen of Morgagni or the esophageal hiatus can mimic a mediastinal mass on plain chest X-ray. However, careful history and further radiological evaluation should readily differentiate these abnormalities from true mediastinal lesions.

METASTATIC DISEASE

Lymphadenopathy from metastatic lung cancer is probably the most common abnormality encountered in the mediastinum. The mediastinal lymph nodes can also be involved with metastatic disease from a variety of other sources, including colon and rectal cancers, head-and-neck malignancies, testicular tumors, and lymphoma. The diagnosis of metastatic carcinoma is usually straightforward, with a known or suspected primary lesion readily identifiable elsewhere. Furthermore, metastatic disease typically presents as multiple enlarged lymph nodes, rather than as a solitary mass that would be more consistent with a primary mediastinal lesion. Evaluation of suspected metastatic disease is usually made with mediastinoscopy or, increasingly, positron emission tomography.

Primary Mediastinal Lesions

NEUROGENIC TUMORS

Neurogenic tumors can arise from cells of the nerve sheath, the autonomic ganglia, or the paraganglion system and can be either benign or malignant (Table 43.4). Young children are much more likely to have a malignant tumor (neuroblastoma), whereas older children and adults are more likely to have benign lesions (ganglioneuromas and neurilemmomas, respectively).[43,54–56] Most neurogenic tumors present as incidental findings and are asymptomatic, but symptoms can arise from either local or systemic effects. Local effects are predominantly pain and paresthesias caused by erosion into the vertebral column or chest wall or impingement of nerve roots. Neurological deficits such as Pancoast's or Horner's syndrome may also be present. Systemic effects are uncommon, and are a consequence of the rare tumor that produces either catecholamines or vasoactive intestinal polypeptide (VIP). Evaluation by MRI can be helpful for determination of intraspinal extension and for planning resection. Ultimately, the determination of whether to use surgical, adjuvant, or neoadjuvant therapies is determined by the particular extent and origin of the neurogenic tumor.

THYMUS

MYASTHENIA GRAVIS

Myasthenia gravis (MG) is an autoimmune disorder of neuromuscular transmission that is characterized by progressive loss of skeletal muscle strength with sustained activity. Antibodies against the acetylcholine receptor (AChR) can be found in 80% of patients with the clinical syndrome,[57,58] and are presumed to mediate the disease by attenuating signal intensity across the neuromuscular junction and hence the strength of muscular contractions. Thymomas are found in approximately 13% of patients presenting with MG and in 21% of those undergoing thymectomy for MG.

Primary medical therapy is with acetylcholinesterase inhibitors to increase acetylcholine concentration at the neuromuscular junction, and with steroids and cytotoxic drugs to suppress the anti-AChR immune response. Plasmapheresis can be used for severe disease.[59] Although well established as appropriate therapy, the precise role of thymectomy in the management of patients with MG is debated between neurologists and surgeons. This controversy is difficult to resolve because there are no prospective studies comparing medical therapy alone to medical therapy plus thymectomy, and because in some patients the disease may stabilize, improve, or even undergo spontaneous complete remission.

THYMOMA

Thymoma is the most common neoplasm of the anterior mediastinum and the most common mediastinal lesion in adults. It is rare in children. Most thymomas are found incidentally and are asymptomatic (Fig. 43.4). Most thymomas are well encapsulated and are clinically benign. However, evidence of either gross or microscopic capsular invasion portends malignant behavior and a less favorable prognosis. Metastases occur late and predominantly through contiguous spread to pericardium and pleura, although pulmonary metastases are seen occasionally. The Masaoka system (Table 43.5) is used most often to stage thymomas because it reflects the prognostic significance of capsular invasion. Treatment for thymoma is primarily surgical, with complete resection being the critical factor in determining long-term survival.[60–63] Although no definitive prospective comparisons are available, review of the available literature supports the use of multimodality therapy for advanced-stage thymoma.

Because thymoma tends to be slow growing and tends not to metastasize hematogenously, surgery also plays an important role in the management of patients with unresectable, metastatic, or recurrent disease. In the setting of unresectable disease, survival is better for those patients undergoing debulking procedures compared to biopsy alone.[60,61,63–65] Reresection of recurrent or metastatic disease has also been shown to improve long-term survival.[60,63,66]

OTHER THYMIC TUMORS

A variety of rare tumors can arise in the thymus gland. Often confused with thymomas, thymic carcinomas are distinct neoplasms with malignant cytological features that are clinically more aggressive than thymomas.[67,68] They often present with extensive local invasion, and imaging reveals areas of necrosis, hemorrhage, calcification, or cyst formation.[69] There is a high incidence of extrathoracic metastases and the prognosis is very poor. Chemotherapy and radiation therapy

TABLE 43.4. Neurogenic Tumors and Their Origin.

Origin	Benign	Malignant
Nerve sheath	Neurilemmoma (schwannoma) Neurofibroma	Malignant schwannoma (neurosarcoma)
Sympathetic ganglia	Ganglioneuroma	Ganglioneuroblastoma Neuroblastoma
Paraganglion system	Paraganglioma (pheochromocytoma) Chemodectoma	Malignant paraganglioma Malignant chemodectoma

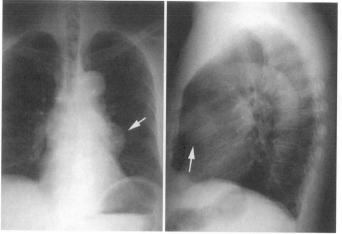

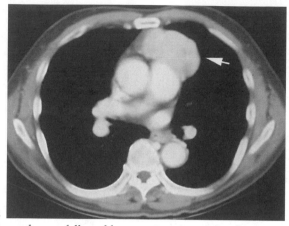

FIGURE 43.4. Chest X-rays (**A**) and CT (**B**) of a 58-year-old man who presented with a 1-week history of a nonproductive cough. Images revealed an anterior mediastinal mass (*arrows*) consistent with thymoma. FNA confirmed the diagnosis, and the patient received induction chemotherapy followed by resection. At surgery, the tumor was confined to the anterior compartment without invasion into adjacent pleura or pericardium. Pathology revealed a Masaoka stage II epithelial-type thymoma, with microscopic invasion of the tumor capsule.

are of no demonstrable benefit, and treatment is wide excision if possible. Thymic carcinoid tumors are more common in men than women and are strongly associated with the multiple endocrine neoplasia syndromes.[70,71] Carcinoid syndrome has not been reported with thymic carcinoids, but they can produce ACTH and cause Cushing's syndrome.[71] The octreoscan may be helpful in making the diagnosis.[70] Treatment is by complete resection. Adjuvant radiation therapy has been used to control residual disease, but this is of no proven benefit. Thymolipoma is a very rare anterior mediastinal mass of mesenchymal origin. It is benign and should be resected to confirm the diagnosis and to prevent complications from growth.[72] Thymic cyst is a descriptive term that refers to a variety of lesions which can be of congenital, inflammatory, or neoplastic origin. Occasionally, thymic cysts are seen following therapeutic responses to medical treatment of germ cell tumors or thymoma.

GERM CELL TUMORS

Less than 5% of all germ cell tumors are found in the mediastinum. They are thought to arise from primordial germ cells that migrate from the urogenital ridge into the mediastinum and thymus gland during embryogenesis, and almost all are found in the anterior compartment. Approximately half of all mediastinal germ cell tumors are benign (teratomas). The peak incidence is during the second, third, and fourth decades of life. Malignant tumors are further classified as either seminomas or nonseminomatous lesions, and are much more common in men than women.[73] The treatment of malignant germ cell tumors is primarily nonsurgical. Seminomas are very responsive to chemotherapy and radiotherapy and have a good prognosis, but NSGCT respond less well and carry a less-favorable prognosis. Clinical presentation, radiographic appearance, and serology suggest the diagnosis. Serum AFP and β-HCG levels should be determined for all young male patients with anterior mediastinal masses, and if negative, FNA, open biopsy, or excisional biopsy should be considered.

LYMPHOMA

Primary lymphomas of the mediastinum occur predominantly in the anterior compartment and are classified as either Hodgkin's disease or non-Hodgkin's lymphoma. Hodgkin's disease is a malignant tumor of B-cell origin and refers to a single disease, whereas the designation of non-Hodgkin's lymphoma refers to a large collection of lymphoblastic malignancies. Non-Hodgkin's lymphomas are further subdivided into indolent and aggressive forms. The incidence of Hodgkin's disease has a bimodal age distribution with peak occurrences between 20 and 30 years of age and over 50 years of age. In contrast, the incidence of non-Hodgkin's lymphomas increases with age. Hodgkin's disease is characterized by local or contiguous spread and is more likely to involve the mediastinum. Non-Hodgkin's lymphomas are more diffuse, tend to be disseminated at the time of diagnosis, and less commonly involve the mediastinum. Because non-Hodgkin's lymphomas are approximately six times more common than Hodgkin's disease overall, they account for approximately two-thirds of all primary mediastinal lymphomas despite the greater propensity for Hodgkin's disease to involve the mediastinum.[55,56,74]

Mediastinal lymphomas usually present with symptoms. Rapidly growing tumors can produce cough, dyspnea, chest pain, stridor, and superior vena cava syndrome. Systemic

TABLE 43.5. The Masaoka Staging System for Thymoma.

Stage	Definition
I	Macroscopically—completely encapsulated Microscopically—no capsular invasion
II	Macroscopic invasion into surrounding fatty tissue or mediastinal pleura Microscopic invasion into capsule
III	Macroscopic invasion into neighboring organ (i.e., pericardium, great vessels, or lung)
IVA	Pleural or pericardial dissemination
IVB	Lymphogenous or hematogenous metastasis

Source: Masaoka et al. 1981.[91]

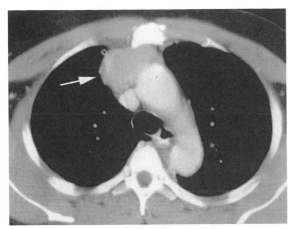

FIGURE 43.5. Anterior mediastinal lymphoma. A 38-year-old man with a strong family history of lymphoma presented with cervical spinal cord compression from tumor. Symptoms responded rapidly to steroids, and CT of the chest revealed an anterior mediastinal mass (*arrow*). Anterior mediastinoscopy confirmed the diagnosis of non-Hodgkin's lymphoma.

symptoms are also common. Weight loss, fever, and drenching night sweats are included in the staging criteria and are referred to as "B" symptoms. (The "A" classification indicates an absence of well-defined generalized symptoms.) Imaging typically demonstrates a large, heterogeneous, and irregularly shaped anterior mediastinal mass (Fig. 43.5). The surgeon's role in managing patients with mediastinal lymphoma is primarily to obtain tissue for diagnosis. Traditionally, needle biopsies have provided inadequate material and tissue architecture with which to distinguish among the various types of lymphoma. Because subtyping can be critical for planning therapy, more tissue is often required. If extrathoracic nodes are not available for biopsy, anterior mediastinoscopy is typically the procedure of choice (because most of these tumors are in the anterior and not visceral compartment). Cervical mediastinoscopy is performed if paratracheal or subcarinal nodes are involved. The need for surgical biopsies is declining, however, because the use of immunohistochemistry for cell-surface markers is increasingly able to subtype lymphomas from FNA specimens alone.[75] Lymphomas are staged based on the number and location of involved nodal regions and involvement of extralymphatic organs. Stage I disease is defined as disease limited to a single nodal region, and stage II disease involves two or more regions on the same side of the diaphragm. Disease present on both sides of the diaphragm, in the spleen, or in extralymphatic organs is classified as stage III, and disseminated disease is stage IV.

Congenital Cysts

True cystic lesions of the mediastinum are considered congenital rather than neoplastic abnormalities, and can be divided into four major categories based on location and histological features of the cyst lining. Foregut cysts are derived from the primitive foregut structures that give rise to the lung and proximal digestive tract. They are lined either by respiratory or digestive tract epithelium and are classified as either bronchogenic or duplication cysts, respectively. Cysts lined by normal mesothelium are termed pleuropericardial cysts, and are usually found at the cardiophrenic angle.

Neurenteric cysts are found in the paravertebral sulcus and are derived from the meninges or dura. Some mediastinal cysts do not have a distinctive lining and by default are lumped into a generic category imaginatively termed "unclassified." Cystic hygromas are congenital cystic masses that present in children and are typically located at the base of the neck and into the chest. These hygromas are more accurately termed lymphangiomas and are classified as mesenchymal tumors rather than as congenital cysts of the mediastinum.

Bronchogenic cysts are the most common form of congenital mediastinal cyst, constituting as many as 75% of this category in some series.[76] Congenital cysts of the mediastinum are typically benign, although an occasional case report suggests the possibility of malignant degeneration.[77,78] The incidence of symptoms is highly variable between series, and may be as low as 30% or as high as 90%.[76,79–83] In general, symptoms are recognized as more common in the pediatric population.[82] Local effects from the size of the lesion are the most common cause of symptoms, and patients present with cough, stridor, dyspnea, or chest discomfort. Larger cysts may produce dysphagia. Uncommonly, cysts become infected, either by hematogenous spread or as a consequence of communication with the airway. Duplication cysts that are lined with gastric mucosa may ulcerate and bleed. If the ulcer erodes through the cyst wall, presentation can be with hemoptysis, hematemesis, hemothorax, or pleural abscess.[76] Rapid increase in the size of the cyst from bleeding can lead to acute onset of mass-effect symptoms.

Definitive diagnosis of mediastinal cysts depends ultimately on histological examination of the cyst lining, but imaging can provide important and sometimes diagnostic clues. Although CT is used most often, MRI may be more helpful because its multiplanar imaging capabilities can facilitate identification of subtle communications between the cyst and the airway or pericardium. Endoscopic ultrasound has been used to diagnose duplication cysts,[84] and may be helpful for planning resection. Duplication cysts lined with gastric mucosa demonstrate activity with ^{99}Tc scintigraphy.

Definitive treatment of mediastinal cysts is resection.

Mesenchymal Tumors

Because the mediastinum contains a wide variety of tissues of mesenchymal origin, an extraordinary spectrum of mesenchymal tumors have been found there. These tumors occur in men and women with equal incidence, and approximately half are malignant. As with other mediastinal lesions, some are asymptomatic and discovered incidentally, whereas others may cause symptoms by mass effect or local invasion. The clinical course and management of mesenchymal tumors of the mediastinum is similar to that of mesenchymal tumors elsewhere in the body and is not detailed here.

Castleman's Disease

Also known as giant lymph node hyperplasia, Castleman's disease is a benign disorder of lymphoid proliferation that is often localized to the mediastinum and tends to occur in women in their third and fourth decades.[85,86] It usually presents as a solitary mass, but may be multicentric, and has been associated with HIV infection and Kaposi's sarcoma. Castleman's disease is usually asymptomatic, but it is characterized by progressive enlargement of nodal tissue and can produce compression of mediastinal structures. Although the lesion is benign, the course of the disease may be fatal.[86,87] Resection is the primary mode of therapy, but can be challenging because of diffuse contiguous nodal involvement and extensive vascularity.[88] Radiation therapy has been recommended for patients with unresectable and multifocal disease.[86]

References

Descending Necrotizing Mediastinitis

1. Wheatley MJ, Stirling MC, Kirsh MM, et al. Descending necrotizing mediastinitis: transcervical drainage is not enough. Ann Thorac Surg 1990;49:780–784.
2. Corsten MJ, Shamji FM, Odell PF, et al. Optimal treatment of descending necrotising mediastinitis. Thorax 1997;52:702–708.
3. Brunelli A, Sabbatini A, Catalini G, et al. Descending necrotizing mediastinitis. Surgical drainage and tracheostomy. Arch Otolaryngol Head Neck Surg 1996;122:1326–1329.
4. Estrera AS, Landay MJ, Grisham JM, et al. Descending necrotizing mediastinitis. Surg Gynecol Obstet 1983;157:545–552.
5. Kiernan PD, Hernandez A, Byrne WD, et al. Descending cervical mediastinitis. Ann Thorac Surg 1998;65:1483–1488.
6. Marty-Ane CH, Alauzen M, Alric P, et al. Descending necrotizing mediastinitis. Advantage of mediastinal drainage with thoracotomy. J Thorac Cardiovasc Surg 1994;107:55–61.
7. Moncada R, Warpeha R, Pickleman J, et al. Mediastinitis from odontogenic and deep cervical infection. Anatomic pathways of propagation. Chest 1978;73:497–500.
8. Alsoub H, Chacko KC. Descending necrotising mediastinitis. Postgrad Med J 1995;71:98–101.
9. Brook I, Frazier EH. Microbiology of mediastinitis [published erratum appears in Arch Intern Med 1996;156(10):1112]. Arch Intern Med 1996;156:333–336.
10. Blomquist IK, Bayer AS. Life-threatening deep fascial space infections of the head and neck. Infect Dis Clin North Am 1988;2:237–264.

Postoperative Mediastinitis

11. Kustal A, Ibrisim E, Catav Z, et al. Mediastinitis after open heart surgery. Analysis of risk factors and management. J Cardiovasc Surg 1991;32:38–41.
12. Satta J, Lahtinen J, Raisanen L, et al. Options for the management of poststernotomy mediastinitis. Scand Cardiovasc J 1998;32:29–32.
13. Loop FD, Lytle BW, Cosgrove DM, et al. J. Maxwell Chamberlain Memorial Paper. Sternal wound complications after isolated coronary artery bypass grafting: early and late mortality, morbidity, and cost of care. Ann Thorac Surg 1990;49:179–186; discussion 186–187.
14. Milano CA, Kesler K, Archibald N, et al. Mediastinitis after coronary artery bypass graft surgery. Risk factors and long-term survival. Circulation 1995;92:2245–2251.
15. Trouillet JL, Chastre J, Fagon JY, et al. Use of granulated sugar in treatment of open mediastinitis after cardiac surgery. Lancet 1985;2:180–184.
16. Farinas MC, Gald Peralta F, Bernal JM, et al. Suppurative mediastinitis after open-heart surgery: a case-control study covering a seven-year period in Santander, Spain. Clin Infect Dis 1995;20:272–279.
17. El Oakley R, Paul E, Wong PS, et al. Mediastinitis in patients undergoing cardiopulmonary bypass: risk analysis and midterm results. J Cardiovasc Surg 1997;38:595–600.
18. Taylor GJ, Mikell FL, Moses HW, et al. Determinants of hospital charges for coronary artery bypass surgery: the economic con-

sequences of postoperative complications. Am J Cardiol 1990;65:309–313.
19. Lopez-Monjardin H, de-la-Pena-Salcedo A, Mendoza-Munoz M, et al. Omentum flap versus pectoralis major flap in the treatment of mediastinitis. Plast Reconstr Surg 1998;101:1481–1485.
20. Munoz P, Menasalvas A, Bernaldo de Quiros JC, et al. Postsurgical mediastinitis: a case-control study. Clin Infect Dis 1997;25:1060–1064.
21. Jones G, Jurkiewicz MJ, Bostwick J, et al. Management of the infected median sternotomy wound with muscle flaps. The Emory 20-year experience. Ann Surg 1997;225:766–776; discussion 776–778.
22. Szerafin T, Vaszily M, Peterffy A. Granulated sugar treatment of severe mediastinitis after open-heart surgery. Scand J Thorac Cardiovasc Surg 1991;25:77–80.
23. Acinapura AJ, Godfrey N, Romita M, et al. Surgical management of infected median sternotomy: closed irrigation vs. muscle flaps. J Cardiovasc Surg 1985;26:443–446.
24. Breatnach E, Nath PH, Delany DJ. The role of computed tomography in acute and subacute mediastinitis. Clin Radiol 1986;37:139–145.
25. Misawa Y, Fuse K, Hasegawa T. Infectious mediastinitis after cardiac operations: computed tomographic findings. Ann Thorac Surg 1998;65:622–624.
26. Browdie DA, Bernstein RV, Agnew R, et al. Diagnosis of post-sternotomy infection: comparison of three means of assessment [published erratum appears in Ann Thorac Surg 1991;52(4):900] [see comments]. Ann Thorac Surg 1991;51:290–292.
27. Bitkover CY, Gardlund B, Larsson SA, et al. Diagnosing sternal wound infections with ^{99m}Tc-labeled monoclonal granulocyte antibody scintigraphy. Ann Thorac Surg 1996;62:1412–1416; discussion 1416–1417.
28. Newman LS, Szczukowski LC, Bain RP, et al. Suppurative mediastinitis after open heart surgery. A case control study of risk factors. Chest 1988;94:546–553.
29. Bitkover CY, Gardlund B. Mediastinitis after cardiovascular operations: a case-control study of risk factors [see comments]. Ann Thorac Surg 1998;65:36–40.
30. Grover FL, Johnson RR, Marshall G, et al. Impact of mammary grafts on coronary bypass operative mortality and morbidity. Department of Veterans Affairs Cardiac Surgeons. Ann Thorac Surg 1994;57:559–568; discussion 568–569.
31. Ringelman PR, Vander Kolk CA, Cameron D, et al. Long-term results of flap reconstruction in median sternotomy wound infections. Plast Reconstr Surg 1994;93:1208–1214; discussion 1215–1216.
32. Scully HE, Leclerc Y, Martin RD, et al. Comparison between antibiotic irrigation and mobilization of pectoral muscle flaps in treatment of deep sternal infections. J Thorac Cardiovasc Surg 1985;90:523–531.

Fibrosing Mediastinitis

33. Mole TM, Glover J, Sheppard MN. Sclerosing mediastinitis: a report on 18 cases. Thorx 1995;50:280–283.
34. Sherrick AD, Brown LR, Harms GF, et al. The radiographic findings of fibrosing mediastinitis. Chest 1994;106:484–489.
35. Urschel HC Jr, Razzuk MA, Netto GJ, et al. Sclerosing mediastinitis: improved management with histoplasmosis titer and ketoconazole. Ann Thorac Surg 1990;50:215–221.
36. Mathisen DJ, Grillo HC. Clinical manifestation of mediastinal fibrosis and histoplasmosis. Ann Thorac Surg 1992;54:1053–1057; discussion 1057–1058.
37. Dines DE, Payne WS, Bernatz PE, et al. Mediastinal granuloma and fibrosing mediastinitis. Chest 1979;75:320–324.
38. Rholl KS, Levitt RG, Glazer HS. Magnetic resonance imaging of fibrosing mediastinitis. AJR (Am J Roentgenol) 1985;145:255–259.

39. Dunn EJ, Ulicny KS, Wright CB, et al. Surgical implications of sclerosing mediastinitis: a report of six cases and review of the literature. Chest 1990;97:338–346.

40. Kalweit G, Huwer H, Straub U, et al. Mediastinal compression syndromes due to idiopathic fibrosing mediastinitis—report of three cases and review of the literature. Thorac Cardiovasc Surg 1996;44:105–109.

Superior Vena Cava Syndrome

41. Ahmann FR. A reassessment of the clinical implications of the superior vena caval syndrome. J Clin Oncol 1984;2:961–969.

42. Nieto AF, Doty DB. Superior vena cava obstruction: clinical syndrome, etiology, and treatment. Curr Probl Cancer 1986;10:441–484.

Mediastinal Lesions

43. Bower RJ, Kiesewetter WB. Mediastinal masses in infants and children. Arch Surg 1977;112:1003–1009.

44. Hunerbein M, Ghadimi BM, Haensch W, et al. Transesophageal biopsy of mediastinal and pulmonary tumors by means of endoscopic ultrasound guidance. J Thorac Cardiovasc Surg 1998;116:554–559.

45. Zafar N, Moinuddin S. Mediastinal needle biopsy. A 15-year experience with 139 cases. Cancer (Phila) 1995;76:1065–1068.

46. Powers CN, Silverman JF, Geisinger KR, et al. Fine-needle aspiration biopsy of the mediastinum. A multi-institutional analysis. Am J Clin Pathol 1996;105:168–173.

47. Singh HK, Silverman JF, Powers CN, et al. Diagnostic pitfalls in fine-needle aspiration biopsy of the mediastinum. Diagn Cytopathol 1997;17:121–126.

48. Shabb NS, Fahl M, Shabb B, et al. Fine-needle aspiration of the mediastinum: a clinical, radiologic, cytologic, and histologic study of 42 cases. Diagn Cytopathol 1998;19:428–436.

49. Sanders LE, Rossi RL, Shahian DM, et al. Mediastinal goiters. The need for an aggressive approach. Arch Surg 1992;127:609–613.

50. Moron JC, Singer JA, Sardi A. Retrosternal goiter: a six-year institutional review. Am Surg 1998;64:889–893.

51. Katlic MR, Grillo HC, Wang CA. Substernal goiter. Analysis of 80 patients from Massachusetts General Hospital. Am J Surg 1985;149:283–287.

52. Sand ME, Laws HL, McElvein RB. Substernal and intrathoracic goiter. Reconsideration of surgical approach. Am Surg 1983;49:196–202.

53. Allo MD, Thompson NW. Rationale for the operative management of substernal goiters. Surgery (St. Louis) 1983;94:969–977.

54. Davis RD Jr, Oldham HN Jr, Sabiston DC Jr. Primary cysts and neoplasms of the mediastinum: recent changes in clinical presentation, methods of diagnosis, management, and results. Ann Thorac Surg 1987;44:229–237.

55. Azarow KS, Pearl RH, Zurcher R, et al. Primary mediastinal masses. A comparison of adult and pediatric populations. J Thorac Cardiovasc Surg 1993;106:67–72.

56. Massie RJ, Van Asperen PP, Mellis CM. A review of open biopsy for mediastinal masses. J Paediatr Child Health 1997;33:230–233.

57. Seybold ME. Myasthenia gravis. A clinical and basic science review. JAMA 1983;250:2516–2521.

58. Olanow CW, Wechsler AS, Roses AD. A prospective study of thymectomy and serum acetylcholine receptor antibodies in myasthenia gravis. Ann Surg 1982;196:113–121.

59. Gracey DR, Howard FM Jr, Divertie MB. Plasmapheresis in the treatment of ventilator-dependent myasthenia gravis patients. Report of four cases. Chest 1984;85:739–743.

60. Blumberg D, Port JL, Weksler B, et al. Thymoma: a multivariate analysis of factors predicting survival. Ann Thorac Surg 1995;60:908–913; discussion 914.

61. Nakahara K, Ohno K, Hashimoto J, et al. Thymoma: results with complete resection and adjuvant postoperative irradiation in 141 consecutive patients. J Thorac Cardiovasc Surg 1988;95:1041–1047.

62. Cohen DJ, Ronnigen LD, Graeber GM, et al. Management of patients with malignant thymoma. J Thorac Cardiovasc Surg 1984;87:301–317.

63. Regnard JF, Magdeleinat P, Dromer C, et al. Prognostic factors and long-term results after thymoma resection: a series of 307 patients. J Thorac Cardiovasc Surg 1996;112:376–384.

64. Cowen D, Richaud P, Mornex F, et al. Thymoma: results of a multicentric retrospective series of 149 non-metastatic irradiated patients and review of the literature. FNCLCC trialists. Federation Nationale des Centres de Lutte Contre le Cancer. Radiother Oncol 1995;34:9–16.

65. Mornex F, Resbeut M, Richaud P, et al. Radiotherapy and chemotherapy for invasive thymomas: a multicentric retrospective review of 90 cases. The FNCLCC trialists. Federation Nationale des Centres de Lutte Contre le Cancer [published erratum appears in Int J Radiat Oncol Biol Phys 1995;33(2):545]. Int J Radiat Oncol Biol Phys 1995;32:651–659.

66. Regnard JF, Zinzindohoue F, Magdeleinat P, et al. Results of re-resection for recurrent thymomas. Ann Thorac Surg 1997;64:1593–1598.

67. Blumberg D, Burt ME, Bains MS, et al. Thymic carcinoma: current staging does not predict prognosis. J Thorac Cardiovasc Surg 1998;115:303–308; discussion 308–309.

68. Suster S, Moran CA. Thymic carcinoma: spectrum of differentiation and histologic types. Pathology 1998;30:111–122.

69. Quagliano PV. Thymic carcinoma: case reports and review. J Thorac Imaging 1996;11:66–74.

70. Satta J, Ahonen A, Parkkila S, et al. Multiple endocrine neoplastic-associated thymic carcinoid tumour in close relatives: octreotide scan as a new diagnostic and follow-up modality. Two case reports. Scand Cardiovasc J 1999;33:49–53.

71. de Montpreville VT, Macchiarini P, Dulmet E. Thymic neuroendocrine carcinoma (carcinoid): a clinicopathologic study of fourteen cases. J Thorac Cardiovasc Surg 1996;111:134–141.

72. Moran CA, Rosado-de-Christenson M, Suster S. Thymolipoma: clinicopathologic review of 33 cases [see comments]. Mod Pathol 1995;8:741–744.

73. Temes R, Chavez T, Mapel D, et al. Primary mediastinal malignancies: findings in 219 patients. West J Med 1999;170:161–166.

74. Whooley BP, Urschel JD, Antkowiak JG, et al. Primary tumors of the mediastinum. J Surg Oncol 1999;70:95–99.

75. Hughes JH, Katz RL, Fonseca GA, et al. Fine-needle aspiration cytology of mediastinal non-Hodgkin's nonlymphoblastic lymphoma. Cancer (Phila) 1998;84:26–35.

76. Nobuhara KK, Gorski YC, La Quaglia MP, et al. Bronchogenic cysts and esophageal duplications: common origins and treatment. J Pediatr Surg 1997;32:1408–1413.

77. Okada Y, Mori H, Maeda T, et al. Congenital mediastinal bronchogenic cyst with malignant transformation: an autopsy report. Pathol Int 1996;46:594–600.

78. Bierhoff E, Pfeifer U. Malignant mesothelioma arising from a benign mediastinal mesothelial cyst. Gen Diagn Pathol 1996;142:59–62.

79. Cioffi U, Bonavina L, De Simone M, et al. Presentation and surgical management of bronchogenic and esophageal duplication cysts in adults. Chest 1998;113:1492–1496.

80. Cuypers P, De Leyn P, Cappelle L, et al. Bronchogenic cysts: a review of 20 cases. Eur J Cardiothorac Surg 1996;10:393–396.

81. Ge F, Liao Q, Xiao S, et al. Diagnosis and surgical treatment of bronchogenic cysts. Chin Med Sci J 1995;10:61–62.

82. Ribet ME, Copin MC, Gosselin B. Bronchogenic cysts of the mediastinum. J Thorac Cardiovasc Surg 1995;109:1003–1010.

83. Aktogu S, Yuncu G, Halilcolar H, et al. Bronchogenic cysts: clin-

icopathological presentation and treatment. Eur Respir J 1996;9: 2017–2021.

84. Geller A, Wang KK, DiMagno EP. Diagnosis of foregut duplication cysts by endoscopic ultrasonography. Gastroenterology 1995;109:838–842.

85. Kim JH, Jun TG, Sung SW, et al. Giant lymph node hyperplasia (Castleman's disease) in the chest [see comments]. Ann Thorac Surg 1995;59:1162–1165.

86. Bowne WB, Lewis JJ, Filippa DA, et al. The management of unicentric and multicentric Castleman's disease: a report of 16 cases and a review of the literature. Cancer (Phila) 1999;85:706–717.

87. Shahidi H, Myers JL, Kvale PA. Castleman's disease. Mayo Clin Proc 1995;70:969–977.

88. Pandya A, Baumgartner FJ, Nguyen D, et al. Thoracic Castleman's disease: implications for resection [letter; comment]. Ann Thorac Surg 1998;65:302–303.

89. Davis RW, Oldham HN, Sabiston DC. The mediastinum. In: Sabiston DC, Spencer FC, eds. Surgery of the Chest, Vol. 1. Philadelphia: Saunders, 1995:576–612.

90. Shields TW. Primary lesions of the mediastinum and their investigation and treatment. In: Shields TW, ed. General Thoracic Surgery, Vol. 2. Malvern, PA: Williams & Wilkins, 1994;1724–1769.

91. Masaoka A, Monden Y, Nakahara K, et al. Follow-up study of thymomas with special reference to their clinical stages. Cancer (Phila) 1981;48:2485–2492.

Congenital Heart Disease

Carl L. Backer and Constantine Mavroudis

Epidemiology

Congenital heart defects occur in approximately 5 to 8 of every 1000 live births.[1] The etiology of these defects is multifactorial in nature with both genetic and environmental influences. There are some clear associations with chromosomal abnormalities, in particular Down syndrome with atrioventricular canal defects, Turner's syndrome with coarctation of the aorta, Noonan syndrome with pulmonary stenosis and atrial septal defect, and Williams syndrome with supravalvar aortic stenosis. If a family has one child with a congenital heart defect, the risk of having a second child with congenital heart disease is 1.8%.[2] The risk of having a child with congenital heart disease to a parent with congenital heart disease is between 2% and 14%, depending on the specific lesion.[3,4]

Clinical Presentation and Diagnosis

In general, children with congenital heart defects present in one of two ways: children with left-to-right shunts present with congestive heart failure, and children with right-to-left shunts present with cyanosis (Table 44.1). There are also mild defects in which the child is clinically asymptomatic but has a cardiac murmur. The diagnosis is based on the history, physical examination, chest X-ray, electrocardiogram, echocardiogram, and cardiac catheterization.

Patients with a pure left-to-right shunt have increased pulmonary blood flow and present with symptoms of congestive heart failure. These symptoms are failure to thrive, recurrent upper respiratory tract infections, and sweating with feeding. Signs of heart failure include tachypnea, tachycardia, and hepatomegaly. These patients have pulmonary hypertension, and if left untreated they can develop pulmonary vascular obstructive disease. With progression of this pulmonary vascular disease, the pulmonary vascular resistance steadily increases and the actual amount of left-to-right shunting decreases. Eventually a point is reached at which the patient becomes cy-

anotic and has what is called Eisenmenger syndrome. At this point, operation to close the intracardiac defect may not help the patient and may actually prove fatal as the child may develop irreversible right ventricular failure. This complication can be prevented by early operative repair.

Patients with intracardiac or extracardiac obstructive lesions may be asymptomatic or present with signs of congestive heart failure. In particular, patients with coarctation of the aorta and interrupted aortic arch may present with severe heart failure and cardiovascular collapse at the time of ductus closure. In fact, there is a group of lesions in which the patient is essentially dependent on a ductus arteriosus for either pulmonary blood flow, systemic blood flow, or mixing of blood (Table 44.2). Management of these infants has been greatly enhanced by the use of prostaglandin E_1 (PGE$_1$) therapy.[5] PGE$_1$ maintains the patency of the ductus arteriosus, and for these critically ill infants can provide either the pulmonary blood flow, systemic blood flow, or mixing that they require for survival. By stabilizing these patients with pharmacological management of the ductus, they can undergo complete diagnostic evaluation and elective therapeutic intervention after resolution of hypoxia, acidosis, and ventricular failure.

Patients with a congenital cardiac lesion causing cyanosis can have either a pure right-to-left shunt with decreased pulmonary blood flow or a complex lesion where there is actually both increased pulmonary blood flow and cyanosis. The most common overall cause of cyanotic heart disease is tetralogy of Fallot, but many of these patients do not present until several months of age when they develop progressive hypertrophy of the right ventricular outflow tract.

Surgical Management

Palliation

The two most commonly used palliative procedures are the systemic-to-pulmonary artery shunts and pulmonary artery

TABLE 44.1. Presentation and Classification of Congenital Heart Disease.

Congestive Heart Failure
Left-to-Right Shunt
(increased pulmonary blood flow)
  Patent ductus arteriosus
  Atrial septal defect
  Ventricular septal defect
  Atrioventricular canal
  Truncus arteriosus
  Aortopulmonary window
Cyanosis
Right-to-Left Shunt
(decreased pulmonary blood flow)
  Tetralogy of Fallot

  Tricuspid atresia

  Pulmonary atresia
    With intact ventricular septum
    With ventricular septal defect
  Hypoplastic left heart syndrome
Miscellaneous
  Anomalous origin of the left coronary artery from the pulmonary artery
  Corrected transposition of the great arteries
  Ebstein's anomaly
  Vascular rings

Obstructive Lesions

  Aortic stenosis
  Mitral stenosis
  Pulmonic stenosis
  Coarctation of the aorta
  Interrupted aortic arch

Complex Lesions

  Transposition of the great arteries
    With intact ventricular septum
    With ventricular septal defect
  Total anomalous pulmonary venous
    connection
  Cor triatriatum

---

banding. Systemic-to-pulmonary artery shunts provide for increased pulmonary blood flow in patients with a right-to-left shunt and decreased pulmonary blood flow. Pulmonary artery banding is used for patients with increased pulmonary blood flow secondary to a left-to-right shunt.

Modified Blalock–Taussig Shunt

The most commonly used systemic to pulmonary artery shunt is the modified Blalock–Taussig shunt (Fig. 44.1). Other shunts that are now essentially of historical interest only are the Potts,[6] Waterston,[7] and Cooley[8] shunts.

Pulmonary Artery Banding

Pulmonary artery banding was first described for patients with truncus arteriosus (Fig. 44.2). The goal is to reduce the pulmonary artery pressure distal to the band to less than half of the systemic pressure. At the same time the child's oxygen saturations must be monitored to ensure that they do not drop excessively. Current indications for pulmonary artery banding would include multiple ventricular septal defects (Swiss cheese ventricular septal defect) and patients with excessive pulmonary blood flow and single ventricle physiology without evidence of subaortic stenosis.

TABLE 44.2. Ductal-Dependent Lesions.

For pulmonary blood flow
  Pulmonary atresia
  Tricuspid atresia
  Severe tetralogy of Fallot

For systemic blood flow
  Hypoplastic left heart syndrome
  Interrupted aortic arch
  Severe coarctation of the aorta

For mixing of blood
  Transposition of the great arteries

Left-to-Right Shunt

Patent Ductus Arteriosus

A patent ductus arteriosus is a persistent communication of the normal fetal connection between the pulmonary artery and the descending thoracic aorta (Fig. 44.3). In patients without other congenital heart defects, this creates a left-to-right shunt. In premature infants, it can cause severe congestive

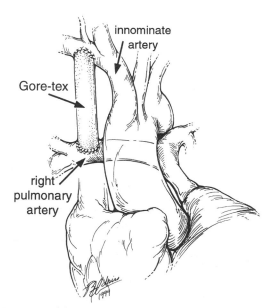

FIGURE 44.1. Modified Blalock–Taussig shunt. This shunt is a Gore-Tex interposition graft between the subclavian artery and the pulmonary artery. The subclavian artery originates from the innominate artery and acts as the regulator of the amount of flow into the shunt. This shunt can be performed through either a thoracotomy incision or a median sternotomy. The shunt shown is in place in a patient with tetralogy of Fallot.

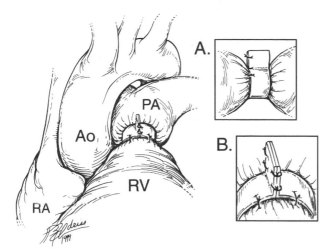

FIGURE 44.2. Pulmonary artery band. Band illustrated is a Teflon-impregnated Dacron band. The band is placed through either a left thoracotomy or a median sternotomy incision. It encircles the pulmonary artery (PA) and is constricted with multiple sutures as illustrated in **inset A** to progressively restrict flow into the pulmonary artery. A pressure monitoring catheter is usually inserted in the distal pulmonary artery during tightening of the band. The band is fixed to the adventitia of the pulmonary artery (**inset B**) to prevent distal migration of the band. **AO**, aorta; **RA**, right atrium; **RV**, right ventricle.

heart failure and respiratory distress syndrome. In older children, the patient may be clinically asymptomatic but have a "machinery-type" murmur. In premature infants the indication for surgical closure is congestive heart failure causing respiratory distress. In older children, simply having a ductus that is audible is an indication for closure. These children are at risk of subacute bacterial endocarditis, aortic aneurysm, pulmonary artery aneurysm, and aortic dissection. Operative ductus closure is usually performed through a left thoracotomy. The technique used to close a ductus in premature infants is simple ligation (Fig. 44.3); in older children, we prefer to use the technique of division and oversewing (Fig. 44.3).

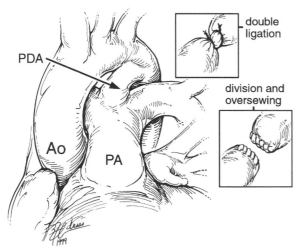

FIGURE 44.3. Patent ductus arteriosus (PDA), exposed through a median sternotomy incision. A PDA may also be approached through a left thoracotomy. The **upper inset** illustrates a double ligation to close the ductus. The **lower inset** shows the ductus divided with the two stumps oversewn. **AO**, aorta; **PA**, pulmonary artery.

This technique ensures complete division of the ductus without the potential for recanalization that can occur in about 3% to 5% of patients that have simple ligation. Transcatheter coil occlusion has been shown to be as effective and less costly than surgical closure for small PDAs if silent residual leaks are not considered clinically significant.[9] Our current approach is to recommend coil occlusion for the smaller ductus and surgical division and oversewing for the large ductus.

ATRIAL SEPTAL DEFECT

An atrial septal defect is a hole in the intraatrial septum that causes a left-to-right shunt. Repair is usually via pericardial patch or direct suture closure. The degree of shunting is determined by the size of the atrial septal defect and the right and left ventricular compliance. Patients with an atrial septal defect are often asymptomatic, but on physical examination have a fixed split second heart sound and may have a systolic murmur of relative (physiological) pulmonary stenosis. The electrocardiogram will demonstrate right ventricular hypertrophy and the chest X-ray cardiomegaly. Any patient who has an audible murmur and documented atrial septal defect by echocardiography is a candidate for surgical closure. Patients with an atrial septal defect are at risk of atrial arrhythmias, right ventricular dysfunction, pulmonary hypertension, and congestive heart failure. Without surgical intervention, the mean age of death in patients with an atrial septal defect is 36 years.[10] Atrial septal defects are classified as ostium secundum (80%), sinus venosus (10%), and ostium primum (10%).

Ostium secundum defects are a simple opening in the atrial septum. Ostium primum and sinus venosus defects are more complex. Ostium primum defects are also called partial atrioventricular canal defects, and these patients also have a cleft in the mitral valve that must be closed to prevent mitral insufficiency. Sinus venosus defects have partial anomalous pulmonary venous drainage of the right superior pulmonary vein to the superior vena cava. Percutaneous transcatheter techniques are becoming more and more successful for small–to moderate–sized ostium secundum defects.

VENTRICULAR SEPTAL DEFECT

A ventricular septal defect is a hole located in the interventricular septum. The degree of left-to-right shunting across the ventricular septal defect is determined by the size of the defect and the pulmonary vascular resistance. Defects are categorized by their location in the interventricular septum (Fig. 44.4). Ventricular septal defects can be further subdivided into two categories, restrictive and nonrestrictive. Nonrestrictive ventricular septal defects are the same size as or larger than the aortic valve annulus. These patients have high pulmonary artery pressure and present with severe congestive heart failure. Left untreated, these patients will develop the Eisenmenger syndrome. These patients should undergo elective closure of the ventricular septal defect at 3 to 6 months of age. In patients with a restrictive ventricular septal defect, the defect is smaller than the aortic valve annulus. Pulmonary artery pressures are less than systemic. These patients may be managed medically unless they meet the following surgical indications: (1) pulmonary to systemic flow ratio greater than 1.5:1; (2) aortic valve prolapse; (3) aortic valve insufficiency; (4) prior episode of endocarditis; (5) conal ventricular septal defect.

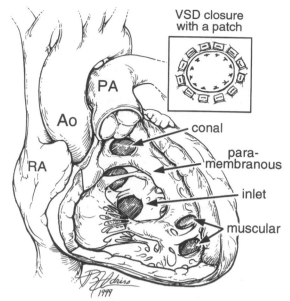

FIGURE 44.4. Ventricular septal defect. A cutaway view of the interventricular septum as it would be seen through a median sternotomy with the anterior right ventricle removed. The four main types of ventricular septal defects are illustrated. Their location within the interventricular septum gives rise to their name. Most ventricular septal defects are closed through the right atrium and through the tricuspid valve. Conal defects are approached through the pulmonary artery. Most ventricular septal defects are closed with a Dacron or Gore-Tex patch, which can be anchored either with interrupted pledgeted sutures (as shown) or with running suture technique. In our experience the interrupted pledgeted suture technique is associated with a lower incidence of residual ventricular septal defects. *RA*, right atrium; *AO*, aorta; *PA*, pulmonary artery.

ATRIOVENTRICULAR CANAL

Atrioventricular canal or endocardial cushion defects involve deficiencies of the atrial septum, ventricular septum, and atrio-ventricular valves. Infants with a complete atrioventricular canal defect usually have severe pulmonary hypertension and present in congestive heart failure. More than 80% of patients with atrioventricular canal defect have trisomy 21 (Down syndrome). We recommend intracardiac repair of atrioventricular canal defects at the age of 6 months.

TRUNCUS ARTERIOSUS

Truncus arteriosus is a complex lesion in which a single arterial trunk emanates from the ventricular mass of the heart. The systemic, coronary, and pulmonary circulations all arise from this single trunk. Nearly all these children have a large ventricular septal defect. They have systemic pulmonary artery pressures and present with severe congestive heart failure in the first several weeks to months of life. Currently, we recommend neonatal repair of truncus arteriosus at the time of diagnosis. The repair involves the use of cardiopulmonary bypass with hypothermia and cardioplegia, detachment of the pulmonary artery from the truncus, ventricular septal defect closure, and placement of a conduit from the right ventricle to the pulmonary artery (Fig. 44.5); this is commonly called a Rastelli procedure.

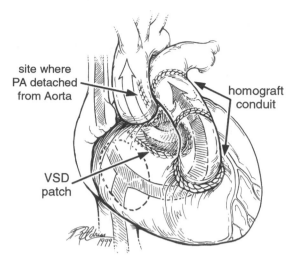

FIGURE 44.5. Rastelli procedure for truncus arteriosus: completed repair of a patient with truncus arteriosus. The pulmonary artery (*PA*) has been detached from the ascending aorta and the resultant opening closed primarily. A homograft conduit has been inserted from the right ventricle (*RV*) to the pulmonary artery. Finally, the ventricular septal defect (*VSD*) has been closed with a patch. *Open curved arrows* illustrate the flow of blood from the superior and inferior vena cava through the tricuspid valve, into the RV, through the conduit, and into the pulmonary artery. Blood from the left atrium is deflected by the ventricular septal defect patch from the LV into the ascending aorta.

AORTOPULMONARY WINDOW

Aortopulmonary window is a very rare congenital lesion where there is a communication between the proximal ascending aorta and the main pulmonary artery. These babies have severe pulmonary hypertension and are at high risk for pulmonary vascular obstructive disease. We recommend neonatal repair of these patients with a patch placed within the aorta to separate the blood flow in the great arteries and baffle the pulmonary artery flow into the right pulmonary artery.

Right-to-Left Shunt

TETRALOGY OF FALLOT

Tetralogy of Fallot is the most common cause of cyanotic heart disease. The four components of tetralogy of Fallot are ventricular septal defect, pulmonary stenosis, right-ventricular hypertrophy, and an overriding aorta. These children usually present with cyanosis within the first several weeks to months of life. Chest X-ray classically shows decreased pulmonary vascularity and a "boot-shaped" heart; 30% of these patients have an aortic arch positioned on the right side. Indications for surgery are hypercyanotic or "tet" spells, progressive polycythemia, or oxygen saturation less than 80% in room air.

TRICUSPID ATRESIA

Patients born with tricuspid atresia have no development of the tricuspid valve and as a result no communication between the right atrium and right ventricle. All the blood that returns to the right atrium from the inferior and superior vena cava must traverse an atrial septal defect to the left atrium and then pass through the left ventricle and out to the systemic circulation. Some of these patients have a small ventricular septal defect that gives rise to a small pulmonary artery. If a ventricular septal defect is not present, these patients may be reliant on a patent ductus arteriosus for pulmonary blood flow. The eventual surgical repair of patients with tricuspid atresia is a Fontan type of operation. The Fontan operation separates the systemic and pulmonary circulations in a patient with one ventricle. Because there is no functioning right ventricle, the systemic venous return is connected directly to the pulmonary artery and the single ventricle becomes the systemic ventricle. Unlike many other pediatric cardiac procedures, the Fontan operation cannot be performed on neonates because of their normally high pulmonary vascular resistance. It is only after about 1 to 2 years of age that the pulmonary vascular resistance is low enough to allow the Fontan operation to be performed.

PULMONARY ATRESIA WITH INTACT VENTRICULAR SEPTUM

Pulmonary atresia refers to complete closure of the pulmonary valve. In many of these patients, the pulmonary valve leaflets are fused. If there is an intact ventricular septum, there is no outlet for the blood within the right ventricle. Because of the small amount of blood flowing into the right ventricle there is usually hypoplasia of the right ventricle. These patients are dependent on pulmonary blood flow through a patent ductus arteriosus. Medical management utilizes intravenous infusion of PGE, which will keep the ductus open and medically stabilize the patient. Diagnosis is usually made by echocardiogram and the precise surgical decision making is based on a cardiac catheterization, which is used to evaluate the size of the right ventricle and the anatomy of the pulmonary arteries.

We recommend operation through a median sternotomy with pulmonary valvotomy on cardiopulmonary bypass and placement of a modified Blalock–Taussig shunt to provide for adequate pulmonary blood flow. Following the initial procedure, the patient is observed to see how the right ventricle grows. The patients that have a very small right ventricle go on to a Fontan-type procedure. In patients where the right ventricle remains between 30% to 60% of predicted normal, the repair involves both atrial septal defect closure and placement of a bidirectional Glenn.[11] The bidirectional Glenn decompresses the volume load on the right ventricle. Those patients who have adequate growth of the right ventricle can undergo atrial septal defect closure and shunt ligation and division, which is a biventricular repair.

PULMONARY ATRESIA WITH VENTRICULAR SEPTAL DEFECT

These infants have fusion of the pulmonary valve cusps and a large ventricular septal defect. Although some of these patients have a distinct ductus arteriosus filling the pulmonary arteries, approximately 50% do not have confluent pulmonary arteries but instead have pulmonary blood flow originating from multiple aortopulmonary collateral arteries from the descending thoracic aorta. These babies present with cyanosis, which may or may not improve after prostaglandin infusion because of the small size or absence of a ductus arteriosus. In these patients, cardiac catheterization is necessary to define the pulmonary artery anatomy and the origins of the multiple aortopulmonary collateral arteries. Initial surgical intervention is usually directed at establishing pulmonary blood flow with either a shunt, right-ventricular outflow tract patch, or right ventricular to pulmonary artery homograft.

Complex Cyanotic Lesions

TRANSPOSITION OF THE GREAT ARTERIES

Transposition of the great arteries is the most common cause of cyanosis from a cardiac condition in the neonate. Patients with transposition of the great arteries have two parallel circulations. The aorta and coronary arteries originate from the right ventricle and the pulmonary artery and ductus arteriosus arise from the left ventricle. In one circuit, the oxygenated blood returning from the lungs flows into the left atrium and ventricle, is ejected into the pulmonary artery, and recirculates back to the left atrium. In the other circuit the unoxygenated blood returning to the right atrium goes into the right ventricle and is ejected out the aorta to recirculate back to the right atrium. With these two parallel circulations, infants with transposition are dependent upon mixing of blood at either the atrial, ventricular, or ductal levels for initial survival.

Infants with transposition usually present with cyanosis in the first 24 h of life. The electrocardiogram shows right-ventricular hypertrophy; the chest radiograph shows a narrow superior mediastinum (because of the anteroposterior relationship of the great vessels), increased pulmonary blood flow, and a cardiac silhouette (in relation to the diaphragm) that looks like an egg on its side. The diagnosis is made by two-dimensional echocardiography. Most patients do not go to cardiac catheterization unless there is a question of a coronary artery anomaly, coarctation, or ventricular septal defect that is not accurately assessed by the echocardiogram. The initial stabilization of the child with transposition begins with the administration of PGE_1; this maintains patency of the ductus arteriosus and allows mixing of blood at that level. However, some patients will not have enough mixing with PGE_1 infusion and may require an atrial septostomy. This is done percutaneously with a balloon catheter, either at the bedside under echo guidance or in the cardiac catheterization laboratory under fluoroscopy. The catheter is advanced into the left atrium, the balloon is inflated, and when the balloon is pulled back into the right atrium the atrial septum is torn open.[12] This procedure allows for mixing of blood at the atrial level. In the current era most patients with transposition of the great arteries then undergo a definitive repair, which is an arterial switch operation in the first or second week of life. If the child presents after approximately 3 to 4 weeks of age, primary repair is no longer possible because the ventricular muscle mass will have "thinned out" and is no longer capable of supporting the systemic circulation that is required after the arterial switch operation. In these patients, the left ventricle must be "retrained" to prepare for an arterial switch by first banding the pulmonary artery.

The arterial switch operation involves "switching" the great vessels and moving the coronary arteries. This operation is done with cardiopulmonary bypass, hypothermia, and cardioplegic arrest of the heart. The ductus arteriosus is ligated and divided. The atrial communication created by septostomy is closed and the arterial switch operation is performed. The great vessels are transected and "switched," anastomosing the aorta to the left ventricular outflow tract and the main pulmonary artery to the right ventricular outflow tract. The coronary arteries are transferred from the right-ventricular outflow tract to the left-ventricular outflow tract. When the arterial switch operation is completed, the left ventricle gives rise to the aorta and the coronary arteries and the right ventricle gives rise to the pulmonary artery.

TOTAL ANOMALOUS PULMONARY VENOUS CONNECTION

In this anomaly, there is no direct communication between the pulmonary veins and the left atrium. The common pulmonary vein instead finds a route to the heart via either the cardinal, umbilical, or systemic venous channels. These patients require either a large patent foramen ovale or an atrial septal defect for survival. These babies have equal oxygen saturations in all four cardiac chambers and the great vessels. They present with cyanosis and congestive heart failure. Chest X-ray reveals a normal heart size with a "ground-glass"-type appearance of the lung fields. Echocardiogram reveals right-ventricular diastolic overload and a free space posterior to the left atrium. Color Doppler flow can be used to demonstrate the morphology and flow patterns in the anomalous vein. Most of these babies are referred for cardiac surgical repair without a cardiac catheterization. Babies that have stenosis or obstruction of the venous drainage may present with extreme cyanosis and hypotension. These patients are surgically repaired at the time of diagnosis.

HYPOPLASTIC LEFT HEART SYNDROME

Hypoplastic left heart syndrome is a severe congenital heart defect in which the child does not have a functioning left ventricle. This syndrome is thought to be caused by premature closure of the patent foramen ovale in utero. These patients have aortic valve atresia or severe aortic stenosis with mitral valve atresia or severe mitral stenosis. There is hypoplasia of the left ventricle and ascending aorta, and most of these patients have a coarctation. Because the left ventricle is too small to support the systemic circulation, they are candidates for either cardiac transplantation or preparation for a Fontan operation later in life. These babies present in the first week of life with cyanosis, tachypnea, and, when the ductus arteriosus closes, cardiovascular collapse. Electrocardiogram shows severe right-ventricular hypertrophy with diminished left-ventricular forces. Diagnosis is readily established by two-dimensional and color Doppler echocardiography; most patients do not require cardiac catheterization for the diagnosis.

The medical management of a child with hypoplastic left heart syndrome before operative intervention is quite important. The child is placed on prostaglandin E_1 as soon as the diagnosis is made. This medication maintains patency of the ductus arteriosus and thus provides a route for coronary and systemic blood flow. It is important to keep the child on very low or no oxygen support despite low saturation to maintain the systemic cardiac output.

Until the early 1980s this syndrome was a fatal lesion. The first successful series of palliative operations were reported by Norwood and colleagues on a group of patients operated on between 1979 and 1981.[13] This operation has three components: (1) an atrial septectomy to provide complete mixing of blood at the atrial level, (2) an anastomosis with patch augmentation between the proximal transected main pulmonary artery and the ascending and descending aorta, and (3) a modified Blalock–Taussig shunt to provide for pulmonary blood flow. This operation establishes single-ventricle circulation with pulmonary blood flow maintained through a shunt. The operative mortality of this procedure was initially more than 50%. With refinements in technique, the mortality is now 15% to 20%.

An alternative approach to staged palliation is orthotopic cardiac transplantation with extensive aortic arch reconstruction. Unfortunately only 70% to 80% of infants placed on the waiting list for heart transplants will receive a heart.[14]

Obstructive Lesions

AORTIC STENOSIS

Congenital aortic stenosis is an obstruction of flow between the left ventricle and the ascending aorta. There are four congenital types of aortic stenosis: supravalvular, valvular, discrete subvalvular, and hypertrophic muscular subaortic stenosis. Many of these babies have associated lesions including coarctation of the aorta, supravalvar mitral ring, and parachute mitral valve (Shone's syndrome).[15] The most common type of aortic stenosis is valvular aortic stenosis secondary to a bicuspid aortic valve. If the aortic stenosis is severe, these patients will present in infancy with congestive heart failure and diminished peripheral pulses. Older children present with exercise intolerance, angina, and syncope. Diagnosis is obtained by echocardiography.

Recently surgeons have become quite interested in using the Ross operation, not necessarily as the first operation for aortic stenosis, but as the second operation when the aortic stenosis reoccurs after initial aortic valvotomy or balloon valvuloplasty. The Ross operation involves harvesting the pulmonary valve from the patient as an autograft, resecting the aortic valve, and then implanting the pulmonary valve into the aortic annulus.[16] This technique necessitates reimplanting the coronary arteries into the sinuses of the harvested pulmonary autograft. To replace the pulmonary valve, a pulmonary valve homograft is selected and sutured between the right ventricle and the main pulmonary artery. The Ross operation is now performed at many centers with a very low mortality.

MITRAL STENOSIS

Congenital mitral stenosis patients often have other congenital heart defects such as coarctation of the aorta or ventricular septal defect. Mitral stenosis is divided into four anatomical types: (1) typical congenital mitral stenosis, (2) hypoplastic congenital mitral stenosis, (3) supramitral ring, and (4) parachute mitral valve. Surgical options include simple valvotomy, excision of the supravalvular ring, and mitral valve replacement.

PULMONIC STENOSIS

Pulmonic stenosis is caused by partial fusion of the pulmonary valve cusps. Depending on the degree of valve fusion, these children may present with cyanosis in the newborn period or may be completely asymptomatic and present later in life with a systolic murmur. Isolated pulmonic stenosis is now being treated successfully in the cardiac catheterization laboratory with percutaneous transcatheter balloon dilatation in nearly all cases.[17]

COARCTATION OF THE AORTA

Coarctation of the aorta is one of the most common obstructive lesions found in children. It is defined as a hemodynamically significant narrowing of the aorta usually found in the descending thoracic aorta just distal to the left subclavian artery. The clinical presentation of the child with coarctation depends on the severity of stenosis and whether or not the blood flow to the lower extremities is dependent on the ductus arteriosus. Infants with coarctation who have closure of a ductus that is supplying blood to the lower extremities will develop cardiovascular collapse when the ductus closes. These children present with poor perfusion of the lower extremities, acidosis, and renal failure. They also may have severe congestive heart failure because the outflow from the left ventricle is severely obstructed by the coarctation. A chest radio-graph in this situation shows cardiomegaly with signs of congestive heart failure.

Older children with a coarctation and even some adults may be asymptomatic. They are usually found to have hypertension in the upper extremities on routine physical examination, often for a school exam. On further evaluation, they are noted to have diminished or absent femoral pulses. Older patients are at risk for bacterial endocarditis, rupture of the aorta, hypertension leading to cerebral vascular accidents, and coronary artery disease. For older patients with a coarctation, the mean age at death is 35 years.[18]

Neonates that present with coarctation are resuscitated with a PGE_1 infusion that opens the ductus arteriosus and the coarctation site itself, restoring blood flow to the lower half of the body. Medical therapy for several days with PGE_1 allows time for resolution of acidosis and renal insufficiency. These children may then be operated on electively in good physiological condition. Our operative procedure of choice for these infants is currently resection of the coarctation site and ductal tissue with extended end-to-end anastomosis. For older patients with coarctation, we currently recommend Gore-Tex patch aortoplasty.

INTERRUPTED AORTIC ARCH

Interrupted aortic arch is physiologically similar to severe coarctation, but in these babies there is complete loss of continuity between the ascending and descending aorta. The blood flow to the descending thoracic aorta is through a patent ductus arteriosus. Most of these patients also have a ventricular septal defect.

These patients present with cardiovascular collapse when the ductus arteriosus closes. They are acidotic, oliguric, and in a low perfusion state. Similarly to a severe coarctation, these patients are medically managed with PGE_1 infusion to open the patent ductus arteriosus. The child is intubated, placed on mechanical ventilation, and given inotropic support to improve peripheral perfusion. The diagnosis is made by echocardiography.

There are two approaches to interrupted aortic arch. The "two-stage" approach is with an initial palliation with repair of the arch and pulmonary artery banding followed by a later procedure to close the ventricular septal defect and remove the pulmonary artery band. The more preferred approach currently is to perform primary repair of the ventricular septal defect and the aortic arch.

Miscellaneous Lesions

ANOMALOUS ORIGIN OF THE LEFT CORONARY ARTERY FROM THE PULMONARY ARTERY

This anomaly is a very rare, usually isolated, congenital lesion. The left coronary artery originates from the pulmonary artery, creating left coronary artery insufficiency. In these patients the blood supply to the left coronary artery distribution is from right coronary artery collaterals. These patients present with severe congestive heart failure. A chest radiograph shows cardiomegaly and the electrocardiogram shows signs of myocardial ischemia or infarction. Echocardiography is diagnostic and reveals an enlarged right coronary artery, a hypokinetic dilated left ventricle, and severe mitral insufficiency. Patients presenting with a picture such as this are referred directly for operative repair. The current preferred surgical therapy for anomalous origin of the left coronary artery from the pulmonary artery is to reimplant the anomalous left coronary artery into the ascending aorta.[19]

CORRECTED TRANSPOSITION OF THE GREAT ARTERIES

Corrected transposition of the great arteries is a very unusual anomaly in which there are two errors in the connections within the heart. Unlike simple transposition, these patients have the blood flow of the pulmonary and systemic circulations in series. However, the right ventricle is the systemic pumping chamber and the left ventricle is the pumping chamber of the pulmonary circulation. Blood flow from the right atrium goes into a morphological left ventricle from which it is directed to the pulmonary artery. The left atrial flow returns to a morphological right ventricle from which it flows out to the aorta. Many of these patients have an associated ventricular septal defect and pulmonary stenosis. Many of these patients will develop complete atrioventricular heart block spontaneously. Surgical options for these patients include (1) closure of the ventricular septal defect and pulmonary valvotomy, (2) a Mustard procedure combined with a Rastelli procedure to make the left ventricle the systemic pumping chamber and the right ventricle the pulmonary pumping chamber,[20] and (3) a double-switch operation combining a Mustard operation with an arterial switch procedure.[21] The latter two operations are more complex than the first, but make the left ventricle the systemic pumping chamber that is less likely to undergo late deterioration.

EBSTEIN'S ANOMALY

Ebstein's anomaly is an abnormal formation of the tricuspid valve in which the tricuspid valve is displaced downward into the right ventricle. Most of these patients have an associated atrial septal defect and may have pulmonary stenosis. These patients can present either with cyanosis at birth or later in life with congestive heart failure. Approximately 20% of these patients have an accessory connection that can cause tachycardia. Diagnosis is by echocardiography, but cardiac catheterization may be required to determine precisely the right-ventricular size and the anatomy of the pulmonary circulation. Infants that present with severe cyanosis and cardiomegaly may require neonatal conversion to a single ventricle-type physiology. Older patients that present with congestive heart failure are usually treated by atrial septal defect closure and tricuspid valvuloplasty.

VASCULAR RINGS

The term vascular ring refers to a group of congenital anomalies in which there is a developmental abnormality in the aortic arch system that causes compression of the trachea and esophagus. The two true vascular rings are the double aortic arch and the right aortic arch with left ligamentum and retroesophageal left subclavian artery. These patients have a complete ring of blood vessels around the trachea and esophagus. These children typically present with noisy respirations, a brassy cough similar to a seal's bark, cyanosis, apnea, or respiratory distress. In older children dysphagia for solid foods may be noticed. Diagnosis is suggested by the chest radigraph, which may reveal the location of the aortic arch to be abnormal. The best initial diagnostic step is a barium swallow examination, which will reveal persistent filling defects in the esophagus if there is a true vascular ring present. Further definition of the anatomy of the ring if considered necessary can be obtained with either CT or MRI imaging. Angiography is reserved for only those patients who have an associated congenital cardiac anomaly. For many of these infants the diagnosis is suggested by bronchoscopic examination, which is commonly performed in patients with noisy respirations or respiratory distress. Operative repair is recommended for all patients with clinical symptoms and evidence of a vascular ring. The vascular structures are divided between vascular clamps with oversewing of the stumps similar to the technique described for patent ductus arteriosus.[22]

References

1. Clark EB. Epidemiology of congenital cardiovascular malformations. In: Emmanouilides GC, Riemenschneider TA, Allen HD, Gutesell HP, eds. Moss and Adams' Heart Disease in Infants, Children and Adolescents, 5th Ed. Baltimore: Williams & Wilkins 1995;1:60–70.
2. Boughman JA, Berg KA, Astemborski JA, et al. Familial risks of congenital heart defect assessed in a population-based study. Am J Med Genet 1987;26:839.
3. Nora JJ, Nora AH. Recurrence risks in children having one parent with a congenital heart disease. Circulation 1976;53:701–702.
4. Whittemore R, Hobbins JC, Engle MA. Pregnancy and its outcome in women with and without surgical treatment of congenital heart disease. Am J Cardiol 1982;50:641.
5. Heymann MA, Berman W, Rudolph AM, Whitman V. Dilatation of the ductus arteriosus by prostaglandin E_1 in aortic arch abnormalities. Circulation 1979;59:169–173.
6. Potts WJ, Smith S, Gibson S. Anastomosis of the aorta to a pulmonary artery. JAMA 1946;132:627–631.
7. Waterston DJ. Treatment of Fallot's tetralogy in infants under the age of 1 year. Rozhl Chir 1962;41:181.
8. Cooley DA, Hallman GL. Intrapericardial aortic-right pulmonary arterial anastomosis. Surg Gynecol Obstet 1966;122:1084–1086.
9. Prieto LR, DeCamillo DM, Konrad DJ, et al. Comparison of cost and clinical outcome between transcatheter coil occlusion and surgical closure of isolated patent ductus arteriosus. Pediatrics 1998;101:1020–1024.
10. Campbell M. Natural history of atrial septal defect. Br Heart J 1970;32:820–826.
11. Muster AJ, Zales VR, Ilbawi MN, Backer CL, Duffy CE, Mavroudis C. Bidirectional cavopulmonary anastomosis with right ventricle-pulmonary artery continuity (pulsatile bidirectional Glenn) for hypoplastic right ventricle. J Thorac Cardiovasc Surg 1993;105:112–119.
12. Rashkind WJ, Miller WW. Creation of an atrial septal defect without thoracotomy: a palliative approach to complete transposition of the great arteries. JAMA 1966;196:991.
13. Norwood WI, Lang P, Castaneda AR, Campbell DN. Experience with operations for hypoplastic left heart syndrome. J Thorac Cardiovasc Surg 1981;82:511–519.
14. Chiaverelli M, Gundry SR, Razzouk AJ, Bailey LL. Cardiac transplantation for infants with hypoplastic left-heart syndrome. JAMA 1993;270:2944–2947.
15. Shone JD, Sellers RD, Anderson RC, et al. The developmental complex of "parachute mitral valve," supravalvular ring of left atrium, subaortic stenosis, and coarctation of aorta. Am J Cardiol 1963;11:714–725.
16. Ross DN. Replacement of aortic and mitral valves with a pulmonary autograft. Lancet 1967;2:956–958.
17. Caspi J, Coles JG, Benson LN, et al. Management of neonatal critical pulmonic stenosis in the balloon valvotomy era. Ann Thorac Surg 1990;49:273–278.
18. Campbell M. Natural history of coarctation of the aorta. Br Heart J 1970;32:633–640.
19. Backer CL, Stout MJ, Zales VR, et al. Anomalous origin of the left coronary artery: A 20-year review of surgical management. J Thorac Cardiovasc Surg 1992;103:1049–1058.
20. Ilbawi MN, DeLeon SY, Backer CL, et al. An alternative approach to the surgical management of physiologically corrected transposition with ventricular septal defect and pulmonary stenosis or atresia. J Thorac Cardiovasc Surg 1990;100:410–415.
21. Yagihara T, Kishimoto H, Isobe F, et al. Double switch operation in cardiac anomalies with atrioventricular and ventriculoarterial discordance. J Thorac Cardiovasc Surg 1994;107:351–358.
22. Backer CL, Ilbawi MN, Idriss FS, DeLeon SY. Vascular anomalies causing tracheoesophageal compression: review of experience in children. J Thorac Cardiovasc Surg 1989;97:725–731.

45

Adult Heart Disease

Todd K. Rosengart, William de Bois, and Nicola A. Francalancia

Cardiopulmonary Bypass (CPB) and Myocardial Preservation

Principles of CPB

The primary purpose of cardiopulmonary bypass is to provide the cardiac surgeon with a bloodless and motion-free operative field. This aim is accomplished by temporarily interrupting the function of the heart and lungs by physiologically substituting a "heart-lung machine" in their place. The "cardiopulmonary bypass" provided by the heart-lung machine (bypass circuit) permits complete cessation of cardiopulmonary activity while allowing the flow of oxygenated blood and preservation of adequate tissue perfusion and organ function systemically. Viewed simplistically, cardiopulmonary bypass is accomplished by pumping blood through an extracorporeal circuit, the primary features of which are the allowance of gas and heat exchange.

The circuit by which CPB is provided consists basically of a set of specialized tubing called cannulae, which are inserted into the heart or great vessels to access the circulation, a reservoir, which collects the blood, an arterial pump, and an oxygenator, which provides heat and gas exchange (Fig. 45.1). Commonly added to this system are filters, air emboli safety devices, a myocardial protection system, and a mechanism for hemodynamic monitoring.

Because the performance of CPB necessitates blood flow over a large surface area of artificial materials, a critical feature of this procedure is the administration of heparin, an anticoagulant that prevents the blood from clotting in the CPB circuit. Adequate levels of anticoagulation are monitored throughout CPB, typically utilizing a simple test known as the activated clotting time (ACT). At the completion of CPB, the heparin is reversed by the administration of protamine, a heparin antagonist.

Strategic Variables in CPB

BLOOD PRESSURE AND FLOW RATES

Because acidosis and lactate production increase in adults when normothermic flow rates are less than 1.6 l/min/m² or 50 ml/kg/min, flow rates employed during hypothermia and normothermia commonly range from approximately 1.5 to 2.5 l/min/m². Although most centers maintain a minimum arterial pressure of 50 mmHg, the optimal arterial perfusion pressure required to maintain nominal tissue perfusion is unknown.

HYPOTHERMIA

The utilization of systemic and cardiac hypothermia to decrease tissue metabolism and enable lower perfusion rates has been a critical component of the performance of CPB. It is estimated that oxygen consumption decreases about 7% per each 1°C decrease in temperature. Systemic hypothermia thus provides a "margin of error" in providing adequate tissue perfusion during CPB.

Most CPB procedures employ moderate hypothermia (28°–32°C) to allow a decrease in CPB flow rates and enhance the safety of CPB. Acceptable cooling rates are approximately 1°C per 1 to 2 min. Rewarming at the end of CPB to a temperature of 36°C is accomplished in an analogous fashion at a rate of 1°C per 3 to 5 min. Temperature gradients during warming are maintained at no greater than 10°C.

BLOOD GAS MANAGEMENT

Gas exchange is another variable that can be regulated during CPB. This is accomplished with a "blender" that controls the diffusion of ventilatory gases, oxygen and air, into the blood, and carbon dioxide out of the blood as it passes through

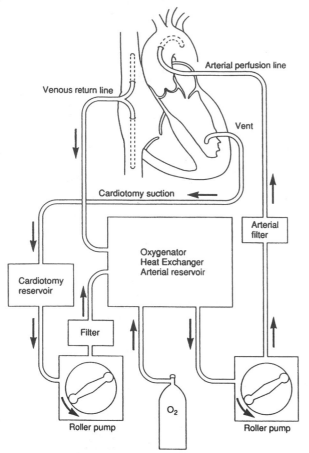

FIGURE 45.1. Schematic representation of the critical components of a cardiopulmonary bypass circuit. (After Callaghan JC, Wartak J. Open Heart Surgery: Theory and Practice. New York: Praeger Press, 1986, with permission.)

the oxygenator. Blood levels of respiratory gases are typically maintained close to normal values, with the exception of PO_2, which is maintained in the range of 150 to 300 mmHg.

The CPB Circuit

CANNULAE

The ascending aorta is the most common site for arterial cannulation and return of blood from the heart-lung machine to the systemic circulation. In previous years and in selected cases today (such as aortic aneurysm surgery), femoral cannulation has been commonly used. Venous cannulae, typically inserted in the right atrium or cavae, provide venous supply and inflow to the CPB circuit, usually by simple gravity drainage.

OXYGENATOR

The oxygenator is attached to a gas source via a gas blender, which allows precise titration of both oxygen percentage and gas flow (and thus blood oxygen and carbon dioxide content, respectively). A heat exchanger is incorporated into the oxygenator and allows warming and cooling of the blood as it passes through this part of the CPB circuit.

PUMPS

There are a minimum of four pumps on the heart-lung console; these include the arterial, ventricular vent, cardiotomy suction, and cardioplegia pumps. These are commonly either a roller or centrifugal pump. The roller pump is a volume-displacement pump that provides output in direct relation to the rotation of the rollers and as a result provides accurate blood flow.

Cardioplegia

As it is often necessary for the surgeon to operate on a still and bloodless field, the heart is typically arrested and blood flow excluded from the heart during the specific portion of open-heart surgery in which cardiac pathology is corrected surgically, whether that be the performance of a valve replacement or a coronary artery bypass. To thus isolate the heart from the systemic circulation, an aortic cross-clamp is placed across the ascending aorta between the heart and the systemic arterial perfusion cannula (Fig. 45.2).

Myocardial protection is typically provided by administration of a cold solution that chemically arrests the heart (cardioplegia), which is injected into the coronary circulation immediately following aortic cross-clamping. Ideally, cardioplegia causes an immediate but reversible myocardial arrest that minimizes expenditure of myocardial energy reserves

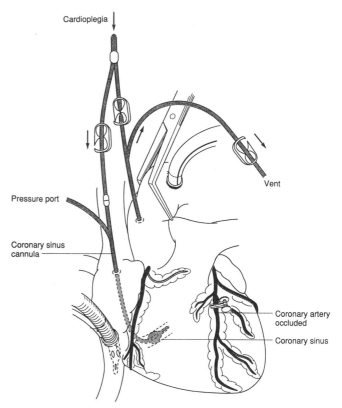

FIGURE 45.2. Typical configuration for antegrade cardioplegia delivery via catheter in aortic root proximal to systemic cannula and aortic cross-clamp, and retrograde cardioplegia delivery via a coronary sinus catheter. (Reproduced with permission from Partington MT, et al. Studies of retrograde cardioplegia. I. J Thorac Cardiovasc Surg 1989;97:613.)

once normal coronary blood flow has been halted by the aortic cross-clamp. After removal of the aortic cross-clamp, the cardioplegic solution is washed out with warm systemic blood, and cardiac rhythm and function return. Cardioplegia may be administered in an antegrade fashion into either the aortic root or directly into the coronary ostia, or in a retrograde fashion into the coronary sinus.

Although there are many different cardioplegia formulations, potassium is the common ingredient. Cardiac asystole induced by potassium cardioplegia alone reduces myocardial oxygen utilization by 90%. Other ingredients added to cardioplegia solution to help improve myocardial protection may include (1) buffers, such as sodium bicarbonate or tromethamine, a buffer (THAM); (2) respiratory substrates such as oxygen, glucose, and Krebs cycle intermediates such as glutamate or aspartate; (3) coronary vasodilators such as nitroglycerin; and (4) membrane stabilizers such as steroids, magnesium, calcium channel blockers, or O_2 radical scavengers.

Conduct of CPB

After incision has been made and appropriate exposure obtained, sufficient heparin is administered (usually 3–4 mg/kg) to produce an activated clotting time of at least 400 to 450 s. The ascending aorta is cannulated. Venous return is obtained from a cannula inserted into the right atrium or, for mitral valve or right heart surgery, two cannulae each inserted into one of the venae cavae, with total venous bypass provided by caval snares. Drainage by gravity from the venous cannulae goes into a venous reservoir chamber. The blood passes through the oxygenator, undergoes gas and heat exchange, as appropriate, and is finally pumped back into the body, usually with a Debakey-type roller pump or Bio-Medicus centrifugal pump (see Fig. 45.1).

Once CPB is established and all other appropriate preparations made as needed for the specific surgical procedures, the heart is arrested by cross-clamping the ascending aorta and injecting about 10 to 15 ml/kg of a cold potassium cardioplegic solution (potassium concentration, 30–35 mEq/l) at 4° to 6°C into the aortic root. Myocardial temperatures are usually maintained at 10° to 20°C, with reinjections of cold cardioplegic solution about every 20 min as protection during the ischemic cross-clamp period. After completion of the cardiac intervention, the cross-clamp is removed, the heart is allowed to resume a normal rhythm, and, after full rewarming, CPB is discontinued and the cannulae removed.

Complications Associated with CPB

Catastrophic complications potentially associated with CPB include protamine reactions, oxygenator failures, line disruptions, air embolism, and blood reactions, among other events.

Metabolic derangements associated with CPB affect nearly every aspect of biochemical homeostasis, and include perturbations in the coagulation and fibrinolytic cascades, immunosuppression, upregulation of stress hormones such as epinephrine and the adrenocorticoids, and activation of leukocytes and inflammatory mediators such as complement and the interleukins. Anemia, thrombocytopenia, and depletion of clotting factors can lead to immediate or delayed risks of bleeding and cardiac tamponade. Hyperthermia and leukocytosis are also common following CPB and are thus not useful as guides to infection.

Hypothermia and a metabolic acidosis, in part resulting from the washout of regions that were poorly perfused during hypothermia, are commonly seen for the first several hours post-CPB. Sodium and water retention normally seen in surgical patients is exacerbated by the metabolic derangements associated with CPB, and a 5% increase in weight can be expected postbypass. Physiological diuresis is usually assisted by the administration of exogenous diuretic agents.

One of the most prevalent side effects of CPB is pulmonary dysfunction, which is most severe through the first 3 days after operation but which may persist for 7 to 10 days. Therapy consists of diuresis, pulmonary toilet, and ventilatory support until appropriate extubation parameters are met.

Moderate to severe renal dysfunction can occur in 7% of patients, with transient azotemia in an additional 20% of patients.[1] Preoperative LV function and renal function, age, duration of CPB, and postoperative LV function are significant risk factors. Maintenance of a brisk urine output in the perioperative period with the use of diuretics may help prevent acute tubular necrosis.

The development of transient deterioration in intellectual ability or other neurological dysfunction has been reported to occur in 7% to 25% of patients undergoing CPB, with a smaller incidence of permanent or fixed local defects.[2] The risk of neurological dysfunction appears to be related to age, preexistent neurological dysfunction, and total cardiopulmonary bypass time. Asymptomatic carotid bruits do not appear to impose an additional risk of neurological events in the absence of hemodynamically significant carotid stenoses.

Jaundice, acalculous cholecystitis, pancreatitis, gastrointestinal bleeding, peptic ulcer disease, intestinal ischemia, and other acute abdominal complications can also occur with increased frequency following CPB compared to other surgical procedures, occurring in almost 1% of patients after open-heart surgery.[3] The pathophysiology of these complications may in part be related to poor organ perfusion during nonpulsatile cardiopulmonary bypass, or the occurrence of atheromatous embolization. Treatment is specific to the given complication.

Coronary Artery Disease

The surgical treatment of coronary artery disease (CAD) represents one of the greatest and most far reaching accomplishments in the recent history of medical therapy. The advent of coronary artery bypass grafting (CABG) as an operation performed more than 300,000 times annually in the United States has had an immeasurable impact on patient well-being and health care today.

Coronary Anatomy and Physiology

The coronary vasculature typically consists of three major arteries, found on or just below the epicardial surface of the heart, that give rise to several major branches, all of which also typically lie in an epicardial or subepicardial position before dividing into numerous intramyocardial branches. The right coronary artery and left (main) coronary artery are the two first branches of the aorta and arise from ostia that are found within the corresponding sinuses of Valsalva, gentle dilatations of the aorta just above the aortic valve, the configurations of which are thought to enhance flow into these ostia.

The branching patterns of both the primary coronary arteries are highly variable. The right coronary artery (RCA), coursing in the right atrioventricular groove, frequently gives off an infundibular branch, which may anastamose with the left anterior descending (LAD) arising from the left main coronary artery; a sinoatrial branch, which supplies the sinus node; and one or several acute marginal branches supplying the right ventricle. The majority of individuals exhibit a "right-dominant" pattern. In this configuration, the RCA continues beyond the crux of the heart (the juncture of the AV and interventricular grooves) in the posterior interventricular groove as the posterior descending artery (PDA). The PDA sends septal perforators into the interventricular septum that anastamose with corresponding branches of the LAD. Alternatively, a minority of patients exhibit a "left dominant" system (Fig. 45.3), in which branches of the circumflex artery from the left main reach the crux, while the remainder of patients demonstrate a "co-dominant" pattern in which both the RCA and left circumflex supply the crux.

The left coronary artery courses posterior to the pulmonary artery from its origin in the aorta for approximately 1 cm as the left main coronary artery before it divides into a LAD branch and a circumflex (CX) branch, which travel in the anterior interventricular groove and the left atrioventricular groove, respectively. The LAD continues down to the apex of the heart, where it may anastamose with the distal PDA, and contributes a series of septal perforating vessels, which anastamose with perforators from the PDA. Diagonal branches from the LAD course obliquely toward the left (obtuse) margin of the heart and supply the anterior left ventricle; obtuse marginal branches correspondingly arise from the circumflex and supply the posterior left ventricle.

The venous drainage of the heart feeds into a system of

epicardial vessels that predominantly run along with the corresponding coronary artery. These coronary veins drain primarily into the great cardiac vein, and ultimately into the coronary sinus, which empties into the right atrium. The thebesian veins represent an alternative deep venous drainage system that empties directly into the cardiac chambers, predominantly the right ventricle.

PHYSIOLOGY OF CORONARY BLOOD FLOW

Because intramyocardial pressures are greatest during systolic contraction and because the coronary ostia are somewhat obstructed by the opening of the aortic valve leaflets during this interval, pressure gradients favor a unique pattern of intracoronary blood flow that occurs primarily during diastole. Myocardial perfusion is also characterized by a flow gradient during systole such that perfusion of the subendocardium actually ceases during this interval because wall tension is greatest in this area. Conversely, diastolic blood flow is greatest to the subendocardium, thereby equalizing blood flow across the myocardium.

It has been estimated that the heart consumes 4% of total body oxygen consumption, while making up only 0.2% of total body weight.[4] Myocardial oxygen extraction ratios may therefore typically be as high as 70% at rest and up to 80% with exercise, and coronary sinus (myocardial venous) saturation levels are consequently the lowest of any organ.

Because of the extent of oxygen extraction at rest, it is obvious that little reserve is available during periods of peak increased myocardial oxygen demand to enhance myocardial oxygen delivery by way of increased oxygen extraction. The heart is therefore dependent on increased blood flow to meet this demand. This increased coronary blood flow is provided in part by an overall increase in systemic cardiac output, but is also provided dramatically by biochemical regulation of coronary vascular resistance.

Biochemical mediators generated by myocardial hypoxia and ischemia that induce coronary vasodilation include nitric oxide, hydrogen and potassium ions, carbon dioxide, and adenosine. Other locally produced hormonal products that are also involved in coronary vasoregulation include bradykinin, epinephrine, norepinephrine, and prostaglandins, among other substances. In the event that an adequate increase in perfusion is not provided by these mechanisms, the heart can also meet energy demands by adapting into an anaerobic glycolytic metabolic pathway that produces less ATP but requires less oxygen than oxidative catabolism. This anaerobic pathway generates lactate, which can be measured in increased quantities in the coronary sinus during ischemic intervals.

Pathogenesis of CAD

Atherosclerosis remains the leading cause of coronary artery disease and the leading cause of death in the Western world.[4–7] Coronary vasospasm, caused by idiopathic processes or by the intake of vasoreactive substances such as cocaine, is the most common of several other, far less prevalent causes of myocardial ischemia. Congenital anomalies in coronary anatomy, such as origin of the left coronary system from the right ostia or the pulmonary artery, represent other causes of myocardial ischemia. As opposed to atherosclerosis, these other processes uncommonly lead to myocardial infarction.

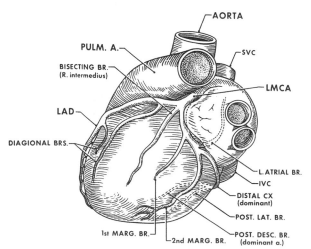

FIGURE 45.3. Lateral view of the left coronary artery system in a left-dominant configuration. Note the major divisions of the left main artery: the left anterior descending (LAD) and the circumflex (CX). In this left-dominant anatomy, the circumflex contributes the posterior descending artery. (Reproduced with permission.)

The pathophysiology of atherosclerotic coronary artery disease is related to the obstruction of the coronary artery lumen by an atheromatous plaque enlarging from within the coronary arterial wall.[4,6,7] Atheromatous lesions typically develop gradually over decades, beginning in the early years of life, where they may be represented by a simple fatty streak. A more advanced, subintimal atheromatous plaque is typically comprised of a central lipid core covered by a fibrous cap. The mature lesion is characteristically a complex mass of cholesterol and cholesterol esters, extracellular matrix components and smooth muscle cells, inflammatory cells such as macrophages, and fibroblasts that have proliferated or been recruited by biochemical perturbations in the vessel wall. The nature of the lesion can change abruptly if intraplaque hemorrhage and plaque rupture occurs, causing acute vessel closure.[8]

Atherosclerotic lesions typically develop in the proximal one-third to one-half of the epicardial vasculature, but may be found more distally at branch points or in the RCA system. Fortuitously, the anatomical localization of CAD to the proximal coronary vasculature typically allows reconstruction by interventional therapies (such as angioplasty and coronary artery bypass) into relatively normal distal vasculature. In contrast, the coronary arteries of diabetic or other patients with advanced disease may be extensively diseased and friable or calcified and inelastic throughout and may not be amenable to conventional therapies.

RISK FACTORS

A large number of risk factors for coronary disease have been identified, the most important of which are hypercholesterolemia, hypertension, smoking, and family history. Reduction of these risk factors, by such measures as diet, weight loss, blood pressure control, cessation of tobacco use, and lifestyle modulation, have most likely contributed significantly to the decreased incidence of fatalities from CAD during the past two decades.

Pathophysiology and Clinical Presentation of CAD

ANGINA PECTORIS

Myocardial ischemia typically occurs only with coronary artery obstruction equivalent to at least a 50% reduction of the diameter (equal to 75% reduction of the cross-sectional area) of the arterial lumen. Angina pectoris may present with classical symptoms, crushing substernal pressure that radiates to the left arm, or as "anginal equivalents," such as throat pain, shortness of breath, or other atypical symptoms, and is typically precipitated by events such as exercise, eating, or stress that increase cardiac activity and thus myocardial oxygen demand. Angina can typically be relieved by cessation of the stress event or with nitroglycerin, a vasodilator that increases coronary blood flow and decrease wall stress, although other conditions such as esophageal spasm may also respond favorably to nitroglycerin.

Severe coronary artery stenoses that greatly compromise flow through the coronary lumen may result in unstable angina, which is defined as angina that occurs with a recent (2-month) trend of increasing frequency or severity, or rest (preinfarction) angina, which occurs without provocation. Al-

ternatively, Prinzmetal or atypical angina may also occur at rest, but as a result of coronary spasm.[9] Coronary vasospasm typically occurs at or near a site of a fixed atherosclerotic lesion, and may occur as a result of plaque ulceration or thrombosis, or as a result of smooth muscle cell spasm caused by local production of serotonin, thromboxane, or other vasoactive substances.

Some patients, typically those with diabetes mellitus, may conversely experience silent ischemia without symptomotology. These patients may be at an increased risk for a catastrophic cardiac event because of the lack of an "early warning system" of angina that allows the halting of provocative stress events and thus the limitation of myocardial ischemia.

Electrocardiographic (ECG) confirmation of myocardial ischemia is essential in confirming that chest pain or related symptomotology in fact represents a myocardial ischemic event. Typical ECG changes consistent with ischemia include ST-segment depression or T-wave inversion. Diagnostic management of the stable patient presenting with angina may include assessment of myocardial flow reserves by one of several provocative tests that induce ischemia by increasing myocardial oxygen demand (Fig. 45.4). Abnormal responses to these screening tests, or a presentation of rest or unstable angina, most likely should result in the performance of coronary angiography that will permit the exact identification of coronary pathology. A presentation of rest or unstable angina will also most likely necessitate interventional therapy, as discussed next.

MYOCARDIAL INFARCTION (MI)

While ischemia can usually be viewed as a graded result of gradual lumen encroachment by a progressively enlarging atheromatous plaque, myocardial infarction typically results from total or near-total occlusion of an epicardial coronary artery by plaque rupture or intraluminal thrombosis.[8] Cholesterol emboli may cause downstream occlusions as well.

Although myocardial contractility is severely diminished within a few minutes of the cessation of blood flow, subsequent myocardial injury is fully reversible for up to 20 min following the onset of ischemia. After about 1 h of profound ischemia, isolated myocyte necrosis progresses to confluent subendocardial necrosis, which then spreads toward the subepicardium. Transmural infarction characteristically ensues after 6 h of coronary occlusion.

An acute coronary occlusion that results in transmural infarction in the region supplied by the occluded vessel is typically diagnosed in the setting of protracted angina or associated symptoms such as nausea, diaphoresis or shortness of breath, and appropriate ECG changes. Development of ST elevation and subsequent ST normalization, T-wave inversion, and, importantly, Q waves, can be anticipated in the ECG leads corresponding to the site of a transmural infarction. In contrast, a subendocardial infarction is typically caused by episodes of perfusion–demand mismatch in a territory supplied by a subtotally occluded or partially collateralized vessel, and is characterized by ST depression, T-wave inversion, and the absence of a Q wave.

Laboratory confirmation of MI is made by demonstration of a rise in serum markers of myocardial injury, most notably creatinine phosphokinase (CPK) in association with a prominent myocardial (MB) fraction. CPK-MB fractions typically

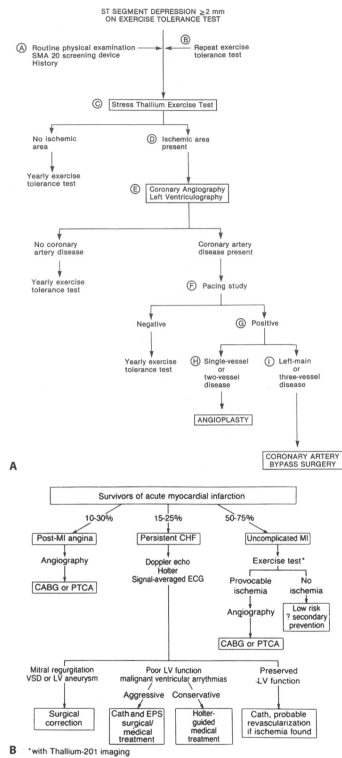

FIGURE 45.4. Typical algorithms for workup of patients with (**A**) stable ischemia pattern, or (**B**) following acute myocardial infarction. (Reproduced with permission from Cohn LH, et al. Decision Making in Cardiothoracic Surgery. Toronto: BC Decker, 1987.)

rise within a few hours after MI and peak 8 to 24 h later. Increases in lactate dehydrogenase (LDH) typically peak over the succeeding 48 to 72 h. Recently, the use of blood troponin assays has been espoused as a more rapid and accurate means of diagnosing MI.[10]

Sudden cardiac death due to ventricular arrhythmias will occur immediately or within the first 24 to 48 h after MI in 20% of patients. This complication can usually be treated or prevented with acute antiarrhythmic medications, and the risk of this complication characteristically resolves within 48 h.

ISCHEMIC CARDIOMYOPATHY

The combination of a series of small infarcts alone or in combination with one or several larger MIs may lead to progressive loss of viable myocytes and degeneration of ventricular contractility. Alternatively, myocytes that are viable but nonfunctioning or "hibernating" due to inadequate blood supply may also contribute to LV dysfunction.[11] The development of heart failure in this setting has been termed ischemic cardiomyopathy. Heart failure may be characterized by fatigue and/or shortness of breath with exertion or even at rest, caused by, respectively, diminished cardiac output (forward failure) and increased left ventricular end diastolic pressure (LVEDP), which is transmitted back into the pulmonary circulation and results in pulmonary congestion (backward failure).

Medical Treatment of CAD

The improvement of coronary blood flow and the decrease of myocardial oxygen demands are the cornerstones of medical therapy for CAD. Efficacy of medical therapy can usually be judged on the basis of relief of angina. The three major drug groups used to treat myocardial ischemia are the nitrates which cause vascular smooth muscle cell relaxation and dilitation, beta blockers which decrease heart rate and contractility, and calcium channel blockers which cause arterial vasodilation, as well as the anticholesterol medications used to limit, halt, or reverse the progression of atherosclerotic plaques.

Progression from an ischemic pattern to an infarction event typically signifies acute coronary thrombosis and is treated by prompt administration of a thrombolytic agent such as urokinase, streptokinase, or tissue plasminogen activator (TPA), with or without heparin. A number of studies have demonstrated that these agents dramatically decrease the mortality associated with acute MI[12–16] if given within 6 h of the onset of symptoms. Contraindications to thrombolytic therapy include anemia, recent surgery or bleeding diatheses, such as peptic ulcer disease, or a recent cerebrovascular accident (CVA).

Percutaneous transluminal coronary angioplasty (PTCA), whereby the atherosclerotic coronary plaque can be dilated by a balloon catheter placed over a guidewire under fluoroscopic guidance via a peripheral artery, together with the more recent introduction of coronary stent technology and sophisticated poststent antiplatelet therapy, represent critically important tools in the treatment of CAD.[17–21] Recent studies in fact suggest better outcomes in patients with acute MI with this interventional therapy than with thrombolytic therapy.[22,23]

Surgical Treatment of CAD

INDICATIONS FOR CABG VERSUS PTCA

Three major trials comparing coronary artery bypass graft (CABG) to medical therapy for CAD were conducted in the 1970s during the early days of coronary surgery: the Coronary

TABLE 45.1.

The Coronary Artery Bypass Trials.

Study	Number of patients	Years of enrollment	Operative mortality (%)	Five-year survival[a]	
				Medical	Surgical
VA Cooperative[26]	686	1972–1974	5.8	64[b]	80[b]
European Cooperative Surgical Study[27–29]	768	1973–1976	3.3	82	94
Coronary Artery Surgery Study (CASS)[24]	780	1974–1979	1.4	74	92

[a]For patients with LVEF > 50%, triple-vessel disease, Class III–IV.

[b]30-month survival for patients with left main disease.

Source: Modified from Cohn LH. Coronary artery disease and the indications for coronary revascularization. In: Baue AE, Geha AS, Hammond, et al., eds, Glenn's Thoracic and Cardiovascular Surgery, Fifth Edition, New York: McGraw-Hill Companies, 1991.

Artery Surgery Study (CASS), the VA study, and the European study[24–29] (Table 45.1). These studies represent the cornerstone of the accepted indications for CABG to this day, despite the fact that the relevance of these studies has been limited by the subsequent evolution of surgical techniques, including the increased use of the internal mammary artery (IMA) as a bypass graft, the decreased operative mortality rates characteristic of current CABG surgery, and limitations in the designs of these studies, including high crossover rates, nonuniformity of data collection, and inclusion–exclusion criteria that do not reflect current indications.

Significant coronary obstruction was generally defined in these studies as at least a 50% narrowing in luminal diameter on coronary angiography, and extent of disease was defined as "single, double or triple vessel disease" based upon the number of major coronary artery territories (LAD, CX, or RCA) involved. Based upon long-term survival rates for CABG versus medical therapy in these studies, coronary bypass surgery became indicated for patients with more than 50% narrowing of the left main coronary artery, patients with triple-vessel disease and evidence of left-ventricular dysfunction, or patients with angina and double-vessel disease including the proximal LAD (Table 45.2). In contrast, no survival benefit was conferred by CABG in patients with lesser degrees of single- or double-vessel disease, and medical treatment or interventional therapy (PTCA/stent) has become indicated for these cases.

PTCA with stenting, as appropriate, can be expected to be initially successful in more than 90% of appropriately selected patients with a 1-3% complication rate.[19–21,30] Contraindications to PTCA/stenting generally include left main disease and complex or calcified lesions, especially those that occur at branch points.

The Duke study of PTCA versus CABG summarized the field as follows[31]: (1) increasing extent of CAD decreases survival whatever the intervention, although to a greater extent with medical therapy compared with CABG; (2) the greatest differences in survival between groups are found in patients with the greatest extent of disease; (3) CABG improves survival compared with medical therapy in patients with at least 95% stenosis of the LAD, and survival increases with increasing severity of CAD; (4) CABG improves survival compared to PTCA in patients with at least "double-vessel" disease with 95% stenosis of the proximal LAD.

OPERATIVE PROCEDURE

PREOPERATIVE MANAGEMENT

Aside from the preoperative considerations common to any surgical procedure, obligatory preoperative assessments for CABG include an examination of coronary anatomy in terms of the severity of the stenoses and suitability of the distal vessels for bypass, determination of left-ventricular ejection fraction, and presence or absence of valvular heart disease. This information can be gathered from the cardiac catheterization,

TABLE 45.2. Indications for Coronary Artery Bypass Graft (CABG).

Anatomical/physiological indications
    Left main stenosis >50%
    Three-vessel disease with impaired LV function
    Three-vessel disease with normal LV function but with inducible ischemia on physiological testing
    Two-vessel disease including proximal LAD
    Cardiogenic shock with appropriate angiographic indications
    Positive physiological studies or significant coronary stenosis before major cardiac or noncardiac surgery
    Congenital coronary anomalies associated with sudden death

Clinical indications
    Unstable or Class III–IV angina refractory to medical therapy (including PTCA/stenting)
    Postinfarction angina with appropriate angiographic indications
    Failed PTCA with acute ischemia/hemodynamic instability
    Acute myocardial infarction <6 h with thrombolytic/PTCA therapy contraindicated

Source: Modified from Bojar RM. Adult Cardiac Surgery. Blackwell Science, Inc.: Boston, 1992, with permission.

with the addition of echocardiography, if needed. Additional useful information in terms of the presence of a calcified or extensively atherosclerotic aorta can be obtained from chest X-ray (CXR), cath, or transesophageal echo, and may influence operative risk and the approach to cannulation and clamping of the aorta.

The severity of the coronary stenoses alerts the surgical team as to the risk of hemodynamic instability or arrhythmias during induction; the ejection fraction similarly determines the likelihood of a difficult postbypass course and the potential need for pharmacological or mechanical ventricular support. To help enhance perioperative hemodynamic stability, cardiac medications, including any prescribed antiplatelet agents, are usually continued up to the time of surgery.

The nature of the coronary disease including the extent of distal disease may suggest the need for additional length of conduit and specify the quality and type of conduit needed; for example, an IMA is more likely than a poor-quality saphenous vein to remain patent when grafted to a small, diffusely diseased LAD.

Determination of the presence of a symptomatic bruit or symptoms of carotid disease is a critical component of the preoperative evaluation. Such findings generally indicate the need for Doppler ultrasound to evaluate the carotid and cerebral vasculature and will possibly warrant carotid surgery in the presence of severe stenoses or symptomatology. With moderate disease, higher on-bypass perfusion pressures may be indicated.[32]

Finally, as with any open-heart procedure, bleeding parameters and potential for coagulopathy should be assessed because of the need for intraoperative heparinization and the coagulopathy sometimes associated with CPB. Patients with significant respiratory compromise should be considered for preoperative pulmonary care, cigarette smoking should be discontinued if possible, and attention should be directed toward improving the nutritional status of the patient.

STANDARD OPERATIVE TECHNIQUE

Routine hemodynamic monitoring usually includes the use of an arterial pressure measuring line, a pulmonary artery (Swan–Ganz) catheter (a central venous line can be substituted in low-risk patients), and a urinary bladder catheter. Adequate oxygenation and maintenance of a stable blood pressure, avoiding hypotension or hypertension, are critical to avoiding ischemia during the initial anesthetic induction period. Nitrates and/or beta blockers may be useful in this setting. Rarely, in the high-risk patient, such as those with a severe left main obstruction or with severely compromised ventricular function, an intraaortic balloon pump (IABP) may be placed to provide cardiac support.

With a standard approach, the heart is exposed through a median sternotomy, followed by systemic heparinization and aortic and atrial cannulation, as described previously. Conduit for performing the bypass is harvested simultaneously to the initial stages of accessing the heart, and may include preparing one or both internal mammary arteries, saphenous vein, or radial arteries. Alternative, lesser utilized conduits include lesser saphenous vein, cephalic vein, gastroepiploic artery, inferior epigastric artery, or cadaveric vein, although the use of these latter conduits is usually limited by poor patency or technical difficulties with use. The use of the radial artery has also recently been popularized.

CPB is initiated once appropriate conduit is harvested. Once

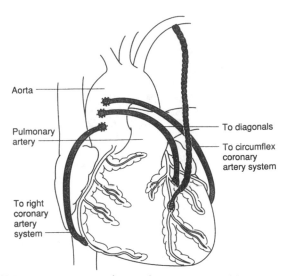

FIGURE 45.5. Depiction of typical arrangement of bypass grafts in patient undergoing coronary artery bypass surgery, including left internal mammary artery to the left anterior descending and saphenous vein grafts. (Reproduced with permission from Greenfield LO, et al. Surgery, Second Edition. Philadelphia: Lippincott-Raven, 1997.)

bypass has been initiated, the surgeon usually identifies and marks the coronary arteries selected for grafting from preoperative angiographic studies. To institute cardiac arrest, the aorta is cross-clamped and approximately 10 to 15 ml/kg of a cardioplegic solution is delivered via the aortic cardioplegia catheter, sometimes with supplemental retrograde cardioplegia delivered via a coronary sinus catheter. This step is usually supplemented by topical cooling and systemic hypothermia to 28° to 32°C.

Once the heart is arrested, distal anastamoses are typically performed by making a linear arteriotomy approximately 6 mm in length in the appropriate coronary artery (Fig. 45.5). Occasionally, distal coronary artery disease is so diffuse or severe that an endarterectomy is performed, in which the atherosclerotic core of the coronary is excised. Graft occlusion or vessel restenosis appears to be more common with this technique compared with standard grafting, and coronary endarterectomy is therefore not routinely performed.

The heart is allowed to rewarm with cross-clamp removal once the distal anastamoses are completed. Once the proximal anastamoses are completed and hemostasis verified, the patient is then weaned from CPB, heparin is reversed with protamine, and the cannulae are removed. Temporary epicardial atrial and ventricular pacing wires are placed, and the sternum reapproximated with stainless steel wires.

OFF PUMP CORONARY ARTERY BYPASS (OPCAB)

In performing an OPCAB or "beating heart" procedure, either through a partial or complete median sternotomy or through a mini-thoracotomy, anastamoses on the coronary arteries are performed utilizing one of several available types of stabilizing devices with occlusive coronary snares or an intracoronary shunt placed to limit blood flow into the area of the anastamosis. The LAD and diagonal coronary arteries are most easily approached with the OPCAB technique. The heart lung machine is not used with OPCAB and cardiopulmonary function is maintained throughout the procedure. Approximately 20% of coronary bypass procedures in the United States are today permormed "off-pump."

"HEARTPORT"

The "Heartport" technique approaches the heart through a limited anterior thoracotomy and utilizes femoral arterial and venous or other direct access cannulae, with the use of an intraaortic balloon occluder to deliver cardioplegia and arrest the heart. Long-term results are still awaited, but patency results appear to be similar to standard technique.[33]

REOPERATIONS

Compared to first-time cardiac procedures, reoperations pose a number of technical challenges that include avoiding myocardial injury when redividing the sternum and dissecting through scar tissue, provision of adequate myocardial preservation despite the presence of diffuse atherosclerotic disease, and finding appropriate target vessels in the absence of appropriate landmarks and surface features. These risks result in an approximate threefold increase in mortality for reoperations compared to previous procedures.

POSTOPERATIVE CARE

One of the primary focuses of the postoperative care of any patient undergoing open-heart surgery must be the maintenance of a cardiac output sufficient to provide adequate systemic perfusion. To facilitate this care, the patient's first 12 to 24 h following open-heart surgery are usually spent in an intensive care unit with a pulmonary artery catheter, arterial line, and urinary bladder catheter in place to assist monitoring.

In the usual event of an uncomplicated postoperative course, patients may be extubated within 6-12 h of surgery, and with "fast-track" protocols now may be extubated within a few hours of surgery.[34] Care following the first 12 to 24 h usually includes pharmacological diuresis to eliminate fluid accumulation that is a by-product of CPB, aggressive pulmonary toilet, and progressive ambulation. Most patients are discharged on beta blockers, nitrates, digoxin (to help prevent atrial arrythmias, which occur in 25%–30% of patients), and aspirin, as well as antiulcer medications to avoid stress gastrointestinal bleeds.

Given the coagulopathy associated with CPB and the need for full systemic heparinization during CPB, excessive bleeding is a unique and critical potential complication following open-heart surgery. High-dose epsilon aminocaproic acid (Amikar) or aprotinin are often utilized intraoperatively in low- and high-bleeding-risk patients, respectively, to minimize the coagulopathy associated with CPB.[35] Bleeding is assessed by chest tube output postoperatively, and algorithms exist to treat with coagulation factors as appropriate. Usually, bleeding in excess of 100 ml/h after the first several hours requires transfusion of platelets, followed by fresh frozen plasma if bleeding persists. Bleeding in excess of 1000 ml in primary operations requires return to the OR (Fig. 45.6). In the absence of significant bleeding, most surgeons utilize low-dose aspirin starting immediately postoperatively to enhance graft patency rates. This precaution may be particularly important in OPCAB patients in whom coagulation function is not depressed by the effects of CPB.

Elevation of central venous pressure in the setting of low cardiac output, falling systemic blood pressures, or decreased urine output may indicate cardiac tamponade from accumulation of blood in the pericardium. A central venous pressure above 20 mmHg and/or echocardiographic evidence of pericardial fluid with or without right-ventricular compression are typical but not pathognomonic signs of tamponade, and tamponade can occur without these findings. The diagnosis of postoperative cardiac tamponade invariably requires urgent reexploration.

Occasionally, large pericardial effusions can also be associated with postcardiotomy syndrome, an inflammatory process that presents with unexplained fevers or leukocytosis, chest pain, pericardial friction rub, or diffuse ST/T wave changes. This syndrome can usually be treated with nonsteroidal antiinflammatory agents or steroids, but can also necessitate pericardial drainage.

Aside from the complications associated with CPB itself, other complications associated with CABG include sternal or leg wound infections and mediastinitis.

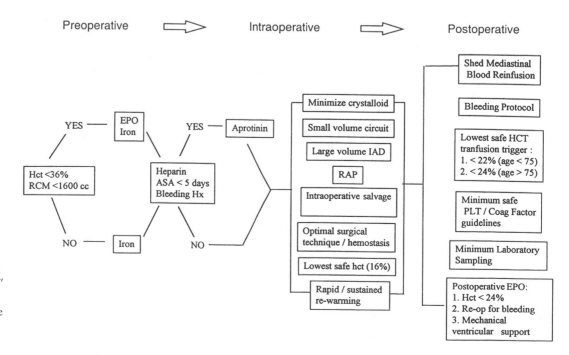

FIGURE 45.6. Algorithm for blood conservation utilizing a "multimodality approach." (Reproduced with permission from Helm RE, Rosengart TK, Klemperer JD, et al. Comprehensive multimodality blood conservation: 100 consecutive CABG operations without transfusion.[35])

OUTCOMES

A number of large databases have been established that accurately allocate the risk associated with CABG as a function of a large number of patient risk parameters. Left-ventricular ejection fraction remains one of the most significant of the many risk factors assigned a relative value in predicting the outcome of CABG. The presence of congestive heart failure or shock were among the leading predictors of operative mortality in multivariate logistic regression analysis. Acuity of operations, female gender, the presence of renal failure or previous neurological events, or the need to perform additional procedures such as mitral valve replacement are other significant risk predictors for operative mortality following CABG. Reoperation is an important predictor of operative mortality, probably both because of the increased incidence of incomplete revascularization in these cases, itself a short- and long-term survival risk factor, but also because of attendant risk factors including acuity of operation, ejection fraction, advanced patient age, and more advanced atherosclerotic disease.[36,37] The risk of inadvertent embolization from diseased grafts and the risk of myocardial injury during dissection through scar tissue are perceived but unproven risks in the reoperative setting as well.

LONG-TERM OUTCOME

The main benefits of CABG include the relief of angina refractory to medical therapy and, as demonstrated in the original CABG trials, increased survival. It should be noted that although patients with the most severe angina receive the greatest benefit in terms of symptomatic relief and improvement in quality of life, the degree of preoperative angina is generally unrelated to survival benefits. Patients with silent ischemia, for example, can be expected to have survival benefits similar to those with symptoms.

Most CABG trials have demonstrated short-term angina relief in greater than 90% of patients. In contrast, because of graft attrition and progression of native vessel disease, only 50% of patients receiving saphenous vein grafts alone are ischemia free at 10 years and only 15% are symptom free at 15 years.[38] In contrast, IMA patency rates are 95% at 1 year, 94% at 8 years, and 85% at 10 years.[39] With increased use of the internal mammary artery, at least 70% of patients can be expected to be symptom free at 10 years.[39] It is therefore anticipated that the long-term benefits of CABG will improve with greater use of the internal mammary artery and other arterial conduits in the years to come. Long-term results with arterial conduits other than the left IMA have, however, been somewhat mixed.

Long-term survival post CABG in the three original prospective CABG trials was 58% at 11 years in the VA study, 71% at 12 years in the European study, and 87% at 8 years in the CASS study. Long-term survival at 8 years was better for CABG than medical therapy in the CASS study in patients with appropriate indications, such as those with decreased ejection fraction and triple-vessel disease, but those differences dissipated at longer follow-up, probably because of the attrition of saphenous grafts.

The survival rate for primary CABG patients has more recently been reported to be 90% at 5 years, 80% at 10 years, and 60% at 15 years. In contrast, a recent study of long-term survival of medically treated patients from the CASS study

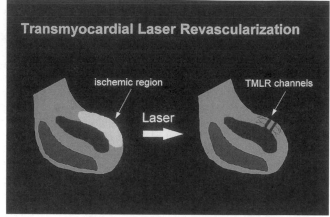

FIGURE 45.7. Schematic of conceptual basis of transmyocardial laser revascularization (TMR), with transmural channels and/or laser-induced neovasculature contributing to perfusion of ischemic territory.

revealed a 12-year survival of only 40% in the presence of triple-vessel disease.[40]

Nonbypass Revascularization

Apart from traditional means of revascularizing the myocardium via direct coronary artery grafting beyond major epicardial obstructions, recent techniques providing "biological revascularization" are under investigation. The first of these techniques, transmyocardial laser revascularization (TMR), which was approved by the FDA in 1998, is thought to provide oxygenated blood from the left ventricle to the ischemic myocardium through transmural channels lased in the area of ischemia (Fig. 45.7).[41] In actuality, it remains controversial whether TMR channels remain patent, or whether TMR in fact is upregulating the expression of endogenous growth factors that induce new blood vessel formation, or angiogenesis.[42,43] As an alternative to TMR, a number of investigators are attempting to enhance collateral development by instilling one of several known growth factors, or angiogens, that have been demonstrated to induce angiogenesis.[44-46]

Other Complications of CAD

Mechanical complications of myocardial infarction include free wall rupture of the ventricle, papillary muscle rupture, ventricular septal defect, formation of ventricular aneurysm, and mitral valvular regurgitation caused by postinfarction conformational changes in the mitral apparatus. These changes may each occur in the acute period following myocardial infarction or develop in the chronic remodeling phase of infarct healing. Surgical intervention is usually indicated when clinical manifestations such as tamponade, congestive heart failure, or arrhythmias present and lead to further diagnostic evaluation.

Valvular Heart Disease

Anatomy of the Cardiac Valves

The two atrioventricular valves, the right-sided tricuspid valve and the left-sided bicuspid, or mitral valve, so named

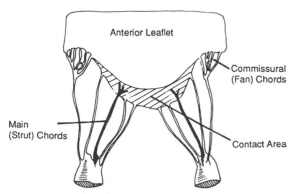

FIGURE 45.8. Schematic of the anatomical makeup of the atrioventricular valves, including the papillary muscles (*bottom*), chordae, and leaflets, as represented by the anterior leaflet of the mitral valve. (Reproduced with permission from Baue AE, Geha AS, Holland GL, et al., eds. Glenn's Thoracic and Cardiovascular Surgery, Fifth Edition. New York: McGraw-Hill Companies, 1991.)

because of the number of their constituent leaflets, prevent reflux of blood from the ventricle to the atrium during ventricular systole. Each valve is made up of a collagenous core lined by endocardium. The leaflets, or cusps, of each valve are continuous with the surrounding annulus fibrosus and meet at attachments called commissures. The chordae tendinae tether the free edges of each of the valve leaflets to the intraventricular papillary muscles, thus preventing reflux during ventricular contraction.

The tricuspid valve consists of a large anterior leaflet, a posterior leaflet at the right margin of the heart, and a smaller, septal leaflet attached to the interventricular septum. The mitral valve consists of a large anterior (aortic) leaflet and a smaller posterior (mural) leaflet (Fig. 45.8). The anterior and posterior mitral valve leaflets are in continuity with the posterior wall of the aorta and the posterior wall of the heart and the AV groove, respectively.

The two anatomically similar semilunar valves, the aortic and pulmonic, bridge the outlets of the two ventricles. "Semilunar" describes the shape of the three valvules, or cusps, comprising the valve overlying the valve orifice. The valvules are attached at their base to the valve annulus, and are attached to each other at the commissures. As opposed to the complex AV valve apparatus, the aortic and mitral leaflets and their annuli comprise the entirety of the valve structure. The left and right coronary sinuses, found above the corresponding valve cusp, give rise to the left and right coronary arteries via ostia in these sinuses, while the third, noncoronary sinus is located posteromedially. Important surgical relationships are the positions of the left and noncoronary cusps of the aortic valve, which are in continuity with the anterior mitral valve leaflet, and the right cusp, which is situated atop the interventricular septum and the conduction system.

Pathology of Valvular Heart Disease

Rheumatic heart disease (RHD) has until recently been the most common cause of heart valve dysfunction and the most common cause of multivalvular disease, but with more pervasive medical therapy of streptococcal infections, the incidence of RHD is undergoing continual decline. RHD most commonly affects the mitral valve, and is by far the most

TABLE 45.3. Prevalent Etiologies of Valvular Heart Disease.

Mitral Stenosis
  Valvular
    Rheumatic disease
    Nonrheumatic disease
      Infective endocarditis
      Congenital mitral stenosis
      Single papillary muscle (parachute valve)
      Mitral annual calcification
  Supravalvular
    Myxoma
    Left atrial thrombus

Mitral Insufficiency
  Valvular
    Rheumatic fever
    Endocarditis
    Systemic lupus erythematosis
    Congenital
      Cleft leaflet (isolated)
      Endocardial cushion defect
    Connective tissue disorders
  Annular
    Degeneration
    Dilation
  Subvalvular
    Chordae tendinae
      Endocarditis
      Myocardial infarction
      Connective tissue disorder
      Rheumatic disease
    Papillary muscle
      Dysfunction or rupture
      Ischemia or infarction
      Endocarditis
      Inflammatory disorder
    Malalignment
      Left ventricular dilation
      Cardiomyopathy

Aortic Stenosis[a]
  Acquired
    Rheumatic disease
    Degenerative (fibrocalcific) disease
      Tricuspid valve
      Congenital bicuspid valve
    Infective endocarditis
  Congenital
    Tricuspid valve with commissural fusion
    Unicuspid unicommissural valve
    Hypoplastic annulus

Aortic Insufficiency
  Valvular
    Rheumatic disease
    Congenital
    Endocarditis
    Connective tissue disorder (Marfan's)
  Annular
    Connective tissue disorders (Marfan's)
    Aortic dissection
    Hypertension
    Inflammatory disease (e.g., ankylosing spondylitis)

[a]Excludes subvalvular and supravalvular processes.

common cause of mitral stenosis (Table 45.3). Nonrheumatic etiologies now supercede RHD as the most common cause of heart valve insufficiency.

Pathophysiology and Clinical Presentation

Dramatic changes in cardiac structure and function that compensate for the volume and pressure overload stresses im-

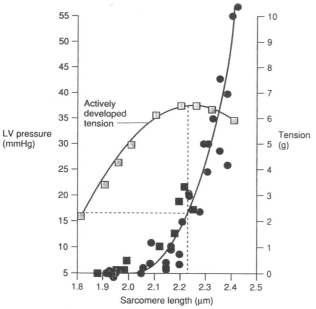

FIGURE 45.9. The Frank–Starling curve. Left-ventricular contractility (pressure or tension) increases as a function of volume loading (sarcomere length) at end diastole. *Lower curve* depicts resting ventricular pressures, representing ventricular compliance relationship. (After Spotnitz JH, Sonnenblick FH, Spiro D. Relationship of ultrastructure to function in the intact heart: sarcomere structure relative to pressure volume curves of the intact left ventricles of dog and cat. Circ Res 1996;18:57, with permission.)

posed on the heart by valvular dysfunction allow individuals with progressing valvular heart disease to persist in an asymptomatic state for many years. The mechanisms that compensate for the hemodynamic derangements associated with valvular heart disease include atrial and/or ventricular chamber enlargement, shifts along the pressure–function relation [Frank–Starling curve (Fig. 45.9)], myocardial hypertrophy, and increased adrenergic stimulation.

Eventually, pressure and volume stresses exceed the reserves provided by the cardiac compensatory mechanisms, and congestive heart failure (CHF) ensues. Heart failure may be characterized by fatigue and/or shortness of breath with exertion or even at rest, caused by, respectively, diminished cardiac output (forward failure) and increased LVEDP, which is transmitted back into the pulmonary circulation and results in pulmonary congestion (backward failure).

Mitral Stenosis

Hemodynamic sequelae of mitral stenosis develop only with reduction of the normal mitral valve orifice area (4–6 cm²) to an area of 2 cm². Critical mitral stenosis develops at an orifice area of 1 cm². Changes in cardiac output result in a disproportionate change in transmitral gradient and LA pressure. Increased loading of the atrium caused by the pressure gradient imposed by MS eventually results in LA dilatation. Atrial fibrillation (AF) eventually develops as a consequence of atrial dilatation and associated fibrosis and disorganization of atrial fibers, which leads to disparate atrial conduction times and refractory periods. These abnormalities allow the develop-

ment of ectopic foci and reentrant circuits that ultimately degenerate into supraventricular tachyarrhythmias and AF.

As opposed to the effects of MS on atrial function, mitral stenosis does not generally cause left-ventricular compromise. When cardiac output is reduced, it is usually caused by decreased preload because of slow filling through the stenotic valve rather than depressed myocardial contractility. In longstanding mitral stenosis, however, pulmonary artery (PA) pressure can exceed systemic pressure. At PA pressures greater than 70 mmHg, impedance to the right heart outflow frequently results in right-sided heart failure, which may be associated with right-ventricular dilation, tricuspid insufficiency, and even pulmonic insufficiency. Further decreases in left heart preload result, and a low cardiac output syndrome can develop.

Aortic Stenosis

The pathophysiological sequelae of aortic valve stenosis develop with a decrease in the normal aortic valve orifice size (2.6–3.5 cm²) to an area of 1 cm². Pressure loading of the ventricle caused by valvular obstruction leads to myocardial sarcomere replication and myocardial hypertrophy. Eventually, myocardial hypertrophy leads to significantly decreased ventricular compliance, increased LVEDP, and pulmonary congestion.

Angina pectoris develops in two-thirds of patients with severe aortic stenosis. Syncope occurs in 25% of symptomatic aortic stenosis patients and is probably due to arterial hypotension and decreased cerebral perfusion caused by the presence of a flow limiting obstruction. Finally, heart failure develops in patients with AS once maximal LV hypertrophy is achieved. Failure develops as an adequate pressure gradient and systolic ejection across the stenotic aortic orifice can no longer be maintained. Right-sided heart failure follows as pulmonary hypertension causes an increase in right-sided afterload. Death occurs in 10% to 20% of patients secondary to congestive heart failure. Sudden death, possibly secondary to arrhythmia, is responsible for mortality in most of the remainder of cases.

Aortic Insufficiency

As opposed to the pressure-loading strain of aortic stenosis, aortic insufficiency produces a volume-loading strain on the left ventricle, caused by the regurgitant flow returning through the aortic root. The volume-loaded ventricle empties more efficiently and completely than normal, as dictated by the principles of the Frank–Starling curve, compensating somewhat for the net loss of forward cardiac output corresponding to the regurgitant fraction. Increased diastolic loading of the ventricle eventually results in excessive LV chamber enlargement.

LV compliance remains relatively high until late in the course of AI, despite the degree of ventricular hypertrophy present, and LVEDP remains low. Ultimately, however, gradual myocardial decompensation progresses in patients with AI, often before the onset of symptoms. Limitations in cardiac output ultimately produce symptoms of fatigue and weakness when stroke volume plateaus with end-stage disease. At this point, any additional regurgitant flow cannot be ejected. LVEDP rises, net forward flow decreases, and cardiac failure ensues.

MITRAL REGURGITATION

Because LV chamber pressure exceeds LA pressure well before it reaches aortic root pressure, up to one-half of the ejected LV volume can be ejected through the incompetent mitral valve before the aortic valve has even opened. Thus, as with AI, MR results in the net forward flow of only a portion of the ejected ventricular end-diastolic volume. Unlike AI, systolic unloading of the LV into the low-pressure atrium allows enhanced ventricular emptying during systole. "Normal" ejection fractions and fractional shortening ratios in MR patients may thus actually reflect severe LV dysfunction. With progression, dilatation of the left atrium and ventricle causes dilatation of the mitral valve orifice, which interferes with proper coaptation of the mitral valve leaflets and worsening MR. Eventually, a point of maximal systolic ejection is reached and increasing regurgitant diastolic filling of the ventricle in the face of fixed forward ejection results in an increase in end-diastolic volumes. A cycle of deterioration in function and worsening MR eventually ensues, and pulmonary hypertension, pulmonary hypertrophy, and right-ventricular dysfunction may develop as well.

RIGHT-SIDED AND COMBINED VALVULAR DYSFUNCTION

Right-sided valvular disease is similar to left-sided disease in terms of the pathophysiology of these processes, except that elevated right-atrial pressure results in systemic venous hypertension rather than pulmonary congestion. Right-sided dysfunction may thus be manifested by ascites, jaundice, and other stigmata of cirrhosis, as well as peripheral edema or abdominal swelling.

Tricuspid regurgitation, the predominant form of right-sided valve pathology, is primarily caused by the right-ventricular dilatation secondary to left-sided disease and develops in a manner analogous to similar mechanisms causing MR. Tricuspid stenosis, although rarely seen, can produce symptoms of systemic venous hypertension with a tricuspid valve gradient as small as 5 mmHg. Significant hemodynamic sequelae of pulmonary valve dysfunction are rare in the setting of acquired heart disease.

Diagnosis of Valvular Heart Disease

Despite the recent introduction of advanced diagnostic techniques, the initial assessment of patients with valvular heart disease still depends on a careful history and physical examination, which will reveal important information regarding not only the kind of valvular disease present, but also the severity, duration, and prognosis of the dysfunction. Data obtained from the chest roentgenogram and 12-lead electrocardiogram (ECG); M-mode, two-dimensional (2-D), and color Doppler echocardiography; the flow-directed PA catheter; and, ultimately, cardiac catheterization provide additional data.

Auscultation is a critical diagnostic tool for detecting and differentiating between the various forms of valvular dysfunction. The midsystolic murmur of aortic stenosis produced by turbulent, high-velocity flow across the narrowed aortic valve is heard best at the base of the heart and usually radiates to both carotid arteries. MR is characterized by a constant, blowing holosystolic murmur characteristically heard best at the apex and usually radiating to the axilla. A high-

pitched, decrescendo *diastolic* murmur that is best heard in expiration at the left sternal border with the patient leaning forward is found in patients with AI. In contrast, an opening snap, accentuated S1, and a diastolic rumble with presystolic accentuation heard best at the apex is diagnostic of MS (although the auscultory findings of MS may vary widely). Finally, the pansystolic murmur of tricuspid regurgitation is localized more to the left lower sternal border and tends to increase with inspiration (Carvallo sign) compared with the other systolic murmurs.

Objective electrocardiographic data provide further evidence of the extent of valvular heart disease by demonstration, for example, of increased QRS voltage or an LV strain pattern associated with LV hypertrophy, left-axis deviation secondary to ventricular chamber enlargement, or "p" wave changes with or without a hypertrophic pattern indicative of LA enlargement.

The routine posteroanterior and lateral chest roentgenograms may provide nonspecific information about valvular calcification, cardiac chamber enlargement, and pulmonary congestion that may help in assessing the physiological impact of valvular heart disease. Radionuclide scintography yields visual and numeric data regarding cardiac function that can be assessed serially to follow progression of disease. Of all the noninvasive studies now available, however, cardiac echocardiography has revolutionized the diagnosis of valvular heart disease. M-mode and 2-D echocardiography allow real-time assessment of chamber size, wall thickness, and valve appearance and motion. 2-D echo with color Doppler overlay now provides physiological data at the bedside regarding blood flow across stenotic or regurgitant valves.

Cardiac catheterization still remains the only methodology allowing direct and exact measurement of intracardiac pressures and valve gradients. Pressure gradients across stenotic valves are determined by pullback of the catheter from one chamber to the next or, preferably, by simultaneous pressure measurements with catheters placed in each chamber. Valve cross-sectional areas are determined by the Gorlin equations. These equations are derived from basic hydrodynamic equation, flow = pressure/resistance.

Medical Management of Valvular Heart Disease

CONGESTIVE HEART FAILURE

Enhancement of cardiac function in patients with congestive failure secondary to valvular dysfunction is directed toward optimizing the three primary determinants of ventricular function: preload, afterload, and myocardial contractility (see Fig. 45.9). Increased preload, or ventricular filling, is an important compensatory mechanism in patients with ventricular failure in that increased volume loading of the ventricle in end-diastole shifts ventricular contractility rightward on the Frank–Starling curve. On the other hand, this increase in preload, which is produced by a decrease in water clearance by the kidney, comes at the expense of an increase in total body water and increased total intravascular volume, which in turn may result in edema formation and pulmonary congestion. Excessive preload is therefore lowered with diuretics, such as furosemide, and venodilator agents, such as nitroglycerin, and can effectively improve the symptoms of

CHF as well as myocardial performance. Excessive reduction in preload, however, deprives the ventricle of filling volumes needed to maintain effective contraction and thus must be avoided. Careful clinical and hemodynamic monitoring of the patient after implementation of therapy is thus mandatory.

Afterload reduction is directed toward lowering the resistance against which the heart must eject, and is thus especially effective in patients with decreased cardiac output in the setting of increased systemic vascular resistance. Afterload reduction with vasodilator agents may also be optimally applied to enhance pressure gradients to the periphery in patients with AI or MR, although these patients may already have experienced an intrinsic decrease in vascular tone.

Afterload reduction can be accomplished with rapidly acting intravenous or oral arterial vasodilators, such as nitroprusside and hydralazine, respectively, or the angiotensin-converting enzyme inhibitors, represented by captopril and enalapril. In the same regard, vasoconstrictor agents such as norepinephrine bitartrate (Levophed) are generally contraindicated because they tend to increase afterload and exacerbate lesions such as AI.

Inotropic agents, which shift the ventricular function curve upward and to the left (see Fig. 45.9), produce more stroke work at any given level of filling, are another important class of drugs for treating heart failure. Improvement in cardiac function allows decreased ventricular filling and creates a greater cardiac reserve because the ventricle is able to function at a lower point on the Frank–Starling curve. Decreased levels of LVEDP lead to decreased pulmonary congestion and symptomatic improvement. Commonly used inotropes include digitalis, dopamine, dobutamine, and the newer agents, amrinone and milrinone.

Surgical Treatment of Valvular Disease

INDICATIONS FOR INTERVENTIONAL THERAPY

Intervention therapy for patients with valvular heart disease is generally indicated on demonstration of deterioration in ventricular function or development of progressing or refractory symptomotology. An inappropriate delay in definitive therapy can result in an increase in operative mortality and in diminished cardiac and functional improvement postoperatively.

The timing of surgery for aortic stenosis is well defined, as based upon the natural history of this disease. Mean survival after the onset of angina is about 5 years; with syncope, it is 3 years, and with heart failure, 2 years. Symptomatic patients with significant uncorrected aortic stenosis have 25% 1-year and 50% 2-year mortality rates.[47] Half these deaths are sudden. Operation is thus usually indicated for any symptoms, including emboli, as well as for a transvalvular gradient greater than or equal to 50 mmHg, and a calculated valve area less than or equal to $0.8 \text{ cm}^2/\text{m}^2$.

Intervention in individuals with MS is similarly usually indicated for "critical" mitral valve stenosis (mitral valve orifice less than $1 \text{ cm}^2/\text{m}^2$) or for any patient with symptoms. Systemic emboli, especially if recurrent, are also an indication for operation. Other parameters include a mean mitral valve gradient of 12 to 15 mmHg and an end-diastolic gradient of 8 to 10 mmHg. The onset of atrial fibrillation has also been suggested as an indication for intervention because prolonged atrial fibrillation seems to worsen the prognosis for patients with mitral stenosis. On the other hand, early operation does not appear to improve long-term survival in asymptomatic patients.

Symptoms may not develop until after irreversible myocardial dysfunction has occurred in patients with AI or MR, and thus the appropriate timing of intervention in these individuals is significantly more challenging than in patients with stenotic lesions. Proposed indications for operation for regurgitant lesions utilize noninvasive technologies such as radionuclide scanning and echo that allow serial assessments of LV function in attempting to guide intervention to the onset of LV dysfunction. For AI, these criteria include an end-systolic LV diameter larger than 55 mm and fractional shortening less than 30%, ejection fraction below 50%, and increases in LVEDV.[48] Along these same lines, operation may be indicated for severe AI, as indicated by a diastolic blood pressure of 50 mmHg, even in the asymptomatic patient. Similar criteria established for the timing of operation in MR patients include an ejection fraction less than 55%, or fractional shortening less than 30% with an end-diastolic diameter of 75 mm and an end-systolic diameter of 50 mm.[49]

Analogous to the indications for left-sided disease, correction of tricuspid valve stenosis is recommended for a tricuspid valve gradient of at least 5 mmHg or for the rare patient with symptomatic disease. Correction of isolated tricuspid regurgitation is usually indicated only in the presence of severe, symptomatic disease with clear physical stigmata.

OPTIONS IN INTERVENTIONAL THERAPY

Percutaneous balloon valvuloplasty is a new technique in which a high-pressure balloon catheter introduced via the femoral artery is inflated across a stenotic valve to dilate the obstructing lesion. Initial and intermediate-term results have been favorable for selected cases of mitral stenosis with limited valvular and subvalvular calcification and fibrosis, as determined by a standardized echocardiographic scoring system.[50] In contrast, percutaneous aortic balloon valvuloplasty suffers from a relatively high complication and recurrence rate, and is only occasionally indicated as a bridging technique in critically ill patients.[51]

For patients with critical mitral stenosis in whom balloon valvuloplasty is not indicated, open mitral commissurotomy can be successfully performed if there is limited calcification, leaflet stiffness, chordal fusion, or associated MR. Commissurotomy carries up to a 20% chance of reoperation within 5 years and a 60% chance at 10 years, but avoids the potential complications of a valve prosthesis during that time.[52] Although excellent long-term results can be expected in appropriately selected patients with degenerative pathology, results are less satisfactory for rheumatic and ischemic etiologies, and repair in these cases must be selected cautiously.

Finally, tricuspid valve annuloplasty is the preferred treatment for significant secondary tricuspid regurgitation, with valve replacement reserved for severe or primary disease. In summary, except for the specific instances just cited, correction of valvular heart disease nearly always requires replacement of the diseased valve with a valve prosthesis or heterograft.

PROSTHETIC VALVES

The ideal prosthetic heart valve should be durable, nonthrombogenic, resistant to infection, and technically easy to insert; it should possess an optimal hemodynamic profile and it should be subjectively acceptable to the patient. Despite the large number of valves that have been designed and introduced clinically over the past four decades, the ideal valve has not yet been developed. The two major classes of valves—the mechanical and the tissue valves (xenograft [porcine or bovine] or homograft [cadaveric human])—can be viewed as representing strengths in durability versus low thrombogenicity, respectively.

Based upon the relative advantages and disadvantages, mechanical valves are recommended for most patients. Tissue valves are generally preferred if life expectancy is less than 10 to 15 years, if there is a contraindication to coumadin administration, such as the presence of a known coagulation defect, history of gastrointestinal bleeding or similar source of potential bleeding, if there is a likelihood of exposure to potential trauma, or if pregnancy is anticipated. Tissue valves are also considered if there are technical considerations at the time of operation that favor tissue valve implantation, such as a friable or heavily calcified annulus. Finally, tissue valves are usually used for tricuspid valve replacement because of the risk of thrombotic complications associated with the use of mechanical valves in this position.

OPERATIVE PROCEDURES FOR VALVULAR DISEASE

PREOPERATIVE CARE

Careful preoperative preparation of the patient about to undergo heart valve replacement can have important consequences in terms of eventual patient morbidity and mortality. Screening for occult infectious processes such as dental abscesses is critical to prevent contamination of the valvular prosthesis and prosthetic valve endocarditis. As with any open-heart procedure, the potential for coagulopathy should be assessed because of the need for intraoperative heparinization and, specific for valve surgery, postoperative anticoagulation. Intractable or potentially recurrent gastrointestinal tract bleeding, in particular, will represent a contraindication to mechanical valve implantation.

As with any operative procedure, patients with significant respiratory compromise should be considered for preoperative pulmonary care, cigarette smoking should be discontinued, and attention should be directed toward improving the nutritional status of the patient. Finally, preoperative enhancement of cardiac function can significantly improve operative mortality; therefore, treatment of congestive failure in the preoperative period should be pursued actively.

SURGICAL TECHNIQUE

A median sternotomy is the standard approach to the heart for open valve surgery, whether it be for repair or replacement, allowing excellent exposure. Excellent exposure to the mitral valve can also be obtained by way of a standard or small ("mini") thoracotomy incision (aided by femoral vascular access techniques), as has been popularized by the recent interest in "minimally invasive" procedures. After institution of CPB and cardioplegic cardiac arrest, the specific valvular pathology is approached.

MITRAL VALVE REPAIR

A mitral commissurotomy is performed by incising the fused commissures to a point a few millimeters from the valve an-

nulus, ensuring that attachments to the chordae tendinae are left intact to prevent iatrogenic mitral insufficiency. The chordae and even the papillary muscle can similarly be divided to improve valve mobility.

Mitral reconstruction for insufficiency most commonly involves mitral annuloplasty, with plication of an enlarged annulus, usually onto a prosthetic ring.[53,54] Mitral reconstruction can also be accomplished utilizing a variety of additional techniques. The most commonly performed of the "tailoring" repairs is quadrangular resection of an enlarged mural leaflet. Triangular resection of the anterior leaflet, shortening of elongated chordae, transposition of mural leaflet chordae to the aortic (anterior) leaflet, and chordal replacement with PTFE sutures are the most commonly performed of a variety of other techniques.[53–57]

VALVE REPLACEMENT

Mitral valve replacement has historically consisted of excising the diseased valve some 3 to 4 mm from the annulus and division of the chordae at their junction with the papillary muscles or through the papillary heads. Heavily calcified valves can present difficulties in excision. Many surgeons now preserve the posterior leaflet or at least some of the chordae to the posterior annulus, especially for nonrheumatic MR, due to theoretical consideration that maintaining the internal left-ventricular architecture will help preserve LV function.[58]

After valve removal and appropriate debridement of calcium to allow passage of sutures into relatively compliant tissue, the valve orifice is sized with a plastic sizer. While a valve size of at least 25 mm is required to allow adequate transmitral flow, oversizing can lead to outflow tract obstruction, AV groove or posterior wall rupture, or prosthetic dysfunction.

Aortic valve replacement is performed in a similar fashion (Fig. 45.10).

Surgery is then completed as per other open-heart procedures. The patient is separated from CPB, protamine is given to neutralize the remaining heparin dose, cannulae are removed, atrial and ventricular epicardial pacing wires are placed in the event that they are needed for transient bradycardia or heart block, and appropriate chest tubes are placed.

POSTOPERATIVE CARE

The postoperative course of patients after valve surgery is in many ways similar to that of any patient undergoing operation, with similar neuroendocrine responses to the stress of surgery, and essentially identical to that for patients undergoing coronary artery bypass. Aside from these considerations, complications specifically related to the prosthetic valve implants are the primary and potentially most catastrophic complication associated with valvular heart surgery.

IMPLANT-RELATED COMPLICATIONS

With appropriate anticoagulant therapy, mechanical prosthetic valves such as the bileaflet valve enjoy freedom from structural failure rates of at least 99% per year. Mechanical valve dysfunction is today predominantly the result of valve thrombosis. Thromboembolic complications associated with mechanical valve implantation occur at a rate of approximately 1% to 2%/year.[59] Lifelong anticoagulation therapy, however, is mandated for all mechanical valve implants to avoid an excessive thromboembolic complication rate, and

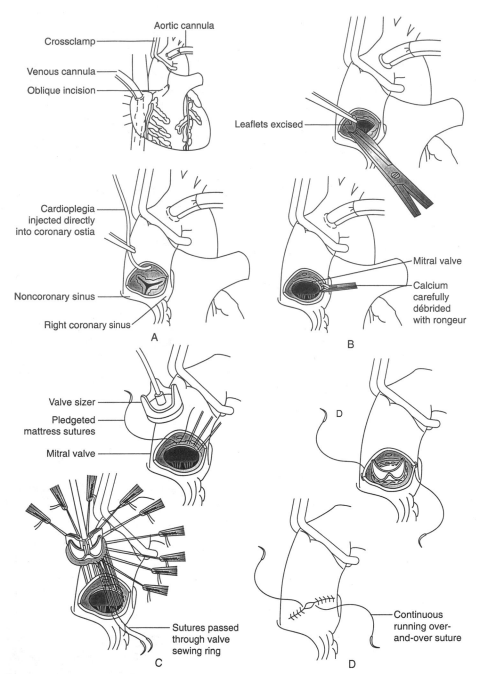

FIGURE 45.10. Aortic valve replacement.
A. Approach to aortic valve via aorta.
B. Valve excision. **C**. Suturing of valve prosthesis. **D**. Aortotomy closure. (Reproduced with permission from Greenfield LO, et al. Surgery, Second Edition. Philadelphia: Lippincott-Raven, 1977.)

carries an additional 1% to 2%/year risk of bleeding complications and a 0.17% mortality rate.[59]

Bioprosthetic implants generally do not require anticoagulation, except for mitral bioprosthetic implants in the presence of atrial fibrillation, which carry an increased thromboembolic risk. It should be noted, however, that approximately 10% of patients with tissue valves in the aortic position and up to 40% to 60% of patients with bioprosthetic valves in the mitral position eventually require anticoagulant therapy, thus partially negating the benefit of a tissue valve implant.[59]

Bleeding complications should be treated as appropriate for the specific event, by cessation of coumadin therapy, and by administration of fresh frozen plasma and/or vitamin K, as appropriate, with continuation of anticoagulant therapy as

soon as possible, but preferably within 1 week. It should be noted that vitamin K administration makes subsequent anticoagulation more difficult, and should thus be avoided if appropriate. In the event of planned or unanticipated surgical intervention, it should be noted that coumadin therapy can be replaced with intravenous heparin anticoagulation, which can then probably be safely interrupted for 24 to 48 h perioperatively. Finally, a planned or unanticipated pregnancy while on coumadin therapy can adequately be managed by transitioning to subcutaneous heparin, or possibly oral heparin analogues, during the first and third trimesters to avoid coumadin teratogenicity and peripartum hemorrhage during these respective intervals.

Hemolysis is another potential complication of valve implantation, most likely to occur with a prosthesis in the aortic position, with small valve sizes, and in the presence of a periprosthetic leak, especially in the mitral position. Hemolysis can be great enough to produce clinically apparent jaundice and require transfusion, but usually resolves with time. Valve replacement may be required, especially if a periprosthetic leak exists.

Finally, infection may occur in 1% to 2% of prosthetic valve implants, typically in the aortic position, representing 15% to 30% of all cases of endocarditis. Endocarditis occurring less than 2 months postoperatively ("early" endocarditis) may be related to a break in sterile technique or contamination from skin flora, whereas late endocarditis is usually related to a bacteremic episode. *Staphylococcus epidermidis, S. aureus,* or the gram-negative rods are the most common inciting organisms in early cases, while strep is more commonly seen in late endocarditis. Patients with prosthetic valves are therefore cautioned to strictly adhere to the recommended guidelines for antibiotic prophylaxis if invasive procedures such as endoscopy or dental procedures are planned.

The chief cause of death from endocarditis is congestive heart failure, and thus evidence of hemodynamic compromise in this setting is an important indication for operation. Operation generally consists of complete excision of the infected valve apparatus, debridement and closure of any abscess, and valve re-replacement.

SURGICAL RESULTS

OPERATIVE MORTALITY

The overall operative mortality rate for valve replacement ranges from 5% to 12%.[60-63] Ejection fraction less than 30%, emergent surgery, reoperations, concomitant coronary bypass grafting, and mitral regurgitation were independent mortality predictors in a retrospective study.

HEMODYNAMIC AND LATE RESULTS

Left-ventricular chamber size, wall thickness, and LV mass generally tend to decrease as early as 7 to 10 days postoperatively after correction of valvular heart disease.[64-66] These changes can be related to decreases in afterload and wall stresses related to decreased diastolic filling and improved systolic emptying related to elimination of excessive regurgitant volumes or valvular obstruction, in the case of insufficiency and stenotic lesions, respectively.

Excellent functional improvement can also generally be expected for nearly all patients undergoing correction of valvular heart disease. Preoperative left-ventricular function, and the type and durability of surgical correction, with attendant complication rates, are the primary predictors of long-time event-free survival. Significant LV dysfunction, in fact, can result in up to a 50% decrease in the 5-year survival rates and extent of functional improvement in patients undergoing valve replacement.

FREEDOM FROM REOPERATION

Aside from operative mortality rates, functional improvement, and thromboembolic and hemorrhagic complication rates, one remaining parameter by which valve surgery must be judged is the freedom from reoperation rate. In general, this is primarily a consideration for heterograft implants, as this rate is less than 1%/year for mechanical implants. In a recent report of 589 patients with a mean age of 67 ± 11 years undergoing bovine pericardial aortic valves implants, freedom from reoperation at 10 years was 97% ± 2% and freedom from valve-related failure was 96% ± 4%, however, suggesting that previous considerations regarding the limited durability of tissue valve implants may become less significant.[67]

Similarly encouraging results have recently been reported for mitral valve repair.[68-72] The overall 5-year freedom from reoperation for mitral valve repair has recently been reported at 90%, while 15-year freedom from reoperation has been reported at 87%.

In summary, encouraging recent trends have been reported with the use of mitral valve repair, bovine pericardial valves, and, in selected cases, aortic homograft implants in terms of long-term freedom from reoperation and other complications. In other cases where mechanical implants are required, long-term durability can be expected, although at the expense of a persistent annual risk of thromboembolic and anticoagulant-related complications.

References

1. Gailuinas P Jr, Chawla R, Lazarus JM, et al. Acute renal failure following cardiac operations. J Thorac Cardiovasc Surg 1980; 79:241.
2. Branthwaite MA. Prevention of neurological damage during open heart surgery. J Thorac Surg 1975;30:258–264.
3. Lawhorne TW, Davis WL, Smith GW. General surgical complications after cardiac surgery. Am J Surg 1978;136:254.
4. Falk E. Unstable angina with fatal outcome: dynamic coronary thrombosis leading to myocardial infarction and/or sudden death. Circulation 1985;712:699–708.
5. Kuller LH. AHA symposium/epidemiology meeting: atherosclerosis. Circulation 1993;87:II34–II37.
6. Ross R, Glomset JA. The pathogenesis of atherosclerosis. New Engl J Med 1976;295:369.
7. Davies MJ. A macro and micro view of coronary vascular insult in ischemic heart disease. Circulation 1990;82(Suppl II):II38–II46.
8. Fuster V. Mechanisms leading to myocardial infarction: insights from studies of vascular biology. Circulation 1994;90:2126–2146.
9. Prinzmetal M, et al. Angina pectoris: a variant form of angina pectoris. Am J Med 1959;27:375.
10. Mair J, Artner-Dworzak E, Leichleitner P, et al. Cardiac troponin in diagnosis of acute myocardial infarction. Clin Chem 1991; 37:845–852.
11. Rahimtoola SH. The hibernating myocardium. Am Heart J 1989; 117:211–221.
12. European Cooperative Study for Streptokinase Treatment in Acute Myocardial Infarction. Streptokinase in acute myocardial infarction. N Engl J Med 1979;301:797–802.
13. The ISAM Study Group. A prospective trial of intravenous streptokinase in acute myocardial infarction (ISAM): mortality, morbidity, and infarct size at 21 days. N Engl J Med 1986;314:1465–1471.
14. Chesebro JH, Knatterud G, Roberts R, et al. Thrombolysis in myocardial infarction (TIMI) trial, phase I: a comparison between intravenous tissue plasminogen activator and intravenous streptokinase. Circulation 1987;76:142–154.
15. Dalen JE, Gore JM, Braunwald E, et al. Six and twelve month follow-up of the phase I thrombolysis in myocardial infarction (TIMI) trial: the TIMI investigators. Am J Cardiol 1988;62:179–185.
16. The European Myocardial Infarction Project. Prehospital thrombolytic therapy in patients with suspected acute myocardial infarction. N Engl J Med 1993;329:383–389.
17. Gruentzig AR. Transluminal dilation of coronary artery stenosis (letter). Lancet 1978;1:263.
18. Myler RD, Shaw RE, Stertzer SH, et al. Unstable angina and coronary angioplasty. Circulation 1990;82(Suppl II):II88–II95.

19. Landau C, Lange RA, Hillis RD. Percutaneous transluminal coronary angioplasty. N Engl J Med 1994;330:981–993.

20. Laham RJ, Ho KKL, Baim DS, Kuntz RE, Cohen DJ, Carozza JP. Multivessel Palmaz-Schatz stenting: early results and one year outcome. J Am Coll Cardiol 1997;30:180–185.

21. Fishman DL, Leon MB, Baim DS, et al. A randomized comparison of coronary-stent placement and balloon angioplasty in the treatment of coronary artery disease. N Engl J Med 1994;331:496–501.

22. Grines CL, Browne KE, Marco J, et al. for the Primary Angioplasty in Myocardial Infarction Study Group. A comparison of immediate angioplasty with thrombolytic therapy for acute myocardial infarction. N Engl J Med 1993;328:673–679.

23. Zijlstra F, deBoer MJ, Hoorntje JC, Reiffers S, Reiber JH, Surypantra H. A comparison of immediate angioplasty with intravenous streptokinase in acute myocardial infarction. N Engl J Med 1993;328:680–684.

24. National Heart, Lung and Blood Institute Coronary Artery Surgery Study. Principal investigators of CASS and their associates. Circulation 1981;63(suppl I):I1–I81.

25. Deter K, Peduzzi P, Murphy M, et al. Effect of bypass surgery on survival in patients in low- and high-risk subgroups delineated by the use of simple clinical variables. Circulation 1981;63:1329–1338.

26. The Veterans Administration Coronary Artery Bypass Surgery Cooperative Study Group. Eleven year survival in the Veterans Administration randomized trial of coronary bypass surgery for stable angina. N Engl J Med 1984;311:333–339.

27. European Coronary Surgery Study Group. Long-term results of prospective randomised study of coronary artery bypass surgery in stable angina pectoris. Lancet 1982;2:1173–1180.

28. Varnauskas E, European Coronary Surgery Study Group. Twelve-year follow-up of survival in the randomized European Coronary Surgery Study. N Engl J Med 1988;319:332–337.

29. Varnauskas E, European Coronary Surgery Study Group. Survival, myocardial infarction, and employment status in a prospective randomized study of coronary bypass surgery. Circulation 1985;72(suppl V):V90–V101.

30. Cutlip DE, Leon MB, Ho KK, et al. Acute and nine-month clinical outcomes after "suboptimal" coronary stenting: results from the STent Anti-thrombotic Regimen Study (STARS) registry. J Am Coll Cardiol 1999;34:698–706.

31. Jones RH, Kesler K, Phillips HR, et al. Long-term survival benefits of coronary artery bypass grafting and percutaneous transluminal angioplasty in patients with coronary artery disease. J Thorac Cardiovasc Surg 1996;111:1013–1025.

32. Gold JP, Charlson ME, Williams-Russo P, et al. Improvement of outcomes after coronary artery bypass: a randomized trial comparing intraoperative high versus low mean arterial pressure. J Thorac Cardiovasc Surg 1995;110:1302–1304.

33. Reichenspurner H, Gulielmos V, Wunderlich J, et al. Port-access coronary artery bypass grafting with the use of cardiopulmonary bypass and cardioplegic arrest. Ann Thorac Surg 1998;65:413–419.

34. Engelman RM, Rousou JA, Flack JE III, et al. Fast-track recovery of the coronary bypass patient. Ann Thorac Surg 194;58:1742–1746.

35. Helm RE, Rosengart TK, Klemperer JD, et al. Comprehensive multimodality blood conservation: 100 consecutive CABG operations without transfusion. Ann Thorac Surg 1998;65:125–136.

36. Rosengart TK, Krieger K, Lang S, et al. Reoperative coronary artery bypass surgery: improved preservation of myocardial function with retrograde cardioplegia. Circulation 1993;88:330–335.

37. Machiraju VR. Redo Cardiac Surgery in Adults. Southampton, NY: CME Network Publishing, 1997.

38. Bourassa MG, Enjalbert M, Campeau L, Lesperance J. Progression of atherosclerosis in coronary arteries and bypass grafts: ten years later. Am J Cardiol 1984;53:102C–107C.

39. Grondin CM, Campeau L, Lesperance J, et al. Comparison of late changes in internal mammary artery and saphenous vein grafts in two consecutive series of patients 10 years after operation. Circulation 1984;70(suppl I):208–212.

40. Emond M, Mock MB, Davis KB, et al. Long-term survival of medically treated patients in the coronary artery surgery study (CASS) registry. Circulation 1994;90:2645–2657.

41. Horvath K. Clinical studies of TMR with the CO_2 laser. In: Rosengart TK and Sanborn TA eds. The Journal of Clinical Laser Medicine and Surgery 1997;15(6):281–286.

42. Mack CA, Patel SR, Magovern CJ, Crystal RG, Rosengart TK. Myocardial angiogenesis: biology and therapy. In: Transmyocardial Revascularization. Whittaker P, Abala G, eds. Direct GS myocardial Revascularization: History, Methodology, Technology. Norwell, MA: Kluwer Academic, 1999.

43. Mack CA, Patel SR, Rosengart TK. Myocardial angiogenesis as a possible mechanism for TMLR efficacy. In: Rosengart TK and Sanborn TA, eds. The Journal of Clinical Laser Medicine and Surgery 1997;15(6):275–279.

44. Rosengart TK, Patel SR, and Crystal RG. Therapeutic angiogenesis: protein and gene therapy delivery strategies. J Cardiovasc Risk 1999;6:29–40.

45. Mack CA, Patel SR, Schwarz EA, et al. Biologic bypass with the use of adenovirus-mediated gene transfer of the complementary deoxyribonucleic acid for vascular endothelial growth factor 121 improves myocardial perfusion and function in the ischemic porcine heart. J Thorac Cardiovasc Surg 1998;115:168–177.

46. Schumaker B, Percher P, von Specht BU, Stegman T. Induction of neoangiogenesis in ischemic myocardium by human growth factors. Circulation 1998;97:645–650.

47. Chizner MA, Pearle DL, deLeon AC Jr. The natural history of aortic stenosis in adults. Am Heart J 1980;99:419.

48. Bonow RO, Rosing DR, Kent KM, et al: Timing of operation for chronic aortic regurgitation. Am J Cardiol 1982;50:325–336.

49. Assey ME, Spann JF Jr. Indications for heart valve replacement. Clin Cardiol 1990;13:81–88.

50. Turi ZG, Reyes VP, Raju BS, et al. Percutaneous balloon valvuloplasty versus closed commissurotomy for mitral stenosis: a prospective, randomized trial. Circulation 1991;83:1179.

51. Smerida NG, Ports TA, Merrick SH, Rankin DS. Balloon aortic valvuloplast as a bridge to aortic valve replacement in critically ill patients. Ann Thorac Surg 1993;55:914–918.

52. Hejjer JJ, Wann LS, Weyman AE, Dillon JC, Feigenbaum H. Long term changes in mitral valve area after successful mitral commissurotomy. Circulation 1979;59:443.

53. Carpentier A. Cardiac valve surgery: the "French correction." J Thorac Cardiovasc Surg 1983;86:323–337.

54. Deloche A, Jebara VA, Relland JYM, et al. Valve repair with Carpentier techniques: the second decade. J Thorac Cardiovasc Surg 1990;99:990–1002.

55. Carpentier AF, Lessana A, Relland JYM, et al. The "Physio-Ring": an advanced concept in mitral valve annuloplasty. Ann Thorac Surg 1993;55:860–863.

56. Cosgrove DM, Arcidi JM, Rodriguez L, Stewart WJ, Powell K, Thomas JD. Initial experience with the Cosgrove-Edwards Annuloplasty System. Ann Thorac Surg 1995;60:499–504.

57. David TE, Omran A, Armstrong, et al. Long-term results of mitral valve repair for myxomatous disease with and without chordal replacement with expanded polytetrafluorothylene. J Thorac Cardiovasc Surg 1998;115:1279–1286.

58. Lillehei CW, Levy MJ, Bonnabeau RC. Mitral valve replacement with preservation of papillary muscles and chordae tendinae. J Thorac Cardiovasc Surg 1964;47:532–543.

59. Edmunds LH Jr. Thromboembolic complications of current cardiac valve prostheses. Ann Thorac Surg 1981;34:96.

60. Christakis GT, Weisel RD, David TE, et al. Factors of operative survival after valve replacement. Circulation 1988;78(suppl I):I25.

61. Klodas E, Enriquez-Sarano M, Tajik AJ, et al. Optimizing timing of surgical correction in patients with severe aortic regurgitation: role of symptoms. J Am Coll Cardiol 1997;30:746–752.

62. Blackstone EH, Kirklin JW. Death and other time-related events after valve replacement. Circulation 1985;72:753.

63. Duarte IG, Murphy CO, Kosinski AS, et al. Late survival after valve operation in patients with left ventricular dysfunction. Ann Thorac Surg 1997;64:1089–1095.

64. Bonow RO. Left ventricular structure and function in aortic valve disease. Circulation 1989;79:966.

65. Dhuikuri H. Effects of mitral valve replacement on left ventricular function in mitral regurgitation. Br Heart J 1983;49:328–333.

66. Crawford MH, Souchek J, Oprian CA, et al. Determinants of survival and left ventricle performance after mitral valve replacement. Circulation 1990;81:1173–1181.

67. Auport MR, Sirinelli AL, Diermont FF, et al. The last generation of pericardial valves in the aortic position: ten year follow-up in 589 patients. Ann Thorac Surg 1996;61:615–620.

68. Galloway AC, Colvin SB, Baumann FG, et al. Long-term results of mitral valve reconstruction with Carpentier techniques in 148 patients with mitral insufficiency. Circulation 1998;78(suppl I):I97–I105.

69. Gillinov MA, Cosgrove DM, Lytle BW, et al. Reoperation for failure of mitral valve repair. J Thorac Cardiovasc Surg 1997;113:467–475.

70. Duran CG. Repair of anterior mitral leaflet chordal rupture or elongation (the flipover technique). J Cardiac Surg 1986;1:161–166.

71. Galloway AC, Colvin SB, Baumann FG, et al. A comparison of mitral valve reconstruction with mitral valve replacement: intermediate term results. Ann Thorac Surg 1989;47:655.

72. Spencer FC, Galloway AC, Gross EA, et al. Recent developments and evolving techniques of mitral valve reconstruction. Ann Thorac Surg 1998;65:307–313.

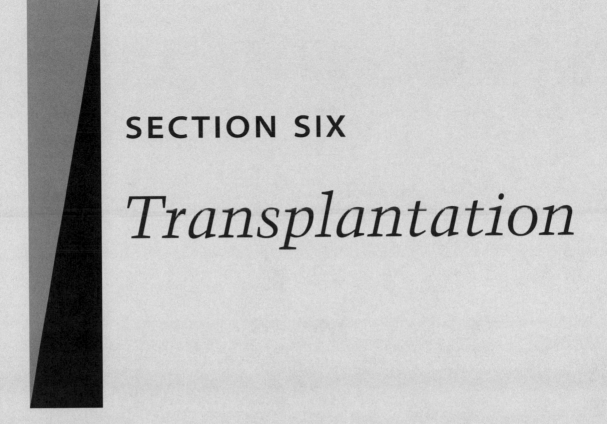

SECTION SIX

Transplantation

46

Immunology of Transplantation

Allan D. Kirk

General Considerations and Terminology

At the most basic level, rejection involves recognition of a tissue that is foreign in a context that is perceived to be appropriate for a defensive response. Put another way, all rejection responses involve something on the graft that is recognized as foreign, some component of the immune system which recognizes it, and something that defines the context of the foreign object as worthy of the immune system's attention. To begin to describe these fundamental aspects of rejection, a rudimentary vocabulary is required.

The word *antigen* is used to describe a molecule or tissue that can be recognized by the immune system. An *epitope* is the portion of the antigen, generally a carbohydrate or peptide moiety, that actually serves as the binding site for a receptor of the immune system. Thus, antigens contain one or many epitopes. Each is bound by one of two types of lymphocyte receptors: the *T-cell receptor* (TCR) of T cells, or the *antibody* (or *immunoglobulin*) of B cells. In general, a TCR or antibody binds to only one epitope and each cell expresses a single type of antigen receptor. These receptors allow a given lymphocyte to "see" and respond to only one epitope, and thus establish the *specificity* of an immune response. The signal from these receptors to the lymphocyte on which they reside defines immune recognition.

The context or appropriateness of an immune response is governed by another set of receptors on lymphocytes called *costimulation* receptors. These receptors bind irrespective of the epitope and allow the lymphocyte to determine whether the specific signal generated by the antigen receptor should evoke a response. By having separate signals for specificity and appropriateness, the immune system can carefully regulate its response to be active when a pathogenic threat is present and inactive as the threat subsides.

Given the myriad of surface receptors involved in lymphocyte function, the descriptive names that are frequently given to a newly discovered molecule are unwieldy. Thus, as new molecules are characterized, they are assigned a "cluster of differentiation" (CD) number. This nomenclature is vital to any discussion of complex cellular interactions.

Organs transplanted between genetically nonidentical individuals of the same species are termed *allografts*. Antigens from these grafts are thus *alloantigens*, and immunity toward these antigens is known as *alloreactivity*. The word *homograft* was used in earlier literature to describe allografts. The degree to which an allograft shares antigens with the recipient is referred to as the *histocompatibility* of the graft. This term generally refers to the similarity of a cluster of genes on chromosome 6 known as the *major histocompatibility complex* (MHC, also known as HLA in humans). Thus, transplant antigens are unique, genetically encoded characteristics of an individual. Basically, two different classes of MHC gene products are produced, termed *class I* and *class II*. The importance of MHC gene products stems from their *polymorphism*. Unlike most genes, which are identical within a given species, polymorphic gene products differ in detail while still conforming to the same basic structure. Thus, polymorphic MHC proteins from one individual are foreign alloantigens to another individual. Allografts that are matched to their recipient at HLA are referred to as *HLA-identical* allografts, and those matched at half of the HLA loci are termed *haplo-identical*. Note that HLA-identical allografts still differ genetically and are to be distinguished from *isografts*. Isografts are organs transplanted between identical twins, are immunologically inconsequential, and thus do not reject. *Xenografts* are organs transplanted from one species to another and were formerly described as *heterografts*.

Physiological Immunity

Two distinct but complementary arms of the immune system have evolved in vertebrates to combat disease: the *innate* and *acquired* immune systems. They differ in their fundamental responsibilities.

The innate immune system recognizes *general* motifs that

have, through selective evolutionary pressure, come to represent universally pathological states to our species (ischemia, necrosis, trauma, and certain nonhuman cell surfaces).[1] Innate recognition leads to prompt and direct attempts to remove the offending entity. Innate mechanisms of defense are thus direct and require little in the way of regulation. The likelihood that self-reactive innate immunity will occur is low because the molecules that trigger innate processes have been defined by their stark differences from normal tissues.

In contrast, the acquired immune system recognizes *specific* pathogens through antigen binding. Antigen binding leads to carefully regulated destruction of the antigen-expressing tissue. Obviously, a large number of receptors are required to specifically distinguish the seemingly endless array of pathogens. Highly specific receptors must also respond to very minor differences in antigen structure. With a large and varied assemblage of receptors, the potential for cross-reactivity with self is high. This system must therefore be under constant regulation to prevent autoimmunity. Acquired responses are therefore characterized by many regulatory steps designed to prevent autoimmune attack and uncontrolled lymphocyte proliferation. Clearly, an immune system tailor made for one individual will be perturbed when it encounters tissues from another individual. This reaction is the cause of allograft rejection.

Physiological Innate Immunity

The innate immune system uses protein receptors encoded in the germ line (passed from one individual to its offspring) to identify foreign or aberrant tissues.[1] These receptors can exist on cells, such as macrophages, neutrophils, and natural killer cells, or free in the circulation, as is the case for complement.[1–3] They are limited in specificity but are broadly reactive against common components of pathogenic organisms, for example, lipopolysaccharides on gram-negative organisms or other glycoconjugates. Thus, *the receptors of innate immunity are the same from one individual to another within a species* and, in general, do not play a role in the recognition of a foreign graft. They may, however, come into play when an injured tissue (e.g., one that has been made ischemic and moved from one individual to another) is present.

Once activated, the innate system performs two vital functions. It initiates cytolytic pathways for the destruction of the offending organism, primarily through the complement cascade. It also communicates the encounter to the acquired immune system for a more specific response through by-products of complement activation and through the function of phagocytic cells.

Complement plays a central role in many innate responses.[4] In a process known as alternative pathway complement activation, C3, the central activating enzyme of the complement cascade, can be activated when carbohydrates lacking sialic acid (a sugar moiety that is not found in most bacteria but is common on human cells) are encountered. One of the cleaved fragments of C3, C3b, is released and binds to the invader, flagging it as foreign, a process known as *opsonization*. C3a, another product of C3 activation, acts to recruit neutrophils to the site, while C3d enhances the immunogenicity of the organism, making it more likely to stimulate a dendritic cell to present the antigen to T cells. C3 activation also leads to formation of the membrane attack complex (MAC). This product is the result of activated C3 catalyzing the activation of C5, which in turn catalyzes the polymerization of C6, C7, C8, and C9, forming the MAC, a pore embedded in the foreign cell that results in disruption of the membrane and lysis.

Macrophages and dendritic cells not only engulf foreign cells that have been bound by complement, but also those identified through receptors for foreign carbohydrates (e.g., mannose receptors).[5] This tissue is broken down and presented to the acquired immune system using molecules of the MHC so that specific T cells can be activated and aid in the attack. Acquired immunity can also reciprocally activate the innate system. In a pathway known as the classical complement activation cascade, antigen-bound antibody can bind to the complement molecule C1q, which in turn becomes activated and activates C3. C3 activation products then proceed toward the MAC and serve chemoattractant functions, as described for the alternative pathway.

Physiological Acquired Immunity

The hallmark of acquired immunity is *specific* recognition and elimination of cells. Highly specialized receptors for distinguishing infected and transformed cells from normal tissues have evolved to facilitate this goal. The altered cell is recognized as a specific entity, not just as nonself, and a record of that encounter is retained for more rapid response to future encounters, a phenomenon known as immunological memory.[6]

THE GENETICS AND STRUCTURAL CHARACTERISTICS OF ANTIGEN RECEPTORS

Two cell types have evolved with the ability to specifically bind to antigen: T cells and B cells (Fig. 46.1). Their receptors

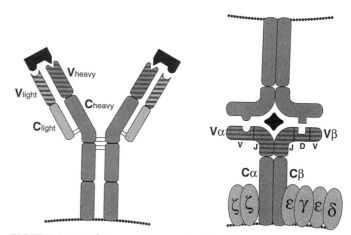

FIGURE 46.1. The general structure of antigen receptors. The two receptor types used by cells of the acquired immune system for specific recognition of antigen. The B-cell antigen receptor (*left*) is an antibody molecule made up of two identical light chains disulfide bonded to two identical heavy chains, thus forming two identical sites for binding soluble antigen. The T-cell antigen receptor (*right*) is associated with a five-chained signal transduction unit called CD3 (shown as the subunits $\zeta_2\epsilon_2\gamma\delta$). It has a single antigen binding site for recognition of a processed peptide antigen bound to an MHC molecule. *Striped areas* represent the regions of most structural variability. (From Kirk AD, Sollinger HW. Transplant immunology and immunosuppression. In: Schwartz S, ed. Principles of Surgery, 7th Ed. 1998. Used with permission.)

are similar in genetic development but differ in the types of antigens they bind. T-cell antigen receptors bind peptide antigens that have been processed by cells and combined with MHC molecules, while B-cell antibodies bind antigens in their native conformation on an invading pathogen or free in the extracellular fluid. T-cell receptors (TCR) are fixed, while antibodies can be secreted and act at locations remote from the cell.

THE T-CELL RECEPTOR

The formation of the TCR is fundamental to the understanding of its function.[7,8] T cells are formed in the fetal liver and bone marrow and migrate to the thymus during the first trimester of fetal development. At this stage, they have no TCR or accessory molecules. Upon entering the thymus, T cells undergo a remarkable rearrangement of the DNA that encodes the TCR.[9] Two recombination-activating genes, RAG-1 and RAG-2, drive this series of genetic deletions and splicing events.[10,11] Four distinct loci (α and δ on chromosome 14, and β and γ on chromosome 7), each made up of a highly polymorphic variable (V), junctional, and/or diversity (J and D, respectively) region, and a well-conserved constant (C) region, are involved. The recombination event randomly joins C, V, D, and J regions together to form a functional α, β, γ, or δ chain.

It is important to note that, regardless of the genes used, individual cells recombine to express a TCR with a single specificity. The rearrangements occur randomly, resulting in a population of T cells capable of binding 10^9 different specificities, essentially all combinations of MHC and peptide.

To avoid the release of autoreactive T cells, developing cells undergo a process following recombination known as thymic selection.[12,13] Cells initially interact with the MHC-expressing cortical thymic epithelium. If binding does *not* occur to self-MHC, the cells are useless to the individual, as they would be unable to bind to and survey cells in the periphery for foreign antigen. Thus, all nonbinding cells undergo apoptosis, or programmed self-destruction, a process called positive selection. Cells surviving positive selection then move to the thymic medulla and lose either CD4 or CD8. If binding to self-MHC in the medulla occurs with an unacceptably high affinity, apoptosis again results; this is called negative selection. The only cells released into the periphery are those that can bind self-MHC without activation. Any foreign peptide encountered will alter the affinity that has been preordained in the thymus, resulting in the initial events of T-cell activation. Likewise, MHC molecules that were not part of the T-cell's thymic education will bind the TCR with unacceptable affinity. This phenomenon defines alloreactivity.

In addition to thymic selection, it is now clear that mechanisms exist for peripheral modification of the T-cell repertoire.[14] Much of this is in place for removal of T cells following an immune response and downregulation of activated clones. A molecule known as Fas (CD98) is expressed on activated T cells.[15] Under appropriate conditions, binding of this molecule to its ligand leads to apoptosis. Complementing this deletional method to TCR repertoire control are nondeletional mechanisms that selectively anergize (make unreactive) specific T-cell clones. One prominent receptor group mediating this function is the CD28:B7 pair.[16] TCR binding only leads to activation if the costimulatory molecule CD28 is bound to its ligand B7, generally found on antigen-presenting cells (APCs). In the absence of binding, the cell is turned off until exogenous IL-2 is added. Thus, TCR binding that occurs to self in the absence of appropriate antigen presentation or active inflammation fails to lead to self-reactivity.

T-CELL ACTIVATION

T cells recognize and destroy cells of the body that make peptide products of mutation or viral infection. They do not recognize these peptide antigens unless they are presented by a self-cell. Molecules of the MHC perform this presentation. By requiring that T cells only respond to antigen encountered when it is physically embedded in self-cells, the body avoids having its T cells constantly activated by soluble molecules.

Because the number of potential antigens is high, and the likelihood is that self-antigens vary minimally from foreign antigens, the nature of the TCR-binding event has evolved such that a single interaction with an MHC molecule is not sufficient to cause activation. In fact, a T cell must register a signal from approximately 8000 TCR–ligand interactions with the same antigen before a threshold of activation is reached.[17–19]

The binding between the TCR and MHC is governed by *accessory molecules* that improve the TCR-binding affinity and regulate the type of cell that the T cell can "see."[20,21] Parenchymal cells express class I MHC molecules. These class I molecules display peptides from within (e.g., peptides from normal cellular processes or from internal viral replication).[22,23] T cells responsible for surveying parenchymal cells express the accessory molecule CD8, a molecule that binds to class I, and will only stabilize a TCR interaction with a class I-presented antigen. Thus, CD8$^+$ T cells evaluate parenchymal cells and mediate most of the destruction of altered cells. They have been termed cytotoxic T cells.

Hematopoietic cells express class II MHC molecules in addition to class I. Class II molecules display peptides that have been phagocytized from surrounding extracellular spaces and are thus more appropriate for the presentation of newly acquired antigen.[22,23] Cells initiating an immune event need to have access to this newly processed antigen. The accessory molecule stabilizing the TCR–class II interaction is called CD4. Thus, under physiological conditions, CD4$^+$ T cells are first alerted to an invasion of the body by hematopoietic *antigen-presenting cells* (APC) that present their newly devoured antigen in a class II molecule (Fig. 46.2). These cells are free to present antigen without evoking a cytotoxic response from cytotoxic CD8$^+$ T cells (remember that the new antigen will not be presented in class I because it is not internally derived). CD4$^+$ cells recognize dendritic cells and macrophages that have an antigen. They then signal back to the APC to activate CD8$^+$ cells to search the body for cells that have been infected by this invader. Thus, APCs alert CD4$^+$ T cells, and CD4$^+$ T cells then endow APCs with the ability to martial CD8$^+$ T cells and "license them to kill."[24,25] This process is mediated through upregulation of *costimulation molecules*. CD8$^+$ T cells then survey parenchymal cells for the offending antigen in the context of MHC class I and kill those cells found to be expressing the antigen from within.

When the TCR is bound to an MHC molecule and the proper accessory molecule stabilizes its binding, it transmits its signal to the cell by initiating the activity of intracyto-

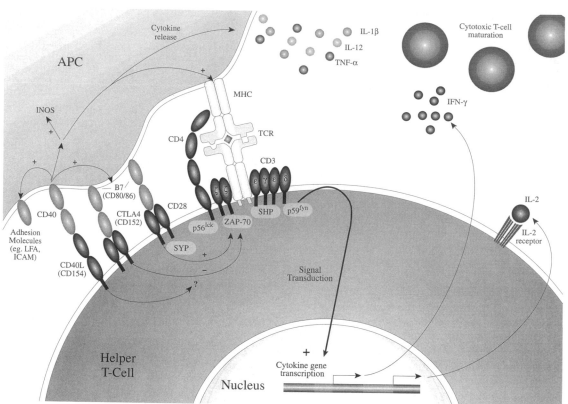

FIGURE 46.2. T-cell interactions with an antigen-presenting cell (APC). The T-cell receptor (TCR) binds to an MHC molecule (class II is shown). This event is stabilized by an accessory molecule (CD4). The costimulatory molecule CD40 upregulates the expression of the APC costimulation molecules, inducing many critical APC functions. Costimulatory molecule binding is shifted away from the neg-

ative regulation by CTLA4 to positive regulation by CD28. This potentiates signal transduction by the TCR through CD3 and in turn induces IL-2 and interferon-γ synthesis. IL-2 works in an autocrine loop to force the cell into a division cycle. Interferon-γ works in concert with APC-derived cytokines to facilitate cytotoxic T-cell maturation.

plasmic protein tyrosine kinases (PTKs) (Fig. 46.3).[26,27] Repetitive binding signals combined with the appropriate costimulation eventually activate phosphokinase-γ (PLC-γ1), which in turn hydrolyzes the membrane lipid phosphatidyl inositol biphosphate (PIP_2), thereby releasing inositol triphosphate (IP_3) and diacyl glycerol (DAG).[28–30] IP_3 binds to the endoplasmic reticulum, causing a release of calcium that induces calmodulin to bind to and activate calcineurin. Calcineurin dephosphorylates the critical cytokine transcription factor NF-AT, prompting it, with the transcription factor NF-κB, to initiate transcription of cytokines including IL-2. IL-2 is then released and binds to the T cell in an autocrine loop, potentiating DAG activation of protein kinase C (PKC). PKC is important in activating many gene regulatory steps critical for cell division.

T-Cell-Mediated Cytotoxicity

Physiological cytotoxicity is mediated by CD8[+] T cells because they bind to the class I MHC of all nucleated cells. Killing occurs either by a Ca^{2+}-dependent secretory mechanism or a Ca^{2+}-independent mechanism that requires direct cell contact.[31]

Antibody

Antibody, also called immunoglobulin (Ig), is formed in B cells much the same way the TCR is in T cells, although maturation occurs in the bone marrow, and not in the thymus, and

continues in the periphery.[9,32] Five different heavy chain loci (μ, γ, α, ε, δ) on chromosome 14, and two light chain loci (κ on chromosome 2, and λ on chromosome 2), each with V, D and/or J, and C regions, are brought together randomly by the RAG-1 and RAG-2 apparatus to form a functional antigen receptor. Antibodies have a basic structure of four chains, two of which are identical heavy chains and two of which are identical light chains (see Fig. 46.1). The heavy-chain usage defines the Ig type as being IgM, IgG, IgA, IgE, or IgD. This structure forms two identical antigen-binding sites brought together on a common region known as the Fc portion of the antibody. The Fc portion is critical in the process of opsonization. It is bound by Fc receptors on phagocytic cells of the innate immune system, facilitating phagocytic destruction of the antigen and processing of antigenic peptides. The Fc portion of IgM and some classes of IgG also serve to activate complement. The mechanism for regulating B-cell tolerance remains a subject of intense investigation.[33]

Unlike the TCR, the Ig loci undergo continued alteration after B-cell stimulation to improve the affinity and functionality of the secreted antibody. In an alteration known as isotype switching, Ig genes change their initial heavy-chain gene usage from the IgM type (used for initial and baseline responses against common carbohydrate antigens) to one of four types, each of which provides heightened specialization for a given purpose.[34] IgG becomes the most significant soluble mediator of opsonization and is clearly the dominant antibody resulting from allostimulation. IgA is formed for mu-

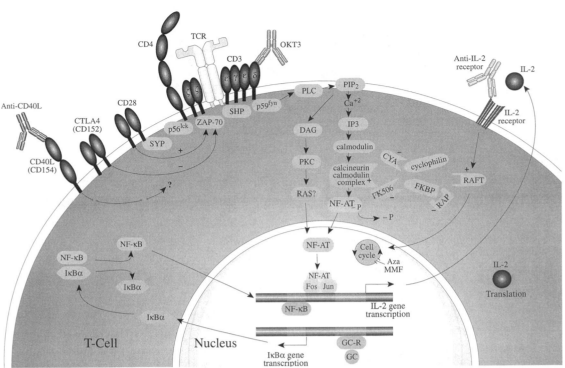

FIGURE 46.3. T-cell receptor activation signal transduction and the sites of action of various immunosuppressants. The TCR binding facilitates kinase activity by CD3 and CD4 (or CD8). The costimulatory molecules CD28, CD152, and CD154 determine the relative potency of these signals. TCR signal transduction proceeds via a calcium-dependent dephosphorylation of NF-AT, which enters the nucleus and acts in concert with NF-κB to facilitate cytokine gene expression. IL-2 works in an autocrine loop to force the cell into a division cycle. Cyclosporine (CyA) and tacrolimus (FK506) both block this signal transduction by blocking the calcineurin/calmodulin-potentiating proteins cyclophilin and FKBP, respectively. This step limits the access of NF-AT to the nucleus. Rapamycin (RAP) blocks the IL-2 receptor signal transduction by blocking the interaction of RAFT and FKBP. Steroids increase IκBα synthesis and limit the ability of NF-κB to enter the nucleus. Azathioprine (Aza) and mycophenolate mofetil (MMF) interrupt the cell cycle by interfering with nucleic acid metabolism. Monoclonal antibodies (OKT3, anti-IL-2 receptor, and anti-CD40L) interrupt key surface interactions required for T-cell function.

cosal immune responses, IgE for mast cell-mediated immunity, and IgD as a primary cell-bound antibody form.

B-CELL ACTIVATION

B cells recognize antigen in its native form without the requirement for processing and presentation on MHC molecules.[35] When antigen is bound by two surface antibodies, the antibodies are brought together on the cell surface in a process known as cross-linking; this is the event that stimulates B-cell activation, proliferation, and differentiation into a plasma cell. Like the T cell, the threshold for B-cell activation is high. B cells also can internalize antigens bound to surface antibodies and process them for presentation to T cells. As such, B cells can bind antigen in circulation and initiate a T-cell response to respond to antigen incorporated into tissues of the body.

In addition to being secreted following exposure to an antigen, antibody can be present as part of a natural repertoire in circulation for initial response to common pathogens.[36] Antigen exposure generally leads to B-cell affinity maturation and isotype switching, and produces high-affinity IgG antibodies. Naturally occurring antibodies, however, are generally IgM antibodies with low affinity and are generally thought to respond to a broad array of carbohydrate epitopes found on many common bacterial pathogens. Natural antibody is responsible for ABO blood group antigen responses and discordant xenograft rejection.

ANTIBODY-MEDIATED CYTOTOXICITY

Antibody facilitates both the destruction and removal of antigenic cells. Once bound to an antigen, antibody serves as an anchoring site for the complement component C1q, as described.[4] Antibody can also serve as an opsonin directly. Most phagocytic cells have receptors for the Fc portion of IgG and actively engulf antibody-coated targets in a process known as antibody-dependent cellular cytotoxicity (ADCC).

CYTOKINES

The entire immune process is dependent on cell-to-cell communication. While receptor interactions can serve this purpose between two cells, soluble mediators of communication are required to facilitate the amplification of the response. *Cytokines* (also known as interleukins [IL]) (see Table 46.1) are polypeptides that are released by many cell types and activate or suppress adjacent cells.[37] They are particularly fundamental to the interactions between CD4+ T cells and APCs. The prototypical cytokine of T-cell activation is IL-2.[38] It has been suggested that T cells, once activated, develop into one of two phenotypes based on cytokine expression. T cells mediating cytotoxic responses, such as delayed-type hypersensitivity, express IL-2, IL-12, IL-15, and IFN-γ and have been called Th1 cells. T cells supporting the development of humoral or eosinophilic responses express IL-4, IL-5, IL-10, and IL-13 and have been called Th2 cells.

TABLE 46.1. Properties of Some Human Cytokines.

Cytokine	Alternative name	Source(s)	Target cell type(s)	Action(s)
IFN-α and IFN-β	—	Activated T cells, endothelial cells, macrophages, fibroblasts	Activated T and B cells, NK and LAK cells	Induces antiviral state, antitumor activity, induces fever, increases class I and II MHC expression, stimulates activated B-cell differentiation and proliferation and NK activity, inhibits T and LAK cell activity
IFN-γ	—	Activated T cells, LAK cells	Activated and resting B and plasma cells, NK, endothelial, and LAK cells, macrophages	Induces antiviral state, antitumor activity, induces fever, increases class I and II MHC expression, stimulates activated B-cell differentiation and proliferation and NK and LAK activity, activates macrophages and endothelial cells, stimulates IgG2a isotype switch
TGF-β	—	T cells, macrophages, NK cells	Monocytes, fibroblasts	Chemotactic for fibroblasts and monocytes, induces extracellular matrix remodeling, repair and fibrosis, induces B-cell differentiation and isotype switching, T-cell proliferation and angiogenesis
TNF	—	Activated T cells, LAK cells, macrophages	Resting T, activated T and B cells, plasma, stem, and endothelial cells, eosinophils, fibroblasts, macrophages	Induces antiviral state, antitumor activity, induces fever, increases class I MHC expression, activates macrophages, granulocytes, eosinophils, and endothelial cells, chemotactic and angiogenic activity
IL-1	Endogenous pyrogen	Activated T and B cells, LAK cells, endothelial cells, macrophages, fibroblasts	Resting T and B cells, activated T and B cells, plasma, stem, and endothelial cells, eosinophils, fibroblasts, macrophages	Induces antiviral state, antitumor activity, induces fever, stimulates activated B-cell differentiation and proliferation, activates and stimulates proliferation of T cells, activates granulocytes and endothelial cells, stimulates hematopoiesis
IL-2	T-cell growth factor	Activated T cells, LAK cells	Activated T cells, activated and resting B cells, NK and LAK cells, macrophages	Activates macrophages, T, NK, and LAK cells, stimulates differentiation of activated B cells, stimulates proliferation of activated B and T cells, induces fever
IL-3	Multi-CSF	Activated T cells	Stem cells, activated B cells, eosinophils	Stimulates hematopoiesis, activated B-cell proliferation, and eosinophil activity
IL-4	B-cell-stimulating factor-1	Activated T cells	Activated T cells, activated and resting B cells, plasma LAK cells, macrophages	Activates macrophages, T and B cells, stimulates differentiation of activated B and T cells, induces IgE receptors on B cells, stimulates IgE and IgG1 isotype switch
IL-5	B-cell growth factor-2	Activated T cells	Activated and resting B cells, plasma cells, eosinophils	Stimulates IgA isotype switch and eosinophil activity
IL-6	B-cell-stimulating factor-2, B-cell-differentiating factor, interferon-β₂	Activated T cells, endothelial cells, fibroblasts, macrophages	Activated T, resting B, and stem cells	Activates T cells, stimulates activated B-cell differentiation and activated T- and B-cell proliferation
IL-7	—	Activated T cells	Activated T and resting B cells	Stimulates activated T-cell and resting B-cell proliferation
IL-8	—	Activated T cells	Granulocytes	Stimulates granulocyte activity, chemotactic activity
IL-9	—	Activated T cells	T cells	Stimulates T-cell proliferation
IL-10	—	Macrophages, B and T cells	Macrophages, B and T cells	Inhibits macrophage cytokine release, induces B-cell differentiation and isotype switching, induces class II expression, T-cell stimulation
IL-11	—	Bone marrow stromal cells	Hematopoietic stem cells	Stimulates megakaryocyte and B lineage stem cell maturation
IL-12	—	NK cells and macrophages	T cells	Induces T-cell maturation and cytotoxic activity
G-CSF	—	Endothelial cells, fibroblasts, macrophages	Granulocytes	Stimulates granulocyte activity and hematopoiesis
M-CSF	—	Macrophages	Macrophages	Activates macrophages
GM-CSF	—	Endothelial cells, fibroblasts, activated T cells	Stem cells, granulocytes, macrophages, eosinophils	Activates macrophages, stimulates granulocyte and eosinophil activity and hematopoiesis

IFN, interferon; TGF, transforming growth factor; TNF, tumor necrosis factor; IL, interleukin; CSF, colony-stimulating factor; LAK, lymphokine-activated killer; NK, natural killer.

Cytokines are secreted polypeptides that mediate autocrine and paracrine cellular communication but do not bind antigen. They include those compounds previously termed interleukins and lymphokines.

Source: Based on the consensus cytokine chart of the British Cytokine Group. Burke F, Naylor MS, et al. The cytokine wall chart. Immunol Today 1993;14:165.

COSTIMULATION

As mentioned, TCR binding is not usually sufficient to cause a T-cell response. Rather, receptor–ligand pairs known as costimulation molecules determine how the T cell will respond[39,40] (Fig. 46.4). Costimulatory molecules include the T-cell-based molecules CD28 and CTLA4 (CD152) (Fig. 46.2). In general terms, CD28 binding permits the TCR signal to lead to activation while CTLA4 binding directs the TCR signal to induce anergy. The ligands for CD28 and CTLA4 are the B7 molecules (CD80, CD86).

An additional costimulation molecule pair is CD40, a molecule found on endothelium, dendritic cells (DCs), and other APCs, and its T-cell-based ligand CD40L (CD154)[41,42] (Fig. 46.4). CD40 binding is required for APCs to stimulate a cytotoxic T-cell response.

Many other adhesion molecules (ICAM, selectins, integrins, etc.) control the movement of immune cells through the body, monitor their trafficking to specific areas of inflammation, and nonspecifically strengthen the TCR–MHC binding interaction.[43,44] They differ from costimulation molecules in that they enhance the interaction of the T cell with its antigen without influencing the quality of the TCR response. Almost all are upregulated by cytokines released during T-cell and endothelial activation.

Transplant Immunity

The Genetics and Structural Characteristics of Transplant Antigens

The antigens primarily responsible for human allograft rejection are those encoded by the HLA region of chromosome 6.[45] The polymorphic proteins encoded by this locus include class I molecules (HLA-A, -B, and -C) and class II molecules (HLA-DR, -DP, and -DQ). Class I genes with limited polymorphism (E, F, G, H, and J) are not currently typed and are not considered here. Although other polymorphic genes, referred to as minor histocompatibility antigens, exist in the genome, they are not covered in this section. The blood group antigens of the ABO system must also be considered polymorphic transplant antigens, and their biology is critical to humoral rejection.

Each class I molecule is encoded by a single polymorphic gene that is combined with the nonpolymorphic protein β_2-microglobulin (β_2M, from chromosome 15) for expression.[21,22] Class II molecules are made up of two chains, α and β, and individuals differ not only in the alleles represented at each locus, but also in the number of loci present in the HLA class II region.[46] As the HLA sequence varies, the ability of various peptides to bind to the molecule and be presented for T-cell recognition changes. Teleologically, this extreme diversity is thought to improve the likelihood that a given pathogenic peptide will fit into the binding site of these antigen-presenting molecules, thus preventing a single viral agent from evading detection by T cells of an entire population.[47,48]

While the structure of HLA is complex, the clinical importance of the region with respect to transplantation is easily understood by simple Mendelian genetics. Recombination within the locus is uncommon, occurring in approximately 1% of molecules. The HLA type of the offspring is therefore predictable. The unit of inheritance is the haplotype, which consists of one chromosome 6 and, therefore, one copy of each class I and class II locus (HLA-A, -B, -C, -DR, -DP, and -DQ). The genetics of HLA is particularly important in understanding clinical living-related donor (LRD) transplantation. Each child inherits one haplotype from each parent; therefore, the chance of siblings being HLA identical is 25%. Haploidentical siblings occur 50% of the time and completely nonidentical or HLA-distinct siblings 25% of the time.

The Biology of Transplant Antigens

The physiological role of MHC molecules is twofold: to provide a mechanism for T-cell inspection of parenchymal cells and to provide an interface between APCs and T cells. Class I

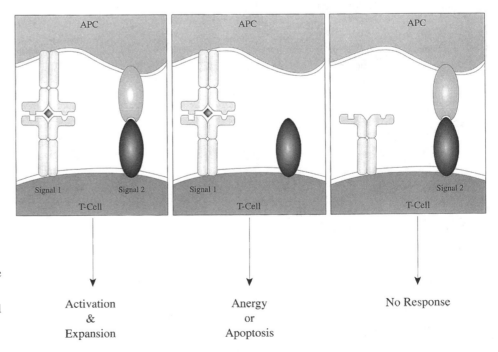

FIGURE 46.4. T-cell costimulation. T-cell responses depend on two signals; signal one is given by antigen through the TCR and signal two is given by costimulatory receptors. Both are required for activation. Signal one alone leads to T-cell anergy or death. Signal two has no independent effect.

Activation & Expansion

Anergy or Apoptosis

No Response

molecules serve the first role, while class II molecules serve the second. It is important to reiterate, however, that organ transplantation is not a physiological process, but rather an artificial situation. Thus, T-cell responses to either class of MHC molecule can generate a rejection episode.

When an inappropriate peptide is detected, CD4$^+$ T cells release cytokines to activate APCs to recruit CD8$^+$ cells into the area to inspect nearby cells for intracytoplasmic presence of the offending peptide. B cells are also stimulated to release antibody to bind the offending peptide and aid in its clearance by the innate immune system. The cytokines released by CD4$^+$ cells, particularly interferon-γ, also induce expression of class II molecules on local cells and increase expression of class I molecules locally.[49] This reaction increases the chance that infected cells will be detected. In the case of transplanted organs, ischemic injury at the time of transplantation accentuates the potential for T-cell activation by upregulation of both class I and class II molecules.[50] Surgical trauma and ischemia also upregulate class II (as well as B7 and other adhesion molecules) on all cells of an allograft, making antigen more abundant. If rejection can be prevented until the cells of the graft can return to their baseline state of antigen expression, the chance of a T cell encountering foreign antigen in sufficient density to become activated is greatly reduced. This alteration is the primary reason that immunosuppression is heavily administered in the immediate postoperative period and tapered to lower, less toxic levels over time.

Clinical Definition of Transplant Antigens

Closely matched transplants are less likely to be recognized and rejected than are similar grafts differing at the MHC. Historically, MHC match has been defined using two assays: the lymphocytotoxicity assay and the MLC.[51,52] Both assays define MHC epitopes but do not comprehensively define the entire antigen or the exact genetic disparity involved. Techniques now exist for precise genotyping that distinguishes the nucleotide sequence of an individual's MHC.

Matching is only temporally feasible before cadaveric renal transplantation and living-related allografts. Some centers now use HLA typing to dictate pancreas allocation as well. Other organs are MHC typed retrospectively. As would be predicted, the incidence of acute rejection declines with decreasing MHC disparity.[53] However, any mismatch puts the patient at risk for T-cell-mediated graft destruction and mandates T-cell-specific immunosuppression. As immunosuppression has improved, the relative importance of MHC matching, even for renal allotransplantation, has decreased. Now, when determining the destination of an organ, significant emphasis is also placed on the recipient's physical condition and time on the waiting list.

Mechanisms of Allograft Rejection

T-Cell-Mediated Rejection

T cells are the primary mediators of acute allograft rejection.[54–56] T cells can respond to transplant antigens either directly, through TCR binding to foreign MHC molecules expressed on transplanted tissues in the presence of donor costimulation, or indirectly, by encountering self-APCs that have phagocytosed alloantigens and processed them for presentation on self-MHC. It is also probable that recipient T cells can bind to donor APCs, particularly dendritic cells, activating them and allowing them to direct recipient cytotoxic T-cell maturation. Regardless of the source of the activating MHC, however, the ensuing internal T-cell events proceed as described for physiological T-cell function.

Initial T-cell binding to a donor APC or endothelial cell is nonspecific and mediated by adhesion molecules.[44] These molecules, including ICAM-1, VCAM-1, LFA-1, and other integrin family molecules, are all upregulated upon donor cell activation. The result is a graft that is poised to report its injured status to the recipient.

Once nonspecific adhesion has formed, MHC recognition can occur. The costimulatory environment of the donor tissue is affected by many factors, most of which are related to the mechanics of transplantation. MHC class II is upregulated, as are many nonspecific adhesion molecules.[50]

Once T-cell activation occurs, cytokines, particularly IL-2 and interferon-γ (IFN-γ) from T cells and IL-12 from APCs, create a potent milieu recruiting other T cells into the response and potentiating clonal expansion.[37,58–60] B-cell activation is also mediated through cytokine secretion. Cytokines are responsible for many of the systemic symptoms of fever and malaise that can be associated with severe graft rejection.

In the late phases of rejection, the inflammatory response recruits cells with nonspecific cytotoxic activity to the organ. Although cytotoxicity is best mediated by CD8$^+$ cells, in the artificial situation presented by allotransplantation, both CD4$^+$ and CD8$^+$ cells have been shown to mediate cytotoxicity.[57] It is now clear that, following activation, non-MHC-restricted, T-cell-mediated cytotoxicity occurs in addition to MHC-directed killing.[59] This reaction allows the utilization of T cells activated in the area of inflammation but without a TCR specific to the antigen to take part in protective or, in the case of transplant rejection, detrimental immunity. It is likely that this additional promiscuous killing is spurred forward by a failure to eliminate the antigen. This type of activity is induced by high concentrations of IL-2, which may be relevant in the local milieu of a rejecting allograft.

Antibody-Mediated Rejection

Although acute rejection is always the result of T-cell recognition and activation, most acute rejections are accompanied by an antibody response.[61] In addition, antibody can be the primary mediator of two types of rejection: hyperacute rejection and acute vascular rejection. Furthermore, antibody formed during the course of an allograft rejection remains in the circulation even after the acute event has been successfully controlled. Many investigators believe that chronic exposure to donor-specific antibody can have progressively damaging effects on the graft and contribute significantly to chronic rejection.

Donor-specific antibody has multiple effects on the graft. Direct cell lysis occurs as a result of classical pathway complement activation. Antibody opsonization increases the phagocytic uptake of donor antigen, and as such increases the antigen presentation to the recipient immune system. Antibody also directly alters the activation status of the endothelial cell. This change leads to cellular retraction and exposure of the underlying matrix, which in turn potentiates platelet activation and aggregation. Endothelial activation also alters its usually anticoagulant environment in favor of a procoagulant one.[62,63] The result is microvascular thrombosis, a hallmark for antibody-mediated graft rejections.

Clinical Rejection Syndromes

Hyperacute Rejection

Hyperacute rejection (HAR) is caused by donor-specific antibody present in the recipient's serum at the time of transplantation.[61] The antibody is not a result of the transplant but rather is a result of prior sensitization to donor antigens or to antigens that are sufficiently similar to those of the donor to elicit cross-reactivity. Presensitization is usually the result of prior transplant, transfusion, or pregnancy. HAR develops in the first minutes to hours following graft reperfusion. Antibodies bind to the donor tissue, initiating complement-mediated lysis, endothelial cell activation, a procoagulant state, and immediate graft thrombosis.

While there is no treatment for hyperacute rejection, a thorough understanding of its cause has resulted in its avoidance through the use of two preoperative screening tests, namely the lymphocytotoxic crossmatch and ABO blood group typing. These two tests identify donor-to-recipient combinations in which HAR would likely occur.

The crossmatch is performed by mixing cells (generally nonactivated T cells that express class I but not class II MHC antigens on their surface) from the donor with serum from the recipient. Lysis of the donor cells indicates that antibodies directed against the donor are present in the recipient serum; this is called a *positive* test result. A positive test can result from IgG or IgM antibodies. In general, only detection of IgG antibodies directed against class I MHC molecules represents a positive test and an absolute contraindication to transplantation. Preoperative verification of proper ABO matching and a negative crossmatch effectively prevent hyperacute rejection in 99.5% of transplants. Many variations of the crossmatch exist.[64,65]

As one might expect, the sensitization status of a patient can change over time. New exposures through transfusions can lead to new antibody formation. Existing sensitivities can wane with prolonged time on the waiting list. Thus, serum from patients awaiting transplantation is frequently screened against a battery of random donor cells to assess their level of sensitization. The screening assay is known as the panel reactive antibody assay, or PRA. A nonsensitized patient has a PRA of 0%; in other words, that patient's serum lyses 0% of randomly selected cells. The chance of that patient having a positive crossmatch is very low. Patients who have had multiple exposures to other human tissues have higher reactivity to random cells. As their PRA rises, the likelihood of their receiving an organ that elicits a negative crossmatch diminishes.

A delayed variant of HAR known as vascular rejection is also mediated by humoral factors.[66] Vascular rejection occurs when offending alloantibodies exist in circulation at levels undetectable by the crossmatch assay, even though presensitization has taken place. Frequently this is seen in a patient with a high PRA that decreases with time. Serum tested at the time of the transplant is negative, but serum from an archived sample is positive. Reexposure leads to restimulation of the memory B cells responsible for the donor-specific antibodies. The result is initial graft function, followed by rapid deterioration on or about postoperative day 3. Enhanced immunosuppression with steroids, combined with nonspecific antibody depletion with plasmapheresis, or administration of nonspecific immunoglobulin (to bind effector cell Fc receptors and complement in circulation and competitively divert them from antibody bound to the graft) is occasionally successful in reversing vascular rejection.

Acute Rejection

T cells cause acute rejection.[54–57] Acute rejection can occur at any time after the first 4 postoperative days, but is most common in the first 6 months post transplant. It evolves over a period of days to weeks, and is the inevitable result of an allotransplant unless immunosuppression directed against T cells is employed. To initiate acute rejection, T cells bind alloantigen via their TCR directly, or following phagocytosis of donor tissue and representation of MHC peptides by self-APC. This then leads to cell activation, as described. The result is a massive infiltration of the graft of T cells (Fig. 46.5), with destruction of the organ through direct cytolysis and endothelial perturbation leading to thrombosis.

Prompt recognition of acute rejection is imperative because prolonged rejection leads to recruitment of multiple arms of the immune system that do not respond to T-cell-specific therapies. In addition, graft damage, particularly for kidney, pancreas, and heart, is generally accompanied by a permanent loss of function that is proportional to the magnitude of involvement. Most acute rejection episodes for patients on modern immunosuppression are asymptomatic until the secondary effects of organ dysfunction occur. By this time, the rejection is well entrenched and difficult to reverse. For this reason, monitoring for acute rejection must be intense, particularly during the first year following transplantation. Generally, unexplained graft dysfunction should

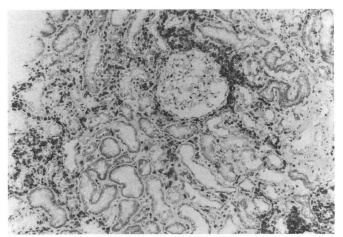

FIGURE 46.5. The histology of acute rejection. A photomicrograph of a renal biopsy with T cells stained dark (immunoperoxidase technique) shows infiltration of the kidney with activated T cells and renal tubular damage. (From Kirk AD, Sollinger HW. Transplant immunology and immunosuppression. In: Schwartz S, ed. Principles of Surgery, 7th Ed. 1998. Used with permission.)

prompt biopsy and evaluation for the lymphocytic infiltration and graft parenchymal necrosis characteristic of acute rejection.

Like HAR resulting from humoral presensitization, T-cell presensitization will result in an accelerated form of cellular rejection mediated by memory T cells. It occurs within 3 days of transplant and is usually accompanied by a significant humoral response.

Chronic Rejection

Unlike acute and hyperacute rejection, chronic rejection (CR) remains poorly understood.[67,68] Its onset is insidious, occurring over a period of months to years, and because the pathophysiology is not well defined, it remains untreatable. Heightened immunosuppression is not effective in reversing or retarding the progression of chronic rejection. Thus, its distinction from acute rejection by biopsy is important. CR tends to be poorly defined even by histological criteria. Regardless of the organ involved, it is characterized by parenchymal replacement by fibrous tissue and with a relatively sparse lymphocytic infiltrate. It is likely that the cumulative effects of mild subclinical immune recognition by several limbs of the immune system, and the resulting exposure to soluble factors, including fibrogenic cytokines, eventually take their toll on the graft.

Immunosuppression

The redundancy and plasticity of the immune system has to date prevented any single agent from specifically preventing graft destruction. In addition, as allograft recognition is mediated by an immune system formed for the detection and elimination of pathogens, manipulations altering this system do so at the expense of a vital defense network. Thus, no immunosuppressive intervention is allograft specific, or, put another way, all drugs preventing allograft loss put the recipient at increased risk for infection or malignancy. Rational, selective use of several immunosuppressive agents acting through different synergistic mechanisms is required to successfully prevent rejection without completely removing the body's defense.

For all organs, it is clear that the events occurring at the time of the initial antigen exposure are the most critical in establishing a lasting state of immune unresponsiveness. For this reason, immunosuppression is extremely intense in the early postoperative period and tapered thereafter. This initial conditioning of the recipient's immune system is known as *induction* immunosuppression. It usually involves deletion of the T-cell response completely and as such cannot be maintained indefinitely without lethal consequences. Medications used to prevent acute rejection for the life of the patient are called *maintenance* immunosuppressants. These agents tend to be well tolerated acutely if dosed appropriately, but all have chronic side effects. Immunosuppressants used to reverse an acute rejection episode are called *rescue* agents. They are generally the same as those agents used for induction therapy.

Corticosteroids

Corticosteroids, in particular glucocorticosteroids, remain a central tool in the prevention and treatment of allograft rejection. Used alone at maintenance doses, they are ineffective in preventing allograft rejection, but used in combination with other agents, they significantly improve graft survival. When used in higher doses they effectively rescue acute cellular rejection. Although steroids have a desirable immunosuppressive effect, they can contribute significantly to morbidity of transplantation.

Glucocorticosteroids bind to an intracellular receptor after nonspecific uptake into the cytoplasm (see Fig. 46.3). The receptor–ligand complex then enters the nucleus, where it acts as a DNA-binding protein and increases the transcription of several genes. The most commonly used form of steroid is prednisone or its intravenous substitute, methylprednisolone.

Antiproliferative Agents

AZATHIOPRINE

The antimetabolite azathioprine (Aza) was the first immunosuppressive pharmaceutical used in organ transplantation and remains a part of many maintenance protocols.[69–71] Aza undergoes hepatic conversion first to 6-mercaptopurine (6-MP), and then to 6-thio-inosine monophosphate (6-tIMP). These derivatives, in turn, inhibit DNA synthesis by alkylating DNA precursors and inducing chromosomal breaks through interference with DNA repair mechanisms. In addition, they inhibit the enzymatic conversion of IMP to AMP and GMP. The primary effect is to deplete the cell of adenosine. The effects of Aza are relatively nonspecific. It acts not only on proliferating lymphocytes and PMNs, but on all rapidly dividing cells. As such, its primary toxicity is directed at the bone marrow, gut mucosa, and liver. Aza is relatively ineffective alone and has no efficacy as a rescue agent. It does effectively inhibit rejection when given as a maintenance agent in combination with steroids and a calcineurin inhibitor.

MYCOPHENOLATE MOFETIL

Mycophenolate mofetil (MMF) inhibits inosine monophosphate dehydrogenase, and thus prevents a critical step in RNA and DNA synthesis, exploiting a critical difference between lymphocytes and other body tissues, including PMNs, to produce relatively lymphocyte-specific immunosuppressive effects. MMF blocks the proliferative response of both T and B cells, inhibits antibody formation, and prevents the clonal expansion of cytotoxic T cells.

MMF decreases the rate of biopsy-proven rejection and the need for antilymphocyte agents in rescue therapy compared to Aza.[72,73] As such, MMF has replaced Aza in patients with high risk of rejection.

Calcineurin Inhibitors

CYCLOSPORINE

The T-cell-specific immunosuppressive drug cyclosporine A (CyA) is a cyclic endecapeptide isolated from the fungus *Tolypocladium inflatum gams*.[74,75] Its mechanism of action is mediated primarily through its ability to bind to the cytoplasmic protein cyclophilin (Cn)[75] (see Fig. 46.5). The CyA–Cn complex binds with high affinity to the calcineurin–calmodulin complex and, in doing so, blocks its role in the calcium-dependent phosphorylation and activation of the transcription-regulating factor NF-AT. This prevents the transcription of the IL-2 gene. Cellular cytotoxicity is also probably interrupted through calcineurin inhibition. The transcription of other genes critical for T-cell activation is also altered. However, once IL-2 is present in the graft cytokine milieu, CyA is ineffective. Cyclosporine therefore works solely as a maintenance agent and is ineffective as a rescue agent.

TACROLIMUS

Tacrolimus, previously described investigationally as FK-506, is a macrolide produced by *Streptomyces tsukubaensis*. Tacrolimus, like CyA, blocks the effects of NF-AT, prevents cytokine transcription, and arrests T-cell activation[76] (Fig. 46.3). The intracellular target is an immunophilin protein distinct from cyclophilin known as FK-binding protein (FK-BP); thus, the effect is additive to that of CyA. As such, the use of tacrolimus with CyA produces prohibitive toxicity. Like CyA, the effects of tacrolimus are relatively T-cell specific, but in addition to its role as a maintenance agent, tacrolimus has also shown promise as a rescue agent.[77] Tacrolimus has been shown to be extremely effective for liver transplantation and has become the drug of choice for many centers.

Antilymphocyte Preparations

ANTILYMPHOCYTE GLOBULIN

Antilymphocyte globulin (ALG) is produced by inoculating heterologous species with human lymphocytes, collecting the plasma, and purifying the IgG fraction. The resulting preparation, known as a polyclonal antibody preparation, contains antibodies directed against many antigens on lymphocytes. Thymocytes rather than lymphocytes are sometimes used as the immunogen, and antibodies formed from this process are known as antithymocyte globulin (ATG). The most commonly inoculated species is the rabbit, and thymoglobulin (SangStat, Inc., Fremont, CA) is the most widely used preparation.

Antibodies in ALG coat multiple epitopes on the T cell.[78,79] This has many effects, including promoting T-cell clearance through complement-mediated lysis and opsonin-induced phagocytosis, as well as limiting the ability of the T cell to generate an effective TCR signal by internalization of key surface receptors. In addition, the antibodies cross-link several key molecules, including adhesion and costimulation molecules[79]; this has the effect of impairing or altering signals generated by these receptors and either preventing activation or possibly leading to an anergic phenotype. The overall result is to functionally remove the primary effector cells required for acute rejection during critical times post transplantation.

When used as an induction agent, T-cell depletion reduces the possibility that T-cell-mediated antigen recognition will occur when the graft is in its most vulnerable state. When ALG is used as a rescue agent, antigen recognition has already occurred and the beneficial effects of ALG are likely related solely to its ability to destroy cytotoxic T cells.

OKT3

Although polyclonal antibody preparations have many binding specificities, monoclonal antibodies have a single specific

target antigen. The first, and for years only, commercially available monoclonal antibody preparation for use in organ transplantation was Orthoclone OKT3 (Muromonab; Ortho Pharmaceuticals, Raritan, NJ). This murine monoclonal antibody is directed at the signal transduction subunit on human T cells (CD3)[80] (see Fig. 46.3).

There are several ways in which OKT3 is thought to have its effect.[80,81] The CD3 determinant, as described earlier, is a cluster of transmembrane proteins found on the surface of all mature T lymphocytes. When OKT3 binds to CD3, it leads to internalization of the TCR receptor complex, thus preventing antigen recognition and TCR signal transduction. In addition, T-cell opsonization and clearance by the reticuloendothelial system occur. Following the administration of OKT3, there is a rapid decrease in the number of circulating CD3$^+$ lymphocytes. Effect is minimal on T cells residing in the thymus, lymph nodes, or spleen. Following several days of administration, there is a return of T cells expressing the accessory binding molecules CD4 and CD8 but lacking the T-cell receptor. These "blind" T cells remain incapable of binding to antigen. In addition to interfering with the generation of cytotoxic T cells and the modulation of cell-surface proteins, OKT3 blocks the cytotoxic activity of already activated T cells; this is the result of inappropriate activation and degranulation that results when the CD3 is bound by OKT3. This reaction is perhaps its most important function, but leads to its substantial side effect profile. Pan-activation of the body's T cells leads to transient activation and systemic cytokine release, similar to the effect of the superantigen staphylococcal exotoxin, the etiological agent for toxic shock syndrome. As such, administration of OKT3 leads to profound, systemic cytokine release syndrome that can result in hypotension, pulmonary edema, and fatal cardiac myodepression. In approximately 2% of patients, the inflammatory response manifests itself as aseptic meningeal inflammation. Administration of high-dose methylprednisolone before OKT3 administration is required to blunt this adverse response, but it is rarely avoided altogether. The syndrome abates with subsequent dosages as the target cells available for degranulation become consumed or exhausted.

Much like ATG, OKT3 was first used as a rescue agent to treat acute renal allograft rejection.[82,83] It is greatly superior to conventional steroid therapy in reversing rejection and, consequently, in improving allograft survival. However, its side effects and the limiting nature of the antimurine antibody response have limited its use to steroid-resistant rejection. Use of OKT3 in induction immunosuppressive protocols for kidney transplants is also common in some centers.

ANTI-IL-2 STRATEGIES

Two new monoclonal antibodies have recently been approved for use in renal transplantation: daclizumab (Zenapax; Roche Pharmaceuticals, Nutley, NJ), and basiliximab (Simulect; Novartis Pharmaceuticals, Basel, Switzerland).[84-86] Both are directed against CD25, the high-affinity chain of the IL-2 receptor (Fig. 46.3). The design of these agents represents significant attempts to achieve the therapeutic benefits of ALG or OKT3 without the toxicity through rational molecular engineering. Targeting this receptor has many potential advantages. It is only present on activated T cells, and thus the effects are limited to those T cells that have become activated in the face of an allotransplant. Theoretically, only allograft-specific cells are affected, leaving T cells with physiological specificity undisturbed. It should be pointed out, however, that because alloreactivity is the result of cross-reactivity, even removal of alloreactive cells might remove cells with important specificity against pathogenic antigens. An additional benefit of anti-CD25 therapy is that it is monoclonal and the binding of its target does not precipitate a T-cell signal which induces cytokine release. Thus, no acute side effects occur. Both anti-CD25 antibodies function as induction agents only.

New Immunosuppressive Agents

RAPAMYCIN

Rapamycin is a macrolide antibiotic derived from *Streptomyces hygroscopicus*.[87–89] Structurally, rapamycin is very similar to tacrolimus, and they antagonize each other's biological activity. Both interact with the cytoplasmic protein FK-BP, but rapamycin does not affect calcineurin activity.[90–92] As a result, rapamycin does not inhibit the expression of NF-AT or IL-2 expression. Rather, it impairs signal transduction by the IL-2 receptor (IL-2R). Rapamycin has been shown to dramatically prolong allograft survival in multiple animal models and has recently been approved for use in humans as a maintenance immunosuppressant.

DEOXYSPERGUALIN

The antitumor antibiotic spergualin was isolated from *Bacillus laterosporus* in 1981. Its derivative deoxyspergualin (DSG) was shown to have strong antiproliferative and immunosuppressant properties.[93] Although the mechanism of DSG is not completely understood, there is evidence that it is immunosuppressive via a predominantly anti-APC effect.[94] DSG has been shown to effectively prolong allograft survival in many animal models.[93] Early clinical studies suggest it will be effective in renal transplantation.[95]

BREQUINAR

Brequinar sodium (BQR) is a new immunosuppressive agent that selectively inhibits both T- and B-cell proliferation. It functions by inhibiting the enzyme dihydroorotate dehydrogenase, thus interfering with de novo pyrimidine synthesis. As with MMF, BQR inhibits lymphocyte DNA synthesis and interrupts the rejection process at the level of clonal expansion.[96] Prolongation of heart, kidney, and liver allografts has been shown in several experimental models, and the effects of BQR are synergistic with CyA. Primary side effects are related to leukopenia.

Tolerance

Physicians have long dreamed of a method that would allow for organs to be transplanted and specifically accepted as self-organs. Since the middle of this century, it has been clear that one *acquires* the ability to respond to certain antigens and not respond to others. More recently, it has become apparent that tolerance to self-tissues is rarely absolute, is closely regulated, and is probably *maintained* by repetitive exposure to self-antigen in a context that fosters T-cell anergy rather than

T-cell activation. Several investigators are now aggressively pursuing means to apply the body's natural ability to acquire and maintain tolerance to transplanted organs rather than relying on toxic immunosuppression for graft survival. Extraordinary success has been achieved in animals using several techniques, the most promising of which are T-cell ablation, mixed chimerism, and costimulation blockade. Early human trials are being contemplated.

Xenotransplantation

Transplantation has now become the treatment of choice for most end-stage diseases of most solid organs. Unfortunately, the indications for organ replacement have expanded at a rate far exceeding the available donor supply. Those that do receive one generally must wait a significant amount of time, during which they undergo deterioration in their fitness for surgery. Many investigators are now examining the feasibility of xenotransplantation to improve the availability of organs.[97] In general, there are two types of xenografts, discordant (from distantly related species) and concordant (from closely related species). The immunology of these two types of xenografts differs markedly, and their use in humans will require considerable advances in immunosuppressive technology.

References

1. Fearon DT, Locksley RM. The instructive role of innate immunity in the acquired immune response. Science 1996;272:50–53.
2. Wright SD, Ramos RA, Tobias PS, et al. CD14, a receptor for complexes of lipopolysaccharide (LPS) and LPS binding protein. Science 1990;249:1431–1433.
3. Dempsey PW, Allison MED, Akkaraju S, et al. C3d of complement as a molecular adjuvant: bridging innate and acquired immunity. Science 1996;271:348–350.
4. Baldwin WM, Pruitt SK, Brauer RB, et al. Complement in organ transplantation. Transplantation 1995;59:797–808.
5. Hart DNJ. Dendritic cells: unique leukocyte populations which control the primary immune response. Blood 1997;90:3245–3287.
6. Ahmed R, Gray D. Immunological memory and protective immunity: understanding their relation. Science 1996;272:54–60.
7. Davis MM, Bjorkman PJ. T-cell antigen receptor genes and T-cell recognition. Nature 1988;334:395–402.
8. Cooper MD. B lymphocytes: normal development and function. N Engl J Med 1987;317:1452–1457.
9. Gill JI, Gulley ML. Immunoglobulin and T-cell receptor gene rearrangement. Hematol Oncol Clin North Am 1994;8:751–770.
10. Oettinger MA, Schatz DG, Gorka C, Baltimore D. RAG-1 and RAG-2, adjacent genes that synergistically activate V(D)J recombination. Science 1990;248:1517–1523.
11. McBlane JF, van Gent DC, et al. Cleavage at a V(D)J recombination signal requires only RAG1 and RAG2 proteins and occurs in two steps. Cell 1995;83:387–395.
12. Kappler JW, Marrack P. T cell tolerance by clonal elimination in the thymus. Cell 1987;49:273–280.
13. Bevan MJ. In thymic selection, peptide diversity gives and takes away. Immunity 1997;7:175–178.
14. Fowlkes BJ, Ramsdell F. T-cell tolerance. Curr Opin Immunol 1993;5:873–879.
15. Itoh N, Yonehara S, Ishii A, et al. The polypeptide encoded by the cDNA for human cell surface antigen Fas can mediate apoptosis. Cell 1991;66:233–243.
16. June CH, Bluestone JA, Nadler LM, Thompson CB. The B7 and CD28 receptor families. Immunol Today 1994;15:321–331.
17. Rothenberg EV. How T cells count. Science 1996;273:78–79.

18. Viola A, Lanzavecchia A. T-cell activation determined by T-cell receptor number and tunable thresholds. Science 1996;273:104–106.

19. Kumagai N, Benedict SH, Mills GB, et al. Requirements for the simultaneous presence of phorbol esters and calcium ionophores in the expression of human T lymphocyte proliferation-related genes. J Immunol 1987;139:1393–1399.

20. Saizawa K, Rojo J, Janeway CA Jr. Evidence for a physical association of CD4 and the CD3: alpha:beta T-cell receptor. Nature 1987;328:260–263.

21. Leahy DJ, Axel R, Hendrickson WA. Crystal structure of a soluble form of the human T cell coreceptor CD8 at 2.6 Å resolution. Cell 1992;68:1145–1162.

22. Germain RN. MHC-dependent antigen processing and peptide presentation: providing ligands for T lymphocyte activation. Cell 1994;76:287–299.

23. Monaco JJ. Structure and function of genes in the MHC class II region. Curr Opin Immunol 1993;5:17–20.

24. Ridge JP, Di Rosa F, Matzinger P. A conditioned dendritic cell can be a temporal bridge between a CD4+ T-helper and a T-killer cell. Nature 1998;393:474–478.

25. Lanzavecchia A. License to kill. Nature 1998;393:413–414.

26. Plas DR. Johnson R, Pingel JT, et al. Direct regulation of ZAP-70 by SHP-1 in T-cell antigen receptor signaling. Science 1996;272:1173–1176.

27. Marengere LEM, Waterhouse P, Duncan GS, et al. Regulation of T-cell receptor signaling by tyrosine phosphatase SYP associated with CTLA-4. Science 1996;272:1170–1173.

28. Crabtree GR. Contingent genetic regulatory events in T lymphocyte activation. Science 1989;243:355–361.

29. Ullman KS, Northrop JP, Verweij CJ, Crabtree GR. Transmission of signals from the T lymphocyte antigen receptor to the genes responsible for cell proliferation and immune function: the missing link. Annu Rev Immunol 1990;8:421–452.

30. Siegel JN, June CH. Signal transduction in T cell activation and tolerance. In: New Concepts in Immunodeficiency Diseases. New York: John Wiley and Sons, Gupta S and Griscelli C, eds. 1993;85–129.

31. Berke G. The CTL's kiss of death. Cell 1995;81:9–12.

32. Hozumi N, Tonegawa S. Evidence for somatic rearrangement of immunoglobulin genes coding for variable and constant regions. Proc Natl Acad Sci U S A 1976;73:3628–3632.

33. Zouali M. B-cell superantigens: implications for selection of the human antibody repertoire. Immunol Today 1995;16:399–405.

34. Jung S, Rajewsky K, Radbruch A. Shutdown of class switch recombination by deletion of a switch region control element. Science 1993;259:984–987.

35. Cambier JC, Pleiman CM, Clark MR. Signal transduction by the B-cell antigen receptor and its coreceptors. Annu Rev Immunol 1994;12:457–486.

36. Takeuchi Y, Porter CD, Strahan KM, et al. Sensitization of cells and retroviruses to human serum by (α1-3) galactosyltransferase. Nature 1996;379:85–88.

37. Arai KI, Lee F, Miyajima A, et al. Cytokines: coordinators of immune and inflammatory responses. Annu Rev Biochem 1990;59:783–836.

38. Waldmann T, Tagaya Y, Bamford R. Interleukin-2, interleukin-15, and their receptors. Int Rev Immunol 1998;16:205–226.

39. Allison JP, Krummel MF. The yin and yang of T-cell costimulation. Science 1995;270:932–933.

40. Chambers CA, Allison JP. Co-stimulation in T cell responses. Curr Opin Immunol 1997;9:396–404.

41. Larsen CP, Pearson TC. The CD40 pathway in allograft rejection, acceptance, and tolerance. Curr Opin Immunol 1997;9:641–647.

42. Harlan DM, Kirk AD. Anti-CD154 therapy to prevent graft rejection. Graft 1998;1:63–70.

43. Butcher EC, Picker LJ. Lymphocyte homing and homeostasis. Science 1996;272:60–66.

44. Fuggle SV, Koo DDH. Cell adhesion molecules in clinical renal transplantation. Transplantation 1998;65:763–769.

45. Campbell RD, Trowsdale J. Map of the major histocompatibility complex. Immunol Today 1993;14:349–352.

46. Brown JH, Jardetzky T, Gorga JC, et al. 3-dimensional structure of the human class II histocompatibility antigen HLA-DR1. Nature 1993;364:33–39.

47. Parham P, Ohta T. Population biology of antigen presentation by MHC class I molecules. Science 1996;272:67–74.

48. Nowak MA, Bangham CRM. Population dynamics of immune responses to persistent viruses. Science 1996;272:74–79.

49. Halloran PF, Madrenas J. Regulation of MHC transcription. Transplantation 1990;50:725–738.

50. Gerritsen ME, Bloor CM. Endothelial cell gene expression in response to injury. FASEB 1993;7:523–533.

51. Bach F, Hirschhorn K. Lymphocyte interaction: a potential histocompatibility test in vitro. Science 1964;143:813–814.

52. Terasaki PI, McClelland JD. Microdroplet assay of human serum cytotoxins. Nature 1964;204:998–1000.

53. Cecka JM, Terasaki PI. The UNOS scientific renal transplant registry. In: Cecka JM, Terasaki PI, eds. Clinical Transplants 1995. Los Angeles: UCLA Tissue Typing Laboratory, 1996;1–18.

54. Halloran PF, Broski AP, Batiuk TD, et al. The molecular immunology of acute rejection: an overview. Transpl Immunol 1993;1:3–27.

55. Suthanthiran M. Acute rejection of renal allografts: mechanistic insights and therapeutic options. Kidney Int 1997;51:1289–1304.

56. Burdick JF. An anatomy of rejection. Transplant Rev 1991;5:81–90.

57. Kirk AD, Ibrahim MA, Bollinger RR, et al. Renal allograft infiltrating lymphocytes: a prospective analysis of in vitro growth characteristics and clinical relevance. Transplantation 1992;53:329–338.

58. Krams SM, Falco DA, Villaneuva JC, et al. Cytokine and T-cell receptor gene expression at the site of allograft rejection. Transplantation 1992;53:151–156.

59. Kirk AD, Bollinger RR, Finn OJ. Rapid, comprehensive analysis of human cytokine mRNA and its application to the study of acute renal allograft rejection. Hum Immunol 1995;43:113–128.

60. Dallman MJ, Clark GJ. Cytokines and their receptors in transplantation. Curr Opin Immunol 1991;3:729–734.

61. Baldwin III WM, Pruitt SK, Sanfilippo F, et al. Alloantibodies: basic and clinical concepts. Transplant Rev 1991;5:100–119.

62. Saadi S, Platt JL. Transient perturbation of endothelial integrity induced by natural antibodies and complement. J Exp Med 1995;181:21–31.

63. Bach FH, Winkler H, Ferran C, et al. Delayed xenograft rejection. Immunol Today 1996;17:379–384.

64. Gebel HM, Lebeck LK. Crossmatch procedures used in organ transplantation. Clin Lab Med 1991;11:603–620.

65. Talbot D. The flow cytometric crossmatch in perspective. Transplant Immunol 1993;1:155–162.

66. Colvin RB. The pathogenesis of vascular rejection. Transplant Proc 1991;23:2052–2055.

67. Paul LC. Chronic renal transplant loss. Kidney Int 1995;47:1491–1499.

68. Almond PS, Matas A, Gillingham KJ, et al. Risk factors for chronic rejection in renal allograft recipients. Transplantation 1993;55:752–757.

69. Hitchings GH, Elion GB, Falco EA, et al. Antagonists of nucleic acid derivatives, I: the lactobacillus casei model. J Biol Chem 1950;183:1.

70. Hitchings GH, Elion GB. Chemical suppression of the immune response. Pharmacol Rev 1963;15:365.

71. Calne RY, Murray JE. Inhibition of rejection of renal homografts in dogs with Burroughs-Wellcome 322. Surg Forum 1961;12:118.

72. Sollinger HW, Deierhoi MH, Belzer FO, et al. RS-61443: a phase

I clinical trial and pilot rescue study. Transplantation 1992;53:428–432.

73. Sollinger HW, US Renal Transplant Mycophenolate Mofetil Study Group. Mycophenolate mofetil for the prevention of acute rejection in primary cadaveric renal allograft recipients. Transplantation 1995;60:225–232.

74. Borel JF, Feurer C, Gubler HU. Biological effects of cyclosporine A: a new antilymphatic agent. Actions and Agents 1976;6:468–475.

75. Kahan BD. Role of cyclosporine: present and future. Transplant Proc 1994;26:3082–3087.

76. Fruman DA, Klee CB, Bierer BE, Burakoff SJ. Calcineurin phosphatase activity in T lymphocytes is inhibited by FK506 and cyclosporin A. Proc Natl Acad Sci U S A 1992;89:3686–3690.

77. Starzl TE, Fung JJ, Venkataramanan, et al. FK-506 for liver, kidney, and pancreas transplantation. Lancet 1989;334:1000–1004.

78. Gaber AO, First MR, Tesi RJ, et al. Results of the double-blind, randomized, multicenter, phase III clinical trial of Thymoglobulin versus Atgam in the treatment of acute graft rejection episodes after renal transplantation. Transplantation 1998;66:29–37.

79. Merion RM, Howell T, Bromberg JS. Partial T-cell activation and energy induction by polyclonal antithymocyte globulin. Transplantation 1998;65:1481–1489.

80. Wilde MI, Goa KL. Muromonab CD3: a reappraisal of its pharmacology and use as prophylaxis of solid organ transplant rejection. Drugs 1996;51:865–894.

81. Delmonico FL, Cosimi AB. Monoclonal antibody treatment of human allograft recipients. Surg Obst Gynecol 1988;166:89–98.

82. The Ortho Multicenter Transplant Study Group. A randomized clinical trial of OKT3 monoclonal antibody for acute rejection of cadaveric renal transplants. N Engl J Med 1985;313:337–342.

83. Light JA, Khawand N, Aquino A, et al. Quadruple immunosuppression: comparison of OKT3 and Minnesota antilymphocyte globulin. Am J Kidney Dis 1989;14:10–13.

84. Soulillou JP, Le Mauff B, Olive D, et al. Prevention of rejection of kidney transplants by a monoclonal antibody directed against interleukin 2. Lancet 1987;1:1339–1342.

85. Nashan B, Moore B, Amlot P, et al. Randomised trial of basiliximab versus placebo for control of acute cellular rejection in renal allograft recipients. Lancet 1997;350:1193–1198.

86. Vincenti F, Kirkman R, Light S, et al. Interleukin-2 receptor blockade with daclizumab to prevent acute rejection in renal transplantation. N Engl J Med 1998;338:161–165.

87. Segal SN, Baker H, Vezina C, et al. Rapamycin (AY-22,989), a new antifungal antibiotic, II: fermentation, isolation and characterization. J Antibiot (Tokyo) 1975;28:727–732.

88. Martel RR, Klicius J, Galet S. Inhibition of the immune response by rapamycin, a new antifungal antibiotic. Can J Physiol Pharmacol 1977;55:48–51.

89. Baker H, Sidorowicz A, Sehgal SN, Vezina C. Rapamycin (AY-22,989), a new antifungal antibiotic, III: In vitro and in vivo evaluation. J Antibiot 1978;31:539–545.

90. Molnar-Kimber KL. Mechanism of action of rapamycin (Sirolimus, Rapamune). Transplant Proc 1996;26:964–969.

91. Dumont FJ, Melino MR, Staruch MJ, et al. The immunosuppressive macrolides FK-506 and rapamycin act as reciprocal antagonists in murine T cells. J Immunol 1990;144:1418–1424.

92. Dumont FJ, Staruch MJ, Koprak SL, et al. Distinct mechanisms of suppression of murine T-cell activation by the related macrolides FK-506 and rapamycin. J Immunol 1990;144:251–258.

93. Kaufman DB. 15-Deoxyspergualin in experimental transplant models: a review. Transplant Proc 1996;28:868–870.

94. Ramos EL, Nadler SG, Grasela DM, Kelly SL. Deoxyspergualin: mechanism of action and pharmacokinetics. Transplant Proc 1996;28:873–875.

95. Gores PF. Deoxyspergualin: clinical experience. Transplant Proc 1996;28:871–872.

96. Cramer DV. Brequinar sodium. Transplant Proc 1996;26:960–963.

97. Auchincloss H Jr, Sachs DH. Xenogeneic transplantation. Annu Rev Immunol 1998;16:433–470.

Principles of Organ Preservation

J.E. Tuttle-Newhall and Pierre-Alain Clavien

Organ preservation is the ability to maintain ex vivo organ viability in addition to the capacity to restore normal organ function at the time of restitution of physiological blood flow.[1] It is currently the basis upon which clinical and research models of organ transplantation rely. Clinically, when the organ does not regain normal function rapidly after implantation surgery and reperfusion, there is either delayed graft function (DGF) or primary nonfunction (PNF). DGF by definition is impaired function that eventually returns to normal. On the other hand, graft PNF indicates complete failure of the organ to restore function or the inability to sustain life. In the clinical setting, DGF occurs in 10% to 15% of all liver grafts and 30% to 50% of cadaveric kidneys transplanted within 24 h of cold preservation.[2] In heart, lung, or liver transplants, DGF can have devastating results in the individual patient, with prolonged ICU and hospital stays and possible long-term effects on organ function. PNF of vital organs results in death of the patient unless a retransplant is rapidly performed.

In the laboratory, organs can be preserved in the University of Wisconsin (UW) preservation solution for as long as 72 h with 100% immediate graft function in some animal models.[3] Although the phenomenon of DGF is often blamed upon hypothermic preservation techniques that are currently used in clinical organ transplants, it is clear that other variables are critical, such as donor, recipient, and specific immunological conditions. To reduce the incidence of DGF and PNF, it is paramount to understand the mechanisms of graft injury during preprocurement, ex vivo transport, and subsequent reperfusion.

Mechanisms of Preservation Injury

To reduce the incidence of DGF and PNF, it is important to understand the types of injuries that occur at the cellular level. In the discussion of preservation and reperfusion injury, there are four different time periods that should be examined:[1] prepreservation, cold preservation, rewarming, and reperfusion. While the prepreservation time period is distinct, the other three time periods are interrelated and codependent, making up the classic ischemia–reperfusion interval.

Prepreservation

Injury to solid organs can occur before the procurement process. Nonimmune-mediated processes may be very important to both short- and long-term patient and graft outcomes. On reviewing the current United Network of Organ Sharing (UNOS) database, immediate function and long-term graft survival are superior in grafts from living donors compared to those procured from classic cadaveric sources. Organ disease present in the donor either may be incompatible with graft survival after transplantation, such as severe hepatic steatosis, or may result in transmissible diseases, such as hepatitis C or B. Brain death triggers specific injuries in the cadaveric donor. Until recently, brain death in itself has not been considered a significant risk factor in the prepreservation period.[4] The phenomena of brain death cause severe and profound derangements of the hemodynamic and endocrine systems as well as striking structural changes in the organs themselves. This chain of events may set the stage for the activation of various pathways at the cellular level, thereby triggering mechanisms of injury that may lead to increased immunogenicity and magnify preservation and reperfusion injuries.

Ischemic Injury

The current clinical methods used to preserve organs for ex vivo transport and later implantation in a suitable recipient are based on the suppression of metabolism by hypothermia at the time of removal from the donor. Organs are made tolerant to hypothermia by removing blood and replacing it with solutions designed to limit the physiological consequences of hypothermic preservation. In addition to cellular injury sustained during hypothermia, there are also organ-specific homeostatic mechanisms that are perturbed in ways that prime them for augmentation of injury during reperfusion. Hypothermia decreases the cellular metabolic rate and the rate at which cellular enzyme systems function. When the temperature is decreased from normothermia, 37°C, to 0° to 4°C, there is a 12- to 13-fold decrease in metabolism.[5] Cellular metabolism in the cold, however, does not cease completely.

Although hypothermia is essential to organ preservation, residual cellular energy requirements exceed the capacity of the cell to generate energy from anaerobic metabolism; this in turn leads to decreased intracellular energy, ATP, and adenosine diphosphate (ADP) levels as demonstrated in several laboratory models.[6] In clinical transplantation, the period of warm ischemia during implantation may lead to further decrease in intragraft ATP, which is thought to be a marker of graft viability. Thus, one mechanism of ischemic hypothermic injury in all cells is the loss of mitochondrial respiration and the resulting depletion in ATP.[7]

As a consequence of the energy debt created during hypothermic conditions, several other intracellular events occur. Due to the use of anaerobic metabolism, there is an increase in intracellular acidosis secondary to lactate accumulation. The result of this acidosis, however, is unclear. After a critical period of ischemia, reperfusion precipitates irreversible injury. Reperfusion injury to several cell lines and experimental models was precipitated by a rapid return to physiological pH, the phenomenon described as a "pH paradox." In this paradox, the cell injury and death are not from the acidosis caused by anaerobic metabolism but rather from the rapid return to normal pH during reperfusion.[8]

Another mechanism of cell injury in the cold is cell swelling. This is caused by inhibition of Na^+/K^+-ATPase in hypothermic conditions, resulting in intracellular accumulation of Na^+. This in turn leads to influx of Cl^- while K^+ exits the cell. With the decrease of the osmotic effect of the intracellular ions, there is an influx of water and resulting cell swelling.[9]

Finally, based on theory and pharmacological intervention studies, it was initially hypothesized that reactive oxygen intermediates played a large role in the initial cellular injury that occurred at the time of reperfusion.[7] Nonetheless, further and recent investigations into this phenomenon have failed to prove that reactive oxygen intermediates play a large role in cellular injury.[10,11]

Preservation Solution

Successful ex vivo transport and reimplantation of graft organs is dependent upon the ability of the graft to survive hypothermic preservation. As such, preservation strategies have sought to optimize the components of the original cold storage Collins and Euro-Collins solutions. Based upon basic knowledge about hypothermic cellular injury, Belzer and Southard described the characteristics of the ideal preservation solution[5]: (1) it must contain substrates to regenerate high-energy phosphate compounds; (2) it must have an alkaline pH to counteract acidosis; (3) it must contain materials to prevent injury from reactive oxygen intermediates; and

TABLE 47.1. Components of University of Wisconsin Solution.

Component	Amount (mmol/l)
KH_2PO_4	25
$MgSO_4$	5
Raffinose	30
Pentafraction (HES)	50 (g/l)
Penicillin	200,000 U/l
Insulin	40 U/l
Dexamethasone	16 (mg/dl)
K Lactobionate	100
GSH	3
Adenosine	5
Allopurinol	1
Na	25
K	125

GSH, glutathione; HES, hydroxyethyl starch.

(4) it must minimize cell swelling in hypothermic conditions. As a consequence, University of Wisconsin (UW) solution contains several agents thought to facilitate storage of the liver, pancreas, and other organs such as heart and lung (Table 47.1). It is also the only solution that is effective for prolonged preservation of isolated transplantable cells such as pancreatic islet cells.[12–14]

Reperfusion Injury

During the ischemic phase of the injury, particularly in the liver, some cells are more sensitive to injury than others. The key to limiting the degree of preservation injury to cells is to restore normal physiological blood flow as soon as possible, that is, to limit the duration of hypothermic and normothermic ischemia (see Table 47.2 for optimal cold ischemia times for specific organs). The mechanism of reperfusion injury is multifactorial and not completely mechanistically defined, but it revolves around activation of specific cell types (e.g. neutrophils), expression of certain cell markers (especially cell adhesion molecules), increased production of specific cell mediators (such as TNF-α, IL-1, and interferon-γ), microvascular perfusion failure (both obstructive and regulatory), and programmed cell death (apoptosis). Mechanisms of cell death are diagrammed in Figure 47.1.

TABLE 47.2.

Optimal Cold Ischemia Time for Different Organs Based on Level of Evidence.

Organ	Cold ischemia time (in UW)	Evidence
Kidney	<24 h	II[79]
Kidney/pancreas	<21 h	II[80]
Liver	<12 h	II[81]
Lungs	4–6 h	I[82,83]
Heart	4 h	I[84]

Source: Adapted from Pita (1997),[15] Stratta (1997),[16] Klar (1998),[17] Serrick (1998),[18] Binns (1996),[19] and Schmid (1997).[20]

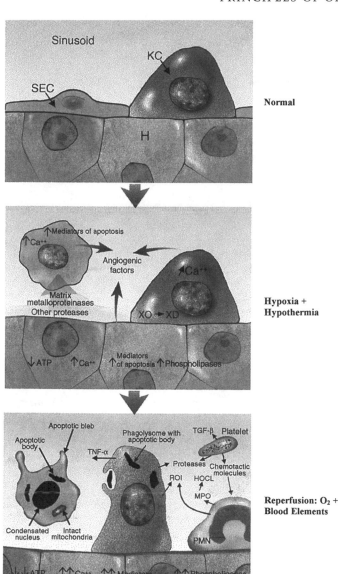

FIGURE 47.1. Potential mechanisms of injury during cold preservation and reperfusion.

Prevention of Ischemia Reperfusion Injury

As discussed, preservation injury is the result of combined effects of brain death and cold and warm ischemia as well as reperfusion. There is no one single event that has yet been identified as more critical than any other, thus limiting focused attempts at attenuating the entire process. It is clear that preservation injury can be obviated or significantly limited by using living donors or limiting storage times. Specific donor qualities, reactive oxygen intermediates, soluble mediators of inflammation, specific cell types, or preconditioning may be manipulated to hinder or prevent preservation injury (Fig. 47.1).

References

1. Clavien PA, Harvey RC, Strasberg SM. Preservation and reperfusion injuries in liver allografts. Transplantation (Baltimore) 1992;53:957–978.
2. Southard J, Belzer F. Organ preservation. Annu Rev Med 1995;46:235–247.
3. Wahlberg JA, Lover R, Landegaard L, Southard JH, Belzer FO. 72-hour preservation of the canine pancreas. Transplant Proc 1987;43:5–8.
4. Pratschke J, Wilhelm MJ, Kuska M, et al. Brain death and its influence on donor organ quality and outcome after transplantation. Transplantation 1999;67:343–348.
5. Belzer FO, Southard JH. Principles of solid-organ preservation by cold storage. Transplantation 1988;45.673–676.
6. Boudjema K, Lindell SL, Southard JH, Belzer FO. The effects of fasting on the quality of liver preservation by simple cold storage. Transplantation 1990;50:943–948.
7. Jaeschke H. Preservation injury: mechanisms, prevention and consequences. J Hepatol 1996;25:774–780.
8. Bond JM, Herman B, Lemasters JJ. Protection by acidotic pH against anoxia/reoxygenation injury to rat neonatal cardiac myocytes. Biochem Biophys Res Commun 1991;179:798–803.
9. Raison J. The influence of temperature-induced phase changes on the kinetics of respiratory and other membrane associated enzyme systems. J Bioenergetics 1973;4:285–290.
10. Engerson TD, McKelvey TG, Rhyne DB, Boggio EB, Synder SJ, Jones HP. Conversion of xanthine dehydrogenase to oxidase in ischemic rat tissue. J Clin Invest 1987;79:1564–1570.
11. de Groot H, Littaurer A. Reoxygenation injury in isolated hepatocytes: cell death precedes conversion of xanthine dehydrogenase to xanthine oxidase. Biochem Biophys Res Commun 1988;155:278–282.
12. Jeevanandam V, Auteri JS, Marboe CC, et al. Extending the limits of donor heart preservation: a trial with UW solution. Transplant Proc 1991;23:697–698.
13. Kawahara K, Ikari H, Hisano H, et al. Twenty-four hour canine lung preservation using UW solution. Transplantation 1991;51:584–587.
14. Zucker PF, Bloom AD, Strasser S, et al. Successful cold storage preservation of canine pancreas with UW-1 solution prior to islet isolation. Transplantation 1988;48:168–170.
15. Pita S, F V, A A, et al. The role of cold ischemia on graft survival in recipients of renal transplants. Transplant Proc 1997;29:3596–3697.
16. Stratta R. Donor age, organ import, and cold ischemia: effect on early outcomes after simultaneous kidney pancreas transplantation. Transplant Proc 1997;29:3291–3292.
17. Klar E, Angelescu M, Zapletal C, et al. Definition of cold ischemia time without reduction of graft quality in clinical liver transplantation. Transplant Proc 1998;30:3683–3685.
18. Serrick C, Giaid A, Reis A, Shennib H. Prolonged ischemia is associated with more pronounced rejection in the lung allograft. Ann Thorac Surg 1997;63:202–208.
19. Binns OAR, Delima N, Buchanan S, et al. Both blood and crystalloid-based extracellular solutions are superior to intracellular solutions for lung preservation. J Thorac Cardiovasc Surg 1996;112:1515–1526.
20. Schmid C, Heemann U, Tilney NL. Factors contributing to the development of chronic rejection in heterotopic rat heart transplantation. Transplantation 1997;64:222–228.

Kidney Transplantation and Dialysis Access

Stuart J. Knechtle

In the United States, more than 200,000 patients undergo dialysis and 70,000 patients have functioning kidney transplants.[1] The prevalence of end-stage renal disease (ESRD) is increasing at 7% to 9% annually, making it likely that more than 350,000 patients with ESRD will be cared for in the United States by the year 2010. The annual incidence of ESRD is 242 cases per million population, although Blacks have a disproportionately high incidence (758 per million population per year) as compared with Whites (180 per million population per year).[1] Diabetes accounts for 35% of newly diagnosed cases of ESRD, making it the most common cause of renal failure, followed by hypertension (30%). Other causes of ESRD include glomerulopathy, cystic and interstitial renal disease, and obstructive uropathy.

The average annual mortality from ESRD is 25% among patients being treated with dialysis.[1] This death rate is 25% to 50% higher than in Japan and Europe,[2] perhaps due to acceptance of older patients with more coexisting conditions for dialysis in the United States. The 1-year mortality of renal transplant patients is 6% for cadaveric recipients and 3% for living-donor kidney recipients. With both dialysis and transplantation, deaths are primarily caused by cardiovascular disease (50%), infection (15%), and malignancy (10%).[3,4]

Should Patients Be Dialyzed or Transplanted?

In patients with known renal disease in whom end-stage renal failure gradually approaches, there is time to anticipate and plan renal replacement therapy. If such a patient is fortunate to have a living donor, a renal transplant can be planned to occur when the recipient's renal failure reaches the critical point at which replacement therapy is necessary to control fluid volume or potassium. Such is the ideal setting, where transplantation occurs as primary treatment without the need for dialysis and where the availability of a living donor removes the indefinite waiting period for a cadaveric donor. It is necessary to wait until the serum cre-

atinine is at least 3 mg/dl to be able to monitor kidney transplant function. The relative proportion of patients with renal failure proceeding directly to renal transplantation without dialysis has varied over time at the University of Wisconsin but averages 39% for recipients of living-donor kidneys and 12% for cadaveric recipients. Early referral for transplantation is largely responsible for this shift and is to be encouraged. Increasing reliance on living donation is also responsible and to be encouraged. Factors influencing waiting time for cadaveric renal transplantation include the patient's blood type (with B blood type waiting the longest), panel reactive antibody (PRA), the rate of cadaveric organ donation, and the size of the waiting list. PRA measures recipient sensitization; the higher the PRA, the more difficult it is to locate immunologically compatible donors. A previous transplant, blood transfusion, or pregnancy may lead to allosensitization, raising the PRA. Often, patients initially present in end-stage renal failure and must begin renal replacement therapy immediately. Hemodialysis or peritoneal dialysis can be started immediately and can be used as either definitive therapy when appropriate or as a bridge to cadaveric or living-donor renal transplantation. Patients with contraindications to renal transplantation (Table 48.1) are treated with dialysis.

Prospective studies comparing the costs, quality of life, and the expected length of life of patients on hemodialysis, peritoneal dialysis, and with renal transplants have been done[5–8] and serve as the basis of the following conclusions: quality of life with a renal transplant is superior to quality of life on peritoneal dialysis which in turn is superior to quality of life on hemodialysis. Despite the greater initial cost of renal transplantation compared to dialysis, cost-effectiveness studies have shown that if the renal transplant functions for at least 2.5 years, the transplant becomes less expensive than dialysis.[7]

Patient survival rates can be compared between hemodialysis, peritoneal dialysis, and renal transplantation overall as well as by specific disease etiology. On average, the annual mortality among patients being treated with dialysis is nearly 25%[1] but depends on disease etiology. Diabetics with

TABLE 48.1. Contraindications to Renal Transplantation.

Cancer present

Active infection

Severe liver disease

Severe lung disease

Severe heart disease

Noncompliance with medical therapy

Active alcohol or substance abuse

Advanced systemic disease (amyloidosis, hemochromatosis)

Advanced age (relative)

Severe obesity (relative)

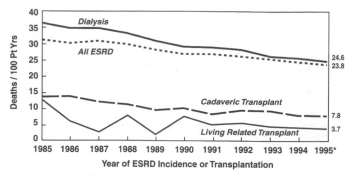

FIGURE 48.1. Death rates based on adjusted Kaplan–Meier estimates, by modality and year of ESRD incidence or of transplantation. Calculation of death rates starts at day 91 following onset of ESRD for dialysis patients and continues through 1 year plus 90 days (censored at first transplant), and starts on the day of transplant for transplanted patients. For each category (dialysis, all ESRD, cadaveric transplant, living-related transplant), death rates are adjusted by age, race, sex, and primary cause of ESRD (diabetes, hypertension, glomerulonephritis, other) to the distribution of the corresponding category of the 1994 incident cohort (level II evidence).[1]

renal failure who are treated with dialysis have a 2-year survival of 30% while those treated with renal transplantation have a 2-year survival of 70%. Figure 48.1 shows comparative survival rates for all ESRD patients and patients treated with cadaveric and living-related renal transplantation. There is a clear benefit of renal transplantation when measured by survival. ESRD patients who are waiting for a suitable living donor or cadaver donor kidney or who have a contraindication to transplantation are maintained with dialysis.

What Type of Dialysis Access Is Best?

Vascular Access

The subcutaneous arteriovenous fistula described by Brescia and Cimino provides the most successful long-term vascular access for chronic hemodialysis. Subsequent developments have included saphenous vein grafts, bovine grafts, and expanded polytetrafluoroethylene (PTFE) grafts. Because of their availability and durability, PTFE grafts have been adopted as the standard prosthetic material when a Cimino fistula is not technically feasible.

Angioaccess for Hemodialysis

An estimated 2% to 5% of patients hospitalized develop acute renal failure, which most often resolves.[9] The mortality in critically ill patients with acute renal failure remains high, at 40% to 70%.[10] Such patients may require renal replacement therapy, either with hemodialysis or with continuous thera-

pies such as slow continuous ultrafiltration or continuous venovenous hemofiltration or continuous venovenous hemodiafiltration. Temporary dialysis access for replacement therapy of this nature can be provided by percutaneous catheters, which are typically placed in the femoral, subclavian, or internal jugular veins. These double-lumen dialysis catheters allow blood to be withdrawn from a proximal port and reinfused through a distal port such that admixture of blood from these two ports is minimized. Placement of these dialysis catheters follows the principles of central catheter placement and currently depends on the use of a modified Seldinger technique.

Arteriovenous Fistulas

BRESCIA–CIMINO FISTULA

Successful long-term hemodialysis is best achieved using a primary AV fistula, which has a 3-year patency rate of 70%.[11] The Cimino fistula utilizing autologous vein and artery has a low complication rate relative to fistulas involving prosthetic material (Table 48.2).[12] The principal limitation of a Cimino fistula is that many patients, especially those with chronic illness, have had numerous percutaneous venous

TABLE 48.2.

Vascular Access for Hemodialysis Complication-Free Function (Level III Evidence).

Time since implant (years)	Cimino-Brescia (%)	Bovine heterograft (%)	Gore-Tex vascular graft (%)
1	88	54	61
2	77	30	37
3	67	16	22
4	59	9	14
5	51	5	8

Based on assumption of exponential distribution of interval between two complications.

Source: Mehta (1991).[12]

catheters and blood draws and do not have a patent cephalic vein. In addition, some cephalic veins are of inadequate size to permit enough flow for technically successful hemodialysis. The radial artery to cephalic vein side-to-side or end-to-side anastomosis is the optimal choice because the limited size of the radial artery limits flow such that high-output cardiac failure is not a problem. This fistula requires 4 to 6 weeks to mature, meaning that the cephalic vein enlarges, thickens, or arterializes, permitting safe cannulation. The more proximal fistula between the brachial artery and basilic or cephalic vein may develop into such a high-flow fistula that high-output cardiac failure develops, requiring fistula takedown.

PTFE GRAFTS

For patients with a brachial artery or cephalic vein inadequate to permit placement of a Cimino fistula, a forearm loop PTFE graft is the next best choice. A PTFE graft 6 mm in diameter is used because adequate flow is achieved with this diameter and high-output cardiac failure is not a risk. Other locations for a PTFE graft are the upper arm and the thigh. Complications of PTFE graft placement include edema of the involved limb and a higher thrombosis and infection rate compared to autologous AV fistulas. In addition, patients with peripheral vascular disease, most typically diabetics, the elderly, and smokers, may develop a significant arterial steal syndrome from a PTFE graft.

Peritoneal Dialysis: Surgical Aspects

Approximately 10% of patients with end-stage renal failure are on peritoneal dialysis,[1] which provides a better quality of life relative to hemodialysis, although relatively less efficient dialysis. Patients must be able to care for their dialysis catheter adequately and to perform the exchanges themselves or with available assistance. Catheter insertion can be performed under local anesthesia using either an infraumbilical or supraumbilical incision, inserting the catheter into the pelvis, and tunneling the catheter subcutaneously to an exit site on the abdominal wall.

Patients who develop catheter sepsis can be treated with antibiotics, both systemically and through the peritoneal dialysis (PD) catheter; however, fungal catheter infections and bacterial infections not responsive to antibiotics generally require catheter removal. Culturing of enteric organisms, especially more than one enteric organism, should raise suspicion of perforation of the GI tract.

Renal Transplantation

Patient Selection

Because of increasingly successful outcomes in renal transplantation, indications have expanded continually and the average age of renal transplant recipients has risen progressively. Patients interested in pursuing renal transplantation should be screened appropriately for coronary artery disease because renal failure itself, as well as hypertension, hyperlipidemia, smoking, and family history of heart disease, is a risk factor for accelerated coronary atherosclerosis. A high proportion of patients in renal failure have multiple risk factors. Noninvasive screening using thallium stress tests are generally satisfactory, reserving cardiac catheterization for patients with positive findings by radionuclide imaging. Careful attention should be paid to addressing cardiac risk factors because cardiovascular disease accounts for the vast majority of deaths following renal transplantation. Coronary angioplasty or revascularization may be appropriate before renal transplantation.

Frequently patients are referred with renal failure of unknown etiology. While a biopsy is in some instances performed, it is only helpful if the patient's underlying disease carries a significant risk of recurrence in the transplanted kidney. This risk should be explained to the patient as well as their potential living donor. Table 48.3 lists the diseases that recur most commonly following renal transplantation.[13]

Bilateral native nephrectomy is not indicated in most patients undergoing renal transplantation and is not helpful from

TABLE 48.3. Recurrent Diseases in the Kidney Transplant.

Systemic diseases	Primary renal diseases
Systemic lupus erythematosus	Focal and segmental glomerulosclerosis
Hemolytic uremic syndrome	IgA nephropathy
Schönlein–Henoch purpura	Membranoproliferative glomerulonephritis type I
Diabetes mellitus	Membranoproliferative glomerulonephritis type II
Monoclonal gammopathies and mixed cryoglobulinemia	Membranous glomerulonephritis
Essential mixed cryoglobulinemia	Anti-GBM disease
Multiple myeloma	
Waldenström macroglobulinemia	
Light-chain deposition disease	
Fibrillary glomerulonephritis	
Wegener granulomatosis	
Primary hyperoxaluria type I	
Cystinosis	
Fabry disease	
Sickle cell disease	
Systemic sclerosis (scleroderma)	
Alport syndrome	

Source: Ramos et al. (1994).[13]

an immunological standpoint.[14] Appropriate indications for bilateral native nephrectomy include recurrent pyelonephritis with significant risk of infection post transplantation; polycystic kidney disease with significant hematuria, pain, or infected cysts; or a mass in the kidney suspicious of malignancy.

PATIENTS WITH MALIGNANCY

Because immunosuppression favors the development and recurrence of malignancies, patients with solid tumors are generally not transplanted unless they are free of disease at least 2 years following curative surgical excision.

INFECTION

Patients with infections of any kind should have the infection treated completely before undergoing renal transplantation. Patients with recurrent antibiotic-resistant urinary tract infections and reflux with or without chronic pyelonephritis should be considered for pretransplant bilateral native nephrectomy.

COMPLIANCE

Noncompliance with drug therapy, blood draws for lab testing, or follow-up visits is likely to lead to failure of a renal transplant whether it is due to financial or nonfinancial reasons. Therefore, pretransplant assessment of compliance is crucial, although admittedly difficult. Patients who have lost a renal transplant as a result of noncompliance and who request retransplantation must be carefully screened. Often a period of several months of hemodialysis convinces them to remain compliant the second time.

Immunological Considerations

TISSUE TYPING

All patients being considered for renal transplantation undergo tissue typing to determine their HLA class I and class II types. Because acute rejection is mediated predominantly by T lymphocytes, which recognize MHC class I and II, it is logical and compelling to optimize the matching of MHC antigens between donor and recipient.[15] Because of the substantial polymorphism of HLA (the human MHC) and because of the significant impact of HLA matching on renal transplant outcome, HLA typing is one criterion for donor–recipient selection.[16]

ANTIDONOR ANTIBODY

Before performing a renal transplant, recipient serum is tested against donor lymphocytes to assess the presence of preformed antidonor antibody. Termed a crossmatch test, this can be done either by using a standard NIH method or by flow cytometry. Renal transplantation in the setting of a positive crossmatch test is contraindicated because the risk of hyperacute rejection is greater than 85%.[17,18] The risk of hyperacute rejection in the setting of a negative T-cell crossmatch is close to 0%.

ABO MATCHING

A donor–recipient pair must be ABO compatible. Otherwise, hyperacute rejection mediated by complement-fixing preformed natural antibody is very likely.

Procurement and Preservation of Cadaver Kidneys

Any patient who has been declared brain dead or is to be withdrawn from life support is a potential multiorgan (including kidney) donor. Brain death is defined as complete and irreversible loss of all brain and brainstem function and presents clinically as apnea, brainstem areflexia, and cerebral unresponsiveness. Table 48.4 lists criteria for brain death.[19]

Evaluation of a potential kidney donor includes obtaining history on the mechanism of death, length of time during cardiac and/or pulmonary arrest, duration of hypotension, vasopressor use, and donor social and medical history. Laboratory evaluation includes serum creatinine, BUN, electrolytes, hemoglobin, WBC, arterial blood gas, urinalysis, prothrombin time/partial thromboplastin time, ABO typing, and viral screening including hepatitis B, hepatitis C, HIV, HTLV-1, and CMV. Table 48.5 lists contraindications to cadaveric kidney donation.[19]

USE OF THE MARGINAL DONOR

Table 48.6 summarizes the number of patients awaiting cadaveric renal transplantation, the number of cadaveric donors, the number of kidneys recovered from these donors, and the number of kidneys transplanted in the United States in 1996.[20] The distribution of waiting times for cadaveric renal transplants is listed in Table 48.7.[20] Because only about one-fourth of patients on the waiting list are transplanted each year, there continues to be an interest in expanding the donor pool to make kidney transplantation available to more needy recipients. Increasing experience with marginal donors who do not meet one of the relative contraindications listed in Table 48.5 suggests that these kidneys ultimately function well.[19] Marginal donors may include those with glomerulosclerosis less than 15%, nonbeating hearts, or elevated serum creatinine levels.

Donor Management

Following declaration of brain death, it is crucial for the donor to receive appropriate medical management to optimize successful organ recovery. Increased intracranial pressure following head injury or cerebrovascular accident results in a massive catecholamine release in an effort to compensate for cerebral ischemia by increasing systemic pressure.[21] However, after the brain becomes necrotic, catecholamine levels drop to less than 10% of baseline within hours.[22] Such patients have

---

TABLE 48.4. Criteria for Brain Death.

Prerequisite
  All appropriate diagnostic and therapeutic procedures have been performed, and the patient's condition is irreversible. The patient is free of sedative drugs or hypothermia.

Criteria (to be present for 30 min at least 6 h after the onset of coma and apnea)
  1. Coma
  2. Apnea (no spontaneous respirations)
  3. Absent cephalic reflexes (pupillary, corneal, oculoauditory, oculovestibular, oculocephalic, cough, pharyngeal, and swallowing)

Confirmatory tests
  Absence of cerebral blood flow by radionuclide brain scan
  Absence of electrical activity by electroencephalogram

Source: Van der Werf et al. (1998).[19]

TABLE 48.5. Absolute and Relative Contraindications to Cadaveric Kidney Donation.

Absolute	Relative
Malignancy outside central nervous system	Age >60 year
Prolonged warm ischemia	Age <6 years
Long-standing hypertension	Mild hypertension
Hepatitis B surface antigen	Hepatitis C virus
Sepsis	Prolonged cold ischemia
Intravenous drug abuse	Acute tubular necrosis
Human immunodeficiency virus	Donor diabetes

Source: Van der Werf et al. (1998).[19]

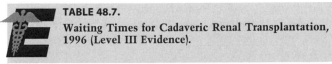

TABLE 48.7.

Waiting Times for Cadaveric Renal Transplantation, 1996 (Level III Evidence).

Time	N	Percent (%)
0–6 months	7,757	22.4
6–12 months	6,385	18.4
1–2 years	8,783	25.4
2–3 years	5,026	14.5
3–5 years	4,279	12.4
5–9 years	1,876	5.4
>9 years	540	1.6
Total	34,646	

Source: U.S. Scientific Registry (1997).[20]

often been managed by a strategy of dehydration to minimize brain edema. These factors in combination often result in a hemodynamically unstable donor who is vasodilated. Most brain-dead donors also develop diabetes insipidus, which exacerbates hypovolemia. Diabetes insipidus is managed by replacing urine output (ml/ml) with hypotonic crystalloid solution. When urine output exceeds 200 ml/h, vasopressin (Pitressin) is administered at a dose of 40 units/l at 120 ml/h for 15 min and repeated every 4 h. Alternatively, desmopressin (DDAVP) can be given at a dose of 1 to 2 μg every 8 h.

It is important to maintain the donor's body temperature. Systolic blood pressures are maintained above 100 mmHg using blood or crystalloid resuscitation as appropriate to maintain a hematocrit of 25% to 30%. Dopamine, norepinephrine, phenylephrine, and epinephrine infusions may be necessary. In summary, the goal of preoperative and intraoperative donor management is to maintain adequate intravascular volume, tissue oxygenation, and normothermia.

Donor Nephrectomy

Donor nephrectomy involves adequate mobilization of the organ, ureter, and associated vasculature. Donors are given heparin and phentolamine prior to eventual vascular division and flushing of the organ with University of Wisconsin (UW) storage solution. The kidney is kept on ice once it has been removed.

Recipient Operation

Regardless of the source of the donor kidney, the preferred site for implantation of the kidney in the recipient is the right pelvis, heterotopically implanting the kidney on the right-sided iliac vessels. The right is preferable to the left because

the iliac vein is more superficial, but some surgeons place a right kidney on the left and a left kidney on the right to keep the renal pelvis anterior to the renal vessels should the pelvis need to be accessed. The peritoneum is reflected medially and the common, external, and internal iliac artery and vein are exposed. The donor renal vein is anastomosed end-to-side to either the right external iliac vein, common iliac vein, or inferior vena cava. The donor renal artery is anastomosed end-to-side to the right common or external iliac artery. An alternative is to anastomose the renal artery end-to-end to the divided internal iliac artery. Following completion of the vascular anastomoses, the kidney is reperfused. The ureter is then anastomosed to the bladder. Figure 48.2 shows the completed kidney transplant procedure. The patient may be administered furosemide (100 mg) and mannitol (12.5 g) to encourage diuresis. However, if no diuresis ensues, intraoperative and postoperative management is aimed at maintaining euvolemia, an adequate hemoglobin concentration, normal blood pressure, and good oxygen delivery. Primary nonfunction resulting from donor factors, preservation injury, or recipient immune response will not respond to diuretics. Patients with initial good function following renal trans-

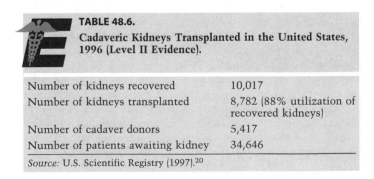

TABLE 48.6.

Cadaveric Kidneys Transplanted in the United States, 1996 (Level II Evidence).

Number of kidneys recovered	10,017
Number of kidneys transplanted	8,782 (88% utilization of recovered kidneys)
Number of cadaver donors	5,417
Number of patients awaiting kidney	34,646

Source: U.S. Scientific Registry (1997).[20]

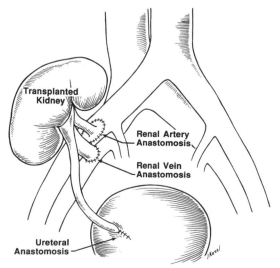

FIGURE 48.2. Completed kidney transplant procedure showing vascular anastomoses to iliac vessels and ureteroneocystostomy.

plantation have a better outcome than patients who experience ATN and require dialysis posttransplant.[16] A native nephrectomy is generally not performed at the time of renal transplantation.

Postoperative Complications and Their Management

THROMBOSIS

Renal artery or renal vein thromboses are rare (<1% incidence), but are devastating because they almost always result in loss of the renal allograft as their recognition and treatment with thrombectomy are generally not performed rapidly enough (within an hour of occurrence). The diagnosis is made by sudden drop in urine output and an ultrasound showing no flow through the renal artery or vein. Alternatively, a radionuclide technetium-99/hippuran scan may demonstrate no blood flow to the kidney. The patient should return to the operating room for transplant nephrectomy because the acutely thrombosed kidney will ultimately cause fever and systemic illness unless removed. Thrombosis occurring years after kidney transplantation as a result of gradual rejection is not clinically apparent and does not require transplant nephrectomy.

URINE LEAK/OBSTRUCTION

A urine leak following renal transplantation presents with local pain and tenderness over the kidney, falling urine output, rise in creatinine, and an ultrasound showing a fluid collection around the kidney. Alternatively, a radionuclide scan demonstrates extravasation of urine into the retroperitoneum. This complication should be managed surgically in an urgent manner by opening the transplant incision and repairing the leak. The diagnosis of urinary obstruction is made most directly by ultrasound showing hydronephrosis. If the cause of obstruction is bladder outlet obstruction or neurogenic bladder dysfunction, this should resolve with Foley catheter placement and repetition of the renal transplant ultrasound 24 h later. If hydronephrosis persists despite decompression of the bladder with Foley catheter, a percutaneous nephrostomy tube can be placed in the renal pelvis by an invasive radiologist. A Whitaker test may be performed by infusing saline through the nephrostomy tube and measuring pressures. Pressures should be less than 12 cm H_2O. A ureterogram can be performed by injecting dye through the nephrostomy tube to identify the site of obstruction. Short strictures, most commonly at the site of the ureteroneocystostomy, can be balloon dilated and stented using the percutaneous nephrostomy as access. However, longer strictures are generally caused by ischemic injury of the transplant ureter and consequent fibrosis and require surgical repair.

LYMPHOCELE

Because of the retroperitoneal dissection involved in the renal transplant procedure, lymphatics in this area may be disrupted and leak a significant amount of lymph into the potential space surrounding the renal transplant. If such a fluid collection becomes substantial, it may compress the adjacent iliac vein, causing leg edema, and ultimately compress the transplant ureter, causing urinary obstruction. The diagnosis is made clin-

ically by a swollen leg on the side of the kidney transplant and a rise in the serum creatinine. The diagnosis is confirmed by ultrasound demonstrating a substantial (i.e., >4 cm in diameter) fluid collection adjacent to the kidney with hydronephrosis. Although percutaneous drainage and injection of sclerosing agents have been attempted, these methods are generally unsuccessful, and surgical repair is indicated.

ACUTE REJECTION/RUPTURED KIDNEY

Severe acute rejection may result in graft loss if it is unresponsive to antirejection therapy. Severe acute rejection may be manifested by a swollen tender kidney with marked enlargement of the kidney by ultrasound. A severely swollen kidney is at high risk for rupture, especially if percutaneously biopsied. Therefore, ultrasound should be performed before attempting to biopsy the kidney, and if it is markedly enlarged, the biopsy should be aborted. A ruptured kidney is diagnosed clinically by a fall in the hematocrit and a tender enlarged kidney. This is a surgical emergency and should be managed by opening the transplant incision, evacuating hematoma, and obtaining hemostasis by wrapping the kidney in a material such as Surgicell. Remarkably, most of the kidneys do not need to be removed and can be salvaged by this technique combined with antirejection therapy.

A severe acute rejection episode unresponsive to antirejection therapy may also progress to thrombosis of the kidney; this can be diagnosed by radionuclide imaging study showing absent blood flow to the kidney. Kidneys undergoing severe acute rejection with graft loss in this manner should be removed because the necrotic kidney will cause systemic illness and fever.

RENAL ARTERY STENOSIS/PSEUDOSTENOSIS

Transplant renal artery stenosis can be diagnosed clinically by extreme sensitivity to cyclosporine or FK506 therapy. Because these drugs cause constriction of the renal afferent arteriole, when this occurs in series with a proximal renal artery stenosis the patient's creatinine may rise precipitously following cyclosporine or FK506 administration. Such patients also commonly present with fluid retention, a rise in serum creatinine, and worsening hypertension. The diagnosis requires either a renal transplant arteriogram or a gadolinium MRI. If the patient's serum creatinine has not been chronically elevated (>3.0 mg/dl), this lesion is worth repairing quickly to restore normal renal function.

Living Donor

Living donors are screened for overall health to assure that they are at low risk for a general anesthetic and a major surgical procedure. Second, they must have no evidence of risk factors for renal failure such as hypertension, diabetes, or underlying kidney disease. Serum BUN and creatinine are measured, although a glomerular filtration rate (GFR) test is not routinely done. Urinalysis is checked to rule out proteinuria or hematuria. Blood type compatibility, tissue typing, and crossmatching are assessed. Finally, an arteriogram or a spiral CT scan is performed to identify the vascular anatomy of the kidneys and to assess for presence of multiple renal arteries. The kidney with the least number of arteries is generally chosen for removal. The advantage of the spiral CT is that it also screens for a renal parenchymal mass. Alternatively, an IVP and arteriogram can be done to accurately delineate the vascular anatomy and collecting system of the donor.

Donors are usually adults between the ages of 18 and 60 years, although older donors have been used successfully and minors may be used as well. Although most donors have traditionally been blood relatives of the recipient, a substantial number of living-unrelated renal transplants have been done. Both open and laparoscopic donor nephrectomy techniques have been used.

Medical Complications and Their Management

DIAGNOSIS OF RENAL DYSFUNCTION

Table 48.8 lists the differential diagnosis of renal transplant dysfunction, dividing causes into early and late and subdividing early complications into surgical (covered earlier) and medical. Acute rejection is the most common cause of early graft dysfunction. Its diagnosis can be accurately based on histological evaluation of a needle biopsy.

Although a successfully treated rejection episode may result in a return of the serum creatinine to baseline levels, patients who have one or more rejection episodes are at increased risk of graft loss compared to patients without rejection.[16] Repeated episodes of acute rejection appear to increase the risk of chronic rejection. Initial good function of a kidney transplant also favors a successful long-term outcome.[16] Patients who require dialysis posttransplant have poorer graft survival compared to patients not dialyzed posttransplant.[16]

Urinary tract infection is the most common infection occurring following renal transplantation and occasionally is accompanied by transplant pyelonephritis causing a rise in serum creatinine. Hypovolemia may cause a rise in creatinine and can be related to dehydration from vomiting, diarrhea, or glucosuria in poorly controlled diabetics. Excessive use of diuretics may also be responsible.

Cyclosporine nephrotoxicity results from vasoconstriction of afferent arteriole of the kidney, which in turn leads to hypertension. Acute cyclosporine toxicity, which is often as-

sociated with a trough level greater than 300 ng/dl in whole blood is reversible with a reduction in cyclosporine dose.

Chronic rejection remains one of the unsolved problems in renal transplantation. It is defined histologically by interstitial fibrosis, neointimal hyperplasia with narrowing of the arteriolar lumen, and a characteristic glomerulopathy with reduplication of the glomerular basement membrane seen on silver stain. There is no effective treatment for chronic rejection, and it generally leads to inexorable deterioration of graft function. Its cause remains poorly defined but probably includes specific and nonspecific immunological injury as well as nonimmunological causes. Despite improvements in immunosuppressive therapy over the past 25 years with a marked reduction in graft loss due to acute rejection, there has not been a coincident decline in the rate of chronic rejection of long-surviving renal allografts.[16]

Cardiovascular Disease

Fifty percent of deaths in renal transplant patients are caused by cardiovascular disease, making it the most common cause of death following transplantation.[4] Transplant patients commonly have multiple risk factors for cardiovascular disease, including hypertension, hyperlipidemia, and diabetes. Many patients also have a smoking history and family history of cardiovascular disease. Improving long-term patient survival requires intensive management of cardiovascular factors. Table 48.9 lists the advantages and disadvantages of antihypertensive drugs in transplant recipients. Patients with difficult-to-control hypertension who are on three or more antihypertensive drugs may benefit from native nephrectomy.

Hyperlipidemia

Posttransplant hyperlipidemia is manifested by increased or unchanged triglyceride and high-density lipoprotein (HDL) levels and by increased low-density lipoprotein (LDL) and total cholesterol levels.[23] Patients treated with tacrolimus have lower LDL and total cholesterol levels than patients treated with cyclosporine. Pharmacological therapy of hyperlipidemia is problematic in renal transplant patients because of potential side effects. Table 48.10 lists agents useful in managing hyperlipidemia in renal transplant patients. Close monitoring of side effects is necessary with these agents.

Infection

During the first month post transplant, infections are most commonly of bacterial origin and related to urinary tract infection, line sepsis, pneumonia, or wound infection. Between 30 and 90 days, fever not caused by bacterial infection is most often due to CMV infection. Prophylaxis with acyclovir or ganciclovir significantly reduces the incidence of posttransplant CMV infection, and these drugs are used to effectively treat infection as well.

Routine prophylaxis with trimethoprim-sulfamethoxazole (TMP-SMX) has made *Pneumocystis carinii* infection rare in transplant patients. Prophylaxis is continued for 1 year after transplantation. After the first 6 months following successful renal transplantation, opportunistic infections become less likely.

TABLE 48.8. Differential Diagnosis of Renal Transplant Dysfunction.

Surgical/mechanical	Medical
Early	Early
Lymphocele	Acute rejection
Urine leak	Ureteral obstruction
Renal artery stenosis	Delayed graft function
Vascular thrombosis	Acute cyclosporine/tacrolimus nephrotoxicity
	Prerenal/volume contraction
	Drug toxicity
	Infection
	Recurrent disease
Late	Late
Ureteral obstruction	Acute or chronic rejection
Renal artery stenosis	Cyclosporine nephrotoxicity, drug toxicity
	Volume contraction
	Infection
	De novo/recurrent disease

TABLE 48.9. Advantages and Disadvantages of Antihypertensive Drugs in Transplant Recipients.

Class	Advantages and indications	Potential side effects
Diuretics	Salt-sensitive hypertension	Hyperuricemia Adverse impact on lipids
Beta-blockers	Large selection Selective agents preferred	Adverse impact on lipids (some) Relative contraindication in diabetes and vascular disease
Alpha-blockers	Young patients Clonidine useful in diabetic patients	Postural hypotension (first dose) Rebound hypertension with clonidine
Calcium channel blockers	Improve renal blood flow May ameliorate cyclosporine nephrotoxicity Nifedipine/isradipine preferred	Verapamil and diltiazem increase cyclosporine levels
ACE inhibitors	Native kidney hypertension	May precipitate renal failure Anemia with enalapril

TABLE 48.10. Pharmacological Agents Useful in Posttransplant Hyperlipidemia.

Drug	Side effects	Recommendations
Cholestyramine/colestipol	Poor compliance May interfere with drug absorption	Schedule doses 1–2 h after immunosuppressive therapy
Niacin	Hepatotoxicity Hyperuricemia Hyperglycemia Flushing	Monitor closely Aspirin to prevent flushing
Gemfibrozil inhibitors	Hepatotoxicity Myositis	Do not use with HMG-CoA inhibitors Monitor hepatic enzymes
HMG-CoA inhibitors	Hepatotoxicity Myositis	Do not use with gemfibrozil Low dose preferred

Malignancy

Skin cancers occur 100 times more commonly in renal transplant patients compared to the general population because of immunosuppressive therapy. Infection with papillomavirus may be related, as is significant sun exposure. Infection with Epstein–Barr virus (EBV) may lead to posttransplant lymphoproliferative disease (PTLD), particularly in patients on high doses of immunosuppressive drugs. PTLD presents with fever and adenopathy with or without graft dysfunction. Successful treatment requires early diagnosis based on EBV serologies and histological evaluation of lymphoid tissue and, most recently, PCR-based DNA analysis. Withdrawal of immunosuppressive drugs is the most important step in therapy.

Kidney transplant patients do not appear to be at increased risk for carcinomas of solid tissue.[24]

Outcomes

The United Network for Organ Sharing (UNOS) compiles the national data on transplant statistics from U.S. centers. The following results summarize national data for renal transplantation.[20]

Table 48.11 lists 1-, 3-, and 5-year graft survival of cadaver-donor kidney transplants and living-donor kidney transplants. Both graft and patient survival are included. Apparent from

TABLE 48.11.

Graft and Patient Survival Rates at 1, 3, and 5 Years (Level II Evidence).

	1-year survival			3-year survival			5-year survival	
	N$_{94-95}$	%	SE	N	%	SE	%	SE
Cadaveric donor								
Graft survival	14,326	86.6	0.3	54,332	72.1	0.2	61.9	0.3
Patient survival	14,330	94.7	0.2	54,341	88.1	0.2	81.4	0.2
Living donor								
Graft survival	5,606	93.3	0.3	18,428	85.2	0.3	77.4	0.4
Patient survival	5,610	97.9	0.2	18,434	94.7	0.2	91.2	0.3

Survival rates were computed using the Kaplan–Meier method.
Source: U.S. Scientific Registry (1997).[20]

these results is the substantial benefit of living-donor kidney transplants compared to cadaver donor transplants.

Recipients who require dialysis within the first week post-transplant had lower graft and patient survival rates at all time points than those who did not require dialysis. Graft survival rates for the dialysis group were 80% at 1 year and 53% at 5 years post transplant, compared with 91% at 1 year and 67% at 5 years post transplant for the nondialysis group.

In 1995, the 1-year graft survival rate for cadaver kidney transplants was 87%; the 1-year patient survival rate were 95%. Patient survival rates for recipients with diabetes was lower at all time points than for recipients with any other diagnosis. Cadaver kidney transplants with a zero HLA-mismatch had the highest graft survival rates at all time points.

The influence of race on renal transplant outcomes is demonstrated by the relatively poorer graft survival among Black recipients. Conversely, Asian recipients had better graft survival rates than any other race.

References

1. US renal data system. In: USRDS 1997 Annual Data Report. Bethesda, Md: The National Institute of Health, National Institute of Diabetes and Digestive and Kidney Diseases, 1997.
2. Friedman EA. End-stage renal disease therapy: an American success story. JAMA 1996;275:1118–1122.
3. Pastan S, Bailey J. Dialysis therapy. N Engl J Med 1998;338:1428–1437.
4. Knechtle SJ, Pirsch JD, D'Alessandro AM, et al. Renal transplantation at the University of Wisconsin in the cyclosporine era. In: Terasaki PI, Cecka JM, eds. Clinical Transplants 1993. Los Angeles: UCLA Tissue Typing Laboratory, 1994:211–218.
5. Laupacis A, Keown P, Pus N, et al. A study of the quality of life and cost-utility of renal transplantation. Kidney Int 1996;50:235–242.
6. Evans RW, Manninen DL, Dugan MK, et al. The Kidney Transplant Health Insurance Study: Final Report. Seattle: Battelle Human Affairs Research Centers, 1990.
7. Russell JD, Beecroft ML, Ludwin D, et al. The quality of life in renal transplantation—a prospective study. Transplantation 1992;54:656–660.
8. Krmar RT, Eymann A, Ramirez JA, et al. Quality of life after kidney transplantation in children. Transplantation 1997;64:540–541.
9. Thadhani R, Pascual M, Bonventre JV. Acute renal failure. N Engl J Med 1996;334:1448–1460.
10. Manns M, Sigler MH, Teehan BP. Continuous renal replacement therapies: an update. Am J Kidney Dis 1998;32:185–207.
11. Williams RA, Hollander L, Benyon RS, et al. Principles of vascular access surgery. In: Wilson SE, Veith FJ, Hobson RW, Williams RA, ed. Vascular Surgery: Principles and Practice. New York: McGraw-Hill, 1987:857–872.
12. Mehta S. Statistical summary of clinical results of vascular access procedures for hemodialysis. In: Sommer BG, Henry ML, eds. Vascular Access for Hemodialysis—II. W.L. Gore Associates, Inc., Precept Press, 1991:145–157.
13. Ramos EL, Tisher CC. Recurrent diseases in the kidney transplant. Am J Kidney Dis 1994;24:142–154.
14. Odorico JS, Knechtle SJ, Rayhill SC, et al. The influence of native nephrectomy on the incidence of recurrent disease following renal transplantation for primary glomerulonephritis. Transplantation 1996;61:228–234.
15. Sayegh MH, Turka LA. The role of T-cell costimulatory activation pathways in transplant rejection. N Engl J Med 1998;338:1813–1821.
16. Cecka JM. The UNOS Scientific Renal Transplant Registry—ten years of kidney transplants. In: Cecka JM, Terasaki PI, eds. Clinical Transplants 1997. Los Angeles: UCLA Tissue Typing Laboratory, 1998:1–14.
17. Kissmeyer-Nielsen F, Olsen S, Petersen VP, et al. Hyperacute rejection of kidney allografts, associated with pre-existing humoral antibodies against donor cells. Lancet 1966;2:662–665.
18. Patel R, Terasaki PI. Significance of the positive crossmatch test in kidney transplantation. N Engl J Med 1969;280:735–739.
19. Van der Werf WJ, D'Alessandro AM, Hoffmann RM, et al. Procurement, preservation, and transport of cadaver kidneys. Surg Clin North Am 1998;78:41–54.
20. 1997 Annual Report of the U.S. Scientific Registry for Transplant Recipients and the Organ Procurement and Transplantation Network—Transplant Data 1988–1996. Richmond, Va: UNOS, and Rockville, Md: Division of Transplantation, Office of Special Programs, Health Resources and Services Administration, US Department of Health and Human Services, 1997.
21. Chen EP, Bittner HB, Kendall SW, et al. Hormonal and hemodynamic changes in a validated animal model of brain death. Crit Care Med 1996;24:1352–1359.
22. Novitzky D, Wicomb WN, Cooper DKC, et al. Electrocardiographic, hemodynamic and endocrine changes occurring during experimental brain death in the chacma and baboon. J Heart Transplant 1984;4:63–69.
23. Markell MS, Friedman EA. Hyperlipidemia after organ transplantation. Am J Med 1989;87(5N):61N–67N.
24. Penn I. Cancers complicating organ transplantation. N Engl J Med 1990;323:1767–1769.

49

Pancreas Transplantation

Robert C. Harland

Diabetes mellitus is a systemic disease that currently affects 6% of the population and ranks as the third most common disease.[1] For insulin-deficient (Type 1) diabetics, exogenous insulin administration is required to avoid hyperglycemia and ketoacidosis. The progression of some of the complications of diabetes can be slowed by intensive control of hyperglycemia. Transplantation of a vascularized pancreas allograft is currently the only therapy that reliably establishes a euglycemic state without the need for exogenous insulin therapy, normalizing the glycosylated hemoglobin level in previously hyperglycemic type I diabetics.

Anatomy and Physiology

The pancreas is a mixed exocrine and endocrine organ with the majority of its mass composed of acinar cells that secrete bicarbonate and digestive enzymes. Scattered throughout the gland are 1 to 2 million endocrine cells in clusters called the islets of Langerhans. These cells arise as part of the APUD (amine precursor uptake and decarboxylation) system. Within these clusters, beta cells provide insulin, alpha cells secrete glucagon, and delta cells are a source of somatostatin. Additional cells located in islets secrete other hormones, including pancreatic polypeptide, gastrin, and vasoactive intestinal peptide.[2] The ability to provide only the endocrine tissue for a diabetic patient without the surrounding exocrine tissue is attractive, but islet cell transplantation until recently, has met with limited success.

Recipient Selection

The initial challenge of clinical pancreas transplantation is the selection of appropriate recipients. The rate of development of diabetic complications is variable, as is their severity, making it difficult to discern which patients might benefit from pancreas transplantation. At this point in time, the

risks of the surgical procedure combined with the long-term risk and cost of immunosuppressive medications has largely limited the application of pancreas transplantation to those patients with established secondary diabetic complications. The most common of these is diabetic nephropathy, which occurs in 40% to 50% of type I diabetics. The ability to treat end-stage diabetic nephropathy with renal transplantation, either before or simultaneously with pancreas transplantation, has resulted in most pancreas transplants' (>90%) being performed in diabetics who have significant renal involvement.[3]

The majority of these patients undergo simultaneous pancreas and kidney transplantation (SPK). Simultaneous transplantation confers the economic benefits of only one transplant procedure and the associated hospitalization. Furthermore, the ability to detect (by monitoring the serum creatinine) and diagnose (by renal biopsy) rejection easily allows early antirejection therapy and reduces immunological pancreas graft loss. Finally, the observation that pancreas graft survival is consistently better in SPK recipients compared to recipients of pancreas transplants alone may be due to the relatively immunosuppressed state induced by uremia.[4]

An increasing number of type I diabetics with nephropathy undergo pancreas transplantation at some time after successful kidney transplantation.[3] As more patients are listed for SPK transplantation and waiting times increase, many patients with a suitable living donor may opt for immediate renal transplantation with a subsequent "pancreas after kidney" (PAK) transplant. This strategy allows elective transplantation utilizing a living donor kidney, with the benefit of better immediate and long-term renal function. Monitoring for pancreas transplant rejection can be more challenging in PAK transplants, but improved immunosuppression and alternative monitoring methods have led to graft survival that is close to that seen in SPK transplant recipients.[3]

Currently, less than 5% of pancreas transplants are performed in patients who have only mild renal impairment or normal renal function. These pancreas transplant alone (PTA) procedures are most often performed in patients with demonstrated progressive secondary complications such as neuropathy (autonomic and/or peripheral), proliferative retinopathy, or early nephropathy (proteinuria with a serum creatinine clearance ≥60) and labite glucose control.

Pretransplant Evaluation

The presence of a chronic systemic disease mandates a thorough, multidisciplinary pretransplant evaluation of all potential pancreas transplant recipients. This workup should include testing to document an insulin-deficient state, a determination of the patient's ability to withstand a major operation, and an assessment of the social and psychological state of the patient with attention to the potential for noncompliance. Specific attention should be given to the cardiovascular evaluation, which should include routine noninvasive cardiac testing. Coronary angiography is performed for indications such as symptomatic cardiac disease, a positive smoking history, age over 45 years, duration of diabetes over 25 years, or a history of peripheral or cerebrovascular disease.[5] The presence of coronary disease is not an absolute contraindication to transplantation, although revascularization with angioplasty or coronary artery bypass grafting may first be required to safely undergo the transplant procedure.[6]

Cadaver Donor Selection, Preservation, and Preparation

Cadaver donors in the age range of 8 to 50 years without a history of diabetes or pancreatic trauma have generally been utilized for pancreas transplantation. Simultaneous procurement of the liver, kidneys, and other organs can occur in essentially all donors despite vascular anomalies.[7,8] En bloc procurement of liver and pancreas with back-table dissection can avoid in situ manipulation and assist in the identification of aberrant anatomy to preserve the arterial blood supply of all transplanted organs. Preservation with an intra-arterial infusion of University of Wisconsin (UW) solution (Viaspan®, Dupont) is universally used in North America; this allows safe cold storage for at least 24 h without compromise of graft function.[9]

Living Donor Versus Cadaveric Donor Pancreas Transplantation

Experience with living-donor, segmental pancreas transplantation is largely limited to the University of Minnesota. While the risk of immunological graft loss is less than that seen with cadaver pancreas transplants, the incidence of graft loss to thrombosis was much greater (18.5%) in living donor transplants, most likely due to the segmental nature of the living donor transplant with a relatively low blood flow. This, combined with the potential morbidity for the donor (including a risk of glucose intolerance), has limited the enthusiasm for living-donor transplantation.[10]

Operative Procedure

Back-Table Preparation

Topical hypothermia is maintained in a bath of UW solution while the arterial supply of the pancreas is reconstructed. Usually, a Y-graft of donor iliac artery is utilized to join the superior mesenteric artery and the splenic artery of the pancreas graft. The portal vein is generally left quite short (1–2 cm) to avoid kinking and subsequent thrombosis. The staple lines on the duodenum are oversewn, as are the mesenteric vascular branches on the anterior surface of the pancreas.

Systemic Venous Drainage Versus Portal Venous Drainage

The pancreas is usually transplanted in the right iliac fossa to the mobilized iliac vein or inferior vena cava. The Y-graft of donor iliac artery is anastomosed to the iliac artery (Fig. 49.1). In this position the donor duodenum can easily be attached to the bladder to drain the exocrine output of the pancreas.

More physiological insulin secretion might be observed with venous outflow from the pancreas to the portal system. To accomplish this, the portal vein of the transplanted pancreas is anastomosed to a branch of the superior mesenteric vein inferior to the transverse mesocolon. Arterial inflow is accomplished by attaching the iliac Y-graft to the iliac artery or to the aorta (Fig. 49.2); this allows more physiological glucose control, avoiding the hyperinsulinemia observed in systemically drained transplants. The attachment of the venous outflow of the pancreas to the portal system may also confer an immunological advantage.

Bladder Drainage Versus Enteric Drainage of Exocrine Secretions

One of the significant milestones in successful pancreas transplantation was the demonstration that outcome with bladder drainage of the exocrine output of the pancreas was superior

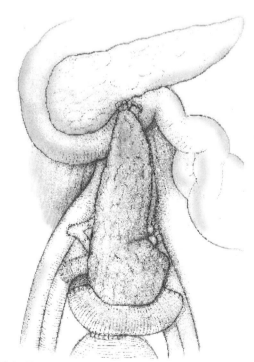

FIGURE 49.1. Pancreas transplant in the right lower quadrant with systemic venous drainage to the iliac vein and exocrine drainage via duodenocystostomy.

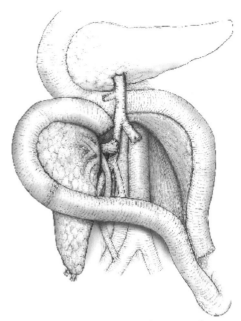

FIGURE 49.2. Pancreas transplant with venous drainage to the portal system via the superior mesenteric vein and enteric drainage of exocrine secretions to a Roux-en-Y limb of jejunum.

to enteric drainage.[11] This finding was attributed to a decreased risk of infection and the ability to monitor the pancreas transplant with urinary amylase secretion. Bladder-related complications, however, led to increased interest in enteric drainage of the pancreatic secretions. Currently, nearly half of pancreas transplants performed in the United States utilize the enteric drainage technique, which also allows the option of portal venous drainage of the transplant with improved glucose control while avoiding hyperinsulinemia. There is no demonstrable difference in infection rates or graft survival when data on the two methods are compared in SPK recipients.

Immunosuppression

When comparing SPK transplant recipients to recipients of kidney transplants alone, several series demonstrated a 50% to 100% increase in the incidence of acute rejection episodes.[12,13] The use of either a polyclonal or monoclonal anti-T-cell induction agent was shown to be effective in improving the outcome of both the kidney and the pancreas in such transplants, despite the increased rate of acute rejection.[14] Incremental improvements in graft survival have been observed with the introduction of newer, more potent agents. This is especially true with the addition of mycophenolate mofetil to the immunosuppressive armamentarium. Many centers now base therapy on the more potent calcineurin agent, tacrolimus, even obviating the use of an antilymphocyte induction agent. Clinical observations suggest that even better results will be observed with the use of IL-2 receptor-blocking agents. Both daclizumab and basiliximab have been effective in reducing the incidence of acute rejection episodes in renal allotransplantation, and trials using these agents in pancreas transplant recipients are under way.

Complications

Graft Thrombosis

The most common cause of early graft loss is thrombosis, which occurs in 5% to 19% of pancreas transplants.[15] Thrombosis usually presents with a rise in the serum glucose. The serum amylase may or may not be elevated. A nuclear medicine blood flow scan or Doppler ultrasonography documents a lack of blood flow to the transplanted organ. At reoperation, infarction of the pancreas is observed and requires transplant pancreatectomy. In most centers aspirin therapy is utilized as a preventive measure. Hemorrhagic complications have been seen with routine use of more aggressive anticoagulation.

Pancreatitis and Exocrine Leaks

Graft pancreatitis is observed in as many as one-third of recipients and may be associated with prolonged preservation times or an elevated serum amylase in the donor. The etiology of pancreatitis may be related to preservation injury or reflux of bladder contents. In severe cases, a picture very similar to that seen in native pancreatitis can be seen, including fever, hypovolemia, and renal dysfunction. Intraabdominal fluid collections may develop and can lead to intraabdominal abscesses.

Similarly, a leak of exocrine secretions from the transplanted duodenum or its anastomosis to either the bladder or recipient intestine can lead to intraabdominal fluid collections that contain digestive enzymes. One or more abdominal explorations may be required if percutaneous drainage does not result in rapid improvement.[16] At exploration, attempted repair of the leak and drainage of the area may be attempted, but graft pancreatectomy is the most reliable way of improving the patient's health and should be applied early in unstable patients or in those with significant intraabdominal infection.

Rejection

Symptoms of pancreas transplant rejection can include fever and graft tenderness. The serum amylase and lipase may be elevated and, in bladder-drained transplants, urinary amylase excretion will decrease. These findings are relatively sensitive but are not very specific for rejection.

For those patients undergoing SPK, the best indicator of rejection is evidence of renal dysfunction. In more than 75% of cases, rejection is observed in both the pancreas and kidney transplanted from the same donor. Percutaneous core biopsies and fine-needle aspiration of the pancreas transplant, as well as transduodenal biopsies via the cystoscope, have all been performed and provide adequate tissue on which to make therapeutic decisions.[17]

Treatment of acute rejection episodes consists of an initial trial of methylprednisolone boluses given for 3 to 5 days. If the patient fails to have an adequate response, then treatment with a monoclonal or polyclonal antilymphocyte agent, is initiated and continued for 7 to 14 days. Most rejection episodes can now be reversed without significant long-term graft dysfunction.

Recurrence of Autoimmune Islet Destruction

The universal use of immunosuppression for allografts explains why recurrence of diabetes has not been observed in patients receiving pancreatic allografts.

Urological Complications

A wide variety of urological complications are observed following bladder-drained pancreas transplantation. These include hematuria, urinary tract infections, leak from the duodenocystostomy, urethritis, urethral strictures, and disruptions.

The majority of these complications can be treated conservatively with bladder catheter drainage and appropriate medical care. Persistent or recurrent symptoms should be treated with operation, usually conversion from bladder drainage to enteric drainage. This may be done relatively early following transplantation to treat a leak from the bladder with a reasonable assurance of graft salvage. Overall, 10% to 30% of patients with a bladder-drained pancreas transplant require conversion to enteric drainage at some point following transplantation.[3]

Outcome

Patient and Pancreas Graft Survival

The International Pancreas Transplant Registry (IPTR) has collected results of clinical pancreas transplantation. Improved graft survival has been seen over the past decade in U.S. transplants reported to the IPTR. The ability to promptly detect rejection in the transplanted kidney and the additional immunosuppression of the uremic state have both been utilized as explanations why SPK recipients enjoy better graft survival than PAK or PTA recipients (Table 49.1). Bladder drainage of exocrine secretions from the pancreatic allograft was associated with better graft survival in all categories of pancreas transplants in the past.[18] The most recent era, however, demonstrates no significant difference in graft survival whether bladder drainage or enteric drainage is initially performed. For solitary pancreas transplants, however, there may still be a deleterious effect of enteric drainage, at least in the PAK category. The majority of this difference appears to be due to a higher incidence of technical failures, especially graft thrombosis, in enteric-drained transplants.

The type of maintenance immunosuppression also influences graft outcome with improved graft survival seen with the use of one or both of the newer immunosuppressive agents (mycophenolate mofetil, tacrolimus). This is observed in all categories of pancreas transplants. Recipient age has an effect on patient, pancreas, and kidney graft survival in SPK recipients, with older (≥45 years) patients experiencing lower survival rates at 1 year. This effect is not observed in PAK or PTA recipients, perhaps because of the restriction of these more "elective" transplants to healthier diabetics with fewer comorbidities.

The beneficial effect of a very well matched donor–recipient combination has been demonstrated in pancreas transplantation as in kidney transplantation.

Benefits of Pancreas Transplantation

PROTECTION FROM NEPHROPATHY

Diabetics who are recipients of a functioning renal allograft eventually develop recurrent diabetic nephropathy, which can be observed histologically as early as 18 months following transplantation. The subsequent performance of a successful pancreas transplant can reverse or prevent this finding.[19,20]

DIABETIC NEUROPATHY

Both peripheral and autonomic neuropathy have consistently shown improvement following pancreas transplantation, as has been documented by nerve conduction studies,[21] cardiorespiratory reflexes, and studies of gastric emptying.

RETINOPATHY

Many of the diabetics who undergo pancreas transplantation have severe visual impairments, making it difficult to assess the beneficial effect of transplantation. Short-term studies have shown no significant improvement in diabetic retinopathy in patients who undergo transplantation.[22] In the presence of a long-term functioning pancreas allograft, however, retinopathy tended to stabilize, while continued deterioration in vision was observed in patients whose grafts had failed.[23]

QUALITY OF LIFE

Kidney transplantation alone or in combination with pancreas transplantation has been shown to provide an improved quality of life for recipients as measured by the patients.[24]

Islet Cell Transplantation

Only a small percentage of the cells comprising the pancreas (the islets of Langerhans) are necessary for glucose homeostasis. The remainder of the tissue is composed of exocrine tissue that not only provides little useful function in the diabetic recipient, but also is responsible for many of the serious complications of pancreas transplantation. The ability to transplant only the cellular elements providing endocrine function is therefore attractive and has been the focus of intense research efforts for more than 30 years. Successful islet transplantation would decrease the morbidity of transplantation, potentially increasing the number of patients who might

TABLE 49.1.

Outcome of U.S. Cadaveric Pancreas Transplants Performed between January 1, 1994, and November 1, 1998, According to Type of Transplant.

Type of transplant	Patient survival (%)		Pancreas graft survival (%)	
	1 year	3 year	1 year	3 year
Simultaneous pancreas-kidney	94	90	83	78
Pancreas after kidney	95	88	71	55
Pancreas transplant alone	95	94	64	52

Source: International Pancreas Transplant Registry (IPTR) Department of Surgery, University of Minnesota, Minneapolis, MN.

benefit from this method of therapy. Recent success with islet transplantation has been seen with newer immunosuppressive regimens and transplantation of islets from more than one donor.[25]

References

1. Harris M, Hadden WC, Knowles WC, Bennett PH. Prevalence of diabetes and impaired glucose tolerance and plasma glucose levels in the US population aged 20–74 years. Diabetes 1987;36: 523–534.

2. Munger B. Morphologic characterization of islet cell diversity. In: Cooperstein S, Watkins D, eds. The Islets of Langerhans: Biochemistry, Physiology, and Pathology. New York: Academic Press, 1981:3–34.

3. Gruessner AC, Sutherland DER. Analysis of United States and non-US pancreas transplants as reported to the International Pancreas Transplant Registry (IPTR) and to the United Network for Organ Sharing (UNOS). Clinical Transplants 1998. Los Angeles: UCLA Tissue Typing Laboratory, 1999:1–19.

4. Sollinger HW, Ploeg RJ, Eckhoff DE, et al. Two hundred consecutive simultaneous pancreas-kidney transplants with bladder drainage. Surgery 1993;114:736–744.

5. Stratta RJ, Taylor RJ, Larsen JL, Cushing K. Pancreas transplantation. Int J Pancreatol 1995;17:1–13.

6. Schweitzer EJ, Anderson L, Kuo PC, et al. Safe pancreas transplantation in patients with coronary artery disease. Transplantation 1997;63:1294–1299.

7. Bunzendahl H, Ringe B, Meyer HJ, Gubernatis G, Pichlmayr R. Combination harvesting procedure for liver and whole pancreas. Transpl Int 1988;1:99–102.

8. Dunn DL, Morel P, Schlumpf R, et al. Evidence that combined procurement of pancreas and liver grafts does not affect transplant outcome. Transplantation 1991;51:150–157.

9. Belzer FO, D'Alessandro AM, Hoffman RM, et al. The use of UW solution in clinical transplantation. Ann Surg 1992;215: 579–585.

10. Seaquist ER, Robertson RP. Effects of hemipancreatectomy on pancreatic alpha and beta cell function in healthy human donors. J Clin Invest 1992;89:1761–1766.

11. Gruessner AC, Sutherland DER. Pancreas transplants for United States and non-US cases as reported to the International Pancreas Transplant Registry (IPTR) and to the United Network for Organ Sharing (UNOS). Clinical Transplants 1997. Los Angeles: UCLA Tissue Typing Laboratory, 1998:40–45.

12. Sollinger HW, Stratta RJ, D'Alessandro AM, Kalayoglu M, Pirsch JD, Belzer FO. Experience with simultaneous pancreas-kidney transplantation. Ann Surg 1988;208:475–483.

13. Rosen B, Frohnert PP, Velosa JA, et al. Morbidity of pancreas transplant during cadaveric renal transplantation. Transplantation 1991;51:123–127.

14. Stratta RJ, Taylor RJ, Lowell JA, et al. OKT3 induction in 100 consecutive pancreas transplants. Transplant Proc 1994;55:509–516.

15. Sutherland DER, Gruessner A. Pancreas transplantation as reported to the United Network for Organ Sharing and analyzed by the International Pancreas Transplant Registry. Clinical Transplants 1995. Los Angeles: UCLA Tissue Typing Laboratory, 1996:49.

16. Troppman C, Gruessner MS, Dunn DL, Sutherland DER, Gruessner RWG. Surgical complications requiring early relaparotomy after pancreas transplantation. Ann Surg 1998;227: 255–268.

17. Drachenberg CB, Papadimitriou JC, Klassen DK, et al. Evaluation of pancreas transplant needle biopsy. Transplantation 1997; 63:1579–1586.

18. Gruessner AC, Sutherland DER. Pancreas transplants for United States and non-US cases as reported to the International Pancreas Transplant Registry (IPTR) and to the United Network for Organ Sharing (UNOS). Clinical Transplants 1997. Los Angeles: UCLA Tissue Typing Laboratory, 1998:40–45.

19. Bohman S-O, Wilsczek H, Tyden G, Jaremko G, Lundgren G, Groth CG. Recurrent diabetic nephropathy in renal allografts placed in diabetic patients and protective effect of simultaneous pancreatic transplantation. Transplant Proc 1987;19:2290–2293.

20. Wilczek HE, Jaremko G, Tyden G, Groth CG. Evolution of diabetic nephropathy in kidney grafts: evidence that a simultaneously transplanted pancreas exerts a protective effect. Transplantation 1995;59:51–57.

21. Muller-Felber W, Landgraf R, Scheuer R, et al. Diabetic neuropathy 3 years after successful pancreas and kidney transplantation. Diabetes 1993;42(10):1482–1486.

22. Wang Q, Klein R, Moss SE, et al. The influence of combined kidney-pancreas transplantation on the progression of diabetic retinopathy: a case series. Ophthalmology 1994;101:1071–1076.

23. Sutherland DER, Kendall DM, Moudry KC, et al. Pancreas transplantation in nonuremic, Type I diabetic recipients. Surgery 1988;104:453–464.

24. Gross CR, Limwattananon C, Matthees BJ. Quality of life after pancreas transplantation: a review. Clin Transplant 1998;12: 351–361.

25. Ryan EA, Lakey JR, Rajotte RV, et al. Clinical outcomes and insulin secretion after islet transplantation with the Edmonton protocol. Diabetes 2001;50(4):710–719.

Transplantation of the Liver and Intestine

Douglas W. Hanto, James F. Whiting, and John F. Valente

Liver Transplantation

Indications, Contraindications, and Timing

GENERAL INDICATIONS

Liver transplantation is indicated in children and adults who develop acute fulminant liver failure or chronic, advanced, irreversible liver disease after alternative medical and surgical treatments have been exhausted and the patients are approaching the terminal phase of their illness. More specifically, liver transplantation is indicated when (1) the patient has end-stage liver disease with a life expectancy of 12 months or less and currently has no medical or surgical alternatives to a liver transplant; (2) the expected mortality of the patient's liver disease is greater than the expected mortality of liver transplantation; (3) the patient has a high likelihood for a successful outcome with an improved quality of life; (4) the patient and the family are capable of understanding the indications, potential benefits, risks, and potential complications of liver transplantation; and (5) the patient is believed to be compliant and able to adhere to the follow-up medical regimen, including taking medications indefinitely.

Specific disease indications for liver transplantation include alcoholic liver disease, chronic active hepatitis (B, C, or autoimmune), cholestatic liver disease (primary biliary cirrhosis (PBC), primary sclerosing cholangitis (PSC), secondary biliary cirrhosis [Caroli's disease, choledochal cyst, trauma, operative bile duct injury/stricture/necrosis, nonalcoholic steatohepatitis (NASH)], cryptogenic cirrhosis, fulminant liver failure (acetaminophen overdose, hepatitis, ischemia, idiosyncratic drug toxicity), Budd–Chiari syndrome, benign neoplasms, extrahepatic biliary atresia or hypoplasia, metabolic diseases (α_1-antitrypsin deficiency, Crigler–Najjar disease, type I, Byler's disease, glycogen storage disease [IA and IV], Wilson's disease, hemochromatosis, tyrosinemia, ornithine transcarbamylase deficiency, galactosemia, etc.), congenital hepatic fibrosis, and cystic fibrosis. Relative indications for liver transplantation include hepatocellular carcinoma (stage I and II), slow-growing metastatic leiomyosarcoma, metastatic neuroendocrine tumors including carcinoids, and hemanigoendotheliomas. The most common indications for liver transplantation in adults are illustrated in Table 50.1 and for children in Table 50.2.

CONTRAINDICATIONS

Absolute contraindications include advanced uncorrectable cardiac or pulmonary disease, severe irreversible pulmonary hypertension, hypotension requiring vasopressor support, recent intracranial hemorrhage, irreversible neurological impairment, human immunodeficiency virus (HIV) infection, uncontrolled sepsis, extrahepatic malignancy with the exception of skin cancer and some neuroendocrine tumors, inability to comply with the posttransplant regimen, and active substance abuse. Relative contraindications include stage III or IV hepatocellular carcinoma, HBV–DNA-positive and HBeAg-positive hepatitis B, cholangiocarcinoma, and age over 70 years.

TIMING

Determining the optimal timing for liver transplantation has been and remains difficult.

Preoperative Evaluation and Management

EVALUATION

Patients undergoing evaluation as potential liver transplant candidates may do so as an outpatient or inpatient depending on the disease and its severity. This is a multidisciplinary evaluation that begins with a complete history, physical examination, routine laboratory studies, chest X-ray, and electrocardiogram. All patients need current hepatitis serological results (A, B, C), viral serology [herpes simplex virus (HSV), cytomegalovirus (CMV), Epstein-Barr virus (EBV), HIV, and varicella zoster virus (VZV)], infectious serology (RPR, toxoplasmosis, rubella), alpha-fetoprotein (AFP), CA19-9 (in pa-

TABLE 50.1. Indications for Liver Transplantation in Adults (1987–1995).

Disease	n (%)
Hepatitis C	3,454 (19.6)
Alcoholic liver disease	3,225 (18.3)
Alcoholic + hepatitis C	527 (3.0)
Unspecified (cryptogenic)	1,911 (10.8)
Primary biliary cirrhosis	1,828 (10.4)
Primary sclerosing cholangitis	1,635 (9.3)
Acute hepatic necrosis	1,066 (6.0)
Hepatitis B	921 (5.2)
Autoimmune hepatitis	900 (5.1)
Malignant neoplasms[a]	724 (4.1)
Metabolic diseases[b]	685 (3.9)
Benign neoplasms	79 (0.5)
Miscellaneous[c]	258 (1.5)
Total	17,729

[a]HCC (267 = 1.5%); HCC + cirrhosis (233 = 1.3%).

[b]α1-antitrypsin (253 = 1.4%); Wilson's disease (167 = 1%); hemachromatosis (169 = 1%).

[c]Budd–Chiari (180 = 1%).

Source: Belle SH, Beringer KC, Detre KM. Recent findings concerning liver transplantation in the United States. In: Cecka JM, Terasaki PI, editors. Clinical Transplants 1996. UCLA Tissue Typing Laboratory, 1996:15–29.

tients with suspected cholangiocarcinoma or PSC), and ABO and HLA typing along with determination of panel reactive antibody (PRA) status. A CAT (computerized axial tomography), MRI (magnetic resonance imaging), or MRA (magnetic resonance angiography) of the liver is performed for vessel patency, liver volume, and to rule out liver tumors. A dental evaluation, Pap smear, mammogram in women more than 40 years of age, and prostate-specific antigen (PSA) in men more than 40 years are required. Other studies that are obtained less frequently, depending on the patient's history and disease, include upper GI endoscopy, pulmonary function tests with arterial blood gases, colonoscopy in patients over 40 years, echocardiogram, dipyridamole stress thallium study, cardiac catheterization with coronary angiography, and psychiatric evaluation for all patients with a history of substance abuse, alcohol abuse, or psychiatric illness. If portal vein occlusion is suspected on MRI, visceral angiography is neces-

TABLE 50.2. Indications for Liver Transplantation in Children (1987–1995).

Disease	n (%)
Biliary atresia	1638 (53.3)
Metabolic diseases	415 (13.5)
Acute hepatic necrosis	340 (11.1)
Cholestatic liver disease (cirrhosis)	110 (3.6)
Other cirrhosis	225 (7.3)
Malignant neoplasms	71 (2.3)
Miscellaneous	266 (8.7)
Total	3113

Source: Belle SH, Beringer KC, Detre KM. Recent findings concerning liver transplantation in the United States. In: Cecka JM, Terasaki PI, editors. Clinical Transplants 1996. UCLA Tissue Typing Laboratory, 1996:15–29.

sary to clearly define the patency of the superior mesenteric vein, splenic vein, and portal vein. Appropriate consultations from physicians in cardiology, pulmonary disease, neurology, and infectious disease are obtained as needed.

LISTING

Patients are listed on the computerized national waiting list through the United Network for Organ Sharing (UNOS) as Status 1, Status 2A, Status 2B, Status 3, or Status 7, depending on their medical condition. Patients are listed as Status 1 if they have acute fulminant liver failure with a life expectancy without a liver transplant of less than 7 days. Patients with primary nonfunction of a transplanted liver, hepatic artery thrombosis within 7 days of transplant, or acute decompensated Wilson's disease are also listed as Status 1. Patients listed as Status 2A must be in an intensive care unit with acute decompensated chronic liver failure with a life expectancy of less than 7 days and a long-term prognosis with a successful liver transplant equal to that of a patient with acute fulminant liver failure. Status 2B patients must have a Child–Turcotte–Pugh (CTP) score greater than or equal to 10 (i.e., Child's C) or a CTP score greater than 7 and meet one of the following medical criteria: (1) unresponsive active variceal hemorrhage; (2) hepatorenal syndrome; (3) spontaneous bacterial peritonitis; (4) refractory ascites/hydrothorax. Status 3 patients require continuous medical care as outpatients and have a CTP score greater than or equal to 7. Status changes are not justified for short hospitalizations for intercurrent problems. Patients listed as Status 7 are inactive.

MANAGEMENT AFTER LISTING

Once a patient is listed for liver transplantation, it can be several months before the transplant is performed. During this period, close patient follow-up and careful management of complications of the liver disease is mandatory to maintain the patient in optimal medical condition for transplantation to reduce morbidity and mortality.

Patients admitted to the hospital with acute fulminant liver failure or decompensation of chronic liver disease require urgent inpatient evaluation and listing for liver transplantation if indicated. The principles of management of patients with acute fulminant liver failure are similar to the principles for patients with primary nonfunction after transplantation and include protection against and treatment of cerebral edema to maintain cerebral perfusion pressure; maintenance of other organ system function (cardiovascular, respiratory, renal); protection against complications of coagulopathy; prevention of sepsis; and prevention of hypoglycemia. A full transplant evaluation is completed as quickly as possible, and patients are activated on the UNOS waiting list if they are acceptable candidates.

Donor Selection and Liver Procurement

DONOR SELECTION

Donor selection and liver procurement are critical to prevent primary nonfunction (PNF) or delayed primary function of the transplanted liver and to prevent disease transmission. When a donor liver is offered for a listed recipient, ABO and size compatibility are the first two criteria that need to be met.

Primary nonfunction of liver allografts occurs in 5% to 15% of cases, requires urgent retransplantation, and is a significant course of morbidity and mortality after liver transplantation.[1-3] Donor risk factors for primary nonfunction include prolonged cold and warm ischemia, severe macrovesicular steatosis, ABO incompatibility, donor age over 50 years, elevated donor transaminase levels, prolonged intensive care unit stay, increased bilirubin, and the need for vasopressors in the donor.[1-7] Because there continues to be a critical shortage of cadaver livers and patients continue to die on the waiting list, many centers are now using livers that previously were discarded and have thereby expanded the donor pool. Liver preservation with University of Wisconsin (UW) solution has allowed the cold ischemia time to be extended from 6 to 8 h with Euro-Collins solution to nearly 24 h. This change has allowed wider sharing of livers, especially for critically ill patients, more elective transplants, and more time to better prepare the recipient.

Another goal of proper donor selection is to prevent transmission of disease, particularly hepatitis B, C, HIV, and malignancy, and careful screening and serological testing of donors is performed. The donor pool can be expanded further, however, by the use of HBsAg−, HBcAb+, HBIgM− donors that have a low risk of transmitting HBV to kidney recipients[8] but a 30% to 50% chance of transmitting HBV to an unmodified liver recipient.[9] Livers from these donors are currently being transplanted into HBsAb+ recipients along with HBIG prophylaxis with the expectation that the risk of the recipient becoming HBsAg+ is minimal.

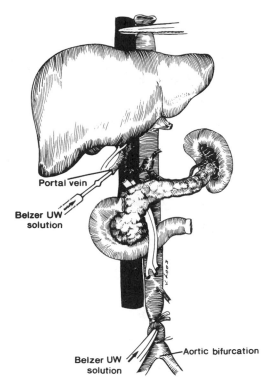

FIGURE 50.1. Perfusion of the liver, kidneys, and pancreas via a cannula in the aorta and a cannula in the portal vein. The vena cava is vented in the right chest. (Reprinted from Sollinger,[125] with permission.)

LIVER PROCUREMENT: STANDARD TECHNIQUE

The donor operation is performed through a midline incision from the suprasternal notch to the symphysis pubis. Several teams are involved in retrieval of the heart, lungs, pancreas, kidneys, and occasionally small bowel. The liver and abdominal cavity should be thoroughly examined to exclude any unsuspected infections, malignancies, or other disease processes that would preclude organ retrieval. A Tru-cut needle biopsy of the liver is obtained for frozen section to rule out severe steatosis, hepatitis, or other abnormalities. The liver is mobilized, and the lesser sac exposed.

The vasculature is examined. A replaced left hepatic artery (R-LHA) arising from the left gastric artery (LGA) occurs in approximately 17% of donors. The porta hepatis should be inspected to identify a replaced right hepatic artery (R-RHA) arising from the superior mesenteric artery (SMA) that occurs in approximately 19% of donors. The aorta should be mobilized so that clamps can be placed above the celiac axis, which allows perfusion of the liver and kidneys without perfusing the heart, and between the celiac axis and SMA (or below the SMA if a R-RHA is present), which allows continued perfusion of the kidneys while the liver is being removed.

The portal vein (PV), splenic vein (SV) and superior mesenteric vein (SMV) are mobilized and isolated. If the pancreas is not being retrieved, the SV is ligated, and a portal perfusion cannula is secured in the SV. If the pancreas is being retrieved, the portal perfusion cannula is placed in the inferior mesenteric vein. The common bile duct (CBD) is ligated and the biliary tree irrigated with saline.

The patient is systemically heparinized and the distal aorta is ligated. A perfusion catheter is inserted and secured in the aorta. In coordination with the cardiac retrieval team, the supraceliac aorta is cross-clamped and infusion of cold UW solution through the aortic and portal cannulae is begun (Fig. 50.1). The vena cava is vented in the right chest by incising the inferior vena cava at the junction with the right atrium. Surface cooling of the liver, pancreas, and kidney is achieved by placing cold slush solution in the abdomen. The liver can then be removed. Before transplantation into the recipient, the cadaver donor liver must be prepared on the back table.

LIVER PROCUREMENT: RAPID FLUSH TECHNIQUE

The technique just described is the traditional procedure for liver procurement. The "rapid flush" technique minimizes the amount of dissection before flushing with preservation solution.[10] Although some surgeons use this technique or a variant routinely, it is most applicable in an unstable donor from whom the expeditious removal of the liver is necessary or in non-heart-beating donors.

LIVER PROCUREMENT: NON-HEART-BEATING DONORS

Liver transplantation from non-heart-beating donors (NHBD) has been reported in 13 cases.[11,12] This technique has not achieved widespread acceptance because of the logistics of retrieving organs from non-heart-beating donors and concerns about long warm ischemia times and increased risk of primary nonfunction. With greater experience, however, NHBD could be an important source of viable livers, increasing the donor pool by 5% to 10%.

LIVER PROCUREMENT: IN SITU SPLITTING

Cadaveric split liver transplantation, in which the liver is split on the back table into a left lateral segment graft (segments II and III) and a right lobe graft including the caudate lobe and medial segment of the left lobe (segments I, IV, V, VI, VII, and VIII) for transplantation into two recipients, was first reported in 1988.[13] The inferior patient and graft survival rates (60% and 43%, respectively), the high incidence of biliary complications (27%), and ischemic necrosis of the medial segment of the left lobe made this procedure unacceptable.[13] Subsequently, it has been shown that these complications can be reduced by split-

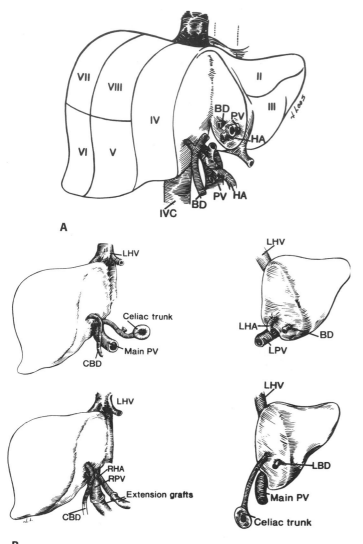

A

B

FIGURE 50.2. (A) Diagrammatic representation of in situ liver splitting in heart-beating cadaver donors. The left hepatic artery, left portal vein, left hepatic vein, and left hepatic duct are isolated. The liver is then split to the right of the falciform ligament between segments II and III and segment IV. *HA*, hepatic artery; *PV*, portal vein; *HV*, hepatic vein; *BD*, bile duct; *IVC*, inferior vena cava. **(B)** Diagrammatic representation of each split graft. The top left view shows the right graft with the celiac trunk, main PV, CBD, and IVC. The top right shows the left graft with the divided left hepatic artery (LVA), BD, left portal vein (LPV), and left hepatic vein (LHV). The bottom left view shows a right graft with the divided right hepatic artery (RHA), right portal vein (RPV), CBD, and IVC. The bottom right shows the left graft with the main PV and celiac trunk. (Adapted with permission from Busuttil.[184])

ting the liver in situ in heart-beating cadaver donors using the technique for procurement of the left lateral segment from a living donor (Fig. 50.2).[14–16] This technique results in a reduction in cold ischemic damage to the grafts, avoidance of the biliary tract complications, and the ability to assess the viability of the medial segment.

Recipient Management and Operative Procedure

INTRAOPERATIVE MANAGEMENT

Several major events occur during a liver transplant that require attention. During the recipient hepatectomy, it is critical to carefully replace ongoing blood loss and to maintain normal fluid, electrolyte, and coagulation studies. After initiation of venovenous bypass and just before removing the liver, additional replacement is usually necessary because of a decrease in venous return that occurs when portal and vena caval blood return to the heart is interrupted. Increasing the venovenous bypass flow rate after the liver is removed is usually helpful. During the anhepatic phase, while hemostasis is achieved in the retroperitoneum and the liver is sewn in place, careful attention to hemodynamic changes, electrolyte abnormalities (hypocalcemia and hyperkalemia), and coagulation abnormalities (decreased fibrinogen, increased PT) is important, and correction of any abnormalities accomplished. Before unclamping the liver, additional calcium, sodium bicarbonate, and fluid or blood products are administered. After the liver is unclamped, there can be a brief period of hyperkalemia, hypocalcemia, metabolic acidosis, depressed cardiac output and hypotension, pulmonary hypertension and right ventricular dysfunction, and fibrinolysis that require correction.

RECIPIENT HEPATECTOMY

A bilateral subcostal skin incision with a midline extension to the xiphoid process is used. There are three options for completing the hepatectomy, depending on the procedure to be performed. In the traditional procedure in which the recipient vena cava is removed as part of the liver with the patient on venovenous bypass, the infrahepatic vena cava is completely mobilized from the level of the renal veins to the suprahepatic vena cava. Alternatively, the infrahepatic and suprahepatic vena cavae can simply be isolated enough to allow clamping and the back wall of the vena cava left in place when the liver is excised. A third option is to divide the hepatic veins (HV) entering the liver posteriorly from the anterior surface of the inferior vena cava and the liver dissected off the vena cava. The inferior vena cava is left in situ, which eliminates the need for venovenous bypass. The donor suprahepatic vena cava is then sewn into the confluence of the HV ("piggyback").[17]

VENOVENOUS BYPASS

The advantages of venovenous bypass include maintenance of venous return and splanchnic venous drainage during the anhepatic phase with improved hemodynamic stability and reduction in mesenteric edema, improved renal perfusion, and provision of additional time to obtain hemostasis in the retroperitoneum, for placement of vascular grafts, and for performance of vascular anastomoses.[18,19] Many surgeons use venovenous bypass selectively or not at all with comparable results.[19–21]

CADAVER DONOR TRANSPLANT

The suprahepatic vena caval anastomosis is performed first as an end-to-end anastomosis (Fig. 50.3). The donor infrahepatic vena caval anastomosis is then performed while infusing 1 l of cold lactated Ringer's solution through the PV cannula. The PV anastomosis is completed end-to-end with a loosely tied corner ("growth stitch") to allow expansion of the PV after unclamping.[22]

There are several techniques for performing the arterial anastomosis, depending on the size of the vessels and the arterial anatomy. It can be performed as an end-to-end anastomosis between the recipient proper HA and the donor common HA. Alternatively, the donor common HA can be sewn end-to-side to the junction of the common HA and the GDA. After completion of the vascular anastomoses, the clamps are removed sequentially. First, the PV clamp is removed and the liver perfused, followed by the suprahepatic vena cava clamp, HA clamp, and inferior vena cava clamp. Hemostasis is obtained and the patient is taken off venovenous bypass.

The bile duct is usually reconstructed as an end-to-end choledochocholedochostomy using interrupted absorbable sutures. Traditionally this has been performed over a T-tube brought out through a separate choledochotomy. However, because 10% to 15% of patients develop a bile duct leak after T-tube removal, some centers have eliminated the use of T-tubes with comparable results.[23–25]

An alternative method for liver transplantation is the "piggyback" technique.[17] This technique involves leaving the recipient vena cava in situ and mobilizing the liver off the inferior vena cava by dividing all the hepatic veins entering the posterior aspect of the liver. Only the left, middle, and right hepatic veins are left in place. A clamp is placed across the hepatic veins and the confluence of the veins opened. The donor infrahepatic vena cava is oversewn on the back table, eliminating one anastomosis, and the donor suprahepatic vena cava is sewn end-to-end to the confluence of the recipient hepatic veins. Venovenous bypass is not required. In addition, there is significantly less blood loss as a result of avoiding dissection posterior to the vena cava where bleeding from retroperitoneal collaterals can be encountered.[17]

REDUCED-SIZE LIVER TRANSPLANTATION

Reduced-size liver transplants were developed to relieve the scarcity of suitable cadaveric grafts for pediatric recipients, most of whom are less than 2 years of age.[26] Reduced size grafts include reduced-size cadaveric grafts, split-liver grafts (discussed earlier), and living-related grafts (discussed later). Reduced-size liver transplants are as effective as full-sized grafts, with a 1-year survival of approximately 80%.[26]

Living-Related Donor Liver Transplantation

THE LIVING DONOR

Briefly, donors should be between 18 and 55 years of age; an immediate family member and genetically related to the recipient; ABO compatible with the recipient; and without medical problems that would increase their surgical risk. The family psychosocial support systems must be adequate as determined by a psychiatric and social work evaluation. The donor should have a normal history, physical examination, hematological and serum chemistry profile, along with normal kidney and liver function tests. An EKG and CXR are obtained and should be normal. The donor must have negative hepatitis B, C, and HIV serological tests.

The anatomical suitability of the liver for living donation must then be determined. This involves the use of CT scanning to exclude mass lesions and to document the liver volume of the left lateral segment, left lobe, and right lobe. Preoperative arteriography is usually performed to define the arterial anatomy. Endoscopic retrograde cholangiopancreatography (ERCP) is occasionally performed to delineate the biliary anatomy but is not routine. A percutaneous liver biopsy may be required in some cases.

Size matching is critically important. The healthy native liver is 2% to 3% of body weight, but the minimum amount of transplanted liver needed to survive is estimated to be approximately 25% of the recipient's ideal liver mass.[27,28] Following transplantation, the allograft and native liver remnant demonstrate differential growth rates to achieve the ideal liver volume for both recipient and donor within 1 to 3 months.[29]

THE RECIPIENT

INDICATIONS

The indications for living-related liver transplantation are essentially the same as those for cadaver liver transplantation. Most recipients are children with biliary atresia or acute fulminant liver failure.[30]

SURGICAL TECHNIQUE

The recipient operation is similar to the cadaveric reduced-size liver transplant except for the need for interposition grafts for hepatic artery and portal vein reconstruction.

RESULTS

Current survival rates are best in ABO-compatible, elective transplants in recipients 15 years old or younger.[31] Long-term graft survival is 75% to 80%.[31,32] The incidence of retransplantation, usually due to arterial thrombosis, is 5% to 10%.

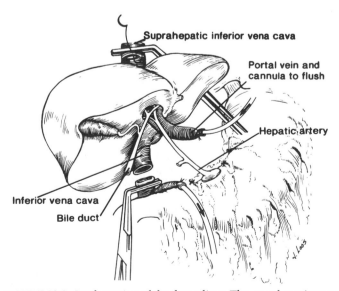

FIGURE 50.3. Implantation of the donor liver. The suprahepatic vena caval anastomosis is performed first, followed by the infrahepatic vena cava, portal vein, hepatic artery, and common bile duct.

There appears to be little immunological benefit to living-related liver transplantation.

COMPLICATIONS

The technical complications associated with living-related liver transplantation are now comparable to other liver transplant procedures in children.

ADULT RECIPIENTS

The use of living-related donor segmental allografts in adult recipients has been limited by the amount of liver available in left lobe and left lateral segment grafts.

Postoperative Surgical Complications

VASCULAR COMPLICATIONS

HEPATIC ARTERY

Hepatic artery (HA) complications include stenosis, thrombosis, pseudoaneurysm, mycotic aneurysm, and hepatic artery rupture. HA stenosis occurs in approximately 5% of patients and is usually diagnosed within the first 3 months posttransplant.[33] The major risk factor for anastomotic HA stenosis has been shown to be flow at the time of transplant.[33] HA thrombosis (HAT) in the early posttransplant period is a significant cause of graft loss in adult and pediatric cadaver and pediatric living-related liver transplantation. The incidence of HAT is approximately 3% to 5% in adults.[34–36]

Hepatic artery pseudoaneurysms are rare (0.2%–0.9%), usually occur at the anastomosis, are often infected, and may rupture and cause fatal hemorrhage, making early diagnosis and treatment imperative.[36–38]

PORTAL VEIN

Portal vein thrombosis (PVT) occurs post transplant in 10% to 8% of liver transplant recipients.[32,39–42] PVT may lead to liver failure, requiring retransplantation, or to recurrent portal hypertension. Portal vein stenosis is uncommon, but can usually be managed with angioplasty.

BILIARY TRACT COMPLICATIONS

Biliary tract complications occur in 15% to 20% of liver transplant recipients and include anastomotic leaks and strictures, leaks from T-tube exit sites, leaks after T-tube removal, and obstruction from sludge, stones, or stents, and biliary fistula from stent migration.[32,43–49] Approximately two-thirds of biliary tract complications occur in the first 4 weeks post transplant.[48,50] Late complications are primarily anastomotic and intrahepatic strictures.

Immunosuppression

The optimal immunosuppressive regimen after liver transplantation has yet to be established. There are several immunosuppressive drugs, polyclonal antibodies, and monoclonal antibodies currently available, and have been described elsewhere in this book.

IMMUNOSUPPRESSIVE PROTOCOLS

In general, immunosuppressive protocols are referred to as "induction" (utilizing polyclonal or monoclonal antibodies at the time of transplant) or "non-induction", and as "double"- (e.g. prednisone and CsA or FK506), "triple"- (e.g., AZA or MMF, prednisone, and CsA or FK506) or "quadriple"- (e.g., AZA or MMF, prednisone, CsA or FK506, and ATGAM, OKT3, basiliximab, or daclizumab) therapy.

NONINDUCTION PROTOCOLS

Most centers that prefer noninduction protocols (the majority) have used either FK506 and steroids or Neoral (a microemulsion formulation of cyclosporine), steroids, and azathioprine. However, recent data have demonstrated a further reduction in the incidence of rejection by using mycophenolate mofetil (MMF) with either FK506 and steroids or Neoral and steroids.[51–53] In one study the incidence of rejection was decreased from 45% in the FK506 and steroids group to 26% in the MMF, FK506, and steroid group ($p = 0.03$).[51] There was no difference in the incidence of CMV infections, and MMF appeared to be FK506 sparing, leading to improved renal function. The data for MMF and Neoral are inconclusive, however, because of small numbers of patients.[52] Another advantage of MMF may be that it will allow the earlier discontinuation of steroids.[54]

INDUCTION PROTOCOLS

The use of polyclonal or monoclonal antibody induction in liver transplantation has been primarily in the setting of posttransplant renal failure where delayed introduction of FK506 or cyclosporine is desired. Some centers, however, have used induction based on the decreased incidence of rejection in kidney transplant recipients treated with quadruple-therapy induction protocols.[55–58] OKT3 has historically been the monoclonal antibody of choice, but more recent interest has centered on the use of the chimeric anti-CD25 mAb, basiliximab, and the humanized anti-CD25 mAb, daclizumab, primarily because of their longer half-life and absence of significant side effects. Data with basiliximab are only available in kidney transplant recipients in whom it has been used with Neoral and steroids. The incidence of rejection was 29.8% in one study[59] and 28% in a second study,[60] with no increase risk of infectious complications. Daclizumab has also been studied in renal transplant recipients with similar results.[61–63]

CONCLUSIONS

Noninduction protocols result in comparable patient and graft survival rates to induction protocols. Although noninduction protocols were previously associated with a greater risk of rejection, the introduction of MMF into triple-therapy protocols may effectively address this disadvantage. Induction will still be useful in patients requiring delayed introduction of Neoral or FK506 posttransplant and may be more effective in allowing the reduction in dose of other immunosuppressive drugs, thereby decreasing their side effects.

Liver Allograft Rejection

DIAGNOSIS

The presumptive diagnosis of rejection can often be made on the basis of clinical and laboratory studies. Studies such as liver function tests, immunological monitoring parameters, radiologic studies, drug levels, and fine-needle aspirates may provide useful information, but the standard against which all studies are compared is the biopsy. Biopsy can confirm the diagnosis and determine the severity of rejection and, therefore, provide important information for therapy and prognosis.

HYPERACUTE REJECTION

Hyperacute rejection, first described in renal allograft recipients, is mediated by anti-HLA (donor-specific lymphocytotoxic) antibodies or by isohemagglutinins directed against donor AB blood group antigens. However, in comparison to the heart or kidney, the liver is less susceptible to antibody-mediated rejection both in experimental animals and in humans. The time course of hyperacute rejection of the liver is longer (3–7 days), perhaps related to the liver's large capacity to absorb antibodies. Histologically, hyperacute rejection in the liver is characterized by a predominantly centrilobular infiltrate of polymorphonuclear leukocytes and by aggregates of fibrin within and around the walls and lumina of the central veins and, subsequently, small arteries, leading to hemorrhagic necrosis and infarction.[64] Clinically, hyperacute rejection should be suspected in patients with recent transfusions associated with a rise in anti-HLA antibodies as measured by an increase in panel-reactive antibodies (PRA) around the time of transplantation. No prospective studies have been performed, but the most current and best retrospective data demonstrate a positive T-cell crossmatch is associated with a decrease in the early liver allograft survival rate (peak at 6 months) that disappears at 2 years posttransplant.[65] More than one-third of patients undergoing ABO-incompatible transplants may develop antibody-mediated rejection leading to graft failure,[66] but the risk may be reduced by plasmapheresis, splenectomy, and intensive immunosuppression.[67,68]

ACUTE REJECTION

Acute hepatic allograft rejection is extremely common, occurring in 30% to 75% of recipients, depending on the type of induction immunosuppression used.[69] Clinical features include a decrease in bile output and change in color and consistency from a thin, clear, golden yellow to a thicker, dark green. Elevated liver function tests may include elevated transaminases, alkaline phosphatase, or bilirubin, alone or in combination. Rejection can be difficult to diagnose clinically, however, because the differential diagnosis of abnormal liver function tests is broad, including preservation injury, ischemia, viral infection, bacterial cholangitis, bile duct obstruction, and recurrent disease. Therefore, a biopsy is usually obtained when acute rejection is suspected or any time the etiology of elevated hepatic function tests is in question. Other studies useful in determining the etiology of elevated liver function tests include cholangiography, duplex ultrasonography of the hepatic vasculature, and, if necessary, hepatic arteriography.

Acute rejection is histologically characterized by three features: (1) a portal mononuclear infiltrate (primarily small lymphocytes, but also variable numbers of eosinophils and polymorphonuclear leukocytes; (2) bile duct epithelial damage and infiltration by small lymphocytes; and (3) subendothelial inflammation of portal or terminal hepatic veins (endothelialitis).[64–78] The diagnosis of rejection requires at least two of these histopathological findings (mixed portal infiltrate and bile duct damage) and biochemical evidence of liver damage. The diagnosis is even more assured if more than 50% of the bile ducts are damaged or if unequivocal endothelialitis is demonstrated.

The Liver Transplantation Database has analyzed the incidence, risk factors, and impact on outcome of acute rejection in the largest number of patients to date.[69] The percentage of recipients who developed a first, second, and third episode of acute rejection in the first year posttransplant were 65%, 20%, and 4%, respectively. Within the first 6 weeks posttransplant, 48% of recipients developed at least one acute rejection episode with the median time to rejection of 8 days. The risk of rejection is 10% to 20% greater for noninduction protocols with cyclosporine and steroids or tacrolimus and steroids, compared to quadruple therapy utilizing cyclosporine, steroids, azathioprine, and antilymphocyte globulin or monoclonal antibody therapy. Risk factors shown to be associated with the development of acute rejection include underlying liver disease (acute fulminant hepatic failure, hepatitis B, and autoimmune chronic active hepatitis), younger age of recipient, lower Karnofsky score, serum creatinine below 2.0 mg/dl, lack of edema, renal failure, or ascites, fewer HLA-DR matches, donor age, and cold ischemia time greater than 15 h. These data suggest that healthier recipients, recipients poorly HLA-matched with the donor, and recipients of livers that are more predisposed to liver injury are at greater risk for developing acute rejection. When the impact of acute rejection on patient and graft survival is analyzed, it has been shown that patient and graft survival rates are better in patients with acute rejection because the highest incidence of rejection is in the healthiest recipients. Adjusting for these risk factors, acute rejection was not shown to have a significant effect on patient or graft survival rates. This finding is in direct contrast to kidney transplantation, where acute rejection episodes have been shown to correlate with poorer patient and graft survival rates.[79,80]

CHRONIC REJECTION

Chronic rejection is a slowly progressive immunological process characterized by increasing cholestasis with an elevation in alkaline phosphatase, γ-glutamyl transpeptidase, or 5'-nucleotidase and eventually bilirubin that occurs in about 5% to 10% of liver allografts,[81,82] although the incidence appears to be decreasing.[83] Histologically it is characterized by obliterative vasculopathy and loss of bile ducts ("vanishing duct syndrome" or "paucity of bile ducts") involving more than 50% of the portal triads. Risk factors for chronic rejection include donor–recipient histocompatibility differences, positive crossmatch, frequency of acute rejection episodes, long ischemia time, chronic viral hepatitis, and cytomegalovirus (CMV) infection.[84] Chronic rejection does not usually occur before 2 months posttransplant and usually develops following an unresolved acute rejection episode, after multiple acute rejection episodes, or slowly over many years in patients with a history of remote acute rejection episodes or no apparent episodes of acute rejection. Chronic rejection is not always irreversible, and bile duct regeneration can occur.

TREATMENT

Treatment of rejection with corticosteroids can be accomplished by a short course of intravenous methylprednisolone boluses (e.g., 250–500 mg/day for 3–5 days) or by an increase in the oral prednisolone dose (e.g., 2 mg/kg/day) with a tapering schedule over 2 to 4 weeks. The current incidence of steroid resistant rejection is 5% to 10% and is probably decreasing as immunosuppression improves. Treatment of steroid-resistant rejection is usually with OKT3 mAb (5 mg/day for 7 days) or ATGAM, but MMF and FK506 have both been used to rescue patients with steroid and OKT3 resistant rejection.[85–88]

Infections

The incidence and severity of infections after liver transplantation are influenced by the type, intensity, and duration of immunosuppression, by the incidence of technical complications, and by the infectious diseases that the patient encounters in the hospital and community.[89] More than 60% to 80% of liver transplant recipients will have at least one infection after transplant with an overall incidence of 1.5 to 1.7 infections per patient, an incidence that is similar in induction and noninduction series.[90–93] Recent series in the current era of antibiotic, antiviral, and antifungal prophylaxis document 70% of posttransplant infections are bacterial, 20% are viral, and 10% are fungal.[89,92] Although early series reported an infection-related mortality rate to 40%,[94–97] current series report a mortality rate of less than 10%[92] to 22%.[98] Posttransplant infections can be classified by the time period after transplantation in which they are most likely to occur, whether they are bacterial, viral, fungal, or protozoal, and by the clinical disease they cause. Most infections occurring in the first month are bacterial or fungal and related to the surgical procedure, including intraabdominal infections, cholangitis, pneumonitis, urinary tract infections, wound infections, and central venous catheter infections. From 1 to 6 months after transplant, viral infections including CMV, HSV, and EBV are most common, although late fungal infections may occur. After 6 months, the risk of infection is low.[89]

BACTERIAL INFECTIONS

Risk factors for the development of bacterial infections include length of operation (>12 h), multiple abdominal operations, retransplantation, pretransplant bilirubin 12 mg/dl or more, length of antibiotic therapy posttransplant (>5 days), and intraoperative transfusions (>25 units of packed red cells and >30 units of fresh frozen plasma).[92,94,99] The most common diagnoses include wound infections, intraabdominal infections (peritonitis, hepatic and extrahepatic abscesses, and cholangitis), pneumonias, urinary tract infections, central venous catheter infections, and bacteremias. Prophylaxis of bacterial infections usually involves perioperative administration of a third-generation cephalosporin along with ampicillin or vancomycin or ampicillin-sulbactam as a single agent for gram-positive and gram-negative coverage.[92] Some centers use selective bowel decontamination protocols involving the administration of oral nystatin, gentamicin, and polymyxin.[97]

VIRAL INFECTIONS

The most important viral infections after liver transplantation include CMV, EBV, HSV, and varicella zoster virus (VZV). HSV infections are uncommon posttransplant because of the widespread use of ganciclovir and acyclovir prophylaxis. The diagnosis can be made by physical examination, endoscopy and biopsy, liver biopsy, bronchoscopy, and culture of vesicular lesions. Serology is rarely helpful. Intra-

venous or oral acyclovir is effective therapy in most patients. CMV infection and disease occur in up to 50% and 25% of liver transplant recipients, respectively, as either primary or reactivation infections.[100,101] The diagnosis can be made by culture or by biopsy (viral inclusions, monoclonal antibody staining for CMV antigens, or in situ hybridization). Ganciclovir is the most effective treatment. EBV infection occurs in 5% to 10% of liver transplant recipients as a primary or reactivation infection.[102] These patients respond to intravenous acyclovir and reduction in immunosuppression. VZV infections occur as primary or reactivation infections. The diagnosis of VZV is made on the basis of physical examination with the classic cutaneous vesicular lesions, by culture, by Tzanck smear of scrapings from skin lesions, or by biopsy. Intravenous acyclovir is used for treatment of disseminated VZV along with a reduction in immunosuppression. Intravenous or oral acyclovir may be used for herpes zoster infections, depending on the severity of the disease.

FUNGAL INFECTIONS

Invasive fungal infections have been reported to occur in 24% to 42% of liver transplant recipients, with the most frequent organisms being *Candida* species, followed by *Aspergillus* species.[92,96–98,103,104] Eighty percent occur in the first month posttransplant. The mortality rate from fungal infections has varied from 22% to 69%,[97,104–107] but recent series have shown a significant decrease in incidence and mortality.[92,98,104] Several risk factors have been identified, including preoperative administration of steroids and antibiotics, urgent clinical status at the time of transplantation, renal insufficiency (serum creatinine >3.0 mg/dl), high Pugh risk score, prolonged duration of surgery, requirement for intraoperative transfusion, method of biliary reconstruction, steroid use posttransplant, early fungal colonization (within 3 days after transplant), bacterial infections posttransplant, prolonged antibiotic use posttransplant, retransplantation, reintubation, and vascular complications.[103–105,108] Prophylaxis with nystatin or clotrimazole is effective in preventing oral candidiasis (thrush) and esophagitis posttransplant, but is less effective in preventing invasive fungal infections. Prophylaxis with low-dose systemic amphotericin has been effective in decreasing the risk of invasive fungal infections, but nephrotoxicity limits its use.[109] Fluconazole has also been shown to be superior to nystatin in decreasing posttransplant fungal infections and is used now in many centers.[110]

PROTOZOAL INFECTIONS

Pneumocystis carinii causes dyspnea, fever, and cough associated with diffuse bilateral interstitial pulmonary infiltrates. The diagnosis is usually made by the identification of the organism using the methenamine silver stain on bronchoalveolar lavage fluid or by transbronchial or open-lung biopsy. Treatment with trimethoprim-sulfamethoxazole or pentamidine is usually effective.

Intestinal Transplantation

In an era in which graft survival rates for heart, lung, liver, kidney, and pancreas transplantation approach or exceed 90% at 1 year,[111] routine success of intestinal transplantation remains elusive, with 1-year graft survival rates of less than 70% and total parenteral nutrition (TPN) -free graft survival even less.[112,113] Moreover, the accompanying morbidity is high, primarily related to a high incidence of rejection and infection.[112,113] The information presented draws heavily from clinical series and data available from the International Intestinal Transplant Registry (IITR) that constitute a total of approximately 260 intestinal transplants.[112,113] There are no comparative trials to evaluate at this time.

Indications

Intestinal transplantation is a potential alternative to permanent TPN in cases of chronic intestinal failure. Combined liver-intestinal transplantation should be considered whenever end-stage liver disease accompanies intestinal failure, whether as a result of chronic TPN administration or as a result of other etiologies.[114,115] With improvements in TPN administration, it remains controversial as to when a patient with isolated intestinal failure and good hepatic function should be considered for isolated intestinal transplantation in light of the currently reported graft and patient survival rates. Clearly, patients with limited venous access or who are doing poorly on TPN should be considered.

The most common cause of intestinal failure leading to transplantation is short bowel syndrome as a result of surgical resection. Malabsorption syndromes, most notably microvillus inclusion disease, and motility disorders, most commonly intestinal pseudoobstruction, make up the next most common indications. Tumors, including desmoids, and gastrinomas, which may require almost total intestinal evisceration, also account for a significant (5%–15%) percentage of cases in most series.[115–117] Retransplantation after primary graft failure accounted for 6% of the transplants in the international registry series.

Surgical Technique

DONOR OPERATION

Evaluation of the possible intestinal organ donor is the same as for any other cadaver organ donor. Size matching is critical in intestinal transplantation, especially if a multivisceral transplant is planned. Acceptable donors for patients at risk for abdominal domain problems should be 20% to 40% smaller than the recipient by body weight.[114] The surgical techniques of intestinal and multivisceral procurement have been well described elsewhere and follow standard principles of organ procurement.[118–120] The acceptable limits of cold preservation for human intestinal allografts have not yet been determined. Short cold ischemic times of less than 12 h have generally been considered desirable.[121] Figures 50.4 and 50.5 demonstrate a composite and isolated graft, respectively.

RECIPIENT OPERATION

In general, arterial supply is from the aorta, and venous drainage is to the recipient superior mesenteric vein or portal vein. Drainage to the inferior vena cava has been described without short-term ill effects.[114] An ostomy is established to provide access for biopsies of the allograft, although reestablishing gastrointestinal continuity either proximally or distally need not be delayed.

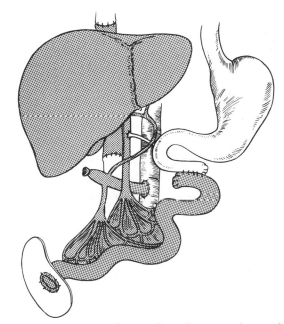

FIGURE 50.4. Composite liver and small intestinal transplant.

Outcomes and Management

PATIENT SURVIVAL

Patient and graft survival rates are lower for recipients of composite liver-intestinal and multivisceral grafts than for recipients of isolated intestines alone.[112,113] The effect of different etiologies, recipient age, or other clinical variables on survival has not yet been clearly elucidated, although data from the IITR suggest that center size and the era in which transplantation was undertaken might be important.[113]

One- and 3-year patient survival rates, as reported by the IITR, are 83% and 47%, respectively, for isolated intestinal grafts, 66% and 40% for liver-intestine grafts, and 59% and 43% for multivisceral grafts.[112,113] The most common causes of death were sepsis and multiorgan failure, together accounting for 91% of mortality.

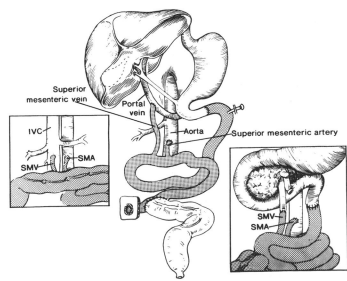

FIGURE 50.5. Isolated small-intestinal transplant.

Graft Survival

One- and 3-year graft survival rates as reported by the IITR are 53% and 31%, respectively, for isolated intestinal grafts, 58% and 39% for liver-intestine grafts, and 41% and 36% for multivisceral grafts.[112,113] It should be noted that graft survival does not equate with freedom from TPN in all cases; between 10% and 20% of survivors continue to need some form of parenteral nutritional support.[113]

Immunosuppression and Immunological Surveillance

Immunologically, intestinal transplantation is unique as compared to other solid-organ grafts for several reasons. First, enterocytes in intestinal allografts constitutively express MHC class II antigens. In other organ allografts, expression of these immunologically important proteins is limited to cells of lymphoid origin or activated endothelial and parenchymal cells. The importance of this is not entirely clear, but it may be one reason for the difficulty experienced in controlling the host immune response to intestinal transplantation. Second, the mesenteric nodes and gut-associated lymphoid tissue transferred with the graft at transplantation constitute an enormous load of immunocompetent cells capable of inducing graft-versus-host reactions.[114] Third, the intestine is obviously not a sterile organ and the heavy colonization of microorganisms probably put recipients at risk for both translocation and systemic sepsis. Rejection rates can be higher than 90%,[113,116] and graft loss due to rejection is prevalent.[112,113]

Early reports of intestinal transplantation were invariably performed under cyclosporine immunosuppression.[112,114] In recent years there has been general agreement that immunological results are improved with the use of FK506,[112,115] and virtually all recent reports have emphasized the use of this immunosuppressive drug in conjunction with steroids and/or azathioprine or MMF.

Treatment of rejection consists of steroid boluses, increasing FK506 levels, the addition of another agent such as MMF, and/or the administration of OKT3.[114–116]

Nutritional and Electrolyte Management

Careful attention to fluid and nutritional needs is mandatory. Both osmotic and secretory diarrheas are common, and fluid and electrolyte losses in the stool can be considerable.[114,117] Conversion from parenteral to enteral nutrition is often slow and difficult. Intestinal motility is disrupted, and studies of explanted intestinal allografts demonstrate an absence of extrinsic neural fibers,[122] although functional studies of recipients have shown the resumption of near-normal motility patterns in more than 50% of patients several months post-transplant.[123] Low-fat, elemental formulas are usually used initially as mesenteric lymphatics have been disrupted during transplantation. Gradually, the feeding can be advanced to more nutritionally complex formulas.

Conclusions

The key to improvement in future results of intestinal transplantation is better understanding and control of the host immune response. Several new immunosuppressive agents that will be entering the commercial market in the next several years may prove useful. Nutritional modification of the immune response is an exciting area just now being seriously investigated that may have special significance in intestinal transplantation.[124] A better understanding of the processes leading to allograft rejection will be gleaned from ongoing experimental work.

References

1. Ploeg RJ, D'Alessandro AM, Knechtle SJ, et al. Risk factors for primary dysfunction after liver transplantation—a multivariate analysis. Transplantation 1993;55:807–813.
2. Mor E, Klintmalm GB, Gonwa TA, et al. The use of marginal donors for liver transplantation: a retrospective study of 365 liver donors. Transplantation 1992;53:383–386.
3. Ploeg RJ, D'Alessandro AM, Hoffman RM. Impact of donor factors and preservation on function and survival after liver transplantation. Transplant Proc 1993;25:3031.
4. Strasberg SM, Howard TK, Molmenti EP, Hertl M. Selecting the donor liver: risk factors for poor function after orthotopic liver transplantation. Hepatology 1994;20:829–838.
5. Gaffey MJ, Boyd JC, Traweek ST, et al. Predictive value of intraoperative biopsies and liver function tests for preservation injury in orthotopic liver transplantation. Hepatology 1997;25:184–189.
6. Adam R, Reynes M, Johann M, et al. The outcome of seatotic grafts in liver transplantation. Transplant Proc 1991;23:1538–1540.
7. D'Alessandro AM, Kalayoglu M, Sollinger HW, et al. The predictive value of donor liver biopsies for the development of primary nonfunction after orthotopic liver transplantation. Transplantation 1991;51:157–163.
8. Satterthwaite R, Ozgu I, Shidban H, et al. Risks of transplanting kidneys from hepatitis B surface antigen-negative, hepatitis B core antibody-positive donors. Transplantation 1947;64:432–435.
9. Wachs M, Amend WJ, Ascher NL, et al. The risk of transmission of hepatitis B from HBsAg−, HBcAb+, HBIgM− organ donors. Transplantation 1995;59:230–234.
10. Emre S, Schwartz ME, Miller CM. The donor operation. In: Busuttil RW, Klintmalm GB, eds. Transplantation of the Liver. Philadelphia: WB Saunders Co, 1996:392–404.
11. D'Alessandro AM. The non-heart-beating donor. Graft 1998;1: 23–24.
12. D'Alessandro AM, Hoffman RM, Knechtle SJ, et al. Successful extrarenal transplantation from non-heart-beating donors. Transplantation 1995;59:977–982.
13. Emond JC, Whitington PF, Thistlethwaite JR, et al. Transplantation of two patients with one liver: analysis of a preliminary experience with "split-liver" grafting. Ann Surg 1990;212:14–22.
14. Rogiers X, Malago M, Gawad K, et al. In situ splitting of cadaveric livers: the ultimate expansion of a limited donor pool. Ann Surg 1996;224:331–341.
15. Goss JA, Yersiz H, Shackleton CR, et al. In situ splitting of the cadaveric liver for transplantation. Transplantation 1997;64: 871–877.
16. Busuttil RW, Goss JA. Split liver transplantation. Ann Surg 1999;229:313–321.
17. Busque S, Esquivel CO, Concepcion W, So SKS. Experience with the piggyback technique without caval occlusion in adult orthotopic liver transplantation. Transplantation 1998;65:77–82.
18. Shaw BW Jr, Martin DJ, Marquez JM, et al. Venous bypass in clinical liver transplantation. Ann Surg 1984;200:524–534.
19. Grande L, Rimola A, Cugat E, et al. Effect of venovenous bypass on perioperative renal function in liver transplantation: results of a randomized, controlled trial. Hepatology 1996;23:1418–1428.
20. Wall WJ, Grant DR, Duff JH, Kutt JL, Ghent CN, Block MS. Liver transplantation without venous bypass. Transplantation 1987;43:56–61.

21. Chari RS, Gan TJ, Robertson KM, et al. Venovenous bypass in adult orthotopic liver transplantation: routine or selective use? J Am Coll Surg 1998;186:683–690.

22. Starzl TE, Iwatsuki S, Shaw BW Jr. A growth factor in fine vascular anastomoses. Surg Gynecol Obstet 1984;159:164–165.

23. Rolles K, Dawson K, Novell R, Hayter B, Davidson B, Burroughs A. Biliary anastomosis after liver transplantation does not benefit from T tube splintage. Transplantation 1994;57:402–404.

24. Rouch DA, Emond JC, Thistlethwaite JR Jr, Mayes JT, Broelsch CE. Choledochostomy without a T tube or internal stent in transplantation of the liver. Surg Gynecol Obstet 1990;170: 239–244.

25. Vougas V, Rela M, Gane E, et al. A prospective randomised trial of bile duct reconstruction at liver transplantation: T tube or no T tube? Transpl Int 1996;9:392–395.

26. Malago M, Rogiers X, Broelsch CE. Reduced size hepatic allografts. Annu Rev Med 1995;46:507–512.

27. Lo CM, Fan ST, Chan JKF, Wei W, Lo RJW, Lai CL. Minimum graft volume for successful adult-to-adult living donor liver transplantation for fulminant hepatic failure. Transplantation 1996;62:696–698.

28. Lo CM, Chan KL, Fan ST, et al. Living donor liver transplantation: The Hong Kong experience. Transplant Proc 1996;28:2390–2392.

29. Kawasaki S, Makuuchi M, Ishizone S, Matsunami H, Terada M, Kawarazaki H. Liver regeneration in recipients and donors after transplantation. Lancet 1992;339:580–581.

30. Hattori H, Higuchi Y, Tsuji M, et al. Living-related liver transplantation and neurological outcome in children with fulminant hepatic failure. Transplantation 1998;65:686–692.

31. Kiuchi T, Tanaka K. Living related donor liver transplantation: status quo in Kyoto, Japan. Transplant Proc 1998;30:687–691.

32. Goss JA, Shackleton CR, McDiarmid SV, et al. Long-term results of pediatric liver transplantation: an analysis of 569 transplants. Ann Surg 1998;228:411–428.

33. Abbasoglu O, Levy MF, Vodapally MS, et al. Hepatic artery stenosis after liver transplantation—incidence, presentation, treatment, and long term outcome. Transplantation 1997;63:250–255.

34. Merion RM, Burtch GD, Ham JM, Turcotte JG, Campbell DA Jr. The hepatic artery in liver transplantation. Transplantation 1989;48:438–443.

35. Busuttil RW, Shaked A, Millis JM, et al. One thousand liver transplants: the lessons learned. Ann Surg 1994;219:490–499.

36. Langnas AN, Marujo W, Stratta RJ, Wood RP, Shaw BW. Vascular complications after orthotopic liver transplantation. Am J Surg 1991;161:76–83.

37. Madariaga J, Tzakis A, Zajko AB, et al. Hepatic artery pseudoaneurysm ligation after orthotopic liver transplantation—a report of 7 cases. Transplantation 1992;54:824–828.

38. Tobben PJ, Zajko AB, Sumkin JH, et al. Pseudoaneurysms complicating organ transplantation: roles of CT, duplex sonography, and angiography. Radiology 1988;169:65–70.

39. Lerut J, Tzakis AG, Bron K, et al. Complications of venous reconstruction in human orthotopic liver transplantation. Ann Surg 1987;205:404–414.

40. Wozney P, Zajko AB, Bron KM, Point S, Starzl TE. Vascular complications after liver transplantation: a 5-year experience. AJR 1986;147:657–663.

41. Burke GW III, Ascher NL, Hunter D, Najarian JS. Orthotopic liver transplantation: nonoperative management of early, acute portal vein thrombosis. Surgery 1988;104:924–928.

42. Davidson BR, Gibson M, Dick R, Burroughs A, Rolles K. Incidence, risk factors, management and outcome of portal vein abnormalities at orthotopic liver transplantation. Transplantation 1994;57:1174–1177.

43. Colonna JO II, Shaked A, Gomes AS, et al. Biliary strictures complicating liver transplantation: incidence, pathogenesis, management, and outcome. Ann Surg 1992;216:344–352.

44. Lebeau G, Yanaga K, Marsh JW, et al. Analysis of surgical complications after 397 hepatic transplantations. Surgery 1990;170: 317–322.

45. Stratta RJ, Wood RP, Langnas AN, et al. Diagnosis and treatment of biliary tract complications after orthotopic liver transplantation. Surgery 1989;106:675–684.

46. Heffron JG, Emond JC, Whitington PF, et al. Biliary complications in pediatric liver transplantation: a comparison of reduced-size and whole grafts. Transplantation 1992;53.391–395.

47. D'Alessandro AM, Kalayoglu M, Prisch JD, et al. Biliary tract complications after orthotopic liver transplantation. Transplant Proc 1991;23:1956–1990.

48. Vallera RA, Cotton PB, Clavien P-A. Biliary reconstruction for liver transplantation and management of biliary complication: overview and survey of current practices in the United States. Liver Transplant Surg 1995;1:143–152.

49. Egawa H, Uemoto S, Inomata Y, et al. Biliary complications in pediatric living related liver transplantation. Surgery 1998;124: 901–910.

50. Greif F, Bronsther OL, Van Thiel DH, et al. The incidence, timing, and management of biliary tract complications after orthotopic liver transplantation. Ann Surg 1994;219:40–45.

51. Eckhoff DE, McGuire BM, Frenette LR, Contreras JL, Hudson SL, Bynon JS. Tacrolimus (FK506) and mycophenolate mofetil combination therapy versus tacrolimus in adult liver transplantation. Transplantation 1998;65:180–187.

52. Fisher RA, Ham JM, Marcos A, et al. A prospective randomized trial of mycophenolate mofetil with neoral or tacrolimus after orthotopic liver transplantation. Transplantation 1998;66:1616–1621.

53. Jain B, Hamad I, Rakela J, et al. A prospective randomized trial of tacrolimus and prednisone versus tacrolimus, prednisone and mycophenolate mofetil in primary adult liver transplant recipients. Transplantation 1998;66:1395–1398.

54. Stegall MD, Wachs M, Everson G, et al. Prednisone withdrawal 14 days after liver transplantation with mycophenolate. Transplantation 1997;64:1755–1760.

55. Wall WJ, Ghent CN, Roy A, McAlister VC, Grant DR, Adams PC. Use of OKT3 monoclonal antibody as induction therapy for control of rejection in liver transplantation. Dig Dis Sci 1995; 40:52–57.

56. McDiarmid SV, Millis MJ, Terasaki PI, Ament ME, Busuttil RW. OKT3 prophylaxis in liver transplantation. Dig Dis Sci 1991;36: 1418–1426.

57. Fung J, Starzl T. Prophylactic use of OKT3 in liver transplantation: a review. Dig Dis Sci 1991;36:1427–1430.

58. Whiting JF, Fecteau A, Martin J, Bejarano PA, Hanto DW. Use of low-dose OKT3 as induction therapy in liver transplantation. Transplantation 1998;65:577–580.

59. Nashan B, Moore R, Amlot P, Schmidt AG, Abeywickrama K, Soulillou JP. Randomized trial of basiliximab versus placebo for control of acute cellular rejection in renal allograft recipients. Lancet 1997;350:1193–1198.

60. Kahan BD, Rajagopalan PR, Hall M. Reduction of the occurrence of acute cellular rejection among renal allograft recipients treated with basiliximab, a chimeric anti-interleukin-2-receptor monoclonal antibody. Transplantation 1999;67:276–284.

61. Ekberg H, Backman L, Tufveson G, Tyden G. Zenapax (Daclizumab) reduces the incidence of acute rejection episodes and improves patient survival following renal transplantation. Transplant Proc 1999;31:267–268.

62. Vincenti F, Kirkman R, Light S, et al. Interleukin-2-receptor blockade with daclizumab to prevent acute rejection in renal transplantation. N Engl J Med 1998;338:161–165.

63. Nashan B, Light S, Hardie IR, Lin A, Johnson JR. Reduction of acute renal allograft rejection by daclizumab. Daclizumab double therapy study group. Transplantation 1999;67:110–115.

64. Hanto DW, Snover DC, Noreen HJ, et al. Hyperacute rejection

of a human orthotopic liver allograft in a presensitized recipient. Clin Transplant 1987;1:304–310.

65. Doyle HR, Marino IR, Morelli F, et al. Assessing risk in liver transplantation: special reference to the significance of a positive cytotoxic crossmatch. Ann Surg 1996;224:168–177.

66. Gugenheim J, Samuel D, Reynes M, Bismuth H. Liver transplantation across ABO blood group barriers. Lancet 1990;336:519–523.

67. Fecteau AH, Alonso M, Valente JF, Whiting JF, Hanto DW. No immunological graft losses after ABO incompatible liver transplant utilizing plasmaphaeresis, splenectomy, cyclosporine and OKT3. Transplantation (submitted)

68. Mor E, Skerrett D, Manzarbeitia C, et al. Successful use of an enhanced immunosuppressive protocol with plasmapheresis for ABO-incompatible mismatched grafts in liver transplant recipients. Transplantation 1995;59:986–990.

69. Wiesner RH, Demetris AJ, Belle SH, et al. Acute hepatic allograft rejection: incidence, risk factors, and impact on outcome. Hepatology 1998;28:638–645.

70. International Working Party. Terminology for hepatic allograft rejection. Hepatology 1995;22:648–653.

71. Knechtle SJ, Kolbeck PC, Tsuchimoto S, Coundouriotis A, Sanfilippo AP, Bollinger RR. Hepatic transplantation into sensitized recipients: demonstration of hyperacute rejection. Transplantation 1987;43:8–12.

72. Demetris AJ, Jaffe R, Tzakis A, et al. Antibody-mediated rejection of human orthotopic liver allografts: a study of liver transplantation across ABO blood group barriers. Am J Pathol 1988;132:489–502.

73. Ratner L, Phelan D, Brunt EM, Mohanakumar T, Hanto DW. Probable antibody-mediated failure of two sequential ABO-compatible hepatic allografts in a single recipient. Transplantation 1993;55:814–819.

74. Bird G, Friend P, Donaldson P, et al. Hyperacute rejection in liver transplantation: a case report. Transplant Proc 1989;21:3742–3744.

75. Flye MW, Duffy BF, Phelan DL, Ratner LE, Mohanakumar T. Protective effects of liver transplantation on a simultaneously transplanted kidney in a highly sensitized patient. Transplantation 1990;50:1051–1053.

76. Starzl TE, Demetris AJ, Todo S, et al. Evidence for hyperacute rejection of human liver grafts: the case of the canary kidneys. Clin Transplant 1989;3:37–45.

77. Eid A, Moore SB, Wiesner RH, DeGoey SR, Nielson A, Krom RAF. Evidence that the liver does not always protect the kidney from hyperacute rejection in combined liver-kidney transplantation across a positive lymphocyte crossmatch. Transplantation 1990;50:331–334.

78. Demetris AJ, Batts KP, Dhillon AP, et al. Banff schema for grading liver allograft rejection: an international consensus document. Hepatology 1997;25:658–663.

79. Lindholm A, Ohlman S, Albrechtsen D, Tulveson G, Persson H, Persson NH. The impact of acute rejection episodes on long-term graft function and outcome in 1347 primary renal transplants treated by 3 cyclosporine regimens. Transplantation 1993;56:307–315.

80. Tesi RJ, Henry ML, Elkhammas EA, Ferguson RM. Predictors of long-term primary cadaveric renal transplant survival. Clin Transplant 1993;7:345–352.

81. Wiesner RH, Ludwig J, van Hoek B, Krom RAF. Current concepts in cell-mediated hepatic allograft rejection leading to ductopenia and liver failure. Hepatology 1991;14:721–729.

82. Freese DK, Snover DC, Sharp HL, Gross CR, Savick SK, Payne WD. Chronic rejection after liver transplantation: a study of clinical, histopathological and immunological features. Hepatology 1991;13:882–891.

83. Pirsch JD, Kalayoglu M, Hafez GR, D'Alessandro AM, Sollinger HW, Belzer FO. Evidence that the vanishing bile duct syndrome is vanishing. Transplantation 1990;49:1015–1018.

84. Lautenschlager I, Hockerstedt K, Jalanko H, et al. Persistent cytomegalovirus in liver allografts with chronic rejection. Hepatology 1997;25:190–194.

85. U.S. Multicenter FK 506 Liver Study Group. Use of Prograf (FK506) as rescue therapy for refractory rejection after liver transplantation. Transplant Proc 1993;25:679–688.

86. Millis JM, Woodle ES, Piper JB, et al. Tacrolimus for primary treatment of steroid-resistant hepatic allograft rejection. Transplantation 1996;61:1365–1369.

87. Woodle ES, Perdrizet GA, So SKS, White HM, Marsh JW. FK506 rescue therapy for hepatic allograft rejection: experience with an aggressive approach. Clin Transplant 1995;9:45–52.

88. Hebert MF, Ascher NL, Lake JR, et al. Four-year follow-up of mycophenolate mofetil for graft rescue in liver allograft recipients. Transplantation 1999;67:707–712.

89. Fishman JA, Rubin RH. Infection in organ transplant recipients. N Engl J Med 1998;338:1741–1751.

90. European FK506 Multicentre Liver Study Group. Randomised trial comparing tacrolimus (FK506) and cyclosporin in prevention of liver allograft rejection. Lancet 1994;344:423–428.

91. The US Multicenter FK506 Liver Study Group. A comparison of tacrolimus (FK 506) and cyclosporine for immunosuppression in liver transplantation. N Engl J Med 1994;331:1110–1115.

92. Whiting JF, Rossi SJ, Hanto DW. Infectious complications after OKT3 induction in liver transplantation. Liver Transplant Surg 1997;3:563–570.

93. Hadley S, Samore MH, Lewis WD, Jenkins RL, Karchmer AW, Hammer SM. Major infectious complications after orthotopic liver transplantation and comparison of outcomes in patients receiving cyclosporine or FK506 as primary immunosuppression. Transplantation 1995;59:851–859.

94. Kusne S, Dummer JS, Singh N. Infections after liver transplantation: an analysis of 101 consecutive cases. Medicine 1988;67:132–143.

95. Colonna JO, Winston DJ, Brill JE, et al. Infectious complications in liver transplantation. Arch Surg 1988;123:360–364.

96. Ascher NL, Stock PG, Bumgardner GL, Payne WD, Najarian JS. Infection and rejection of primary hepatic transplant in 93 consecutive patients treated with triple immunosuppressive therapy. Surg Gynecol Obstet 1988;167:474–484.

97. Paya CV, Hermans PE, Washington JA, et al. Incidence, distribution, and outcome of episodes of infection in 100 orthotopic liver transplantations. Mayo Clin Proc 1989;64:555–564.

98. Wade JJ, Rolando N, Hayllar K, Philpott-Howard J, Casewell MW, Williams R. Bacterial and fungal infections after liver transplantation: an analysis of 284 patients. Hepatology 1995;21:1328–1336.

99. George DL, Arnow PM, Fox AS. Bacterial infection as a complication of liver transplantation. Rev Infect Dis 1991;13:387–396.

100. Winston DJ, Wirin D, Shaked A, Busuttil RW. Randomised comparison of ganciclovir and high-dose acyclovir for long-term cytomegalovirus prophylaxis in liver transplant recipients. Lancet 1995;346:69–74.

101. Gane E, Saliba F, Valdecasas GJC, O'Grady J, Pescovitz MD, Lyman S. Randomised trial of efficacy and safety of oral ganciclovir in the prevention of cytomegalovirus disease in liver-transplant recipients. Lancet 1997;350:1729–1733.

102. Hanto DW. Classification of Epstein-Barr virus-associated posttransplant lymphoproliferative diseases: implications for understanding their pathogenesis and developing rational treatment strategies. Ann Rev Med 1995;46:381–394.

103. Tollemar J, Ericzon BG. Invasive Candida albicans infections in orthotopic liver graft recipients: incidence and risk factors. Clin Transplant 1991;5:306–312.

104. Collins LA, Samore MH, Roberts MS, et al. Risk factors for in-

vasive fungal infections complicating orthotopic liver transplantation. J Infect Dis 1994;170:644–652.

105. Castaldo P, Stratta RJ, Wood RPM, et al. Clinical spectrum of fungal infections after orthotopic liver transplantation. Arch Surg 1991;126:149–156.

106. Wajszcuzuk CP, Dummer JS, Ho M, et al. Fungal infections in liver transplant recipients. Transplantation 1985;40:347–353.

107. Nieto-Rodriguez JA, Kusne S, Manez R, et al. Factors associated with the development of candidemia and candidemia-related death among liver transplant recipients. Ann Surg 1996;223:70–76.

108. Patel R, Portela D, Badley AD, et al. Risk factors of invasive Candida and non-Candida fungal infections after liver transplantation. Transplantation 1996;62:926–934.

109. Mora NP, Klintmalm G, Solomon H, Goldstein RM, Gonwa TA, Husberg BS. Selective amphotericin B prophylaxis in the reduction of fungal infections after liver transplant. Transplant Proc 1992;24:154–155.

110. Lumbreras C, Cuervas-Mons V, Jara P, del Palacio A, Turrion S, Barrios C. Randomized trial of fluconazole versus nystatin for the prophylaxis of Candida infection following liver transplantation. J Infect Dis 1996;174:583–588.

111. UNOS. UNOS graft and patient survival rates. In: UNOS 1996 Annual Report. Washington, DC: US Department of Health & Human Services, 1997:144.

112. Grant D. Current results of intestinal transplantation. Lancet 1996;347:1801–1803.

113. International Intestinal Transplant Registry, 1997. http:/www.iitr.on.ca/itr/.

114. Asfar S, Zhong R, Grant D. Small bowel transplantation. Surg Clin North Am 1994;74:1197–1210.

115. Abu-Elmagd K, Reyes J, Todo S, et al. Clinical intestinal transplantation: new perspectives and immunologic considerations. J Am Coll Surg 1998;186:512–527.

116. Tzakis AG, Weppler D, Khan MF, et al. Mycophenolate mofetil as primary and rescue therapy in intestinal transplantation. Transplant Proc 1998;30:2677–2679.

117. Langnas AN, Shaw BW, Jr., Antonson DL, et al. Preliminary experience with intestinal transplantation in infants and children. Pediatrics 1996;97:443–448.

118. Williams JW, Sankary HN, Foster PF, Lowe J, Goldman GM. Splanchnic transplantation: an approach to the infant dependent on parenteral nutrition who develops irreversible liver disease. JAMA 1989;261:1458–1462.

119. Starzl TE, Todo S, Tzakis A, et al. The many faces of multivisceral transplantation. Surg Gynecol Obstet 1991;172:335–344.

120. Sindhi R, Fox IJ, Heffron T, Shaw BW Jr, Langnas AN. Procurement and preparation of human isolated small intestinal grafts for transplantation. Transplantation 1995;60:771–773.

121. Tesi RJ, Jaffe BM, McBride V, Haque S. Histopathologic changes in human small intestine during storage in Viaspan organ preservation solution. Arch Pathol Lab Med 1997;121:714–718.

122. Sugitani A, Reynolds JC, Todo S. Immunohistochemical study of enteric nervous system after small bowel transplantation in humans. Dig Dis Sci 1994;39:2448–2456.

123. Mousa H, Bueno J, Griffiths J, et al. Intestinal motility after small bowel transplantation. Transplant Proc 1998;30:2535–2536.

124. Alexander JW. Specific nutrients and the immune response. Nutrition 1995;11:229–232.

125. Sollinger HW, Vernon W, D'Alessandro AM, Kalayoglu M, Stratta RJ, Belzer FO. Combined liver and pancreas procurement with Belzer-UW solution. Surgery 1989;106:685–691.

Lung Transplantation

Christine L. Lau and R. Duane Davis, Jr.

Lung transplantation has become the preferred treatment for end-staged pulmonary disease. The 1-, 3-, and 5-year actuarial survival rates for all lung transplants are approximately 70%, 55%, and 40%, respectively.[1] Donor organ shortage remains a critical problem, and efforts to increase the number of available organs include the use of marginal donors, increased public campaigns regarding donation, and living lobar transplantation. Additionally, alternatives to lung transplantation, for example, lung volume reduction surgery for chronic obstructive pulmonary disease (COPD), may be used as an alternative to or a bridge until transplantation.[2–4] Major causes of mortality remain primary graft failure and infections, and chronic rejection and novel strategies are being devised to address these devastating issues.

Recipient Selection

The international guidelines for selection of pulmonary transplant recipients have been agreed upon jointly by transplant physicians and surgeons representing the International Society for Heart and Lung Transplantation (ISHLT), the American Thoracic Society, the American Society of Transplant Physicians, the European Respiratory Society, and the Thoracic Society of Australia and New Zealand.[5] The general guidelines are listed in Table 51.1.

Disease-Specific Guidelines

The actual measured degree of pulmonary insufficiency required for lung transplant consideration is disease specific.[6] Before being considered for pulmonary transplantation, patients with COPD should have maximization of medical therapy consisting of bronchodilator therapies and oxygen therapy. Consideration should be given to lung volume reduction surgery in patients with appropriate criteria (heterogeneous emphysema, apical disease). Generally, in patients with COPD, the forced expiratory volume in 1 s (FEV_1) should be less than or equal to 25% predicted and not reversible, although most patients actually have FEV_1 less than 20% predicted at the time of transplantation. Progressive deterioration as evidenced by hypercarbia ($PaCO_2 \geq 55$ mmHg), increasing oxygen requirement, or the development of worsening pulmonary hypertension[5] indicates decreased survival, suggesting the need for transplantation.

Patients with septic lung diseases (cystic fibrosis, bronchiectasis) presenting with FEV_1 30% or less of predicted or rapidly progressive disease despite optimal medical management should be evaluated for potential lung transplantation. Progressive disease is indicated by increasing number of hospitalizations, rapid decline in FEV_1, massive hemoptysis, or increasing weight loss.[5] Patients with septic lung diseases require double-lung transplantation.

Patients with idiopathic pulmonary fibrosis (IPF) should be evaluated for transplantation when they become symptomatic. IPF is associated with the highest mortality while waiting for transplantation.[7] For this reason in the United States, potential recipients with pulmonary fibrosis are credited with 90 days at transplant listing.[8] In addition to symptomatic presentation, physiological parameters may be utilized, including a fall in vital capacity to below 60% to 70% predicted or a fall in diffusion capacity to below 50% to 60% predicted, as requirements for transplant evaluation. If the pulmonary fibrosis is part of a systemic disease process, the systemic symptoms should be under control and preferably in remission.[5] Patients with IPF requiring transplantation usually undergo single-lung transplants, but may undergo double-lung placement if care is taken to prevent oversizing of the donor lungs.

Patients with pulmonary hypertension were previously considered for lung transplantation early in the course of their disease because of the poor outcome of this disease process. Recently, with the use of intravenous prostacyclin (Flolan), and other pulmonary vasodilators an improvement in pulmonary artery pressures and relief of symptoms is seen in more than 80% of patients undergoing a therapeutic trial.[9]

TABLE 51.1. Absolute or Relative Criteria for Recipient Selection.

End-stage pulmonary disease

Maximization of medical therapy

Functional limitations (NYHA class III or IV)

Life expectancy anticipated <2 years

Life expectancy and quality of life anticipated to be improved
following pulmonary transplantation

Without significant comorbid diseases
    Symptomatic osteoporosis
    Severe musculoskeletal disease
    Other major organ dysfunction
        Creatinine clearance <50 mg/ml/min
        Untreatable coronary artery disease or left-ventricular
        dysfunction

HIV-negative/no active hepatitis B/C

Proven smoking cessation for 6 months

Without alcohol or drug addiction

Medically compliant

Single lung transplants ≤65 years of age

Bilateral lung transplants ≤60 years of age

Without active or recent malignancy (within 2 years) except basal/
    squamous skin cancers and some cases of bronchioloalveolar
    lung cancer

Inadequate nutrition <70% IBW

Morbid obesity >130%

Ambulatory with oxygen if required

Systemic steroids <15 mg prednisone/day

Psychosocial stability

Completion of pulmonary rehabilitation

Adequate support

Source: Davis et al. (1995)[6]; McCurry et al. (1997)[47]; Lau et al. (1998).[48]

Transplantation may be delayed so long as patients remain
clinically stable on Flolan.

After initial evaluation, patients with end-stage lung disease who are being evaluated for lung transplantation undergo
extensive preoperative testing to assess their overall medical
condition as well as the severity of their lung disease. The
transplant evaluation consists of the tests shown in Table 51.2.
In potential recipients more than 40 years of age, cardiac
catheterization is performed. Laboratory tests consisting of general blood work (including creatinine clearance and liver panel),

TABLE 51.2. Studies Obtained During Lung Transplant Evaluation.

Full lung function tests

Exercise performance measured by a standardized test, such as a
    6-min walk

Electrocardiogram

Echocardiogram

High-resolution computed tomography (CT) of the thorax in
    patients with parenchymal disease, pleural disease or previous
    thoracic surgical procedures

Stress echocardiogram—such as dobutamine, dobutamine positron
    emission tomography, and sestamibi—or coronary angiograms in
    patients at high risk for coronary artery disease

A 24-h creatinine clearance

Liver function studies

Source: Maurer JR, Frost AE, Estenne M, Higenbottam T, Glanville AR. International guidelines for selection of lung transplant candidates. J Heart and
Lung Transplantation 1998;17:705. Reprinted with permission.

blood typing, and immunological determination of preformed
antibodies are done. Excluding patients with pulmonary vascular diseases and congenital heart disease, potential recipients
are required to complete pulmonary rehabilitation to improve
cardiac conditioning before transplantation. Consults with psy-
chiatry, nutrition, social work, and financial are obtained. Before listing for lung transplantation, patients need to have
shown abstinence from smoking for at least 6 months. Potential transplant recipients should be without significant comorbid diseases.

Adequate nutrition preoperatively is particularly important to address. A recent analysis of data from the Toronto
group demonstrates a body mass index (BMI) greater than 27
is associated with an increased risk of postoperative death
(odds ratio, 4.6), and a BMI less than 17 similarly increases
the risk of postoperative death (odds ratio, 3.6).[10] Dietary consultation and oral supplements may suffice, but the placement of a percutaneous endoscopic gastrostomy tube for tube
feedings before transplantation may also prove useful.

Noncutaneous malignancy, unless more than 5 years from
diagnosis and curative treatment, remains a contraindication
(except in certain cases of bronchioloalveolar lung cancer).[11]
Prior thoracic surgery may increase the technical difficulty,
with greater risk of hemorrhage and nerve injury, but is not
a contraindication to lung transplantation. Active infection
outside the thorax is a contraindication to transplantation.

Donor Selection

Careful selection of donors is required (Table 51.3). The
donor's medical history is obtained, with particular emphasis
and attention paid to the donor's age, cause of death, timing
of death, smoking history, and prior thoracic procedures. ABO
incompatibility between donor and recipient, HIV positivity,
active malignancies, and active hepatitis infections remain absolute contraindications to donor lung procurement. Histo-

TABLE 51.3. Criteria of Donor Lung Suitability.

Preliminary
    Age <60 years
    ABO compatibility
    Chest roentgenogram
        Clear
        Allows estimate of size match
    History
        Smoking ≤ 20 pack-years
        No significant trauma (blunt, penetrating)
        No aspiration/sepsis
        Gram stain and culture data if prolonged intubation
        No prior cardiac/pulmonary operation
    Oxygenation
        Arterial oxygen tension ≥ 300 mm Hg, on inspired oxygen
            fraction of 1.0, 5 cm H_2O positive end-expiratory pressure
    Adequate size match

Final assessment
    Chest roentgenogram shows no unfavorable changes
    Oxygenation has not deteriorated
    Bronchoscopy shows no aspiration or mass
    Visual/manual assessment
        Parenchyma satisfactory
        No adhesions or masses
        Further evaluation of trauma

Source: Adapted with permission from the Society of Thoracic Surgeons.
Annals of Thoracic Surgery 1993;56:1409.

compatibility antigen (HLA) matching currently is not performed between donor and recipient before transplantation.

The primary reasons why lungs from a multiorgan donor are not suitable for transplantation are pulmonary contusions, pulmonary sepsis, and pulmonary edema.[12]

Operative Procedure

Donor Harvest

A median sternotomy provides excellent exposure to both lungs. The superior vena cava is encircled doubly with silk sutures and the inferior vena cava is encircled. The next step is encirclement of the pulmonary artery and aorta by exposure and dissection of the pulmonary artery window. Following completion of the thoracic dissection and before placement of the IV cannula, the patient is heparinized. The ascending aorta and main pulmonary artery are then cannulated for cardioplegia and pulmonary flush. Following this, a bolus dose of prostaglandin E_1 (PGE_1) is given directly into the pulmonary artery adjacent to the placement of the pulmonary artery catheter. Immediately after the PGE_1, the superior vena cava is ligated, and the inferior vena cava is divided, allowing the right heart to decompress. The aorta is cross-clamped, cardioplegia is initiated, and the left atrial appendage is incised, allowing the left side of the heart to decompress. The pulmonary flush is initiated and consists of several liters (50–75 ml/kg) of either University of Wisconsin or modified Eurocollins solution at 4°C.

After completion of the pulmonary flush and the cardioplegia, the cardiac team extracts the heart. Once the heart is carefully removed from the table, and the pulmonary team proceeds with the en bloc lung removal.[13]

Complete encirclement of the trachea is substantially easier now that the great vessels have been divided. The contents of the thoracic cavity are removed en bloc to prevent injury to the membranous trachea, pulmonary arteries, and pulmonary veins. Completion esophagectomy is performed with a GIA stapler, the thoracic aorta is transected, and the lungs are removed en bloc.

Implantation into Recipient

All recipients should have complete hemodynamic monitoring including a Swan–Ganz catheter. Transesophageal echocardiography is routinely performed and should be available. Double-lumen endotracheal intubation is performed for adults, followed by replacement with a single-lumen tube at the completion of the procedure. For children and small adults, routine cardiopulmonary bypass is utilized.[14]

For single-lung transplantation, the choice of side of transplant is based on several factors, but when possible, the side with the poorest function determined by preoperative ventilation perfusion scanning is transplanted, provided the presence of a normal thoracic cavity. The standard incision is the posterolateral thoracotomy. In patients with pulmonary hypertension with profound hypoxia or hypercarbia, the right side is preferred, which enables easier placement of cannulas for cardiopulmonary bypass. A pneumonectomy is performed via standard technique.

The donor lung is placed within the recipient's chest cavity covered by a cold lap pad. The bronchial anastomosis is usually performed first. Following this, the pulmonary artery of the donor and recipient are aligned in proper orientation and trimmed to prevent excessive length and possible kinking of the pulmonary artery postoperatively. The anastomosis is performed end-to-end. Finally, the left atrial cuff of the donor containing the superior and inferior pulmonary veins is anastomosed to the recipient's left atrium.[14] Following completion of the transplantation and closure of the incision, bronchoscopy is performed before leaving the operating room to check for adequacy of the bronchial anastomosis.

Postoperative Care

Immediately postoperatively patients are transported intubated to the intensive care unit for constant monitoring. Once stabilized, a standard ventilator pressure support weaning protocol is initiated. All attempts are made to limit mean airway pressures to prevent barotrauma to the new anastomosis. In single-lung transplant patients with COPD, zero or minimal positive end-expiratory pressure (PEEP) is used, along with prolonged expiratory phase of ventilation to prevent stacking of breaths and air-trapping in the native lung. The patient should be turned to the lateral position with the transplanted side up to maintain optimal function of the graft. Only rarely is it necessary to use a dual-lumen endotracheal tube to prevent hyperinflation of the native lung with subsequent compression of the transplanted lung. The smaller-diameter lumens of double-lumen tubes do not allow easy suctioning or bronchoscopy. Furthermore, maintaining the desirable position of these tubes is more difficult and subsequent lobar atelectasis may occur with malposition.

Postoperatively, a quantitative lung perfusion scan to assess for adequate patency and graft flow is usually performed. Typically, mismatch between perfusion and ventilation occurs more commonly in single-lung transplant recipients. If a lobar or greater perfusion defect is appreciated, further interrogation for the cause should be undertaken either by catherization or operative exploration.

Careful fluid management is necessary to avoid substantial transplant lung edema, and usually negative fluid balance is attempted within the first 48 h. Adequate urine output is carefully maintained with combinations of blood, colloid, diuretics, and dopamine at 2 to 3 $\mu g/kg/min$. Before extubation, patients undergo bronchoscopy to ensure adequate clearance of secretions. Following extubation, the apical chest tubes are removed in the absence of an air leak, commonly within 48 h postoperatively. Because of the frequent occurrence and reoccurrence of pleural effusions postoperatively, especially in bilateral lung transplant candidates, the basal chest tubes remain for several days, usually being removed on postoperative day 5 to 7 (chest tube drainage, <150 ml/24°).

Vigorous chest physiotherapy, postural drainage, inhaled bronchodilators, and frequent clearance of pulmonary secretions by endotracheal suctioning are required in the postoperative care of these patients. In patients with early allograft dysfunction requiring prolonged intubation, early tracheostomy allows easier mobility and better patient comfort, oral hygiene, and clearance of pulmonary secretions.

Adequate pain control is a necessity to prevent atelectasis from poor chest movement and inadequate coughing effort secondary to postthoracotomy incisional pain. An epidural catheter typically is used to provide this relief.

Most institutions prefer that transplant recipients undergo scheduled surveillance bronchoscopies with bronchoalveolar lavage (BAL) and transbronchial lung biopsies (TBBx); however, some perform only diagnostic bronchoscopies with BAL and transbronchial biopsies based on clinical indication.[15] There have been no randomized trials addressing which approach is optimal. Samples from the BAL are routinely sent for cytology, Gram's, KOH, and AFB stains and immunostains for respiratory viruses, herpes simplex virus, and CMV. Additionally bacterial, mycobacterial, fungal, and viral cultures are performed. Open-lung biopsies are performed on occasion when necessary and may be particularly useful in later time points.[16]

Immunosuppression

The initial immunosuppression protocol utilized at Duke University Medical Center consists of triple therapy including cyclosporine, azathioprine, and corticosteroids. The role of newer immunosuppressive agents in lung transplantation is still being defined.

Infection Prophylaxis

Table 51.4 shows the infection prophylaxis regimen utilized at Duke University Medical Center.

Postoperative Complications

Anastomotic Complications

Anastomotic complications including dehiscence, stenosis, and malacia are rare in lung transplant recipients today because of improvement in anastomotic techniques, improvement in pulmonary preservation, and improved care in pre-serving collateral circulation during harvesting. However, when these airway complications occur they often are initially detected by bronchoscopy and are a result of anastomotic ischemia and/or infection. Treatment is surgical repair if the anastomosis is technically inadequate. When a dehiscence occurs as a result of ischemia and necrosis at the suture line, it may present as the development of massive air leak or mediastinal emphysema in the early posttransplant period. If the dehiscence remains localized, it usually will heal by granulation and reepithelialization so long as adequate drainage of the dehiscence is maintained, which may on occasion require external drainage. Persistent air leaks are treated by chest tube placement.

Late complications from airway ischemia, infection, and dehiscence include bronchial stricture or malacia and may present as stridor and wheezing. Bronchoscopic assessment confirms the diagnosis. Bronchial stenosis and bronchomalacia can be successfully treated with serial balloon dilatation in the case of bronchial stenosis and stent placement in cases of refractory bronchial stenosis and bronchomalacia.

Primary Graft Failure

Primary graft failure (PGF) is believed to represent the extreme of severe reperfusion injury to the donor lung. Clinically, PGF is initially characterized by pulmonary edema with the radiologic findings of patchy infiltrates progressing to diffuse consolidation. The incidence of PGF varies depending on institutional definition between 13% and 35% of transplants.[17] Mortality from primary graft failure is high, with one series reporting 60% of patients dying before hospital discharge.[17]

Treatment of primary graft failure is usually supportive with continued mechanical ventilation, positive end-expiratory pressure, and high levels of inspired oxygen. Inhaled nitric oxide has been proven to improve oxygenation and cardiopulmonary performance in patients experiencing severe reperfusion injury.[18] Extracorporeal membrane oxygenation

TABLE 51.4. Infection Prophylaxis Regimen at Duke University Medical Center.

Bacterial	7–10 day course (or until invasive lines are removed) of antimicrobial prophylaxis consisting of ceftazidime and vancomycin; modified depending on results of cultures obtained from donor and recipient before transplantation		
Viral	CMV donor positive/recipients positive Ganciclovir 5 mg/kg i.v. every 12 h for 2 weeks followed by 5 mg/kg/day for 2 weeks	Donor positive/recipient negative CMV hyperimmune globulin (CytoGam) at 150 mg/kg per dose for a total of 5 doses over 8 weeks and ganciclovir 5 mg/kg i.v. every 12 h for 4 weeks followed by oral ganciclovir 1g TID indefinitely	Donor negative/recipient negative CMV negative and leuko-reduced packed red blood cells if transfusion is required
Fungal	Aerosolized liposomal amphotericin B as part of an ongoing study and/or mycostatin suspension for first 6 months		
Pneumocystis carinii pneumonia	Trimethoprim/sulfamethoxazole three times a week or monthly, aerosolized pentamidine if allergic to sulfa		
Miscellaneous	Unless specific contraindication, pneumococcal vaccine before lung transplantation, and yearly influenza vaccines after transplantation; hepatitis B series vaccine; if seronegative for varicella, then varicella vaccine		

may be required when refractory hypoxemia persists despite adequate mechanical ventilation and nitric oxide.

Acute Rejection

Acute rejection of the lung allograft is expected to occur in the first couple of months and usually weeks post transplant. In 60% of the transplant recipients, the first episode of acute rejection occurs in the first 6 months post transplant. Normally symptomatic episodes present with dyspnea, hypoxemia, low-grade fever, and moderate leukocytosis and can be difficult to differentiate from early infection. The chest radiograph findings of diffuse perihilar interstitial infiltrates along with these clinical findings further suggests rejection, but importantly can occur with infection also. Bronchoscopy with transbronchial biopsies and BAL can be helpful in confirming the diagnosis and ruling out infection. A uniform grading system for classification of pulmonary transplant rejection is based on histological criteria found on biopsy, recognizing that injury occurs to the vasculature and the airways in both acute and chronic graft rejection (see Table 51.5). Although vascular and airway inflammation are recognized in defining acute rejection, the consensus is more uniform on treatment of the perivascular inflammation while much less agreement exists on treatment of peribronchial inflammation.

Acute rejection is usually treated with i.v. methylprednisolone, 500 to 1000 mg each day for 3 days. Usually there is improvement in symptoms and radiographic findings within 8 to 12 h. Often this is followed with a steroid taper. Treatment of steroid refractory acute rejection is not uniform. A trial of cytolytic therapy is often initiated with either a polyclonal antibody such as antilymphocyte globulin or a monoclonal antibody such as OKT3 (antibody to CD3 receptor on lymphocytes). Other regimens have been attempted, but no controlled trials have been performed, with reported studies having small numbers of patients and varying degrees of success.

Chronic Rejection

Bronchiolitis obliterans is the histological finding of chronic rejection in the lung allograft. It is characterized by dense eosinophilic scar formation and fibrosis of the small airways. The presentation of chronic rejection is often subtle, and the

TABLE 51.5. Grading of Acute Pulmonary Allograft Rejection.

A. Acute rejection	
Grade 0	None
Grade 1	Minimal
Grade 2	Mild
Grade 3	Moderate
Grade 4	Severe
B. Airway inflammation	
With or without	
Lymphocytic bronchitis/bronchiolitis	
May grade	
Grade 0	None
Grade 1	Minimal
Grade 2	Mild
Grade 3	Moderate
Grade 4	Severe
Grade X	Ungradable

Source: Adapted from Yousem SA, Berry GJ, Cagle PT, et al. Revision of the 1990 working formulation for the classification of pulmonary allograft rejection: lung rejection study group. J Heart Lung Transplant 1996;15:2.

first sign may be a drop in FEV_1 on routine testing. The pathological diagnosis can be very difficult to make especially on TBBx because of the nonuniformity of areas involved, and open-lung biopsy, although occasionally beneficial, is usually not performed.

Treatment of patients with bronchiolitis obliterans syndrome (BOS) or BO rarely reverses the lung dysfunction. Several therapies have been attempted, including increasing standard immunosuppression regimens, cytolytic therapy, inhaled steroids, aerosolized CyA, methotrexate, tacrolimus, MMF, total lymphoid irradiation, photopheresis, and plasmapheresis; a few have resulted in stabilization of the patients pulmonary status but generally treatment is disappointing.[19–32] Despite attempts to reverse or stabilize the patients pulmonary status, progression of the chronic rejection process occurs, and retransplantation has been used with moderate success.

Infectious Complications

BACTERIAL

Bacterial infections are most common in the early posttransplant period and remain the primary cause of mortality in the early posttransplant period.[33] Gram-negative pathogens such as *Pseudomonas* spp., *Klebsiella*, and *Haemophilus influenzae* are responsible for most early posttransplant bacterial pneumonias, but gram-positive organisms such as *Staphylococcus aureus* are also causes.

VIRAL

Cytomegalovirus disease is the most commonly seen infectious postoperative complication, reportedly affecting between 13% and 75% of transplant patients depending on definitions of CMV disease and use of CMV prophylaxis.[34,35] Confirmation of the diagnosis of CMV disease is by demonstration of CMV inclusion bodies or positive immunoperoxidase stain on tissue biopsies. The routine use of ganciclovir prophylaxis delays the onset and severity of CMV infections in most patients.[36] Most CMV infections respond to 14 to 21 days of i.v. ganciclovir.

Most commonly isolated non-CMV viruses included herpes simplex virus (HSV), rhinovirus, and parainfluenza viruses. Less frequently isolated viruses were respiratory syncytial virus, influenza virus, adenovirus, and varicella zoster virus. HSV, parainfluenza, adenovirus, varicella zoster, and respiratory syncytial virus were associated with a greater clinical severity of illness.

FUNGAL

Fungal infections are a major problem after lung transplantation and occur early and late post transplant. *Candida albicans* is commonly isolated posttransplant, but usually represents colonization[33]; however, it may also be invasive.[37] *Aspergillus* spp. can also represent colonization, but more often the presence of these organisms is more serious. Reports of other fungal infections such as *Histoplasma*, *Coccidiomycosis*, *Zygomycetes*, and *Cryptococcus* are less common.[33]

OTHER

Mycobacterium tuberculosis and atypical *Mycobacterium* species have been seen in lung transplant recipients. *Pneu-*

mocystis carinii pneumonia is only rarely seen because of adequate prophylaxis with trimethoprim-sulfamethoxazole. Other uncommon organisms isolated and reported include *Actinomyces*, *Mucormycosis*, and *Nocardia*.[33,38]

Posttransplant Malignancies

Posttransplant lymphoproliferative disorder (PTLD) caused by Epstein–Barr virus occurs in 6.2% to 9.4% of the lung transplant population and generally is seen 6 months or longer after transplantation, more commonly in the transplanted lung.[39] In the lung transplant population, the development of PTLD is associated with a 40% mortality. The clinical course of PTLD varies from relatively benign to an aggressive non-Hodgkin's lymphoma picture. Treatment is based on the stage and progression of disease. Initially a trial of reduction of immunosuppression is attempted, particularly with disease limited to the allograft. Although chemotherapy has been used in patients with widespread disease or who have progression of disease, treatment-related mortality is considerable. The role of immunotherapy for aggressive disease holds promise.

Results

Over the past 15 years, almost 5000 single-lung transplants and more than 3000 double-lung transplants have been performed. According to the ISHLT registry data, the most common indication for single-lung transplantation is emphysema, accounting for 44%, followed by IPF (21%), alpha-1-antitrypsin deficiency (11%), PPH (5%), retransplant (3%), CF (2%), and miscellaneous (14%). For double-lung transplantation, the largest pretransplant diagnosis is cystic fibrosis, which represents 34% of the cases. Other indications for double-lung transplantation include emphysema (18%), miscellaneous (18%), alpha-1-antitrypsin deficiency (11%), PPH (10%), IPF (7.5%), and retransplantation (2%).

Actuarial survival rate for lung transplants were 70%, 55%, and 40% at 1, 3, and 5 years respectively for all lung transplants reported to ISHLT as of March 1998.[1] According to the ISHLT, median survival for bilateral recipients was 4.5 years and for single-lung recipients was 3.6 years.

Quality of Life

Multiple studies have addressed quality of life in lung transplant recipients.[40–44] Improvement in quality of life is seen posttransplant and usually becomes evident after 3 to 6 months. Pretransplant psychological status appears to affect posttransplant quality of life and adjustment.[41]

Living-Related and Nonrelated Lobar Transplantation

Living lobar transplantation using a lobe from two separate donors has been successfully used mostly in cystic fibrosis patients but also in other recipients.[45,46] Morbidity from lobectomy is low in the donors. In the recipients undergoing lobar transplants with cystic fibrosis, the 1-year survival is 73.8%, and in the recipients with other lung diseases the 1-year survival is 75%.[46] One report comparing outcomes between living lobar and cadaveric lung transplantation in children concluded that living lobar transplants were preferred in children.

References

1. Hosenpud JD, Bennett LE, Keck BM, Fiol B, Boucek MM, Novick RJ. The Registry of the International Society for Heart and Lung Transplantation: fifteenth official report—1998. J Heart Lung Transplant 1998;17:656–668.
2. Zenati M, Keenan RJ, Landreneau RJ, Paradis IL, Ferson PF, Griffith BP. Lung reduction as bridge to lung transplantation in pulmonary emphysema. Ann Thorac Surg 1995;59:1581–1583.
3. Zenati M, Keenan RJ, Sciurba C, et al. Role of lung reduction in lung transplant candidates with pulmonary emphysema. Ann Thorac Surg 1996;62:994–999.
4. Bavaria JE, Pochettino A, Kotloff RM, et al. Effect of volume reduction on lung transplant timing and selection for chronic obstructive pulmonary disease. J Thorac Cardiovasc Surg 1998;115:9–18.
5. Maurer JR, Frost AE, Estenne M, Higenbottam T, Glanville AR. International guidelines for selection of lung transplant candidates. J Heart Lung Transplant 1998;17:703–709.
6. Davis RD, Pasque MK. Pulmonary transplantation. Ann Surg 1995;221:14–28.
7. Hosenpud JD, Bennett LE, Keck BM, Edwards EB, Novick RJ. Effect of diagnosis on survival benefit of lung transplantation for end-stage lung disease. Lancet 1998;351:24–27.
8. UNOS. UNOS policy 3.7.5.1: Allocation of Thoracic Organs, Waiting Time Accrual for Lung Candidates with Idiopathic Pulmonary Fibrosis (IPF). Richmond, VA: UNOS, 1997.
9. McLaughlin VV, Genthner DE, Panella MM, Rich S. Reduction in pulmonary vascular resistance with long-term epoprostenol (prostacyclin) therapy in primary pulmonary hypertension. N Engl J Med 1998;338:273.
10. Gutierrez C, Chaparro C, Hutcheon M, Chan C, Keshavjee S. Male gender a risk factor for short term mortality after lung transplant. Chest 1998;114:395.
11. Etienne B, Bertocchi M, Gamondes J-P, Wiesendanger T, Brune J, Mornex J-F. Successful double-lung transplantation for bronchioloalveolar carcinoma. Chest 1997;112:1423–1424.
12. Follette DM, Rudich SM, Babcock WD. Improved oxygenation and increased lung donor recovery with high-dose steroid administration after brain death. J Heart Lung Transplant 1998;17:423–429.
13. Sundaresan S, Trachiotis GD, Aoe M, Patterson GA, Cooper JD. Donor lung procurement: assessment and operative technique. Ann Thorac Surg 1993;56:1409–1413.
14. Patterson GA, Cooper JD. Lung transplantation. In: Pearson FG, Deslauriers J, Ginsberg RJ, et al., eds. Thoracic Surgery. Vol 1. New York: Churchill Livingstone, 1995:931–959.
15. Kukafka DS, O'Brien GM, Furukawa S, Criner GI. Surveillance bronchoscopy in lung transplant recipients. Chest 1997;111:377–381.
16. Chaparro C, Maurer JR, Chamberlain DW, Todd TR. Role of open lung biopsy for diagnosis in lung transplant recipients: ten-year experience. Ann Thorac Surg 1995;59:928–932.
17. Christie JD, Bavaria JE, Palevsky HI, et al. Primary graft failure following lung transplantation. Chest 1998;114:51–60.
18. Date H, Triantafillou AN, Trulock EP, Pohl MS, Cooper JD, Patterson GA. Inhaled nitric oxide reduces human lung allograft dysfunction. J Thorac Cardiovasc Surg 1996;111:913–919.
19. Snell GI, Esmore DS, Williams TJ. Cytolytic therapy for the bronchiolitis obliterans syndrome complicating lung transplantation. Chest 1996;109:874–878.
20. Kesten S, Rajagopalan N, Maurer J. Cytolytic therapy for the treatment of bronchiolitis obliterans syndrome following lung transplantation. Transplantation 1996;61:427–430.
21. Speich R, Boehler A, Russi EW, et al. A case report of a double-

blind, randomized trial of inhaled steroids in a patient with lung transplant bronchiolitis obliterans. Respiration 1997;64:375–380.

22. Iacono AT, Keenan R, Duncan SR, et al. Aerosolized cyclosporine in lung recipients with refractory chronic rejection. Am J Respir Crit Care Med 1996;153:1451–1455.

23. Dusmet M, Maurer J, Winston T, Kesten S. Methotrexate can halt the progression of brochiolitis obliterans syndrome in lung transplant recipients. J Heart Lung Transplant 1996;15:948–954.

24. Reichenspurner H, Meiser BM, Kur F, et al. First experience with FK506 for treatment of chronic pulmonary rejection. Transplant Proc 1995;27:2009.

25. Kesten S, Chaparro C, Scavuzzo M, et al. Tacrolimus as rescue therapy for bronchiolitis obliterans syndrome. J Heart Lung Transplant 1997;16:905–912.

26. Speich R, Boehler A, Thurnheer R, Weder W. Salvage therapy with mycophenolate mofetil for lung transplantation bronchiolitis obliterans: importance of dosage. Transplantation 1997;64:533–535.

27. Whyte RI, Rossi SJ, Mulligan MS, et al. Mycophenolate mofetil for obliterative bronchiolitis syndrome after lung transplantation. Ann Thorac Surg 1997;64:945–949.

28. Diamond DA, Michalski JM, Lynch JP, Trulock EP. Efficacy of total lymphoid irradiation for chronic allograft rejection following bilateral lung transplantation. Int J Radiat Oncol 1998;41:795–800.

29. Slovis BS, Loyd JE, LE King J. Photopheresis for chronic rejection of lung allografts. N Engl J Med 1995;332:962.

30. Karamachandani K, McCabe M, Simpson KP, et al. Photopheresis in the management of bronchiolitis obliterans syndrome (BOS) following lung transplantation. Am J Respir Crit Care Med 1997;155:A276.

31. Achkar A, Laaban JP, Andreu G, et al. Extracorporeal photohemotherapy (ECP) for bronchiolitis obliterans (BO) after heart-lung (HTLx) and lung transplantation (LTx). Am J Respir Crit Care Med 1997;155:A277.

32. Nepomuceno DJ, Simpson KP, McCabe MA, et al. Plasmapheresis in the treatment of chronic rejection/BOS following lung transplantation. Am J Respir Crit Care Med 1997;155:A389.

33. Chaparro C, Kesten S. Infections in lung transplant recipients. Clin Chest Med 1997;18:339–351.

34. Ettinger NA, Bailey TC, Trulock EP, et al. Cytomegalovirus infection and pneumonitis: impact after isolation lung transplantation. Am Rev Respir Dis 1993;147:1017–1023.

35. Gutierrez CA, Chaparro C, Drajden M, Winton T, Kesten S. Cytomegalovirus viremia in lung transplant recipients receiving ganciclovir and immune globulin. Chest 1998;113:924–932.

36. Soghikian MV, Valentine VG, Berry GJ, Patel HR, Robbins RC, Theodore J. Impact of ganciclovir prophylaxis on heart-lung transplant recipients. J Heart Lung Transplant 1996;15:881–887.

37. Palmer SM, Perfect JR, Howell DN, et al. Candidal anastomotic infection in lung transplant recipients: successful treatment with a combination of systemic and inhaled antifungal agents. J Heart Lung Transplant 1998;17:1029–1033.

38. Bassiri AG, Girgis RE, Theodore S. Actinomyces odontolyticus thoracopulmonary infections: Two cases in lung and heart-lung transplant recipients and review of the literature. Am J Respir Crit Care Med 1995;152:374–376.

39. Aris RM, Maia DM, Neuriner IP, et al. Post-transplantation lymphoproliferative disorder in the Epstein-Barr virus-naive lung transplant recipient. Am J Respir Crit Care Med 1996;154:1712–1717.

40. Ramsey SD, Patrick DL, Lewis S, Albert RK, Raghu G, The University of Washington Medical Center Lung Transplant Study Group. Improvement in quality of life after lung transplantation: a preliminary study. J Heart Lung Transplant 1995;14:870–877.

41. Cohen L, Littlefield C, Kelly P, Maurer J, Abbey S. Predictors of quality of life and adjustment after lung transplantation. Chest 1998;113:633–644.

42. Limbos MM, Chan CK, Kesten S. Quality of life in female lung transplant candidates and recipients. Chest 1997;112:1165–1174.

43. Gross CR, Raghu G. The cost of lung transplantation and the quality of life post-transplant. Clin Chest Med 1997;18:391–403.

44. Ramsey SD, Patrick DL, Albert RK, Larson EB, Wood DE, Raghu C. The cost-effectiveness of lung transplantation: a pilot study. Chest 1995;108:1594–1601.

45. Barbers RG. Cystic fibrosis: bilateral living lobar versus cadaveric lung transplantation. Am J Med Sci 1998;315:155–160.

46. Starnes VA, Barr ML, Schenkel FA, et al. Experience with living-donor lobar transplantation for indications other than cystic fibrosis. J Thorac Cardiovasc Surg 1997;114:917–922.

47. McCurry KR, Iacono AT, Dauber JH, et al. Lung and heart-lung transplantation at the University of Pittsburgh. Clin Transplants 1997;11:209–218.

48. Lau CL, Palmer SM, D'Amico TA, Tapson VF, Davis RD. Lung transplantation at Duke University Medical Center. Clin Transpl 1998;12:327–340.

52

Heart Transplantation

Daniel Kreisel and Bruce R. Rosengard

Donor Issues

The clinical success of cardiac transplantation for patients suffering from end-stage heart failure has led to an increased demand for heart donors. Currently, one-third of patients listed for transplantation die while awaiting a suitable donor organ. The availability of donor organs is presently the primary limiting factor to cardiac transplantation. As in the case of abdominal organs, a common approach has been to extend the acceptance criteria for hearts. Donor parameters such as advanced age, high-dose inotropic support, seropositivity for hepatitis C, size and gender mismatch, echocardiographic abnormality, and prolonged cold ischemic time have been reconsidered as contraindications to organ usage. Certain criteria such as donor seropositivity for HIV, intractable ventricular dysrhythmias, extracranial malignancy, documented prior myocardial infarction, severe coronary artery or valvular disease, and death from carbon monoxide poisoning with a blood carboxyhemoglobin level greater than 20% remain absolute contraindications.

Recipient Issues

Pulmonary Hypertension

Pulmonary hypertension in heart transplant recipients most commonly arises as a consequence of long-standing left-ventricular dysfunction. An elevated pulmonary vascular resistance is the primary risk factor for right heart failure in the perioperative period. Right heart failure is thought to occur as a result of the sudden increase in right-ventricular afterload when a heart is implanted into a patient with pulmonary hypertension. Hence, evaluation of the severity and the reversibility of pulmonary hypertension with serial right heart catheterization is a critical component of heart transplant candidate selection.[1] Patients with reversible pulmonary hypertension can safely undergo heart transplantation because

pulmonary artery pressures normalize after implantation of a graft with normal left-ventricular function.

The introduction of inhaled nitric oxide into clinical practice has made an enormous impact on the perioperative management of patients with elevated pulmonary vascular resistance as a result of long-standing left heart failure. One question that remains unanswered is whether nitric oxide would allow programs to transplant patients with higher degrees of pulmonary vascular resistance. Careful study is required before routine recommendations for a pulmonary vascular resistance cutoff can be made.

Diabetes Mellitus

Diabetic patients are often excluded from transplantation because of the systemic consequences of long-standing disease and an increased baseline susceptibility to infections, which is exacerbated by immunosuppressive therapy. Because high-dose corticosteroids make blood sugar control in diabetics extremely difficult, this increases the infectious risk in the perioperative period. The high prevalence of atherosclerosis in the diabetic population increases the risk of peripheral vascular complications. Last, the nephrotoxicity of cyclosporine and tacrolimus in the setting of diabetic nephropathy can lead to frank renal failure. At the same time, the increased incidence of coronary artery disease and cardiomyopathy in diabetics results in a significant number of potential heart transplant recipients in this patient population.

Improvements in immunosuppression, leading to reduced doses of corticosteroids, as well as refinements in operative and perioperative management have led an increasing number of centers to consider selected diabetic patients for cardiac transplantation.

Dual Listing

In 1991, cardiologists and cardiothoracic surgeons from the University of California at Los Angeles proposed an "alternate" recipient list as an approach to maximize the utilization of marginal donor hearts and thereby expand the number of organ recipients.[2] The guiding principle behind their method was matching the higher-risk patients with the higher-risk donors. High-risk candidates constituted patients over the age of 65 years and those who were being considered for a third heart transplant. Criteria that defined marginal donors included ventricular dysfunction requiring high-dose inotropic support, wall motion abnormalities on echocardiography, coronary artery disease, donor age greater than 55 years, a history of cardiac risk factors (e.g., smoking), and prolonged ischemia time. In the UCLA series, there was no significant difference between this patient population and "standard" heart transplant recipients with respect to length of stay in the intensive care unit, duration of hospitalization, postoperative cardiac function, frequency of acute rejection, incidence of infectious complications, or actuarial survival at 1 year. The early outcomes of the UCLA group justified the "alternate" list as a potential approach to expand the recipient population to include patients who would otherwise not be considered for this lifesaving procedure.

Elderly

Age greater than 60 years has traditionally been considered to be an exclusion criterion for heart transplantation, based on several studies that found advanced age adversely influences outcome.[3,4] However, a recent series of heart transplants in patients >65 years old showed that survival rates at a mean follow-up period of 3.2 years were comparable to a cohort of younger heart transplant recipients.[5] In addition, the quality of life indices of the elderly patient group were quite satisfactory.

Ventricular Assist

Temporary circulatory support with ventricular-assist devices (VADs) has become a well-established treatment option for patients awaiting cardiac transplantation. Recent studies demonstrate that transplantation after mechanical support offers satisfactory outcomes to a population of patients who otherwise would have faced certain death.[6] However, bridge-to-transplant patients, who have usually suffered hemodynamic deterioration with consequent end-organ dysfunction, have a lower overall survival rate after heart transplantation than nonbridged controls. Despite continuous advances in this field, mechanical vetricular assistance is associated with the potential for several complications that can preclude transplantation.

As more data become available, it is likely that VAD patients may need to be considered for dual listing because they represent a "high-risk" group.

Surgical Issues

Bicaval versus Biatrial

Orthotopic heart transplantation is usually performed using one of two different techniques (Figs. 52.1–52.5). The biatrial

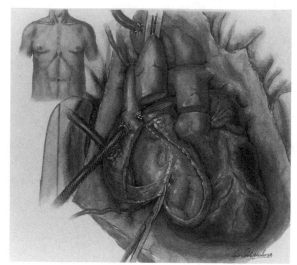

FIGURE 52.1. Recipient cardiectomy for standard heart transplantation.

technique developed by Shumway and Lower, which is considered to be the standard method, involves performing the recipient cardiectomy by removing the ventricles at the AV groove and then trimming the atria, leaving a cuff of atrial wall behind. The recipient heart is implanted using four anastomoses: the left and right atria, the pulmonary artery, and the aorta.

The alternative method is termed bicaval orthotopic heart transplantation. In most cases, bicaval implantation is performed with a left-atrial anastomosis, identical to that performed using the standard biatrial technique. Thus, the procedure requires five anastomoses. Total orthotopic heart transplantation involves complete excision of the recipient heart except for two pulmonary venous cuffs and two caval cuffs. Bilateral pulmonary venous anastomoses and individual anastomoses of the cavae are performed during implan-

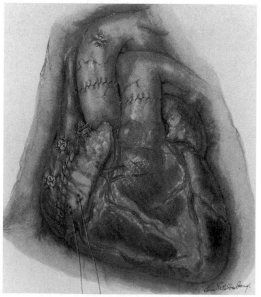

FIGURE 52.2. Graft after completed implantation.

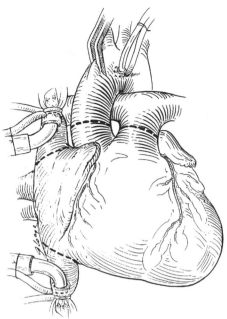

FIGURE 52.3. Incision lines for recipient cardiectomy in bicaval heart transplantation.

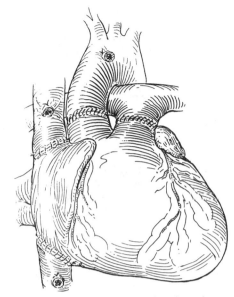

FIGURE 52.5. Graft after completed implantation.

tation, for a total of six anastomoses. For this reason, total orthotopic transplantation has not gained widespread application.

Several nonrandomized studies have demonstrated improved atrial function,[7,8] a reduction in atrial arrhythmias,[9,10] fewer left-atrial thrombi,[11] and improved tricuspid and mitral valve function with the bicaval procedure.[12] However, these

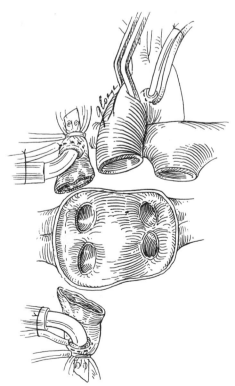

FIGURE 52.4. Completion of recipient cardiectomy.

echocardiographic findings have yet to be correlated to clinical endpoints.

Cardioplegia

The need to expand the donor pool has led to a renewed interest in improving techniques for myocardial protection. Remote procurement of cardiac allografts is greatly limited by the lack of methods for prolonged myocardial preservation. The incidence of primary graft failure that occurs as a result of suboptimal preservation techniques is still unacceptably high. Although primary nonfunction of the graft may not be life threatening in kidney transplantation, the heart transplant recipient depends on immediate function of the allograft. Unlike the case with kidneys and livers, there is great variability among heart transplant centers with respect to preservation methods. Research has focused on methods of cardioplegic induction, efficacy of different cardioplegic solutions, choice of the transport medium and storage modalities, and reperfusion strategies.

In most cases, antegrade cardioplegia is administered through the aortic root during the procurement. Traditionally, cardioplegia has consisted of cold, high-potassium crystalloid solutions, which lead to a quick diastolic arrest of the heart. However, in the routine practice of cardiac surgery, investigators have described improved myocardial protection by using blood-based cardioplegia. Several theoretical advantages exist for using blood-based cardioplegia for donor hearts. As compared to crystalloid solutions, blood cardioplegia provides osmotic support that reduces myocardial edema, excellent buffering capacity that minimizes intracellular acidosis, free radical scavengers, and improved rheological properties. In addition, blood cardioplegia can provide oxygen for aerobic metabolism, although this effect is minimized when the solution is delivered at low temperatures. Favorable results with induction of cardiac arrest in the donor with cold blood cardioplegia as compared to a cold crystalloid solution have been reported.[13]

Reperfusion is the final component of perservation of the cardiac allograft. Controversial areas include the composition, temperature, and infusion pressure of reperfusion solutions. Common regimens include intermittent doses of cold blood or cold oxygenated crystalloid cardioplegia during graft implantation and delivery of a warm, blood-based solution before release of the aortic cross-clamp. Important characteristics of the ideal reperfusion solution are the capacity for oxygen delivery, the provision of substrate, the maintenance of asystole with high concentrations of potassium, and normothermic conditions to enhance anabolism and cellular repair. The goal is to facilitate metabolic recovery and thus improve early graft function. Ultimately, single-dose, antegrade, crystalloid cardioplegia remains the standard in clinical practice and is very unlikely to change due to the simplicity of the approach.

Heterotopic Auxiliary Heart Transplantation

The first human heterotopic heart transplantation was performed by Barnard and Losman in 1974.[14] The donor heart is implanted in parallel by anastomosing donor and recipient atria and great vessels. Cooper[15] summarized the limited indications for this procedure: (1) patients in whom recovery of the native myocardium is possible; (2) situations in which the function of the donor heart is considered inadequate to maintain the recipient's cirulation alone (undersized donors, long ischemic intervals, etc.); (3) recipients with elevated pulmonary vascular resistance; (4) situations requiring a bridge to orthotopic heart transplantation; and (5) certain cases of severe angina that are unresponsive to medical therapy or myocardial revascularization where left-ventricular function is preserved. Because several reports suggest that undersized donor hearts implanted heterotopically are not detrimental to long-term allograft function, it is generally thought that fixed pulmonary hypertension in the recipient is the only absolute indication for heterotopic heart transplantation.[16] Heterotopic heart transplantation brings with it a unique set of complications, which may contribute to slightly worse outcomes as compared to orthotopic heart transplantation. Over the past 5 years, heterotopic auxiliary heart transplants have been performed worldwide with a 1-year survival of 71% as compared to a 1-year survival rate of 91% for orthotopic transplants. However, as heterotopic auxiliary heart transplantation is reserved for selected high-risk situations, it is not clear that the procedure is, in fact, any less successful or any more morbid. Complications of the heterotopic procedure include an increased risk of pulmonary infections due to obstructive atelectasis of the right lower lobe, an increased high risk of thromboembolic events from thrombus formation in the native heart, and mitral regurgitation in donor and native hearts. Auxiliary heart transplantation remains an acceptable option in certain, selected clinical situations.

Postoperative Management: ICU Phase

Inotropic Support

Right-ventricular dysfunction is a common occurrence in the early posttransplant period that requires the administration of pulmonary vasodilators and inotropes. Isoproterenol, a pure β-agonist, is a positive inotrope and chronotrope that also re-duces right-ventricular afterload by dilating the pulmonary arterial tree. It is a first-line agent and is used prophylactically by virtually all surgeons and intensivists for the transplant recipient. The dose is titrated to a heart rate of 90 to 120. Low-dose dopamine is also frequently administered routinely to increase heart rate and splanchnic and renal perfusion in hope of mitigating the toxicity of cyclosporine or tacrolimus. Other inotropes or vasoconstrictors are often added, depending on the clinical situation. Pulmonary hypertension often necessitates the use of milrinone, amrinone, or enoximone. However, the peripheral vasodilating effects of these agents often limits their utility, particularly in patients who have been managed for long periods of time on ACE inhibitors. Inhaled nitric oxide, which is selective for the pulmonary vasculature by dint of its route of administration, has become an essential component in postoperative management.[17] In addition to perioperative right heart dysfunction, the other common hemodynamic derangement in the postoperative period is a low systemic vascular resistance due to a combination of the effects of cardiopulmonary bypass and chronic therapy with ACE inhibitors. Alpha agonists such as phenylephrine and norepinephrine have traditionally been used as vasoconstrictors. Recently, the use of vasopressin has been popularized by several groups.[18] The primary advantage of vasopressin is that it increases systemic vascular resistance without altering myocardial oxygen demand.

Pacing

The transplanted heart is devoid of autonomic innervation and has a resting heart rate of approximately 100 beats per minute. Although bradyarrhythmias are common in the early postoperative period, tachyarrhythmias are far less common and are often associated with acute allograft rejection. As the sinus node usually resumes normal function within 3 weeks, the majority of these cases respond well to pharmacological agents or temporary pacing via epicardial wires. In most series, the incidence of perioperative nodal dysfuntion requiring permanent pacing is approximately 5%.

Pulmonary Hypertension

Failure of the right ventricle in the immediate and the early postoperative period accounts for nearly half of all cardiac complications following heart transplantation. It can be associated with inability to separate the patient from cardiopulmonary bypass and represents one of the major risk factors for death. In recipients with elevated pulmonary vascular resistance, the etiology of right-ventricular dysfunction is the abrupt increase in afterload at the time of the operation, aided and abetted by ischemia–reperfusion injury. To avert acute graft failure, it is imperative to effectively control the recipient's hemodynamics immediately after discontinuation of cardiopulmonary bypass. There are several agents in clinical use that dilate the pulmonary vasculature and thus lower the pulmonary vascular resistance and, hence, reduce right-ventricular afterload. The pulmonary vasodilators differ in their selectivity of action and therefore in their systemic side effects. These include intravenous sodium nitroprusside, prostacyclin, prostaglandin E$_1$, and inhaled nitric oxide. Comparative studies suggest that the high degree of pulmonary selectivity makes inhaled nitric oxide the preferred treatment for pulmonary hypertension in the postoperative phase.

Immunosuppression

The lack of a generally accepted guideline and newly emerging regimens lead to divergent policies at different heart transplant centers. Controversies are not just limited to maintenance immunosuppression but extend to monitoring for rejection and treatment of rejection episodes.

Induction Therapy

There is great controversy in the literature with respect to the necessity for induction therapy with cytolytic agents in heart tranplantation. Induction therapy refers to the administration of cytolytic agents for 7 to 14 days in the immediate postoperative period. The principal cytolytics in clinical use include the polyclonal agents horse, antithymocyte globulin (ATGAM), rabbit antithymocyte globulin (Thymoglobulin), and the murine monoclonal antibody OKT3.

The use of cytolytic induction therapy is most advantageous in patients who have preexisting renal dysfunction. Early postoperative administration of cyclosporine in such patients leads to oliguria or anuria and, consequently, poor outcome.[19] Cytolytics postpone the need to begin cyclosporine until hemodynamic parameters improve and the effects of cardiopulmonary bypass resolve, thus reducing the toxic effects of the drug. Induction therapy is also beneficial in heart recipients who are at a higher risk for acute rejection (e.g., retransplantation candidates or presensitized patients). Several investigators have suggested that the use of induction therapy may permit subsequent discontinuation of steroids.[20] Finally, there is controversy whether induction therapy has any impact on later episodes of rejection.

The risk of infection and the question of an association with lymphoproliferative disorders are the main arguments against the use of cytolytic induction therapy. However, the available data are rather inconclusive.

Mycophenolate Mofetil versus Azathioprine

Mycophenolate mofetil inhibits de novo purine synthesis. Mycophenolate mofetil was designed to exert preferential effects on both B- and T lymphocytes, because lymphocytes lack the salvage pathway for purine synthesis. This selective action may represent an advantage of mycophenolate mofetil over azathioprine, which inhibits both the de novo and the salvage pathways of purine biosynthesis and thereby suppresses erythropoiesis and neutrophil production, in addition to blocking lymphopoiesis. Favorable results of an uncontrolled, nonrandomized phase I trial of the efficacy and safety of mycophenolate mofetil in heart transplant recipients were published in 1993.[21]

More recently, a randomized multicenter double-blind trial comparing the efficacies of mycophenolate mofetil and azathioprine in 650 heart transplant recipients additionally receiving cyclosporine and corticosteroids as maintenance immunosuppressants has been reported.[22] Patients who were treated with mycophenolate mofetil had higher 1-year survival rates as well as higher rates of freedom from allograft rejection at 6 months. Overall, substitution of mycophenolate mofetil for azathioprine in maintenance immunosuppression appeared beneficial, although the differences are not dramatic and a substantial number of patients are unable to tolerate the drug because of GI toxicity.

Cyclosporine versus Tacrolimus

Tacrolimus has been shown to be 10- to 100-fold more potent than cyclosporine at inhibiting the activation of alloreactive T lymphocytes when compared on a molar basis. The spectrum of adverse effects resembles that of cyclosporine, including nephrotoxicity, central nervous system toxicity, hypertension, and gastrointestinal disturbances. Three recent randomized trials have compared the efficacy of cyclosporine and tacrolimus in preventing acute rejection in heart transplant recipients.[23–25] The studies demonstrated equivalent survival rates and incidences of acute rejection. The primary differences noted were the distribution of drug-related complications. Nephrotoxicity was slightly more frequent in patients treated with tacrolimus. Moreover, tacrolimus was frequently associated with hyperglycemia. In contrast, cyclosporine was associated with higher incidences of hypertension and hypercholesterolemia. Neurotoxocity was equivalent.

Steroids

Triple-drug immunosuppression with cyclosporine, azathioprine, and corticosteroids after heart transplantation has been shown to be associated with improvements in short- and long-term survival.[26] The ability of this combination to significantly reduce the incidence of acute rejection has made it the most commonly used regimen in both the adult and the pediatric populations.

Approaches to decrease morbidity from steroid use have varied from late weaning many months posttransplant[27] to protocols that exclude steroids entirely from maintenance immunosuppression. In one report, patients who were withdrawn from steroids had a higher incidence of allograft rejection, but also had a decrease in infectious complications and a reduction in bone loss. The authors concluded that even in the absence of induction therapy early withdrawal from steroids was safe for the majority of patients.

Given the significant morbidity associated with their use, it is likely that efforts to aggressively wean steroids are warranted.

Endomyocardial Biopsy

The routine use of postoperative surveillance endomyocardial biopsies has contributed to an overall increase in survival after cardiac transplantation. Biopsy allows allograft rejection to be detected and therefore treated before the onset of hemodynamically significant graft dysfunction. Because allograft rejection is most common early after transplantation, endomyocardial biopsies have been traditionally performed weekly for the first month and progressively less frequently thereafter. Despite ongoing attempts to develop noninvasive techniques to monitor allograft rejection, transvenous endomyocardial biopsy has remained the gold standard for diagnosis of rejection. However, because this is an invasive, expensive procedure, the utility of continuning with biopsies more than 1–2 years following transplant has been questioned. Thus, policies for routine surveillance biopsy vary by both indication and patient risk factors.

Rejection Therapy

Cardiac allograft rejection accounts for approximately one-third of all deaths related to the procedure. Treatment of rejection episodes depend on histological grade and on clinical symptoms. The rationale to treat even mild acute cardiac rejection without hemodynamic compromise early and aggressively stems from the beliefs that low-grade rejection is a precursor to high-grade rejection and that repetitive episodes of untreated low-grade rejection can compromise long-term cardiac function and may predispose to cardiac allograft vasculopathy. This notion that low-grade rejection portends high-grade rejection is supported by the observation that increasing immunosuppression in patients with low-grade rejection prevents progression to moderate rejection on subsequent biopsies.[28]

A variety of both pharmacological and nonpharmacological strategies can be employed for the treatment of allograft rejection. Corticosteroids have been used most commonly to treat episodes of cellular rejection with or without hemodynamic compromise. Policies differ with respect to dose, route of administration, and tapering after the bolus therapy. Other small molecule immunosuppressants can reverse acute rejection. Tacrolimus has been shown to reverse steroid-resistant acute rejection. Moreover, if substituted for cyclosporine in the maintenance regimen, it will also prevent recurrent acute rejection. Methotrexate, a folic acid analogue that inhibits the biosynthesis of purine, has been utilized successfully in the treatment of recurrent cellular rejection in heart transplant recipients receiving triple-drug immunosuppression.[29] However, unlike tacrolimus, methotrexate does not decrease the risk of subsequent rejection episodes.

Cytolytic therapy has been the preferred treatment for steroid-resistant, hemodynamically significant, and acute vascular rejection for many years. The success of this ranges from 17–90%.

The main nonpharmacological modalities for the treatment of allograft rejection are photopheresis and total lymphoid irradiation. Photopheresis is an immunomodulatory therapy in which the patient's mononuclear cells are treated with 6-methylpsoralen, a photosensitizing agent, and subsequently exposed to ultraviolet A ex vivo. After photoexposure, these cells are then returned to the patient. It is postulated that these cells stimulate a suppressor response by altering of antigen presentation. Initially used in the treatment of cutaneous T-cell lymphoma, the indications for photopheresis were expanded to several autoimmune diseases and more recently to bone marrow and solid-organ transplantation. Although its specific mechanisms of action have not been clearly elucidated, preliminary results from animal experiments and small clinical series are encouraging. Several authors have demonstrated that photopheresis can reverse steroid-resistant, cytolytic-resistant, or recurrent acute rejection.[30–32] Photochemotherapy also can reduce panel reactive antibodies in multiparous women or candidates for retransplantation.[33] Last, prophylactic photopheresis clearly reduces the incidence of acute rejection and may help prevent allograft vasculopathy.[34,35]

Complications

Infections

The drug-induced immunosuppressive state in solid-organ recipients places this population at risk for life-threatening infections. The risk of infectious complications following heart transplantation is one of the leading causes of morbidity and mortality, as is clearly illustrated by the fact that more than two-thirds of all heart transplant recipients develop at least one infectious episode within the first year after the operation. Among heart transplant recipients, infections are responsible for 18% of early and 38% of late mortality. The type of infection depends on several factors including the patient's environment, the time period that has elapsed since the operation, and the net state of immunosuppression. Bacterial infections are common in the perioperative period (0–6 months post transplant) and warrant aggressive work-up and expeditious treatment. Opportunistic infections (fungal, parasitic, viral) tend to occur later in the postoperative course.

The primary controversy that exists with regard to management of infectious complications after heart transplantation involves the choice between expectant and prophylactic management for CMV. We support aggressive prophylaxis in all circumstances of donor or recipient seropositivity with intravenous ganciclovir during the hospitalization, followed by oral ganciclovir on discharge. We extend therapy with intravenous ganciclovir to 6 weeks for seronegative recipients of seropositive organs. Currently, we use hyperimmune globulin only for those patients with severe symptomatic CMV.

Cardiac Allograft Vasculopathy

The major cause for late morbidity and mortality is cardiac allograft vasculopathy, which is a pathological process distinct from atherosclerotic coronary artery disease. The disease process is not just limited to the epicardial coronary arteries but also involves intramyocardial arterioles, venous structures, and the great vessels of the allograft. Cardiac allograft vasculopathy is diffuse in nature, begins distally and progresses proximally, and is characterized by concentric proliferation of the intima. The pathological anatomy is associated with abnormalities in the vasodilatory response of the coronary circulation.[36] The precise etiology remains under investigation. To date, the only definitive therapy for this potentially fatal late complication of cardiac transplantation remains retransplantation.

Retransplantation

The question of cardiac retransplantation involves both ethical and scientific issues. Although it is the only possible life-saving intervention for an individual patient, society is faced with a scarcity of donor organs. There are no universal guidelines, and health care professionals must make this difficult decision on a case-by-case basis because a decision for retransplantation will deny a potential recipient access to a transplant. The outcome after retransplantation is generally worse than after a primary transplant. The Stanford group reported a 1-year survival rate of 49% and a 5-year survival rate of 24% for retransplanted patients, while in the case of primary transplants these figures were 82% and 62%, respectively.[37]

Indications for retransplantation in the early postoperative period are usually allograft failure on the basis of nonimmunological factors (ischemia, high PVR, etc.) or immune-mediated injury. There are several isolated reports in the literature of favorable outcomes where patients were bridged for several hours with assist devices for nonimmunological primary graft failure before a second heart became available. Because patients with immediate or early primary cardiac allograft failure are generally hemodynamically unstable, the urgency of the situation oftens leads to acceptance of marginal hearts for this already high-risk group. As a result, a recent study found that three of four patients who underwent retransplantation for primary graft failure died within 2 weeks of the operation.[38] The main indication for cardiac retransplantation is for cardiac allograft vasculopathy in the late postoperative period. This patient population has more favorable outcomes after retransplantation. In the Stanford series, the 1-year and 5-year survival rates for patients who underwent retransplantation for graft atherosclerosis were 69% and 34%, respectively. Although these results are clearly inferior to primary transplants, they are not poor enough to clearly contraindicate retransplantation in this subgroup of patients.

References

1. Stein JH, Neumann A, Preston LM, et al. Echocardiography for hemodynamic assessment of patients with advanced heart failure and potential heart transplant recipients. J Am Coll Cardiol 1997;30:1765–1772.
2. Stevenson LW, Warner SL, Steimle AE, et al. The impending crisis awaiting cardiac transplantation: modeling a solution based on selection. Circulation 1994;89:450–457.
3. Anguita M, Arizon JM, Valles F, et al. Influence on survival after heart transplantation of contraindications seen in transplant recipients. J Heart Lung Transplant 1992;11:708–715.
4. Miller LW, Kubo SH, Young JB, et al. Report of the consensus conference on candidate selection for heart transplantation—1993. J Heart Lung Transplant 1995;14:562–571.
5. Frazier OH, Macris MP, Duncan JM, et al. Cardiac transplantation in patients over 60 years of age. Ann Thorac Surg 1997;64:1866–1867.
6. Masters RG, Hendry PJ, Davies RA, et al. Cardiac transplantation after mechanical circulatory support: a Canadian perspective. Ann Thorac Surg 1996;61:1734–1739.
7. Traversi E, Pozzoli M, Grande A. The bicaval anastomosis technique for orthotopic heart transplantation yields better atrial function than the standard technique: an echocardiographic automatic boundary detection study. J Heart Lung Transplant 1998;17:1065–1074.
8. Blanche C, Nessim S, Quartel A, et al. Heart transplantation with bicaval and pulmonary venous anastomoses. A hemodynamic analysis of the first 117 patients. J Cardiovasc Surg 1997;38:561–566.
9. Brandt M, Harringer W, Hirt SW, et al. Influence of bicaval anastomoses on late occurrence of atrial arrhythmia after heart transplantation. Ann Thorac Surg 1997;64:70–72.
10. Rothman SA, Jeevanandam V, Combs WG, et al. Eliminating bradyarrhythmias after orthotopic heart transplantation. Circulation 1996;(suppl 9):II178–II182.
11. Bouchart F, Derumeaux G, Mouton-Schleifer D, et al. Conventional and total orthotopic cardiac transplantation: a comparative clinical and echocardiographical study. Eur J Cardiothorac Surg 1997;12:555–559.
12. Aleksic I, Freimark D, Blanche C, et al. Resting hemodynamics after total versus standard orthotopic heart transplantation in patients with high preoperative pulmonary vascular resistance. Eur J Cardiothorac Surg 1997;11:1037–1044.
13. Luciani GB, Faggian G, Forni A, et al. Myocardial protection during heart transplantation using blood cardioplegia. Transplant Proc 1997;29:3386–3388.
14. Barnard CN, Losman JG. Left ventricular bypass. South African Med J 1975;49:303–312.
15. Cooper DK, Novitzky D, Becerra E, et al. Are there indications for heterotopic heart transplantation in 1986? A 2- to 11-year follow-up of 49 consecutive patients undergoing heterotopic heart transplantation. Thor Cardiovasc Surgeon 1986;34:300–304.
16. Baumgartner WA. Heterotopic transplantation: is it a viable alternative? Ann Thorac Surg 1992;54:401–402.
17. Chester AH, Birks EJ, Yacoub MH. Role of nitric oxide following cardiac transplantation. J Hum Hypertens 1998;12:883–887.
18. Argenziano M, Chen JM, Choudri AF, et al. Management of vasodilatory shock after cardiac surgery: identification of predisposing factors and use of a novel pressor agent. J Thorac Cardiovasc Surg 1998;116:973–980.
19. Wahlers T. Cytolytic induction therapy in heart and lung transplantation: the protagonist opinion. Transplant Proc 1998;30:1100–1103.
20. Keogh A, Macdonald PO, Harvison A, et al. Initial steroid-free versus steroid-based maintenance therapy and steroid withdrawal after heart transplantation: two views of the steroid question. J Heart Lung Transplant 1992;11:421–427.
21. Ensley RD, Bristow MR, Olsen SL, et al. The use of mycophenolate mofetil (RS-61443) in human heart transplant. Transplantation 1993;56:75–82.
22. Kobashigawa J, Miller L, Renlund D, et al. A randomized active-controlled trial of mycophenolate mofetil in heart transplant recipients. Transplantation 1998;66:507–515.
23. Meiser BM, Uberfuhr P, Fuchs A, et al. Single-center randomized trial comparing tacrolimus and cyclosporine in the prevention of acute myocardial rejection. J Heart Lung Transplant 1998;17:782–788.
24. Reichart B, Meisr B, Vigano M, et al. European multicenter tacrolimus (FK506) heart pilot study: one-year-results—European tacrolimus multicenter heart study group. J Heart Lung Transplant 1998;17:775–781.
25. Pham SM, Kormos RL, Hattler BG, et al. A prospective trial of tacrolimus (FK506) in clinical heart transplantation: intermediate-term results. J Thorac Cardiovasc Surg 1996;111:764–772.
26. Olivari MT, Jesse ME, Baldwin BJ, et al. Triple-drug immunosuppression with steroid discontinuation by six months after heart transplantation. J Heart Lung Transplant 1995;14:127–135.
27. Kobashigawa JA, Stevenson LW, Brownfield ED, et al. Initial success of steroid weaning late after heart transplantation. J Heart Lung Transplant 1992;11:428–430.
28. Kobashigawa JA, Stevenson LW, Moriguchi J, et al. Randomized study of high dose oral cyclosporine therapy for mild acute cardiac rejection. J Heart Lung Transplant 1989;8:53–58.
29. Bourge RC, Kirklin JK, White-Williams C, et al. Methotrexate pulse therapy in the treatment of recurrent acute heart rejection. J Heart Lung Transplant 1992;11:1116–1124.
30. Dall'Amico R, Livi U, Milano A, et al. Extracorporeal photochemotherapy as adjuvant treatment of heart transplant recipients with recurrent rejection. Transplantation 1995;60:45–49.
31. Costanzo-Nordin MR, Hubbell EA, O'Sullivan EJ, et al. Photophoresis versus corticosteroids in the therapy of heart transplant rejection: preliminary clinical report. Circulation 1992;86(suppl 5):11242–11250.

32. Costanzo-Nordin MR, Hubbell EA, O'Sullivan EJ, et al. Successful treatment of heart transplant rejection with photophoresis. Transplantation 1992;53:808–815.

33. Rose EA, Barr ML, Xu H, et al. Photochemotherapy in human heart transplant recipients at high risk for fatal rejection. J Heart Lung Transplant 1992;11:746–759.

34. Barr ML, Meisser BM, Eisen HJ, et al. Photophoresis for the prevention of rejection in cardiac transplantation: photophoresis transplantation study group. N Engl J Med 1998;339:1744–1751.

35. Ross HJ, Gullestad L, Pak J, et al. Methotrexate of total lymphoid radiation for treatment of persistent or recurrent allograft cellular rejection: a comparative study. J Heart Lung Transplant 1997;16:179–189.

36. Kofoed KF, Czernin J, Johnson J, et al. Effects of cardiac allograft vasculopathy on myocardial blood flow, vasodilatory capacity, and coronary vasomotion. Circulation 1997;95:600–606.

37. Smith JA, Ribakove GH, Hunt SA, et al. Heart retransplantation: the 25-year experience at a single institution. J Heart Lung Transplant 1995;14:832–839.

38. Schnetzler B, Pavie A, Dorent R, et al. Heart retransplantation: a 23-year single-center clinical experience. Ann Thorac Surg 1998;65:978–983.

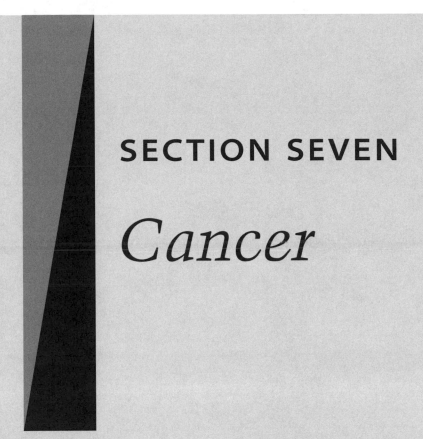

Cancer

53

Diseases of the Breast

Helen A. Pass

Clinical Evaluation of the Breast Patient: History and Risk Assessment

In addition to a history taken as part of a standard medical evaluation, there are a variety of items specific to the evaluation of patients with benign and malignant breast diseases. The patient's age, age at menarche, age of menopause, and history of menstrual irregularities should be determined. Age at first pregnancy, number of pregnancies, and history of breastfeeding contribute to breast cancer risk assessment. Evaluation of the medication history should focus upon past and present use as well as duration of use of oral contraceptives and hormone replacement therapies. A past history of breast complaints and interventions or radiation exposure must be documented. A family history of breast, ovarian, and prostate cancer should be sought.

In the evaluation of a patient with a breast mass, one needs to evaluate when and how it was found, if it has changed since its discovery, timing relative to menstrual cycle, and if it is painful. Similarly, complaints of breast pain need to be correlated with timing of menstrual cycles and aggravating factors identified. Nipple discharge should be classified as unilateral versus bilateral, spontaneous versus induced, and characterized by color and consistency (bloody, milky, yellow, or clear). Concern regarding the possibility of cancer should prompt inquiry of constitutional symptoms such as fatigue, weight loss, or bone pain.

Risk Assessment

As with other malignancies, an assessment for the development of breast cancer is important to define populations that may benefit from early and more aggressive screening programs or preventive interactions. The average American female's lifetime risk of developing breast cancer is 11% and her risk of death from breast cancer is 3% to 4%. Numerous factors have been implicated (Table 53.1) including reproductive or hormonal history, dietary fat or alcohol use, a per-

sonal or family history of breast cancer, a past history of benign proliferative breast disease (especially if associated with atypia), and a history of radiation exposure. Nevertheless, more than two-thirds of women diagnosed with breast cancer have no identifiable risk factor.

Management of the High-Risk Patient

Screening Guidelines

Risk factor assessment is imprecise at best, but certain high-risk populations can be identified. As previously mentioned, women with a personal history of atypia, radiation exposure, or family history of breast and/or ovarian cancer are at increased risk for the development of breast cancer. Additionally, a personal history of breast cancer or lobular carcinoma in situ increases risk and thereby influences screening recommendations.

For women with a personal history of breast cancer, follow-up is determined by time from diagnosis. Physical examination should be performed every 3 to 4 months within the first 2 years from diagnosis, biannually from 2 until 5 years, and annually thereafter. Mammography should be obtained annually. Other laboratory and radiologic evaluation should be determined by stage at presentation. Women with lobular carcinoma in situ have twice-yearly clinical breast examinations and annual mammography. Those with atypia may be followed annually with both clinical breast examination and mammography.

Women with a significant radiation exposure or family history may benefit from earlier screening as proposed by Lynch.[1] Patients with an autosomal dominant pattern of transmission of breast cancer, including those with a BRCA1[2,3] mutation, should have twice-yearly physical examination (see Familial/Hereditary Breast Cancer section). Screening mammograms should be obtained annually or semiannually beginning 10 years younger than the youngest affected relative, or no

TABLE 53.1. Factors Associated with Increased Risk for the Development of Breast Cancer.

Increasing age

Age at menarche ≤ 11 years

Age at menopause ≥ 55 years

Age at first pregnancy ≥ 30 years

Nulliparity

Absence of lactation

Use of hormone replacement therapy or fertility regimens

Prior breast biopsy with benign proliferative disease, atypia, or lobular carcinoma in situ

Family history of breast, ovarian, or prostate cancer

Known carrier of BRCA1 or 2 mutation

Personal history of breast cancer

History of thoracic radiation

Alcohol consumption

Controversial

Prior abortion

High fat diet

Obesity

---

later than 35 years. The lifetime risk for the development of breast cancer in a known *BRCA1* or *BRCA2* carrier has been estimated at between 60% and 80%.[4,5] *BRCA1* mutations are linked to the development of breast, ovarian, and prostate cancers[6] whereas *BRCA2* families have an increased incidence of male and female breast cancers.[7,8] Undoubtedly, practice recommendations will change as more is learned about the natural history of these patients.

Chemoprevention

One of the most important new advances for the treatment of the high-risk patient has been the demonstrated benefit of tamoxifen as a chemopreventive agent in women at high risk. The National Surgical Adjuvant Breast and Bowel Project P-1 Study (NSABP-P1) demonstrated a 49% reduced risk of invasive breast cancer in high-risk women randomized to tamoxifen versus placebo.[9] High-risk women were defined as those with a history of lobular carcinoma in situ, a 5-year predicted risk for breast cancer of at least 1.66% as defined by the Gail Model, or 60 years of age or older. The findings of the NSABP-P1 study are consistent with tamoxifen's demonstrated benefit in lowering the incidence of contralateral breast cancer in women with a previous history of breast cancer,[10] prolonging survival when used as a postoperative adjuvant in women with stage I or II disease,[11] and efficacy with or without chemotherapy in the treatment of advanced breast cancer.[12] The authors were careful to point out that even though tamoxifen prevented the occurrence of breast cancer in a substantial number of patients over the duration of the study, there was no evidence to support the assumption that carcinogenesis was inhibited or that tumors were permanently prevented.

A new NSABP chemoprevention trial, P-2, will compare the benefits and side effects of tamoxifen versus raloxifene in a prospective randomized fashion. Raloxifene is a selective estrogen receptor modulator (SERM) that has been used primarily to treat osteoporosis. To date, it has not been shown to cause an increased incidence of secondary malignancies,

especially endometrial cancer, and therefore has a more attractive toxicity profile than tamoxifen. Its value as a treatment for established breast cancer, an adjuvant agent, or a chemopreventive agent is still unknown but probable given its mechanism of action. It is clear that, as newer agents with fewer detrimental effects become available, more women will become candidates for chemoprevention.

Prophylactic Mastectomy

It is likely that the indications for prophylactic mastectomy will continue to evolve as the long-term outcomes of both chemoprevention and genetic testing become better defined. There are currently no absolute indications for prophylactic mastectomy, and decisions are best made on a case-by-case basis.

Any discussion about prophylactic mastectomy must be prefaced by the caveat that the efficacy of the procedure is not established. There are no prospective, randomized controlled trials of prophylactic mastectomy and therefore no accurate data regarding the magnitude of risk reduction with this procedure. Even with great attention to operative detail, it is impossible to guarantee removal of all breast tissue, and therefore it is also impossible to guarantee eradication of all subsequent risk of the development of breast cancer. If prophylactic surgery is chosen, the operation should be a bilateral total simple mastectomy with sacrifice of the nipple–areolar complex. This may be performed in a skin-sparing manner, with or without immediate reconstruction. Subcutaneous mastectomy leaves an unacceptable amount of breast tissue beneath the nipple–areolar complex and therefore is not a satisfactory operative option.

Various patients may be considered for prophylactic mastectomies. The most common indications include hereditary breast cancer (i.e., *BRCA1* or -2 carriers), strong family history of breast cancer, a personal history of lobular carcinoma in situ, or a personal history of atypia combined with a family history of breast cancer. Softer criteria include women with unduly high anxiety about cancer development (after appropriate psychiatric counseling and screening), women in whom clinical or radiographic surveillance is difficult, and patients with contralateral breast cancer.

The best study to date regarding the efficacy of bilateral prophylactic mastectomy is a retrospective study of the outcome of 639 women with a family history positive for breast cancer who underwent the procedure.[13] After a median follow-up of 14 years, prophylactic mastectomy was associated with a 90% reduction in the incidence and risk of death from breast cancer as compared to the untreated sisters. Thus, for select women bilateral prophylactic mastectomy remains a valid treatment option.

Screening Recommendations

Breast cancer screening relies upon the triad of self-breast examination (SBE), clinical breast examination (CBE) by a trained examiner, and screening mammography.

SELF BREAST EXAMINATION (SBE)

Only two prospective randomized trials of SBE have been conducted to date. A randomized population-based SBE trial of more than 120,000 women ages 40 to 64 has been conducted in St. Petersburg since 1985. At interim analysis, there was no difference in mortality or demonstration of a stage-shift at presentation between the group that received personalized SBE training and calendars versus the no-intervention "control" population.[14] Similarly, a randomized trial of SBE in Shanghai failed to demonstrate a reduction in breast cancer mortality or a trend toward earlier detection in the SBE group.[15] It is important to remember that, because of the insufficient data to recommend for or against SBE, current practice patterns should not be changed until additional and longer-term data are available.

CLINICAL BREAST EXAMINATION (CBE)

Accurate interpretation of the clinical breast examination (CBE) can be difficult. In a study of 15 patients with malignant lesions evaluated by four experienced surgeons, the diagnostic accuracy of concordance for the need for biopsy was only 73%.[16] Nevertheless, CBE should be viewed as a complementary modality to mammography because up to 10% of breast cancers are mammographically occult.

Physical examination of the breast should ideally be performed the week after menses when there is the least tenderness and engorgement. The breast examination begins with inspection in both the sitting and supine positions. While sitting, the patient should be evaluated with the hands relaxed at the sides, and with the arms raised overhead tensing the pectoralis muscles. Skin changes including dimpling, retraction, asymmetry, edema, and/or erythema should be noted. Cervical, supraclavicular, and axillary nodal basins should be evaluated bilaterally. If palpable nodes are discovered, the location, number, size, mobility, consistency, and tenderness should be recorded. Examination of the breast is best performed in the supine position with the patient's ipsilateral hand behind her head. Each breast should be systematically palpated including the axillary tail. Areas of abnormality are best described according to their location on a clock face with the nipple at the center. Size, tenderness, borders, consistency, and mobility also need to be documented. Evaluation of the nipple–areolar complex skin changes, nipple discharge, and subareolar masses complete the CBE. If latent nipple discharge is expressed, the location and number of involved ducts as well as the color and character of the drainage should be noted.

Evaluation of multiple mammographic screening trials has led to the conclusion that breast physical examination accounts for 50% to 67% of the value of CBE and mammography.[17] For example, in the Canadian National Breast Screening Study (NBSS2) only 44% of the cancers were found by mammography alone[18]; therefore, CBE and mammography should be viewed and employed as complementary modalities.

Mammography: The Screening Trials and Surveillance Recommendations

Mammography remains the cornerstone of early detection programs for breast cancer. Multiple trials have demonstrated a reduction in breast cancer mortality as a result of mammographic screening of women over 50, and more recent analyses have now shown a statistically significant benefit for women 40 to 49 years old. Because not all agencies have taken the most recent trial results into account, screening recommendations vary among organizations (Table 53.2). The American Cancer

TABLE 53.2. Screening Recommendations of Various National Organizations.

American Cancer Society[65]

Age	SBE	CBE	MMG
20–39	Monthly	Every 3 years	Diagnostic
40–49	Monthly	Annually	Annually
50+	Monthly	Annually	Annually

National Cancer Institute[66,67]

Age	SBE	CBE	MMG
Under 40	Seek expert medical opinion if high risk	Seek expert medical opinion if high risk	Seek expert medical opinion if high risk
40–49	Monthly	With regular health care	Every 1–2 years
50–69	Monthly	Every 1–2 years with mammogram	Every 1–2 years

American College of Radiology[68]

Age	SBE	CBE	MMG
40+		Annually	Annually

American College of Obstetricians and Gynecologists[69]

Age	SBE	CBE	MMG
40–49	Monthly	Annually	Every 1–2 years
50+	Monthly	Annually	Annually

American Academy of Family Physicians[70]

Age	SBE	CBE	MMG
40–49	Receive counseling about risk and benefits	Receive counseling about risk and benefits	Receive counseling about risk and benefits
50+		Every 1–2 years	Every 1–2 years

US Preventive Health Service Task Force[71]

Age	SBE	CBE	MMG
Under 50/FH negative		No screening	None
Under 50/FH positive		Every 1–2 years (optional)	Every 1–2 years
50–69		Every 1–2 years (optional)	Every 1–2 years
70+ and healthy		Every 1–2 years (optional)	Every 1–2 years

SBE, self breast examination; CBE, clinical breast examination; MMG, mammogram; FH, family history.

Ages are in years.

Society, however, is the most current in its recommendations, which include monthly SBE and annual CBE, as well as annual mammography for all women 40 years or older.

The eight randomized and four nonrandomized trials have varied greatly. Analysis of all trials, except NBSS2, demonstrated a reduction in breast cancer mortality for women who received mammographic screening. More cancers were detected in the screened group; however, this did not translate into a decrease in the relative risk of dying of breast cancer in the NBSS2. A meta-analysis of six of the eight randomized trials of breast cancer screening were performed for the International Workshop on Screening for Breast Cancer convened by the National Cancer Institute in 1993. Overall, a 30% reduction in breast cancer mortality was attributed to the effects of screening for women age 50 to 69 years.[19] As a result of this analysis, the NCI consensus recommendation was to perform CBE annually with mammography every 1 to 2 years in women over 50 years.

To summarize, the data support that annual screening mammography can reduce breast cancer mortality and therefore should be incorporated into an overall strategy of SBE, CBE, and radiologic screening. Because 10% of palpable cancers are mammographically occult, all modalities must be incorporated into a comprehensive screening policy. Nevertheless, mammography remains the cornerstone because the 10-year survival for cancers detectable only by mammography nears 95%. The most common reason identified for failure to undergo annual mammography has been failure of the women's physician to recommend screening. All health care professionals should incorporate SBE instructions, CBE annually at the time of health maintenance examination, and recommendation for annual screening mammography in women of the appropriate age.

Diagnostic Mammography

Although screening mammography is performed in an asymptomatic woman, diagnostic mammography is obtained in a woman with a palpable abnormality, breast complaints, or lesion identified on screening. Mammographic abnormalities include densities, calcifications, or both. The most worrisome radiologic features include spiculated masses (Fig. 53.1), mass with associated microcalcifications, and linear branching calcifications (Fig. 53.2). Overall, about one-third of nonpalpable lesions discovered on mammography prove to be malignant. In abnormalities for which no biopsy is recommended, short-term mammographic follow-up must be obtained. The American College of Radiology has adopted standard definitions and established six mammographic categories (Table 53.3).[20] These definitions assist patients and their physicians in treatment planning.

Management of Nonpalpable, Mammographic Abnormalities

The widespread use of screening mammography has resulted in the increased detection of clinically occult breast lesions. Approximately 5% to 10% of all screened women require additional radiologic evaluation after a screening study.

Wire localization excisional breast biopsy has been, until recently, the routine method for the diagnosis of the nonpalpable, mammographically detected, breast lesion (Fig. 53.3).

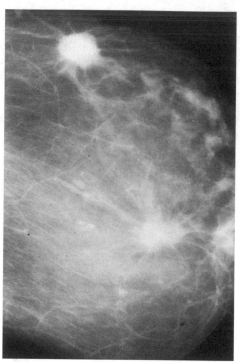

FIGURE 53.1. Mammogram demonstrating two spiculated masses characteristic of breast cancer. (Courtesy of M. Helvie, M.D.)

A specimen radiograph must be performed to confirm the adequacy of excision (Fig. 53.4).

Mammogram-guided percutaneous stereotactic biopsy has several advantages over core biopsy. It is faster, produces less scarring and breast deformity by limiting tissue removal, requires shorter convalescence, and is less costly. Diagnostic costs can be reduced at least 50% by performing stereotactic core versus open surgical biopsies.

Contraindications to stereotactic core biopsy include both patient-related and technical considerations. The patient must be able to lie unmoving in the prone position for as long as 45 min. Patients with significant anxiety, clinical arthritis, chronic cough, or severe kyphosis may not be able to meet this restriction. Technically, lesions located close to the chest

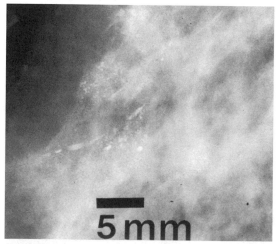

FIGURE 53.2. Mammogram demonstrating linear branching microcalcifications suspicious for cancer. (Courtesy of M. Helvie, M.D.)

TABLE 53.3. American College of Radiology BIRADS Classification.

BIRADS classification	Interpretation	Follow-up
0: Assessment is incomplete	Finding on screening evaluation; more workup is needed	Complete the radiologic evaluation
1: Negative	Normal	Annual mammography after 40
2: Benign finding	No evidence of malignancy, but a characteristic benign lesion found (i.e., implant, cyst, intramammary lymph node)	Annual mammography after 40
3: Probably benign finding	Risk of malignancy 1%–2%	Short-term (4–6 month) mammographic follow-up
4: Suspicious abnormality	Lesion does not have absolute malignant characteristics, but a definite probability of cancer exists	Biopsy recommended
5: Highly suggestive of malignancy	High probability of breast cancer	Biopsy required

wall, in the axillary tail, very superficial, or in small breasts that compress to less than 3 cm must be excluded from core biopsy.

If pathological concordance with image characteristics is obtained, the specificity and sensitivity of core biopsy is greater than 90%.[21,22] Cases of atypical ductal hyperplasia (ADH) diagnosed by core biopsy should undergo reexcision with wire localization because approximately 50% of lesions diagnosed as ADH by core will be found to have carcinoma at excisional biopsy.[23,24] Similarly, complete excision is necessary to confirm the diagnosis of radial scar.

The ABBI (Automated Breast Biopsy Instrumentation) is an automated surgical biopsy device whose utility remains undefined. The procedure is performed under mammographic guidance. After stereotactic localization, a skin incision just large enough to admit a 5-, 10-, or 20-mm circular scalpel is made. In a single pass, under local anesthesia, a large cylinder of tissue is removed. Unlike core biopsy, the soft tissue defect requires cautery for hemostasis and suture closure. Advantages of this technique are purported to include a continuous, nonfragmented specimen that aids in pathological diagnosis, and less tissue removal than standard wire localization. The goal is ultimately to provide diagnosis and therapy in one procedure.

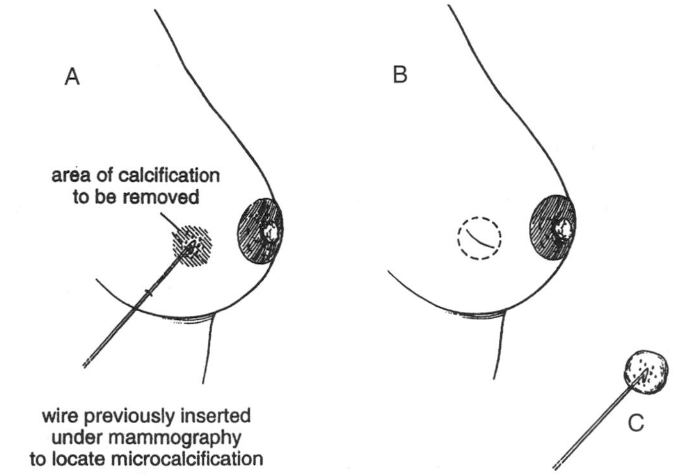

Benign Breast Disease

It is estimated that one of every two women will see a physician for a breast complaint during her life.[25] Although breast cancer is the most common malignancy of American women, 80% to 90% of clinical evaluations for breast disorders are for benign conditions. Thus, the goal in the evaluation of a patient with an abnormal clinical breast examination is to avoid missing the diagnosis of a malignancy while providing reassurance for benign conditions.

Abnormal Clinical Breast Examination

The initial step in the evaluation of a dominant mass is to determine degree of suspicion (Fig. 53.5). Breast cancer generally presents as a hard, nontender, irregular mass; however, it is impossible to rule out cancer by clinical evaluation alone. Low suspicion lesions in premenopausal women may be observed through one cycle. Complete resolution implies that the mass was a cyst.

A dominant mass that occurs in a postmenopausal woman, persists for one or more cycles in a premenopausal woman, or is suspicious requires additional evaluation. Either fine-needle aspiration (FNA) or urgent radiologic evaluation within 1 week is appropriate; however, there are some

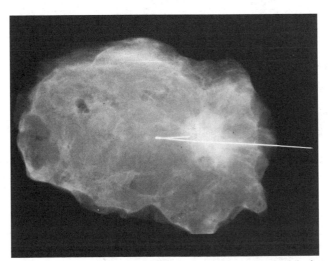

FIGURE 53.3. Wire localization breast biopsy. **A.** A hook wire is placed under mammographic guidance. **B.** Abnormal area is encompassed by excisional biopsy using the wire as a guide. **C.** Specimen and wire are sent for confirmatory mammogram and pathological examination.

FIGURE 53.4. Specimen mammogram demonstrates removal of area with microcalcifications. (Courtesy of M. Helvie, M.D.)

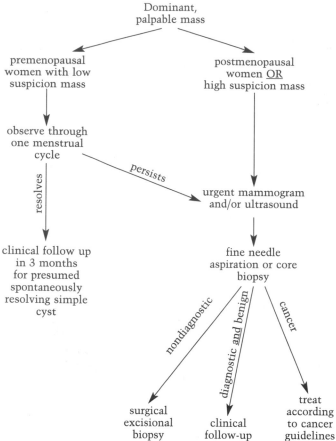

FIGURE 53.5. Algorithm for the management of a dominant palpable mass.

advantages in obtaining imaging studies first. FNA results in tissue disruption and even when performed by experienced physicians may result in hematoma formation significant enough to interfere with radiographic imaging. Additionally, mammography will ultimately be required to evaluate the remainder of the ipsilateral breast parenchyma and contralateral breast if a malignancy is diagnosed. In the ideal setting, same-day imaging followed by FNA would be performed. Importantly, a negative mammogram in the setting of a clinically dominant mass should not delay biopsy because 10% of cancers are radiologically occult.

Specific Entities

Cyst

If a cyst is suspected clinically or documented sonographically, an FNA can be both diagnostic and therapeutic. Determination that a palpable mass is a cyst is impossible by physical examination alone, but sonography can confirm the diagnosis. Cysts may be classified as simple or complex based upon their appearance on ultrasound. A simple cyst is a round, well-circumscribed, smooth-walled structure that is hypoechoic, without internal echoes, and has enhanced through transmission. A complex cyst has central septations, indistinct margins, or internal echoes.

The pathogenesis of cyst formation is not well understood; however, cyst formation is undoubtedly influenced by ovarian hormones. Cysts often suddenly appear midmenstrual cycle then spontaneously regress with the onset of menses. Cysts most commonly occur after age 35. The incidence of cystic disease increases steadily until menopause, when cysts are rare except in women on hormone replacement therapy. Therefore, any lesion presumed to be a cyst in a postmenopausal woman not on hormone replacement therapy must be proven to be fluid filled by needle aspiration. Intracystic carcinoma, however, is very rare.

Fibrocystic Breast Disease

Cysts may occur as solitary, grossly visible abnormalities called macrocysts or as clusters of multiple microscopic cysts. Fibrocystic breast disease is a generalized process of microscopic cyst formation, often accompanied by breast nodularity, with stromal proliferation. Ovarian hormones are again implicated, and fibrocystic changes seem to represent an exaggerated response of the breast epithelium. Whereas pain is not an indication for surgical therapy, a dominant mass, even in the setting of fibrocystic changes, requires confirmation by aspiration or biopsy. Women with biopsy-proven atypical ductal or lobular hyperplasia have a 4.4-fold increased cancer risk. If this is combined with a positive family history, the risk increases to 9 fold. Women with nonproliferative fibrocystic breast disease do not have a demonstrable increased breast cancer risk.

Mastalgia

Breast pain (*mastalgia* or *mastodynia*) is one of the most common breast symptoms. The etiology is poorly understood, but again hormonal causes are suggested. Women with irregular ovulatory cycles, immediately premenstrual, or on hormone replacement therapy often report breast pain. Furthermore, cyclic mastalgia usually resolves at menopause.

Mastalgia should be characterized as cyclic or noncyclic. Cyclical mastalgia varies in intensity throughout the menstrual cycle. It is most severe immediately before menstruation, then resolves with the onset of menses. It is the most frequent type, may occur unilaterally or bilaterally, as a burning sensation or sharp pain, and occasionally may radiate to the arm, scapula or abdomen. Cyclic mastalgia is more responsive to therapy and usually spontaneously resolves with menopause.

Noncyclic mastalgia bears no relationship to the menstrual cycle. It may be continuous or intermittent, is more commonly unilateral and sharp in character, and often occurs in the fourth decade. Chest wall musculoskeletal abnormalities (i.e., costochondritis) may mimic noncyclic mastalgia.

In the absence of findings on physical examination and mammography, treatment consists of reassurance and conservative measures. Breast pain in the absence of palpable or mammographic abnormality rarely represents carcinoma. One-half to one-third of women achieve significant improvement in their symptoms with conservative measures such as caffeine elimination, nicotine and alcohol reduction, as well as change to a better-fitting or more supportive brassiere. Anecdotally, vitamin E has been purported to be beneficial.

Nipple Discharge

Evaluation of a patient with nipple discharge should begin with an attempt to classify it as physiological, pathological, or galactorrhea. While frightening for the patient, nipple discharge usually has a benign etiology. Only 6% to 12% of patients with nipple discharge have carcinoma.[26,27] The likelihood of carcinoma is increased if the discharge is bloody.

Pathologic nipple discharge is unilateral, spontaneously arising from one duct. The drainage may be clear, brownish, or bloody. Benign intraductal papilloma is the most common cause of bloody nipple discharge. In the absence of another lesion, ductogram may be pursued (Fig. 53.6). Galactography may provide a surgical road map by identifying an intraluminal filling defect consistent with an intraductal papilloma. An approximate distance from the nipple, and in cases of diffuse papillomatosis extent of ductal involvement, can be determined by ductogram and this information may alter surgical treatment. Additionally, ductogram may identify diffusely dilated subareolar ducts consistent with duct ectasia.

Gynecomastia

Gynecomastia is hypertrophy of male breast tissue. Pubertal hypertrophy occurs during adolescence whereas senescent hypertrophy occurs in the elderly. Imbalance in the testosterone to estrogen ratio has been implicated in both forms. In puberty, estrogen levels may rise before testosterone production, and in the elderly testosterone levels may fall with maintenance of physiological estrogen levels. This relative hormonal imbalance accounts for the bimodal prevalence of gynecomastia. Several commonly used medications can exacerbate senescent gynecomastia including cimetidine, thiazides, digoxin, theophylline, phenothiazines, androgens or estrogens, and marijuana. Management of gynecomastia involves identification and correction of the underlying cause. If any question exists regarding the benignity of the condition, biopsy may be required.

Breast Infection and Abscess

Breast infections are broadly categorized as lactational versus nonpuerperal, and mastitis versus abscess. Puerperal mastitis is thought to originate from the reflux of bacteria into the milk-containing breast by the nursing infant. Treatment involves oral antibiotics to cover gram-positive cocci, local heat or ice packs, and frequent nursing or pumping to prevent engorgement.

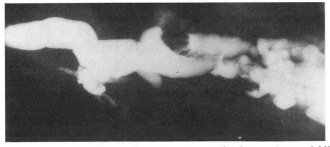

FIGURE 53.6. Ductogram demonstrating multiple intraluminal filling defects. (Courtesy of M Helvie, MD.)

Nonlactational mastitis is often a complication of duct ectasia, an irregular dilatation of the subareolar ducts. The ducts fill with secretions, debris, and keratin, and chronic inflammation results. Manifestations of this periductal mastitis include nipple discharge, recurrent subareolar abscesses, mammary fistula (Zuska's disease), and nipple retraction. These infections are more likely to be polymicrobial with a mix of gram-positive cocci and skin anaerobes. Treatment involves broad-spectrum oral antibiotics, analgesics, and local comfort measures.

Once abscess formation occurs therapy must include surgical incision and drainage. Breast abscesses in lactating women rarely present with a fluctuant mass because of the dense fibrous septa. Clinically, these women present with fever, leukocytosis, and point tenderness. Ultrasonography can be confirmatory. Incision and drainage should be performed under general anesthesia because it is too painful to adequately break up the loculations under local anesthesia. Breastfeeding must be discontinued because the cavity should be left open and packed. The wall of the abscess cavity should be biopsied to rule out necrotic cancer as an etiology of the infections, especially in spontaneous abscesses in nonlactating women. Subareolar abscesses can be especially difficult to eradicate and if recurrent may require excision of the entire subareolar duct complex.

Fibroadenoma

Fibroadenoma is a benign, solid lesion composed of both stromal and epithelial elements. Clinically, they are the most common mass in women under 30 years of age, with a peak incidence of 21 to 25 years. They are rubbery, lobulated, well-circumscribed, highly mobile masses on physical examination. Although usually single, multiple fibroadenomas occur in 15% of affected patients. Radiographically, they may have a lobulated appearance suggestive of a fibroadenoma. As with any solid mass, malignancy cannot be excluded on clinical or radiographic criteria alone and tissue confirmation must be obtained. Fibroadenoma growth has not been found to be influenced by oral contraceptive use; however, premenstrual tenderness, and growth with pregnancy and lactation are common features. While fibroadenomas themselves are not thought to have malignant potential, the epithelial elements, like all breast epithelium, are at risk.

Juvenile Fibroadenoma

Juvenile or giant fibroadenomas are fibroadenomas that attain unusually large size (greater than 5 cm) and commonly occur in adolescence. These lesions may display rapid growth, but are benign, and surgery is curative. Histologically, these lesions tend to be more cellular than typical fibroadenomas and must be differentiated from cystosarcoma phyllodes.

Hamartoma

Hamartoma of the breast is a benign lesion best characterized as an adenofibrolipoma. It is an exceptionally soft lesion and may be difficult to appreciate on physical examination even when very sizable. On mammography, it is an easily visualized, well-circumscribed lesion impossible to differentiate from the more common fibroadenoma. If hamartoma is clinically suspected, surgical excision is preferable as well as curative.

Adenoma

Tubular and lactational adenomas are also histologically benign lesions related to fibroadenomas. They are characterized by glandular structures with minimal to absent supporting stromal structures. Clinically and radiographically, they resemble fibroadenomas as well. Lactational adenomas occur during pregnancy and lactation, may increase in size under the influence of gestational hormones, and have secretory differentiation on histological analysis. Again, biopsy is diagnostic and curative.

Papillary Lesions

Solitary intraductal papilloma is the most common papillary breast lesion. They most frequently occur in women 35 to 55 years of age, and usually arise as a single lesion, in a subareolar duct, and are manifest as bloody nipple discharge. Intraductal papillomas occurring in peripheral ducts present as mammographic or palpable masses. Ductography may be helpful, and solitary or central duct excision is the treatment of choice.

Sclerosing Adenosis

Sclerosing adenosis is the benign proliferation of both stromal tissue (sclerosis) associated with an increase in the small terminal ductules (adenosis). It is usually a component of fibrocystic disease and is manifest as microcalcifications found on screening mammogram. Stereotactic core or wire localization biopsy is diagnostic. No further therapy is necessary if this lesion is found as the etiology of microcalcifications on biopsy.

Breast Cancer

Staging

Even though pathological evaluation of the primary breast tumor and axillary lymph node status are the most important determinants of survival, accurate clinical staging is important. Preoperative diagnostic and therapeutic interventions are based on careful assessment of the clinical extent of disease. Many staging classifications exist; however, the TNM system of the American Joint Committee on Cancer (AJCC) and the International Union Against Cancer (UICC) is the one most widely used for breast cancer.[28]

At presentation, a patient's TNM status should be determined (Table 53.4). On staging physical examination primary tumor size and degree of axillary nodal involvement should be estimated. It is recognized that clinical staging of the axilla has a false negative rate of 30%.[29] Furthermore, breast cancer is currently believed to have systemic micrometastases at the time of diagnosis. Nevertheless, some general treatment guidelines can be based on clinical tumor staging.

All patients with invasive breast cancer should have a thorough history and physical examination, chest X-ray, complete blood count, and chemical profile. Asymptomatic stage I or II patients with normal findings on these studies do not require further metastatic evaluation because the likelihood of finding occult metastatic disease has been estimated to be 2% to 3%.

Patients with stage IIIA or B disease, however, should undergo screening bone scan and computed tomography because of the high probability of distant metastases. Additionally, as discussed earlier, neoadjuvant chemotherapy may be appropriate for patients with stage III breast cancer. Metastatic, stage IV disease occurs most frequently in the bone, lung, or liver; however, any nodal or visceral site may become involved.

Noninvasive Breast Carcinomas

Noninvasive or in situ carcinomas are proliferations of malignant epithelial cells confined within the duct or lobule without invasion of the basement membrane. These lesions are classified by cell of origin as ductal carcinoma in situ (DCIS) or lobular carcinoma in situ (LCIS) (see Table 53.5).

Ductal Carcinoma In Situ (DCIS)

DCIS, noninvasive ductal carcinoma, and intraductal carcinoma are the same entities. Before the widespread use of screening mammography, DCIS presented as a palpable mass, nipple discharge, or an incidental finding on biopsy and accounted for 2% of diagnosed malignancies. Today, in some series it represents 30% of all malignancies found by screening.[30] DCIS is thought to be a precursor of invasive carcinoma and therefore once recognized treatment is indicated. Data supporting this position are multiple. First, if left untreated DCIS will progress to invasive carcinoma in up to 50% of women; moreover, the cancers that develop are ductal in origin and occur at the site of the original biopsy. The second piece of evidence that DCIS is a precursor lesion is from recurrence data after breast-conserving therapy. In patients with DCIS treated with lumpectomy, 87% of treatment failures occur at or close to the lumpectomy bed rather than at distant sites.[31] Left untreated, DCIS will progress to invasive ductal carcinoma 30% of the time over 10 years.[32,33]

For many years simple mastectomy was the treatment of choice for DCIS. Currently, breast conservation is deemed an acceptable alternative in select patients. Lumpectomy must be to negative margins, and radiation therapy is routinely advocated. Survival with breast conservation is believed to be equivalent to that with mastectomy. Patient choice is one factor in deciding between breast conservation and mastectomy. Because of the low (2%) risk of axillary involvement, routine axillary lymph node dissection is not performed. Certain patients, however, may benefit from one or more sampling procedures.

Another controversial issue is the omission of radiation therapy in a select subset of well-informed patients with favorable presentations of DCIS. Comedo-type DCIS has prominent intraductal necrosis and is believed to represent a more aggressive form of DCIS. Tumor grade is also of prognostic significance. Some advocate that women with non-comedo DCIS less than 1 cm in size and excised to widely negative margins (approximately 1 cm) may forego radiation.

Based on the only study available, it appears that addition of tamoxifen to standard therapy for DCIS may be warranted in patients without a contradiction to the drug. Extrapolation of this data to women with DCIS treated by mastectomy because of the reduction in contralateral breast cancer risk is tempting, but further studies are necessary to validate the original finding and to specifically address this population.

TABLE 53.4. AJCC Definition of TNM and Stage Groupings for Breast Cancer.

Primary Tumor (T)

Definitions for classifying the primary tumor (T) are the same for clinical and for pathologic classification. If the measurement is made by physical examination, the examiner will use the major headings (T1, T2, or T3). If other measurements, such as mammographic or pathologic measurements, are used, the subsets of T1 can be used. Tumors should be measured to the nearest 0.1 cm increment.

TX	Primary tumor cannot be assessed
T0	No evidence of primary tumor
Tis	Carcinoma *in situ*
Tis (DCIS)	Ductual carcinoma *in situ*
Tis (LCIS)	Lobular carcinoma *in situ*
Tis (Paget's)	Paget's disease of the nipple with no tumor

Note: Paget's disease associated with a tumor is classified according to the size of the tumor.

T1	Tumor 2 cm or less in greatest dimension
T1mic	Microinvasion 0.1 cm or less in greatest dimension
T1a	Tumor more than 0.1 cm but not more than 0.5 cm in greatest dimension
T1b	Tumor more than 0.5 cm but not more than 1 cm in greatest dimension
T1c	Tumor more than 1 cm but not more than 2 cm in greatest dimension
T2	Tumor more than 2 cm but not more than 5 cm in greatest dimension
T3	Tumor more than 5 cm in greatest dimension
T4	Tumor of any size with direct extension to (a) chest wall or (b) skin, only as described below
T4a	Extension to chest wall, not including pectoralis muscle
T4b	Edema (including peau d'orange) or ulceration of the skin of the breast, or satellite skin nodules confined to the same breast
T4c	Both T4a and 4b
T4d	Inflammatory carcinoma

Regional Lymph Nodes (N) (Clinical)

NX	Regional lymph nodes cannot be assessed (e.g., previously removed)
N0	No regional lymph node metastasis
N1	Metastasis to movable ipsilateral axillary lymph node(s)
N2	Metastasis in ipsilateral axillary lymph nodes fixed or matted, or in clinically apparent* ipsilateral internal mammary nodes in the *absence* of clinically evident axillary lymph node metastasis
N2a	Metastasis in ipsilateral axillary lymph nodes fixed to one another (matted) or to other structures
N2b	Metastasis only in clinically apparent* ipsilateral internal mammary nodes and in the *absence* of clinically evident axillary lymph node metastasis
N3	Metastasis in ipsilateral infraclavicular lymph node(s) with or without axillary lymph node involvement, or in clinically apparent* ipsilateral internal mammary lymph node(s) and in the *presence* of clinically evident axillary lymph node metastasis; or metastasis in ipsilateral supraclavicular lymph node(s) with or without axillary or internal mammary lymph node involvement
N3a	Metastasis in ipsilateral infraclavicular lymp nodes(s)
N3b	Metastasis in ipsilateral internal mammary lymph nodes(s) and axillary lymph node(s)
N3c	Metastasis in ipsilateral supraclavicular lymph node(s)

Clinically apparent is defined as detected by imaging studies (excluding lymphoscintigraphy) or by clinical examination or grossly visible pathologically.

Pathologic (pN)[a]

pNX	Regional lymph nodes cannot be assessed (e.g., previously removed, or not removed for pathologic study)
pN0	No regional lymph node metastasis histologically, no additional examination for isolated tumor cells (ITC)

Note: Isolated tumor cells (ITC) are defined as single tumor cells or small cell clusters not greater than 0.2 mm, usually detected only by immunohistochemical (IHC) or molecular methods but which may be verified in H&E stains. ITCs do not usually show evidence of malignant activity e.g., proliferation or stromal reaction.

pN0(i−)	No regional lymph node metastasis histologically, negative IHC
pN0(i+)	No regional lymph node metastasis histologically, positive IHC, no IHC cluster greater than 0.2 mm
pN0(mol−)	No regional lymph node metastasis histologically, negative molecular findings (RT-PCR)[b]
pN0(mol+)	No regional lymph node metastasis histologically, positive molecular findings (RT-PCR)[b]

[a]Classification is based on axillary lymph node dissection with or without sentinel lymph node dissection. Classification based solely on sentinel lymph node dissection without subsequent axillary lymph node dissection is designated (sn) for "sentinel node," e.g., pN0(i +) (sn).
[b]RT-PCR: reverse transcriptase/polymerase chain reaction.

pN1	Metastasis in 1 to 3 axillary lymph nodes, and/or in internal mammary nodes with microscopic disease detected by sentinel lymph node dissection but not clinically apparent**
pN1mi	Micrometastasis (greater than 0.2 mm, none greater than 2.0 mm)
pN1a	Metastasis in 1 to 3 axillary lymph nodes
pN1b	Metastasis in internal mammary nodes with microscopic disease detected by sentinel lymph node dissection but not clinically apparent**
pN1c	Metastasis in 1 to 3 axillary lymph nodes and in internal mammary lymph nodes with microscopic disease detected by sentinel lymph node dissection but not clinically apparent** (If associated with greater than 3 positive axillary lymph nodes, the internal mammary nodes are classified as pN3b to reflect increased tumor burden)
pN2	Metastasis in 4 to 9 axillary lymph nodes, or in clinically apparent* internal mammary lymph nodes in the *absence* of axillary lymph node metastasis
pN2a	Metastasis in 4 to 9 axillary lymph nodes (at least one tumor deposit greater than 2.0 mm)
pN2b	Metastasis in clinically apparent* internal mammary lymph nodes in the *absence* of axillary lymph node metastasis
pN3	Metastasis in 10 or more axillary lymph nodes, or in infraclavicular lymph nodes, or in clinically apparent* ipsilateral internal mammary lymph nodes in the *presence* of 1 or more positive axillary lymph nodes; or in more than 3 axillary lymph nodes with clinically negative microscopic metastasis in internal mammary lymph nodes; or in ipsilateral supraclavicular lymph nodes
pN3a	Metastasis in 10 or more axillary lymph nodes (at least one tumor deposit greater than 2.0 mm), or metastasis to the infraclavicular lymph nodes
pN3b	Metastasis in clinically apparent* ipsilateral internal mammary lymph nodes in the *presence* of 1 or more positive axillary lymph nodes; or in more than 3 axillary lymph nodes and in internal mammary lymph nodes with microscopic disease detected by sentinel lymph node dissection but not clinically apparent**
pN3c	Metastasis in ipsilateral supraclavicular lymph nodes

Clinically apparent is defined as detected by imaging studies (excluding lymphoscintigraphy) or by clinical examination.
**Not clinically apparent* is defined as not detected by imaging studies (excluding lymphoscintigraphy) or by clinical examination.

Distant Metastasis (M)

MX	Distant metastasis cannot be assessed
M0	No distant metastasis
M1	Distant metastasis

Stage grouping

Stage 0	Tis	N0	M0
Stage I	T1*	N0	M0
Stage IIA	T0	N1	M0
	T1*	N1	M0
	T2	N0	M0
Stage IIB	T2	N1	M0
	T3	N0	M0
Stage IIIA	T0	N2	M0
	T1*	N2	M0
	T2	N2	M0
	T3	N1	M0
	T3	N2	M0
Stage IIIB	T4	N0	M0
	T4	N1	M0
	T4	N2	M0
Stage IIIC	Any T	N3	M0
Stage IV	Any T	Any N	M1

*T1 includes T1mic.

Source: Used with permission of the American Joint Committee on Cancer (AJCC), Chicago, IL. The original source for this material is the AJCC Cancer Staging Manual, Sixth Ed. (2002) published by Springer-Verlag New York, www.springer-ny.com.

TABLE 53.5. Comparison of LCIS and DCIS.

	LCIS	DCIS
Age at presentation	Premenopausal	Postmenopausal
Physical examination	Negative	Occasionally palpable mass
Mammogram	Negative	Microcalcifications
Diagnosis	Incidental	Workup of abnormality
Risk	In all breast tissue	At site of diagnosis
Treatment	Observation vs. chemoprevention vs. bilateral prophylactic mastectomy	Lumpectomy plus radiation vs. ipsilateral simple mastectomy Consider tamoxifen

LCIS, lobular carcinoma in situ; DCIS, ductal carcinoma in situ.

Lobular Carcinoma In Situ (LCIS)

Lobular carcinoma in situ (LCIS) is believed to represent a predictor of increased risk of the development of breast cancer rather than a precursor of invasive disease. As seen in Table 53.5, LCIS differs markedly from DCIS. Because it is found incidentally during biopsy for another cause, its true incidence is unknown. However, in a variety of series, LCIS was found in 0.8% to 8.0% of benign breast biopsies.[34–36] It occurs in asymptomatic premenopausal women, and is not manifest by a palpable mass, mammographic microcalcifications, or architectural distortion.

Treatment recommendations for women with LCIS include careful observation as for any high-risk patient, chemoprevention with tamoxifen as per the NSABP-P1 trial, or bilateral prophylactic mastectomies.

Familial/Hereditary Breast Cancer: Molecular Genetics and Syndromes

Families that are characterized by having hereditary breast cancer are distinguished by the following characteristics: (1) early onset of breast cancer, classically less than 45 years of age; (2) an excess of bilateral breast cancer; (3) autonomic dominant inheritance for the cancer; and (4) greater frequency of multiple primary cancers. Lynch is credited with the first description of the hereditary breast ovarian cancer syndrome, by reporting families with two or more first-degree relatives with breast cancer and a variety of other cancer sites.[37]

Breast Cancer Susceptibility Genes

BRCA1

In 1990, Marie-Clare King reported mapping, by segregation analysis, the first breast cancer susceptibility gene (BRCA1) to chromosome 17q21, and this gene was determined to have linkage with the hereditary breast and ovarian cancer syndrome.[38] The majority of these mutations result in a decreased or truncated BRCA1 protein. Overall, the BRCA1 gene confers an 83% risk of breast and 63% risk of ovarian cancer by the age of 70.

A second breast cancer susceptibility gene, BRCA2, was mapped to chromosome 13q12 in 1995.[39] Unlike BRCA1, BRCA2 is associated with male breast cancer and confers only a 10% risk of ovarian cancer. The pathology of BRCA2-associated breast cancers is weighted toward tubular-lobular invasive carcinomas and invasive cribiform carcinomas. These tend to be lower-grade tumors with less proliferation.[40]

Hereditary Breast Cancer Syndromes and High-Risk Groups

Hereditary Breast/Ovarian/Cancer (HBOC) Syndromes

These families have predominantly breast and ovarian cancers, with a lifetime risk of 85% for breast cancer in BRCA1 and BRCA2 carriers and of 40% to 60% for ovarian cancer in BRCA1 carriers.[38] Li-Fraumeni syndrome, Cowden syndrome, Muir syndrome, and ataxia telangectasia are included in this group.

TABLE 53.6. Tissues Resected in Various Types of Mastectomies.

	Skin of entire chest wall (skin grafting required)	Nipple–areolar complex	Breast mound	Pectoralis minor and major muscles	Axillary lymph nodes	Internal mammary lymph nodes
Urban extended radical mastectomy	X	X	X	X	X	X
Halstead radical mastectomy	X	X	X	X	X	
Patey modified radical mastectomy		X	X	Pectoralis minor only	X	
Auchincloss modified radical mastectomy		X	X		X	
Simple mastectomy		X	X			
Subcutaneous mastectomy			X			

TABLE 53.7.

Randomized Trial of Mastectomy versus Breast Conservation (Level I Evidence).

Trial	Reference	Year	n	Randomized	Stage	Design	Median Follow-up	Results
Guy's Hospital	72	1961–1970	376	Yes	T_1N_0 or T_1N_1	WLE + XRT vs. radical mastectomy +XRT	11 years	(1) Treatment deemed inadequate (omission of ALND and low-dose XRT) (2) Higher regional recurrence and lower survival in WLE + XRT group, especially in stage II patients
		1971–1976	250	Yes	T_1N_0	Radical Mastectomy + XRT vs. WLE +XRT		
Gustave-Roussay	73	1972–1979	179	Yes	T_1N_0 or T_1N_1	Tumorectomy + XRT vs. MRM	10 years	No difference in overall survival, local control, distant metastasis, or contralateral breast cancer rate
NCI Milan	74	1973–1980	701	Yes	T_1N_0	Quadrentectomy, ALND, and XRT vs. radical mastectomy	10 years	(1) No difference in local recurrence or survival (2) BCT can be performed in lymph node-positive patients if there is adjuvant chemotherapy
NSABP-B06	75	1976–1984	1843	Yes	T < 4cm N_0	Lumpectomy, ALND, and XRT vs. Lumpectomy/ ALND, vs. MRM	8 years	(1) 10% of patients assigned to BCT-negative margins could not be achieved (2) XRT critically important for local control as breast recurrence occurred in 10% of lumpectomy/XRT vs. 39% of lump alone ($p < 0.001$) (3) No difference in survival thus local recurrence does not predict survival
NCI Bethesda	76	1979–1987	247	Yes		Lumpectomy/ ALND + XRT vs. MRM	8 years	No difference in survival or local control
EORTC	77	1980–1986	148	Yes	I	Lumpectomy/ ALND + XRT vs. MRM	8 years	No difference in survival, local control, or distant recurrence
			755	Yes	II			
Danish Breast Cancer Group	78	1983–1989	905	Yes	I or II	Quadrantecto-my/ALND + XRT vs. MRM	6 years	(1) Identical overall survival (2) Fewer local/regional recurrences in BCT group (NS)

NCI, National Cancer Institute; EORTC, European Organization for Research and Treatment of Cancer; ALND, axillary lymph node dissection; XRT, radiation therapy; MRM, modified radical mastectomy; WLE, wide local excision; BCT, breast conservation treatment; NS, not significant.

LI–FRAUMENI SYNDROME

This syndrome is characterized by families with p53 germline mutations, causing a higher than expected occurrence of sarcomas, breast cancers, brain tumors, lung and laryngeal cancers, leukemias, and adrenal cortical carcinomas.[41] There is autosomal dominant pattern of transmission, and 30% of the tumors occur before 15 years of age; 77% of the women who develop breast cancer with Li–Fraumeni syndrome are between 22 and 45 years, and 25% have bilateral disease.

Treatment of Stage I or II Breast Cancer

Primary Surgical Therapy

Once malignant cells invade the basement membrane of the breast ducts or lobules, the lesion is classified as an invasive or infiltrating cancer. Because of the current belief that invasive cancer is a micrometastatic disease at diagnosis, local therapies are no longer believed to influence long-term survival.

Several nonrandomized[42,43] and two randomized trials[44,45] showed no survival difference for women treated with radical (RM) versus modified radical mastectomy (MRM) (Table 53.6) mastectomies. The initial study from the Alabama Breast Cancer Project randomized stage I, II, or operable stage III women by birth date to RM ($n = 136$) versus MRM ($n = 175$). At 10-year analysis, no difference in survival was demonstrated; however, foreshadowing the breast conservation trials, local control was superior in the RM group.[46] A large trial of 534 women in Manchester, England, which randomized patients with stage I or II cancer in a similar design to RM versus MRM,[44] also failed to demonstrate a difference in disease-free or overall survival. The lack of survival advantage combined with the superior functional and cosmetic results of MRM has made MRM a viable and standard treatment option for all women with operable breast cancer.

Several trials have confirmed that lumpectomy with axillary lymph node dissection plus radiation is as effective as modified radical mastectomy for patients with early-stage breast cancer (Table 53.7). Based on the findings from these

TABLE 53.8. Risk Modulators in Breast Cancer.

	Favorable	Unfavorable	Clinical utility
Tumor grade	I	II or III	Very favorable low-grade tumors (pure tubular, mucinous, or papillary) may not require adjuvant chemotherapy
Estrogen and progesterone receptor	Positive	Negative	The presence of receptors as well as efficacy of tamoxifen results in improved disease-free survival in positive patients
Her-2/neu expression	Negative	Positive	Positive tumors should receive an anthracycline-based chemotherapy regimen
Lymphovascular invasion	Absent	Present	Even in node-negative patients adjuvant chemotherapy should be received
Ploidy	Diploid	Aneuploid	Replaced by S-phase
S-phase percentage	<5%	>5%	May influence borderline patients to receive adjuvant chemotherapy
Ki-67	<20%	>20%	Investigational
p53	<5%	>5%	Investigational

trials as well as the availability of mature results, the National Institutes of Health Consensus Development Conference on the Treatment of Early Breast Cancer issued a consensus statement in 1990.[47] They stated that BCT provided equivalent survival to mastectomy and, because it spared the breast, it is the preferable choice in women with stage I or II tumors.

Surgical Management of the Axilla

The rationale for the performance of axillary lymph node dissection in women with breast cancer is to provide prognostic information, guide adjuvant chemotherapy treatment decisions, and maintain local control. As demonstrated in the NSABP-B04 trial, however, radiation therapy is as effective as axillary dissection in providing local control.[48,49]

The extent and method of axillary dissections that should be performed is currently a controversial topic. As stated earlier, about 30% of patients with a clinically negative axillary examination will have pathologically positive lymph nodes at the time of axillary dissection. Conversely, approximately 30% of women with palpably enlarged lymph nodes will fail to have lymphatic metastases documented at lymph node dissection. Pathological false-negative rates correlate with the extent of lymphadenectomy.[50] Nonanatomic sampling resulted in a 14% to 45% incidence of positive lymph nodes in a completion dissection when the sampled nodes were negative, a 10% to 12% false-negative rate when only level I nodes were dissected, and a 2% to 3% false-negative rate for a formal level I and II lymph node dissection. Thus, the procedure of choice as recommended by the 1991 National Institutes of Health Consensus conference for a standard axillary dissection[51] has become a level I/II dissection. The addition of a level III dissection is reserved for patients with bulky, palpable lymphadenopathy in an attempt to improve local control and not to aid in staging. Other modulators of disease are listed in Table 53.8.

While major complications from axillary lymph node dissection are rare, minor complications are not infrequent and may cause significant morbidity. Major complications include laceration or thrombosis of the axillary vessels and neuropathy secondary to damage to the motor nerves at the axilla. Minor complications include wound infection, seroma formation, intercostal brachial nerve syndrome (pain and paresthesia in an upper arm, shoulder, axilla, and anterior chest wall secondary to sacrifice of the nerve), impaired shoulder mobility, and lymphedema.

In an effort to eliminate routine axillary lymph node dissection without losing the prognostic information obtained, sentinel lymph node dissection (SLND) was developed. The sentinel lymph node (SLN) is defined as the first lymph node to receive lymphatic drainage from the tumor. Injecting vital blue dye, radiolabeled colloid, or both in the vicinity of the primary tumor site identifies the SLN. SLND is much more challenging for breast cancer than melanoma because the breast parenchymal lymphatics are not as much as the dermal lymphatics, and the upper outer quadrant location of most breast cancers can make identification of the SLN with radiocolloid mapping difficult due to the high background activity at the primary tumor site. Nevertheless, in all mappings the SLN is located by injecting a vital blue dye or radioisotope at the location of choice. The blue dye is visually identified leaving the

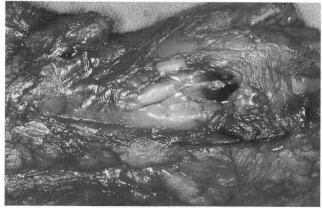

FIGURE 53.7. Lymphatic mapping with vital blue dye. Dissected specimen clearly demonstrates blue afferent lymphatic leading into blue stained sentinel lymph node. (Courtesy of AE Chang, MD.)

periphery of the breast and the afferent lymphatic channel is traced to the blue stained lymph node (Fig. 53.7). When radiocolloid is used, the SLN can be identified by preoperative lymphoscintigraphy, or intraoperatively with a handheld gamma detector. There is no significant difference in success based on protocol implemented. At all major institutions the SLN can be identified in 95% of patients and is accurate in up to 100% of cases. A significant learning curve exists.

Patient selection is also critical. SLND is contraindicated in patients with palpably enlarged axillary lymph nodes, tumors greater than 5 cm, or locally advanced cancer or in patients who have received preoperative neoadjuvant chemotherapy. In each of these scenarios tumor cells may block the lymphatics and accurate mapping may not be possible. Patients who have a large biopsy cavity may be difficult to accurately map, especially if the tumor was small. Because the periphery of the cavity and not the epicenter of the tumor will be mapped, patients with prior significant axillary or breast surgery may also have disrupted lymphatic channels, making accurate mapping impossible. With multiple injections it is technically feasible to map multifocal or multicentric tumors; however, with a mean of two sentinel nodes per tumor it may be more efficient to perform a standard axillary dissection in these patients.

An additional important issue is that SLN mapping, by providing the pathologist with the lymph node most likely to contain disease, may be more sensitive for the detection of metastatic disease. With only one or two lymph nodes to process, a more detailed examination with thin serial sectioning, immunohistochemical staining, or potentially reverse transcriptase polymerase chain reaction (RT-PCR) analysis is possible. In a trial of SLND followed by complete axillary lymph node dissection in 103 patients, the SLN was positive in 42% of the patients by thin serial sectioning and immunohistochemical staining; only 29% of the remainder of the axillary lymph nodes were positive by conventional processing ($p < 0.03$).[52] In a similar study, routine hematoxylin and eosin staining of SLN identified metastatic foci in 32% of the patients; however, with immunohistochemical staining 42% of patients were node positive.[53] Thus, 10% of patients were upstaged.

The prognostic importance of micrometastases has historically been questioned. Currently, the discovery of micrometastases has been proved clinically relevant with poorer survival for patients with micrometastases detected by serial staining,[54] anticytokeratin immunohistochemical staining,[55] and RT-PCR.[56] It is currently recommended that SLN-positive patients undergo formal level I and II lymph node dissection if not already performed.

In summary, axillary dissection provides effective control of axillary disease in patients with stage I or II breast cancer. With the omission of axillary dissection or radiation, axillary relapse is unacceptably high; 16% to 37% of patients with a clinically negative axilla will recur without treatment.[57] Presumably, the relapse rate will be even greater in the presence of clinically palpable nodes. Additionally, in some institutes the number of involved nodes influences the selection of chemotherapeutic regimen. Most importantly, pathological axillary staging remains the most significant prognostic indicator in breast cancer. Sentinel lymph node mapping is a promising technique that may provide similar information with reduced morbidity.

Adjuvant Chemo- or Hormonal Therapy for Lymph Node-Negative Breast Carcinoma

The current paradigm for breast cancer asserts that it is a systemic disease from the time of diagnosis. In patients with lymph node-negative disease, tumor size is the most important prognostic factor for relapse.[58] Patients with tumors less than 1 cm have a favorable prognosis, with greater than 90% 10-year disease-free survival.[58] The National Institutes of Health 1990 Breast Cancer Conference recommended that these patients rarely receive adjuvant chemotherapy.[47]

Patients with node-negative tumors larger than 1 cm, however, have a significant enough risk of relapse that adjuvant systemic therapy is warranted. Almost 25% of stage I and 33% to 44% of stage II node-negative patients will develop recurrent disease.[58]

Adjuvant Chemotherapy for Lymph Node-Positive Breast Carcinoma

Lymph node status is the most important prognostic factor. Multiple studies have demonstrated that adjuvant systemic chemotherapy can prolong disease-free and overall survival in the node-positive patients.[59]

Adjuvant Radiation Therapy

The need for postlumpectomy radiation therapy is absolute. The current controversy centers on the sequencing of adjuvant chemotherapy and radiation after breast conservation. Currently, treatment is frequently individualized on the basis of risk assessment. Sequencing is based on the greatest perceived risk. For patients with a high risk of systemic relapse, chemotherapy precedes radiation; for patients with local control issues (see postmastectomy chest wall radiation, next), radiation may be given first.

Currently, postmastectomy radiation should be performed for women with T3 or T4 primary tumors, four or more positive nodes, or positive margins, and should be considered in premenopausal women with one to three positive nodes based on these studies.

Treatment of Locally Advanced (Stage III) Breast Cancer

Locally advanced breast cancers (LABC) includes patients with tumors greater than 5 cm (T3 lesions), fixed to the chest wall or skin (T4 tumors), and/or those with bulky fixed axillary lymph nodes (N2 disease). Inflammatory cancer is a distinct entity and is discussed separately. For both these situations, neoadjuvant chemotherapy has become the treatment of choice. Furthermore, numerous studies have demonstrated an improvement in survival with multimodal sequential therapy where treatment is initiated with neoadjuvant chemotherapy.

Patients with inflammatory cancer present with brawny induration of the skin, often with peau d'orange (skin edema) and erythema. These changes are caused by tumor embolization of dermal lymphatics. Neoadjuvant chemotherapy produces similar response rates (up to 80%) as in LABC patients. Most patients can then be resected by mastectomy with clear margins. Local control rates up to 70% can now be achieved[60] with a 50% 5-year survival.[61] To achieve these results, surgery must be followed by radiation and chemotherapy.

Treatment of Metastatic (Stage IV) Breast Cancer

Metastatic breast cancer is rarely cured. The median survival of women with stage IV disease is 2 years. Therefore, palliation and prolongation of life are the goals of treatment. Thus, when two therapeutic choices are equally efficacious, the least toxic should be selected.

Treatment of Unusual Presentations of Breast Cancer

Paget's Disease

Paget's disease of the breast is a rare form of in situ carcinoma involving the nipple and is often associated with an underlying invasive or intraductal carcinoma.[62] Clinically it is manifest as eczematoid changes of the nipple with accompanying edema, erythema, pruritis, and nipple discharge. Punch biopsy of the nipple is diagnostic and reveals large cells with prominent nucleoli and pale cytoplasm (Paget's cells). Because of its unusual presentation, there is often a delay in making the diagnosis. The majority of women with Paget's disease have an underlying cancer at the time of diagnosis; therefore, a careful physical examination coupled with a mammogram must be performed. For patients with an associated lesion, mastectomy is the preferred treatment. Axillary lymph node dissection should be performed only if the associated cancer has an invasive component. For patients without palpable breast masses or mammographic densities, breast conservation may be considered. Recent data demonstrate that complete resection of the nipple–areola complex followed by definitive radiotherapy has an acceptable disease-free and overall survival.[63] The prognosis of Paget's disease is that of the underlying cancer, and approaches 100% for patients without an associated invasive cancer.

Occult Breast Cancer Presenting as Axillary Metastases

Although breast cancer presenting with axillary lymphadenopathy without an identifiable primary represents less than 1% of breast cancers, this entity has been recognized since the times of Halstead. Evaluation should include physical examination, focusing on the breast, skin, and thyroid, as well as fecal occult blood testing. Radiologic workup should be limited to mammography, chest X-ray, and possibly bone scan to exclude metastatic disease before therapy. Laboratory evaluation should include a complete blood course, liver function tests, and carcinoembryonic antigen determination.

Women with axillary metastasis from an occult breast primary historically have been treated with mastectomy. The likelihood of identifying an occult primary has decreased as high-resolution mammography has become widely available. As with other breast cancers, there has been a trend toward breast conservation. Some groups advocate axillary lymph node dissection followed by radiation therapy. Overall survival

is the same as for women with stage II cancer in whom a breast primary was identified,[64] reinforcing the prognostic importance of axillary staging. Because of the nodal involvement, adjuvant systemic therapy is recommended for these women.

Breast Cancer During Pregnancy

It used to be believed that breast cancer arising during pregnancy was especially aggressive; however, when stratified by stage, survival is similar to that of nonpregnant women. Delay in diagnosis and treatment resulting in presentation at a later stage is now implicated in the poorer prognosis overall for pregnant women with breast cancer.

Nonepithelial Tumors

PHYLLODES TUMOR (CYSTOSARCOMA PHYLLODES)

Phyllodes tumors are the most common nonepithelial tumors of the breast. Despite the older designation of cystosarcoma, the majority of these lesions are benign. Therefore, "malignant" or "benign" should qualify the diagnosis of "phyllodes tumor the breast."

These tumors exclusively occur in the female breast. They present as large, mobile, well-circumscribed masses that are mammographically indistinguishable from fibroadenomas. They occasionally can grow rapidly. For benign tumors, local excision to widely negative margins is appropriate. Some advocate mastectomy for malignant phyllodes tumors, especially if they are of large size. Because the risk of axillary metastasis is less than 1%, axillary lymph node dissection is not indicated.

Male Breast Cancer

Male breast cancer typically presents as a hard, irregular, nontender, eccentric mass often fixed to the chest wall. It must be distinguished from gynecomastia, which is more commonly bilateral, symmetrical, and retroaereolar. Mammography is extremely helpful in differentiating between the two entities. If any question persists, tissue diagnosis via fine-needle aspiration, core, or surgical biopsy should be undertaken. Almost all male breast cancers are ductal in origin due to the paucity of lobular elements in the male breast. Both ductal carcinoma in situ and Paget's disease have been described.

Traditionally male breast cancer presented at a later stage, often because of delay either in the patient seeking medical care or in diagnosis. Treatment depends on extent of involvement. Often there is invasion of the pectoralis major muscle, necessitating radical mastectomy. For earlier tumors, modified radical mastectomy is the preferred procedure. For close or positive margins, postmastectomy radiation should be added. Breast conservation, while theoretically acceptable, is often not feasible because of the limited amount of tissue of the male breast. If all criteria for breast conservation are met, however, there is no absolute contraindication to its use.

The value of systemic adjuvant chemotherapy has been extrapolated from the large trials on women, and should be considered at least for patients with stage II or greater disease. The majority of patients (80%) are estrogen receptor positive, and treatment with Tamoxifen should be considered in male patients with tumors greater than 1 cm or nodal positivity. Stage for stage, survival curves parallel those of female epithelial breast cancers.

Acknowledgments   Figures 1,2,3, and 7 are reprinted with permission from Breast Care: A Clinical Guidebook for Women's Primary Healthcare Providers, William H. Hindle, Editor. ©1999 Springer-Verlag New York.

References

1. Lynch HT. Introduction to breast cancer genetics. In: Lynch HT, ed. Genetics and Breast Cancer. New York: Van Nostrand Reinhold, 1992:1–13.

2. Miki Y, Swensen J, Shattuck-Eiden D, et al. A strong candidate gene for the breast and ovarian cancer susceptibility gene BRCA1. Science 1994;266:66.

3. Wooster R, Bignell G, Lancaster J, et al. Identification of the breast cancer susceptibility gene BRCA2. Nature 1995;378:789–792.

4. Claus EB, Schildkraut J, Iversen ES Jr, et al. Effect of BRCA1 and BRCA2 on the association between breast cancer risk and family history. J Natl Cancer Inst 1998;90:1824–1829.

5. Brody LC, Biesecker BB. Breast cancer susceptibility genes: BRCA1 and BRCA2. Rev Mol Med 1998;77:208–226.

6. Narod SA, Reuteun J, Lynch HT, et al. Familial breast-ovarian cancer locus on chromosome 17q12-q23. Lancet 1991;338:82–83.

7. Akashi-Tanaka S, Fukutomi T, Tukami A, et al. Male breast cancer in patients with a familial history of breast cancer. Surg Today 1996;26:975–979.

8. Stratton MR, Ford D, Neuhasen S, et al. Familial male breast cancer is not linked to the BRCA1 locus on chromosome 17q. Nat Genet 1994;7:103–107.

9. Fisher B, Costantino JP, Wickerham L, et al. Tamoxifen for the prevention of breast cancer: report of the National Surgical Adjuvant Breast and Bowel Project P1 study. J Natl Cancer Inst 1998;90:1371–1388.

10. Fisher B, Costantino JP, Redmond C, et al. A randomized clinical trial evaluating Tamoxifen in the treatment of patients with node negative breast cancer who have estrogen receptor positive tumors. N Engl J Med 1989;320:479–484.

11. Fisher B, Redmond C, Brown A, et al. Adjuvant chemotherapy with and without Tamoxifen in the treatment of primary breast cancer: 5 year results from the National Surgical Adjuvant Breast and Bowel Project Trial. J Clin Oncol 1986;4:459–471.

12. Mouridsen H, Palshof T, Patterson J, et al. Tamoxifen in advanced breast cancer. Cancer Treat Rev 1978;5:137–141.

13. Hartmann LC, Schaid DJ, Woods JE, et al. Efficacy of bilateral prophylactic mastectomy in women with a family history of breast cancer. N Engl J Med 1999;340:77–84.

14. Semiglazar VF, Moiseyenko VM, Bauli JL, et al. The role of breast self-examination in early breast cancer detection (results of the 5 year USSR/WHO randomized study in Leningrad). Eur J Epidemiol 1992;8:498.

15. Thomas DB, Gao DL, Self SG, et al. Randomized trial of breast self examination in Shanghai: methodology and preliminary results. J Natl Cancer Inst 1997;89:355–365.

16. Boyd NF, Sutherland HF, Fish EB, et al. Prospective evaluation of physical examination of the breast. Am J Surg 1981;142:331.

17. Sox HC Jr. Preventive health services in adults. N Engl J Med 1993;330:1589.

18. Miller AB, Baines CJ, To T, et al. Canadian National Breast Screening Study 2: breast cancer detection and death rates among women 50 to 59 years. Can Med Assoc J 1992;147:1477.

19 Fletcher S, Black W, Harris R, et al. Special article: report of the International Workshop on Screening for Breast Cancer. J Natl Cancer Inst 1993;85:1644.

20. American College of Radiology. Breast Imaging Reporting and Data System (BI-RADS). Reston, VA: American College of Radiology, 1993.

21. Dronkers DJ. Stereotaxic core biopsy of breast lesions. Radiology 1992;183:631–634.

22. Parker SH, Lovin JD, Jobe WE, et al. Nonpalpable breast lesions: stereotactic automated large-core biopsies. Radiology 1991;180:403–407.

23. Jackman RJ, Nowels KW, Shepard MJ, et al. Stereotaxic large-core needle biopsy of 450 nonpalpable breast lesions with surgical correlation in lesions with cancer or atypical hyperplasia. Radiology 1994;193:91–95.

24. Liberman L, Cohen MA, Dershaw DD, et al. Atypical ductal hyperplasia diagnosed at stereotaxic core biopsy of breast lesions: an indication for surgical biopsy. Am J Roentgenol 1995;164:1111–1113.

25. Smith BL, Souba WW. Algorithm and explanation: assessment and management of breast complaints. Common Clin Prob 1995:1–17.

26. Devitt JE. Management of nipple discharge by clinical findings. Am J Surg 1985;149:789.

27. Leis HP Jr, Greene FL, Cammarata A, et al. Nipple discharge: surgical significance. South Med J 1988;81:20.

28. Singletary SE, et al. Breast. In: Greene FL, Page DL, Fleming ID, et al. AJCC Cancer Staging Manual, Sixth Edition. New York, 2002:221–240.

29. Van Lancker M, Goor C, Sacre R, et al. Patterns of axillary lymph node metastasis in breast cancer. Am J Clin Oncol 1995;18:267–272.

30. Frykberg ER, Bland KI. Management of in situ and minimally invasive breast carcinoma. World J Surg 1994;18:45.

31. Fisher B, Costantino JP, Redmond C, et al. Lumpectomy compared with lumpectomy and radiation therapy for the treatment of intraductal breast cancer. N Engl J Med 1993;328:1581–1586.

32. Page DL, Dupont W, Rogers L, Landenberger M. Intraductal carcinoma of the breast: follow up after biopsy only. Cancer 1982;49:751–758.

33. Haagensen CD, Lane N, Lattes R, et al. Lobular neoplasia (so-called lobular carcinoma in situ) of the breast. Cancer 1978;42:737–769.

34. Schwartz G, Feig S, Rosenberg A. Staging and treatment of clinically occult breast cancer. Cancer 1984;53:1379.

35. Wheeler J, Enterline H, Rosenman J. Lobular carcinoma in situ of the breast. Long-term follow-up. Cancer 1974;34:554–563.

36. Frykberg E, Santiago F, Betsill W, O'Brien P. Lobular carcinoma in situ of the breast. Surg Gynecol Obstet 1987;164:285–301.

37. Lynch HT, Krush AJ, Lemon HM, Kaplan AR, Condit PT, Bottomley RH. Tumor variation in families with breast cancer. JAMA 1972;222:1631–1635.

38. Easton DF, Ford D, Bishop DT. Breast and ovarian cancer incidence in BRCA1-mutation carriers: Breast Cancer Linkage Consortium. Am J Hum Genet 1995;56:265–271.

39. Stratton MR, Ford D, Neuhasen S, et al. Familial male breast cancer is not linked to the BRCA1 locus on chromosome 17q. Nat Genet 1994;7:103–107.

40. Marcus JN, Watson P, Page DL, et al. Hereditary breast cancer: pathobiology, prognosis, and BRCA1 and BRCA2 gene linkage [see comments]. Cancer 1996;77:697–709.

41. Li FP, Fraumeni JF Jr. Soft-tissue sarcomas, breast cancer, and other neoplasms: a familial syndrome? Ann Intern Med 1969;71:747–752.

42. Robinson G, Van Heerden J, Payne WEA. The primary surgical treatment of carcinoma of the breast: a changing trend toward modified radical mastectomy. Mayo Clin Proc 1976;51:433–442.

43. Baker R, Montague A, Childs J. A comparison of modified radical mastectomy to radical mastectomy in the treatment of operable breast cancer. Ann Surg 1979;189:553–559.

44. Turner L, Swindell R, Bell W. Radical versus modified radical

mastectomy for breast cancer. Ann R Coll Surg Engl 1981;63:239–243.

45. Maddox W, Carpenter J, Laws H. A randomized prospective trial of radical mastectomy versus modified radical mastectomy in 311 breast cancer patients. Ann Surg 1983;198:207–212.

46. Maddox W, Carpenter J, Laws H, et al. Does radical mastectomy still have a place in the treatment of primary operable breast cancer? Arch Surg 1987;122:1320.

47. NIH Consensus Development Conference Treatment of early-stage breast cancer. NIH Consens Statement 1990;8:1–19.

48. Fisher B, Montague A, Redmond C, et al. Comparison of radical mastectomy with alternatives for primary breast cancer: a first report of results from a prospective randomized clinical trial. Cancer 1977;39:2827.

49. Fisher B, Redmond C, Fisher ER, et al. Ten-year results of a randomized clinical trial comparing radical mastectomy and total mastectomy with or without radiation. N Engl J Med 1985;312:674.

50. Moffat FL Jr, Senofsky GM, Davis K, Clark KC, Robinson DS, Ketcham AS. Axillary node dissection for early breast cancer: some is good, but all is better. J Surg Oncol 1992;51:8–13.

51. NIH Consensus Conference. Treatment of early-stage breast cancer. JAMA 1991;265:391–395.

52. Giuliano AE, Kirgan DM, Guenther JM, Morton DL. Lymphatic mapping and sentinel lymphadenectomy for breast cancer. Ann Surg 1994;220:391–401.

53. Turner RR, Ollila DW, Krasne DL, Giuliano AE. Histopathologic validation of the sentinel lymph node hypothesis for breast carcinoma. Ann Surg 1997;226:271–276.

54. Prognostic importance of occult axillary lymph node micrometastases from breast cancers. International (Ludwig) Breast Cancer Study Group [see comments]. Lancet 1990;335:1565–1568.

55. Trojani M, de M I, Bonichon F, Coindre JM, Delsol G. Micrometastases to axillary lymph nodes from carcinoma of breast: detection by immunohistochemistry and prognostic significance. Br J Cancer 1987;55:303–306.

56. Noguchi S, Aihara T, Motomura K, Inaji H, Imaoka S, Koyama H. Detection of breast cancer micrometastases in axillary lymph nodes by means of reverse transcriptase-polymerase chain reaction: comparison between MUC1 and mRNA and keratin 19 mRNA amplification. Am J Pathol 1996;148:649–656.

57. Danforth DN. The role of axillary lymph node dissection in the management of breast cancer. In: Rosenberg S, Devita V, Hellman S, eds. Principles and Practice of Oncology Updates. Vol. 6. Philadelphia: Lippincott-Raven 1992:1–16.

58. Rosen PP, Groshen S, Kinne DW, Norton L. Factors influencing prognosis in node-negative breast carcinoma: analysis of 767 T1N0M0/T2N0M0 patients with long-term follow-up. J Clin Oncol 1993;11:2090–2100.

59. Jones SE, Moon TE, Bonadonna G, et al. Comparison of different trials of adjuvant chemotherapy in stage II breast cancer using a natural history data base. Am J Clin Oncol 1987;10:387–395.

60. Rouesse J, Friedman S, Sarrazin D, et al. Primary chemotherapy in the treatment of inflammatory breast carcinoma: a study of 230 cases from the Institut Gustave-Roussy. J Clin Oncol 1986;4:1765–1771.

61. Perez CA, Fields JN, Fracasso PM, et al. Management of locally advanced carcinoma of the breast, II: Inflammatory carcinoma. Cancer 1994;74(suppl 1):466–476.

62. Paget J. Disease of the mammary areola preceding cancer of the mammary gland. St Bart Hosp Rep 1874;10:79–89.

63. Pierce LJ, Haffty BG, Solin LJ, et al. The conservative management of Paget's disease of the breast with radiotherapy. Cancer 1997;80:1065–1072.

64. Baron PL, Moore MP, Kinne DW, Candela FC, Osborne MP, Petrek JA. Occult breast cancer presenting with axillary metastases: updated management. Arch Surg 1990;125:210–214.

65. American Cancer Society. Guidelines for the cancer related checkup. http://www.cancer.org/guide/guidchec.html 1997.

66. National Cancer Institute. Breast cancer screening. In: PDQ: detection and prevention. http://cancernet.nci.nih.gov/clinpdq/screening/Screening_for_breast_cancer_Physician.html 1997.

67. National Cancer Advisory Board. National cancer advisory board mammography recommendations for women ages 40–49. http://cancernet.nci.nih.gov/news/ncabrec.htm 1997.

68. American College of Radiology. ACR standard for the performance of screening mammography. http://www.acr.org/departments/stand_accred/standards/pdf_standards/toc.pdf 1997.

69. American College of Obstetricians and Gynecologists. ACOG news release: April 1997 press statement on mammography screening guidelines. http://www.acog.org/from_home/publications/press_releases/nr-mammos.htm 1997.

70. American Academy of Family Physicians. AAFP recommendations for periodic health examination. In: 1996–1997 AAFP Reference Manual: Clinical Policies. http://www.aafp.org/family/policy/camp/14.html 1997.

71. US Preventive Services Task Force. Highlights: US Preventive Services Task Force Guide to Clinical Preventive Services. 2nd ed. http://www.ahcpr.gov/clinic/uspstf.htm 1997.

72. Hayward J. The Guy's trials on "early" breast cancer. World J Surg 1977;1:314.

73. Sarrazin D, Le M, Arriagada R, et al. Ten-year results of a randomized trial comparing a conservative treatment to mastectomy in early breast cancer. Radiother Oncol 1989;14:177.

74. Veronesi U, Saccozzi R, Del Vecchio M, et al. Comparing radical mastectomy with quadrantectomy, axillary dissection, and radiotherapy in patients with small cancers of the breast. N Engl J Med 1981;305:6.

75. Fisher B, Redmond C, Poisson R, et al. Eight-year results of a randomized clinical trial comparing total mastectomy and lumpectomy with or without irradiation in the treatment of breast cancer. N Engl J Med 1989;320:822.

76. Lichter A, Lippman M, Danforth D, et al. Mastectomy versus breast-conserving therapy in the treatment of stage I and II carcinoma of the breast: a randomized trial at the National Cancer Institute. J Clin Oncol 1992;10:976.

77. Van Dongen J, Bartelink H, Fentimen I, et al. Randomized clinical trial to assess the value of breast conserving therapy in Stage I and II breast cancer: EORTC 10801 trial. Monogr J Natl Cancer Inst 1992;11:15.

78. Blichert-Toft M, Rose C, Andersen J, et al. Danish randomized trial comparing breast conservation therapy with mastectomy: six years of life-table analysis. Monogr J Natl Cancer Inst 1992;11:19.

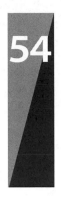

54

Melanoma and Other Cutaneous Malignancies

Vernon K. Sondak and Kim A. Margolin

Cancers of the skin constituted nearly one-half of all cancers diagnosed in 1999, at least 1,000,000 new cases in the United States alone. In fact, the skin is by far the most common primary site for human cancer development.

Melanoma

The incidence of melanoma has climbed steadily since 1930; the rate of this increase is higher than that for any other type of cancer.[1] Because of its relatively young age of onset, melanoma is second only to leukemia in terms of the years of potential life lost per death among all types of malignancy in the United States.[2]

Demographics and Epidemiology

The major etiological factor in the development of most cases of cutaneous melanoma is intermittent, acute exposure to ultraviolet radiation in susceptible individuals who lack adequate protection in terms of pigmentation (acquired or natural).[3]

DISEASE SITES

More than 90% of melanomas are cutaneous lesions,[4] but melanomas also occur in the pigmented cells of the retina (choroidal or ocular melanomas) and on the mucous membranes of the nasopharynx, vulva, and anal canal. In general, these noncutaneous tumors present at a more advanced stage and have a poorer prognosis (Table 54.1).[4] About 2% of melanoma cases present as metastatic disease to regional lymph nodes or distant sites without a known primary.[4]

AGE

The average age at diagnosis is 55 years, with more than three-fourths of all cases arising before age 70.[4]

GENDER

Melanoma is slightly more common in men than in women, with a male to female ratio of approximately 1.2:1. It appears

that women have a slightly better prognosis, stage for stage, compared to men.[4]

RACE

Melanoma is much less common in Blacks, with an annual age-adjusted incidence only 1% of that seen in Caucasians. Asians and Hispanics are similarly at very low risk for melanoma compared to whites.[5]

GEOGRAPHY

Incidence rates of melanoma are highest in areas of the world where fair-skinned Whites live in a very sunny climate near the equator.[6] Thus, Australia and Israel have among the highest melanoma rates in the world.

SPECIFIC RISK FACTORS

ULTRAVIOLET LIGHT
Most dangerous is UVB radiation (wavelength, 290–320 nm), but UVA (320–400 nm) probably also has carcinogenic potential.[7]

SKIN TYPE AND TYPICAL AND ATYPICAL MOLES
Typical moles or benign moles, also called melanocytic nevi, are small (<6 mm), round, uniformly tan or brown, and symmetrical. They are generally raised above the skin surface, as opposed to freckles, which are flat. Patients with many (>25) melanocytic nevi are at increased risk for melanoma development[8,9]; most of these patients are also fair-skinned, light-haired individuals who burn easily and rarely tan.

Atypical moles, also called clinically atypical nevi or dysplastic nevi, are larger (generally >6 mm), asymmetrical, and often raised with a pebbly surface (Fig. 54.1). Although atypical moles are frequently referred to as dysplastic nevi, pathological analysis does not always demonstrate the presence of dysplasia. Otherwise normal individuals with at least one clinically atypical nevus have a 6% lifetime risk of developing melanoma. This risk rises to as high as 80% or more in individuals who have a family history of melanoma in addition to one or more atypical nevi.[10] Even if every atypical mole is sur-

TABLE 54.1. Melanoma 5-Year Survival Rates by Site.

Site	Number of cases	Five-year survival (%)
Cutaneous	23,696	80.8
Ocular	1275	74.6
Unknown primary site	518	29.1
Mucosal	306	25.0
All cases	25,795	78.8

Source: Adapted from Chang AE, Karnell LH, Menck HR. The National Cancer Data Base report on cutaneous and non-cutaneous melanoma: a summary of 84,836 cases from the past decade. Cancer 1998;83:1664–1678.

gically removed, however, the patient remains at increased risk for melanoma development in the remaining normal skin. Therefore, close follow-up is particularly important in those with a family history of melanoma.

Dysplastic nevus syndrome is a familial tendency to develop atypical moles and also melanoma. Familial patients tend to be diagnosed at a younger age and often develop multiple primaries. Studies in several kindreds suggest an autosomal-dominant pattern of inheritance.

Giant congenital nevi are pigmented lesions actually present at birth, as opposed to developing months or years later. Among congenital nevi, only the giant congenital nevus (defined as greater than 20 cm in maximum diameter), a very rare lesion, is a documented precursor to melanoma.[11] Whenever the cosmetic result permits, giant congenital nevi should be excised in early childhood. If complete excision is impossible, even with staged procedures, close follow-up is indicated.

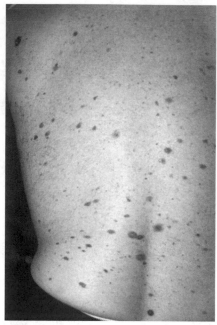

FIGURE 54.1. Clinically atypical moles, also called dysplastic nevi, are large (generally >6 mm), asymmetrical, and have a pebbly surface. They may have various shades of coloration.

Diagnosis and Prognosis

The prognosis for melanoma is directly related to the stage at initial diagnosis. The most commonly used staging system is the TNM system. Table 54.2 illustrates the differences between the previous (1997) version and the present (2002) ver-

TABLE 54.2. Differences Between the Previous (1997) Version and the Present (2002) Version of the Melanoma Staging System.

Factor	Old system	New system	Comments
Thickness	Secondary prognostic factor; thresholds of 0.75, 1.50, 4.0 mm	Primary determinant of T staging; thresholds of 1.0, 2.0, 4.0 mm	Correlation of metastatic risk is a continuous variable
Level of invasion	Primary determinant of T staging	Used only for defining T1 melanomas	Correlation only significant for thin lesions; variability in interpretation
Ulceration	Not included	Included as a second determinant of T and N staging	Signifies a locally advanced lesion; dominant prognostic factor for grouping Stages I, II, and III
Satellite metastases	In T category	In N category	Merged with in-transit lesions
Thick melanomas (> 4.0 mm)	Stage III	Stage IIC	Stage III defined as regional metastases
Dimensions of nodal metastases	Dominant determinant of N staging	Not used	No evidence of significant prognostic correlation
Number of nodal metastases	Not included	Primary determinant of N staging	Thresholds of 1 vs. 2–3 vs. ≥ 4 nodes
Metastatic tumor burden	Not included	Included as a second determinant of N staging	Clinically occult ("microscopic") vs. clinically apparent ("macroscopic") nodal volume
Lung metastases	Merged with all other visceral metastases	Separate category as M1b	Has a somewhat better prognosis than other visceral metastases
Elevated serum LDH	Not included	Included as a second determinant of M staging	
Clinical vs. pathologic staging	Did not account for sentinel node technology	Sentinel node results incorporated into definition of pathologic staging	Large variability in outcome between clinical and pathologic staging; pathologic staging encouraged prior to entry into clinical trials

Source: Adapted from Balch et al.[56]

TABLE 54.3. Five-Year Survival Rates of Pathologically Staged Patients.

	IA	IB	IIA	IIB	IIC	IIIA	IIIB	IIIC
Ta: non-ulcerated melanoma	T1a 95%	T2a 89%	T3a 79%	T4a 67%		N1a N2a 67%	N1b N2b 54%	N3 28%
Tb: ulcerated melanoma		T1b 91%	T2b 77%	T3b 63%	T4b 45%	N1a N2a 52%	N2b N2b N3 24%

T1a, melanoma ≤ 1.0 mm in thickness and level II or III, no ulceration; T1b, melanoma ≤ 1.0 mm in thickness and level IV or V or with ulceration; T2a, melanoma 1.01–2.0 mm in thickness, no ulceration; T2b, melanoma 1.01–2.0 mm in thickness, with ulceration; T3a, melanoma 2.01–4.0 mm in thickness, no ulceration; T3b, melanoma 2.01–4.0 mm in thickness, with ulceration; T4a, melanoma > 4.0 mm in thickness, no ulceration; T4b, melanoma > 4.0 mm in thickness, with ulceration; N1a, clinically occult (microscopic) metastasis in one lymph node; N1b, clinically apparent (macroscopic) metastasis in one lymph node, N2a, clinically occult (microscopic) metastasis in 2–3 regional nodes or intralymphatic regional metastasis without nodal metastasis; N2b, clinically apparent (macroscopic) metastasis in 2–3 regional nodes or intralymphatic regional metastasis without nodal metastasis; N3, metastasis in four or more regional nodes, or matted metastatic nodes, or intransit metastasis or satellite(s) with metastasis in regional node(s).

Source: Adapted from Balch, C.M., et al., Prognostic factors of 17,600 melanoma patients. Validation of the AJCC melanoma staging system. J Clin Oncol, 19;3622–3634, 2001 and Greene, F.L., Page D.L., Fleming, I.D., et al., editors. AJCC Cancer Staging Manual, Sixth Ed. New York: Springer-Verlag. 2002:209–220.

sion of the melanoma staging system that will be implemented on January 1, 2003. If detected early (stage I or II), most cutaneous melanomas can be cured with surgical excision. The prognosis of patients with lymphatic dissemination decreases significantly, and only a minority of patients who develop metastatic disease survive beyond 5 years (Table 54.3).

EARLY DIAGNOSIS OF MELANOMA

DIFFERENTIATION FROM BENIGN MOLES

Early melanomas (Fig. 54.2) may be differentiated from benign moles by assessing for asymmetry, border irregularity, color (variable or very dark), and diameter greater than 6 mm (the so-called ABCDs; see Table 54.4). Other signs of melanoma include itching, bleeding, ulceration, or changes in a preexisting benign mole.

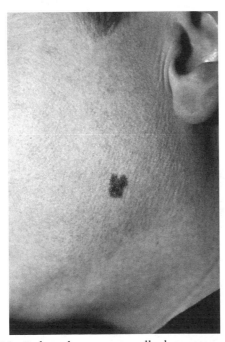

FIGURE 54.2. Early melanomas generally demonstrate asymmetry, border irregularity, dark or variable coloration, and diameter >6 mm.

CLINICALLY ATYPICAL NEVI

Clinically atypical nevi have some, but not all, the features of melanoma: They are generally larger than 6 mm, asymmetrical, and often show border irregularity (see Fig. 54.1). Biopsy of any suspicious skin lesion should be carried out. Patients with too many atypical nevi to excise require careful follow-up.

AMELANOTIC MELANOMA

Most (but not all) melanomas are pigmented. Nonpigmented melanomas are referred to as "amelanotic" melanomas. These are among the hardest types of melanoma to diagnose. A high index of suspicion and a low threshold for conducting biopsies of persistent or suspicious nonpigmented lesions is the only way amelanotic melanomas can be diagnosed at a relatively early stage.

SKIN AND REGIONAL LYMPH NODE EXAMINATION

Total-body skin examination is a critical part of the initial evaluation and subsequent follow-up of patients with melanoma, nonmelanoma skin cancer, or clinically atypical nevi. Because of the common denominator of solar exposure in the causation of most skin cancers, patients with one skin cancer are at significant risk of harboring or developing a second or even multiple skin cancers, often of a different histological type.

All accessible lymph nodes groups (cervical, supraclavicular, axillary, and inguinal regions) should be carefully examined in melanoma patients at the time of presentation and at each follow-up visit. Lymphatic metastasis is the most frequently encountered type of dissemination in melanoma.

BIOPSY TECHNIQUES

When the decision is made to biopsy a suspicious pigmented or nonpigmented skin lesion, several factors must be taken into consideration. First and foremost, the pathologist must receive adequate tissue to permit assessment of all relevant histological features. Also, the initial biopsy should be planned so as not to complicate subsequent surgical treatment.[12] Partial-thickness shave biopsies, cryosurgery, or electrodesic-

TABLE 54.4. Differentiating Melanoma from Benign Moles: the ABCDs.

	Characteristic	Melanoma	Benign moles
A:	Asymmetry	Asymmetrical	Symmetrical
B:	Border irregularity	Irregular, notched	Regular, round
C:	Color	Very dark or variable	Uniform, brown or tan
D:	Diameter	Usually >6 mm	Always <6 mm

cation do not allow for pathological analysis of margins and depth of invasion and should be avoided.

COMPLETE EXCISION

Ideally, most clinically suspicious skin lesions should be biopsied by complete excision using local anesthesia, taking a 1- to 2-mm margin of normal skin and including some subcutaneous fat. Unusually large lesions or those situated in cosmetically sensitive areas, such as the face, may be approached by incisional or punch biopsy.

BIOPSY OF LYMPH NODES

Palpably enlarged lymph nodes suspected of representing melanoma metastasis are initially evaluated by fine-needle aspiration cytology.[13] A positive cytology is grounds for performing a full lymph node dissection. If the cytology is nondiagnostic or negative, or if the node is in a location that precludes aspiration, an open biopsy is appropriate. Sentinel lymph node biopsy is described later in this chapter.

HISTOLOGICAL TYPES OF MELANOMA

Melanomas are classified into four major histological categories. *Superficial spreading melanomas* constitute up to 70% of cutaneous melanomas. They often arise within a preexisting nevus. *Nodular melanomas* represent about 8% to 10% of cutaneous melanomas. They are generally dark blue-black and are more symmetrical and uniform in color than other melanomas. *Lentigo maligna melanomas* also account for about 10% of cutaneous melanomas. They typically occur on the sun-exposed areas of the head and neck and the hands. These lesions arise from a precursor lesion known as lentigo maligna, or Hutchinson's melanotic freckle. *Acral-lentiginous melanomas* occur on the palms, soles, and beneath the nails (subungual melanoma), and make up only 1% of melanoma cases.[4]

GROWTH PHASES OF MELANOMA

The local growth of melanoma has been characterized as occurring in two distinct phases: a radial and a vertical phase.[14] *Radial growth phase* is characterized by melanoma tumor cells extending laterally ("radially") within the epidermis and papillary dermis. *Vertical growth phase* into the deeper layers of skin is associated with increasing nodularity of the lesion and a much greater potential for metastasis.

PATHOLOGICAL STAGING OF MELANOMA

In the absence of distant metastatic disease, the single most important prognostic factor in melanoma is the status of the regional lymph nodes. Currently, 85% of melanoma patients present with clinically normal lymph nodes. In clinically node-negative patients, most investigators have found the microscopic degree of invasion of the melanoma, or *microstage*, to be of critical importance in predicting outcome. Two meth-

ods have been described for microscopic staging of primary cutaneous melanomas.

Clark's levels classify melanomas according to the level of invasion relative to histologically defined landmarks in the skin. Clark's five levels are depicted in Figure 54.3. Clark's levels correlate with prognosis: lesions with deeper levels of invasion have a greater risk of recurrence.

Breslow's thickness is a measurement of the thickness of the primary tumor from the top of the granular layer of the epidermis to the deepest contiguous tumor cell at the base of the lesion using a micrometer in the microscope eyepiece. Many investigators have documented an inverse correlation between the maximum measured tumor thickness and survival. More importantly, several studies have demonstrated that tumor thickness conveys more prognostic information than does Clark's level of invasion.

REGIONAL LYMPH NODE INVOLVEMENT

There is a direct relationship between the thickness of a primary melanoma and the likelihood of metastatic involvement of the regional lymph nodes. The presence of regional lymph node metastases is a poor prognostic sign regardless of the microstage of the primary lesion.

OTHER PROGNOSTIC FACTORS

HISTOLOGIC TYPE

In general, nodular and acral-lentiginous melanomas are significantly thicker at the time of diagnosis than superficial spreading or lentigo maligna melanomas. Thus, even when TNM stage is taken into account, nodular and acral-lentiginous melanomas have a significantly worse prognosis.

SITE OF THE PRIMARY

Several studies have shown that patients with melanomas of the extremities have a better survival rate than patients with

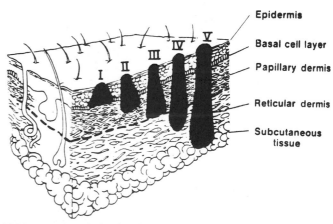

FIGURE 54.3. Clark's levels of invasion for cutaneous melanoma.

lesions arising on the trunk or head and neck. However, this may be because truncal, head, and neck lesions are harder to see, and may present later (thicker).

OTHER PATHOLOGICAL FEATURES

Several pathological characteristics of the primary tumor retain their significance as prognostic factors independent of Breslow's thickness in node-negative melanoma: these include a lymphocytic in filtrate and areas of apparent regression.[14] Ulceration and satellitosis (the presence of satellite nodules of melanoma within 2 cm of the primary) are also indicators of an increased risk of local recurrence after wide excision.[15,16]

GENDER AND AGE

Female gender and age less than 60 years have been found to be independent favorable prognostic factors in many but not all studies.[4,14,17]

Surgical Treatment of Cutaneous Melanoma

Surgery remains the mainstay of treatment for local/regional cutaneous melanoma (TNM stages I–III), and occasionally plays a role in selected patients with stage IV disease as well. Initial surgical management of the patient with clinically localized melanoma involves adequate excision of the primary lesion and, in many cases, staging of the regional lymph nodes.

EXCISION OF THE PRIMARY LESION

The current recommendations for excision margins of cutaneous melanomas are summarized in Table 54.5. Regardless of the recommended width of excision, a histologically negative margin is necessary.

MANAGEMENT OF REGIONAL LYMPH NODES

Melanoma patients with clinical evidence of lymph node involvement but no evidence of distant disease (AJCC clinical stage III) should undergo a fine-needle aspiration cytology or, when necessary, an open biopsy to document the presence of metastatic melanoma. If the cytology or biopsy confirms the presence of nodal involvement in a single node, complete regional lymph node dissection should be carried out.

Recommendations regarding surgical management of patients with clinically negative regional nodes are best made in the context of the thickness of the primary tumor.

Patients with thin melanomas (<1 mm in thickness) have a very low likelihood of nodal involvement (<5%). These patients should undergo periodic physical examinations to detect the rare cases of nodal recurrence.

Melanomas 1 mm to 4 mm in thickness are associated with about a 20% to 25% chance of occult nodal involvement. However, elective dissection of the regional nodes would convert all these cases from outpatient into inpatient procedures requiring general anesthesia, increasing costs and morbidity for all patients while only identifying and treating positive nodes in a minority of the group. Thus, there would have to be substantial evidence of a survival benefit to argue for elective node dissection as routine treatment in this group of patients.

Retrospective data suggested that there was, indeed, a survival benefit for immediate (elective) lymph node dissection at the time of excision of the primary in patients with intermediate-thickness melanoma.[18] These data led to a number of randomized trials in the United States and around the world. The results of those trials argue strongly against the routine use of elective dissection in patients who have intermediate-thickness melanomas and clinically negative lymph nodes. Nonetheless, *staging* of the regional nodes (selective lymphadenectomy) may be of benefit in selecting patients for adjuvant therapy.

Patients with thick melanomas (>4 mm) have a high likelihood of nodal involvement but also have a high incidence of occult systemic metastasis at the time of diagnosis. For this reason, even strong proponents of elective node dissection agree that patients with thick primaries do not benefit from elective removal of clinically negative lymph nodes.[18]

TABLE 54.5.

Current Recommendations for Excision Margins for Cutaneous Melanomas.

Location	Tumor thickness	Recommended margin	Evidence	Reference
Trunk and proximal extremity	≤1 mm	1 cm	Randomized trial[a]	41,42
	1–2 mm	2 cm if able to be closed primarily, otherwise 1 cm	Randomized trials[a]	16,41–43
	2–4 mm	2 cm	Randomized trial[a]	16,43
	>4 mm or with satellitosis	At least 2 cm	Nonrandomized clinical series[b] Accepted surgical practice[c]	44
Head and neck and distal extremity	≤1 mm	1 cm	Randomized trial[a]	41,42
	>1 mm	At least 1 cm	Accepted surgical practice[c]	

[a]Level I evidence.

[b]Level II evidence.

[c]Level III evidence.

Note: Level I evidence is defined as prospective, randomized clinical trials.

Level II evidence is defined as clinical trials without randomization or case-controlled retrospective studies.

Level III evidence is defined as retrospective analyses without case controls, accepted clinical practice, or anecdotal case reports.

SELECTIVE LYMPHADENECTOMY

Recently, a new option for the management of melanoma patients with clinically negative nodes has emerged. It has been shown that the lymphatics from any given spot on the skin drain to a single or at most two or three specific lymph nodes within the regional basin. These initial draining nodes, called the "sentinel" nodes, are almost always the first site of nodal involvement when melanoma spread to the regional nodes. If the sentinel nodes are negative for melanoma, the remaining nodes are also free of involvement in at least 96% of cases.[19] Based on these findings, the technique of selective lymphadenectomy for patients with intermediate and thick melanomas and clinically negative nodes has been proposed. In this strategy, only the sentinel nodes are removed initially, and full lymph node dissection is reserved for patients with involved sentinel nodes. The technique of selective lymphadenectomy has been adopted by a number of surgeons as an alternative to "watch and wait" or routine elective node dissection strategies.

TECHNIQUES OF SELECTIVE LYMPHADENECTOMY

Two techniques are available for identifying the sentinel node draining a cutaneous melanoma. The first involves blue lymphangiogram dye (either isosulfan blue [Lymphazurin] or patent blue) injected intradermally at the site of the primary, followed about 5 min later by an incision over the lymph node basin, and the blue lymphatic channel or channels coursing to the sentinel node are identified and traced until a blue-stained node is identified and removed. This technique allows for identification of the sentinel node at least 80% of the time. The alternative technique involves injection of a radiolabeled colloid solution, which can be done up to 4 h before surgery, combined with intraoperative identification of the sentinel node using a handheld gamma detector. As the radiolabeled technique provides no visual clues to the sentinel node's location, most surgeons combine the two techniques. The combined use of blue lymphangiogram dye plus radiolabeled colloid enables the detection of the sentinel node in more than 98% of cases.[20,21]

Postoperative Follow-up of the Melanoma Patient

The main goals of postoperative followup are to detect treatable (i.e., local-regional) recurrences and new primary tumors in an expeditious fashion. Hence, physical examination plays a more important role than laboratory or radiologic examination.

Melanoma and Pregnancy

When melanoma occurs during pregnancy, a number of unique considerations arise. Hormones, in particular estrogen, stimulate the proliferation of normal melanocytes and there is abundant evidence to suggest they affect melanoma cells as well. Furthermore, melanoma is one of the few malignancies that have been recognized to metastasize to the placenta and even cross the placenta to involve the fetus.[22] While these facts merit careful consideration, the bulk of the available evidence suggests that, stage for stage, the outcome of a pregnant patient with stage I or II melanoma is not different from a nonpregnant patient.[23] Subsequent pregnancy also does not seem to be associated with an adverse outcome.

Surgical Treatment of Noncutaneous Melanomas

Noncutaneous melanomas generally present at a more advanced stage than cutaneous lesions. The site of the lesion greatly affects the approach to the primary tumor and regional lymph nodes.

OCULAR MELANOMA

Prognostic factors for ocular melanoma are not nearly as well characterized as for cutaneous melanomas. Ocular melanomas generally do not have access to lymphatic channels, so regional spread is rarely seen. Treatment options are enucleation or radiotherapy.

ANAL AND VULVAR MELANOMA

Melanomas of the anus and vulva pose challenges in the treatment of both the primary lesion and regional nodes. Excision of primary tumors in these areas should not be overly radical: abdominoperineal resection or radical vulvectomy are unnecessarily deforming and are not associated with improved survival compared to wide local excision. Elective dissection of clinically normal inguinal nodes has never been demonstrated to be of any survival value in either anal or vulvar melanoma.

NASAL OR NASOPHARYNGEAL MELANOMA

Melanomas arising in the nasal or nasopharyngeal mucosa should be conservatively excised, with node dissection reserved for patients who have proven nodal involvement. Because of the difficulty achieving wide, tumor-free margins around the primary site, postoperative radiation is often employed.[24]

Adjuvant Therapy of Cutaneous Melanoma

Although the prognosis for patients with early-stage cutaneous melanoma is quite good, less than 50% of patients with deep primaries (>4 mm) or regional lymph node involvement will be cured by surgery alone. The development of effective adjuvant therapy capable of increasing postsurgical survival has been a long-standing goal of melanoma researchers.

CHEMOTHERAPY AND NONSPECIFIC IMMUNOSTIMULANTS

These agents, including DTIC (dacarbazine), BCG stimulations and levamisole have shown no clear benefit.

INTERFERONS

Studies involving interferon (IFN) γ demonstrated no benefit and actually raised the possibility of a detrimental effect.[25,26] On the other hand, IFN-α has been shown to have antitumor activity in advanced disease.[27] Several randomized trials for stage IIb and III disease demonstrated statistically significant improvements in disease-free and overall survival when interferon-treated patients were compared with observed patients.[28] Regarding patients with stage I and II melanomas, IFN-α treatment was associated with significantly improved relapse-free survival but no overall survival benefit.[29,30]

ADJUVANT VACCINE THERAPY

The idea that a tumor vaccine could prevent recurrence after surgery even if the same vaccine could not induce regression of advanced disease is a compelling one. However, this strategy remains under investigation.

TABLE 54.6.

Potential Roles of Locoregional Radiotherapy in the Management of Melanoma.

Objective of radiotherapy	Indication	Timing	Evidence [references]
Avoid morbidity of surgery in cosmetically sensitive area	Large lesion in surgically difficult site, e.g., lentigo maligna of face	Primary (instead of surgery)	Anecdotal, case reports (level III evidence) [45]
Reduce extent of surgery	Large lesion in surgically difficult site, e.g., sinus	Preoperative or adjunctive following surgery	Anecdotal, accepted clinical practice (level III evidence) [24,46,47]
Reduce locoregional recurrence	Extranodal extension of tumor; multiple positive lymph nodes; ?any positive lymph nodes in the head and neck	Adjunctive following surgery (?during interferon therapy)	Nonrandomized clinical series (level II evidence); small randomized trials have been inconclusive [48–51]

RADIATION THERAPY

The potential roles of radiotherapy in local-regional melanoma are outlined in Table 54.6.

Treatment of Metastatic Melanoma

Stage IV melanoma is associated with a very poor overall prognosis, yet some patients are long-term survivors with aggressive treatment. Surgery, radiation therapy, and systemic treatments all have a role to play. In general, solitary metastases in any location should be considered for resection.

MANAGEMENT OF METASTATIC DISEASE IN SELECTED SITES

IN-TRANSIT SKIN METASTASES

In-transit metastases, that is, cutaneous or subcutaneous nodules arising between the primary site and the regional lymph node basin, are a well-recognized but fairly uncommon site of failure in cutaneous melanoma. A surgical technique developed to treat in-transit metastases, isolation limb perfusion, involves cannulating the artery and vein to an extremity and connecting the cannulas to a cardiopulmonary bypass machine. This procedure effectively isolates the blood flow to that extremity and allows for prolonged perfusion with cytotoxic or biological agents. Most commonly, the chemotherapeutic agent melphalan (L-phenylalanine mustard, Alkeran) has been used. Hyperthermic isolation perfusion with melphalan alone or combined with tumor necrosis factor-α (TNF-α) results in the regression of more than 90% of cutaneous in-transit metastases.[31–33]

CENTRAL NERVOUS SYSTEM

The brain and central nervous system (CNS) are the initial site of metastasis in 12% to 20% of patients with metastatic melanoma. The best outcomes are in patients without other evidence of systemic metastatic disease who develop limited intracranial metastases that can be treated with the combination of surgery and whole-brain radiotherapy.[34] Systemic chemotherapy with nitrosoureas, which penetrate the blood–brain barrier and have some antitumor activity, is occasionally used for recurrent or refractory cases (Table 54.7).[35]

TABLE 54.7.

Management of Central Nervous System Metastases.ᵃ

Site	Characteristics	Recommended therapy	Evidence [references]
Brain	Single or limited number, resectable	Surgical excision followed by whole-brain radiotherapy; stereotactic radiation followed by whole-brain radiotherapy	Prospective, randomized trials (level I evidence); nonrandomized clinical series (level II evidence) [34,52]
Brain	Multiple and/or unresectable	Whole brain radiotherapy	Accepted clinical practice (level III evidence) [53]
Brain	Recurrent	Stereotactic radiation; systemic chemotherapy with nitrosoureas	Nonrandomized clinical series (level II evidence) [35,52]
Spinal cord	Resectable	Resection followed by radiation; radiation alone	Anecdotal, case reports (level III evidence); small randomized trial (level I evidence) [53,54]
Meninges	Diffuse, nonlocalizing neurological findings with positive CSF cytology and/or focal enhancing lesions on CT or MR	Intrathecal chemotherapy or immunotherapy	Anecdotal, case reports (level III evidence) [55]

ᵃAll patients should receive high dose glucocorticoid therapy to be tapered as tolerated based on neurologic symptoms and signs.

Gastrointestinal Tract and Abdominal Viscera

Melanoma has a propensity for metastases involving the gastrointestinal tract. Manifestations that mandate surgical intervention include hemorrhage, obstruction, intussusception, and even perforation. Surgical resection is indicated whenever feasible, even if extraintestinal spread is present that cannot be removed.

Systemic Therapy of Metastatic Melanoma

The systemic therapy of melanoma is one of the most frustrating tasks for the medical oncologist. Strategies include the use of DTIC based chemotherapy, biological therapies (IFN-α, interleukin-2, melanoma vaccines, gene transfer), and combination biochemotherapy. Objective responses may be as high as 15 or 20%. Still, despite great strides in the understanding of tumor biology, immunology, and pharmacology, the treatment of advanced melanoma yields few durable remissions and minimal impact on survival at the cost of considerable toxicity.

Nonmelanoma Skin Cancer

With more than 1 million cases annually in the United States alone, nonmelanoma skin cancer is by far the most common form of human malignancy.[36] Most are basal and squamous cell cancers. For these two tumor types, chronic solar exposure is the predominant etiological factor, with fair-skinned individuals who have had a long history of sun exposure at highest risk. Little is known about the etiologies of other histological types of cutaneous malignancy.

Risk Factors for Nonmelanoma Skin Cancer Development

ACTINIC KERATOSES

Actinic keratoses are scaly, rough, erythematous patches that occur in chronically sun-exposed areas. They are both markers for and precursors to nonmelanoma skin cancer development.

BURNS

Squamous cell cancers occasionally arise in burns or other scars.

XERODERMA PIGMENTOSUM

Xeroderma pigmentosum, a rare congenital disorder in which patients lack the capacity to repair UV-induced DNA damage, is associated with the development of innumerable nonmelanoma skin cancers at a very early age and also with an increased risk of developing melanoma.[37]

IMMUNOSUPPRESSION OR PRIOR HEMATOLOGICAL MALIGNANCY

Nonmelanoma skin cancers and, to a much lesser degree, melanomas are increased in patients who are immunosuppressed or have had previous hematological malignancies.

Histological Types of Nonmelanoma Skin Cancer

BASAL CELL AND SQUAMOUS CELL CARCINOMAS

The two most common types of nonmelanoma skin cancer are basal cell carcinoma and squamous cell carcinoma.

Bowen's disease is the name given to squamous cell carcinoma in situ involving the skin. A rarer, more aggressive skin cancer, presumably arising from the neuroendocrine cells of the skin, is Merkel's cell cancer. Nonmelanoma skin cancers can occur on any part of the skin surface but are largely found on the head and neck, hands, and forearms.

CANCERS ARISING IN THE SKIN APPENDAGES

The skin appendages (e.g., hair follicles and sweat glands) can be the site of origin of adenocarcinomas or apocrine cancers; these are exceedingly rare.

SARCOMAS

The most common primary sarcoma affecting the skin is dermatofibrosarcoma protuberans; leiomyosarcoma, angiosarcoma, and malignant fibrous histiocytoma can also arise entirely within the skin. Generally speaking, cutaneous and subcutaneous sarcomas have a better prognosis than lesions that involve or are deep to the muscular fascia.[38] Angiosarcomas, however, tend to have a poor prognosis even when confined to the skin.

DIFFERENTIATING NONMELANOMA SKIN CANCERS

Basal cell cancers often have a pearly, translucent appearance with a rolled border, whereas squamous cell cancers are often keratinized or ulcerated. Dermatofibrosarcoma protuberans and angiosarcomas present as raised nodules or plaques, and are frequently multifocal. Both often have a purplish or violaceous hue. Merkel's cell cancers present as a raised, ulcerated lesion that can achieve very large size.

NONMELANOMA SKIN CANCERS IN AFRICAN-AMERICANS

The presentations of nonmelanoma skin cancer differ in more deeply pigmented races. Basal cell cancers, which are usually nonpigmented in Whites, are almost always pigmented in Black patients. Most cases of squamous cell cancer of the skin occur on the sun-exposed skin of the head and neck or arms, but in Blacks the majority of cases develop on less exposed areas, such as the legs, often in association with burns.[5]

Surgical Treatment of Nonmelanoma Skin Cancers

Surgery is the mainstay of treatment for nonmelanoma skin cancers, just as for melanoma. Less radical resections than required for melanoma are generally adequate. Because so many nonmelanoma skin cancers occur on cosmetically critical areas, a number of special techniques are used in their removal.

MARGINS OF EXCISION

Excision margins of 0.5 to 1.0 cm are adequate for most nonrecurrent basal and squamous cell cancers, and yield local recurrence rates under 5% provided that histologically negative margins are achieved.

RECURRENT CANCERS AND LESIONS IN DIFFICULT SITES

More sophisticated techniques are required for recurrent skin cancers or those in cosmetically difficult areas, such as the tip of the nose or the eyelid. For these lesions, a variation of Mohs micrographic surgery is frequently employed. This type of surgery is simply a very controlled surgical excision in which the removed tissue is precisely oriented and carefully examined histologically, and serial reexcisions are performed wherever residual disease is noted.[39] After Mohs surgery has achieved complete excision, reconstruction is done by whatever means is appropriate, but often involves skin grafts or local flaps rather than primary closure.

RADIATION THERAPY

Radiation therapy is a potential treatment for skin cancers located in critical sites where surgical excision would be disfiguring. Primary basal and squamous cell cancers treated with radiation have nearly identical cure rates (about 95%) as those treated with surgical excision. Radiation is also employed postoperatively to reduce local recurrence rates after excision of high-grade or recurrent sarcomas of the skin.

TOPICAL AND INTRALESIONAL THERAPY

Occasionally, patients present with numerous skin cancers that would be impossible to resect completely. For these patients, topical chemotherapy with 5-fluorouracil cream can dramatically reduce the number of excisions required. Direct intralesional injections of IFN-α have been reported to successfully treat basal cell cancers.

Management of Recurrent Disease

LOCAL/REGIONAL RECURRENCE

The vast majority of nonmelanoma skin cancers are successfully treated with surgery or primary radiation, with fewer than 5% recurring locally. Of those that do recur locally, at least 80% are cured by further local treatment. Regional lymph node metastases develop in up to 5% of squamous cell cancers and less than 2% of basal cell cancers. There is essentially no role for elective dissections of clinically normal nodes in any form of nonmelanoma skin cancer, but there may be a role for sentinel node biopsy in Merkel's cell cancers.[40]

DISTANT METASTASIS

Distant spread occurs in about 2% of squamous cell cancers and 0.1% of basal cell cancers, most frequently after nodal recurrence. No effective therapy exists for metastatic nonmelanoma skin cancer, although a few reports of scattered temporary responses to chemotherapy exist.

References

1. Wingo PA, Ries LAG, Rosenberg HM, Miller DS, Edwards BK. Cancer incidence and mortality. Cancer 1998;82:1197–1207.
2. Albert VA, Koh HK, Geller AC, Miller DR, Prout MN, Lew RA. Years of potential life lost: another indicator of the impact of cutaneous malignant melanoma on society. J Am Acad Dermatol 1990;23:308–310.
3. Marks R. An overview of skin cancers: incidence and causation. Cancer 1995;75:607–612.
4. Chang AE, Karnell LH, Menck HR. The National Cancer Data Base report on cutaneous and non-cutaneous melanoma: a summary of 84,836 cases from the past decade. Cancer 1998;83:1664–1678.
5. Halder RM, Bridgeman-Shah S. Skin cancer in African Americans. Cancer 1995;75:667–673.
6. Weinstock MA. Issues in the epidemiology of melanoma. Hematol Oncol Clin North Am 1998;12:681–698.
7. Elwood JM, Jopson J. Melanoma and sun exposure: an overview of published studies. Int J Cancer 1997;73:198–203.
8. Holly EA, Kelly JW, Shpall SN, Chiu S-H. Number of melanocytic nevi as a major risk factor for malignant melanoma. J Am Acad Dermatol 1987;17:459–468.
9. Tucker MA, Halpern A, Holly EA, et al. Clinically recognized dysplastic nevi: a central risk factor for cutaneous melanoma. JAMA 1997;277:1439–1444.
10. Greene MH, Clark WH Jr, Tucker MA, Kraemer MH, Elder DE, Fraser MC. High risk of malignant melanoma in melanoma-prone families with dysplastic nevi. Ann Intern Med 1985;102:458–465.
11. Marghoob AA, Schoenbach SP, Kopf AW, Orlow SJ, Nossa R, Bart RS. Large congenital melanocytic nevi and the risk for the development of malignant melanoma: a prospective study. Arch Dermatol 1996;132:170–175.
12. Arca MJ, Biermann JS, Johnson TM, Chang AE. Biopsy techniques for skin, soft-tissue, and bone neoplasms. Surg Oncol Clin North Am 1995;4:157–174.
13. Basler GC, Fader DJ, Yahanda A, Sondak VK, Johnson TM. The utility of fine needle aspiration in the diagnosis of melanoma metastatic to lymph nodes. J Am Acad Dermatol 1997;36:403–408.
14. Clark WH, Elder DE, Guerry D, et al. Model predicting survival in stage I melanoma based on tumor progression. J Natl Cancer Inst 1989;81:1893–1904.
15. León P, Daly JM, Synnestvedt M, Schultz DJ, Elder DE, Clark WH Jr. The prognostic implications of microscopic satellites in patients with clinical stage I melanoma. Arch Surg 1991;126:1461–1468.
16. Karakousis CP, Balch CM, Urist MM, Ross MM, Smith TJ, Bartolucci AA. Local recurrence in malignant melanoma: long-term results of the multiinstitutional randomized surgical trial. Ann Surg Oncol 1996;3:446–452.
17. Balch CM, Soong S, Shaw HM, Urist MM, McCarthy WH. An analysis of prognostic factors in 8500 patients with cutaneous melanoma. In: Balch CM, Houghton AN, Milton GW, Sober AJ, Soong S, ed. Cutaneous Melanoma. 2nd ed. Philadelphia: JB Lippincott Co, 1992:165–187.
18. Balch CM. The role of elective lymph node dissection in melanoma: rationale, results, and controversies. J Clin Oncol 1988;6:163–172.
19. Morton DL, Wen D-R, Wong JH, et al. Technical details of intraoperative lymphatic mapping for early stage melanoma. Arch Surg 1992;127:392–399.
20. Reintgen DS, Brobeil A. Lymphatic mapping and selective lymphadenectomy as an alternative to elective lymph node dissection in patients with malignant melanoma. Hematol Oncol Clin North Am 1998;12:807–821.
21. Bostick P, Essner R, Glass E, et al. Comparison of blue dye and probe-assisted intraoperative lymphatic mapping in melanoma to identify sentinel nodes in 100 lymphatic basins. Arch Surg 1999;134:43–49.
22. Baergen RN, Johnson D, Moore T, Benirschke K. Maternal melanoma metastatic to the placenta. Arch Pathol Lab Med 1997;121:508–511.
23. Mackie RM. Pregnancy and exogenous hormones in patients with cutaneous malignant melanoma. Curr Opin Oncol 1999;11:129–131.
24. Cooper JS. The evolution of the role of radiation therapy in the management of mucocutaneous malignant melanoma. Hematol Oncol Clin North Am 1998;12:849–862.
25. Meyskens FL Jr, Kopecky K, Taylor CW, et al. Randomized trial of adjuvant human interferon gamma versus observation in high-risk cutaneous melanoma. J Natl Cancer Inst 1995;87:1710–1713.
26. Sondak VK, Kopecky KJ, Smith JW II, et al. Is interferon-γ detrimental? results of a Southwest Oncology Group randomized trial of adjuvant human interferon-γ versus observation in malignant

melanoma. In: Salmon SE, ed. Adjuvant Therapy of Cancer VIII, Philadelphia: Lippincott-Raven, 1997:259–272.

27. Legha SS. The role of interferon alfa in the treatment of metastatic melanoma. Semin Oncol 1997;24(suppl 4):S24–S31.

28. Kirkwood JM, Strawderman MH, Ernstoff MS, Smith TJ, Borden EC, Blum RH. Interferon alfa-2b adjuvant therapy of high-risk resected cutaneous melanoma: the Eastern Cooperative Oncology Group trial EST 1684. J Clin Oncol 1996;14:7–17.

29. Pehamberger H, Soyer HP, Steiner A, et al. Adjuvant interferon alfa-2a treatment in resected primary stage II cutaneous melanoma: Austrian Malignant Melanoma Cooperative Group. J Clin Oncol 1998;16:1425–1429.

30. Grob JJ, Dreno B, de la Salmoniere P, et al. Randomised trial of interferon alpha-2a as adjuvant therapy in resected primary melanoma thicker than 1.5 mm without clinically detectable node metastases: French Cooperative Group on Melanoma. Lancet 1998;351:1905–1910.

31. Cumberlin R, De Moss E, Lassus M, Freidman M. Isolation perfusion for malignant melanoma of the extremity: a review. J Clin Oncol 1985;3:1022–1031.

32. Lienard D, Ewalenko P, Delmotte J-J, Renard N, Lejeune FJ. High-dose recombinant tumor necrosis factor alpha in combination with interferon gamma and melphalan in isolation perfusion of the limbs for melanoma and sarcoma. J Clin Oncol 1992;10:52–60.

33. Fraker DL, Alexander HR, Andrich M, Rosenberg SA. Treatment of patients with melanoma of the extremity using hyperthermic isolated limb perfusion with melphalan, tumor necrosis factor, and interferon gamma: results of a tumor necrosis factor dose-escalation study. J Clin Oncol 1996;14:479–489.

34. Patchell RA, Tibbs PA, Regine WF, et al. Postoperative radiotherapy in the treatment of single metastases to the brain: a randomized trial. JAMA 1998;280:1485–1489.

35. Jacquillat C, Khayat D, Banzet P, et al. Final report of the French multicenter phase II study of the nitrosourea fotemustine in 153 evaluable patients with disseminated malignant melanoma including patients with cerebral metastases. Cancer 1990;66:1873–1878.

36. Landis SH, Murray T, Bolden S, Wingo PA. Cancer statistics, 1999. CA Cancer J Clin 1999;49:8–31.

37. Halpern AC, Altman JF. Genetic predisposition to skin cancer. Curr Opin Oncol 1999;11:132–138.

38. Brooks AD, Heslin MJ, Leung DH, Lewis JJ, Brennan MF. Superficial extremity soft tissue sarcoma: an analysis of prognostic factors. Ann Surg Oncol 1998;5:41–47.

39. Swanson NA. Mohs surgery: technique, indications, applications, and the future. Arch Dermatol 1983;119:761–773.

40. Messina JL, Reintgen DS, Cruse CW, et al. Selective lymphadenectomy in patients with Merkel cell (cutaneous neuroendocrine) carcinoma. Ann Surg Oncol 1997;4:389–395.

41. Veronesi U, Cascinelli N, Adamus J, et al. Thin stage I primary cutaneous malignant melanoma. Comparison of excision with margins of 1 or 3 cm. N Engl J Med 1988;318:1159–1162.

42. Veronesi U, Cascinelli N. Narrow excision (1-cm margin): a safe procedure for thin cutaneous melanoma. Arch Surg 1991;126:438–441.

43. Balch CM, Urist MM, Karakousis CP, et al. Efficacy of 2 cm surgical margins for intermediate-thickness melanomas (1–4 mm): results of a multi-institutional randomized surgical trial. Ann Surg 1993;218:262–269.

44. Heaton KM, Sussman JJ, Gershenwald JE, et al. Surgical margins and prognostic factors in patients with thick (>4 mm) primary melanoma. Ann Surg Oncol 1998;5:322–328.

45. Harwood AR. Conventional fractionated radiotherapy for 51 patients with lentigo maligna and lentigo maligna melanoma. Int J Radiat Oncol Biol Phys 1983;9:1019–1021.

46. Johanson CR, Harwood AR, Cummings BJ, Quirt I. 0-7-21 radiotherapy in nodular melanoma. Cancer 1983;51:226–232.

47. O'Brien CJ, Coates AS, Petersen-Schaefer K, et al. Experience with 998 cutaneous melanomas of the head and neck over 30 years. Am J Surg 1991;162:310–314.

48. Ang KK, Peters LJ, Weber RS, et al. Postoperative radiotherapy for cutaneous melanoma of the head and neck region. Int J Radiat Oncol Biol Phys 1994;30:795–798.

49. Strom EA, Ross MI. Adjuvant radiation therapy after axillary lymphadenectomy for metastatic melanoma: toxicity and local control. Ann Surg Oncol 1995;2:445–449.

50. O'Brien CJ, Petersen-Schaefer K, Stevens GN, et al. Adjuvant radiotherapy following neck dissection and parotidectomy for metastatic malignant melanoma. Head Neck 1997;19:589–594.

51. Creagan ET, Cupps RE, Ivins JC, et al. Adjuvant radiation therapy for regional nodal metastases from malignant melanoma: a randomized, prospective study. Cancer 1978;42:2206–2210.

52. Auchter RM, Lamond JP, Alexander E, et al. A multiinstitutional outcome and prognostic factor analysis of radiosurgery for resectable single brain metastasis. Int J Radiat Oncol Biol Phys 1996;35:27–35.

53. Ang KK, Geara FB, Byers RM, Peters LJ. Radiotherapy of melanoma. In: Balch CM, Houghton AN, Sober AJ, Soong S, eds. Cutaneous Melanoma. 3rd ed. St. Louis: Quality Medical Publishing, 1998:389–403.

54. Young RF, Post EM, King GA. Treatment of spinal epidural metastases: randomized prospective comparison of laminectomy and radiotherapy. J Neurosurg 1980;53:741–748.

55. Fathallah-Shaykh HM, Zimmerman C, Morgan H, Rushing E, Schold SC Jr, Unwin DH. Response of primary leptomeningeal melanoma to intrathecal recombinant interleukin-2: a case report. Cancer 1996;77:1544–1550.

56. Balch C, Buzaid AC, Soong SJ, et al. Final version of the AJCC staging system for cutaneous melanoma. J Clin Oncol 2001;19:3635–3648.

57. Balch C, Soong SJ, Gershewald JE, et al. Prognostic factors analysis of 17,600 melanoma patients. Validation of the AJCC melanoma staging system. J Clin Oncol 2001;19:3622–3634.

58. Margolin K, Longmate J, Johnson D, et al. Temozolomide and whole brain irradiation in melanoma metastatic to the brain: a phase II trial of the Cytokine Working Group. J Cancer Res Clin Oncol 2001 (published online).

Soft Tissue Sarcoma

Peter W.T. Pisters

Soft tissue sarcomas comprise a group of relatively rare, anatomically and histologically diverse neoplasms. These tumors share a common embryological origin, arising primarily from tissues derived from the meso-derm. The notable exceptions are neurosarcomas, primitive neuroectodermal tumors, and possibly Ewing's sarcomas, which are believed to arise from tissues of ectodermal origin.

Despite the fact that the somatic soft tissues account for as much as 75% of total body weight, neoplasms of the soft tissues are comparatively rare, accounting for 1% of adult malignancies and 15% of pediatric malignancies. The annual incidence of soft tissue sarcomas in the United States is about 7800 new cases with 4400 deaths annually.[1]

Etiology and Epidemiology

In the United States, the race and sex distribution of adult soft tissue sarcomas approximates that of the U.S. population.[2] No specific etiological agent is identified in the majority of patients with soft tissue sarcoma. There are, however, a number of recognized associations between specific environmental factors and the subsequent development of sarcoma. In clinical practice, the most commonly observed nongenetic predisposing factors are previous irradiation and chronic lymphedema.

A number of genetic conditions are also associated with an increased risk for the development of soft tissue sarcoma. These conditions include neurofibromatosis, Li–Fraumeni syndrome, familial retinoblastoma, and Gardner's syndrome. The most commonly encountered genetically related soft tissue sarcomas occur in patients with neurofibromatosis or Gardner's syndrome.

Pathology

Anatomical Site Distribution

Soft tissue sarcomas have been described at virtually all anatomical sites. The anatomical sites and site-specific histological sub-types of 1182 sarcomas treated at a single referral institution are outlined in Figure 55.1. Approximately one-third to one-half of all soft tissue sarcomas occur in the extremities, where the most common histopathological subtypes are malignant fibrous histiocytoma and liposarcoma. These are the focus of the first part of the chapter. Retroperitoneal sarcomas comprise 15% to 20% of all soft tissue sarcomas, with liposarcoma and leiomyosarcoma being the predominant histological subtypes. These are discussed separately at the end of the chapter. The visceral sarcomas make up an additional 24%, while the head and neck sarcomas comprise approximately 4% of all sarcomas seen at a tertiary care cancer center (Fig. 55.1).

Histological Classification

In broad terms, sarcomas can be classified into neoplasms arising in bone and those arising from the periosseous soft tissue. Sarcomas of the soft tissues can be further grouped into those that arise from viscera (gastrointestinal, genitourinary, and gynecological organs) and those that originate in nonvisceral soft tissues such as muscle, tendon, adipose tissue, pleura, synovium, and connective tissue.

The most universally applied classification scheme for soft tissue sarcoma is based on histogenesis, as outlined in the recent World Health Organization (WHO) classification system for sarcomas.[3] This classification system is reproducible for the better-differentiated tumors. However, as the degree of histological differentiation declines, the determination of cellular origin becomes increasingly difficult. Nonetheless, difficulties in establishing the specific cellular origin have limited clinical importance because the histological subtype is not generally directly related to biological behavior. Important exceptions to this generalization include epithelioid sarcoma, clear cell sarcoma, angiosarcoma, and embryonal rhabdomyosarcoma, all of which have a greater risk of regional lymph node metastasis.[4,5]

Histological Grading

Biologic aggressiveness can be best predicted on the basis of histological grade.[6,7] In careful comparative multivariate

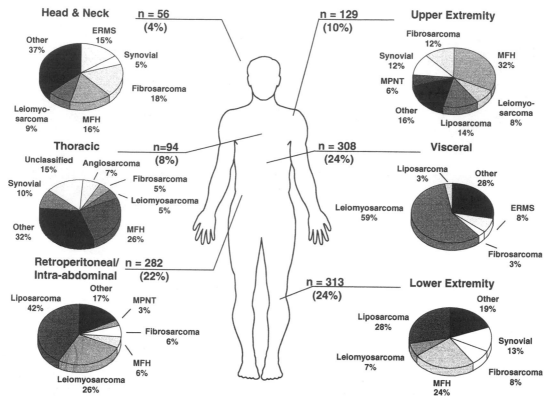

FIGURE 55.1. Anatomical distribution and site-specific histological subtypes of 1182 consecutive patients with soft tissue sarcomas seen at The University of Texas M.D. Anderson Cancer Center (University of Texas M.D. Anderson Cancer Center Sarcoma Database, June 1996–December 1998). MFH, malignant fibrous histiocytoma; ERMS, embryonal rhabdomyasarcoma; MPNT, malignant peripheral nerve sheath tumor.

analyses, histological grade has been the most important prognostic factor in assessing the risk for distant metastasis and tumor-related mortality.[6,7] Several grading systems have been proposed, but there is no consensus regarding the specific morphological criteria that should be employed in the grading of soft tissue sarcomas.

Clinical Presentation and Diagnosis

The majority of patients present with a painless mass, although pain is noted at presentation in up to a third of cases.[2] Delay in diagnosis or sarcomas is common, with the most common incorrect diagnosis for extremity and trunk lesions being hematoma or "pulled muscle."

Physical examination should include an assessment of the size and mobility of the mass. Its relationship to the fascia (superficial versus deep) and nearby neurovascular and bony structures should be noted. A site-specific neurovascular examination and assessment of regional lymph nodes should also be performed.

Imaging

Optimal imaging of the primary tumor is dependent on the anatomic site. For soft tissue masses of the extremities, magnetic resonance imaging (MRI) has been regarded as the imaging modality of choice. However, a recent study that compared MRI and computed tomography (CT) in patients with malignant bone and soft tissue tumors showed no specific ad-

vantage of MRI over CT.[8] For pelvic lesions, the multiplanar capability of MRI may provide superior single-modality imaging. In the retroperitoneum and abdomen, CT usually provides satisfactory anatomical definition of the lesion. More invasive studies such as angiography or cavography are almost never required for the evaluation of soft tissue sarcomas.

Biopsy

Biopsy of the primary tumor is essential for most patients presenting with soft tissue masses. In general, any soft tissue mass in an adult that is asymptomatic or enlarging, is larger than 5 cm, or persists beyond 4 to 6 weeks should be biopsied. The preferred biopsy approach is generally the least invasive technique required to allow a definitive histological diagnosis and assessment of grade. In most centers, core needle biopsy provides satisfactory tissue for diagnosis[9–11] and has been demonstrated to result in substantial cost savings compared to open surgical biopsy.[11] Needle tract tumor recurrences after percutaneous biopsy are rare but have been reported.[12] A practical approach for biopsy and staging of the patient who presents with a primary extremity soft tissue mass is outlined in Figure 55.2.

Staging

The relative rarity of soft tissue sarcomas, the anatomical heterogeneity of these lesions, and the presence of more than 30 recognized histological subtypes of variable grade have made

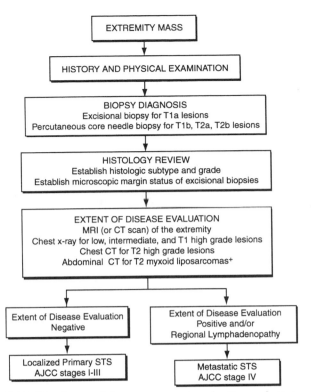

FIGURE 55.2. Approach for pretreatment evaluation and staging of the patient with a primary extremity soft tissue mass. *AJCC*, American Joint Commission on Cancer. (From Pisters PWT. Ann Surg Oncol 1998;5:464–472, with permission.)

TABLE 55.1. American Joint Commission on Cancer/International Union Against Cancer Staging System for Soft Tissue Sarcomas.

T1		≤5 cm		
T1a		Superficial to muscular fascia		
T1b		Deep to muscular fascia		
T2		>5 cm		
T2a		Superficial to muscular fascia		
T2b		Deep to muscular fascia		
N1		Regional nodal involvement		
G1		Well differentiated		
G2		Moderately differentiated		
G3		Poorly differentiated		
G4		Undifferentiated		
Stage I	G1, 2	T1a, b, T2a,b	N0	M0
Stage II	G3, 4	T1a, b, T2a,b	N0	M0
Stage III	G3, 4	T2b	N0	M0
Stage IV	Any G	Any T	N1	M0
	Any G	Any T	Any N	M1

Source: Used with the permission of the American Joint Committee on Cancer (AJCC) Chicago, IL. The original source for this material is the AJCC Cancer Staging Manual, Sixth Ed. (2002) published by Springer-Verlag New York, www.springer-ny.com.

it difficult to establish a functional system that can accurately stage all forms of this disease. The recently revised staging system (6th edition) of the American Joint Committee on Cancer (AJCC) and the International Union Against Cancer (UICC) is the most widely employed staging system for soft tissue sarcomas.[13] Four distinct histological grades are recognized, ranging from well differentiated to undifferentiated. Histological grade and tumor size are the primary determinants of clinical stage (Table 55.1). The system is designed to optimally stage extremity tumors but is also applicable to torso, head and neck, and retroperitoneal lesions; it should not be used for sarcomas of the gastrointestinal tract.

Prognostic Factors

Conventional Clinicopathological Factors

Multiple studies have shown an adverse prognostic significance of large (≥5 cm), high grade, deeply located tumors. Results of regression analyses for these and other factors using the endpoints of local recurrence, distant recurrence (metastasis), and disease-specific survival are shown in Table 55.2. Note that patients with a constellation of adverse prognostic factors for local recurrence are not necessarily at increased risk for distant metastasis or tumor-related death.

Potential Molecular Prognostic Factors

Specific molecular parameters evaluated for prognostic significance have included p53,[14] mdm2,[14] Ki-67,[14] altered ex-

pression of the retinoblastoma gene product (pRb)[15,16] in high-grade sarcomas, and the presence of SYT-SSX fusion transcripts in synovial sarcoma[17] or EWS-FL11 fusion transcripts in Ewing's sarcoma.[18,19] Complete discussion of the extensive literature on molecular prognostic factors in sarcoma is beyond the scope of this chapter. Of these, Ki-67 score seems most likely to have prognostic significance. Still, although specific cellular and molecular parameters have been identified as having independent prognostic significance, there is presently no consensus on how these prognostic factors should be utilized in clinical practice.

Treatment of Localized Primary Soft Tissue Sarcoma

Surgery

Surgical resection remains the cornerstone of therapy for localized primary soft tissue sarcoma. Currently, at least 90% of patients with localized extremity sarcomas can undergo limb-sparing procedures with postoperative external beam radiotherapy (EBRT) and chemotherapy (e.g. doxorubicin, cyclophosphamide, and methotrexate).[20,21] Most surgeons consider definite major vascular, bony, or nerve involvement as relative indications for amputation. Complex en bloc bone, vascular, and nerve resections with interposition grafting can be undertaken, but the associated morbidity is high. Therefore, for a few patients with critical involvement of major bony or neurovascular structures, amputation remains the only surgical option but offers the prospect of prompt rehabilitation with excellent local control and survival.[22] Given the low (2%–3%) prevalence of lymph node metastasis in adults with sarcomas,[4,5] there is no role for routine regional lymph node dissection.

TABLE 55.2. Multivariate Analysis of Prognostic Factors in Patients with Extremity Soft Tissue Sarcoma.

Endpoint	Adverse prognostic factor	Relative risk
Local recurrence	Fibrosarcoma	2.5
	Local recurrence at presentation	2.0
	Microscopically positive surgical margin	1.8
	Malignant peripheral nerve sheath tumor	1.8
	Age >50 years	1.6
Distant recurrence	High grade	4.3
	Deep location	2.5
	Size 5.0–9.9 cm	1.9
	Leiomyosarcoma	1.7
	Nonliposarcoma histology	1.6
	Local recurrence at presentation	1.5
	Size ≥10.0 cm	1.5
Disease-specific survival	High grade	4.0
	Deep location	2.8
	Size ≥10.0 cm	2.1
	Malignant peripheral nerve sheath tumor	1.9
	Leiomyosarcoma	1.9
	Microscopically positive surgical margin	1.7
	Lower-extremity site	1.6
	Local recurrence at presentation	1.5

Adverse prognostic factors identified are independent by Cox regression analysis.
Source: Pisters et al.,[6] by permission of *Journal of Clinical Oncology.*

Surgery Alone

Although the majority of patients with extremity soft tissue sarcoma should receive pre- or postoperative radiotherapy (see following section), recent reports suggest that radiotherapy may not be required for selected patients with completely resected, small (probably ≤5 cm), primary soft tissue sarcomas.[23–27]

Preoperative or Postoperative Radiotherapy

Data from two phase III trials[28,29] have confirmed several retrospective reports suggesting that conservative (limb sparing) surgery combined with radiotherapy results in superior local control compared to surgery alone for patients with localized soft tissue sarcoma. Patients with high-grade tumors receive chemotherapy as well. Radiotherapy can be administered preoperatively, postoperatively, or by interstitial techniques (brachytherapy). No one route has proven superior, although head-to head trials are underway. Still, despite the improvement in local recurrence, there has been no demonstrable survival benefit using this modality.[30–32]

Postoperative Chemotherapy

EFFICACY OF POSTOPERATIVE CHEMOTHERAPY

Despite two decades of randomized trials, the role of postoperative chemotherapy in the management of localized soft tissue sarcoma remains controversial. Level I evidence is found in 12 published randomized trials evaluating postoperative chemotherapy in patients with localized soft tissue sarcoma.[33–46] Each of these trials had a control arm that received surgery (+/− radiotherapy) without postoperative chemotherapy and a group that received surgery plus postoperative systemic therapy with doxorubicin alone or doxorubicin-based combination chemotherapy. Four of the trials reported significantly improved relapse-free survival rates with postoperative chemotherapy, but only 2 of 12 trials found a statisti-

cally significant improvement in overall survival rates. These trials contain recognized deficiencies in design and conduct. The most commonly cited deficiencies relate to the relatively small sample size and to the fact that small differences in survival require relatively large numbers of patients to detect with sufficient statistical power. The statistical tool of meta-analysis is designed to address these deficiencies by examining a group of similarly designed clinical trials. Recently, the Sarcoma Meta-Analysis Collaboration (SMAC) group reported on a comprehensive meta-analysis of the published randomized trials evaluating local therapy plus adjuvant doxorubicin-based chemotherapy versus local therapy alone.[47] This meta-analysis demonstrated statistically significantly improved local and distant recurrence-free survival and disease-free survival rates in patients who received doxorubicin-containing postoperative chemotherapy (Table 55.3). However, there was no statistically significant improvement in overall survival rates in this meta-analysis of individual patient data. As a significant improvement in survival with postoperative chemotherapy has not been detected with these advanced statistical techniques, it appears reasonable to conclude that if such a benefit exists, it must be quite small.

Given these findings, most investigators agree that postoperative chemotherapy should not be given to patients with low-grade sarcomas because of their inherently low rates of systemic disease spread.

Preoperative Chemotherapy

Preoperative chemotherapy has specific theoretical advantages over postoperative treatment. First, preoperative chemotherapy provides an in vivo test of chemosensitivity. Patients whose tumors show objective evidence of response are presumed to be the subset who will benefit most from further postoperative systemic treatment. In contrast, it is assumed that the population of nonresponding patients defined by this in vivo assessment will derive minimal or no benefit from further chemo-

TABLE 55.3.

Sarcoma Meta-Analysis Collaboration Group's Meta-Analysis of Randomized Doxorobucin-Based Postoperative Chemotherapy in Soft Tissue Sarcoma.

Endpoint	Hazard ratio	Absolute benefit	p value
Local recurrence-free interval	0.74	6% (75% → 81%)	0.024
Distant recurrence-free interval	0.69	10% (60% → 70%)	0.0003
Overall recurrence-free interval	0.69	13% (45% → 58%)	0.000008
Overall recurrence-free survival	0.74	11% (40% → 51%)	0.00008
Overall survival	0.87	5% (50% → 55%)	0.087

Source: Tierney et al.,[47] by permission of Lancet.

postoperative therapy and can therefore be spared its toxicity. A second theoretical advantage of preoperative chemotherapy is that it treats occult micrometastatic disease as soon after the cancer diagnosis as possible. This may prevent the development of chemoresistance by isolated clones of metastatic cells or prevent the postoperative growth of micrometastases. Finally, chemotherapy-induced cytoreduction may permit a less radical and consequently less morbid surgical resection than would have been required initially. In patients with large soft tissue sarcomas of the extremities, cytoreduction may reduce the morbidity of limb-salvage surgical procedures and possibly even allow patients who might otherwise have required an amputation to undergo limb-salvage surgery. Nonetheless, despite these theoretical advantages, the exact benefit of preoperative chemotherapy remains unclear.

Combined Preoperative Chemotherapy and Radiotherapy

The benefit of this approach remains largely investigational.

Hyperthermic Isolated Limb Perfusion

Hyperthermic isloated limb perfusion (HILP) is an investigational technique that has been evaluated for the treatment of extremity soft tissue sarcomas in the setting of (1) locally advanced extremity lesions amenable only to amputation used in an attempt to preserve the limb, and (2) locally advanced extremity lesions with synchronous pulmonary metastases, for which HILP is employed in an effort to preserve a functional extremity for the short survival anticipated in the setting of stage IV disease. A multicenter phase II trial has evaluated a series of 55 patients with radiologically unresectable extremity soft tissue sarcomas treated with HILP using high-dose tumor necrosis factor-α, interferon-γ, and melphalan.[48] A major tumor response was seen in 87% of patients: complete responses in 20 (36%) and partial responses in 28 (51%). Limb salvage was achieved in 84% of patients. Regional toxicity was limited, and systemic toxicity was minimal to moderate. There were no treatment-related deaths. This approach is presently being further evaluated in ongoing trials in Europe.

Treatment of Sarcoma Patients at Specialty Centers

Recent data on other tumor types have demonstrated improved outcomes for patients requiring complex treatment who are treated at specialty centers.[49,50] Similar data confirm the same phenomenon in soft tissue sarcoma.[51,52]

Treatment of Locally Recurrent Soft Tissue Sarcoma

Incidence of Local Recurrence

Despite optimal multimodality therapy, at least 20% to 30% of soft tissue sarcoma patients will develop locally recurrent disease, with a median disease-free interval of 18 months.[6,53]

Surgery and Radiotherapy

Locally recurrent disease generally presents as a nodular mass or series of nodules arising in the surgical scar or radiation port. Treatment approaches for patients with locally recurrent soft tissue sarcoma need to be individualized based on local anatomical constraints and the limitations on present treatment options imposed by prior therapies. In general, all patients with locally recurrent sarcoma should be evaluated for reresection of their local recurrence. The results of such "salvage surgery" are good, with two-thirds of patients experiencing long-term survival.[54,55]

If no prior radiotherapy was employed, adjuvant radiation should be utilized after surgery for locally recurrent disease. If subtherapeutic or low-dose radiation was previously employed, patients may be candidates for additional adjuvant radiation by external-beam or brachytherapy approaches. Patients who have had a full course of prior radiation should be managed on an individual basis.

Relationship Between Local Control and Survival

Whether local control impacts overall survival for patients with soft tissue sarcoma remains unclear and highly controversial.[56–60] None of the currently available prospective randomized data support the hypothesis that better local control enhances survival in patients with sarcoma.

Treatment of Metastatic Soft Tissue Sarcoma

The most common site of metastasis from soft tissue sarcoma of the extremity is the lungs. Indeed, the lungs are the only site of recurrence in approximately 80% of all patients with metastases from primary extremity and trunk soft tissue sarcomas.[53,61] Primary visceral and gastrointestinal sarcomas also commonly metastasize to the liver. Extrapulmonary metastases are uncommon forms of first metastasis and usually occur as a late manifestation of widely disseminated disease.[53] The median survival after development of distant metastases is 11.6 months.[62]

Surgical Resection

Multiple investigators have reported their experience with pulmonary metastasectomy for metastatic soft tissue sarcoma in adults.[63–72] Three-year survival rates following thoracotomy for pulmonary metastasectomy range from 23% to 54%. Adverse prognostic factors for patients with pulmonary metastases, as determined by univariate and multivariate analyses, include short disease-free interval and tumor doubling time, the number (>3) of pulmonary nodules on preoperative chest CT, and, most significantly, incomplete pulmonary resection or inability to resect all disease. In selecting patients to undergo pulmonary metastatectomy, the following criteria are generally agreed: (1) the primary tumor is controlled or is controllable, (2) there is not extrathoracic disease, (3) the patient is a medical candidate for thoracotomy and pulmonary resection, and (4) complete resection of all disease appears possible.[73] With careful patient selection, the morbidity of thoracotomy can be limited to the subset of patients who are most likely to benefit from this aggressive treatment approach.

Chemotherapy

Soft tissue sarcoma patients with unresectable pulmonary metastases or extrapulmonary metastatic disease have a generally poor prognosis and usually are best treated with systemic chemotherapy or supportive care. A number of agents including cyclophosphamide, dactinomycin, and vincristine have been studied and have produced response rates between 5% and 10%.[74,75] Doxorubicin was the first and remains the most active single chemotherapeutic agent in soft tissue sarcoma.[76–80] A variety of schedules and doses have been employed,[77,78,81] with objective overall response rates of approximately 25% in the advanced disease setting.[82] Unfortunately, however, there is little difference in survival rates between responders and nonresponders to chemotherapy.

Treatment of Retroperitoneal Sarcomas

Presentation and Pretreatment Evaluation

Retroperitoneal sarcomas are relatively uncommon, accounting for approximately 15% of all sarcomas (see Fig. 55.1). The most common histological subtypes are liposarcoma and leiomyosarcoma (Fig. 55.1). Nearly 80% of patients present with an abdominal mass, and 50% of patients report pain at the time of presentation.[83] Patients commonly describe nonspecific gastrointestinal symptoms. Other commonly noted symptoms include neurological symptoms (primarily sensory) in 27% and weight loss in 7%.[83,84] These tumors often grow to substantial size before the patient's nonspecific complaints are evaluated or an abdominal mass is noted on physical examination.

The differential diagnosis for a retroperitoneal mass is relatively limited when soft tissue neoplasms are considered as a group. Physical examination should include a testicular examination in men to evaluate the possibility of a primary testicular neoplasm. Laboratory tests should include the common serum markers for germ cell tumors, beta-human chorionic gonadotropin, and alpha-fetoprotein. If physical examination is suggestive of malignancy or biochemical markers are elevated, testicular ultrasonography should be performed. This modality may obviate laparotomy for patients with metastatic testicular tumors and allow for identification of primary retroperitoneal germ cell tumors.

CT and MRI are the primary methods used to image retroperitoneal tumors.[85–87] These modalities allow for assessment of the consistency of the mass (cystic or solid components, associated necrosis), precise anatomical location of the mass, and the extent of any regional disease and for confirmation of function of the kidneys. CT of the abdomen and pelvis usually provides images satisfactory for treatment planning. Occasionally, MRI with flow-sensitive gradient sequence imaging may be helpful in defining vascular anatomy for surgical planning. For patients with an abnormal chest radiograph, chest CT should be performed to exclude the possibility of metastatic disease.

In general, preoperative biopsy is not necessary when surgical resection is planned for a resectable primary retroperitoneal mass. However, there are specific circumstances in which biopsy of primary retroperitoneal masses should be performed. These include (1) clinical suspicion of lymphoma or germ cell tumor, (2) tissue diagnosis for preoperative treatment, (3) tissue diagnosis of radiologic unresectable disease, and (4) suspected retroperitoneal or intraabdominal metastasis from another primary tumor. In the main, however, for patients for whom exploratory laparotomy is planned, surgical resection or intraoperative incisional biopsy (for unresectable lesions) is the best means of establishing a tissue diagnosis of a potentially resectable retroperitoneal mass.

Surgical Resection

Surgical resection with negative margins remains the standard primary treatment for patients with localized retroperitoneal sarcoma. Because en bloc multiorgan resection may be required to achieve negative margins, all patients should have preoperative bowel preparation and assessment of bilateral renal function by CT. Resectability rates in recent series combining patients with primary and recurrent retroperitoneal sarcomas range from 25% to 95%. The ability to achieve complete surgical resection (resection of all gross tumor) is a function of presentation—primary lesions are more likely to be completely resected than are locally recurrent retroperitoneal sarcomas, and the ability to achieve complete resection declines as the number of local recurrences increases (Fig. 55.3). The most common reasons for unresectability are the presence of major vascular involvement (aorta or vena cava), peritoneal implants, or distant metastases.[83] Resection of adjacent retroperitoneal or intraabdominal organs, frequently the kidney, colon, or pancreas, is required in the majority (50%–80%) of cases to permit complete resection.[83,88,89] Partial resections or debulking procedures have been performed, but there is no evidence that partial resection improves survival.[83,89]

The survival of patients with retroperitoneal sarcoma is

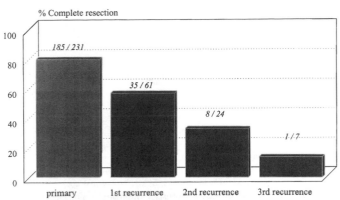

% Complete resection

FIGURE 55.3. Rate of initial complete resection for 231 patients presenting with primary retroperitoneal sarcoma and rates of complete resection for subsequent local recurrences stratified by recurrence number. The number of patients who underwent complete resection divided by those undergoing attempted resection is indicated above each bar. The ability to achieve complete tumor resection declined as the number of recurrences increased. (From Lewis et al.,[90] by permission of *Annals of Surgery.*)

largely related to clinical presentation: the median disease-specific survivals of patients with primary disease, locally recurrent disease, and metastatic disease are 72 months, 28 months, and 10 months, respectively. The median survival of patients with incompletely resected retroperitoneal sarcomas is 18 months and is comparable to that of patients who do not undergo resection.[90]

Local recurrence is a significant problem, with recurrence rates of 40–50% or higher. Thus, improving local control for patients with retroperitoneal sarcoma remains one of the most clinically significant challenges.

Postoperative follow-up strategies are based on the continuing risk for local failure and the difficulties inherent in detecting recurrent disease by clinical criteria alone. Serial CT or MRI should be utilized for follow-up as detection of recurrent retroperitoneal sarcoma by physical examination of identification of symptoms is unreliable. There are no published data to make specific follow-up recommendations, but because many patients develop late (>5 years) recurrence, it is clear that follow-up should continue at least 10 years after initial treatment.[91,92] Any sign of recurrent disease should be investigated promptly because complete resection of recurrent disease is often possible and is associated with 5-year survival rates of 50% or greater.[83,93]

In univariate and multivariate analyses, adverse prognostic factors for retroperitoneal sarcomas include incomplete surgical resection, high histologic grade, tumor size (>10 cm), and fixation to adjacent retroperitoneal structures other than neurovascular bundles or bone.

Postoperative Radiation Therapy and Chemotherapy

Postoperative EBRT has been shown to reduce local recurrence rates for extremity and superficial trunk sarcomas. However, gastrointestinal or neural toxicities often limit the delivery of sufficient radiation doses to the retroperitoneum. Currently, there is no consensus on the role of postoperative EBRT following complete resection of retroperitoneal sarcomas. Preoperative EBRT and intraoperative radiation therapy

(IORT) both show promise, but at this time remain largely investigational.

Retrospective studies have not demonstrated any benefit to preoperative[94] or postoperative[83,95,96] doxorubicin-based chemotherapy for retroperitoneal sarcomas, and so the routine use of chemotherapy in these patients cannot be supported.

References

1. Landis SH, Murray T, Bolden S, et al. Cancer statistics, 1999. CA J Clin 1999;49:8–31.
2. Lawrence W Jr, Donegan WL, Natarajan N, et al. Adult soft tissue sarcomas. a pattern of care survey of the American College of Surgeons. Ann Surg 1987;205:349–359.
3. Weiss SW, Sobin LH. Histologic typing of soft tissue tumors. 2nd ed. Berlin: Springer-Verlag 1994.
4. Fong Y, Coit DG, Woodruff JM, et al. Lymph node metastasis from soft tissue sarcoma in adults: analysis of date from a prospective database of 1772 sarcoma patients. Ann Surg 1993; 217:72–77.
5. Weingrad DN, Rosenberg SA. Early lymphatic spread of osteogenic and soft-tissue sarcomas. Surgery 1978;84:231–240.
6. Pisters PWT, Leung DHY, Woodruff J, et al. Analysis of prognostic factors in 1041 patients with localized soft tissue sarcomas of the extremities. J Clin Oncol 1996;14:1679–1689.
7. Coindre JM, Terrier P, Bui NB, et al. Prognostic factors in adult patients with locally controlled soft tissue sarcoma. A study of 546 patients from the French Federation of Cancer Centers Sarcoma Group. J Clin Oncol 1996;14:869–877.
8. Panicek DM, Gatsonis C, Rosenthal DI, et al. CT and MR imaging in the local staging of primary malignant musculoskeletal neoplasms: report of the Radiology Diagnostic Oncology Group. Radiology 1997;202:237–246.
9. Heslin MJ, Lewis JJ, Woodruff JM, et al. Core needle biopsy for diagnosis of extremity soft tissue sarcoma. Ann Surg Oncol 1997;4:425–431.
10. Ball AB, Fisher C, Pittam M, et al. Diagnosis of soft tissue tumours by Tru-Cut biopsy. Br J Surg 1990;77:756–758.
11. Skrzynski MC, Biermann JS, Montag A, et al. Diagnostic accuracy and charge-savings of outpatient core needle biopsy compared with open biopsy of musculoskeletal tumors. J Bone Joint Surg Am 1996;78:644–649.
12. Schwartz HS, Spengler DM. Needle tract recurrences after closed biopsy for sarcoma: three cases and review of the literature. Ann Surg Oncol 1997;4:228–236.
13. Pollock RE. Soft Tissue Sarcoma. In: Greene FL, Page DL, Fleming ID, et al. eds. AJCC Staging Manual, Sixth Ed. New York: Springer-Verlag 2002:193–200.
14. Heslin MJ, Cordon-Cardo C, Lewis JJ, et al. Ki-67 detected by MIB-1 predicts distant metastasis and tumor mortality in primary, high grade extremity soft tissue sarcoma. Cancer 1998;83: 490–497.
15. Cance WG, Brennan MF, Dudas ME, et al. Altered expression of the retinoblastoma gene product in human sarcomas. N Engl J Med 1990;323:1457–1462.
16. Karpeh MS, Brennan MF, Cance WG, et al. Altered patterns of retinoblastoma gene product expression in adult soft-tissue sarcomas. Br J Cancer 1995;72:986–991.
17. Kawai A, Woodruff J, Healey JH, et al. SYT-SSX gene fusion as a determinant of morphology and prognosis in synovial sarcoma. N Engl J Med 1998;338:153–160.
18. Zoubek A, Dockhorn-Dworniczak B, Delattre O, et al. Does expression of different EWS chimeric transcripts define clinically distinct risk groups of Ewing tumor patients? J Clin Oncol 1996; 14:1245–1251.
19. de Alava E, Kawai A, Healey JH, et al. EWS-FLII fusion tran-

script structure is an independent determinant of prognosis in Ewing's sarcoma. J Clin Oncol 1998;16:1248–1255.

20. Williard WC, Collin CF, Casper ES, et al. The changing role of amputation for soft tissue sarcoma of the extremity in adults. Surg Gynecol Obstet 1992;175:389–396.

21. Brennan MF, Casper ES, Harrison LB, et al. The role of multimodality therapy in soft-tissue sarcoma. Ann Surg 1991;214:328–337.

22. Yang JC, Rosenberg SA. Surgery for adult patients with soft tissue sarcomas. Semin Oncol 1989;16:289–296.

23. Karakousis CP, Proimakis C, Walsh DL. Primary soft tissue sarcoma of the extremities in adults. Br J Surg 1995;82:1208–1212.

24. Geer RJ, Woodruff J, Casper ES, et al. Management of small soft-tissue sarcoma of the extremity in adults. Arch Surg 1992;127:1285–1289.

25. Rydholm A, Gustafson P, Rooser B, et al. Limb-sparing surgery without radiotherapy based on anatomic location of soft tissue sarcoma. J Clin Oncol 1991;9:1757–1765.

26. Healey B, Corson JM, Demetri GD, et al. Surgery alone may be adequate treatment for select stage IA–IIIA soft tissue sarcomas [abstract]. Proc Am Soc Clin Oncol 1995;14:517.

27. Respondek P, Pollack A, Feig BW, et al. Prospective trial of conservative surgery and selective use of radiotherapy for AJCC T1 extremity and trunk soft tissue sarcomas [abstract]. Sarcoma 1997;1:219.

28. Yang JC, Chang AE, Baker AR, et al. A randomized prospective study of the benefit of adjuvant radiation therapy in the treatment of soft tissue sarcomas of the extremity. J Clin Oncol 1998;16:197–203.

29. Pisters PWT, Harrison LB, Leung DHY, et al. Long-term results of a prospective randomized trial of adjuvant brachytherapy in soft tissue sarcoma. J Clin Oncol 1996;14:859–868.

30. Barkley HT Jr, Martin RG, Romsdahl MM, et al. Treatment of soft tissue sarcomas by preoperative irradiation and conservative surgical resection. Int J Radiat Oncol Biol Phys 1988;14:693–699.

31. Lindberg RD, Martin RG, Romsdahl MM, et al. Conservative surgery and postoperative radiotherapy in 300 adults with soft-tissue sarcomas. Cancer 1981;47:2391–2397.

32. Suit HD, Mankin HJ, Wood WC, et al. Treatment of the patient with stage M0 soft tissue sarcoma. J Clin Oncol 1988;6:854–862.

33. Bui NB, Maree D, Coindre JM, et al. First results of a prospective randomized study of CYVADIC adjuvant chemotherapy in adults with operable high risk soft tissue sarcoma [abstract]. Proc Am Soc Clin Oncol 1989;8:318.

34. Bramwell VHC, Rouesse J, Steward W, et al. Adjuvant CYVADIC chemotherapy for adult soft tissue sarcoma—reduced local recurrence but no improvement in survival: a study of the European Organization for Research and Treatment of Cancer Soft Tissue and Bone Sarcoma Group. J Clin Oncol 1994;12:1137–1149.

35. Glenn J, Sindelar WF, Kinsella T, et al. Results of multimodality therapy of resectable soft-tissue sarcomas of the retroperitoneum. Surgery 1985;97:316–325.

36. Glenn J, Kinsella T, Glatstein E, et al. A randomized, prospective trial of adjuvant chemotherapy in adults with soft tissue sarcomas of the head and neck, breast, and trunk. Cancer 1985;55:1206–1214.

37. Edmonson JH, Fleming TR, Ivins JC, et al. Randomized study of systemic chemotherapy following complete excision of nonosseous sarcomas. J Clin Oncol 1984;2:1390–1396.

38. Edmonson JH. Role of adjuvant chemotherapy in the management of patients with soft tissue sarcomas. Cancer Treat Rep 1984;68:1063–1066.

39. Eiber FR, Giuliano AE, Huth JF, et al. A randomized prospective trial using postoperative adjuvant chemotherapy (Adriamycin) in high-grade extremity soft-tissue sarcoma. Am J Clin Oncol 1988;11:39–45.

40. Alvegard TA, Sigurdsson H, Mouridsen H, et al. Adjuvant chemotherapy with doxorubicin in high-grade soft tissue sarcoma: a randomized trial of the Scandinavian Sarcoma Group. J Clin Oncol 1989;7:1504–1513.

41. Picci P, Bacci G, Gherlinzoni F, et al. Results of a randomized trial for the treatment of localized soft tissue tumors (STS) of the extremities in adult patients. In: Ryan JR, Baker LO, eds. Recent concepts in sarcoma treatment. Dordrecht: Kluwer Academic Publishers, 1988:144–148.

42. Antman K, Amato D, Lerner H. Eastern Cooperative Oncology Group and Dana-Farber Cancer Institute/Massachusetts General Hospital study. In: Jones S, Salmon S, eds. Adjuvant Therapy of Cancer. 4th ed. Orlando: Grune & Stratton, 1984:611–620.

43. Antman K, Anato D, Lerner H, et al. Adjuvant doxorubicin for sarcoma: data from the Eastern Cooperative Oncology Group and Dana-Farber Cancer Institute/Massachusetts General Hospital studies. Cancer Treat Symp 1985;3:109–115.

44. Antman K, Suit H, Amato D, et al. Preliminary results of a randomized trial of adjuvant doxorubicin for sarcomas: lack of apparent difference between treatment groups. J Clin Oncol 1984;2:601–608.

45. Antman K, Amato D, Pilepich M, et al. A preliminary analysis of a randomized Intergroup (SWOG, ECOG, CALBG, NCOG) trial of adjuvant doxorubicin for soft tissue sarcomas. In: 5th ed. Orlando: Grune & Stratton, 1987:725–734.

46. Omura GA, Blessing JA, Major F, et al. A randomized clinical trial of adjuvant Adriamycin uterine sarcomas: a Gynecologic Oncology Group study. J Clin Oncol 1985;3:1240–1245.

47. Tierney JF. Adjuvant chemotherapy for localised resectable soft-tissue sarcoma of adults: meta-analysis of individual data. Lancet 1997;350:1647–1654.

48. Eggermont AMM, Shraffordt Koops H, Lienard D, et al. Isolated limb perfusion with high-dose tumor necrosis factor-α in combination with interferon-γ and melphalan for nonresectable extremity soft tissue sarcomas: a multicenter trial. J Clin Oncol 1996;14:2653–2665.

49. Begg CB, Cramer LD, Hoskins WJ, et al. Impact of hospital volume on operative mortality for major cancer surgery. JAMA 1998;280:1747–1751.

50. Birkmeyer JD, Finlayson SR, Tosteson AN, et al. Effect of hospital volume on in-hospital mortality with pancreaticoduodenectomy. Surgery 1999;125:250–256.

51. Clasby R, Tilling K, Smith MA, et al. Variable management of soft tissue sarcoma: regional audit with implications for specialist care. Br J Surg 1997;84:1692–1696.

52. Gustafson P, Dreinhofer KE, Rydholm A. Soft tissue sarcoma should be treated at a tumor center: a comparison of quality of surgery in 375 patients. Acta Orthop Scand 1994;65:47–50.

53. Potter DA, Glenn J, Kinsella T, et al. Patterns of recurrence in patients with high-grade soft-tissue sarcomas. J Clin Oncol 1985;3:353–366.

54. Singer S, Antman K, Corson JM, et al. Long-term salvageability for patients with locally recurrent soft-tissue sarcomas. Arch Surg 1992;127:548–553.

55. Midis GP, Pollock RE, Chen NP, et al. Locally recurrent soft tissue sarcoma of the extremities. Surgery 1998;123:666–671.

56. Stotter AT, Ahern RP, Fisher C, et al. The influence of local recurrence of extremity soft tissue sarcoma on metastasis and survival. Cancer 1990;65:1119–1129.

57. Barr LC, Stotter AT, A'Hern RP. Influence of local recurrence on survival: a controversy reviewed from the perspective of soft tissue sarcoma. Br J Surg 1991;78:648–650.

58. Rooser B, Gustafson P, Rydholm A. Is there no influence of local control on the rate of metastases in high-grade soft tissue sarcoma? Cancer 1990;65:1727–1729.

59. Gustafson P, Rooser B, Rydholm A. Is local recurrence of minor importance for metastases in soft tissue sarcoma? Cancer 1991;67:2083–2086.

60. Lewis JJ, Leung D, Heslin M, et al. Association of local recurrence with subsequent survival in extremity soft tissue sarcoma. J Clin Oncol 1997;15:646–652.

61. Brennan MF. The surgeons as a leader in cancer care: lessons learned from the study of soft tissue sarcoma. J Am Coll Surg 1996;182:520–529.

62. Billingsley KG, Lewis JJ, Leung DH, et al. Multifactorial analysis of the survival of patients with distant metastasis arising from primary extremity sarcoma. Cancer 1999;85:389–395.

63. Creagan ET, Fleming TR, Edmonson JH, et al. Pulmonary resection for metastatic nonosteogenic sarcoma. Cancer 1979;44:1908–1912.

64. Casson AG, Putnam JB, Natarajan G, et al. Five-year survival after pulmonary metastasectomy for adult soft tissue sarcoma. Cancer 1992;69:662–668.

65. Gadd MA, Casper ES, Woodruff JM, et al. Development and treatment of pulmonary metastases in adult patients with extremity soft-tissue sarcoma. Ann Surg 1993;218:705–712.

66. Huth JF, Holmes EC, Vernon SE, et al. Pulmonary resection for metastatic sarcoma. Am J Surg 1980;140:9–16.

67. McCormack PM, Martini N. The changing role of surgery for pulmonary metastases. Ann Thorac Surg 1979;28:139–145.

68. Morrow CE, Vassilopoulos PP, Grage TB. Surgical resection for metastatic neoplasms of the lung: experience at the University of Minnesota Hospitals. Cancer 1980;45:2981–2985.

69. Mountain CF, McMurtney MJ, Hermes KE. Surgery for pulmonary metastasis: a 20-year experience. Ann Thorac Surg 1984;38:323–330.

70. Pastorino U, Valente M, Gasparini M, et al. Lung resection for metastatic sarcomas: total survival from primary treatment. J Surg Oncol 1989;4:275–280.

71. Rizzoni WE, Pass HI, Wesley MN, et al. Resection of recurrent pulmonary metastases in patients with soft-tissue sarcomas. Arch Surg 1986;121:1248–1252.

72. van Geel AN, Pastorino U, Jauch KW, et al. Surgical treatment of lung metastases: the European Organization for Research and Treatment of Cancer-Soft Tissue and Bone Sarcoma Group study of 255 patients. Cancer 1996;77:675–682.

73. McCormack P. Surgical resection of pulmonary metastases. Semin Surg Oncol 1990;6:297–302.

74. Jacobs EM. Combination chemotherapy of metastatic testicular germinal cell tumors and soft part sarcomas. Cancer 1970;25:324–332.

75. Greenhall MJ, Magill GB, DeCosse JJ, et al. Chemotherapy for soft tissue sarcoma. Surg Gynecol Obstet 1986;162:193–198.

76. O'Bryan RM, Baker LH, Gottlieb JE, et al. Dose response evaluation of adriamycin in human neoplasia. Cancer 1977;39:1940–1948.

77. Schoenfeld DA, Rosenbaum C, Horton J, et al. A comparison of Adriamycin versus vincristine and Adriamycin, and cyclophosphamide versus vincristine, actinomycin-D, and cyclophosphamide for advanced sarcoma. Cancer 1982;50:2757–2762.

78. O'Bryan RM, Luce JK, Talley R, et al. Phase II evaluation of Adriamycin in human neoplasia. Cancer 1973;32:1–8.

79. Cruz AB Jr, Thames EA Jr, Aust JB, et al. Combination chemotherapy for soft-tissue sarcomas: a phase III study. J Surg Oncol 1979;11:313–323.

80. Creagan ET, Hahn RG, Ahmann DL, et al. A clinical trial of Adriamycin (NSC 123127) in advanced sarcomas. Oncology 1977;34:90–91.

81. Borden EC, Amato DA, Rosenbaum C, et al. Randomized comparison of three Adriamycin regimens for metastatic soft tissue sarcomas. J Clin Oncol 1987;5:840–850.

82. Gottlieb JA, Baker LH, O'Bryan RM, et al. Adriamycin (NSC-123127) used alone and in combination for soft tissue and bony sarcoma. Cancer Chemother Rep 1975;6(part 3):271–282.

83. Jaques DP, Coit DG, Hajdu SI, et al. Management of primary and recurrent soft-tissue sarcoma of the retroperitoneum. Ann Surg 1990;212:51–59.

84. Alvarenga JC, Ball AB, Fisher C, et al. Limitations of surgery in the treatment of retroperitoneal sarcoma. Br J Surg 1991;78:912–916.

85. Neifeld JP, Walsh JW, Lawrence W Jr. Computed tomography in the management of soft tissue tumors. Surg Gynecol Obstet 1982;155:535–540.

86. Sundaram M, McLeod RA. MR imaging of tumor and tumor like lesions of bone and soft tissue. AJR Am J Roentgenol 1990;155:817–824.

87. Manaser BJ, Ensign MF. Imaging of musculoskeletal tumors. Semin Oncol 1991;18:140–149.

88. Dalton RR, Donohue JH, Mucha P Jr, et al. Management of retroperitoneal sarcomas. Surgery 1989;106:725–733.

89. McGrath PC, Neifeld JP, Lawrence W Jr, et al. Improved survival following complete excision of retroperitoneal sarcomas. Ann Surg 1984;200:200–204.

90. Lewis JJ, Leung D, Woodruff JM, et al. Retroperitoneal soft-tissue sarcoma: analysis of 500 patients treated and followed at a single institution. Ann Surg 1998;228:355–365.

91. Heslin MJ, Lewis JJ, Nadler E, et al. Prognostic factors associated with long-term survival for retroperitoneal sarcoma: implications for management. J Clin Oncol 1997;15:2832–2839.

92. Catton CN, O'Sullivan B, Kotwall C, et al. Outcome and prognosis in retroperitoneal soft tissue sarcoma. Int J Radiat Oncol Biol Phys 1994;29:1005–1010.

93. Karakousis CP, Velez AF, Gerstenbluth R, et al. Resectability and survival in retroperitoneal sarcomas. Ann Surg Oncol 1996;3:150–158.

94. Storm FK, Eilber FR, Mirra J, et al. Retroperitoneal sarcomas: a reappraisal of treatment. J Surg Oncol 1981;17:1–7.

95. Bevilacqua RG, Rogatko A, Hajdu SI, et al. Prognostic factors in primary retroperitoneal soft-tissue sarcomas. Arch Surg 1991;126:328–334.

96. Karakousis CP, Velez AF, Emrich LJ. Management of retroperitoneal sarcomas and patient survival. Am J Surg 1985;150:376–380.

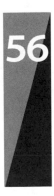

56

Head and Neck Malignancies

Carol R. Bradford

Head and neck cancer accounts for 4% of all new cancer cases and 2% of all cancer deaths in the United States annually. Survival rates have not significantly improved over the past three decades despite improvements in diagnosis and local management. Development of second primary tumors remains a major threat to long-term survival in patients initially cured of head and neck squamous cell carcinoma (HNSCC).[1] In addition to the problem of long-term survival in the face of second primary risk, HNSCC patients also face tremendous quality-of-life effects following definitive treatment. New strategies for the management of HNSCC are desperately needed.

Etiology and Epidemiology

Tobacco and Alcohol Exposure

Approximately 90% of head and neck cancers occur after exposure to known carcinogens, specifically tobacco and alcohol. Tobacco is a carcinogen that initiates a linear dose–response carcinogenic effect in which duration is more important than intensity of exposure.[2] In heavy smokers, roughly 15 years must pass before the risk approximates the level of nonsmokers. Smokeless tobacco and betel nut significantly elevate the risk of oral cavity cancers.

Alcohol is an equally important promoter of carcinogenesis and is a contributing factor in at least 75% of HNSCC.[3] The major clinical significance is that it potentiates the carcinogenic effect of tobacco at every level of tobacco use.

Viruses

Viral agents have been implicated in the pathogenesis of oral, laryngeal, and nasopharyngeal carcinomas. Increasing data has emerged supporting a role for human papilloma virus (HPV) in the development of head and neck neoplasms. There is also a strong epidemiological link between Epstein–Barr virus and nasopharyngeal carcinoma (NPC).

Diet

Considerable evidence suggests that vitamin A and β-carotene play a protective role in epithelial neoplasia.[4–6]

Radiation

Apparently, there is no strong association between exposure to ionizing radiation and development of squamous carcinoma of the head and neck.

Occupation

Exposure to nickel refining, woodworking, and leather working are risk factors for adenocarcinomas of the sinonasal region.[7–8]

Anatomy

The term "cancer of the head and neck" is most commonly applied to those cancers arising from the mucosal surfaces of the upper aerodigestive tract. Other relevant sites include the nose and paranasal sinuses as well as the salivary glands (major and minor).

Oral Cavity

The oral cavity includes the lips, buccal mucosa, anterior or oral tongue (two-thirds), floor of mouth, hard palate, as well as the upper and lower alveolar ridges and retromolar trigone (Fig. 56.1).

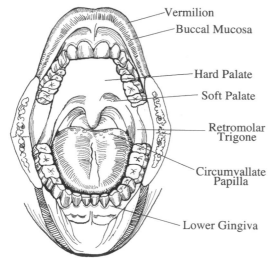

FIGURE 56.1. Oral cavity includes lips, floor of mouth, anterior two-thirds of tongue, buccal mucosa, hard palate, upper and lower alveolar ridge, and retromolar trigone.

Pharynx

The pharynx is a musculomembranous tube extending from the skull base to the cervical esophagus. The muscular support is from the superior, middle, and inferior constrictor muscles as well as other muscles arising from the styloid process and skull base. The pharynx can be subdivided into three distinct sites: the nasopharynx, oropharynx, and hypopharynx (Fig. 56.2).

Larynx

The larynx is composed of a mucosally covered cartilaginous framework (the thyroid and cricoid cartilages). The larynx is divided into three anatomically distinct regions: the supraglottis, the glottis, and the subglottis (Fig. 56.3).

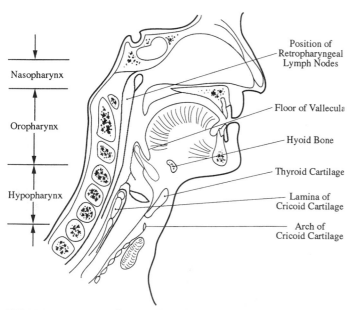

FIGURE 56.2. Sagittal view of the face and neck depicting the subdivisions of the pharynx as described in the text.

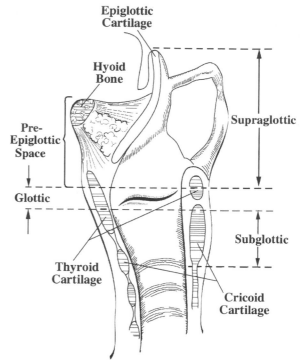

FIGURE 56.3. Sagittal view of the larynx depicting the subdivisions of the larynx. The preepiglottic space is that area anterior to the epiglottis bordered by the hyoid bone superiorly and the thyrohyoid membrane and superior rim of the thyroid cartilage anteriorly.

Neck

Anatomical considerations in the treatment of cancers of the head and neck must include a thorough understanding of the neural, vascular, and lymphatic structures of the neck. There are 10 major groups of lymph nodes in the head and neck: these include the occipital, mastoid, parotid, submandibular, facial, submental, sublingual, retropharyngeal, anterior cervical, and lateral cervical lymph node groups. Primary and secondary echelon lymph node drainage has been determined for each major site in the head and neck (Fig. 56.4).

Pathology

More than 90% of head and neck cancers are squamous cell carcinomas. Features reflecting aggressive behavior include presence of lymphatic invasion, perineural invasion, lymph node metastasis, and extracapsular spread (penetration of tumor through the capsule of the involved lymph node).[9] The presence of extracapsular spread in cervical lymph node metastasis has been associated with decreased disease-free and overall survival.[10]

Diagnosis

Early identification and treatment of squamous cell carcinomas of the upper aerodigestive tract is the most important component in reducing mortality from this devastating disease. Physicians and dentists must harbor a high index of suspicion and a low threshold for biopsy of any mucosal abnormality such as leukoplakia (a white patch) or erythroplasia (a red patch).[11]

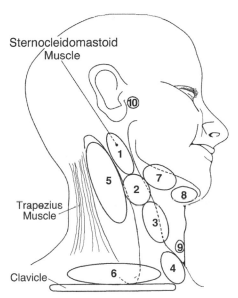

FIGURE 56.4. Depicted is a guide to usual lymphatic drainage patterns for head and neck malignancies as it pertains to usual patterns of early metastases. The primary lesions are listed under each level. (1) Superior jugular nodes: (a) nasopharynx, (b) base of tongue, (c) palatine tonsil, (d) parotid gland, and (e) larynx. (2) Subdigastric lymph nodes: (a) palatine tonsil, (b) tongue and other intraoral structures, (c) larynx, (d) oro- and hypopharynx, and (e) paranasal sinuses. (3) Middle jugular nodes: (a) larynx, (b) cervical esophagus, (c) hypopharynx, and (d) thyroid. (4) Inferior jugular nodes: (a) thyroid, (b) larynx, and (c) cervical esophagus. (5) Posterior cervical triangle (spinal accessory): (a) nasopharynx, (b) thyroid, and (c) posterior wall of hypopharynx (occasionally). (6) Supraclavicular: (a) lung, (b) breast, (c) virtually any head and neck primary, and (d) other locations below cavicles. (7) Submandibular: (a) intraoral primary (floor of mouth, buccal mucosa) and (b) submandibular salivary gland. (8) Submental: (a) lip, (b) anterior floor of mouth and alveolar ridge, (c) buccal mucosa and (d) breast. (9) Cricothyroid (delphian): (a) larynx and (b) thyroid. (10) Preauricular: (a) parotid salivary gland, (b) external auditory canal, (c) skin of lateral face, temple region, and scalp, and (d) genitourinary tract.

Dysphagia, odynophagia, referred otalgia, hoarseness, mucosal abnormalities, weight loss, and neck mass are the most common presenting complaints of HNSCC.[12] Unilateral serous otitis media is a sign of nasopharyngeal carcinoma. Nasal cavity or paranasal sinus neoplasms commonly present with unilateral nasal polyps, nasal obstruction, or epistaxis. A firm unilateral neck mass is cancer until proven otherwise. In an adult, 80% of firm neck masses represent cancer and most are cervical metastasis from HNSCC.

Most commonly, occult or unknown primaries responsible for cervical metastasis arise in the nasopharynx, tongue base, tonsil, or hypopharynx. Random biopsies from these sites are recommended in the setting of unknown primary with cervical metastasis. Fine-needle aspiration cytology of suspicious neck masses has greatly reduced the necessity of open cervical node biopsy for diagnosis of squamous cell carcinoma.

Staging

Staging criteria for cancers arising in the upper aerodigestive tract, paranasal sinuses, and salivary glands have been developed by the American Joint Council on Cancer (AJCC). The stage groupings for head and neck cancer are based upon T (primary tumor) stage, N (regional nodal status) stage, and M

TABLE 56.1. AJCC Definition for Regional Lymph Node (N) Staging for Head and Neck Cancer.

NX	Regional lymph nodes cannot be assessed
N0	No regional lymph node metastasis
*N1	Metastasis in a single ipsilateral lymph node, 3 cm or less in greatest dimension
*N2	Metastasis in a single ipsilateral lymph node, more than 3 cm but not more than 6 cm in greatest dimension; or in multiple ipsilateral lymph nodes, none more than 6 cm in greatest dimension; or in bilateral or contralateral lymph nodes, none more than 6 cm in greatest dimension
*N2a	Metastasis in a single ipsilateral lymph node more than 3 cm but no more than 6 cm in greatest dimension
*N2b	Metastasis in multiple ipsilateral lymph nodes, none more than 6 cm in greatest dimension
*N2c	Metastasis in bilateral or contralateral lymph nodes, none more than 6 cm in greatest dimension
*N3	Metastasis in a lymph node more than 6 cm in greatest dimension

*Note: A designation of "U" or "L" may be used to indicate metastasis above the lower border of the cricoid (U) or below the lower border of the cricoid (L).

Source: Used with permission of the American Joint Committee on Cancer (AJCC), Chicago, Illinois. The original source for this material is the AJCC Cancer Staging Manual, Sixth Ed. (2002) published by Springer-Verlag New York, www.springer-ny.com.

(distant metastasis). The regional lymph node staging for nasopharyngeal carcinoma varies slightly (Tables 56.1–56.3).

Treatment

General Principles

Surgery, with or without radiation therapy, is the mainstay of treatment for most head and neck cancers. Stage I and II tumors (T1N0M0 or T2N0M0) are typically treated with a single modality, either radiation therapy or surgery.[13] Stage III and IV tumors require a combined modality approach, typically surgery plus radiation therapy. Chemotherapy plus radiation therapy can be offered to patients with advanced cancers of the larynx or hypopharynx as an alternative to surgery plus radiation based upon the results of large, randomized, multiinstitutional trials. Surgical salvage of nonresponders or persistent/recurrent tumors is essential to not decrease overall survival rates in patients treated with organ preservation strategies.

The workup of a newly diagnosed head and neck cancer patient should include a complete history and physical examination, including a comprehensive head and neck examination. Biopsy should be performed of the primary and/or neck mass either in the office setting or in the operative room at the time of formal endoscopy. Triple or panendoscopy has traditionally been defined as direct laryngoscopy, full-length esophagoscopy, and bronchoscopy, although many head and neck surgeons per-

TABLE 56.2. AJCC Definition for Distant Metastasis (M) Staging for Head and Neck Cancer.

MX	Distant metastasis cannot be assessed
M0	No distant metastasis
M1	Distant metastasis

Source: Used with permission of the American Joint Committee on Cancer (AJCC), Chicago, Illinois. The original source for this material is the AJCC Cancer Staging Manual, Sixth Ed. (2002) published by Springer-Verlag New York, www.springer-ny.com.

TABLE 56.3. Clinical Tumor Stage Grouping for Head and Neck Cancer.

Stage I	T1	N0	M0
Stage II	T2	N0	M0
Stage III	T3	N0	M0
	Any T	N1	M0
Stage IV	T4	N0	M0
	T4	N1	M0
	Any T	N2	M0
	Any T	N3	M0
	Any T	Any N	M1

Source: Data from the 1997 AJCC Cancer Staging Manual.[22]

form only direct laryngoscopy and cervical esophagoscopy as part of the staging workup. A preoperative chest X-ray is indicated as is a barium esophagram, particularly if rigid esophagoscopy is planned. Further radiologic studies such as panorex and neck CT are ordered as indicated for primary tumor evaluation and/or extent of cervical adenopathy.[13]

Surgical Principles

Wide surgical resection for primary squamous cell carcinoma of the head and neck generally can be interpreted as resection of tumor with 1- to 2-cm margins, often with frozen section control of surgical margins. In conservation laryngeal surgery, much narrower surgical margins are acceptable.

Surgical management of the neck is an evolving science. In general terms, when the risk of occult nodal metastasis exceeds 25% to 30%, selective nodal dissection is recommended, particularly when postoperative radiation therapy is not planned. Selective neck dissection refers to any type of cervical lymphadenectomy where there is preservation of one or more lymph node groups removed by radical neck dissection.[14] In addition, if the surgeon must enter the neck to resect the primary tumor, a selective neck dissection is recommended.

Surgical management of the N1 neck is controversial. Some surgeons perform selective neck dissection and others perform modified neck dissection. Modified radical neck dissection refers to the excision of all lymph node stations routinely removed by radical neck dissection with preservation of one or more nonlymphatic structures; that is, spinal accessory nerve, internal jugular vein, and sternocleidomastoid muscle.[14] Modified or radical neck dissection is indicated for N2 or N3 nodal disease.

Radiation Therapy Principles

Radiation therapy is an effective modality in treating local/regional disease. For early lesions (stage I/II), radiation therapy offers comparable cure rates to surgical excision. Local tumor control rates are generally better with primary surgical resection, but local recurrences after primary radiation can be managed successfully with salvage surgery. Surgical complication rates are increased following radiation therapy. The choice between radiation therapy and surgery as definitive primary treatment depends upon a consideration of treatment morbidity and functional outcome.

For stage III/IV disease (extensive primary tumors or regional metastases), planned combined modality treatment offers improved local/regional control rates. While radiotherapy can be given either preoperatively or postoperatively, postoperative radiation therapy had improved local/regional control rates (65% versus 48%, $p = 0.04$) in a randomized clinical trial of 277 patients with cancers of the oral cavity, oropharynx, larynx, or hypopharynx.[15] Optimally, postoperative radiation therapy should be initiated within 6 weeks of extirpative surgery.[16]

Chemotherapy Principles

Data from many different trials do not demonstrate a survival advantage for use of chemotherapy for HNSCC in any setting compared to standard surgery and/or radiation therapy. Chemotherapy does play a role in the palliation of recurrent or unresectable disease and has proven effective when combined with radiation for organ preservation in trials of larynx and hypopharynx cancer.[17–19] The most active agents in head and neck squamous cell carcinoma are cisplatin or carboplatin and 5-fluorouracil. Several studies have suggested that chemotherapy may have some activity in reduction of distant metastatic rate.[17,20,21]

Natural History and Treatment by Site

Oral Cavity

Tumor growth and treatment affect speech and swallowing, particularly for patients with oral cavity cancers. The current T staging of oral cavity carcinoma is shown in Table 56.4.[22]

The principles of treatment of oral cavity cancers are stage dependent. For early lesions (T1N0, T2N0), excision of the primary tumor with or without a unilateral or bilateral selective (supraomohyoid) neck dissection is usually the treatment of choice.[13] Pathological assessment of the primary and neck contents at risk can be carried out. Postoperative radiation therapy is indicated for close surgical margins, perineural/lymphatic/vascular invasion, multiple positive lymph nodes, and/or extracapsular extension. For resectable advanced oral cavity tumors, combined surgery and postoperative radiation therapy is the standard treatment approach.[13]

TABLE 56.4. Primary Tumor Staging of Oral Cavity and Oropharynx Cancer.

TX	Primary tumor cannot be assessed
T0	No evidence of primary tumor
Tis	Carcinoma *in situ*
T1	Tumor 2 cm or less in greatest dimension
T2	Tumor more than 2 cm but not more than 4 cm in greatest dimension
T3	Tumor more than 4 cm in greatest dimension
T4 (lip)	Tumor invades through cortical bone, inferior alveolar nerve, floor of the mouth, or skin of face, i.e., chin or nose
T4a	(oral cavity) Tumor invades adjacent structures (e.g., through cortical bone, into deep [extrinsic] muscle of tongue [genioglossus, hyoglossus, palatoglossus, and styloglossus], maxillary sinus, skin of face)
T4b	Tumor invades masticator space, pterygoid plates, or skull base and/or encases internal carotid artery

Source: Used with permission of the American Joint Committee on Cancer (AJCC), Chicago, Illinois. The original source for this material is the AJCC Cancer Staging Manual, Sixth Ed. (2002) published by Springer-Verlag New York, www.springer-ny.com.

Lip

Squamous cell carcinoma of the lip is the most common oral cavity cancer. Most occur on the lower lip (90%). Early lesions without neck metastasis can be treated most efficiently with wide excision and closure. Neck dissection is indicated for nodal metastasis. Radiation therapy can be utilized as first-echelon treatment in patients with increased surgical risk or as adjuvant treatment in high-risk tumors. The indications for adjuvant radiation in lip cancers are close or positive margins, perineural/vascular/lymphatic invasion, and recurrent and/or large primary tumors (more than 3 cm).

Tongue

Occult nodal metastasis is present in 30% to 40% of early oral tongue cancers.[23] Therefore, selective neck dissection for all early tongue cancers except the most superficial lesions is advisable. Adequate surgical margins are required for tongue carcinomas, and most early lesions require hemiglossectomy. When tumors extend across the midline or involve the base of tongue, subtotal or total glossectomy may be required.

Floor of Mouth

Surgery is the treatment of choice for most patients with floor of mouth cancer. Because of the occult metastatic rate of 40% (T2) to 70% (T3), patients with lesions greater than 2 cm in diameter should have either selective (supraomohyoid) neck dissection or irradiation of the cervical nodes.[24] This strategy appears to offer a survival advantage for T2–T4 tumors.[25]

Buccal Mucosa

Buccal carcinoma is an uncommon form of oral cavity carcinoma. Early-stage squamous cell carcinoma of the buccal mucosa without bony involvement is best treated with primary radiation therapy. Surgery plus postoperative radiation therapy is the preferred mode of treatment of stage III/IV buccal cancer.

Retromolar Trigone/Alveolar Ridge

Most early tumors of the retromolar trigone or alveolar ridge can be treated effectively with transoral resection including rim mandibulectomy. Advanced lesions require segmental mandibulectomy plus neck dissection (composite resection) and postoperative radiation therapy.

Oropharynx

Oropharyngeal cancers include those of the tonsil, base of tongue, and soft palate and posterior pharyngeal wall. The most common presenting symptom of oropharyngeal cancers is chronic sore throat and referred otalgia. Change in voice, dysphagia, and trismus are later signs. Survival rates for advanced primary lesions are less than 50%. The presence of lymph node metastasis drops survival rates to the 25% range. Generally, T1 or T2 primary tumors of the oropharynx can be treated equally well with surgery or radiation therapy. Because lymphatic drainage of the oropharynx can be bilateral in all sites except lateralized tonsillar primaries, radiation is often an attractive first-treatment approach. Advanced oropharyngeal tumors can be treated with combined modality treatment.

TABLE 56.5. Primary Tumor Staging of Hypopharynx Cancer.

TX	Primary tumor cannot be assessed
T0	No evidence of primary tumor
Tis	Carcinoma *in situ*
T1	Tumor limited to one subsite of hypopharynx and 2 cm or less in greatest dimension
T2	Tumor invades more than one subsite of hypopharynx or adjacent site, or measures more than 2 cm but not more than 4 cm in greatest diameter
T3	Tumor more than 4 cm or with fixation of hemilarynx
T4a	Tumor invades thyroid/cricoid cartilage, hyoid bone, thyroid gland, esophagus, or central compartment soft tissue*
T4b	Tumor invades prevertebral fascia, encases carotid artery, or involves mediastinal structures

*Note: Central compartment soft tissue includes prelaryngeal strap muscles and subcutaneous fat.

Source: Used with permission of the American Joint Committee on Cancer (AJCC), Chicago, Illinois. The original source for this material is the AJCC Cancer Staging Manual, Sixth Ed. (2002) published by Springer-Verlag New York, www.springer-ny.com.

Hypopharynx

Squamous cell carcinoma of the hypopharynx is an aggressive disease with a poor prognosis irrespective of the therapeutic regimen instituted.[26] Stage III and IV squamous cell carcinoma of the hypopharynx has 5-year survival rates of 25% and 5%, respectively.[27] The staging of hypopharynx cancer is based primarily upon the subsite of pharynx involved, the presence of vocal cord fixation, and the extent of lymph node metastasis (Table 56.5). Because of the necessity of removing the larynx as part of the surgical management of most hypopharyngeal cancers, chemotherapy plus radiation therapy approaches have been investigated.

Larynx

Laryngeal tumors may be supraglottic, glottic, or subglottic. The cardinal symptom of laryngeal cancer is hoarseness. Other symptoms include airway obstruction, hemoptysis, odynophagia, otalgia (referred), dysphagia, neck mass, and weight loss. Because of the prominent role the larynx plays in speech, swallowing, and airway, treatment decisions about cancer of the larynx involve significant quality-of-life issues. In general, stage I and II disease can be managed with radiation therapy or conservation surgery. Stage III and IV disease often requires laryngectomy with or without neck dissection plus postoperative radiation therapy or induction chemotherapy plus radiation therapy.

Nasopharynx

NPC accounts for 2% of all HNSCCs in the United States. One-third of patients initially present with a neck mass, and 70% to 75% have enlarged neck nodes at time of presentation. Presenting symptoms may also include epistaxis, nasal obstruction, headache, or unilateral hearing loss. Unilateral serous otitis media is an indication for evaluation of the nasopharynx. A CT and/or MRI are critical for evaluation of base of skull involvement and/or presence of occult lymph nodes. The staging of nasopharyngeal carcinoma is shown in Table 56.6.

The treatment of Stage I/II nasopharyngeal cancer is definitive radiotherapy to the nasopharynx. Surgical resection

TABLE 56.6. Primary Tumor Staging of Nasopharyngeal Cancer.

Primary Tumor (T)

TX	Primary tumor cannot be assessed
T0	No evidence of primary tumor
Tis	Carcinoma *in situ*
T1	Tumor confined to the nasopharynx
T2	Tumor extends to soft tissues
T2a	Tumor extends to the oropharynx and/or nasal cavity without parapharyngeal space extension
T2b	Any tumor with parapharyngeal space extension*
T3	Tumor involves bony structures and/or paranasal sinuses
T4	Tumor with intracranial extension and/or involvement of cranial nerves, infratemporal fossa, hypopharynx, orbit, or masticator space

Source: Used with permission of the American Joint Committee on Cancer (AJCC), Chicago, Illinois. The original source for this material is the AJCC Cancer Staging Manual, Sixth Ed. (2002) published by Springer-Verlag New York, www.springer-ny.com.

even of early-stage disease is difficult because of proximity to the base of skull. Stage III/IV NPC (M0) is treated with concomitant chemotherapy plus radiation. Patients with metastatic disease can be treated with platinum-based combination chemotherapy regimens. If a complete response occurs, definitive radiation therapy may be added.

Paranasal Sinus and Nasal Cavity

Cancers arising in the paranasal sinuses and nasal cavity are relatively rare, accounting for only 0.2% of all human cancers. Approximately two-thirds arise in the maxillary sinus, and one-third arise in the ethmoid sinus. Malignant tumors arising in the frontal or sphenoid sinuses are exceedingly rare. Sinus cancers are associated with woodworking, nickel refining, and inhalation of noxious fumes (nitrosamines, dioxanes), as well as tobacco exposure. Eighty percent are squamous cell carcinomas but other cell types exist: these include adenocarcinoma, esthesioneuroblastoma, sinonasal undifferentiated carcinoma (SNUC), malignant melanoma, lymphoma, and inverting papilloma.

Malignant tumors of the paranasal sinuses often present at a late stage. Most have bony involvement at the time of presentation. Symptoms are often vague and mimic more benign conditions such as sinusitis. Cross-sectional imaging with MRI or CT is mandatory for accurate pretreatment staging of malignant tumors of the sinuses.

Surgical therapy with curative intent is considered in patients without evidence of distant disease who have no medical contraindications, if consistent with a reasonable functional outcome.[13] A recent series suggested that survival rates are better in patients treated with surgery plus postoperative radiation therapy.[28] For patients in whom adequate surgical resection is not consistent with a reasonable functional outcome (i.e., bilateral orbital involvement, extensive intracranial extension), definitive radiation therapy may be employed. In patients with advanced squamous cell carcinoma, esthesioneuroblastoma, and SNUC, an appropriate chemotherapy regimen may be utilized in combination with radiation therapy, surgery, or both.

Salivary Gland Malignancies

Tumors can arise in major or minor salivary glands. The major salivary glands include the parotid gland, submandibular and sublingual glands. Minor salivary glands are distributed throughout the hard palate, base of tongue, and buccal mucosa. Staging of primary salivary gland tumors is based upon size and extraparenchymal extension.

Surgery is the mainstay of treatment in patients with resectable salivary gland cancer. All malignant tumors of the parotid gland warrant total parotidectomy. The facial nerve should be sacrificed only for direct tumor invasion. Patients with high-grade tumors should also undergo selective neck dissection (N0) or modified or radical neck dissection (N+). Postoperative radiotherapy is indicated for all high-grade tumors (any histology except low-grade mucoepidermoid and acinic cell less than 3 cm), close surgical margins, recurrent disease, skin, bone, nerve, or extraparotid involvement, positive nodes, and for gross residual or unresectable disease.[35] Fast-neutron radiation therapy has a role in patients with large, inoperable salivary gland cancers.[29]

References

1. Lippman SM, Hong WK. Second malignant tumors in head and neck squamous cell carcinoma: the overshadowing threat for patients with early-stage disease [editorial]. Int J Radiat Oncol Biol Phys 1989;17:691.
2. Wynder EL, Hoffman D. Tobacco. In: Schottenfield D, Fraumeri JF Jr, eds. Cancer Epidemiology and Prevention. Philadelphia: WB Saunders, 1982:277–292.
3. Blot WJ, McLaughlin JK, Winn DM, et al. Smoking and drinking in relation to oral and pharyngeal cancer. Cancer Res 1998;48:3282.
4. Graham S. Epidemiology of retinoids and cancer. J Natl Cancer Inst 1984;73:1423.
5. Lippman SM, Meyskens FL. Retinoids for the prevention of cancer. In: Moon TE, Micozzi M, eds. Nutrition and Cancer Prevention: The Role of Micronutrients. New York: Marcel Dekker, 1989:243–272.
6. McLaughlin JK, Gridley G, Block G, et al. Dietary factors in oral and pharyngeal cancer. J Natl Cancer Inst 1988;80:1237.
7. Barton RT, Hogeveit AC. Nickel-related cancers of the respiratory tract. Cancer 1980;45:3061.
8. Cann CI, Fried MP, Rotman KJ. Epidemiology of squamous cell cancer of the head and neck. Otolaryngol Clin North Am 1985;18:367.
9. Cooper JS, Pajak TF, Forastiere A. Precisely defining high-risk operable head and neck tumors based on RTOG:85093 and :88–24: targets for postoperative radiochemotherapy? Head Neck 1998;20:588–594.
10. Bradford CR, Wolf GT, Carey TE, et al. Predictive markers for response to chemotherapy, organ preservation, and survival in patients with advanced laryngeal carcinoma. Otolaryngol Head Neck Surg, 1999;121:534–538.
11. Mashberg AL. Erythoplasia vs. leukoplakia in the diagnosis of early asymptomatic oral squamous carcinoma. N Engl J Med 1977;297:109.
12. Jacobs C. The internist in the management of head and neck cancer. Ann Intern Med 1990;113:771.
13. American Society for Head and Neck Surgery and the Society of Head and Neck Surgeons. Cancer of the head and neck: clinical practice guidelines. 1996.
14. Robbins KT, ed. Pocket Guide to Neck Dissection Classifica-

tion and TNM Staging of Head and Neck Cancer. Alexandria, VA: American Academy of Otolaryngology—Head and Neck Surgery Foundation, Inc, 1991.

15. Kramer S, Gelber RD, Snow JB, et al. Combined radiation therapy and surgery in the management of advanced head and neck cancer: final report of the study 73-03 of the Radiation Therapy Oncology Group. Head Neck Surg 1987;10:19.

16. Vikram B, Strong EW, Shah J, et al. Elective postoperative irradiation in stages III and IV epidermioid carcinoma of the head and neck. Am J Surg 1980;140:580.

17. Wolf GT, Hong WK, Fisher SG, et al. Induction chemotherapy plus radiation compared with surgery plus radiation in patients with advanced laryngeal cancer. N Engl J Med 1991;324: 1685–1690.

18. Lefebvre J L, Chevalier D, Luboinski B, et al. Larynx preservation in pyriform sinus cancer: preliminary results of a European Organization for Research and Treatment of Cancer phase III trial. J Natl Cancer Inst 1996;88:890–899.

19. Richard JM, Sancho-Garnier H, Pessey JJ, et al. Randomized trial of induction chemotherapy in larynx carcinoma. Oral Oncology 1998;34:224–228.

20. Schuller DE, Stein DW, Metch B. Analysis of treatment failure patterns: a Southwest Oncology Group study. Arch Otolaryngol Head Neck Surg 1989;115:834–836.

21. Laramore GE, Scott CB, al-Sarraf M, et al. Adjuvant chemotherapy for resectable squamous cell carcinomas of the head and neck: report on Intergroup 0035. Int J Radiat Oncol Biol Phys 1992;23:885–886.

22. American Joint Committee on Cancer. AJCC Cancer Staging Manual. 1997.

23. Spiro RH, Alfonso AE, Farr HW, et al. Cervical node metastases from epidermoid carcinoma of the oral cavity and oropharynx: a critical assessment of current staging. Am J Surg 1974;128: 562.

24. DiTroia JF. Nodal metastases and prognosis in carcinoma of the oral cavity. Otolaryngol Clin North Am 1972;5:333.

25. Baker SR. Malignant neoplasms of the oral cavity. In: Cummings CW, Frederickson JM, Harker LA, et al, eds. Otolaryngology—Head and Neck Surgery. 1st ed. St. Louis: CV Mobsy Co, 1986: 1281–1344.

26. Bradford CR, Esclamado RM, Carroll WR, et al. Analysis of recurrence, complications, and functional results with free jejunal flaps. Head Neck 1994:150–154.

27. Razack M, Sako K, Marchetta F, et al. Carcinoma of the hypopharynx: success and failure. Am J Surg 1977;134:489.

28. Isaacs J, Mooney S, Mendenhall W, et al. Cancer of the maxillary sinus treated with surgery and/or radiation therapy. Am Surg 1990;56:327.

29. Griffin T, Pajak T, Laramore G, et al. Neutron vs. photon irradiation of inoperable salivary gland tumors: results of an RTOG-MRC Cooperative Randomized Study. Int J Radiat Oncol Biol Phys 1988;15:1085.

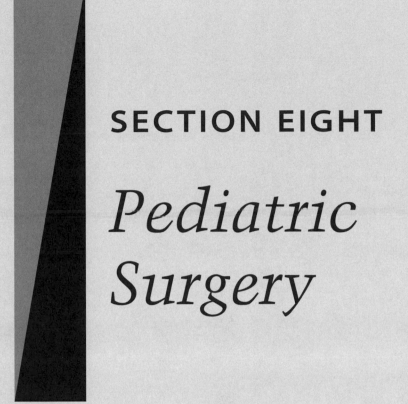

Pediatric Surgery

Craig T. Albanese

Preoperative and Postoperative Management

The neonate, infant, child, and adolescent differ significantly from each other and from the adult. The most distinctive and rapidly changing physiological characteristics occur during the neonatal period as the result of the newborn infant's adaptation to the extrauterine environment, differences in the physiological maturity of individual newborn infants, the small size of these patients, and the demands of growth and development.[1]

Classification

Newborn infants can be classified according to their level of maturation (gestational age) and development (weight).

1. Term infant: The normal full-term infant has a gestational age of 38 weeks or more and a body weight greater than 2500 g.
2. Low birth weight infant (LBW)
   a. Preterm infant: The premature infant has a gestational age less than 38 weeks with a birth weight appropriate for that age.
   b. Small-for-gestational-age infant (SGA): The SGA infant is more than 38 weeks' gestation with a body weight less than 2500 g.
3. Very low birth weight (VLBW) or extremely premature infants: These infants are generally less than 32 weeks gestation with a body weight less than 1500 g. They are also termed the "micropremie."
4. Large-for-gestational age (LGA): Their birth weight is greater than 4000 g if term, or greater than the 90th percentile for gestational age.
5. Postterm infants: These infants have a gestational age of 42 weeks or greater.

PREMATURE INFANT

Premature infants are those born before 38 weeks' gestation with a body weight appropriate for that age. The principal features of prematurity are a head circumference below the 50th percentile, a thin, semitransparent skin, absence of plantar creases, soft malleable ears (little cartilage), absence of breast tissue, undescended testes (testicular descent begins around the 32nd week of gestation) with a flat scrotum; and, in females, relatively enlarged labia minora with small labia majora.

Several physiological abnormalities exist in preterm infants. Apneic and bradycardic episodes are common and may occur spontaneously or as nonspecific signs of problems such as sepsis or hypothermia. Prolonged apnea with significant hypoxemia leads to bradycardia and ultimately to cardiac arrest. All premature infants should therefore have electrocardiographic pulse monitoring with the alarm set at a minimum pulse rate of 90 beats per minute as well as apnea monitoring. The lungs and retinae of preterm infants are very susceptible to high oxygen levels, and even relatively brief exposures may result in various degrees of lung disease [hyaline membrane disease (HMD)] and retinopathy of prematurity (ROP). Thus, infants receiving oxygen therapy require continuous pulse oximetry monitoring, with the alarm limits set between 85% and 92%.

Shunting across a patent ductus arteriosus (PDA) or foramen ovale is not uncommon. The direction of the shunt is determined by body weight as well as the underlying physiological or organic disorder. Generally, most shunts are left to right with resultant cardiac failure. Right-to-left shunts result in hypoxemia and are present in newborns with congenital diaphragmatic hernia, meconium aspiration, and sepsis. Right-to-left shunting is not present in infants less than 1200 g because they lack the vascular musculature necessary to produce pulmonary hypertension.

The premature infant may be unable to tolerate oral feeding because of a weak suck reflex, and intragastric tube feeds or total parenteral nutrition (TPN) may be required. Bilirubin metabolism may be impaired. Compared to term infants, preterm infants have increased requirements for glucose, calcium, and sodium as well as a propensity for hypothermia, intraventricular hemorrhage (IVH), and metabolic acidosis (renal tubular).

VERY LOW BIRTH WEIGHT (VLBW) INFANT

Physiologically, these neonates are similar to the "ordinary" premature infant. However, most (if not all) of the aforementioned problems are either accentuated (electrolyte abnormalities, hypothermia, hyperbilirubinemia) or are found with greater frequency (ROP, IVH, PDA, oxygen requirement with resultant HMD) in this group of extremely fragile infants. Most require several weeks of TPN because of the extreme prematurity of the gastrointestinal (GI) tract as well as its tendency for NEC.

SMALL FOR GESTATIONAL AGE (SGA) INFANT

Although body weight is low, the body length and head circumference of the SGA infant are age appropriate. A SGA infant is the product of a pregnancy complicated by any one of several placental, maternal, or fetal abnormalities that result in intrauterine growth retardation. Compared with a premature infant of equivalent weight, the SGA infant is older and developmentally more mature, and faces different physiological problems. Because of the longer gestational period and resultant well-developed organ systems, the metabolic rate of the SGA infant is much higher in proportion to their body weight. Thus, fluid and caloric requirements are increased. Intrauterine malnutrition results in a relative lack of body fat and decreased glycogen stores and, coupled with their relatively large surface area and high metabolic rate, greatly predispose these newborns to hypothermia and hypoglycemia. Close monitoring of the blood sugar is therefore essential. Polycythemia is common and the hematocrit should be monitored. SGA infants also have an increased risk of meconium aspiration syndrome. Because of the adequate length of gestation, ROP, IVH, and HMD are relatively uncommon.

Metabolic Considerations in the Care of the Newborn Infant

Thermoregulation

Newborn infants are susceptible to heat loss because of their large surface area, low body fat relative to body weight, small mass to act as a heat sink, and high thermoneutral temperature zone. When an infant is exposed to a cold environment, metabolic work increases above basal levels and calories are consumed to maintain body temperature. If prolonged, this leads to depletion of the limited energy reserves and predisposes to hypothermia and increased mortality.

The optimal thermal environment (thermoneutrality) is defined as the range of ambient temperatures in which a baby, at a minimal metabolic cost, can maintain a constant and normal body temperature by vasomotor control. Thermoneutrality is determined by weight, and postnatal age and standard nomograms are used.[2] The neonate's environmental temperature is best controlled by placing the infant in an incubator. In a cold environment such as in the operating room or radiology department, heat loss may be reduced by wrapping the head, extremities, and as much of the trunk as possible in wadding, plastic sheets, or aluminum foil.

Glucose Homeostasis

The fetus receives glucose from the mother by facilitated transplacental diffusion, with very little derived from fetal gluconeogenesis. Following delivery, the limited liver glycogen stores are rapidly depleted (within 2–3 h), and the blood glucose level then depends on the infant's capacity for gluconeogenesis, the adequacy of substrate stores, and energy requirements. Infants at high risk of developing hypoglycemia include LBW (especially SGA) infants, infants of toxemic or diabetic mothers, and infants requiring surgery who are unable to take oral nutrition and who have the additional metabolic stresses of their disease and the surgical procedure. All pediatric surgical patients, particularly neonates, are therefore monitored for hypoglycemia. Intravenous fluids should contain a minimum of 10% dextrose, and if non-dextrose-containing solutions such as blood or plasma are being administered, close monitoring of the blood glucose level is essential.

In contrast, hyperglycemia is commonly a problem of the VLBW infant on TPN due to a diminished insulin response to glucose. Hyperglycemia may lead to IVH, and to renal, water and, electrolyte loss from glycosuria. Prevention is by small and gradual incremental changes in the glucose concentration and infusion rate.

Calcium and Magnesium Homeostasis

Hypocalcemia, defined as serum ionized calcium less than 1.0 mg%, is most likely to occur 24 to 48 h after delivery. LBW infants are at greatest risk (particularly if they are premature), as well as those infants of a complicated pregnancy or delivery (e.g., diabetic mother), or those receiving bicarbonate infusions. Exchange transfusions or the rapid administration of citrated blood may also lead to hypocalcemia. The same infants at risk for hypocalcemia are also at risk for hypomagnesemia.

Blood Volume and Transfusion

Total blood, plasma, and red cell volumes are higher during the first few postnatal hours than at any other time in an individual's life (Table 57.1). Several hours after birth, plasma shifts out of the circulation, and total blood and plasma volume decrease. The high red blood cell volume persists, decreasing slowly to reach adult levels by the seventh postnatal week. Given an infant with a normal blood volume, mild blood loss, defined as less than 10% of blood volume, does not require transfusion. A transfusion of packed red blood cells at a volume of 10 ml/kg usually raises the hematocrit 3% to 4%.

Jaundice

In the fetus, the lipid-soluble, unconjugated (indirect) bilirubin is cleared across the placenta. In the newborn, the ca-

TABLE 57.1. Age-Based Estimation of Blood Volume.

Premature infants	85–100 ml/kg
Term newborns	85 ml/kg
Age >1 month	75 ml/kg
Age 3 months to adult	70 ml/kg

Source: Adapted from Rowe PC, (ed). In: The Harriet Lane Handbook, 11th Ed. Chicago: Year Book Medical, 1987:25.

pacity for conjugating bilirubin is not fully developed and may be exceeded by the bilirubin load. This excess results in transient physiological jaundice, which reaches a maximum at the age of 4 days but returns to normal levels by the sixth day. Usually the maximum bilirubin level does not exceed 10.0 mg/dl.

High serum levels of unconjugated bilirubin may cross the immature blood–brain barrier in the newborn and can act as a neural poison, leading to a condition termed kernicterus. This condition, in its severest form, is characterized by athetoid cerebral palsy and sensorineural hearing loss.

Phototherapy is widely used prophylactically in high-risk infants to decrease the serum bilirubin by photodegradation of bilirubin in the skin to water-soluble products. It is continued until the total serum bilirubin is less than 10.0 mg/dl and falling. Exchange transfusion is indicated when the indirect bilirubin level exceeds 20.0 mg/dl.

Vitamin K

The routine administration of vitamin K to all newborn infants to prevent hypoprothrombinemia and hemorrhagic disease of the newborn is established practice.

Caloric Requirements

The newborn requires a relatively large caloric intake because of the high basal metabolic rate, caloric requirements for growth and development, energy needs to maintain body heat, and the limited energy reserve. Caloric requirements are increased 10% to 25% by surgery, more than 50% by infection, and 150% by burns. The caloric needs of an infant are calculated according to the requirements for basal metabolism plus growth (Table 57.2).

ENTERAL ALIMENTATION

The best means of providing calories is via the GI tract either by mouth, or nasogastric or nasojejunal feeding tube, or through a surgically placed gastrostomy or jejunostomy tube. Gastric feeding is preferable because it allows for normal digestive processes and hormonal responses, a greater tolerance for larger osmotic loads, and a lower incidence of dumping. Breast- or bottlefeeding is preferable for infants, usually more than 32 to 34 weeks gestation, who have a coordinated suck-and-swallow mechanism. Gavage feeding is indicated for infants with an impaired coordinated suck-and-swallow mechanism, or for supplementation for those infants with a high metabolic rate who cannot gain weight with oral feeding alone.

TABLE 57.2. Caloric Requirements of Various Age Groups per 24 h.

Age	Kilocalories per kilogram
Newborn term (0–4 days)	110–120
Low birth weight infant	120–130
3–4 months	100–106
5–12 months	100
1–7 years	90–75
7–12 years	75–60
12–18 years	60–30

TABLE 57.3. Total Parenteral Nutrition Requirements.

Component	Neonate	Six months to 10 years	More than 10 years
Calories (kcal/kg/d)	90–120	60–105	40–75
Fluid (ml/kg/d)	120–180	120–150	50–75
Dextrose (mg/kg/min)	4–6	7–8	7–8
Protein (g/kg/d)	2–3	1.5–2.5	0.8–2.0
Fat (g/kg/d)	0.5–3.0	1.0–4.0	1.0–4.0
Sodium (mEq/kg/d)	3–4	3–4	3–4
Potassium (mEq/kg/d)	2–3	2–3	1–2
Calcium (mg/kg/d)	80–120	40–80	40–60
Phosphate (mg/kg/d)	25–40	25–40	25–40
Magnesium (mEq/kg/d)	0.25–1.0	0.5	0.5
Zinc (mcg/kg/d)	300	100	3 mg/day
Copper (mcg/kg/d)	20	20	1.2 mg/day
Chromium (mcg/kg/d)	0.2	0.2	12 mg/day
Manganese (mcg/kg/d)	6	6	0.3 mg/day
Selenium (mcg/kg/d)	2	2	10–20/day

PARENTERAL NUTRITION

The indications for parenteral feeding include the following: extremely low birth weight infant, surgical GI abnormalities with prolonged postoperative ileus (gastroschisis, necrotizing enterocolitis), short gut syndrome following extensive bowel resection, chronic diarrhea (malabsorption syndrome), inflammatory bowel disease, severe acute alimentary disorders (pancreatitis, necrotizing enterocolitis), chylothorax, intestinal fistulae, and persistent vomiting associated with cancer chemotherapy.[3] The requirements for TPN are detailed in Table 57.3.

FLUID AND ELECTROLYTE MANAGEMENT

Effective fluid and electrolyte management involves (1) calculating the fluid and electrolyte requirements for maintaining metabolic functions, (2) replacing losses (evaporative, third space, external), and (3) considering preexisting fluid deficits or excess (see Table 57.4). Taking these factors into consideration, a tentative program is devised for fluid and electrolyte administration. The patient's response is monitored and the program is adjusted accordingly.[1,4]

General Perioperative Considerations

Gastrointestinal Decompression

The importance of gastric decompression in the surgical newborn cannot be overemphasized. The distended stomach carries the risk of aspiration and pneumonia, and may also impair diaphragmatic excursion, resulting in respiratory distress.

TABLE 57.4. Calculation of Maintenance Fluid Requirements.

Body weight (kg)	Fluid volume/24 h
1–10	100 ml/kg
11–20	1000 ml + 50 ml/each kg over 10 kg
>20	1500 ml + 20 ml/each kg over 20 kg

A double-lumen sump tube, such as the Replogle tube, is preferred, utilizing low continuous suction. If a single-lumen tube is used, intermittent aspiration by syringe or machine is required.

Antimicrobial Therapy

Deficiencies in the immune system of the newborn infant render it vulnerable to major bacterial insults. Prophylactic antimicrobial therapy is advised for infants undergoing major surgery, particularly of the gastrointestinal tract or genitourinary system. Adequate coverage is provided by combining a penicillin (e.g., ampicillin) or first-generation cephalosporin (e.g., cefazolin) with an aminoglycoside (e.g., gentamicin). Clindamicin or metronidazole is added when anaerobic coverage is deemed necessary. Alternatively, single-drug therapy using a broad-spectrum cephalosporin (e.g., cefoxitin) may be appropriate. Antibiotics are commenced before operation and may be discontinued postoperatively at the surgeon's discretion.

Preoperative Blood Sampling

Blood analyses should be restricted to those studies essential for diagnosis and management. The volume of blood drawn for laboratory tests should be documented as these small volumes cumulatively represent significant blood loss in a small infant. Generally, the only "routine" preoperative blood analyses for a neonate consist of a complete blood count with a differential and platelet counts, and a blood specimen for type and crossmatch (in the case of major newborn surgery). Electrolytes in the first 12 h of life simply reflect the mother's electrolytes. Coagulation studies (e.g., PT/PTT) are virtually never indicated.

Preoperative NPO Guidelines

PATIENTS YOUNGER THAN 6 MONTHS

No food or formula 4 h before the procedure. Children may continue to have breast milk and clear liquids (water, pedialyte, glucose water, or apple juice) until 2 h before the procedure.

PATIENTS FROM 6 MONTHS TO 18 YEARS

Nothing to eat or drink after midnight except clear liquids (water, apple juice, pedialyte, plain jello, popsicles, white grape juice), which can be continued until 2 h before the procedure.

PATIENTS OLDER THAN 18 YEARS

Nothing to eat or drink after midnight except clear liquids (water, apple juice, plain jello, popsicles) until 4 h before the procedure.

Bowel Preparation Instructions

The bowel is mechanically cleansed for elective bowel resection. There is varied opinion as to whether a bowel preparation is needed for certain procedures, as well as what to use to accomplish it, and whether to do it at home or in the hospital.

Lateral Neck Masses

The differential diagnosis of a laterally presenting neck mass is extensive and includes branchial cleft remnants, lymphangioma, dermoid cyst, epidermoid cyst, hemangioma, lymphadenitis, leukemia, torticollis, neurofibroma, lipoma, metastatic tumor to the cervical lymph nodes, parotid tumor, and tumors of dentigerous origin. Of these, branchial cleft remnants, lymphangioma (cystic hygroma), and torticollis are discussed.

Branchial Cleft Cysts, Sinuses, and Remnants

The branchial arches develop and partially regress all during the first 6 weeks of life.[5] They are composed of endodermal pouches on the pharyngeal wall and are noted externally by the presence of ectodermal clefts. Cysts developing from branchial structures usually appear later in childhood as opposed to sinuses, fistulae, and cartilagenous remnants. Incomplete sinus tracts are mere dimples in the skin. Approximately 15% are bilateral, and one frequently observes similar lesions in siblings.

Anomalies of the first branchial cleft are rare and often present in adulthood as a small cyst lying close to the parotid gland. During infancy, this anomaly is usually noted as a draining sinus located anterior to the ear. Anomalies of the second branchial cleft are the most common lesions, arising in the mid- or lower neck, along the anterior border of the sternocleidomastoid muscle. A cyst, sinus, or fistula may be present. Anomalies of the third branchial cleft are extremely rare and, like the second branchial cleft remnant, are located along the anterior border of the sternocleidomastoid muscle.

TREATMENT

Rarely are branchial cleft anomalies cosmetically unappealing. Rather, they should be excised early in life, shortly after diagnosis, because repeated infection is quite common, making resection more difficult. When infection occurs, antibiotic therapy and often incision and drainage are indicated. The definitive excision is staged, approximately 6 weeks later, giving the inflammation adequate time to resolve, thus assuring a complete resection. Every effort should be made to excise the entire cyst wall or fistula tract (including the skin punctum, if present) because recurrence and infection are common with incomplete removal.

Lymphangioma (Cystic Hygroma)

These growths are benign, multilobular, multinodular cystic masses lined by endothelial cells. They result from maldevelopment of the lymphaticovenous sacs.[6] Eventually, sequestrations of lymphatic tissue that do not communicate with the normal lymphatic system develop; 50% to 65% appear at birth, and 90% by the second year of life. They are located most commonly in the posterior triangle of the neck (75%); axilla (20%); mediastinum, retroperitoneum, pelvis, and groin (5%). The majority are asymptomatic.

There are two modes of treatment that are chosen on the basis of imaging (CT, MRI) studies: sclerotherapy and excision. Intralesional injection of a sclerosing agent is most effective for unilocular cysts. Examples of agents that have been used are OK-432 (a lyophilized mixture of *Streptococcus pyo-*

genes and penicillin G potassium), and bleomycin.[7,8] surgical resection is an alternative option. The recurrence rate is low (10%) if all microscopic disease is resected. When gross disease is left, recurrence appears in up to 100%.

Cervical Lymphadenitis

Cervical adenitis is an inflammatory enlargement of one or more lymph nodes of the head and neck.[9] There is tenderness, erythema, fever, and leukocytosis. Treatment is with antibiotics, warm compresses, and surgical drainage when the lymph node(s) become fluctuant.

Torticollis

Torticollis occurs in newborns and results from fibrosis and shortening of the sternocleidomastoid muscle, producing a "tumor" in the muscle that causes the face to turn toward the contralateral side and the head to tilt toward the ipsilateral shoulder.[10] Increasing facial and cranial asymmetry results from this abnormal positioning. Passive range-of-motion exercises, coupled with a change in the infant's feeding position, will cure most. The only indication for operation (division of the muscle) is facial hemihypoplasia.

Midline Neck Masses

Midline neck masses usually present in children more than 6 months old and are often thyroglossal duct cysts/sinuses, dermoid/epidermoid inclusion cysts, or goiter. Less common differential diagnoses are: ectopic midline thyroid, pyramidal lobe of the thyroid, thyroid adenoma of the isthmus, carcinoma of the thyroid with a pretracheal nodal metastasis, lipoma, and submental lymphadenitis. In contrast, cervical teratoma and lymphangioma are the most common midline neck masses in the newborn. They are often quite large and may threaten the airway.

Congenital Anomalies of the Lung

Congenital Cystic Adenomatoid Malformation

Congenital cystic adenomatoid malformation (CCAM) are cystic, solid, or mixed intrapulmonary hamartomas that communicate with the normal tracheobronchial tree and do not have an anomalous blood supply.[11] The majority of these lesions are lobar and can be identified prenatally by ultrasound. The prenatal natural history can be quite variable.[12] Some may grow so large and produce such severe mediastinal shift that heart failure and hydrops results. Others may remain the same size, or regress considerably. Asymptomatic children may be observed but resection (pulmonary lobectomy) is recommended since these lesions often become infected and there are case reports of malignant transformation occurring in untreated, long-standing cysts.[13]

Pulmonary Sequestration

This is a relatively normal segment of lung parenchyma, most commonly in the lower left hemithorax, that has an aberrant arterial supply, usually from the infradiaphragmatic aorta, and venous drainage that is either pulmonary or systemic.[14] There is an extralobar variant that has its own investing pleura but no communication with the tracheobronchial tree. Unlike prenatally diagnosed CCAMs, sequestrations rarely grow large enough to produce hydrops and in utero demise. Children with extralobar sequestrations are usually asymptomatic at birth and have been diagnosed either prenatally or by chest radiograph demonstrating a radiopaque mass in the lower hemithorax. Treatment is by excision of the sequestration, which may or may not require lower lobectomy, depending on the degree of inflammation.

Congenital Lobar Emphysema

Congenital lobar emphysema (CLE) consists of hyperinflation of a single lobe, usually the upper or middle lobes.[15] There are a variety of causes such as bronchial obstruction (deficient bronchial cartilage support, redundant mucosa, bronchial stenosis, bronchial compression by anomalous vessels or mediastinal mass, mucus plug), a polyalveolar lobe (large number of abnormal alveoli that are prone to expansion), or hypoplastic emphysema (reduced number of bronchi and alveoli with increased air space size).

Infants with CLE usually do not present with respiratory distress for several days or weeks. Many infants, however, present with mild tachypnea at birth. In only 5% of cases do symptoms develop after 6 months of life. Most of these babies require excision of the affected lobe due to progressive hyperinflation.

Mediastinal Masses

Mediastinal masses are relatively common in infants and children and can be classified according to the compartment of the mediastinum from which they arise.[16] The most common mediastinal mass is a posterior mediastinal neurogenic tumor.

ANTERIOR MEDIASTINAL MASSES

1. Thymic cysts and thymomas are rare and account for 5% of cases.
2. Lymphoma accounts for approximately 10% and is either a Hodgkin's or non-Hodgkin's variety. About 40% to 60% of children with Hodgkin's disease present with an anterior mediastinal mass.
3. In teratoma (15%), the masses may be cystic, solid, and may also be found within the pericardium, and approximately 20% are malignant.
4. Lymphangioma (cystic hygroma) occur in 7% and most commonly extend caudally from the neck into the mediastinum. Rarely, they arise primarily in the mediastinum.

MIDDLE MEDIASTINAL MASSES

1. Bronchogenic cysts (15%): extrapulmonary cysts are located in either the paratracheal or juxtahilar regions. These cysts are three times more common on the right side than on the left.
2. Pericardial cysts are rare, are almost always asymptomatic, and are usually an incidental chest radiograph finding.

POSTERIOR MEDIASTINAL MASSES

1. Neurogenic tumors (see "Childhood Tumors") account for 33%: they include neuroblastoma, ganglioneuroblastoma,

ganglioneuroma, neurofibroma, and neurofibrosarcoma. Common symptoms include respiratory distress (via tracheal or lung compression), Horner's syndrome, and pain.

2. Enterogenous cysts (28%) are esophageal duplications that often contain ectopic gastric tissue.

Congenital Diaphragmatic Hernia

Congenital diaphragmatic hernia (CDH) is a highly lethal and morbid disease that affects 1 in 2000 live births.[17] Anatomically, CDH results from an embryological fusion defect, allowing herniation of intraabdominal contents into the chest. Failure of posterolateral fusion of the various components comprising the diaphragm leads to a persistent pleuroperitoneal canal, the foramen of Bochdalek. The hernia is most common on the left side (90%) with a rate of associated anomalies of 20% (chromosomal abnormalities, neural tube defects, and congenital heart disease). Pulmonary hypoplasia is believed to occur when the developing fetal lungs are compressed by the herniated abdominal viscera, limiting the number of bronchopulmonary generations.[18] Herniation of gut through the diaphragmatic defect prevents normal intestinal rotation and fixation, accounting for the almost universal presence of intestinal rotational anomalies in infants with CDH. The size of the defect ranges from a small slit to complete diaphragmatic agenesis.

The development of symptoms in CDH correlates with the degree of pulmonary hypoplasia and pulmonary hypertension. The abdomen is classically scaphoid. Breath sounds may be absent on the ipsilateral side, and cardiac sounds may be distant. They are usually symptomatic in the delivery room with tachypnea, grunting respirations, retractions, and cyanosis, and may require urgent intubation. The radiographic findings include air-filled loops of bowel in the hemithorax, a paucity of gas within the abdomen, radiopaque hemithorax if the bowel does not contain a significant amount of gas or if the liver occupies the majority of the hemithorax, contralateral mediastinal shift with compression of the contralateral lung, loss of normal ipsilateral diaphragmatic contour, and the nasogastric tube may coil in the hemithorax.

Prenatal diagnosis is occurring more and more frequently and allows the mother and fetus to be referred to an institution where sophisticated perinatal and pediatric surgical units are available. For those fetuses with a severe CDH by ultrasound criteria, intervention before birth is an option and has proven very promising.[19] Treatment includes prompt orotracheal intubation after sedation and paralysis. Avoid bag-mask ventilation, administer 100% oxygen, insert a sump gastric tube (Replogle) and place it on low continuous suction. Monitor pre- and postductal oxygen saturations and treat right-to-left shunting (pulmonary hypertension) as per Table 57.5. Persistent pulmonary hypertension may respond only to extracorporeal membrane oxygenation (ECMO) support.

Repair of the diaphragmatic defect is not a surgical emergency and should be performed once the infant has stabilized and has demonstrated minimal to no pulmonary hypertension (usually >48 h postnatally). Primary diaphragmatic closure using interrupted nonabsorbable sutures can be performed if the defect is small. If the defect is too large for a

TABLE 57.5. Treatment of Pulmonary Hypertension.

Oxygenate	Mechanical ventilation, FiO_2 1.0
Correct acidosis	Hyperventilate
	Sodium bicarbonate (or THAM if retaining CO_2)
Correct malperfusion	Adequate volume replacement as needed
	Inotropic agents: dopamine, dobutamine
Sedation/paralysis	Fentanyl infusion, neuromuscular blockade (vecuronium)
Pulmonary vasodilation	Nitric oxide
Correct hypocalcemia	Intravenous calcium supplements ($CaCl_2$, Ca gluconate)

THAM, Tromethamine.

primary closure, then a prosthetic patch (e.g., Gore-Tex) should be inserted and sutured around the ribs of the posterolateral body wall. The majority of children with CDH who survive the neonatal period and are successfully extubated enjoy relatively normal lives. Recurrent diaphragmatic hernia occurs in 10% to 20% of infants and should be considered in any child with a history of CDH who presents with new GI or pulmonary symptoms.

Foramen of Morgagni Hernia

The foramen of Morgagni (or space of Larrey) represents the junction of the septum transversum, the lateral portion of the diaphragm, and the anterior thoracic wall and allows the passage of the superior epigastric vessels. This anterior diaphragmatic defect accounts for only 2% of diaphragmatic hernias. Typically, children are asymptomatic and the defect is discovered later in life on a chest radiograph taken for reasons unrelated to the hernia. Repair is indicated in the asymptomatic patient because of the risk of bowel incarceration or strangulation.

Eventration of the Diaphragm

Diaphragmatic eventration is an abnormally elevated portion of the diaphragm or, most commonly, hemidiaphragm. It may be congenital (usually idiopathic, but can be associated with congenital myopathies or intrauterine infections) or acquired (as a result of phrenic nerve injury during forceps delivery or thoracotomy).[20] There is a variable absence of diaphragmatic muscle, at which point its distinction from a CDH with a persistant hernia sac is obscure. The elevated diaphragm produces abnormalities of chest wall mechanics with impaired pulmonary function. Respiratory distress and pneumonia are frequent presenting symptoms, although GI symptoms such as vomiting or gastric volvulus may occur.

The diagnosis is made by chest radiograph and confirmed by fluoroscopy or ultrasound, which demonstrates paradoxical movement of the diaphragm during spontaneous respiration. Incidentally discovered small localized eventrations do not need to be repaired. Eventrations that are large or that are associated with respiratory symptoms should be repaired.

Congenital Chest Wall Deformities

Sternal Defects

SIMPLE CLEFT STERNUM

This defect results from a failure of the embryonic sternal bars to unite and fuse, typically involving the manubrium and varying lengths of the body. Patients are usually asymptomatic. Operative correction is performed in the neonatal period, as the chest wall is so pliable, and consists of simple suture approximation of the sternal halves.

CLEFT STERNUM WITH TRUE ECTOPIA CORDIS

Varying degrees of upper sternal cleft are associated with ectopia cordis or a "bare" heart (no investing pericardium) that is located outside the chest wall, via the cleft. This condition is generally incompatible with life due to the severe congenital heart lesion(s).

CLEFT STERNUM WITH THORACOABDOMINAL ECTOPIA CORDIS (PENTALOGY OF CANTRELL)

There are five components to this disorder: minimal distal sternal cleft, ventral diaphragmatic defect (central tendon defect), epigastric abdominal wall defect (omphalocele), CHD, and apical pericardial defect. As the heart is not completely outside the mediastinum and retains most of its investing pericardium, this is not considered true ectopia cordis. The CHD is typically not severe (usually a septal defect). Mortality is appreciable and is related to the huge upper abdominal wall defect and the cardiorespiratory compromise that results from attempted closure.

Pectus Excavatum

This depression deformity is the most common congenital chest wall abnormality, occurring in 1 in 300 live births, with a 3:1 male predominance. It is associated with other musculoskeletal disorders (Marfan's syndrome, Poland's anomaly, scoliosis, clubfoot, syndactylism), and 2% have CHD. There is a familial form. It results from unbalanced posterior growth of costal cartilages that are often fused, bizarrely deformed, or rotated.[21] The body of the sternum secondarily exhibits a prominent posterior curvature, usually involving its lower half (Fig. 57.1). It is identified during infancy in 90%. In general, there is no cardiopulmonary benefit after chest wall repair except in rare instances in which the deformity is extensive. Otherwise, the repair is performed solely to improve appearance.

Pectus Carinatum

This defect is a protrusion deformity, also referred to as pigeon or chicken breast.[22] Approximately 10 times less frequent than depression deformities, it results from overgrowth of costal cartilages, with forward buckling and secondary deformation of the sternum. Atypical and asymmetrical forms with rotation are common. There is a familial form. It is associated with Marfan's disease, neurofibromatosis, Poland's disease, and Morquio's disease. The defect does not affect car-

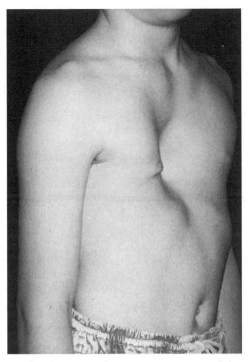

FIGURE 57.1. Adolescent with a pectus excavatum deformity. Note that the most pronounced posterior sternal curvature is in the lower one-half. (Reproduced with permission from R. Shamberger, Congenital chest wall deformities. In: Pediatric Surgery, Fifth Edition, JA O'Neill, MI Rowe, JL Grosfeld, Editors. © 1998 CV Mosby, Co.)

diopulmonary function. Unlike pectus excavatum, the deformity is typically mild or nearly imperceptible in early childhood and becomes increasingly prominent during the rapid growth in early puberty. There is no cardiorespiratory compromise with this deformity, and repair is performed solely for an improved cosmetic appearance.

Congenital Anomalies of the Esophagus

Anomalies of the esophagus, namely esophageal atresia, tracheoesophageal fistula, and their variants, are potentially life threatening in the newborn period.[23] Shortly after birth, the infant with esophageal atresia is noted to have excessive salivation and repeated episodes of coughing, choking, and cyanosis, and attempts at feeding are unsuccessful. Those with an associated tracheoesophageal fistula are prone to gastric reflux into the tracheobronchial tree with resulting chemical tracheobronchitis and pneumonia, especially if they are on mechanical ventilatory support. The diagnosis is confirmed by demonstrating that a small feeding tube coils in the upper esophageal pouch on a plain radiograph. A contrast study is almost never indicated. Bronchoscopy is the most sensitive means of identifying a tracheoesophageal fistula. There is a 50% to 70% incidence of associated anomalies, namely cardiac (PDA, septal defects), gastrointestinal (imperforate anus, duodenal atresia), genitourinary, and skeletal. The VACTERL association (vertebral, anorectal, cardiac, tracheo-esophageal, renal, and limb anomalies) is present in 25% of cases.

These anomalies are classified based on the presence or absence of an esophageal atresia (Fig. 57.2). Esophageal atre-

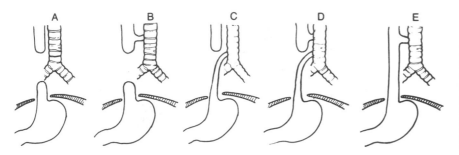

FIGURE 57.2. **A.** Pure (long gap) esophageal atresia. **B.** Esophageal atresia with proximal tracheoesophageal fistula. **C.** Esophageal atresia with distal tracheoesophageal fistula. **D.** Esophageal atresia with proximal and distal fistulae. **E.** Tracheoesophageal fistula without esophageal atresia. (Reproduced with permission from JL Grosfeld, Pediatric surgery. In: Textbook of Surgery. DC Sabiston, Editor. © 1991 WB Saunders Co.)

sia with distal tracheoesophageal fistula (type C) is the most common type (85% of cases).

Treatment begins with stabilization of the child and assessment for associated anomalies. A Replogle sump suction catheter should be placed in the upper esophageal pouch and the head of the bed elevated. An echocardiogram is required to determine the position of the aortic arch as a right-sided arch makes the standard right thoracotomy repair difficult. The goal of operative therapy is to divide and ligate the fistula and repair the atresia in one stage. Staged operations are reserved for extremely premature babies and those with severe anomalies or long gaps between the esophageal pouches.

Gastrointestinal Tract Abnormalities

Gastroesophageal Reflux

Gastroesophageal reflux (GER) is physiological at birth because the lower esophageal sphincter does not mature for approximately 2 months; this accounts for the commonly noted regurgitation (chalazia) during and after feeds in a normal newborn. The symptoms of GER in infants and children are protean.[24] The most common is vomiting, which can cause failure to thrive, aspiration pneumonia, apnea, bronchospasm that is confused with asthma, and laryngospasm which may lead to sudden infant death. The gold standard diagnostic test is lower esophageal 24-h pH monitoring.

Nonoperative treatment is successful in most cases. For infants, thickening the feeds with rice cereal and upright positioning during and shortly after feeding is effective. Persistent symptoms mandate drug therapy with an antacid (e.g., H_2 blocker or proton pump inhibitor). The indications for operation are failure of medical therapy (e.g., recurrent pneumonia), severe esophagitis, Barrett's esophagitis, esophageal stricture, or significant bleeding. The gold standard antireflux surgical procedure is the Nissen complete fundoplication.[25] This can be done laparoscopically.

Pyloric Stenosis

Pyloric stenosis is the most common surgical disorder producing emesis in infancy. The symptoms are of gastric outlet obstruction and are caused by concentric hypertrophy of the pyloric muscle with progressive narrowing of the pyloric canal. The disease evolves postnatally, as it is rare in preterm infants, and symptoms are usually absent in the first week of life. It is usually diagnosed in the first 3 to 6 weeks after birth.

Clinically there is progressive, forceful, nonbilious emesis. The vomiting occurs immediately or within 30 to 45 min of the last feeding and consists of undigested formula with thick curds. Brownish or coffee-ground material may be pres-ent and suggests gastritis. Affected infants are voraciously hungry after vomiting and will eagerly take to the bottle or nurse. The differential diagnosis is overfeeding (most common), formula intolerance, GER, pyloric duplication, antral web, CNS lesion with increased intracranial pressure, and salt-wasting adrenogenital syndrome. Infants are often dehydrated with sunken fontanelles, dry mucous membranes, and poor skin turgor. Jaundice (elevated indirect bilirubin) may be present due to decreased glucuronyl transferase activity. A firm, mobile hypertrophic pylorus, or "olive," is palpated by an experienced examiner in 90% of cases, provided the child is relaxed and the stomach is decompressed. Diagnostic imaging is required only if the olive cannot be palpated. Ultrasonography is the most sensitive test although a negative study is nondiagnostic for other entities. An upper GI contrast study can provide anatomical and functional details. Plain abdominal radiographs are never indicated.

Prolonged vomiting of gastric fluid can result in a hypochloremic, hypokalemic, metabolic alkalosis. Fluid and electrolyte abnormalities are corrected using D_5 0.45% normal saline at 150 to 175 ml/kg/d. Potassium (20 mEq/l) is added after the child voids. The volume of resuscitation fluid is adjusted based on the child's urine output, urine specific gravity, and vital signs.

The timing of operation is dictated solely by the fluid and electrolyte status. Surgery may be undertaken when an adequate amount (1–2 ml/kg/h) of nonconcentrated (specific gravity ≤ 1.012) urine is established and the serum chloride and potassium are corrected. The surgical repair consists of an extramucosal myotomy beginning 1 to 2 mm proximal to the pyloroduodenal junction and extending onto the antrum. Recent series show equally effective results with the laparoscopic approach to pyloric stenosis. Pyloric stenosis never recurs, and there is a uniformly excellent outcome.

Intestinal Obstruction in the Newborn

Because fetuses continually swallow amniotic fluid into their GI tracts and excrete it via the urine, intestinal obstruction may be noted on prenatal ultrasound by the presence of polyhydramnios (increased amniotic fluid level). After birth, vomiting is the principal symptom, and the vomitus is bile stained if the obstruction is distal to the ampulla of Vater. *It is important to note that newborn bilious vomiting is pathological until proven otherwise.* On physical examination, the presence and degree of abdominal distension depends on the level of the obstruction and should be noted. For example, there is no significant distension with duodenal obstruction versus massive distension with colonic obstruction (e.g., Hirschsprung's disease). A careful perineal examination should be performed to assess if an anus is present, patent, and in the normal location. Meconium, the first newborn stool, is passed in the first 24 h of life in 94% of normal full-term infants and by 48 h in 98%. Failure to pass meconium may be indicative of lower GI tract obstruction.

Depending on the plain abdominal radiograph, an upper GI series may or may not be needed before operative intervention. As the plain abdominal radiograph in a newborn cannot differentiate small bowel from large bowel in an infant with multiple distended bowel loops, the most common test in the workup of bilious emesis is the contrast enema. It can be both diagnostic and therapeutic (e.g., wash out a meconium plug).

Duodenal Obstruction

Duodenal obstruction[26] can be complete (e.g., atresia) or partial (e.g., stenosis). The various causes are idiopathic atresia (failure of canalization), annular pancreas, preduodenal portal vein, or peritoneal bands (Ladd's bands) from malrotation. There may also be a mucosal web or diaphragm that can partially (perforated web) or completely obstruct the duodenum. Approximately one-third of babies with duodenal atresia or stenosis have trisomy 21 (Down syndrome). Patients present with bilious emesis and the presence of a "double bubble" on plain abdominal radiographs (Fig. 57.3). Rarely are contrast studies needed preoperatively. Treatment is by duodenoduodenostomy. In contrast, an obstructing duodenal web is excised. Obstruction from Ladd's bands requires simple division of the bands and correction of the malrotation.

Disorders of Intestinal Rotation

Disorders of intestinal rotation are classified in four ways: incomplete rotation (the most common), nonrotation, reversed rotation (the least common), and anomalous mesenteric fixation.[27,28]

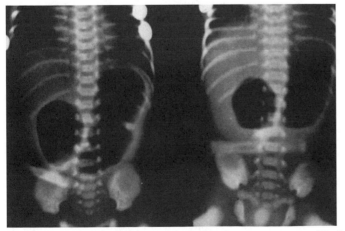

FIGURE 57.3. Plain abdominal radiographs demonstrate a gas-filled stomach and proximal duodenum ("double bubble"), indicative of proximal duodenal obstruction. The radiograph on the *left* was taken with the baby supine, the one on the *right* with the child upright.

Incomplete rotation may affect the duodenojejunal portion, the cecocolic portion, or both. As only partial rotation occurs, the bowel is fixed posteriorly by a relatively narrow mesenteric base that is prone to twisting (volvulus). The partial rotation of the cecum may result in duodenal obstruction by Ladd's bands. These are peritoneal folds that serve to fix the cecum to the posterior body wall; if rotation halts in the right upper quadrant, these bands will stretch out over the duodenum. Incomplete intestinal rotation is managed by division of Ladd's bands, division of any intermesenteric adhesions, straightening the duodenum as much as possible, and placing the cecum on the left side of the abdomen. In essence, one is creating nonrotated intestinal anatomy, much like early fetal life. Appendectomy is advocated based on the abnormal final position of the appendix.

With nonrotation of the intestine, the midgut is "suspended" from the superior mesenteric vessels; the majority of the small intestine lies on the right side of the abdomen, the large bowel on the left. It is often noted in patients with CDH, gastroschisis, and omphalocele. This anatomy is less prone to volvulus compared to the incomplete rotation variant. In reversed rotation, the duodenojejunal bowel rotates varying degrees in a clockwise direction about the SMA. The cecocolic portion may rotate clockwise or counterclockwise, anterior or posterior to the SMA. Anomalous mesenteric fixation accounts for internal mesenteric and paraduodenal hernias. The bowel may rotate normally but fixes to the abdominal wall abnormally. Excessive cephalad rotation of the duodenojejunal portion results in obstruction of the third portion of the duodenum in thin patients (SMA syndrome).

Atresia of the Jejunum, Ileum, and Colon

Unlike duodenal atresia, more distal intestinal atresias are caused not by a failure of canalization but by a mesenteric vascular accident with resultant aseptic resorption of the bowel, usually later in gestation. The spectrum of anomalies ranges from a stenosis or mucosal web (type I), a fibrous cord between two bowel ends (type II), to blind-ending proximal and distal bowel loops with a V-shaped mesenteric defect (type IIIa), and multiple atresias of any kind (type IV).[29] The most common site of atresia is the ileum, followed by the jejunum and the colon. Bilious emesis is uniform. Plain radiographs demonstrating only a few dilated bowel loops are indicative of a proximal obstruction, and a contrast study is not required.

At operation, the distal portion of the proximal blind-ending bowel segment is disproportionally dilated and should be resected because it is functionally abnormal and atonic. There is always a discrepancy in bowel diameter between the proximal and distal ends, so an end-to-side or end-to-oblique anastomosis is necessary.

Duplications of the Gastrointestinal Tract

Duplications are rare congenital cystic abnormalities of the GI tract that have been reported to occur anywhere from the mouth to the anus. They originate on the mesenteric side of the associated alimentary tract and share a common blood supply with the native bowel.[30] Heterotopic gastric mucosa is seen in up to one-third of these lesions and may result in severe ulceration, bleeding, and eventual perforation. Communication with the lumen of the gut is more common with tubular duplications. 85% of duplications are diagnosed before age 2 and 60% by 6 months of age. Vertebral anomalies are seen in 21% of patients, while other congenital anomalies are encountered in 48% of patients with alimentary tract duplications.

The signs and symptoms of alimentary tract duplications are not unique and therefore may be confused with other GI tract pathology. Although many duplications remain 'silent' and are incidentally discovered during an operative procedure, others present with severe GI distress. Abdominal pain and melena are the most common symptoms, and a mobile abdominal mass may be palpated in approximately half of patients. Accumulation of secretion within the duplication can cause intense pain and potential obstruction due to compression of the adjacent bowel lumen. The treatment for the majority of intraabdominal duplications is excision.

Meckel's Diverticulum

A Meckel's diverticulum is present in 1% to 3% of the population and is the most common remnant of the omphalomesenteric duct.[31] It is located 10 to 90 cm from the ileocecal valve and may contain ectopic gastric (most common) or ectopic pancreatic tissue. The lifelong risk of complications is 4%, and 40% of these cases occur in children under 10 years of age. Complications include bleeding (40%), intussusception (20%), diverticulitis or peptic perforation (15%), umbilical fistula (15%), intestinal obstruction (7%), and abscess (3%). Bleeding is the most serious complication and most often occurs in children younger than 5 years. It is often massive, seldom occult. Contrast studies rarely outline the diverticulum. The diagnosis is often made by a technetium-99m pertechnetate scan, which will demonstrate uptake of the tracer by ectopic gastric parietal cells. The sensitivity of the scan is increased with pretreatment by either cimetidine or pentagastrin. Resection can be accomplished by laparotomy or laparoscopically.

Anorectal Anomalies: Imperforate Anus

Anomalies of the rectum develop as a result of the faulty division of the cloaca into the urogenital sinus. The sphincters and levator muscle complex as well as the sacral nerves are affected to varying degrees. Therefore, a "perfect" surgical repair may not result in perfect continence.[32] There is a wide range of anomalies, many of which can be simply classified as either "low" or "high" on the basis of physical examination and imaging studies. Low defects are defined by an orifice that is visible at the perineum but is not in the normal location or is partially covered in the normal location. In males, the orifice is anywhere on the perineum, including the median raphe of the scrotum, or it may simply be a covered anus in which there is an incomplete epithelial membrane over the anus. In females, the orifice is either at the perineal body, fourchette, vestibule, or distal vagina. High defects most often have a fistulous connection to the urethra or bladder neck (males) or the upper vagina (females). The rectum may end blindly in 10% of cases. The most severe of the high deformities is the cloacal anomaly, also termed a persistent urogenital sinus. There is only one visible orifice on the perineum; within it there is a common channel between the vagina and urethra, with the rectum opening into the vagina.

All infants with imperforate anus should be prophylactically treated against a urinary tract infection until a voiding cystourethrogram is obtained that rules out vesicoureteral reflux. Low deformities are treated by perineal anoplasty. Traditionally, a high deformity was treated by a three-staged repair consisting of a divided loop colostomy, a posterior sagittal anorectoplasty 4 to 6 weeks later, and closure of the colostomy several months later.[33] Fistulae to the bladder neck usually require division via laparotomy. Recently, the staged approach has been challenged and a one-staged repair has been performed.[34] In all cases, the neoanus must be dilated for several months to prevent circumferential cicatrix formation.

Meconium Plug and Meconium Ileus

Meconium plug syndrome, or neonatal small left colon syndrome, is believed to result from transient colonic immaturity-related dysmotility. More than 50% of babies are born to diabetic mothers. Infants present with abdominal distention, bilious emesis, and failure to pass meconium. The obstructing plug of meconium is most often located in and around the splenic flexure. The contrast enema, using a water-soluble agent, is both diagnostic and therapeutic. It demonstrates a small left colon and dilated bowel proximal to the meconium filling defects. Persistent symptoms after evacuation of the meconium mandates a suction rectal biopsy to rule out Hirschsprung's disease.

It is important to differentiate meconium plug syndrome from meconium ileus. Meconium ileus results from obstruction of the terminal ileum by abnormal meconium. Of the patients with meconium ileus, 10% to 33% have a family history of cystic fibrosis.[35] The presentation is no different from that of meconium plug syndrome, Hirschsprung's disease, or distal intestinal atresia. Characteristically, the proximal ileum is greatly dilated and contains thick, viscous meconium, while the terminal ileum is collapsed and obstructed by thickly packed round mucous plugs that resemble rabbit stool pellets. Initial treatment is with a hypertonic contrast enema mixed with a mucolytic agent (N-acetylcysteine). This treatment draws hypotonic fluid into the intestinal lumen, so the infant must be kept well hydrated. If this fails to relieve the obstruction, laparotomy is indicated. All patients should be evaluated for cystic fibrosis.

Hirschsprung's Disease

Congenital intestinal aganglionosis (Hirschsprung's disease) results from a failure of craniocaudal migration of neuroblasts that are destined to become the parasympathetic ganglion cells of the intestine. The absence of ganglion cells always begins just proximal to the dentate line, never skips intestinal segments, and extends proximally for varying lengths. In approximately 75%, the disease is limited to the rectosigmoid colon; 5% of cases involve the entire colon (total colonic aganglionosis), and 5% can involve varying lengths of small intestine. The absence of ganglion cells results in a functional obstruction because the affected area fails to relax due to unopposed sympathetic tone. The disease may run in families and is associated with trisomy 21 and congenital heart disease.

The typical neonate with Hirschsprung's disease has bil-

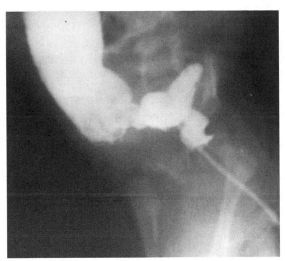

FIGURE 57.4. Lateral view of a contrast enema from a baby with Hirschsprung's disease shows distal rectosigmoid narrowing with proximal dilation of the colon.

ious emesis, abdominal distension, and passes little or no meconium. Rectal examination of the infant may produce an expulsion of stool and air. Short segments of disease may allow a baby to escape diagnosis for weeks, months, or even years. The older patients present with chronic constipation, alternating with diarrhea, and failure to thrive. Untreated Hirschsprung's disease may lead to enterocolitis, characterized by fever, abdominal distension, and foul-smelling watery stools. Enterocolitis is the principal cause of neonatal mortality associated with Hirschsprung's disease.

Plain abdominal radiographs demonstrate dilated loops of bowel. A contrast enema is the imaging test of choice. Typically, it demonstrates a transition zone in which there is proximal colonic dilation and distal narrowing, most evident in the lateral projection (Fig. 57.4). The definitive diagnosis is made by rectal biopsy, where serial sections demonstrate an absence of ganglion cells, hypertrophied nerve trunks, and increased acetylcholinesterase staining.

Traditionally, the surgical treatment was staged and consisted of a leveling colostomy followed several months later by resection of the aganglionic bowel and a pull-through procedure.[36] Recently, there has been a trend toward performing a single-stage procedure (no colostomy) in the newborn period.[37]

Necrotizing Enterocolitis

Necrotizing enterocolitis (NEC) is the most serious and frequent GI disorder of predominantly premature infants, with a median onset at 10 days after birth. The incidence is increasing given the recent therapeutic advancements in neonatal intensive care, which have allowed smaller and smaller babies to survive. Strong evidence exists that infection in a vulnerable host plays the key role in the pathogenesis of NEC.[38] The most common site of involvement is the terminal ileum, followed by the colon.

Clinical findings include abdominal distention; feeding intolerance; palpable abdominal mass; and abdominal wall edema, erythema, and crepitus. Rectal bleeding is frequent but seldom massive.[39] There are a variety of nonspecific clinical findings that suggest physiological instability, such as ap-

nea, bradycardia, hypoglycemia, temperature instability, and lethargy. Plain abdominal radiographs (supine and either left lateral decubitus or cross-table lateral views) may demonstrate pneumatosis, portal vein air, or pneumoperitoneum. There is virtually no role for contrast studies to evaluate the acute disease.

Initial treatment consists of cessation of feeds, broad-spectrum antibiotics, gastric suction, and correction of hypovolemia, acidosis, and electrolyte abnormalities. The only absolute indication for operation is pneumoperitoneum. However, another strategy that is gaining acceptance for those with documented intestinal perforation is bedside peritoneal drainage using a Penrose drain inserted under general anesthesia.[40] In approximately one-third of cases, no further operation will be necessary.

Intussusception

Intussusception (Fig. 57.5) is the most common cause of intestinal obstruction in children under 2 years of age. The peak incidence is at 6 to 12 months, and there is a 3:1 male predominance. It is defined by the telescoping of a segment of proximal bowel (intussusceptum) into the adjacent distal bowel (intussuscipiens). It is typically idiopathic and involves the terminal ileum and right colon (ileocolic intussusception). In most cases, hypertrophied Peyer's patches are noted to be a leading point.

The characteristic clinical presentation is one of crying and drawing the legs upward, alternating with periods of apparent well-being or even lethargy. Reflex vomiting may occur, but vomiting from bowel obstruction is a late finding. Blood and mucus in the stool are noted in one-third of patients and have a characteristic "currant jelly" appearance. A mass may be palpable where the intussusceptum ends. Contrast enema is both diagnostic and therapeutic in more than 90% of

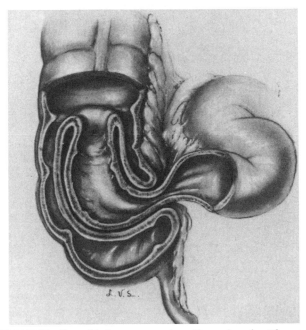

FIGURE 57.5. Ileocolic intussusception. (Reproduced with permission from AA de Lorimier, Pediatric surgery. In: Current Surgical Diagnosis and Treatment, LW Way, Editor. © 1994 Appleton & Lange.)

cases. A successful study reduces the intussusceptum and demonstrates reflux of barium or air into the terminal ileum. The indications for operation are peritonitis, bowel perforation, and inability to completely reduce the intussusceptum using contrast.

Biliary Tract Anomalies

Neonatal Jaundice

Neonatal jaundice is common and physiological for the first 7 to 10 days of life. It is principally due to immaturity of the hepatic enzyme glucuronyl transferase and results in a predominantly indirect hyperbilirubinemia. Jaundice persisting after 2 weeks following birth is pathological, often associated with a rise in the direct bilirubin fraction, and mandates prompt evaluation. The most frequent causes of prolonged jaundice in infancy are biliary atresia, a variety of hepatitides, and choledochal cyst. The differential diagnosis of neonatal jaundice is summarized in Table 57.6.

Biliary Atresia

Biliary atresia is the absence of patent bile ducts draining the liver.[41] The disease is progressive postnatally because infants are rarely born with remarkable jaundice. The extent of ductal involvement may vary greatly. Liver biopsy demonstrates proliferation of the bile canaliculi containing inspissated bile. Over time, the failure to excrete bile out of the liver causes progressive periportal fibrosis and obstruction of the intrahepatic portal veins, resulting in biliary cirrhosis.

Neonates with biliary atresia are usually healthy appearing and active, unlike those with neonatal hepatitis. The urine is dark from bilirubin and the stools are light (acholic). Firm hepatomegaly appears by 4 weeks. Ascites and portal hypertension do not become manifest for several months. Ultrasonography may demonstrate absence or inability to visualize a contracted gallbladder. There is no intrahepatic biliary dilation with biliary atresia. A technetium-99m-labeled iminodiacetate compound (HIDA, DISIDA) scintiscan will demonstrate uptake but no intestinal excretion. Percutaneous liver biopsy may be necessary to distinguish biliary atresia from neonatal hepatitis, although there is considerable histological overlap in advanced cases. Unless the workup has conclusively diagnosed another entity, all children suspected of having biliary atresia should undergo operative cholangiography with the intention of proceeding to exploration of the porta hepatis. Confirmed biliary atresia requires hepatic portoenterostomy (Kasai procedure).[42]

Choledochal Cyst

Choledochal cysts are dilations or diverticuli of all or a portion of the common bile duct. The incidence is estimated from 1 in 13,000 to 1 in 2,000,000.[43] There is a female predominance (3:1), and the cysts are more common in Asians, with a large majority of the reported cases originating from Japan.

Choledochal cysts are classified into one of five subtypes.[44] Type I is a fusiform dilation of the extrahepatic bile duct. Type II is a saccular outpouching of the common bile duct. Type III, referred to as a choledochocels, is a wide-mouth dilation of the common duct at its confluence with the duodenum. Type IV is a cystic dilation of both the intra- and extrahepatic bile ducts. Type V consists of lakes of multiple intrahepatic cysts with no extrahepatic component, and when Type V is associated with hepatic fibrosis, it is termed Caroli's disease. Type I and Type IV are the most common. If left, untreated choledochal cysts may cause cholangitis and cholangiocarcinoma in the long term.

The classic presentation of a choledochal cyst is the triad of abdominal pain, jaundice, and an abdominal mass. However, the complete triad proves to be the exception rather than the rule. Ultrasonography is increasingly responsible for detecting choledochal cysts in the fetus. Neonates more commonly present with asymptomatic jaundice (predominantly direct hyperbilirubinemia) or an abdominal mass. As children grow older the cyst may become painful or infected. In adults, an abdominal mass is rarely appreciated, and patients present more commonly with symptoms of cholangitis or pancreatitis. An ultrasound usually confirms the diagnosis, although radionuclide scanning, MRI, and ERCP (endoscopic retrograde cholangiopancreatography) have also been used.

Historically, choledochal cysts were treated with internal drainage by anastomosis of the cyst wall to the stomach, duodenum, or small bowel. However, internal drainage procedures have an unacceptably high morbidity and the unresected cyst is capable of malignant degeneration. The current gold standard operation consists of complete cyst excision with Roux-en-Y hepaticojejunostomy.

Abdominal Wall Defects

Omphalocele

Omphalocele is a midline abdominal wall defect noted in 1 in 5000 live births. The abdominal viscera (commonly liver and bowel) are contained within a sac composed of peritoneum and amnion, from which the umbilical cord arises at

---

TABLE 57.6. Differential Diagnosis of Neonatal Jaundice.

ABO, Rh, and rare blood group incompatibilities

Breastfeeding

Sepsis

Metabolic disorders
  Alpha-1-antitrypsin deficiency
  Gaucher's disease
  Galactosemia
  Tyrosinemia
  Hypothyroidism
  Cystic fibrosis

Criglar–Najjar syndrome

Gilbert's disease

Hepatitis

Biliary atresia

Choledochal cyst

Inspissated bile syndrome

Parenteral alimentation cholestasis

Alagille's syndrome

Byler's disease

Pyloric stenosis

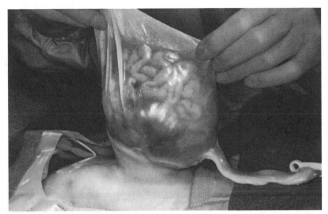

FIGURE 57.6. Neonate with an omphalocele. The liver and bowel herniated through a midline abdominal wall defect and are surrounded by a sac of amnion and chorion from which the umbilical cord emanates.

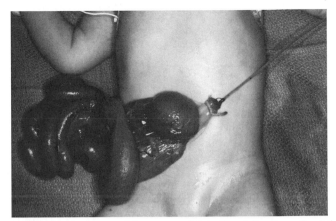

FIGURE 57.7. Neonate with a gastroschisis. The defect is to the right of the umbilical cord and the bowel has no investing sac. Note the edema of the bowel wall and the dilated stomach adjacent to the umbilical cord.

the apex and center[45] (Fig. 57.6). When the defect is less than 4 cm, it is termed a hernia of the umbilical cord and when greater than 10 cm it is termed a giant omphalocele. Associated abnormalities occur in 30% to 70% and include, in descending order of frequency, chromosomal abnormalities (trisomy -13, -18, -21), congenital heart disease, Beckwith–Wiedemann syndrome (hyperinsulinism, gigantism, macroglossia, cloacal exstrophy (hypogastric omphalocele, open hemibladders separated by a vesicointestinal fissure, ambiguous genitalia), pentalogy of Cantrell, and prune belly syndrome (absent abdominal wall muscles, genitourinary abnormalities, cryptorchidism).

After delivery, the omphalocele is covered by placing the baby's lower extremities and torso within a sterile bag (bowel bag) or placing saran wrap around the defect to minimize heat and water loss. Intravenous fluids are administered and nasogastric suction commenced. Emergency operation is not necessary, so a thorough physical examination and workup for associated anomalies is performed. The primary goal of surgery is to return the viscera to the abdominal cavity and close the defect. The success of primary closure is predicated on the size of the defect and the size of the abdominal and thoracic cavities. It is wise to leave the sac in situ because primary closure may not be possible and thus one has maintained the best biological dressing for the viscera. In rare cases, nonoperative treatment is indicated by the presence of a giant omphalocele or severe associated anomalies (e.g., pentalogy of Cantrell). The aim is to allow the sac to dry and form an eschar, allowing epithelialization to occur during the ensuing 16 to 20 weeks. A ventral hernia results, which is repaired electively when the patient is stable.

Gastroschisis

Compared to an omphalocele, a gastroschisis is a much smaller, right paramedian defect without an investing sac[45] (Fig. 57.7). It is twice as common as omphalocele, and the hernia contains gut and pelvic organs but not the liver. Forty percent are in infants who are born prematurely or are small-for-gestational age. The bowel may be edematous, matted, foreshortened, and have extensive fibrin coating or "peel" due to amniotic peritonitis. In both omphalocele and gastroschi-

sis, nonrotation of the gut is common. Unlike omphalocele, associated anomalies are rare. The most common is intestinal atresia (10%–15%).

At delivery, the bowel should be assessed for ischemia from obstructed mesenteric vessels herniating out a small defect or for a volvulus. The infant should be placed on his or her side to prevent "kinking" of the mesentery as it drapes over the abdominal wall. The bowel is covered with a sterile bag and the GI tract decompressed with a gastric tube. Unlike omphalocele, urgent repair is necessary. Unlike infants with omphalocele, those with repaired gastroschisis have a predictably prolonged ileus (2–6 weeks) and require central parenteral nutrition.

Umbilical Hernia

An umbilical fascial defect is very common in newborns. The highest incidence is in preterm infants and those of African-American descent. In most children (95%), a defect less than 1.5 cm will progressively diminish in size and eventually close.[46] This may take months or years. Unlike inguinal hernias, complications (incarceration, strangulation) from umbilical hernias are extremely rare. Repair of the defect is indicated when the defect is larger than 1.5 cm or the child is 4 years or older because defects in these children are not likely to close spontaneously.

Inguinal and Scrotal Disorders

Inguinal Hernia and Hydrocele

Inguinal hernia is a common condition in infancy and childhood.[47] Unlike hernias in adulthood, these hernias result nearly exclusively from a patent processus vaginalis (indirect hernia) and not a weakness in the floor of the inguinal canal (direct hernia). The processus vaginalis follows the descent of the testis into the inguinal canal. Failure of obliteration of the processus may lead to a variety of anomalies including scrotal hernia, inguinal hernia, communicating hydrocele, noncommunicating hydrocele, hydrocele of the spermatic cord, and hydrocele of the tunica vaginalis (Fig. 57.8).

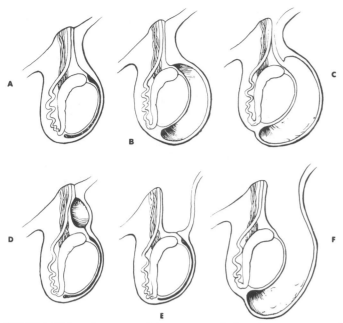

FIGURE 57.8. Spectrum of inguinoscrotal disorders. **A.** Normal anatomy. The processus vaginalis is obliterated and there is a small remnant, the tunica vaginalis, adjacent to the posterior surface of the testis. **B.** Scrotal hydrocele. **C.** Communicating hydrocele. Note the proximal patency of the processus vaginalis. **D.** Hydrocele of the spermatic cord. **E.** Inguinal hernia. **F.** Inguinoscrotal hernia. (Reproduced with permission from MI Rowe, Inguinal and scerotal disorders. In: Essentials of Pediatric Surgery. © 1995 CV Mosby Co.)

The incidence of a clinically detectable inguinal hernia varies with gestational age; 9% to 11% in preterm infants and 3% to 5% for full-term infants. These hernias occur on the right side in 60% (due to later descent of the right testis), on the left in 30%, and bilaterally in 10% and are more common in males. Conditions associated with an increased risk of inguinal hernia include prematurity, family history, abdominal wall defects, cryptorchidism, intersex anomalies, connective tissue disorders, and ascites from any cause (e.g., ventriculoperitoneal shunt, peritoneal dialysis, liver disease). The usual presentation is a nontender mass in the inguinal region. The hernia is often appreciated only when the child strains or cries. One must always locate the position of the testis during an examination for a hernia because an inguinal bulge due to an undescended or retractile testis may be mistaken for a hernia. Commonly, testicular hydroceles are mistaken for hernias. The hallmark of the hydrocele is that one can palpate the normal spermatic cord above the level of the hydrocele. Transillumination is not reliable in the newborn because intestine and fluid transilluminate equally well. It may be difficult to distinguish between a large inguinoscrotal hydrocele and an incarcerated hernia. In general, hydroceles that do not communicate with the peritoneal cavity are physiological and the vast majority resolve within 1 year. Those that persist after 1 year or those which demonstrate changes in size (communicating hydrocele) should be repaired.

All inguinal hernias in children should be repaired shortly after diagnosis to prevent incarceration (nonreducible viscera in the hernia sac), strangulation (vascular compromise to the incarcerated bowel), or injury to the ipsilateral testis from compression of the spermatic cord by the incarcerated bowel. An incarcerated hernia can usually be reduced before surgery.

Historically, it was recommended that all boys under 2 years of age and all girls under 5 years undergo operative exploration of the contralateral inguinal canal in search of a clinically silent patent processus vaginalis.[48] This approach has been replaced, in large part, by laparoscopic exploration.[49,50] The incidence of complications from inguinal hernia repair (recurrence, wound infection, and damage to the spermatic cord) should be 2% or less.

Disorders of the Testes

Cryptorchidism

By the eighth month of gestation, testicular descent should be complete. The incidence of undescended or partially descended testis is 1% to 2% in full-term infants and up to 30% in premature babies. The cryptorchid testis may be located in the inguinal canal, in the peritoneal cavity, or anywhere on the lower abdomen, thigh, and perineum (ectopic testis). The cryptorchid testis may continue to descend into the scrotum for as long as 1 year after birth. Operation is indicated after 1 year because degenerative changes begin to take place in these testes that may impair spermatogenesis and lead to malignant transformation. Additionally, crytorchid testes are more prone to trauma and torsion, often have an associated inguinal hernia, and may cause adverse psychosocial effects. The incidence of testicular cancer in a cryptorchid testis (30 times higher than the normal population) is not lessened by repair, but a scrotal testicle can be more reliably examined for a testicular mass later in life.

Testicular Torsion

Testicular torsion is most frequent in late childhood and early adolescence, although the range is from fetus to adulthood.[51] Anatomically, there are two forms of testicular torsion: intravaginal torsion (bell-clapper deformity) the most common form, and extravaginal torsion, which occurs principally in neonates and in children with an undescended testis (Fig. 57.9). Rarely the testis may twist on a long epididymal mesentery. In children, testicular torsion is either idiopathic or occurs after activity or trauma. There is acute scrotal or testicular pain that may radiate to the lower abdomen. Progressive swelling, edema, and erythema of the hemiscrotum occur. The testicle is exquisitely tender on palpation.

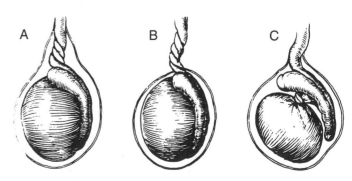

Testicular Torsion

FIGURE 57.9. Three anatomical variants of testicular torsion. **A.** Intravaginal. **B.** Extravaginal. **C.** Torsion around a long epididymal mesentery.

Torsion of the testicular appendices[52] (vestigial Müllerian duct structures) and epididymitis may mimic testicular torsion. With epididymitis, there is often pyuria, voiding symptoms, and fever. Torsion of the testicular appendices often has a gradual onset, and careful palpation may reveal point rather than diffuse tenderness. There may be a visible necrotic lesion on scrotal transillumination (blue dot sign).

The diagnosis of testicular torsion is made principally on clinical grounds. Although one may utilize Doppler ultrasonography and radionuclide scanning to aid in the diagnosis, these tests are time consuming and, in the case of ultrasound, not very specific. If the diagnosis is strongly suspected, the best "test" is operative scrotal exploration. The testicular salvage rate if detorsion is performed within 6 h of symptoms is up to 97% versus less than 10% if greater than 24 h. At operation, the testicle is detorsed and, if viable, it is fixed to the hemiscrotum in three places. The contralateral testicle is at risk for torsion because the testicular anatomy tends to mirror itself, so a contralateral orchiopexy should be performed in all cases. Torsion of the testicular appendices tends to be self-limiting because necrosis and autoamputation usually occur. Treatment is with warm baths, limited activity, and an antiinflammatory agent. If significant pain persists after 2 to 3 days, the appendix has not autoamputated and excision is indicated.

Cutaneous Vascular Anomalies

Hemangiomas

Hemangiomas demonstrate endothelial hyperplasia and are seen in children and adults, but behave differently at different ages. Hemangiomas are much more common than vascular malformations. In the neonatal period, hemangiomas can be subclassified according to their growth phase. A rapid proliferating phase is usually seen during the first few years of life, followed by the involuting phase, which may last several years. Their clinical appearance depends on depth of the lesion.

Fifty percent will involute without treatment by age 5 years, and 70% by 7 years. The remainder will slowly resolve by age 10 to 12 years. Steroid therapy hastens the rate of proliferation of hemangiomas by 30% to 90% and is indicated for complicated lesions (i.e., those causing severe physiological or anatomical abnormalities).

Cutaneous Vascular Malformations

Vascular malformations have normal endothelial cell turnover and tend to grow with the child. These lesions are structural anomalies that are considered errors in vascular morphogenesis. They are usually visible at birth but may take years or even decades to manifest. They are separated into low and high flow variants, and further classified according to the type of vascular channel abnormality: capillary, venous, arterial, and mixed malformations.

Capillary malformations consist of port wine stain (naevus flammeus), naevus flammeus neonatorum (angel's kiss), naevus flammeus nuchae (stork bite, salmon patch), angiokeratomas, and telangiectasias [spider, hereditary hemorrhagic telangiectasia (Rendu-Osler-Weber syndrome)]. They are prone to infection and are treated aggressively with intravenous antibiotics. A compression garment should be used if anatomically feasible. Some lesions can be excised or injected with a sclerosing solution.

Venous malformations have a wide spectrum of appearances ranging from simple varicosities to complex deep lesions that may be located in deeper tissues (e.g., bone, muscle, salivary gland). Pain is often related to thrombosis within the lesion. Radiographic imaging delineates the nature and extent of the lesion (angiogram, CT, MRI). Photocoagulation or YAG laser may be effective for superficial lesions. Resection is the definitive treatment as it can reduce bulk, improve contour and function, and control pain. It is limited by anatomical boundaries, and multiple staged procedures may be required.

Arterial and arteriovenous malformations have multiple small fistulae surrounded by abnormal tissues and can cause high-output cardiac failure; they are most common in the head and neck region (especially intracerebral). There is pain and overlying cutaneous necrosis. Adjacent osseous structures are often destroyed. Selective embolization is used either as palliation or presurgically to limit hemorrhage. Excision, when possible, is the procedure of choice.

Combined vascular malformations and hypertrophy syndromes consist of Klippel–Trenaunay–Weber syndrome (combined capillary–lymphatic venous malformation associated with lower limb hypertrophy), Parkes–Weber syndrome (upper limb arteriovenous shunting), Marffucci's syndrome (low-flow vascular malformations and multiple extremity enchondromas with hypoplastic long bones), and Sturge–Weber syndrome (upper facial port wine stain and vascular anomalies of the choroid plexus and leptomeninges).

Childhood Tumors

Neuroblastoma

Neuroblastoma is the most common tumor in infants less than 1 year of age and the second most common solid tumor of childhood[53] (brain tumors are the most common solid tumor). Approximately 60% of all cases occur in children less than 2 years of age and 97% before age 10 years. The most common site for primary disease is in the abdomen (adrenal), followed by the thorax, pelvis, and occasionally the head and neck.

Symptoms are site specific. The most common is pain (from the primary or metastatic disease). Other symptoms include failure to thrive, malaise, fever, weight loss, and anorexia. Children frequently appear "ill" at the time of diagnosis.

Imaging includes a chest radiograph, skeletal survey, and bone scan. Neuroblastoma is the most common abdominal tumor to demonstrate calcifications (50%) before chemotherapy. The CT scan is instrumental in making the diagnosis and in determining resectability. CT myelography is useful in assessing tumor within the spinal canal and spinal cord compression. MRI is as sensitive as CT scanning in terms of assessing tumor size and resectability, but has the added advantage of being superior to CT in assessing vessel encasement, vessel patency, and spinal cord compression. MRI can also demonstrate bone marrow involvement in selected cases.

TABLE 57.7. International Neuroblastoma Staging System and Estimated Survival Rates.

Stage 1. Localized tumor confined to the area of origin; complete gross excision, with or without microscopic residual disease; identifiable ipsilateral and contralateral lymph nodes negative microscopically. Survival 100%.

Stage 2A. Unilateral tumor with incomplete gross excision; identifiable ipsilateral nonadherent lymph nodes negative microscopically. Survival 80%.

Stage 2B. Unilateral tumor with complete or incomplete gross excision; with positive ipsilateral nonadherent lymph nodes; identifiable contralateral lymph nodes negative microscopically. Survival 70%.

Stage 3. Tumor infiltrating across the midline (vertebral column) with or without regional lymph node involvement; or unilateral tumor with contralateral regional lymph node involvement; or midline tumor with bilateral regional lymph node involvement or extension by infiltration. Survival 40%.

Stage 4. Dissemination of tumor to distant lymph nodes, bone, bone marrow, liver, or other organs (except as defined in stage 4S). Survival 15%.

Stage 4S. Localized primary tumor as defined for stage 1 or 2 with dissemination limited to liver, skin, and/or bone marrow (<10% tumor) in infants younger than 1 year. Survival 85%.

TABLE 57.8. Wilms Tumor Staging System.

Stage I. Tumor limited to kidney and completely excised. The surface of the renal capsule is intact and the tumor was not ruptured before removal. There is no residual tumor.

Stage II. Tumor extends through the perirenal capsule but is completely excised. There may be local spillage of tumor confined to the flank or the tumor may have been biopsied. Extrarenal vessels may contain tumor thrombus or be infiltrated by tumor.

Stage III. Residual nonhematogenous tumor confined to the abdomen: lymph node involvement, diffuse peritoneal spillage, peritoneal implants, tumor beyond surgical margin either grossly or microscopically, or tumor not completely removed.

Stage IV. Hematogenous metastases to lung, liver, bone, brain, etc.

Stage V. Bilateral renal involvement at diagnosis; each kidney should be staged separately.

I^{131}-meta-iodobenzylguanidine nuclear scanning is very sensitive in detecting tumors that concentrate catecholamines and has been useful in the diagnosis of primary, residual, and metastatic disease in patients with neuroblastoma. The staging systems are surgically and anatomically based, and all have prognostic value. The most recent is the International Neuroblastoma Staging System (Table 57.7). The diagnosis rests upon the demonstration of immature neuroblastic tissue obtained by tissue or bone marrow aspirate and biopsy.

Primary excision is attempted whenever possible. Gross total excision is attempted, but negative microscopic tumor margins are not necessary. Tumors that are not safely resectable at diagnosis should be biopsied, along with any visible lymph nodes. Cyclic chemotherapy with or without radiation therapy frequently results in shrinkage and maturation of the tumor, allowing for later attempts at more aggressive resection.

Bone marrow transplantation is used for patients with stage 3 and 4 disease who are high risk by virtue of their age, stage, or biological characteristics of their tumor.[54] Patients receive sublethal doses of chemotherapeutic agents and total body irradiation, then are "rescued" with either allogeneic bone marrow or, more commonly, with purged autologous bone marrow.

Wilms Tumor

Wilms tumor is the most common childhood intraabdominal tumor.[55] Seventy-five percent of children are less than 5 years old; the peak incidence is 2 to 3 years of age. It is associated with aniridia, hemihypertrophy, and the Beckwith–Wiedemann syndrome. The constellation of Wilms tumor, aniridia, genitourinary anomalies, and mental retardation (WAGR syndrome) and the Denys–Drash syndrome (mental retardation, pseudohermaphroditism, renal disease, and Wilms tumor) are associated with a deletion of 11p13.[56]

Children are healthy appearing and present with an asymptomatic abdominal mass. It is not uncommonly detected during the workup of seemingly trivial trauma-induced hematuria. The physical findings are generally limited to a large, nontender mass. Ascites may be present in advanced cases.

There are no specific tumor markers. Imaging is required to determine the extent of the mass, to assess for bilateral disease, venous invasion, and metastases, and to confirm contralateral renal function; this is accomplished with an abdominal ultrasound and a CT scan of the chest and abdomen. The most important determinants of outcome for children are histopathology and tumor stage. Histopathologically, there are two prognostic groups: favorable and unfavorable. Unfavorable types display varying degrees of anaplasia. Staging is based on surgical and pathological aspects of the tumor (Table 57.8).

Surgical excision can often be accomplished without any preoperative treatment. The aim of surgery is to completely remove the tumor (nephrectomy) without spill and determine the stage by virtue of its size, extent, and lymph node involvement. Tumor rupture with gross spillage portends a sixfold increase in risk of local recurrence and requires the use of postoperative external beam radiation. If the tumor is too large for safe resection it is biopsied, along with regional lymph nodes. Chemotherapy with or without radiation therapy usually results in a significant reduction in tumor size and allows subsequent resection. The overall survival is 85%, and most patients will be cured. Survival correlates with stage. The 4-year survival rate with respect to age and histology is presented in Table 57.9.

Rhabdomyosarcoma

Rhabdomyosarcoma is a childhood malignancy that arises from embryonic mesenchyme with the potential to differen-

TABLE 57.9. Four-year Survival for Wilms Tumor.

Stage I/FH: 98%
Stage I–III/UH: 68%
Stage II/FH: 90%–95%
Stage III/FH: 85%–90%
Stage IV/FH: 78%–86%
Stage IV/UH: 52%–58%

FH, favorable histology; UH, unfavorable histology.

TABLE 57.10. Intergroup Rhabdomyosarcoma Study Clinical Group Staging System.

Group I. Localized disease, completely removed
  a. Confined to muscle or organ of origin
  b. Infiltration outside organ or muscle of origin; regional nodes not involved

Group II. Total gross resection with evidence of regional spread
  a. Grossly resected tumor with microscopic residual
  b. Regional disease with involved nodes, completely resected with no microscopic residual
  c. Regional disease with involved nodes, grossly resected, but with evidence of microscopic residual and/or histological involvement of the most distal regional node in the dissection

Group III. Incomplete resection, or biopsy with presence of gross disease

Group IV. Distant metastases

---

tiate into skeletal muscle.[57] It is the most common pediatric soft tissue sarcoma and is the third most common solid malignancy. It accounts for 4% to 8% of all malignancies and 5% to 15% of all solid malignancies of childhood. The age distribution is bimodal; the first peak is between 2 to 5 years and the secondary peak between 15 and 19 years.

The clinical presentation varies with the site of origin of the primary tumor, age, and the presence or absence of metastatic disease. The majority of symptoms are secondary to the effects of tumor compression or the presence of a mass. The most common site is the head and neck region (35%).

Staging as determined by the histological variant, the primary site, and the extent of disease is mandatory as each has an important influence on the choice of treatment and on prognosis. CT or MRI scanning are essential to evaluate the primary tumor and its relationship to surrounding structures. A clinical grouping system was designed by the Intergroup Rhabdomyosarcoma Study Group (IRS) to stratify different extents of disease to compare treatment and outcome results (Table 57.10). It is based upon pretreatment and operative outcome and does not account for the biological differences or the natural history of tumors arising from different primary sites.

The surgical management is site specific and includes complete wide excision of the primary tumor and surrounding uninvolved tissue while preserving cosmesis and function. Incomplete excision (beyond biopsy) or tumor debulking is not beneficial, and severely mutilating or debilitating procedures should not be performed. Tumors not amenable to primary excision should be amply biopsied and then treated with neoadjuvant therapies; secondary excision is then performed and is associated with a better outcome than partial or incomplete excisions.

Liver Neoplasms

Tumors of the liver are uncommon in childhood (2% of all pediatric malignancies). More than 70% of pediatric liver masses are malignant. The majority of hepatic malignancies are of epithelial origin whereas most benign lesions are vascular in nature.[58]

HEPATOBLASTOMA

Hepatoblastomas account for almost 50% of all liver masses in children and approximately two-thirds of malignant tumors.

The most common finding is an asymptomatic abdominal mass or diffuse abdominal swelling in a healthy-appearing child. There may be obstructive GI symptoms secondary to compression of the stomach or duodenum, or acute pain secondary to hemorrhage into the tumor. Physical examination reveals a nontender, firm mass in the right upper quadrant or midline that moves with respiration. Advanced tumors present with weight loss, ascites, and failure to thrive. Alpha-fetoprotein (AFP) is significantly elevated in 90% to 95%.

Abdominal ultrasound demonstrates a solid, usually unilobar (right lobe most common) lesion of the liver but lacks sufficient detail to determine resectability. An abdominal CT scan using intravenous contrast is currently the imaging procedure of choice, both for diagnosis and planning therapy. The definitive diagnosis requires a tissue biopsy.

Complete surgical resection is the major objective of therapy and is the only chance for cure.[59] Approximately 60% of patients have primarily resectable lesions. Hepatic transplantation is used for unresectable disease where chemotherapy has failed to allow complete resection but no demonstrable metastases exist.[60] Long-term follow-up is required before this becomes an accepted alternative treatment. The overall survival for all children with hepatoblastoma is approximately 50%.

HEPATOCELLULAR CARCINOMA

Hepatocellular carcinoma is less common than hepatoblastoma and typically presents in older children and adolescents (median age, 10 years). It is associated with preexisting chronic hepatitis, cirrhosis due to hepatitis B virus, and other causes of childhood cirrhosis. Signs and symptoms consist of an abdominal mass or diffuse swelling, abdominal pain, weight loss, anorexia, and jaundice. The serum AFP level is elevated in 50%, although the absolute levels are lower than in patients with hepatoblastoma. The diagnostic studies, staging, and treatment are similar to hepatoblastoma.[59] Only 15% to 20% of hepatocellular carcinomas are resectable. The overall long-term survival is poor (15%), even for resectable disease. The role of liver transplantation remains unclear.

HEMANGIOMA

This is the most common benign pediatric hepatic lesion.[61] These lesions are solitary (cavernous hemangioma) or multiple (infantile hemangioendothelioma), involving the bulk of the liver. Patients with a solitary hemangioma frequently have no symptoms or present with a mass. Infrequently, intratumor hemorrhage or rupture result in abdominal pain.

The diagnosis is made by red blood cell-labeled radionuclide or dynamic abdominal CT scanning. The CT scan demonstrates increased filling and rapid venous phase from arteriovenous shunting. Angiography is unnecessary, and percutaneous biopsy is contraindicated.

Treatment is not necessary for an asymptomatic child. Patients with congestive heart failure and/or thrombocytopenia are treated with corticosteroids, digoxin, and diuretics. Refractory patients benefit from hepatic artery embolization. External-beam radiation reduces hepatic size and controls symptoms. Their large size and diffuse involvement may preclude resection. Disease limited to one lobe can be surgically removed. Hemangioendotheliomas may undergo malignant degeneration into angiosarcoma.

Hepatic Adenoma

This is a benign lesion that accounts for less than 5% of all pediatric liver tumors.[62] It presents as an asymptomatic mass; occasionally, acute abdominal pain results from tumor rupture and bleeding. Abdominal CT scan demonstrates a well-circumscribed mass, usually confined to the right lobe. AFP levels and liver function tests are normal. The major management problem is the inability to differentiate adenomas from hepatocellular carcinoma. Thus, excision is recommended.

Focal Nodular Hyperplasia

This is a well-circumscribed, nonencapsulated nodular liver mass. It presents as an asymptomatic hepatic mass or abdominal pain (from rupture or bleeding). Ultrasonography and CT scan demonstrate a solid mass, but one cannot differentiate it from an adenoma or malignancy without a biopsy. If the diagnosis can be made by biopsy (percutaneous or open), no further treatment is needed.

Mesenchymal Hamartoma

This is an uncommon benign lesion presenting in the first year of life as an asymptomatic large solitary mass usually confined to the right lobe of the liver.[63] The CT scan demonstrates a well-defined tumor margin and minimal to no contrast enhancement. The treatment is surgical wedge resection; lobectomy is rarely required.

Teratomas

Teratomas are embryonal neoplasms derived from totipotential cells containing tissue from at least two of three germ layers (ectoderm, endoderm, mesoderm). Approximately 80% are found in females. They are typically midline or paraaxial tumors[64] and are distributed in the following regions: sacrococcygeal (57%), gonadal (29%), mediastinal (7%), cervical (3%), retroperitoneal (4%), and intracranial (3%). Other sites are rare. Nongonadal teratomas present in infancy whereas gonadal are seen in adolescence; 21% are malignant.

The serum AFP level is elevated in tumors containing malignant endodermal sinus (yolk sac) elements. Serial AFP levels are a marker for recurrence. β-hCG is produced from those tumors containing malignant choriocarcinoma tissue. Rarely, enough β-hCG is produced to cause precocious puberty. Elevated AFP and β-hCG levels in histologically benign tumors indicate an increased risk of recurrence and malignant transformation, particularly with "immature" benign teratomas. Treatment of these tumors is by complete excision.

References

1. Rowe MI. The newborn as a surgical patient. In: O'Neill JA, Rowe MI, Grosfeld JL, Fonkalsrud EW, Coran AG, eds. Pediatric Surgery, 5th Ed. St. Louis: Mosby-Year Book, 1999:43–57.
2. Sauer PJJ, Dane HJ, Visser HKA. New standards for neutral thermal environment of healthy very low birth weight infants in week one of life. Arch Dis Child 1984;59:18.
3. Taylor L, O'Neill JA Jr. Total parenteral nutrition in the pediatric patient. Surg Clin North Am 1991;71:477.
4. Bell EF, Oh W. Fluid and electrolyte balance in very low birth weight infants. Clin Perinatol 1979;6:139–150.
5. Gray SW, Skandalakis JE. The pharynx and its derivatives. In: Embryology for Surgeons: The Embryological Basis for the Treatment of Congenital Defects. Baltimore: William & Wilkins, 1994:17–64.
6. Ninh TN, Ninh TX. Cystic hygroma in children: A report of 126 cases. J Pediatr Surg 1974;9:2.
7. Tanigawa N, Shimomatsuya T, Takahashi K, et al. Treatment of cystic hygroma and lymphangioma with the use of bleomycin fat emulsion. Cancer (Phila) 1987;60:741–749.
8. Ogita S, Tsuto T, Tokiwa K, et al. Intracystic injection of OK-432: a new sclerosing therapy for cystic hygroma in children. Br J Surg 1987;74:690–691.
9. Bodenstein L, Altman RP. Cervical lymphadenitis in infants and children. Semin Pediatr Surg 1994;3:134–141.
10. Armstrong D, Pickerell K, Fetter B, et al. Torticollis: an analysis of 271 cases. Plast Reconstr Surg 1965;35:14–19.
11. Neilson IR, Russo P, Laberge JM, et al. Congenital adenomatoid malformation of the lung: current management and prognosis J Pediatr Surg 1991;26:975.
12. Stocker JT, Madewell JE, Drake RM. Congenital cystic adenomatoid malformation of the lung. Hum Pathol 1977;8:155–171.
13. Benjamin DR, Cahill JL. Bronchioalveolar carcinoma of the lung and congenital cystic adenomatoid malformation. Am J Clin Pathol 1991;95:889.
14. Lopoo JB, Lipshutz GS, Goldstein R, et al. Fetal pulmonary sequestration: a favorable congenital lung lesion. Obstet Gynecol 1999;94:567–571.
15. Stigers KB, et al. The clinical and imaging spectrum of findings in patients with congenital lobar emphysema. Pediatr Pulmonol 1992;14:160.
16. Grosfel JL, Skinner MA, Rescorla FJ, et al. Mediastinal tumors in children: experience with 196 cases. Ann Surg Oncol 1994; 1:121–127.
17. Puri P. Congenital diaphragmatic hernia. Curr Probl Surg 1994; 31:785–856.
18. Adzick N, Outwater KM, Harrison MR, et al. Correction of congenital diaphragmatic hernia in utero IV: an early gestational fetal lamb model for pulmonary vascular morphometric analysis. J Pediatr Surg 1985;20:673–680.
19. Harrison MR, Mychaliska GB, Albanese CT, et al. Correction of congenital diaphragmatic hernia in utero IX: fetuses with poor prognosis (liver herniation and low lung-to-head ratio) can be saved by fetoscopic temporary tracheal occlusion. J Pediatr Surg 1998;33:1017–1023.
20. Smith CD, Sade RM, Crawford FA, Othersen HB. Diaphragmatic paralysis and eventration in infants. J Thorac Cardiovasc Surg 1986;91:490–497.
21. Ravitch MM. Congenital Deformities of the Chest Wall and Their Operative Correction. Philadelphia: Saunders, 1977.
22. Ravitch MM. Protrusion deformities. In: Pediatric Surgery, 4th Ed. St. Louis: Mosby-Year Book, 1986:578–581.
23. Harmon CM, Coran AG. Congenital anomalies of the esophagus. In: O'Neill JA, Rowe MI, Grosfeld JL, Fonkalsrud EW, Coran AG, eds. Pediatric Surgery, 5th Ed. St. Louis: Mosby-Year Book, 1999:941–967.
24. Boyle J. Gastroesophageal reflux in the pediatric patient. Gastroenterol Clin North Am 1985;18:315.
25. Kazarooni NL, et al. Fundoplication in 160 children under 2 years of age. J Pediatr Surg 1994;29:677.
26. Grosfeld JL, Rescorla FJ. Duodenal atresia and stenosis: reassessment of treatment and outcome based on antenatal diagnosis, pathologic variance, and long-term followup. World J Surg 1993;17:301–309.
27. Rescorla FJ, Shedd FJ, Grosfeld JL, et al. Anomalies of intestinal rotation in childhood. Analysis of 447 cases. Surgery (St. Louis) 1990;108:710.
28. Rotational anomalies and volvulus. In: Rowe MI, O'Neill JA Jr,

Grosfeld JL, Fonkalsrud EW, Coran AG, eds. Essentials of Pediatric Surgery. St. Louis: Mosby-Year Book, 1995:492–500.

29. Grosfeld JL, Ballantine TVN, Showemaker R. Operative management of intestinal atresia based on pathologic findings. J Pediatr Surg 1979;14:368.

30. Ildstad ST, Tollerud DJ, Weiss RG, et al. Duplications of the alimentary tract. Clinical characteristics, preferred treatment, and associated malformations. Ann Surg 1988;208:184–189.

31. St-Vil D, Brandt ML, Panic S, et al. Meckel's diverticulum in children: a 20 year review. J Pediatr Surg 1991;26:1289.

32. Peña A. Posterior sagittal anorectoplasty: results in the management of 332 cases of anorectal malformations. Pediatr Surg Int 1988;3:94–104.

33. Peña A, deVries PA. Posterior sagittal anorectoplasty: important technical considerations and new applications. J Pediatr Surg 1982;17:796.

34. Georgeson K, Inge T, Albanese CT. Minimally invasive repair of high imperforate anus. J Pediatr Surg (in press).

35. Allan DL, Robbie M, Phelan PD, et al. Familial occurrence of meconium ileus. Eur J Pediatr 1981;135:291–292.

36. Rescorla FJ, Morrison AM, Engles D, et al. Hirschsprung's disease: evaluation of mortality and long-term function in 260 cases. Arch Surg 1992;127:934–942.

37. Langer JC, Fitzgerald PG, Winthrop AL, et al. One-stage versus two-stage Soave pull-through for Hirschsprung's disease in the first year of life. J Pediatr Surg 1996;31:33–37.

38. Necrotizing enterocolitis. In: Rowe MI, O'Neill JA Jr, Grosfeld JL, Fonkalsrud EW, Coran AG, eds. Essentials of Pediatric Surgery. St. Louis: Mosby-Year Book, 1995:526–535.

39. Grosfeld JL, Cheu H, Schlatter M, et al. Changing trends in necrotizing enterocolitis. Ann Surg 1991;214:300.

40. Ein SH, Shandling B, Wesson D, Filler RM. A 13-year experience with peritoneal drainage under local anesthesia for necrotizing enterocolitis perforation. J Pediatr Surg 1990;25:1034–1037.

41. Hays DM, Kimura K. Biliary Atresia. Cambridge: Harvard University Press, 1980.

42. Lilly JR, Karrer FM, Hall RJ, et al. The surgery of biliary atresia. Ann Surg 1989;210:289.

43. O'Neill J. Choledochal cyst. Curr Probl Surg 1992;29:365–410.

44. Todani T, Watanabe Y, Narusue M, et al. Congenital bile duct cysts: classification, operative procedures, and review of 37 cases including cancer arising from choledochal cyst. Am J Surg 1977;134:263–269.

45. Meller JL, Reyes HM, Loeff DS. Gastroschisis and omphalocele. Clin Perinatol 1989;16:113.

46. Lassaleta L, Fonkalsrud EW, Tovar J, et al. The management of umbilical hernias in infancy and childhood. J Pediatr Surg 1975;10:405.

47. Grosfeld JL. Current concepts in inguinal hernia in infants and children. World J Surg 1989;13:506.

48. Weber TR, Tracy TF Jr. Groin hernias and hydrocele. In: Ashcraft KW, Holder TM, eds. Pediatric Surgery, 2nd Ed. Philadelphia: Saunders, 1993:562–570.

49. Yerkes EB, Brock JW III, Holcomb GW III, Morgan WM. Laparoscopic evaluation for a contralateral patent processus vaginalis: part III. Urology 1998;51:480–483.

50. Fuenfer MM, Pitts RM, Georgeson KE. Laparoscopic exploration of the contralateral groin in children: an improved technique. J Laparoendosc Surg 1996;1:S1–S4.

51. Williamson RCN. Torsion of the testis and allied conditions. Br J Surg 1976;63:465–476.

52. Skoglund RW, McRoberts JW, Ragde H. Torsion of the testicular appendages: presentation of 43 new cases and a collective review. J Urol 1970;104:604–607.

53. Matthay KK. Neuroblastoma: a clinical challenge and biologic puzzle. CA Cancer J Clin 1995;45:179.

54. Chamberlain RS, Quinones R, Dinndorf P, et al. Complete surgical resection combined with aggressive adjuvant chemotherapy and bone marrow transplantation prolongs survival in children with advanced neuroblastoma. Ann Surg Oncol 1995;2:93.

55. Ritchey ML, Haase GM, Shochat S. Current management of Wilms tumor. Semin Surg Oncol 1993;9:502.

56. Green DM, D'Angio GJ, Beckwith JB, et al. Wilms tumor. CA Cancer J Clin 1996;46:46.

57. Wiener ES. Rhabdomyosarcoma: new dimensions in management. Semin Pediatr Surg 1993;2:47.

58. Weinberg AG, Finegold MJ. Primary hepatic tumors of childhood. Hum Pathol 1983;14:512–537.

59. Wheatley JM, LaQuaglia MP. Management of hepatic epithelial malignancy in childhood and adolescence. Semin Surg Oncol 1993;9:532.

60. Tagge EP, Tagge DU, Reyes J, et al. Resection, including transplantation, for hepatoblastoma and hepatocellular carcinoma: impact on survival. J Pediatr Surg 1992;27:292.

61. Selby DM, Stocker JT, Waclaw IW, et al. Infantile hemangioendothelioma of the liver. Hepatology 1994;20:39.

62. Cherqui D, Rahmouni A, Charlotte F, et al. Management of focal nodular hyperplasia and hepatocellular adenoma in young women: a series of 41 patients with clinical, radiological, and pathological correlations. Hepatology 1995;22:1674.

63. Chandra RS, Kapur SP, Kelleher J, et al. Benign hepatocellular tumors in the young: a clinicopathologic spectrum. Arch Pathol Lab Med 1984;108:168–171.

64. Rescorla FJ. Pediatric germ cell tumors. Semin Pediatr Surg 1999;16:144–158.

Index